MANUAL OF NEONATAL CARE

Seventh Edition

Editors

John P. Cloherty, MD
Associate Clinical Professor
Department of Pediatrics
Harvard Medical School
Boston, Massachusetts;
Associate Neonatologist
Neonatology Program at Harvard
Brigham and Women's Hospital
Beth Israel Deaconess Medical Center
Children's Hospital Boston
Boston, Massachusetts

Eric C. Eichenwald, MD
Associate Professor
Department of Pediatrics
Chief, Division of Neonatology
Vice-Chair, Department of Pediatrics
University of Texas Health Science Center
Children's Memorial Hermann Hospital
Houston, Texas

Anne R. Hansen, MD, MPH
Assistant Professor
Department of Pediatrics
Harvard Medical School
Boston, Massachusetts;
Medical Director, Neonatal Intensive Care Unit
Children's Hospital Boston
Boston, Massachusetts

Ann R. Stark, MD
Professor
Department of Pediatrics - Neonatology
Baylor College of Medicine
Houston, Texas

 Wolters Kluwer | Lippincott Williams & Wilkins
Health
Philadelphia · Baltimore · New York · London
Buenos Aires · Hong Kong · Sydney · Tokyo

Acquisitions Editor: Sonya Seigafuse
Product Manager: Nicole Walz
Vendor Manager: Bridgett Dougherty
Senior Manufacturing Manager: Benjamin Rivera
Marketing Manager: Lisa Lawrence
Design Coordinator: Doug Smock
Production Service: Absolute Service, Inc./Maryland Composition

Printed in China

Library of Congress Cataloging-in-Publication Data

Manual of neonatal care / editors, John P. Cloherty ... [et al.]. — 7th ed.
    p. ; cm.
  Includes bibliographical references and index.
  ISBN 978-1-60831-777-6 (pbk.)
  1. Neonatology—Handbooks, manuals, etc. I. Cloherty, John P.
  [DNLM: 1. Infant, Newborn, Diseases—Handbooks. 2. Intensive Care, Neonatal—Handbooks.
3. Neonatology—methods—Handbooks. WS 39]
  RJ251.M26 2012
  618.92'.01—dc23

                                                                                    2011021093

Care has been taken to confirm the accuracy of the information presented and to describe generally accepted practices. However, the authors, editors, and publisher are not responsible for errors or omissions or for any consequences from application of the information in this book and make no warranty, expressed or implied, with respect to the currency, completeness, or accuracy of the contents of the publication. Application of the information in a particular situation remains the professional responsibility of the practitioner.

The authors, editors, and publisher have exerted every effort to ensure that drug selection and dosage set forth in this text are in accordance with current recommendations and practice at the time of publication. However, in view of ongoing research, changes in government regulations, and the constant flow of information relating to drug therapy and drug reactions, the reader is urged to check the package insert for each drug for any change in indications and dosage and for added warnings and precautions. This is particularly important when the recommended agent is a new or infrequently employed drug.

Some drugs and medical devices presented in the publication have Food and Drug Administration (FDA) clearance for limited use in restricted research settings. It is the responsibility of the health care providers to ascertain the FDA status of each drug or device planned for use in their clinical practice.

To purchase additional copies of this book, call our customer service department at (800) 638-3030 or fax orders to (301) 223-2320. International customers should call (301) 223-2300.

Visit Lippincott Williams & Wilkins on the Internet at LWW.com. Lippincott Williams & Wilkins customer service representatives are available from 8:30 am to 6 pm, EST.

10 9 8 7 6 5 4 3 2 1

We dedicate this edition

to our spouses: Ann, Caryn, Jonathan, and Peter

to our children: Maryann, David, Joan, Neil, Danny, Monica, Tom, Victoria, Anne, Tim, Zachary, Taylor, Connor, Laura, Jonah, Gregory, Oliver, Julian, and Nathalie

to our grandchildren: Chrissy, Elizabeth, Daniel, Patrick, John, Tom, Ryan, Catherine, Sophie, Jack, Eva, Jane, Peter, Nora, Sheila, and James

and to the many babies and parents we have cared for.

Contributors

Elisa Abdulhayoglu, MD
Instructor
Department of Pediatrics
Harvard Medical School
Boston, Massachusetts;
Neonatologist
Department of Neonatology
Newton-Wellesley Hospital
Newton, Massachusetts

Steven A. Abrams, MD
Professor
Department of Pediatrics
Baylor College of Medicine
Houston, Texas;
Attending Physician
Department of Pediatrics
Texas Children's Hospital
Houston, Texas

James M. Adams, MD
Professor
Department of Pediatrics
Baylor College of Medicine
Houston, Texas;
Attending Physician
Neonatology
Texas Children's Hospital
Houston, Texas

Pankaj B. Agrawal, MD, DM, MMSc
Instructor
Department of Pediatrics
Harvard Medical School
Boston, Massachusetts;
Neonatologist
Children's Hospital Boston
Boston, Massachusetts

Katherine W. Altshul, MD
Instructor
Department of Pediatrics
Harvard Medical School
Boston, Massachusetts;
Pediatric/NICU Hospitalist
Division of Newborn Medicine
Brigham and Women's Hospital
Boston, Massachusetts

Diane M. Anderson, PhD, RD
Associate Professor
Department of Pediatrics
Baylor College of Medicine
Houston, Texas;
Neonatal Nutritionist
Department of Pediatrics
Texas Children's Hospital
Houston, Texas

Theresa M. Andrews, RN, CCRN
Staff Nurse III
Neonatal Intensive Care Unit
Children's Hospital Boston
Boston, Massachusetts

John H. Arnold, MD
Associate Professor
Department of Anesthesia
Harvard Medical School
Boston, Massachusetts;
Senior Associate
Anesthesia & Critical Care
Children's Hospital Boston
Boston, Massachusetts

David J. Askenazi, MD, MsPH
Assistant Professor
Department of Pediatrics
University of Alabama at Birmingham
Birmingham, Alabama;
Attending Physician
Division of Nephrology and Transplantation
Children's Hospital of Alabama
Birmingham, Alabama

Muhammad Aslam, MD
Instructor
Department of Pediatrics
Harvard Medical School
Boston, Massachusetts;
Neonatologist
Division of Newborn Medicine
Children's Hospital Boston
Boston, Massachusetts

Carlos A. Bacino, MD
Associate Professor
Department of Molecular and Human
  Genetics
Baylor College of Medicine
Houston, Texas;
Director
Genetics Clinic
Texas Children's Hospital
Houston, Texas

Mandy Brown Belfort, MD, MPH
Instructor
Department of Pediatrics
Harvard Medical School
Boston, Massachusetts;
Attending Neonatologist
Division of Newborn Medicine
Children's Hospital Boston
Boston, Massachusetts

Ann M. Bergin, MB, SCM
Assistant Professor
Neurology
Harvard Medical School
Boston, Massachusetts;
Staff Physician
Neurology
Children's Hospital Boston
Boston, Massachusetts

Kushal Y. Bhakta, MD
Assistant Professor
Department of Pediatrics - Neonatology
University of California
Irvine, California;
Attending Neonatologist
Neonatology
Children's Hospital of Orange Country
Orange, California

Rosalind S. Brown, MD
Associate Professor
Department of Pediatrics
Harvard Medical School
Boston, Massachusetts;
Director, Clinical Trials Research
Division of Endocrinology
Medicine
Children's Hospital Boston
Boston, Massachusetts

Sandra K. Burchett, MD, MSc
Associate Professor
Department of Pediatrics
Harvard Medical School
Boston, Massachusetts;
Clinical Director, Division of Infectious
  Diseases
Associate Physician in Medicine
Children's Hospital Boston
Boston, Massachusetts

Heather H. Burris, MD, PhD
Instructor
Department of Pediatrics
Harvard Medical School
Boston, Massachusetts;
Neonatologist
Department of Neonatology
Beth Israel Deaconess Medical Center
Boston, Massachusetts

Carol Spruill Turnage, MSN, RN,
CNS
Neonatal Clinical Nurse Specialist
Nursing-Neonatal Intensive Care
Texas Children's Hospital
Houston, Texas

Kimberlee Chatson, MD
Instructor
Newborn Medicine
Harvard Medical School
Boston, Massachusetts;
Associate Medical Director Special Care
  Nursery
Winchester Hospital
Winchester, Massachusetts

Chaitanya Chavda, MD
Clinical Fellow
Harvard Program in Newborn Medicine
Boston, Massachusetts

Helen A. Christou, MD
Assistant Professor
Department of Pediatrics
Harvard Medical School
Boston, Massachusetts;
Neonatologist
Division of Newborn Medicine
Brigham and Women's Hospital,
  Children's Hospital
Boston, Massachusetts

John P. Cloherty, MD
Associate Clinical Professor
Department of Pediatrics
Harvard Medical School
Boston, Massachusetts;
Associate Neonatologist
Neonatology Program at Harvard
Brigham and Women's Hospital
Beth Israel Deaconess Medical Center
Children's Hospital Boston
Boston, Massachusetts

William D. Cochran, MD
Associate Clinical Professor (emeritus)
Department of Pediatrics
Harvard Medical School
Boston, Massachusetts;
Senior Associate in Medicine (emeritus)
Newborn Intensive Care Unit
Beth Israel Deaconess Medical Center
Boston, Massachusetts

Elizabeth G. Doherty, MD
Instructor
Department of Pediatrics
Harvard Medical School
Boston, Massachusetts;
Neonatologist
Division of Newborn Medicine
Children's Hospital Boston and Winchester
  Hospital
Winchester, Massachusetts

Caryn E. Douma, MS, RN
Project Manager for the Chief Nursing
  Officer
Administration
Children's Memorial Hermann Hospital
Houston, Texas

Dmitry Dukhovny, MD, MPH
Instructor
Department of Pediatrics
Harvard Medical School
Boston, Massachusetts;
Neonatologist
Department of Neonatology
Beth Israel Deaconess Medical Center
Boston, Massachusetts

Stephanie Dukhovny, MD
Clinical Fellow
Maternal Fetal Medicine/Genetics
Boston University School of Medicine
Boston, Massachusetts;
Division of Maternal-Fetal Medicine
Brigham and Women's Hospital
Boston, Massachusetts

Eric C. Eichenwald, MD
Associate Professor
Department of Pediatrics
Chief, Division of Neonatology
Vice-Chair, Department of Pediatrics
University of Texas Health Science Center
Children's Memorial Hermann Hospital
Houston, Texas

Ayman W. El-Hattab, MBBS
Medical Biochemical Genetics Fellow
Department of Molecular and Human
  Genetics
Baylor College of Medicine
Houston, Texas;
Medical Biochemical Genetics Fellow
Genetics
Texas Children's Hospital
Houston, Texas

**Deirdre M. Ellard, MS, RD, LDN,
CNSD**
Neonatal Dietitian
Department of Nutrition
Brigham and Women's Hospital
Boston, Massachusetts

Caraciolo J. Fernandes, MD
Associate Professor
Department of Pediatrics - Neonatology
Baylor College of Medicine
Houston, Texas;
Medical Director, Transport
Section of Neonatology
Texas Children's Hospital
Houston, Texas

Jennifer Schonen Gardner, PharmD
Neonatal Clinical Pharmacy Specialist
Department of Pharmacy
Texas Children's Hospital
Houston, Texas

Stuart L. Goldstein, MS
Professor
Department of Pediatrics
University of Cincinnati College of Medicine
Cincinnati, Ohio;
Director
Center for Acute Care Nephrology
Cincinnati Children's Hospital Medical Center
Cincinnati, Ohio

James E. Gray, MD, MS
Assistant Professor
Department of Pediatrics
Harvard Medical School
Boston, Massachusetts;
Attending Neonatologist
Department of Neonatology
Beth Israel Deaconess Medical Center
Boston, Massachusetts

Mary Lucia P. Gregory, MD, MMSc
Instructor
Department of Pediatrics
Harvard Medical School
Boston, Massachusetts;
Attending Neonatologist
Department of Neonatology
Beth Israel Deaconess Medical Center
Boston, Massachusetts

Munish Gupta, MD, MMSc
Instructor
Department of Pediatrics
Harvard Medical School
Boston, Massachusetts;
Associate Director, Neonatal Intensive Care Unit
Department of Neonatology
Beth Israel Deaconess Medical Center
Boston, Massachusetts

Anne R. Hansen, MD, MPH
Assistant Professor
Department of Pediatrics
Harvard Medical School
Boston, Massachusetts;
Medical Director, Neonatal Intensive Care Unit
Children's Hospital Boston
Boston, Massachusetts

Linda J. Heffner, MD, PhD
Professor and Chair
Obstetrics and Gynecology
Boston University School of Medicine
Boston, Massachusetts;
Chief
Obstetrics and Gynecology
Boston Medical Center
Boston, Massachusetts

Nancy Hurst
Assistant Professor
Department of Pediatrics
Baylor College of Medicine
Houston, Texas;
Director
Women's Support Services
Texas Children's Hospital
Houston, Texas

Ruth A. Hynes
Staff Nurse III
Neonatal Intensive Care Unit
Children's Hospital Boston
Boston, Massachusetts

Lise Johnson, MD
Instructor
Department of Pediatrics
Harvard Medical School
Boston, Massachusetts;
Medical Director, Well New Born Nurseries
Division of Newborn Medicine
Brigham and Women's Hospital
Boston, Massachusetts

Yvette R. Johnson, MD, MPH
Assistant Professor
Department of Pediatrics
Baylor College of Medicine
Houston, Texas;
Medical Director of the Perinatal Outcomes
Database
Section of Neonatology
Texas Children's Hospital
Houston, Texas

Marsha R. Joselow
Social Worker
Pediatric Advanced Care Team
Children's Hospital Boston and Dana-Farber
Cancer Institute
Boston, Massachusetts

James R. Kasser, MD
Catharina Ormandy Professor of
Orthopaedic Surgery
Harvard Medical School
Boston, Massachusetts;
Orthopaedic Surgeon-in-Chief
Department of Orthopaedic Surgery
Children's Hospital Boston
Boston, Massachusetts

Kirsten A. Kienstra, MD
Assistant Professor
Department of Pediatrics - Neonatology
Baylor College of Medicine
Houston, Texas;
Attending Physician
Neonatology
Texas Children's Hospital
Houston, Texas

Aimee Knorr, MD
Instructor
Department of Pediatrics
Harvard Medical School
Boston, Massachusetts;
Staff Physician Newborn Medicine
Director of Newborn Hearing Screening at
Winchester Hospital
Winchester, Massachusetts

Michelle A. LaBrecque, MSN
Clinical Nurse Specialist
Neonatal Intensive Care Unit
Children's Hospital Boston
Boston, Massachusetts

Aviva Lee-Parritz, MD
Associate Professor
Obstetrics and Gynecology
Boston University, School of Medicine
Boston, Massachusetts;
Vice-Chair
Obstetrics and Gynecology
Boston Medical Center
Boston, Massachusetts

Joseph R. Madsen, MD
Associate Professor
Department of Surgery
Harvard Medical School
Boston, Massachusetts;
Director, Neurodynamics Laboratory
Director, Epilepsy Surgery Program
Neurosurgery
Children's Hospital Boston
Boston, Massachusetts

Lucila Marquez, MD
Clinical Fellow
Department of Pediatrics, Section of
Infectious Diseases
Baylor College of Medicine
Houston, Texas

Camilia R. Martin, MD, MS
Associate Professor
Department of Pediatrics
Harvard Medical School
Boston, Massachusetts;
Associate Director
Neonatal Intensive Care Unit
Beth Israel Deaconess Medical Center
Boston, Massachusetts

Thomas F. McElrath, MD, PhD
Associate Professor
Department of Obstetrics and Gynecology
Harvard Medical School
Boston, Massachusetts;
Division of Maternal-Fetal Medicine
Brigham and Women's Hospital
Boston, Massachusetts

Tiffany M. McKee-Garrett, MD
Assistant Professor
Department of Pediatrics - Neonatology
Baylor College of Medicine
Houston, Texas;
Attending Physician
Texas Children's Hospital
Houston, Texas

Ellis J. Neufeld, MD, PhD
Professor
Department of Pediatrics
Harvard Medical School
Boston, Massachusetts;
Associate Chief
Division of Hematology/Oncology
Children's Hospital Boston
Boston, Massachusetts

Deirdre O'Reilly, MD, MPH
Instructor
Department of Pediatrics
Harvard Medical School
Boston, Massachusetts;
Neonatologist
Division of Newborn Medicine
Children's Hospital Boston
Boston, Massachusetts

Debra Palazzi, MD
Assistant Professor
Department of Pediatric, Section of
  Infectious Diseases
Baylor College of Medicine
Houston, Texas;
Attending Physician
Section of Infectious Diseases
Texas Children's Hospital
Houston, Texas

Mohan Pammi, MD, MRCP
Assistant Professor
Department of Pediatrics - Neonatology
Baylor College of Medicine
Houston, Texas;
Attending Physician
Neonatology
Texas Children's Hospital
Houston, Texas

Lu-Ann Papile, MD
Professor
Department of Pediatrics - Neonatology
Baylor College of Medicine
Houston, Texas;
Attending Physician
Neonatology
Texas Children's Hospital
Houston, Texas

Richard B. Parad, MD, MPH
Associate Professor
Department of Pediatrics
Harvard Medical School
Boston, Massachusetts;
Attending Neonatologist
Division of Newborn Medicine
Brigham and Women's Hospital
Boston, Massachusetts

Frank X. Placencia, MD
Assistant Professor
Department of Pediatrics - Neonatology
Baylor College of Medicine
Houston, Texas;
Attending Physician
Neonatology
Texas Children's Hospital
Houston, Texas

Muralidhar H. Premkumar, MBBS, DNB, MRCPCH
Assistant Professor
Department of Pediatrics - Neonatology
Baylor College of Medicine
Houston, Texas;
Attending Physician
Neonatology
Texas Children's Hospital
Houston, Texas

Karen M. Puopolo, MD, PhD
Assistant Professor
Department of Pediatrics
Harvard Medical School
Boston, Massachusetts;
Attending Physician
Division of Newborn Medicine
Brigham and Women's Hospital
Boston, Massachusetts

Steven A. Ringer, MD, PhD
Associate Professor
Department of Pediatrics
Harvard Medical School
Boston, Massachusetts;
Chief
Division of Newborn Medicine
Brigham and Women's Hospital
Boston, Massachusetts

Matthew Saxonhouse, MD
Attending Neonatologist
Pediatrix Medical Group
Carolinas Medical Center-NE
Concord, New Carolina

Lori A. Sielski, MD
Associate Professor
Department of Pediatrics - Neonatology
Baylor College of Medicine
Houston, Texas;
Director of Newborn Nursery
Department of Pediatrics
Ben Taub General Hospital
Houston, Texas

Steven R. Sloan, MD, MPH
Assistant Professor
Department of Pathology
Harvard Medical School
Boston, Massachusetts;
Blood Bank Medical Director
Department of Laboratory Medicine
Children's Hospital Boston
Boston, Massachusetts

Vincent C. Smith, MD, MPH
Instructor
Department of Pediatrics
Harvard Medical School
Boston, Massachusetts;
Associate Director, Neonatal Intensive Care
  Unit
Department of Neonatology
Beth Israel Deaconess Medical Center
Boston, Massachusetts

Martha Sola-Visner, MD
Assistant Professor
Department of Pediatrics
Harvard Medical School
Boston, Massachusetts;
Neonatologist
Division of Newborn Medicine
Children's Hospital Boston
Boston, Massachusetts

Janet S. Soul, MD, CM, FRCPC
Assistant Professor
Department of Neurology
Harvard Medical School
Boston, Massachusetts;
Director, Clinical Neonatal Neurology
Neurology
Children's Hospital Boston
Boston, Massachusetts

Norman P. Spack, MD
Assistant Professor
Department of Pediatrics
Harvard Medical School
Boston, Massachusetts;
Associate in Endocrinology
Endocrine Division
Children's Hospital Boston
Boston, Massachusetts

Ann R. Stark, MD
Professor
Department of Pediatrics - Neonatology
Baylor College of Medicine
Houston, Texas

Jane E. Stewart, MD
Assistant Professor
Department of Pediatrics
Harvard Medical School
Boston, Massachusetts;
Associate Director
Department of Neonatology
Beth Israel Deaconess Medical Center
Boston, Massachusetts

V. Reid Sutton, MD
Associate Professor
Department of Molecular and Human
  Genetics
Baylor College of Medicine
Houston, Texas;
Genetics
Texas Children's Hospital
Houston, Texas

Linda J. Van Marter, MD, PhD
Associate Professor
Department of Pediatrics
Harvard Medical School
Boston, Massachusetts;
Senior Associate in Newborn Medicine and
  Director of Clinical Research
Division of Newborn Medicine
Children's Hospital Boston
Boston, Massachusetts

Deborah K. VanderVeen, MD
Assistant Professor
Department of Ophthalmology
Harvard Medical School
Boston, Massachusetts;
Associate in Ophthalmology
Department of Ophthalmology
Children's Hospital Boston
Boston, Massachusetts

Louis Vernacchio, MD, MSc
Assistant Clinical Professor
Department of Pediatrics
Harvard Medical School
Boston, Massachusetts;
Division of General Pediatrics
Children's Hospital Boston
Boston, Massachusetts

Ari J. Wassner, MD
Clinical Fellow
Department of Pediatrics
Harvard Medical School
Boston, Massachusetts;
Fellow in Endocrinology
Children's Hospital Boston
Boston, Massachusetts

Gil Wernovsky, MD, FACC, FAPP
Associate Professor
Department of Pediatrics
University of Pennsylvania School of Medicine
Philadelphia, Pennsylvania;
Director
Program Development
Staff Cardiologist
Cardiac Intensive Care Unit
Cardiac Center at the Children's Hospital of
  Philadelphia
Philadelphia, Pennsylvania

Richard E. Wilker, MD
Instructor
Department of Pediatrics
Harvard Medical School
Boston, Massachusetts;
Chief of Neonatology
Department of Pediatrics
Newton-Wellesley Hospital
Newton, Massachusetts

Louise E. Wilkins-Haug, MD, PhD
Associate Professor
Department of Obstetrics and Gynecology
Harvard Medical School
Boston, Massachusetts;
Division Director
Division of Maternal-Fetal Medicine and
  Reproductive Genetics
Brigham and Women's Hospital
Boston, Massachusetts

Gerhard K. Wolf, MD
Assistant Professor of Anesthesia
Harvard Medical School
Boston, Massachusetts;
Associate in Critical Care Medicine
Anesthesia, Division of Critical Care Medicine
Children's Hospital Boston
Boston, Massachusetts

John A. F. Zupancic, MD, ScD
Assistant Professor
Department of Pediatrics
Harvard Medical School
Boston, Massachusetts;
Department of Neonatology
Beth Israel Deaconess Medical Center
Boston, Massachusetts

Preface

This edition of the *Manual of Neonatal Care* has been completely updated and extensively revised to reflect the changes in fetal, perinatal, and neonatal care that have occurred since the sixth edition. In addition, we welcome Anne Hansen from Harvard as a new editor and collaborator.

In the Manual, we describe our current and practical approaches to evaluation and management of conditions encountered in the fetus and the newborn, as practiced in high volume clinical services that include contemporary prenatal and postnatal care of infants with routine, as well as complex medical and surgical problems. Although we base our practice on the best available evidence, we recognize that many areas of controversy exist, that there is often more than one approach to a problem, and that our knowledge continues to grow.

Our commitment to values, including clinical excellence, multidisciplinary collaboration, teamwork, and family-centered care, is evident throughout the book. Support of families is reflected in our chapters on Breastfeeding, Developmental Care, Bereavement, and Decision Making and Ethical Dilemmas.

The Children's Hospital Boston Neonatology Program at Harvard has grown to include 57 attending neonatologists and 18 fellows who care for more than 28,000 newborns delivered annually at the Beth Israel Deaconess Medical Center (BIDMC), the Brigham and Women's Hospital (BWH) (formerly the Boston Lying-In Hospital and the Boston Hospital for Women), Beverly Hospital, Saint Elizabeth's Medical Center, Holy Family Hospital, Good Samaritan Medical Center, South Shore Hospital, and Winchester Hospital. They also care for the 650 neonates transferred annually to the NICU at Children's Hospital Boston for management of complex medical and surgical problems. Fellows in the Harvard Neonatal–Perinatal Fellowship Program train in addition to Children's Hospital at the Beth Israel Deaconess Medical Center, the Brigham and Women's Hospital, and the Massachusetts General Hospital.

This would have been an impossible task without the administrative assistance of Jessica DeNaples and Katie Scarpelli. We also thank Nicole Walz, Sonya Seigafuse, and Ave McCracken of Lippincott Williams & Wilkins for their invaluable help.

We acknowledge the efforts of many individuals to advance the care of newborns and recognize, in particular, our teachers, colleagues, and trainees at Harvard, where the editors trained in newborn medicine and practiced in the NICUs. We are indebted to Clement Smith and Nicholas M. Nelson for their insights into newborn physiology and to Steward Clifford, William D. Cochran, John Hubbell, and Manning Sears for their contributions to the care of infants at the Boston Lying-In Hospital. We thank the former and current directors of the Newborn Medicine Program at Harvard: H. William Taeusch Jr., Barry T. Smith, Michael F. Epstein, Merton Bernfield, Ann R. Stark, Gary A. Silverman, and Stella Kourembanas.

We dedicate this book to Dr. Mary Ellen Avery for her contributions to the care of infants all over the world and to the personal support and advice she has provided to so many, including the editors. We also dedicate this book to the memory of Dr. Ralph D. Feigin for his leadership in academic pediatrics, his support of the highest quality care for infants and children, and his contribution to the training of countless pediatricians. Finally, we gratefully acknowledge the nurses, residents, fellows, parents, and babies who provide the inspiration for and measure the usefulness of the information contained in this volume.

John P. Cloherty, MD
Eric C. Eichenwald, MD
Anne R. Hansen, MD, MPH
Ann R. Stark, MD

Contents

Prenatal Assessment and Conditions

1 **Fetal Assessment and Prenatal Diagnosis** 1
Louise E. Wilkins-Haug and Linda J. Heffner

2 **Diabetes Mellitus** 11
Aviva Lee-Parritz and John P. Cloherty

3 **Thyroid Disorders** 24
Mandy Brown Belfort and Rosalind S. Brown

4 **Preeclampsia and Related Conditions** 39
Thomas F. McElrath

Assessment and Treatment in the Immediate Postnatal Period

5 **Resuscitation in the Delivery Room** 47
Steven A. Ringer

6 **Birth Trauma** 63
Elisa Abdulhayoglu

7 **The High-Risk Newborn: Anticipation, Evaluation, Management, and Outcome** 74
Vincent C. Smith

8 **Assessment of the Newborn History and Physical Examination of the Newborn** 91
Lise Johnson and William D. Cochran

9 **Care of the Well Newborn** 103
Lori A. Sielski and Tiffany M. McKee-Garrett

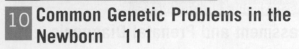

General Newborn Condition

10 **Common Genetic Problems in the Newborn 111**
Carlos A. Bacino

11 **Multiple Births 124**
Yvette R. Johnson

12 **Maternal Drug Abuse, Exposure, and Withdrawal 134**
Katherine W. Altshul

13 **Care of the Extremely Low Birth Weight Infant 154**
Steven A. Ringer

14 **Developmentally Supportive Care 166**
Caroll Spruill Turnage and Lu-Ann Papile

15 **Temperature Control 178**
Kimberlee Chatson

16 **Follow-up Care of Very Preterm and Very Low Birth Weight Infants 185**
Jane E. Stewart and Marsha R. Joselow

17 **Neonatal Transport 192**
Caraciolo J. Fernandes

18 **Discharge Planning 203**
Ruth A. Hynes and Theresa M. Andrews

19 **Decision Making and Ethical Dilemmas 219**
Frank X. Placencia

20 Management of Neonatal End-of-Life Care and Bereavement Follow-up 225
Caryn E. Douma

Fluid Electrolytes Nutrition, Gastrointestinal, and Renal Issues

 21 Nutrition 230
Deirdre M. Ellard and Diane M. Anderson

 22 Breastfeeding 263
Nancy Hurst

23 Fluid and Electrolyte Management 269
Elizabeth G. Doherty

24 Hypoglycemia and Hyperglycemia 284
Richard E. Wilker

25 Abnormalities of Serum Calcium and Magnesium 297
Steven A. Abrams

26 Neonatal Hyperbilirubinemia 304
Mary Lucia P. Gregory, Camilia R. Martin, and John P. Cloherty

27 Necrotizing Enterocolitis 340
Muralidhar H. Premkumar

28 Renal Conditions 350
David J. Askenazi and Stuart L. Goldstein

Respiratory Disorders

29 Mechanical Ventilation 377
Eric C. Eichenwald

30 Blood Gas and Pulmonary Function Monitoring 393
James M. Adams

 31 Apnea 397
Ann R. Stark

32 Transient Tachypnea of the Newborn 403
Kirsten A. Kienstra

33 Respiratory Distress Syndrome 406
Kushal Y. Bhakta

 34 Bronchopulmonary Dysplasia/Chronic Lung Disease 417
Richard B. Parad

35 Meconium Aspiration 429
Heather H. Burris

 36 Persistent Pulmonary Hypertension of the Newborn 435
Linda J. Van Marter

37 Pulmonary Hemorrhage 443
Kirsten A. Kienstra

 38 Pulmonary Air Leak 446
Mohan Pammi

 39 Extracorporeal Membrane Oxygenation 454
Gerhard K. Wolf and John H. Arnold

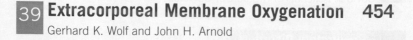

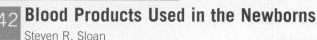

Cardiovascular Disorders

40 Shock 463
Pankaj B. Agrawal

41 Cardiac Disorders 469
Stephanie Burns Wechsler and Gil Wernovsky

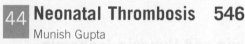

Hematologic Disorders

42 Blood Products Used in the Newborns 529
Steven R. Sloan

43 Bleeding 538
Ellis J. Neufeld

44 Neonatal Thrombosis 546
Munish Gupta

45 Anemia 563
Helen A. Christou

46 Polycythemia 572
Deirdre O'Reilly

47 Neonatal Thrombocytopenia 578
Chaitanya Chavda, Matthew Saxonhouse, and Martha Sola-Visner

Infectious Diseases

48 Viral Infections 588
Sandra K. Burchett

49 Bacterial and Fungal Infections 624
Karen M. Puopolo

50 Congenital Toxoplasmosis 656
Lucila Marquez and Debra Palazzi

51 Syphilis 664
Louis Vernacchio

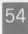
52 Tuberculosis 672
Dmitry Dukhovny and John P. Cloherty

53 Lyme Disease 683
Muhammad Aslam

Neurologic Disorders

54 Intracranial Hemorrhage 686
Janet S. Soul

55 Perinatal Asphyxia and Hypoxic-Ischemic Encephalopathy 711
Anne R. Hansen and Janet S. Soul

56 Neonatal Seizures 729
Ann M. Bergin

57 Neural Tube Defects 743
Joseph R. Madsen and Anne R. Hansen

Bone Conditions

58 Orthopaedic Problems 757
James R. Kasser

59 Osteopenia (Metabolic Bone Disease) of Prematurity 762
Steven A. Abrams

Metabolism

 Inborn Errors of Metabolism 767
Ayman W. El-Hattab and V. Reid Sutton

Sexual Development

 Disorders of Sex Development 791
Ari J. Wassner and Norman P. Spack

Surgery

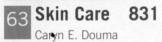 **Surgical Emergencies in the Newborn 808**
Steven A. Ringer and Anne R. Hansen

Dermatology

 Skin Care 831
Caryn E. Douma

Auditory and Ophthalmologic Disorders

 Retinopathy of Prematurity 840
Deborah K. VanderVeen and John A. F. Zupancic

Hearing Loss in Neonatal Intensive Care Unit Graduates 846
Jane E. Stewart and Aimee Knorr

Common Neonatal Procedures

Common Neonatal Procedures 851
Steven A. Ringer and James E. Gray

Pain and Stress Control

67 Preventing and Treating Pain and Stress among Infants in the Newborn Intensive Care Unit 870
Carol Spruill Turnage and Michelle A. LaBrecque

Appendix A: Common Neonatal Intensive Care Unit (NICU) Medication Guidelines 886
Caryn E. Douma and Jennifer Schonen Gardner

Appendix B: Effects of Maternal Drugs on the Fetus 932
Stephanie Dukhovny

Appendix C: Maternal Medications and Breastfeeding 973
Karen M. Puopolo

Index 985

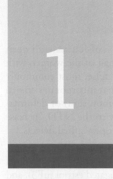

1 Fetal Assessment and Prenatal Diagnosis

Louise E. Wilkins-Haug and Linda J. Heffner

I. GESTATIONAL-AGE ASSESSMENT is important to both the obstetrician and pediatrician and must be made with a reasonable degree of precision. Elective obstetric interventions such as chorionic villus sampling (CVS) and amniocentesis must be timed appropriately. When premature delivery is inevitable, gestational age is important with regard to prognosis, the management of labor and delivery, and the initial neonatal treatment plan.

A. **The clinical estimate** of gestational age is usually made on the basis of the first day of the last menstrual period. Accompanied by physical examination, auscultation of fetal heart sounds and maternal perception of fetal movement can also be helpful.

B. **Ultrasonic estimation** of gestational age. During the first trimester, fetal crown-rump length can be an accurate predictor of gestational age. Crown-rump length estimation of gestational age is expected to be within 7 days of the true gestational age. During the second and third trimesters, measurements of the biparietal diameter (BPD) and the fetal femur length best estimate gestational age. Strict criteria for measuring the cross-sectional images through the fetal head ensure accuracy. Nonetheless, owing to normal biologic variability, the accuracy of gestational age estimated by BPD decreases with increasing gestational age. For measurements made at 14 to 20 weeks of gestation, the variation is up to 11 days; at 20 to 28 weeks, the variation is up to 14 days; and at 29 to 40 weeks, the variation can be up to 21 days. The length of the calcified fetal femur is often measured and used in validating BPD measurements or used alone in circumstances where BPD cannot be measured (e.g., deeply engaged fetal head) or is inaccurate (e.g., hydrocephalus).

II. PRENATAL DIAGNOSIS OF FETAL DISEASE continues to improve. The genetic or developmental basis for many disorders is emerging, along with increased test accuracy. Two types of tests are available: screening tests and diagnostic procedures. Screening tests, such as a sample of the mother's blood or an ultrasound, are noninvasive but relatively nonspecific. A positive serum screening test, concerning family history, or an ultrasonic examination that suggests anomalies or aneuploidy may lead patient and physician to consider a diagnostic procedure. Diagnostic procedures, which necessitate obtaining a sample of fetal material, pose a small risk to both mother and fetus but can confirm or rule out the disorder in question.

A. **Screening by maternal serum analysis** during pregnancy individualizes a woman's risk of carrying a fetus with a neural tube defect (NTD) or an aneuploidy such as trisomy 21 (Down syndrome) or trisomy 18 (Edward syndrome).

1. **Maternal serum alpha-fetoprotein (MSAFP)** measurement between 15 and 22 weeks' gestation screens for NTDs. MSAFP elevated above 2.5 multiples

of the median for gestation age occurs in 70% to 85% of fetuses with open spina bifida and 95% of fetuses with anencephaly. In half of the women with elevated levels, ultrasonic examination reveals another cause, most commonly an error in gestational age estimate. Ultrasonography that incorporates cranial or intracranial signs, such as changes in head shape (lemon sign) or deformation of the cerebellum (banana sign) that are secondary to the NTD, increase the sensitivity of ultrasound for the visual detection of open spinal defects.

2. **Second-trimester aneuploidy screening: MSAFP/triple panel/quad panel.** Low levels of MSAFP are associated with chromosomal abnormalities. Altered levels of human chorionic gonadotropin (hCG), unconjugated estriol (uE3), and inhibin are also associated with fetal chromosomal abnormalities. On average, in a pregnancy with a fetus with trisomy 21, hCG levels are higher than expected and uE3 levels are decreased. A serum panel in combination with maternal age can estimate the risk of trisomy 21 for an individual woman. For women younger than 35 years, 5% will have a positive serum screen, but the majority (98%) will not have a fetus with aneuploidy. However, only approximately 70% of fetuses with trisomy 21 will have a "positive" maternal triple screen (MSAFP, hCG, uE3) compared with 80% with a positive quad screen (MSAFP, hCG, uE3, inhibin). Trisomy 18 is typically signaled by low levels of all markers.

3. **First-trimester serum screening.** Maternal levels of two analytes, pregnancy-associated plasma protein-A (PAPP-A) and hCG (either free or total), are altered in pregnancies with an aneuploid conception, especially trisomy 21. Similar to second-trimester serum screening, these values can individualize a woman's risk of pregnancy complicated by aneuploidy. However, these tests need to be drawn early in pregnancy (optimally at 9–10 weeks) and even if abnormal, detect less than half of the fetuses with trisomy 21.

4. **First-trimester nuchal lucency screening.** Ultrasonographic assessment of the fluid collected at the nape of the fetal neck is a sensitive marker for aneuploidy. With attention to optimization of image and quality control, studies indicate a 70% to 80% detection of aneuploidy in pregnancies with an enlarged nuchal lucency on ultrasonography. In addition, many fetuses with structural abnormalities such as cardiac defects will also have an enlarged nuchal lucency.

5. **Combined first-trimester screening.** Combining the two first-trimester maternal serum markers (PAPP-A and beta hCG) and the nuchal lucency measurements in addition to the maternal age detects 80% of trisomy 21 fetuses with a low screen positive rate (5% in women younger than 35 years). This combined first-trimester screening provides women with a highly sensitive risk assessment in the first trimester.

6. **Combined first- and second-trimester screening for trisomy 21.** Various approaches have been developed to further increase the sensitivity of screening for trisomy 21 while retaining a low screen positive rate. These approaches differ primarily by whether they disclose the results of their first-trimester results.
   a. Integrated screening is a nondisclosure approach, which achieves the highest detection of trisomy 21 (97%) at a low screen positive rate (2%). It involves a first-trimester ultrasound and maternal serum screening in both the first and second trimester before the results are released.
   b. Sequential screening. Two types of sequential screening tools exist. Both are disclosure tests, which means that they release those results indicating a high risk for trisomy 21 in the first trimester, but then go on to further screen either

the entire remaining population in the second trimester (stepwise sequential) or only a subgroup of women felt to be in a medium risk zone (contingent sequential). With contingent sequential screening, patients can be classified as high, medium, or low risk for Down syndrome in the first trimester. Low-risk patients do not return for further screening as their risk of a fetus with Down syndrome is low. When the two types of sequential tests are compared, they have similar overall screen positive rates of 2% to 3%, and both have sensitivities of over 90% for trisomy 21 (stepwise, 95%; contingent, 93%).

7. **Use of ultrasound following serum screening for aneuploidy.** Second-trimester ultrasound targeted for detection of aneuploidy has been successful as a screening tool. Application of second-trimester ultrasound that is targeted to screen for aneuploidy can decrease the *a priori* maternal age risk of Down syndrome by 50% to 60%, as well as the risk conveyed by the second-trimester serum screening. Recently, second-trimester ultrasound following first-trimester screening for aneuploidy has likewise been shown to have value in decreasing the risk assessment for trisomy 21.

B. In women with a **positive family history of genetic disease,** a positive screening test, or at-risk ultrasonographic features, diagnostic tests are considered. When a significant malformation or a genetic disease is diagnosed prenatally, the information gives the obstetrician and pediatrician time to educate parents, discuss options, and establish an initial neonatal treatment plan before the infant is delivered. In some cases, treatment may be initiated *in utero.*

1. **Chorionic villus sampling (CVS).** Under ultrasonic guidance, a sample of placental tissue is obtained through a catheter placed either transcervically or transabdominally. Performed at or after 10 weeks' gestation, CVS provides the earliest possible detection of a genetically abnormal fetus through analysis of trophoblast cells. Transabdominal CVS can also be used as late as the third trimester when amniotic fluid is not available or when fetal blood sampling cannot be performed. Technical improvements in ultrasonographic imaging and in the CVS procedure have brought the pregnancy loss rate very close to the loss rate after second-trimester amniocentesis, 0.5% to 1.0%. The possible complications of amniocentesis and CVS are similar. CVS, if performed before 10 weeks of gestation, can be associated with an increased risk of fetal limb-reduction defects and oromandibular malformations.

   a. Direct preparations of rapidly dividing cytotrophoblasts can be prepared, making a full karyotype analysis available in 2 days. Although direct preparations minimize maternal cell contamination, most centers also analyze cultured trophoblast cells, which are embryologically closer to the fetus. This procedure takes an additional 8 to 12 days.

   b. In approximately 2% of CVS samples, both karyotypically normal and abnormal cells are identified. Because CVS-acquired cells reflect placental constitution, in these cases, amniocentesis is typically performed as a follow-up study to analyze fetal cells. Approximately one-third of CVS mosaicisms are confirmed in the fetus through amniocentesis.

2. **Amniocentesis.** Amniotic fluid is removed from around the fetus through a needle guided by ultrasonic images. The removed amniotic fluid (~20 mL) is replaced by the fetus within 24 hours. Amniocentesis can technically be performed as early as 10 to 14 weeks' gestation, although early amniocentesis (<13 weeks) is associated with a pregnancy loss rate of 1% to 2% and an increased incidence

of clubfoot. Loss of the pregnancy following an ultrasonograph-guided second-trimester amniocentesis (16–20 weeks) occurs in 0.5% to 1.0% cases in most centers, so they are usually performed in the second trimester.

a. Amniotic fluid can be analyzed for a number of compounds, including alpha-fetoprotein (AFP), acetylcholinesterase (AChE), bilirubin, and pulmonary surfactant. Increased levels of AFP along with the presence of AChE identify NTDs with more than 98% sensitivity when the fluid sample is not contaminated by fetal blood. AFP levels are also elevated when the fetus has abdominal wall defects, congenital nephrosis, or intestinal atresias. In cases of **isoimmune hemolysis**, increased levels of bilirubin in the amniotic fluid reflect erythrocyte destruction. Amniotic fluid bilirubin proportional to the degree of hemolysis is dependent upon gestational age and can be used to predict fetal well-being (Liley curve) (see Chap. 26). Pulmonary surfactant can be measured once or sequentially to assess fetal lung maturity (see Chap. 33).

b. Fetal cells can be extracted from the fluid sample and analyzed for chromosomal and genetic makeup.

  i. Among second-trimester amniocentesis, 73% of clinically significant karyotype abnormalities relate to one of five chromosomes: 13, 18, 21, X, or Y. These can be rapidly detected using fluorescent *in situ* hybridization (FISH), with sensitivities in the 90% range.

  ii. DNA analysis is diagnostic for an increasing number of diseases.

    a) For genetic diseases in which the DNA sequence has not been determined, **indirect DNA studies** use restriction fragment length polymorphism (RFLP) for linkage analysis of affected individuals and family members. Both crossing over between the gene in question and the RFLP probe and the need for multiple informative members from a family limit the number of genetic diagnoses that can be made this way.

    b) Direct DNA methodologies can be used when the gene sequence producing the disease in question is known. Disorders secondary to deletion of DNA (e.g., α-thalassemia, Duchenne and Becker muscular dystrophy, cystic fibrosis, and growth hormone deficiency) can be detected by the altered size of DNA fragments produced following a polymerase chain reaction (PCR). Direct detection of a DNA mutation can also be accomplished by allele-specific oligonucleotide (ASO) analysis. If the PCR-amplified DNA is not altered in size by a deletion or insertion, recognition of a mutated DNA sequence can occur by hybridization with the known mutant allele. ASO analysis allows direct DNA diagnosis of Tay-Sachs disease, α- and β-thalassemia, cystic fibrosis, and phenylketonuria.

  iii. DNA sequencing for many genetic disorders has revealed that a multitude of different mutations within a gene can result in the same clinical disease. For example, cystic fibrosis can result from more than 1,000 different mutations. Therefore, for any specific disease, prenatal diagnosis by DNA testing may require both direct and indirect methods.

3. Percutaneous umbilical blood sampling (PUBS) is performed under ultrasonic guidance from the second trimester until term. PUBS can provide diagnostic samples for cytogenetic, hematologic, immunologic, or DNA studies; it can also provide access for treatment *in utero*. An anterior placenta facilitates obtaining a sample close to the cord insertion site at the placenta. Fetal sedation is usually not needed. PUBS has a 1% to 2% risk of fetal loss, along with complications that can lead to a preterm delivery in another 5%.

4. **Preimplantation biopsy or preimplantation genetic diagnosis (PGD).** Early in gestation (at the eight-cell stage in humans), one or two cells can be removed without known harm to the embryo. In women who are at risk for X-linked recessive disorders, determination of XX-containing embryos by FISH can enable transfer of only female embryos through assisted reproduction. Similarly, woman at increased risk for a chromosomally abnormal conception can benefit from preimplantation biopsy. When one member of a couple carries a balanced translocation, only those embryos that screen negative for the chromosome abnormality in question are transferred. Difficulties remain when more cells are needed for molecular diagnoses. An alternative approach is analysis of the second polar body, which contains the same genetic material as the ovum. PGD is also useful for a wide range of autosomal recessive, dominant, and X-linked molecular diagnoses. Preimplantation genetic screening (PGS) to assess preimplantation embryos for aneuploidy is not currently considered to provide reproductive advantage to women of advanced maternal age or poor reproductive histories.

5. **Free fetal DNA in the maternal circulation.** Whereas fetal cells in the maternal circulation can be separated and analyzed to identify chromosomal abnormalities, the limited numbers preclude using this technique on a clinical basis. Development of a noninvasive method of prenatal diagnosis is ideal because it would eliminate the potential procedure-related loss of a normal pregnancy. Analysis of free fetal DNA and RNA, which is present in larger quantities in the maternal circulation, is a reality for a number of conditions, including red blood cell antigens, single gene disorders, and fetal sex. Development of modalities to address the intricacies of the ratios involved in assessing aneuploid conditions is rapidly evolving. Further work is needed to determine the most appropriate signal to sort the smaller fetal fragments of free nucleic acids from the larger body of maternal-free nucleic acids.

III. **FETAL SIZE AND GROWTH-RATE ABNORMALITIES** may have significant implications for perinatal prognosis and care (see Chap. 7). Appropriate fetal assessment is important in establishing a diagnosis and a perinatal treatment plan.

A. **Intrauterine growth restriction (IUGR)** may be due to conditions in the fetal environment (e.g., chronic deficiencies in oxygen or nutrients or both) or to problems intrinsic to the fetus. It is important to identify constitutionally normal fetuses whose growth is impaired so that appropriate care can begin as soon as possible. Because their risk of mortality is increased several-fold before and during labor, IUGR fetuses may need preterm intervention for best survival rates. Once delivered, these newborns are at increased risk for immediate complications including hypoglycemia and pulmonary hemorrhage, so they should be delivered at an appropriately equipped facility.

Intrinsic causes of IUGR include chromosomal abnormalities (such as trisomies), congenital malformations, and congenital infections (e.g., cytomegalovirus or rubella). Prenatal diagnosis of malformed or infected fetuses is important so that appropriate interventions can be made. Prior knowledge that a fetus has a malformation (e.g., anencephaly) or chromosomal abnormality (e.g., trisomy 18) that adversely affects life allows the parents to be counseled before birth of the child and may influence the management of labor and delivery.

1. **Definition of IUGR.** There is no universal agreement on the definition of IUGR. Strictly speaking, any fetus that does not reach his or her intrauterine growth potential is included. Typically, fetuses weighing less than the 10th percentile for gestational age are classified as IUGR; however, many of these fetuses are normal and at the lower end of the growth spectrum (i.e., "constitutionally small").

2. **Diagnosis of IUGR.** Clinical diagnostics detect about two-thirds of cases and incorrectly diagnose it about 50% of the time. Ultrasonography improves the sensitivity and specificity to over 80%. IUGR may be diagnosed with a single scan when a fetus less than the 10th percentile demonstrates corroborative signs of a compromised intrauterine environment such as oligohydramnios, an elevated head–abdomen ratio in the absence of central nervous system pathology, or abnormal Doppler velocimetry in the umbilical cord. Serial scans documenting absent or poor intrauterine growth regardless of the weight percentile also indicate IUGR. Composite growth profiles derived from a variety of ultrasound measurements and repeated serially provide the greatest sensitivity and specificity in diagnosing IUGR.

B. **Macrosomia.** Macrosomic fetuses (>4,000 g) are at increased risk for shoulder dystocia and traumatic birth injury. Conditions such as maternal diabetes, post-term pregnancy, and maternal obesity are associated with an increased incidence of macrosomia. Unfortunately, efforts to use a variety of measurements and formulas have met with only modest success in predicting the condition.

IV. FUNCTIONAL MATURITY OF THE LUNGS is one of the most critical variables in determining neonatal survival in the otherwise normal fetus. A number of tests can be performed on amniotic fluid specifically to determine pulmonary maturity (see Chap. 33).

V. ASSESSMENT OF FETAL WELL-BEING. Acute compromise is detected by studies that assess fetal function. Some are used antepartum, whereas others are used to monitor the fetus during labor.

A. **Antepartum tests** generally rely on biophysical studies, which require a certain degree of fetal neurophysiologic maturity. The following tests are not used until the third trimester; fetuses may not respond appropriately earlier in gestation.

1. **Fetal movement monitoring** is the simplest method of fetal assessment. The mother lies quietly for an hour and records each perceived fetal movement. Although she may not perceive all fetal movements that might be noted by ultrasonic observation, she will record enough to provide meaningful data.

   Fetuses normally have a sleep–wake cycle, and mothers generally perceive a diurnal variation in fetal activity. Active periods average 30 to 40 minutes. Periods of inactivity >1 hour are unusual in a healthy fetus and should alert the physician to the possibility of fetal compromise.

2. **The nonstress test (NST)** is a reliable means of fetal evaluation. It is simple to perform, relatively quick, and noninvasive, with neither discomfort nor risk to mother or fetus.

The NST is based on the principle that fetal activity results in a reflex acceleration in heart rate. The required fetal maturity is typically reached by approximately 32 weeks of gestation. Absence of these accelerations in a fetus who previously demonstrated them may indicate that hypoxia has sufficiently depressed the central nervous system to inactivate the cardiac reflex.

The test is performed by monitoring fetal heart rate (FHR) either through a Doppler ultrasonographic device or through skin-surface electrodes on the maternal abdomen. Uterine activity is simultaneously recorded through a toco-dynamometer, palpation by trained test personnel, or the patient's report. The test result may be reactive, nonreactive, or inadequate. The criteria for a reactive test are as follows: (i) heart rate between 110 and 160, (ii) normal beat-to-beat variability (5 beats/minute [bpm]), and (iii) two accelerations of at least 15 bpm lasting for not less than 15 seconds, each within a 20-minute period. A nonreactive test fails to meet the three criteria. If an adequate fetal heart tracing cannot be obtained for any reason, the test is considered inadequate.

Statistics show that a reactive result is reassuring, with the risk of fetal demise within the week following the test at approximately 3 in 1,000. A nonreactive test is generally repeated later the same day or is followed by another test of fetal well-being.

3. The **contraction stress test (CST)** may be used as a backup or confirmatory test when the NST is nonreactive or inadequate.

The CST is based on the idea that uterine contractions can compromise an unhealthy fetus. The pressure generated during contractions can briefly reduce or eliminate perfusion of the intervillous space. A healthy fetoplacental unit has sufficient reserve to tolerate this short reduction in oxygen supply. Under pathologic conditions, however, respiratory reserve may be so compromised that the reduction in oxygen results in fetal hypoxia. Under hypoxic conditions, the FHR slows in a characteristic way relative to the contraction. FHR begins to decelerate 15 to 30 seconds after onset of the contraction, reaches its nadir after the peak of the contraction, and does not return to baseline until after the contraction ends. This heart rate pattern is known as a *late deceleration* because of its relationship to the uterine contraction. Synonyms are type II deceleration or deceleration of uteroplacental insufficiency.

Similar to the NST, the CST monitors FHR and uterine contractions. A CST is considered completed if uterine contractions have spontaneously occurred within 30 minutes, lasted 40 to 60 seconds each, and occurred at a frequency of three within a 10-minute interval. If no spontaneous contractions occur, they can be induced with intravenous oxytocin, in which case the test is called an *oxytocin challenge* test.

A CST is positive if late decelerations are consistently seen in association with contractions. A CST is negative if at least three contractions of at least 40 seconds each occur within a 10-minute period without associated late decelerations. A CST is suspicious if there are occasional or inconsistent late decelerations. If contractions occur more frequently than every 2 minutes or last longer than 90 seconds, the study is considered a hyperstimulated test and cannot be interpreted. An unsatisfactory test is one in which contractions cannot be stimulated, or a satisfactory FHR tracing cannot be obtained.

A negative CST is even more reassuring than a reactive NST, with the chance of fetal demise within a week of a negative CST being approximately 0.4 per 1,000. If a positive CST follows a nonreactive NST, however, the risk of stillbirth is 88 per 1,000, and the risk of neonatal mortality is also 88 per 1,000. Statistically, about one-third of patients with a positive CST will require cesarean section for persistent late decelerations in labor.

4. **The biophysical profile** combines an NST with other parameters determined by real-time ultrasonic examination. A score of 0 or 2 is assigned for the absence or presence of each of the following: a reactive NST, adequate amniotic fluid volume, fetal breathing movements, fetal activity, and normal fetal musculoskeletal tone. The total score determines the course of action. Reassuring tests (8–10) are repeated at weekly intervals, whereas less-reassuring results (4–6) are repeated later the same day. Very low scores (0–2) generally prompt delivery. The likelihood that a fetus will die *in utero* within 1 week of a reassuring test is approximately the same as that for a negative CST, which is approximately 0.6 to 0.7 per 1,000.

5. Doppler ultrasonography of **fetal umbilical artery blood flow** is a noninvasive technique to assess downstream (placental) resistance. Poorly functioning placentas with extensive vasospasm or infarction have an increased resistance to flow that is particularly noticeable in fetal diastole. Umbilical artery Doppler flow velocimetry may be used as part of fetal surveillance based on characteristics of the peak systolic frequency shift (S) and the end-diastolic frequency shift (D). The two commonly used indices of flow are the systolic:diastolic ratio (S/D) and the resistance index (S–D/S). Umbilical artery Doppler velocimetry measurements have been shown to improve perinatal outcome only in pregnancies with a presumptive diagnosis of IUGR and should not be used as a screening test in the general obstetric population. Absent or reversed end-diastolic flow is seen in the most extreme cases of IUGR and is associated with a high mortality rate. The use of umbilical artery Doppler velocimetry measurements, in conjunction with other tests of fetal well-being, can reduce the perinatal mortality in IUGR by almost 40%. Doppler measurements of the **middle cerebral artery** can also be used in the assessment of the fetus that is at risk for either IUGR or anemia.

B. **Intrapartum assessment of fetal well-being** is important in the management of labor.

1. **Continuous electronic fetal monitoring** is widely used despite the fact that it has not been shown to reduce perinatal mortality or asphyxia relative to auscultation by trained personnel but has increased the incidence of operative delivery. When used, the monitors simultaneously record FHR and uterine activity for ongoing evaluation.

a. The **fetal heart rate (FHR)** can be monitored in one of three ways. The noninvasive methods are ultrasonic monitoring and surface-electrode monitoring from the maternal abdomen. The most accurate but invasive method is to place a small electrode into the skin of the fetal presenting part to record the fetal electrocardiogram directly. Placement requires rupture of the fetal membranes. When the electrode is properly placed, it is associated with a very low risk of fetal injury. Approximately 4% of monitored babies develop a mild infection at the electrode site, and most respond to local cleansing.

b. **Uterine activity** can also be recorded either indirectly or directly. A tocodynamometer can be strapped to the maternal abdomen to record the timing and duration of contractions as well as crude relative intensity. When a more precise evaluation is needed, an intrauterine pressure catheter can be inserted following rupture of the fetal membranes to directly and quantitatively record contraction pressure. Invasive monitoring is associated with an increased incidence of chorioamnionitis and postpartum maternal infection.

c. **Parameters of the fetal monitoring** record that are evaluated include the following:

    i. **Baseline heart rate** is normally between 110 and 160 bpm. The baseline must be apparent for a minimum of 2 minutes in any 10-minute segment and does not include episodic changes, periods of marked FHR variability, or segments of baseline that differ by more than 25 bpm. Baseline fetal bradycardia, defined as an FHR <110 bpm, may result from congenital heart block associated with congenital heart malformation or maternal systemic lupus erythematosus. Baseline tachycardia, defined as an FHR >160 bpm, may result from a maternal fever, infection, stimulant medications or drugs, and hyperthyroidism. Fetal dysrhythmias are typically associated with FHR >200 bpm. In isolation, tachycardia is poorly predictive of fetal hypoxemia or acidosis unless accompanied by reduced beat-to-beat variability or recurrent decelerations.

    ii. **Beat-to-beat variability** is recorded from a calculation of each RR interval. The autonomic nervous system of a healthy, awake term fetus constantly varies the heart rate from beat to beat by approximately 5 to 25 bpm. Reduced beat-to-beat variability may result from depression of the fetal central nervous system due to fetal immaturity, hypoxia, fetal sleep, or specific maternal medications such as narcotics, sedatives, β-blockers, and intravenous magnesium sulfate.

    iii. **Accelerations** of the FHR are reassuring, as they are during an NST.

    iv. **Decelerations** of the FHR may be benign or indicative of fetal compromise, depending on their characteristic shape and timing in relation to uterine contractions.

        a) Early decelerations are symmetric in shape and closely mirror uterine contractions in time of onset, duration, and termination. They are benign and usually accompany good beat-to-beat variability. These decelerations are more commonly seen in active labor when the fetal head is compressed in the pelvis, resulting in a parasympathetic effect.

        b) Late decelerations are visually apparent decreases in the FHR in association with uterine contractions. The onset, nadir, and recovery of the deceleration occur after the beginning, peak, and end of the contraction, respectively. A fall in the heart rate of only 10 to 20 bpm below baseline (even if still within the range of 110–160) is significant. Late decelerations are the result of uteroplacental insufficiency and possible fetal hypoxia. As the uteroplacental insufficiency/hypoxia worsens, (i) beat-to-beat variability will be reduced and then lost, (ii) decelerations will last longer, (iii) they will begin sooner following the onset of a contraction, (iv) they will take longer to return to baseline, and (v) the rate to which the fetal heart slows will be lower. Repetitive late decelerations demand action.

        c) Variable decelerations vary in their shape and in their timing relative to contractions. Usually, they result from fetal umbilical cord compression. Variable decelerations are a cause for concern if they are severe (down to a rate of 60 bpm or lasting for 60 seconds or longer, or both), associated with poor beat-to-beat variability, or mixed with late decelerations. Umbilical cord compression secondary to a low amniotic fluid volume (oligohydramnios) may be alleviated by amnioinfusion of saline into the uterine cavity during labor.

2. **A fetal scalp blood sample for blood gas** analysis may be obtained to confirm or dismiss suspicion of fetal hypoxia. An intrapartum scalp pH above 7.20 with a base deficit <6 mmol/L is normal. Many obstetric units have replaced fetal scalp blood sampling with noninvasive techniques to assess fetal status. FHR accelerations in response to mechanical stimulation of the fetal scalp or to vibroacoustic stimulation are reassuring.

Suggested Readings

Aagaard-Tillery KM, Malone FD, Nyberg DA, et al. Role of second-trimester genetic sonography after Down syndrome screening. *Obstet Gynecol* 2009;114(6):1189–1196.

Alfirevic Z, Gosden CM, Neilson JP. Chorion villus sampling versus amniocentesis for prenatal diagnosis. *Cochrane Database Syst Rev* 2000;(2):CD000055.

American College of Obstetricians and Gynecologists (ACOG). *ACOG Practice Bulletin No. 12: Intrauterine Growth Restriction.* Washington, DC: American College of Obstetricians and Gynecologists; 2000.

American College of Obstetricians and Gynecologists (ACOG). *ACOG Practice Bulletin No. 62: Intrapartum Fetal Heart Rate Monitoring.* Washington, DC: American College of Obstetricians and Gynecologists; 2005.

Antsaklis A, Papantoniou N, Xygakis, A, et al. Genetic amniocentesis in women 20–34 years old: associated risks. *Prenat Diagn* 2000;20(3):247–250.

Ball RH, Caughey AB, Malone FD, et al. First- and second-trimester evaluation of risk for Down syndrome. *Obstet Gynecol* 2007;110(1):10–17.

Malone FD, Canick JA, Ball RH, et al. First-trimester or second-trimester screening, or both for Down's syndrome. *N Engl J Med* 2005;353(19):2001–2011.

Nicolaides KH, Brizot ML, Snijders RJ. Fetal nuchal translucency: ultrasound screening for fetal trisomy in the first trimester of pregnancy. *Br J Obstet Gynaecol* 1994;101(9):782–786.

Pandya PP, Brizot ML, Kuhn P, et al. First-trimester fetal nuchal translucency thickness and risk for trisomies. *Obstet Gynecol* 1994;84(3):420–423.

Platt LD, Greene N, Johnson A, et al. Sequential pathways of testing after first-trimester screening for trisomy 21. *Obstet Gynecol* 2004;104(4):661–666.

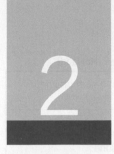

2 Diabetes Mellitus

Aviva Lee-Parritz and John P. Cloherty

I. DIABETES AND PREGNANCY OUTCOME. Improved management of diabetes mellitus and advances in obstetrics, such as ultrasonography and measurement of fetal lung maturity (FLM), have reduced the incidence of adverse perinatal outcome in infants of diabetic mothers (IDMs). With appropriate management, women with good glycemic control and minimal microvascular disease can expect pregnancy outcomes comparable to the general population. Women with advanced microvascular disease, such as hypertension, nephropathy, and retinopathy, have a 25% risk of preterm delivery because of worsening maternal condition or preeclampsia. Pregnancy does not have a significant impact on the progression of diabetes. In women who begin pregnancy with microvascular disease, diabetes often worsens, but in most, the disease return to baseline. Preconception glucose control may reduce the rate of complications to as low as that seen in the general population.

II. DIABETES IN PREGNANCY

A. General principles

1. **Definition.** Diabetes that antedates the pregnancy can be associated with adverse fetal and maternal outcomes. The most important complication is diabetic embryopathy resulting in congenital anomalies. Congenital anomalies are associated with 50% of perinatal deaths among women with diabetes compared to 25% among nondiabetic women. The risk of congenital anomalies is related to the glycemic profile at the time of conception. Women with type 1 and type 2 diabetes are at significantly increased risk for hypertensive disorders, such as preeclampsia, which is potentially deleterious to both maternal and fetal well-being. The White classification is a risk stratification profile based on length of disease and presence of vascular complications (see Table 2.1). Gestational diabetes mellitus (GDM) is defined as carbohydrate intolerance of variable severity first diagnosed during pregnancy, and it affects 3% to 5% of pregnancies.

2. **Epidemiology.** Approximately 3% to 5% of patients with GDM actually have underlying type 1 or type 2 diabetes, but pregnancy is the first opportunity for testing. Risk factors for GDM include advanced maternal age, multifetal gestation, increased body mass index, and strong family history of diabetes. Certain ethnic groups, such as Native Americans, Southeast Asians, and African Americans, have an increased risk of developing GDM.

3. **Pathophysiology for diabetes antedating pregnancy.** In the first half of pregnancy, as a result of nausea and vomiting, **hypoglycemia** can be as much of a problem as **hyperglycemia**. Hypoglycemia, followed by hyperglycemia from counter-regulatory hormones, may complicate glucose control. Maternal hyperglycemia leads to fetal hyperglycemia and fetal hyperinsulinemia, which results in fetal overgrowth. Gastroparesis from long-standing diabetes may be a factor as well. There does not appear to be a direct relation between hypoglycemia alone and

Table 2.1	White Classification of Maternal Diabetes (Revised)
Gestational diabetes (GD):	Diabetes not known to be present before pregnancy
	Abnormal glucose tolerance test in pregnancy
GD diet	Euglycemia maintained by diet alone
GD insulin	Diet alone insufficient; insulin required
Class A:	Chemical diabetes; glucose intolerance before pregnancy; treated by diet alone; rarely seen
	Prediabetes; history of large babies >4 kg or unexplained stillbirths after 28 weeks
Class B:	Insulin-dependent; onset after 20 years of age; duration <10 years
Class C:	C_1: Onset at 10–19 years of age
	C_2: Duration 10–19 years
Class D:	D_1: Onset before 10 years of age
	D_2: Duration 20 years
	D_3: Calcification of vessels of the leg (macrovascular disease)
	D_4: Benign retinopathy (microvascular disease)
	D_5: Hypertension (not preeclampsia)
Class F:	Nephropathy with >500 mg/day of proteinuria
Class R:	Proliferative retinopathy or vitreous hemorrhage
Class RF:	Criteria for both classes R and F coexist
Class G:	Many reproductive failures
Class H:	Clinical evidence of arteriosclerotic heart disease
Class T:	Prior renal transplantation

Note: All classes below A require insulin. Classes R, F, RF, H, and T have no criteria for age of onset or duration of disease but usually occur in long-term diabetes.
Modified from Hare JW. Gestational diabetes. In: *Diabetes complicating pregnancy: The Joslin Clinic Method.* New York: Alan R. Liss; 1989.

adverse perinatal outcome. Throughout pregnancy, **insulin requirements** increase because of the increasing production of placental hormones that antagonize the action of insulin. This is most prominent in the mid–third trimester and requires intensive blood glucose monitoring and frequent adjustment of insulin dosage.

B. **Complications of type 1 and type 2 diabetes during pregnancy**

1. **Differential diagnosis**

   a. **Ketoacidosis** is an uncommon complication during pregnancy. However, ketoacidosis carries a 50% risk of fetal death, especially if it occurs before the third trimester. Ketoacidosis can be present in the setting of even mild hyperglycemia (200 mg/dL) and should be excluded in every patient with type 1 diabetes who presents with hyperglycemia and symptoms such as nausea, vomiting, or abdominal pain.

   b. **Stillbirth** remains an uncommon complication of diabetes in pregnancy. It is most often associated with poor glycemic control, fetal anomalies, severe vasculopathy, and intrauterine growth restriction (IUGR), as well as severe preeclampsia. Shoulder dystocia that cannot be resolved can also result in fetal death.

   c. **Polyhydramnios** is not an uncommon finding in pregnancies complicated by diabetes. It may be secondary to osmotic diuresis from fetal hyperglycemia. Careful ultrasonographic examination is required to rule out structural anomalies, such as esophageal atresia, as an etiology, when polyhydramnios is present.

   d. **Severe maternal vasculopathy**, especially nephropathy and hypertension, is associated with uteroplacental insufficiency, which can result in IUGR, fetal intolerance of labor, and neonatal complications.

III. MANAGEMENT OF DIABETES DURING PREGNANCY

A. **General principles for type 1 or type 2 diabetes.** Management of type 1 or type 2 diabetes during pregnancy begins before conception. Tight glucose control is paramount during the periconceptional period and throughout pregnancy. Optimal glucose control requires coordinated care between endocrinologists, maternal–fetal medicine specialists, diabetes nurse educators, and nutritionists. Preconception glycemic control has been shown to decrease the risk of congenital anomalies to close to that of the general population. However, <30% of pregnancies are planned. Physicians should discuss pregnancy planning or recommend contraception for all diabetic women of childbearing age until glycemic control is optimized.

B. **General principles for gestational diabetes.** In the United States, most women are screened for GDM between 24 and 28 weeks' gestation by a 50-g, 1-hour glucose challenge. A positive result of a blood glucose equal to or greater than 140 mg/dL is followed by a diagnostic 100-g, 3-hour oral glucose tolerance test (GTT). A positive test is defined as two or more elevated values on the GTT. There is a current movement to move to a single diagnostic test, consisting of a 75-g, 2-hour GTT, a method that is used uniformly outside of the United States. Uncontrolled GDM can lead to fetal macrosomia and concomitant risk of fetal injury at delivery. GDM shares many features with type 2 diabetes. Women diagnosed with GDM have a 60% lifetime risk of developing overt type 2 diabetes.

1. **Testing (first trimester) for type 1 and type 2 diabetes**

   a. **Measurement of glycosylated hemoglobin** in the first trimester can give a risk assessment for congenital anomalies by reflecting ambient glucose concentrations during the period of organogenesis.

b. Accurate dating of the pregnancy is obtained by ultrasonography.

c. Ophthalmologic examination is mandatory, because retinopathy may progress because of the rapid normalization of glucose concentration in the first trimester. Women with retinopathy need periodic examinations throughout pregnancy, and they are candidates for laser photocoagulation as indicated.

d. Renal function is assessed by 24-hour urine collection for protein excretion and creatinine clearance. Patients with recent diagnosis of diabetes can have screening of renal function with urine microalbumin, followed by a 24-hour collection if abnormal.

e. Thyroid function should be evaluated.

f. Nuchal translucency and first-trimester serum screening. This is part of routine pregnancy care. It is especially important, as an abnormal nuchal translucency is also associated with structural abnormities, the risk of which is increased in this group of patients.

2. Testing (second trimester) for type 1 and type 2 diabetes

a. Maternal serum screening for neural tube defects is performed between 15 and 19 weeks' gestation. Women with diabetes have a 10-fold increased risk of neural tube defects compared to the general population.

b. All patients undergo a thorough **ultrasonographic survey**, including fetal echocardiography for structural anomalies.

c. Women older than 35 years of age or with other risk factors for fetal aneuploidy are offered **chorionic villus sampling** or **amniocentesis** for karyotyping.

3. Testing (third trimester) for type 1 and type 2 diabetes, GDM

a. Ultrasonographic examinations are performed monthly through the third trimester for fetal growth measurement.

b. Weekly fetal surveillance using nonstress testing or biophysical profiles is implemented between 28 and 32 weeks' gestation, depending on glycemic control and other complications (see Chap. 1).

C. Treatment for all types of glucose intolerance

Strict **diabetic control** is achieved with nutritional modification, exercise, and medications, with the traditional goals of fasting glucose concentration <95 mg/dL and postprandial values <140 mg/dL for 1 hour and 120 mg/dL for 2 hours. Recent data have suggested that in pregnant women, euglycemia may be even lower, with fasting glucose levels in the 60 mg/dL range and postmeal glucose levels <105 mg/dL. Insulin therapy has the longest record of accomplishment of perinatal safety. It has been demonstrated that human insulin analogs do not cross the placenta. More recently, the oral hypoglycemic agent glyburide has been shown to be effective in the management of GDM. Data are emerging that metformin may also be an alternative to achieve glycemic goals during pregnancy.

IV. MANAGEMENT OF LABOR AND DELIVERY FOR WOMEN WITH DIABETES

A. General principles. The risk of spontaneous preterm labor is not increased in patients with diabetes, although the risk of iatrogenic preterm delivery is increased for patients with microvascular disease as a result of IUGR, nonreassuring fetal testing, and maternal hypertension. Antenatal corticosteroids for induction of FLM should be employed for the usual obstetric indications. Corticosteroids can cause temporary hyperglycemia; therefore, patients may need to be managed with continuous intravenous (IV) insulin infusions until the effect of the steroids wears off. **Delivery is planned** for 39 to 40 weeks, unless other pregnancy complications dictate earlier delivery. Elective delivery after 39 weeks does not require FLM testing. Nonemergent delivery before 39 weeks requires documentation of FLM testing using the lecithin–sphingomyelin (L/S) ratio greater than 3.5:1, positive Amniostat (phosphatidyglycerol present), saturated phosphatidylcholine (SPC) greater than 1,000 μg/dL, or mature FLM (see Table 2.2 and Fig. 2.1). Emergent delivery should be carried out without FLM testing. **Route of delivery** is determined by ultrasonography-estimated fetal weight, maternal and fetal conditions, and previous obstetric history. The ultrasonography-estimated weight at which an elective cesarean delivery is recommended is a controversial issue, with the American College of Obstetricians and Gynecologists recommending discussion of cesarean delivery at an estimated fetal weight of greater than 4,500 g due to the increased risk of shoulder dystocia.

B. **Treatment. Blood glucose concentration** is tightly controlled during labor and delivery. If an induction of labor is planned, patients are instructed to take one-half of their usual basal insulin on the morning of induction. During spontaneous or induced labor, blood glucose concentration is measured every 1 to 2 hours. Blood glucose concentration higher than 120 to 140 mg/dL is treated with an infusion of IV short-acting insulin. IV insulin is very short acting, allowing for quick response to changes in glucose concentration. Active labor may also be associated with hypoglycemia, because the contracting uterus uses circulating metabolic fuels. **Continuous fetal monitoring** is mandatory during labor. Cesarean delivery is performed for obstetric indications. The risk of cesarean section for obstetric complications is approximately 50%. Patients with **advanced microvascular disease** are at increased risk for cesarean delivery because of the increased incidence of IUGR, preeclampsia, and nonreassuring fetal status. A history of retinopathy that has been treated in the past is not necessarily an indication for

Table 2.2	Lecithin–Sphingomyelin Ratio, Saturated Phosphatidylcholine Level, and Respiratory Distress Syndrome in Infants of Diabetic Mothers at the Boston Hospital for Women during 1977–1980			
SPC level (mg/dL)	**L/S ratio**			**Mild, moderate, or severe RDS/ total**
	<2.0:1.0	**2.0–3.4:1**	**≥3.5:1.0**	
Not done	0/1	0/12	0/13	0/26 (0%)
≤500	6/6	1/9	1/2	8/17 (47%)
501–1,000	0/2	3/20	1/15	4/37 (11%)
>1,000	0/0	2/22	0/142	2/164 (1.2%)
Total (RDS)	6/9 (67%)	6/63 (10%)	2/172 (1.2%)	14/244 (5.7%)

SPC = saturated phosphatidylcholine; L/S = lecithin/sphingomyelin; RDS = respiratory distress syndrome.

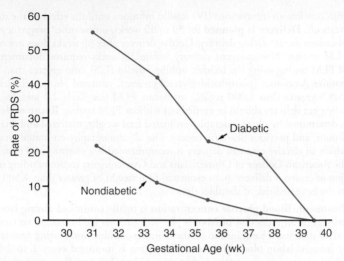

Figure 2.1. Rate of respiratory distress syndrome (RDS) versus gestational age in nondiabetic and diabetic pregnancies at the Boston Hospital for Women from 1958 to 1968. (Reprinted with permission from Robert MF, Neff RK, Hubbell JP, et al. Association between maternal diabetes and the respiratory-distress syndrome in the newborn. *N Engl J Med* 1976;294:357–360.)

cesarean delivery. Patients with active proliferative retinopathy that is unstable or active hemorrhage may benefit from elective cesarean delivery. **Postpartum** patients are at increased risk for hypoglycemia, especially in the postoperative setting with minimal oral intake. Patients with pregestational diabetes may also experience a "honeymoon" period immediately after delivery, with greatly reduced insulin requirements that can last up to several days. Lactation is also associated with significant glucose utilization and potential hypoglycemia, especially in the immediate postpartum period. For women with type 2 diabetes, the use of metformin and glyburide is compatible with breastfeeding.

V. EVALUATION OF INFANTS OF DIABETIC MOTHERS (IDMS)

A. **General principles.** The evaluation of the infant begins **before actual delivery**. If pulmonary maturity is not certain, amniotic fluid can be obtained before delivery through amniocentesis. Fluid may be evaluated by the L/S ratio, FLM testing, or SPC content (see IV.A. and Chap. 33).

B. **Treatment**

1. **After the infant is born**, assessment is made on the basis of Apgar scores to determine the need for any resuscitative efforts (see Chap. 5). The infant should be dried and placed under a warmer. The airway is bulb suctioned for mucus, but the stomach is not aspirated because of the risk of reflex bradycardia and apnea from pharyngeal stimulation in the first 5 minutes of life. A screening physical examination for the presence of major congenital anomalies should be performed, and the placenta should be examined. Glucose level and pH may be determined

on cord blood. In the nursery, **supportive care** should be given while a continuous evaluation of the infant is made. This includes providing warmth, suction, and oxygen as needed while checking vital signs (e.g., heart and respiratory rates, temperature, perfusion, color, blood pressure). Cyanosis should make one consider cardiac disease, respiratory distress syndrome (RDS), transient tachypnea of the newborn, or polycythemia. An examination should be repeated for possible anomalies because of the increased incidence of major congenital anomalies in IDMs. Special attention should be paid to the brain, heart, kidneys, and skeletal system. Reports indicate that IDMs have a 47% risk of significant hypoglycemia, 22% risk of hypocalcemia, 19% risk of hyperbilirubinemia, and a 34% risk of polycythemia; therefore, the following studies are performed:

Blood glucose levels are checked at 1, 2, 3, 6, 12, 24, 26, and 48 hours. Glucose is measured with Chemstrip bG (Bio-Dynamics, BMC, Indianapolis, Indiana). Readings <40 mg/dL should be checked rapidly by a clinical laboratory or by Ames eyetone instrument (Ames Company, Division of Miles Laboratories, Inc., Elkhart, Indiana). The infant is fed orally or given IV glucose by 1 hour of age (see VI. and Chap. 24). **Hematocrit levels** are checked at 1 and 24 hours (see Chaps. 44 and 46). **Calcium levels** are checked if the infant appears jittery or is sick for any reason (see VIII.B. and Chap. 25). **Bilirubin levels** are checked if the infant appears jaundiced (see Chap. 26).

Every effort is made to involve the parents in infant care as early as possible.

VI. HYPOGLYCEMIA IN INFANTS OF DIABETIC MOTHERS (IDMS)

A. **General principles**

1. **Definition.** Hypoglycemia is defined as a blood glucose level <40 mg/dL in any infant, regardless of gestational age and whether or not symptoms are present. Previously, we used a level of <30 mg/dL as the definition of hypoglycemia (see Chap. 24).

2. **Epidemiology.** With <30 mg/dL as the definition, the **incidence of hypoglycemia** in IDMs is 30% to 40%. The onset is frequently within 1 to 2 hours of age and is most common in macrosomic infants.

3. **Pathophysiology.** The pathogenetic basis of **neonatal hypoglycemia in IDMs** is explained by the Pederson maternal hyperglycemia–fetal hyperinsulinism hypothesis. The correlation among fetal macrosomia, elevated HbA_1 in maternal and cord blood, and neonatal hypoglycemia, as well as between elevated cord blood C-peptide or immunoreactive insulin levels and hypoglycemia, suggests that control of maternal blood sugar in the last trimester may decrease the incidence of neonatal hypoglycemia in IDMs. Mothers should not receive large doses of glucose before or at delivery, because this may stimulate an insulin response in the hyperinsulinemic offspring. We attempt to keep maternal glucose level at delivery at approximately 120 mg/dL.

4. Hypoglycemia in small-for-gestational-age (SGA) infants born to diabetic mothers with vascular disease may be due to inadequate glycogen stores; it may also present later (e.g., at 12–24 hours of age). Other factors that may cause hypoglycemia in IDMs are decreased catecholamine and glucagon secretion, as well as inadequate substrate mobilization (diminished hepatic glucose production and decreased oxygenation of fatty acids).

B. Diagnosis

1. **Clinical presentation. Symptomatic, hypoglycemic IDMs** are usually quiet and lethargic rather than jittery. Symptoms such as apnea, tachypnea, respiratory distress, hypotonia, shock, cyanosis, and seizures may occur. If symptoms are present, the infant is probably at greater risk for sequelae. The significance of asymptomatic hypoglycemia is unclear, but conservative management to maintain the blood sugar level in the normal range (>40 mg/dL) appears to be indicated.

2. **Laboratory studies.** Our neonatal protocol is explained in V.B.1. The blood glucose level is measured more often if the infant is symptomatic or has had a low level previously. The blood glucose level is also measured to see the response to therapy.

C. Treatment

1. **Asymptomatic infants with normal blood glucose levels.** In our nursery, we begin **feeding "well" IDMs** by bottle or gavage with dextrose 10% (5 mL/kg body weight) at or before 1 hour of age. Infants weighing <2 kg should have parenteral dextrose starting in the first hour of life. Larger infants can be fed hourly for three or four feedings until the blood sugar determinations are stable. Infants should be switched to formula feeding (20 cal/oz) if the feedings are 2 hours apart or more. This schedule prevents some of the insulin release associated with oral feeding of pure glucose. The feedings can then be given every 2 hours and later every 3 hours, and as the interval between feedings increases, the volume is increased. If by 2 hours of age the blood glucose level is <40 mg/dL despite feeding, or if feedings are not tolerated, as indicated by large volumes retained in the stomach, **parenteral treatment** is necessary.

2. **Symptomatic infants, infants with a low blood glucose level after enteral feeding, sick infants, or infants <2 kg in weight.** The basic treatment element is **IV glucose administration** through reliable access. Administration is usually by **peripheral IV catheter**. Peripheral lines may be difficult to place in obese IDMs, and sudden interruption of the infusion may cause a reactive hypoglycemia in such hyperinsulinemic infants. Rarely, in emergency situations, we have used umbilical venous catheters in the inferior vena cava until a stable peripheral line is placed. Specific treatment is determined by the infant's condition. If the infant is in **severe distress** (e.g., seizure or respiratory compromise), 0.5 to 1.0 g of glucose per kg of body weight is given by an IV push of 2 to 4 mL/kg of 25% dextrose in water (D/W) at a rate of 1 mL/min/kg. For example, a 4-kg infant would receive 8 to 16 mL of 25% D/W over 2 to 4 minutes. This is followed by a continuous infusion at a rate of 4 to 8 mg of glucose per kg of body weight per minute. The concentration of dextrose in the IV fluid depends on the total daily fluid requirement. For example, on day 1, the usual fluid intake is 65 mL/kg, or 0.045 mL/kg/min. Therefore, 10% D/W would provide 4.5 mg of glucose per kg per minute, and 15% D/W would provide 6.75 mg of glucose per kg per minute. In other words, 10% D/W at a standard IV fluid maintenance rate usually supplies sufficient glucose to raise the blood glucose level above 40 mg/dL. However, the concentration of dextrose and the infusion rates are increased as necessary to maintain the blood glucose level in the normal range (Fig. 24.1). The **usual method** in an infant not in severe distress is to give 200 mg of glucose per kg of body weight (2 mL/kg of 10% dextrose) over 2 to 3 minutes. This is followed by a maintenance drip of 6 to 8 mg of glucose per kg per minute (10% dextrose at 80 to 120 mL/kg/day) (Fig. 24.1). **If the infant**

is asymptomatic but has a blood glucose level in the hypoglycemic range, an initial push of concentrated sugar should not be given in order to avoid a hyperinsulinemic response. Rather, an initial infusion of 5 to 10 mL of 10% D/W at 1 mL/min is followed by continuous infusion at 4 to 8 mg/kg/min. Blood glucose levels must be carefully monitored at frequent intervals after beginning IV glucose infusions, both to be certain of adequate treatment of the hypoglycemia and to avoid hyperglycemia and the risk of osmotic diuresis and dehydration. Parenteral sugar should never be abruptly discontinued because of the risk of a **reactive hypoglycemia.** As oral feeding progresses, the rate of the infusion can be decreased gradually, and the concentration of glucose infused can be reduced by using 5% D/W. It is vital to measure blood glucose levels during tapering of the IV infusion. **In difficult cases,** hydrocortisone (5 mg/kg/day intramuscularly in two divided doses) has occasionally been helpful. In our experience, other drugs (epinephrine, diazoxide, or growth hormone) have not been necessary in the treatment of the hypoglycemia of IDMs. In a hypoglycemic infant, **if difficulty is experienced in achieving vascular access,** we may administer crystalline glucagon intramuscularly or subcutaneously (300 μg/kg to a maximum dose of 1.0 mg), which causes a rapid rise in blood glucose levels in large IDMs who have good glycogen stores; the response is not reliable in smaller infants of maternal classes D, E, F, and others. The rise in blood glucose may last 2 to 3 hours and is useful until parenteral glucose can be started. This method is rarely used. The hypoglycemia of most IDMs usually responds to the treatment mentioned earlier and resolves by 24 hours. **Persistent hypoglycemia** is usually due to a continued hyperinsulinemic state and may be manifested by the requirement for glucose use of >8 mg of glucose/kg/min (Fig. 24.1). Efforts should be made to decrease islet cell stimulation (e.g., keeping blood glucose adequate but not high, moving a high umbilical artery line to a low line). **If the hypoglycemia lasts >7 days,** consider other etiologies (see Chap. 24).

VII. RESPIRATORY DISTRESS IN INFANTS OF DIABETIC MOTHERS (IDMS)

A. **General principles**

1. **Epidemiology.** With changes in pregnancy management resulting in longer gestations and more vaginal deliveries, the incidence of RDS in IDMs has fallen from 28% during 1950 to 1960 to 4% in 1990, with the major difference in the incidence of RDS between diabetics and nondiabetics occurring in infants born before 37 weeks' gestation. Most of the deaths from RDS also occur at <35 weeks' gestation in infants who were delivered by cesarean section because of fetal distress or maternal indications.

2. **Etiology.** Besides RDS, causes of respiratory distress are cardiac or pulmonary anomalies (4%), hypertrophic cardiomyopathy, transient tachypnea of the newborn, and polycythemia. Pneumonia, pneumothorax, and diaphragmatic hernia should also be considered. Delayed lung maturity may occur in IDMs because hyperinsulinemia blocks cortisol induction of lung maturation.

B. **Diagnosis**

1. **Laboratory studies** (See Chap. 33 for the differential diagnosis and management of respiratory disorders.)

   a. **Blood gas** analysis should be performed to evaluate gas exchange and the presence of right-to-left shunts.

b. Blood cultures, with spinal-fluid examination and culture, should be taken if the infant's condition permits and infection is a possibility.

2. **Imaging**

a. A **chest x-ray** should be viewed to evaluate aeration, presence of infiltrates, cardiac size and position, and the presence of pneumothorax or anomalies.

b. An **electrocardiogram** and an **echocardiogram** should be taken if **hypertrophic cardiomyopathy** or **a cardiac anomaly** is thought to be present.

VIII. OTHER PROBLEMS FREQUENTLY OBSERVED IN INFANTS OF DIABETIC MOTHERS (IDMS)

A. Congenital anomalies. Congenital anomalies occur more frequently in IDMs than in infants of nondiabetic mothers. As mortality from other causes such as prematurity, stillbirth, asphyxia, and RDS falls, malformations become the major cause of perinatal mortality in IDMs. Infants of diabetic fathers show the same incidence of anomalies as the normal population; therefore, the maternal environment may be the important factor. In the era before modern management, approximately 6% to 10% of pregnancies complicated with diabetes demonstrated a structural abnormality directly related to glycemic control in the period of organogenesis, compared with a usual major anomaly rate of 2% for the general population (see Chap. 10). The most common fetal structural defects associated with maternal diabetes are cardiac malformations, neural tube defects, renal agenesis, and skeletal malformations. Situs inversus also occurs. The central nervous system (anencephaly, meningocele syndrome, holoprosencephaly) and cardiac anomalies make up two-thirds of the malformations seen in IDMs. Although there is a general increase in the anomaly rate in IDMs, no anomaly is specific for IDMs, although half of all cases of caudal regression syndrome (sacral agenesis) are seen in IDMs. There have been several studies correlating metabolic control of diabetes in early pregnancy with **malformations in the IDMs**. Among the more recent studies, that performed by the Joslin Clinic showed a relation between elevated HbA$_1$ in the first trimester and major anomalies in IDMs. The data are consistent with the hypothesis that poor metabolic control of maternal diabetes in the first trimester is associated with an increased risk of major congenital malformations.

B. Hypocalcemia (see Chap. 25). This condition, which is found in 22% of IDMs, is not related to hypoglycemia. The nadir in calcium levels occurs between 24 and 72 hours, and 20% to 50% of IDMs become hypocalcemic, as defined by a total serum calcium level <7 mg/dL. Hypocalcemia in IDMs may be caused by a delay in the usual postnatal rise of parathyroid hormone or vitamin D antagonism at the intestinal level from elevated cortisol and hyperphosphatemia that is due to tissue catabolism.

There is no evidence of elevated serum calcitonin concentrations in these infants in the absence of prematurity or asphyxia. Other causes of hypocalcemia, such as asphyxia and prematurity, may be seen in IDMs. Hypocalcemia in "well" IDMs usually resolves without treatment, and we do not routinely measure serum calcium levels in asymptomatic IDMs. Infants who are sick for any reason—prematurity, asphyxia, infection, respiratory distress—or IDMs with symptoms of lethargy, jitteriness, or seizures that do not respond to glucose should have their serum calcium levels measured. If an infant has symptoms that coexist with a low calcium level, has an illness that delays onset of calcium regulation, or is unable to feed, treatment with calcium may be necessary (see Chap. 25).

C. **Hypomagnesemia** should be considered in hypocalcemia in IDMs because the hypocalcemia may not respond until the hypomagnesemia is treated.

D. **Polycythemia** (see Chap. 46). This condition is common in IDMs. It may be due to reduced oxygen delivery secondary to elevated HbA_1 in both maternal and fetal blood. In SGA infants, polycythemia may be related to placental insufficiency, causing fetal hypoxia and increased erythropoietin. If fetal distress has occurred, there may be a shift of blood from the placenta to the fetus.

E. **Jaundice.** Hyperbilirubinemia (bilirubin >15 mg/dL) is seen with increased frequency in IDMs. Bilirubin production is increased in IDMs as compared with infants of nondiabetic mothers. Bilirubin levels higher than 16 mg/dL were seen in 19% of IDMs at the Brigham and Women's Hospital. Mild hemolysis is compensated for but may cause increased bilirubin production. Insulin causes increased erythropoietin. When measurement of carboxyhemoglobin production is used as an indicator of increased heme turnover, IDMs are found to have increased production as compared with controls. There may be decreased erythrocyte life span because of less deformable cell membranes, possibly related to glycosylation of the erythrocyte cell membrane. Other factors that may account for jaundice are prematurity, impairment of the hepatic conjugation of bilirubin, and an increased enterohepatic circulation of bilirubin as a result of poor feeding. Infants born to well-controlled diabetic mothers have fewer problems with hyperbilirubinemia. The increasing gestational age of IDMs at delivery has contributed to the decreased incidence of hyperbilirubinemia. Hyperbilirubinemia in IDMs is diagnosed and treated as in any other infant (see Chap. 26).

F. **Poor feeding.** This condition is a major problem in IDMs, occurring in 37% of a series of 150 IDMs at the Brigham and Women's Hospital. In our most recent experience (unpublished), it was found in 17% of infants born to mothers with class B to class D diabetes and in 31% of infants born to women with class F diabetes. Infants born to women with class F diabetes are often preterm. There was no difference in the incidence of poor feeding in large-for-gestational-age infants versus appropriate-for-gestational-age infants, and there was no relation to polyhydramnios.

Sometimes, poor feeding is related to prematurity, respiratory distress, or other problems; however, it is often present in the absence of other problems. Poor feeding is a major reason for prolonged hospital stays and parent–infant separation.

G. **Macrosomia.** Macrosomia is defined as a birth weight higher than the 90th percentile or a weight of >4,000 g. The incidence of macrosomia was 28% at the Brigham and Women's Hospital from 1983 to 1984. Macrosomia is not usually seen in infants born to women with class F diabetes. Macrosomia may be linked with an increased incidence of primary cesarean section or obstetric trauma, such as fractured clavicle, Erb palsy, or phrenic nerve palsy as a result of shoulder dystocia. Associations have been found between macrosomia and the following:

1. Third-trimester elevated maternal blood sugar
2. Fetal and neonatal hyperinsulinemia
3. Neonatal hypoglycemia

H. **Myocardial dysfunction.** In IDMs, transient hypertrophic subaortic stenosis resulting from ventricular septal hypertrophy has been reported. Infants may present with heart failure, poor cardiac output, and cardiomegaly. The cardiomyopathy may complicate the management of other illnesses such as RDS. The diagnosis is made using echocardiography, which shows hypertrophy of the ventricular septum, the right anterior ventricular wall, and the left posterior ventricular wall in the absence of chamber dilation. Cardiac output decreases with increasing septal thickness. Most symptoms resolve by 2 weeks of age, and septal hypertrophy resolves by 4 months. Most infants respond to supportive care. Oxygen and furosemide (Lasix) are often needed. Inotropic drugs are contraindicated unless myocardial dysfunction is seen on echocardiography. Propranolol is the most useful agent. The differential diagnosis of myocardial dysfunction that is due to diabetic cardiomyopathy of the newborn includes the following:

1. Postasphyxial cardiomyopathy
2. Myocarditis
3. Endocardial fibroelastosis
4. Glycogen storage disease of the heart
5. Aberrant left coronary artery coming off the pulmonary artery

There is some evidence that good diabetic control during pregnancy may reduce the incidence and severity of hypertrophic cardiomyopathy (see Chap. 41).

I. **Renal vein thrombosis.** Renal vein thrombosis may occur *in utero* or postpartum. Intrauterine and postnatal diagnosis may be made by ultrasonographic examination. Postnatal presentation may include hematuria, flank mass, hypertension, or embolic phenomena. Most renal vein thrombosis can be managed conservatively, allowing preservation of renal tissue (see Chaps. 28, 44, and 62).

J. **Other thromboses** (see Chap. 44)

K. **Small left colon syndrome.** Small left colon syndrome presents as generalized abdominal distension because of inability to pass meconium. Meconium is obtained by passage of a rectal catheter. An enema performed with meglumine diatrizoate (Gastrograffin) makes the diagnosis and often results in evacuation of the colon. The infant should be well hydrated before Gastrograffin is used. The infant may have some difficulties with passage of stool in the first week of life, but this usually resolves after treatment with half-normal saline enemas (5 mL/kg) and glycerine suppositories. Other causes of intestinal obstruction should be considered (see Chap. 62).

IX. TOPICS OF CONCERN TO PARENTS

A. **Genetics.** The parents of IDMs are often concerned about the eventual development of diabetes in their children. There are conflicting data on the incidence of insulin-dependent diabetes in IDMs.

1. In type 1 diabetes, a person in the general population has a <1% chance of developing the disease. If the mother has type 1 diabetes, the risk of the offspring developing the disease is 1% to 4%. If the father has type 1 diabetes, the risk to the offspring is 10%. If both parents have the disease, the risk is approximately 20%.

2. In type 2 diabetes, the average person has a 12% to 18% chance of developing the disease. If one parent has the disease, the risk to offspring is 30%; if both parents have it, the risk is 50% to 60%.

B. **Perinatal survival.** Despite all problems, a diabetic woman has a 95% chance of having a healthy child if she is willing to participate in a program of pregnancy management and surveillance at an appropriate perinatal center.

Suggested Readings

American College of Obstetricians and Gynecologists (ACOG). ACOG Practice Bulletin. Clinical management guidelines for obstetrician–gynecologists. Number 30, September 2001. Gestational diabetes. *Obstet Gynecol* 2001;98:525–538.

American College of Obstetricians and Gynecologists (ACOG). ACOG Practice Bulletin. Clinical management guidelines for obstetrician–gynecologists. Number 60, March 2005. Pregestational diabetes mellitus. *Obstet Gynecol* 2005;105(3):675–685.

American Diabetes Association. Gestational diabetes mellitus. *Diabetes Care Suppl* 2002;25 (suppl 1):S94–S96.

Buchanan TA, Metzger BE, Freinkel N, et al. Insulin sensitivity and B-cell responsiveness to glucose during late pregnancy in lean and moderately obese women with normal glucose tolerance or mild gestational diabetes. *Am J Obstet Gynecol* 1990;162:1008–1014.

Cloherty JP. Neonatal management. In: Brown F, ed. *Diabetes Complicating Pregnancy: The Joslin Clinic Method.* 2nd ed. New York: Wiley-Liss; 1995:169–186.

HAPO Study Cooperative Research Group, Metzger BE, Lowe LP, et al. Hyperglycemia and adverse pregnancy outcomes. *N Engl J Med* 2008;358(19):1991–2002.

Kitzmiller JL, Gavin LA, Gin GD, et al. Preconception care of diabetes: glycemic control prevents congenital anomalies. *JAMA* 1991;265:731–736.

Landon MB. Diabetes in pregnancy. *Clin Perinatol* 1993;20:507.

Landon MB, Langer O, Gabbe SG, et al. Fetal surveillance in pregnancies complicated by insulin-dependent diabetes mellitus. *Am J Obstet Gynecol* 1992;167:617–621.

Langer O, Berkus MD, Huff RW, et al. Shoulder dystocia: should the fetus weighing greater than or equal to 4000 grams be delivered by cesarean section? *Am J Obstet Gynecol* 1991;165:831–837.

Langer O, Conway DL, Berkus MD, et al. A comparison of glyburide and insulin in women with gestational diabetes mellitus. *N Engl J Med* 2000;343(16):1134–1138.

Miller EM, Hare JW, Cloherty JP, et al. Elevated maternal hemoglobin A1c in early pregnancy and major congenital anomalies in infants of diabetic mothers. *N Engl J Med* 1981;304:1331–1334.

Moore LE, Clokey D, Rappaport VJ, et al. Metformin compared with glyburide in gestational diabetes: a randomized controlled trial. *Obstet Gynecol* 2010;115(1):55–59.

Naylor CD, Sermer M, Chen E, et al. Cesarean delivery in relation to birth weight and gestational glucose tolerance: pathophysiology or practice style? Toronto Trihospital Gestational Diabetes Investigators. *JAMA* 1996;275(15):1165–1170.

Parretti E, Mecacci F, Papini M, et al. Third-trimester maternal glucose levels from diurnal profiles in nondiabetic pregnancies: correlation with sonographic parameters of fetal growth. *Diabetes Care* 2001;24(8):1319–1323.

Reece EA, Homko CJ. Infant of the diabetic mother. *Semin Perinatol* 1994;18:459–469.

3 Thyroid Disorders

Mandy Brown Belfort and Rosalind S. Brown

I. THYROID PHYSIOLOGY IN PREGNANCY. Multiple changes occur in maternal thyroid physiology during normal pregnancy.

A. **Increased iodine clearance.** Starting early in pregnancy, increased renal blood flow and glomerular filtration lead to increased clearance of iodine from maternal plasma. Iodine is also transported across the placenta for iodothyronine synthesis by the fetal thyroid gland after the first trimester. These processes increase the maternal dietary requirement for iodine but have little impact on the maternal plasma iodine level or maternal or fetal thyroid function in iodine-sufficient regions such as the United States. To ensure adequate intake, supplementation with 150 mcg per day of iodine is recommended for pregnant and lactating women; of note, many prenatal vitamins lack iodine. In contrast, in regions with borderline or deficient iodine intake, increased iodine clearance and transplacental transfer may lead to decreased thyroxine (T_4) and increased thyroid-stimulating hormone (TSH) levels, as well as increased thyroid gland volume in both the mother and fetus.

B. **Human chorionic gonadotropin (hCG) has weak intrinsic TSH-like activity.** The high circulating level of hCG in the first trimester leads to a small, transient increase in free T_4 accompanied by partial suppression of TSH that resolves by approximately the 14th week of gestation.

C. **Increased thyroxine-binding globulin (TBG) levels** occur early in pregnancy. TBG doubles by mid-gestation then plateaus at a high level. This TBG rise occurs largely as a result of diminished hepatic clearance of TBG from the plasma due to increased estrogen-stimulated sialation of the TBG protein. Estrogen also stimulates TBG synthesis in the liver.

D. **Increased total triiodothyronine (T_3) and T_4 levels** occur from early in gestation as a result of rapidly increasing TBG levels (see I.C.). Free T_4 levels rise much less than total T_4 in early pregnancy (see I.B.), then decline progressively in the second and third trimesters. This physiologic decline is minimal ($<10\%$) in iodine-sufficient regions but may be more pronounced in regions with borderline or deficient iodine intake. Direct free T_4 assays may be affected by TBG and should not be used to monitor maternal thyroid function during pregnancy.

E. **TSH levels decline in the first trimester** in the setting of elevated levels of hCG (see I.B.) and may transiently fall below the normal range for nonpregnant women in approximately 20% of healthy pregnancies. After the first trimester, TSH levels return to the normal, nonpregnant range.

F. **The negative feedback control mechanisms of the hypothalamic-pituitary-thyroid (HPT) axis** remain intact.

G. **Placental metabolism and transplacental passage.** Iodine and TSH-releasing hormone (TRH) freely cross the placenta. The placenta is also permeable to thyroid stimulating and blocking IgG antibodies, as well as antithyroid drugs, but is impermeable to TSH. T_4 crosses the placenta in limited amounts due to inactivation by the type 3 deiodinase (D3) enzyme, which converts T_4 to inactive reverse T_3, rather than to T_3. T_3 is similarly inactivated. In the setting of fetal hypothyroxinemia, maternal–fetal transfer of T_4 is increased, particularly in the second and third trimesters, protecting the developing fetus from the effects of fetal hypothyroidism.

II. MATERNAL HYPERTHYROIDISM. Hyperthyroidism complicates 0.1% to 1% of pregnancies.

A. **Graves' disease** accounts for $\geq$85% of clinical hyperthyroidism in pregnancy. Hyperemesis gravidarum is associated with transient subclinical or mild hyperthyroidism that may be due to the thyroid stimulatory effects of hCG and typically resolves without treatment.

B. **Signs and symptoms of hyperthyroidism** may be nonspecific and include tachycardia, increased appetite, tremor, anxiety, and fatigue. The presence of goiter, ophthalmopathy, and/or myxedema suggests Graves' disease.

C. **Poorly controlled** maternal hyperthyroidism is associated with serious **pregnancy complications**, including spontaneous abortion, preterm delivery, intrauterine growth restriction (IUGR), fetal demise, preeclampsia, placental abruption, thyroid storm, and congestive heart failure (CHF).

D. **Treatment** of maternal hyperthyroidism substantially reduces the risk of associated maternal and fetal complications.

   1. **Antithyroid drugs** are indicated for the treatment of **moderate-to-severe hyperthyroidism**. In the first trimester, propylthiouracil (PTU), rather than methimazole (MMI), is recommended due to possible teratogenic effects of MMI, which has been associated with aplasia cutis congenita, tracheoesophageal fistula, and choanal atresia. Because PTU can cause severe maternal liver dysfunction, in the second trimester, PTU should be switched to MMI. Both PTU and MMI cross the placenta. The fetus is more sensitive than the mother to the effects of antithyroid drugs, so fetal hypothyroidism and goiter can occur even with doses in the therapeutic range for the mother. Clinicians should use the lowest possible dose and monitor closely, aiming to maintain T_4 levels in the high-normal range and TSH levels in the low-normal or suppressed range. **Mild hyperthyroidism** can be monitored without treatment.

   2. **β-adrenergic blocking agents** such as propranolol may be useful in controlling hypermetabolic symptoms; however, long-term use should be avoided due to potential neonatal morbidities, including impaired response to hypoglycemia, hypoxemia, and bradycardia.

   3. **Surgical thyroidectomy** may be necessary to control hyperthyroidism in women who cannot take antithyroid drugs due to allergy or agranulocytosis or in cases of maternal nonadherence to medical therapy.

   4. **Iodine** given at a pharmacologic dose is generally contraindicated because with prolonged use, it can cause fetal hypothyroidism and goiter. However, a short course of iodine in preparation for thyroidectomy appears to be safe, and clinicians may also use iodine in selected cases in which antithyroid drugs cannot be used. **Radioactive iodine** is contraindicated after the first trimester

because it can destroy the fetal thyroid gland, which starts to concentrate iodine at 10 to 12 weeks' gestation.

E. **Fetal and neonatal hyperthyroidism** occurs in approximately 1% to 5% of cases of maternal Graves' disease and results from transplacental passage of TSH receptor–stimulating antibodies. High levels of these antibodies in maternal serum are predictive of fetal and neonatal hyperthyroidism. All pregnant women with Graves' disease should be monitored for fetal hyperthyroidism through serial assessment of fetal heart rate and prenatal ultrasound to detect the presence of fetal goiter and monitor fetal growth. Maternal treatment with antithyroid drugs is effective in treating fetal hyperthyroidism, but if excessive, it can also suppress the fetal thyroid gland and cause hypothyroidism.

F. **Fetal and neonatal hypothyroidism and maternal Graves' disease.** Fetal exposure to PTU or MMI can cause transient hypothyroidism that resolves rapidly and usually does not require treatment (see VI.A.2.a.). In the setting of a history of prior maternal Graves' disease, transplacental passage of TSH receptor–blocking antibodies may cause fetal hypothyroidism. A rare neonatal outcome of maternal Graves' disease is transient pituitary suppression and central hypothyroidism, which may be due to prolonged intrauterine hyperthyroidism. Usually, the serum concentration of TSH receptor–stimulating antibodies is only modestly elevated. Infants of mothers with Graves' disease can present with thyrotoxicosis or hypothyroidism in the newborn period and require close monitoring after birth (see VII.).

III. MATERNAL HYPOTHYROIDISM. Maternal hypothyroidism in pregnancy can be either overt (0.3%–0.5% of pregnancies) or subclinical (2%–3% of pregnancies).

A. **The most common cause of maternal hypothyroidism in iodine-sufficient regions is chronic autoimmune thyroiditis.** Other causes include previous treatment of Graves' disease or thyroid cancer with surgical thyroidectomy or radioablation, drug- and external radiation–induced hypothyroidism, congenital hypothyroidism in the mother, and pituitary dysfunction. Chronic autoimmune thyroiditis is more common in patients with type 1 diabetes mellitus. Rarely, mothers with a prior history of Graves' disease become hypothyroid due to the development of TSH receptor–blocking antibodies.

B. **Signs and symptoms of hypothyroidism in pregnancy** include weight gain, cold intolerance, dry skin, weakness, fatigue, and constipation and may go unnoticed in the setting of pregnancy, particularly in subclinical hypothyroidism.

C. **Unrecognized or untreated hypothyroidism** is associated with spontaneous abortion and maternal complications of pregnancy, including anemia, preeclampsia, postpartum hemorrhage, placental abruption, and need for cesarean delivery. Associated adverse fetal and neonatal outcomes include preterm birth, IUGR, congenital anomalies, fetal distress in labor, and fetal and perinatal death. However, these complications are avoided with adequate treatment of hypothyroidism, ideally from early in pregnancy. **Affected fetuses may experience neurodevelopmental impairments, particularly if both the fetus and the mother are hypothyroid during gestation** (e.g., iodine deficiency, TSH receptor–blocking antibodies).

D. **Women with preexisting hypothyroidism who are treated appropriately typically deliver healthy infants.** Thyroid function tests should be measured as soon as pregnancy is confirmed, 4 weeks later, at least once in the second and third trimesters, and additionally 4 to 6 weeks after any L-thyroxine dose change. The TSH level should be maintained in the low-normal range (<2.5 mU/L), which often requires a T_4 dose 30% to 50% higher than in the nonpregnant state.

E. **Routine thyroid function testing in pregnancy** is currently recommended only for symptomatic women and women with a family history of thyroid disease. Because this strategy detects only two-thirds of women with hypothyroidism, many authors advocate universal screening in early pregnancy; however, this topic remains controversial.

F. **TSH receptor–blocking antibodies** cross the placenta and may cause fetal and transient neonatal hypothyroidism (see VI.A.2.e.).

IV. FETAL AND NEONATAL GOITER

A. **Fetal ultrasound** by an experienced ultrasonographer is an excellent tool for intrauterine diagnosis and monitoring of fetal goiter.

B. **Maternal Graves' disease is the most common cause of fetal and neonatal goiter,** which results most often from fetal hypothyroidism due to PTU or MMI. Fetal and neonatal goiter can also result from fetal hyperthyroidism due to TSH receptor-stimulating antibodies. Antibody-mediated fetal effects can occur in women with active Graves' disease or women previously treated with surgical thyroidectomy or radioablation. Maternal history and serum antibody testing is usually diagnostic. Rarely, cord blood sampling is necessary to distinguish between PTU- or MMI-induced fetal hypothyroidism and TSH receptor-stimulating antibody-induced fetal hyperthyroidism. After delivery, neonates exposed *in utero* to PTU or MMI eliminate the drug rapidly. Thyroid function tests usually normalize by 1 week of age, and treatment is not required.

C. **Other causes of fetal and neonatal goiter** include fetal disorders of thyroid hormonogenesis (usually inherited), excessive maternal iodine ingestion, and iodine deficiency. Goiter resolves with suppression of the serum TSH concentration by L-thyroxine treatment on iodine replacement.

D. **Fetal goiter due to hypothyroidism is usually treated with maternal L-thyroxine administration.** Rarely, treatment with intra-amniotic injections of L-thyroxine in the third trimester is used to reduce the size of fetal goiter and **minimize complications of tracheoesophageal compression,** including polyhydramnios, lung hypoplasia, and airway compromise at birth.

V. THYROID PHYSIOLOGY IN THE FETUS AND NEWBORN

A. The **fetal HPT axis** develops relatively independent of the mother due to the high placental concentration of D3, which inactivates most of the T_4 presented from the maternal circulation (see I.G.).

B. **Thyroid embryogenesis** is complete by 10 to 12 weeks' gestation, by which time the fetal thyroid gland starts to concentrate iodine and synthesize and secrete T_3 and T_4. T_4 and TBG levels increase gradually throughout gestation. Circulating T_3 levels remain low, although brain and pituitary T_3 levels are considerably higher as a result of a local intracellular type 2 deiodinase (D2) enzyme, which converts T_4 to the active isomer T_3. In the setting of fetal hypothyroidism, D2 activity in the brain maintains local T_3 concentration, allowing normal development to proceed.

C. TSH from the fetal pituitary gland increases from mid-gestation. The **negative feedback mechanism of the HPT axis** starts to mature by 26 weeks of gestation. Circulating levels of TRH are high in the fetus relative to the mother, although the physiologic significance is unclear.

D. The ability of the thyroid gland to adapt to exogenous iodine does not mature until 36 to 40 weeks' gestation. Thus, premature infants are more sensitive than are full-term infants to the **thyroid suppressing effects of exogenous iodine.**

E. **Neonatal physiology.** Within 30 minutes after delivery, there is a dramatic surge in serum TSH, with peak levels as high as 80 mU/L at 6 hours of life, followed by a rapid decline over 24 hours, then a slower decline over the first week of life. The TSH surge causes marked stimulation of the neonatal thyroid gland. Serum T_3 and T_4 levels increase sharply and peak within 24 hours of life, followed by a slow decline.

F. In the preterm infant, the pattern of postnatal thyroid hormone change is similar to the pattern seen in the full-term infant, but the TSH surge is less marked, and the T_4 and T_3 responses are blunted. In very preterm infants (<31 weeks' gestation), no surge is seen and, instead, the circulating T_4 level may fall for the first 7 to 10 days. Umbilical cord blood thyroid hormone levels are directly related to gestational age and birth weight (Table 3.1).

VI. CONGENITAL HYPOTHYROIDISM (CH)

A. CH is one of the **most common preventable causes of mental retardation**. The incidence of CH varies globally. In the United States, the incidence is approximately 1:2,500 and appears to be rising. CH is more common among Hispanic (1:1,600) and Asian Indian (1:1,757) infants but less common among non-Hispanic black infants (1:11,000). The female-to-male ratio is 2:1. CH is also more common in infants with trisomy 21, congenital heart disease, and other congenital malformations, including renal, skeletal, gastrointestinal anomalies, and cleft palate. CH may be permanent or transient. Hypothyroxinemia with delayed TSH rise can be caused by permanent or transient conditions.

1. Causes of **permanent CH** (Table 3.2).

   a. **Thyroid dysgenesis.** Abnormal thyroid gland development is the cause of permanent CH in >85% of cases. Thyroid dysgenesis includes aplasia, hypoplasia, and dysplasia; the latter often accompanied by failure to descend into the neck (ectopy). It is almost always sporadic with no increased risk to subsequent siblings. Rarely, thyroid dysgenesis is associated with a genetic abnormality in one of the transcription factors necessary for thyroid gland development (PAX8, TTF-2, NKX2.1). Clinically, infants with thyroid dysgenesis have no goiter, low total and free T_4 levels, elevated TSH, and normal TBG. Thyroglobulin (TG) reflects the amount of thyroid tissue present and is low in aplasia and hypoplasia. Ultrasound and/or thyroid scintiscanning with radioactive iodine (RAI) or pertechnetate (^{99m}Tc) confirms an absent or ectopic thyroid gland.

   b. **Defects in thyroid hormone synthesis and secretion** (thyroid dyshormonogenesis) are responsible for most of the remaining 10% to 15% of permanent CH cases and generally carry a 25% recurrence risk in subsequent siblings. The most common synthetic defect is abnormal thyroid peroxidase activity, which

Table 3.1	Thyroid Hormone Reference Ranges (Mean ±SD) for Full Term and Preterm Neonates			
Gestational age (wks)	Age			
	Birth	7 days	14 days	28 days
Total T$_4$ (mcg/dL)				
23–27	5.4 ±2.0	4.0 ±1.8	4.7 ±2.6	6.1 ±2.3
28–30	6.3 ±2.0	6.3 ±2.1	6.6 ±2.3	7.5 ±2.3
31–34	7.6 ±2.3	9.4 ±3.4	9.1 ±3.6	8.9 ±3.0
≥37	9.2 ±1.9	12.7 ±2.9	10.7 ±1.4	9.7 ±2.2
Free T$_4$ (ng/dL)				
23–27	1.3 ±0.4	1.5 ±0.6	1.4 ±0.5	1.8 ±0.5
28–30	1.4 ±0.4	1.8 ±0.7	1.6 ±0.4	1.7 ±0.5
31–34	1.5 ±0.3	2.1 ±0.6	2.0 ±0.4	1.8 ±0.6
≥37	1.4 ±0.4	2.7 ±0.6	2.0 ±0.3	2.1 ±2.5
Total T$_3$ (ng/dL)				
23–27	19.5 ±14.9	32.6 ±20.2	41.0 ±24.7	63.1 ±27.3
28–30	28.6 ±20.8	56.0 ±24.1	72.3 ±28.0	87.2 ±31.2
31–34	35.2 ±23.4	91.8 ±35.8	109.4 ±41.0	119.8 ±40.1
≥37	59.9 ±34.5	147.8 ±50.1	167.3 ±31.2	175.8 ±31.9
TSH (mU/L)				
23–27	6.8 ±2.9	3.5 ±2.6	3.9 ±2.7	3.8 ±4.7
28–30	7.0 ±3.7	3.6 ±2.5	4.9 ±11.2	3.6 ±2.5
31–34	7.9 ±5.2	3.6 ±4.8	3.8 ±9.3	3.5 ±3.4
≥37	6.7 ±4.8	2.6 ±1.8	2.5 ±2.0	1.8 ±0.9

(continued)

Table 3.1	Thyroid Hormone Reference Ranges (Mean ±SD) for Full Term and Preterm Neonates *(Continued)*			
Gestational age (wks)	**Age**			
	Birth	**7 days**	**14 days**	**28 days**
TBG (mg/dL)				
23–27	0.19 ±0.06	0.17 ±0.04	0.19 ±5.2	0.23 ±0.06
28–30	0.20 ±0.05	0.20 ±0.05	0.21 ±5.2	0.22 ±0.06
31–34	0.24 ±0.08	0.24 ±0.08	0.23 ±7.9	0.23 ±0.08
≥37	0.29 ±0.06	0.34 ±0.11	0.28 ±3.8	0.27 ±0.07

Source: Adapted from Williams FL, Simpson J, Delahunty C, et al. Developmental trends in cord and postpartum serum thyroid hormones in preterm infants. *J Clin Endocrinol Metab* 2004;89(11):5314—5320.

results in impaired oxidation and organification of iodine. Additional reported defects affect other key steps in thyroid hormone synthesis, such as thyroglobulin synthesis, iodine trapping, hydrogen peroxide generation, and tyrosine deiodination. **Pendred syndrome** is characterized by a goiter due to an underlying mild organification defect. It is an important cause of sensorineural deafness, but hypothyroidism rarely occurs in the newborn period. In thyroid dyshormonogenesis, goiter may be present. Total and free T_4 levels are low, TSH is elevated, and TBG is normal. Defects in TG synthesis can be distinguished from other abnormalities in thyroid hormone formation by measurement of serum TG, which is low in TG synthetic defects and high in other thyroid hormone synthetic defects. Unlike in thyroid dysgenesis, thyroid imaging typically reveals a normally placed thyroid gland, which may be of normal size or enlarged.

c. **TSH resistance** is usually caused by mutations in the TSH receptor gene. Rarely, it is due to a loss-of-function mutation in the G-stimulatory subunit that links TSH binding to action (Albright hereditary osteodystrophy). Characteristically, the thyroid gland is small. T_4 is normal or low and TSH is elevated. The severity of the hypothyroidism depends on the degree of resistance.

d. **Central (hypothalamic–pituitary) hypothyroidism** is less common than primary hypothyroidism. Although previously thought to be rare, this condition may be more common than generally appreciated, with an incidence of 1/16,000 to 1/25,000. Affected infants may have other signs of pituitary dysfunction, such as hypoglycemia, microphallus, and midline facial abnormalities. Septo-optic dysplasia is an important cause of central hypothyroidism. Goiter is not present. Total and free T_4 are low, TSH is low or inappropriately normal, and TBG is normal. If central hypothyroidism is suspected, cortisol and growth hormone levels should be measured and a magnetic resonance imaging (MRI) scan done to visualize the hypothalamus and pituitary gland. Failure to identify associated pituitary–hypothalamic defects, particularly adrenocorticotropic and growth hormone deficiencies may lead to substantial morbidity and/or mortality.

2. Causes of **transient CH** (see Table 3.2).

   a. Antithyroid drugs. As discussed in section IV.B., intrauterine exposure to PTU or MMI can cause transient hypothyroidism that typically resolves within 1 week and does not require treatment. The elimination half-life of PTU is 1.5 to 5 hours and of MMI is 4 to 6 hours.

   b. Iodine excess. Neonates may be exposed to excess iodine in the perinatal and/or neonatal period. Preterm infants are particularly susceptible to the thyroid suppressing effects of excess iodine (see V.D.), such as from topical antiseptic solutions (e.g., povidine iodine), radiographic contrast solutions, and drugs (e.g., amiodarone). Iodine is also passed through breast milk and can be excessive in mothers who ingest large amounts of seaweed (e.g., in Japan). Goiter may be present. T_4 is low and TSH is elevated. RAI or ^{99m}Tc uptake is blocked by excess iodine, and ultrasound shows a normally positioned thyroid gland, which may be enlarged.

   c. Worldwide, iodine deficiency is the most common cause of transient hypothyroidism, particularly in preterm infants but is less common in the United States, a generally iodine-sufficient region.

   d. Transient hypothyroxinemia of prematurity is most common in infants born at <31 weeks' gestation. Etiologic factors include hypothalamic–pituitary immaturity (particularly in infants <27 weeks' gestation), acute illness, and medications (e.g., dopamine, steroids). Unlike in primary hypothyroidism, the TSH is inappropriately "normal." Usually, the total T_4 is more affected than the free T_4. Measurement of reverse T_3, which is high in sick euthyroid syndrome but low in hypothyroidism, may be helpful but, frequently, results are not immediately available. Observational studies in premature infants have demonstrated an association of transient hypothyroxinemia with adverse short- and long-term outcomes, including neonatal death, intraventricular hemorrhage, periventricular leukomalacia, cerebral palsy, intellectual impairment, and school failure. However, several randomized trials of routine L-thyroxine supplementation have failed to show a beneficial effect, thus the extent to which low T_4 levels cause these adverse outcomes is unclear. Treatment is controversial but may be most beneficial to infants <27 weeks' gestation.

   e. TSH receptor-blocking IgG antibodies account for 1% to 2% of all cases of CH and occur in 1/180,000 live births, typically in the setting of known maternal autoimmune thyroid disease. These antibodies freely cross the placenta and persist in the neonatal circulation with a half-life of approximately 2 weeks. Both stimulating and blocking antibodies may be present simultaneously and their relative proportions may change over time. Hypothyroidism typically persists for 2 to 3 months and depends on the potency of the blocking activity. Goiter is not present. T_4 is low, TSH is elevated, and TBG is normal. High concentrations of TSH receptor-blocking antibodies are present in maternal and neonatal serum. On thyroid scintiscanning, uptake may be absent, but a normally placed thyroid gland is seen on ultrasound.

   f. Large liver hemangiomas can be associated with severe, refractory hypothyroidism due to expression of D3 activity by the hemangioma. Infants typically present after the newborn period as the hemangioma enlarges. Large doses of L-thyroxine are required for treatment. The hypothyroidism resolves as the hemangioma regresses.

3. **Hypothyroxinemia with delayed TSH elevation (atypical CH)** is often due to recovery from sick euthyroid syndrome but needs to be distinguished from

Table 3.2   Interpretation of Thyroid Function Tests and Imaging Results in Congenital Hypothyroidism and Related Disorders

Cause of hypothyroidism	Total T$_4$	Free T$_4$	TSH	TG	Thyroid imaging	Treatment	Comments
Permanent							
Dysgenesis	↓	↓	↑	↓	Absent, small, or ectopic	Yes	Almost always sporadic
Dyshormonogenesis	↓	↓	↑	*	Normal or ↑	Yes	Usually autosomal recessive
TSH resistance	Normal or ↓	Normal or ↓	↑	↓	Normal or ↓	Depends on severity	Autosomal dominant or recessive
Central (pituitary) hypothyroidism	↓	↓	Normal or ↓	↓	Normal	Yes	Not detected on primary TSH NB screen; may be other pituitary hormone deficiencies
Transient							
Maternal antithyroid medication (PTU, MMI)	↓	↓	↑	Normal or ↑	Normal or ↑	Not usually	Resolves within 1 week
TSH receptor–blocking antibodies	↓	↓	↑	↓	Normal or ↓	Yes	Usually resolves within 2–3 months

							Controversial	
Hypothyroxinemia of prematurity	↓	↓	↓	Normal	Normal	Normal		Some physicians treat infants <27 weeks' gestation
Iodine deficiency	↓	↓	↓	↑	↓	Normal or ↑	Yes†	↓Urinary iodine
Iodine excess	↓	↓	↓	↑	↓	Normal or ↑	Yes	↑Urinary iodine; infants <36 weeks' gestation most susceptible
TBG deficiency	↓	Normal	Normal	Normal	Normal	Normal	No	
Liver hemangioma	↓	↓	↓	↑	↓	Normal	Yes	Rare, usually present after newborn period Requires high L-thyroxine doses

*Absent or ↓ in TG synthetic defect, ↑ in other forms of dyshormonogenesis
†Treat with iodine, not L-thyroxine

transient hypothyroidism, or from a mild form of permanent CH. This condition is most common among very low birth weight infants (<1,500 g, reported incidence 1/250) and low birth weight infants (<2,500 g, reported incidence 1/1,589), and in other critically ill newborns including those with congenital heart disease. Monozygotic twins can also present with delayed TSH rise due to fetal blood mixing before birth. Delayed TSH elevation may be missed on the initial screen, particularly in primary TSH screening programs. Some screening programs require repeat testing at 2 to 6 weeks of age for infants at high risk for delayed TSH elevation and a few require repeat testing for all infants.

B. **Diagnosis.** Over 95% of newborns with CH are asymptomatic at birth, but universal newborn screening allows for early diagnosis and treatment, resulting in an optimal neurodevelopmental outcome. In the United States, 1,600 cases of mental retardation per year are prevented through newborn screening for CH.

1. **Newborn screening for CH** is routine in most developed countries but currently is not performed in many developing countries. It is mandated by law in the United States, where specific screening protocols and cutoff values vary by state. Some programs measure T_4 for the primary screen, followed by TSH when T_4 is low, whereas other programs measure TSH as the primary screen. There are advantages and disadvantages to each approach. A few states measure both T_4 and TSH in the initial screen for all newborns, or for a subset of high-risk newborns, which is an ideal but expensive strategy.

2. In Massachusetts, the primary screening protocol is to measure T_4, followed by TSH measurement for infants whose T_4 is ≤13 mcg/dL or in the lowest 10th percentile for the set of samples run together. Additionally, the TSH level is measured for infants in the NICU, infants weighing <1,500 g, infants with a reported family history or clinical signs of hypothyroidism, or for follow-up of a previously unsatisfactory specimen (e.g., too early, incorrect technique). The screening program considers the TSH level to be elevated if it is ≥25 mU/L for infants <24 hours of age; ≥20 mU/L for infants 24 to 96 hours of age; and ≥15 mU/L for infants >96 hours of age. Infants with abnormal screening test results should be evaluated urgently in consultation with a pediatric endocrinologist (see VI.B.5. and Figure 3.1).

3. A **filter paper blood spot specimen** should be sent from all newborns, optimally at 48 to 72 hours of age but, often, this is not possible due to the practice of early discharge. For infants discharged prior to 48 hours of age, a specimen should be sent prior to discharge. Infants discharged before 24 hours of age should be retested at 48 to72 hours to minimize risk of false negative results. For infants transferred to another hospital, the receiving hospital should send a specimen if it cannot be confirmed that the hospital of birth sent one. For infants <1,500 g birth weight, repeat specimens should be sent at 2, 6, and 10 weeks of age due to the risk of delayed TSH elevation (see VI.A.3.).

4. **If clinical signs of hypothyroidism** are present (prolonged jaundice, constipation, hypothermia, poor tone, mottled skin, poor feeding, large tongue, open posterior fontanel), thyroid function tests should be sent immediately, **even if the initial screen was normal**. Rarely, screening programs miss cases of CH as a result of early discharge, improper or no specimen collection (e.g., hospital transfers, home births, sick or premature neonates), laboratory error, or delayed TSH elevation. Human error in reporting abnormal results can also occur. Primary TSH screening programs may miss infants

with central (pituitary) hypothyroidism. Acquired hypothyroidism will also be missed on newborn screening.

5. **Follow-up of newborn screening for CH** in hospitalized preterm infants is outlined in Figure 3.1. Screening protocols and cutoffs for T_4 and TSH levels vary slightly by screening program (see VI.B.2.).

   a. Any infant with abnormal screening results should be evaluated without delay. Consultation with a pediatric endocrinologist is recommended. Maternal and family history should be reviewed and a physical examination performed. Thyroid function tests should be repeated in serum within 24 hours. Most infants with an initial TSH level >50 mU/L have a permanent form of CH. If the initial TSH is 20 to 40 mU/L, the CH may be transient. If it is not possible to see the patient promptly, therapy should be initiated as soon as the diagnosis is confirmed. If the TSH level is not elevated, the TBG level should be measured to exclude TBG deficiency.

   b. Measurement of **TG level** and **thyroid ultrasound and/or thyroid scanning with RAI or ^{99m}Tc** can help differentiate thyroid dysplasia from defects

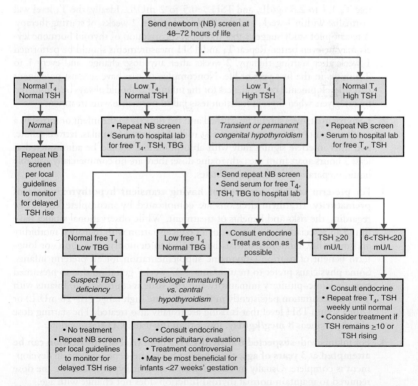

Figure 3.1. Suggested approach to follow-up of newborn screening for hypothyroidism in the hospitalized preterm infant. (Modified from Brodsky D, Ouellette MA, eds. *Primary Care of the Premature Infant.* Philadelphia: Elsevier Saunders; 2008.)

*In the United States, screening protocols and cutoff values vary slightly by state.

in thyroid hormone synthesis, and transient from permanent conditions. These tests are not necessary if transient hypothyroxinemia of prematurity is suspected. Thyroid scanning is useful to detect dysplastic or ectopic thyroid tissue as long as the serum TSH level is >30 mU/L at the time of scanning. **Treatment should not be delayed to perform thyroid scanning.** If scanning cannot be performed within 5 days of diagnosis, it should be deferred until the child is >3 years old, at which time thyroid hormone replacement can be safely discontinued for a brief period of time. Unlike thyroid scintiscan, ultrasound can be performed irrespective of the TSH concentration.

  c. Bone age may be helpful in assessing the severity and duration of intrauterine hypothyroidism but currently is performed less frequently than in the past.

C. **Treatment and monitoring.** An optimal neurodevelopmental outcome depends on early, adequate treatment of CH.

  1. For **infants with suspected transient or permanent CH**, L-thyroxine should be initiated at **10 to 15 mcg/kg/day**, with a higher dose used for infants with the lowest T_4 and highest TSH levels. The goal of treatment is to normalize thyroid hormone levels as soon as possible, with total T_4 in the 10 to 16 mcg/dL range, free T_4 1.4 to 2.3 ng/dL, and TSH >0.5 to 2 mU/L. Ideally, the T_4 level will normalize within 1 week, and the TSH level within 2 weeks, of starting therapy. A recent pilot study suggests that more rapid correction of thyroid hormone levels may be even better. Repeat T_4 and TSH measurements should be performed 1 week after starting therapy, 2 weeks after any dose change, and every 1 to 2 months in the first year of life. Noncompliance can have serious, permanent neurodevelopmental consequences for the infant and should always be considered by caregivers when thyroid function tests fail to normalize with treatment.

  2. **L-thyroxine** tablets should be crushed and fed directly to the infant or mixed in a small amount of juice, water, or breast milk. Soy-based formulas, ferrous sulfate, and fiber interfere significantly with absorption and should be administered at least 2 hours apart from the L-thyroxine dose; there are no commercially available liquid preparations in the United States.

  3. For **preterm infants suspected of having transient hypothyroxinemia of prematurity**, treatment decisions are complicated by incomplete knowledge regarding the risks and benefits of treatment. While observational studies have found an association of a low serum T_4 concentration with increased morbidity and mortality, randomized trials have failed to demonstrate a short- or long-term benefit of routine L-thyroxine supplementation for all preterm infants. Some physicians prefer to treat infants <27 weeks' gestation due to presumed hypothalamic–pituitary immaturity, but this issue is controversial. Infants with TSH concentration persistently in the borderline high range (10–20 mU/L) or with a serum TSH level that is rising are usually also treated. The starting dose of L-thyroxine is **8 mcg/kg/day**, lower than the usual CH starting dose.

  4. For infants with **suspected transient CH**, a brief **trial off medication can be attempted at 3 years of age,** after thyroid hormone-dependent brain development is complete. Usually in infants with transient hypothyroidism, the dose required to maintain normal thyroid function does not change with age.

D. **Prognosis.** With prompt diagnosis and treatment, the neurodevelopmental outcome is excellent for infants with CH. Subtle visuospatial processing, memory, and sensorimotor defects have been reported, particularly in those infants with severe CH, but the clinical significance of these differences is controversial. In contrast, infants who are diagnosed late may have substantial cognitive and behavioral defects ranging from mild to severe, depending on the severity of the CH and the length of delay in starting treatment.

VII. NEONATAL HYPERTHYROIDISM is uncommon, accounting for approximately 1% of hyperthyroidism in childhood and is almost always transient. Most newborns with hyperthyroidism are born to mothers with Graves' disease. Rarely, permanent hyperthyroidism can be caused by an activating mutation of the TSH receptor with autosomal dominant inheritance, a condition that may require thyroid gland ablation.

A. Incidence. The overall incidence of neonatal hyperthyroidism is 1/50,000. Of infants born to mothers with Graves' disease, 1% to 5% develop hyperthyroidism.

B. Pathogenesis. Clinical hyperthyroidism in the neonate results from transplacentally acquired maternal TSH receptor-stimulating antibodies. Rarely, both potent stimulating and blocking antibodies are present simultaneously. Due to differential clearance from the neonatal circulation, infants may present with hypothyroidism and develop thyrotoxicosis later with the disappearance of the more potent thyroid-blocking antibodies that initially masked the thyroid-stimulating antibody effects. Initial hypothyroidism may also be present as a result of the transplacental passage of PTU or MMI and typically resolves within the first week of life.

C. Neonatal hyperthyroidism usually occurs with active maternal disease, but may also occur in infants of mothers who have undergone surgical thyroidectomy or radioablation. These mothers are no longer hyperthyroid but continue to produce thyroid autoantibodies. High maternal serum levels of stimulating antibodies predict the presence of hyperthyroidism in the newborn, but precise values differ depending on the sensitivity of the assay used.

D. Clinical findings. Thyrotoxicosis usually presents toward the end of the first week of life as maternal antithyroid medication is cleared from the neonatal circulation but can occur earlier. Clinical manifestations in the newborn infant include prematurity, IUGR, tachycardia, irritability, poor weight gain, goiter, prominent eyes, hypertension, and craniosynostosis. Arrhythmias and CHF can be life threatening. Rarely, neonatal thyrotoxicosis can present with signs and symptoms suggestive of congenital viral infection, including hepatosplenomegaly, petechiae, fulminant hepatic failure, and coagulopathy. Maternal history, high titers of thyroid-stimulating antibodies, elevation of the total and free T_4 levels, and suppression of TSH are diagnostic.

E. Treatment.

  1. PTU (5–10 mg/kg/day in three divided doses) or **MMI** (0.5–1 mg/kg/day in three divided doses) are used to treat neonatal thyrotoxicosis.

  2. For severe hyperthyroidism, to block the release of T_4 immediately, an **iodine preparation** such as Lugol's solution (potassium iodide, 100 mg/mL) or SSKI (potassium iodide, 1 g/mL) can be given at a dose of 1 drop three times per day for 10 to 14 days.

  3. Propranolol, 2 mg/kg/day in three divided doses, is used to control tachycardia. If CHF develops, propranolol should be discontinued, and treatment with digoxin considered.

  4. Additional therapy may include **prednisone** at 1 to 2 mg/kg/day but is rarely necessary.

5. **Supportive care** maintains adequate oxygenation, fluid balance, calorie and nutrient intake for growth, and temperature regulation.

6. **Treatment course.** Thyroid function tests (free T_4, total T_3, and TSH) are repeated every few days initially, and the dose of antithyroid drug is adjusted to maintain levels within the normal range. Treatment is usually required for 2 to 3 months but may be longer. Once control is gained, the infant can be discharged with close follow-up. Iodine solutions are given until the thyroid function tests normalize. Infants are weaned off propranolol as indicated by the heart rate, and then the dose of PTU or MMI is tapered as allowed by the T_4 level and clinical symptoms.

F. **Prognosis.** Delayed diagnosis and/or inadequate treatment are associated with serious long-term consequences, including craniosynostosis, failure to thrive, developmental delay, and hyperactivity. Older series report a 10% to 20% mortality rate. With early diagnosis and proper treatment, most newborns improve rapidly, and therapy can be withdrawn within 2 to 3 months. Rarely, persistent central hypothyroidism may occur as a result of fetal pituitary exposure to high serum thyroid hormone levels at a critical period in development.

VIII. MATERNAL THYROID MEDICATIONS AND BREASTFEEDING

A. The antithyroid drugs **PTU** and **MMI** are excreted into breast milk but only in small amounts. Breastfeeding is considered safe for mothers taking doses <400 mg per day of PTU or 40 mg per day of MMI.

B. There is **limited transfer of propranolol** into breast milk. It is considered safe to breast feed while taking propranolol.

C. Only minimal amounts of L-thyroxine are transferred to the breast milk, in amounts no different from endogenous T_4 in euthyroid women. Thus, breastfeeding is safe for women taking L-thyroxine replacement.

D. Iodine is excreted into the breast milk, and **the iodine status of the exclusively breast fed infant is dependent on adequate iodine nutrition in the mother**. Even in regions considered iodine sufficient such as the United States, pregnant and lactating women should take 150 mcg per day of supplemental iodine. Of note, many prenatal vitamins do not contain iodine. Preterm infants are particularly susceptible to the thyroid-suppressive effects of excess iodine, which can lead to subclinical hypothyroidism. Excess iodine in the mother can come from the diet (e.g., seaweed) or from exposure to topical antiseptic agents used commonly around labor and delivery such as povidine iodine.

Suggested Readings

American Academy of Pediatrics, Rose SR, Section on Endocrinology and Committee on Genetics, American Thyroid Association, et al. Update of newborn screening and therapy for congenital hypothyroidism. *Pediatrics* 2006;117(6):2290–2303.

Brown RS. Disorders of the thyroid gland in infancy, childhood, and adolescence. Available at: www.thyroidmanager.org. Updated November 2009.

Glinoer D. Thyroid regulation and dysfunction in the pregnant patient. Available at: www.thyroidmanager.org. Updated August 2008.

National Newborn Screening and Genetics Resource Center. Available at: http://genes-r-us.uthscsa.edu/resources/newborn/00/ch4_complete.pdf

Preeclampsia and Related Conditions

Thomas F. McElrath

I. CATEGORIES OF PREGNANCY-ASSOCIATED HYPERTENSIVE DISORDERS

A. **Chronic hypertension.** Hypertension preceding pregnancy or first diagnosed before 20 weeks' gestation.

B. **Chronic hypertension with superimposed preeclampsia.** Worsening hypertension and new-onset proteinuria, in addition to possible concurrent hyperuricemia, thrombocytopenia, or transaminase derangements after the 20th week of pregnancy in a woman with known chronic hypertension.

C. **Pregnancy-induced hypertension.** Hypertension without proteinuria after 20 weeks' gestation.

D. **Preeclampsia.** Hypertension with proteinuria after 20 weeks' gestation.

E. **Eclampsia.** Generalized tonic–clonic seizure activity in a woman with no prior history of a seizure disorder.

II. INCIDENCE AND EPIDEMIOLOGY.
Hypertensive disorders are a major cause of maternal morbidity and mortality, accounting for 15% to 20% of maternal deaths worldwide. In the United States, hypertensive disorders are the second leading cause of maternal mortality after thrombotic/hemorrhagic complications. Beyond 20 weeks' gestation, preeclampsia complicates 5% to 8% of pregnancies, and severe preeclampsia complicates <1% of pregnancies. Eclampsia itself is much less frequent, occurring in 0.1% of pregnancies. Several risk factors have been identified, as outlined in Table 4.1.

III.
Preeclampsia has been called the "disease of theories," and many **etiologies** have been proposed. What is clear, however, is that it is a condition of dysfunction within the maternal endothelium. Increased levels of the soluble receptors *sFLT1* and *endoglin* within the maternal circulation for vascular endothelial growth factor (VEGF) and transforming growth factor-beta (TGF-β), respectively, may be associated with preeclamptic pathology. Higher circulating levels of these soluble receptors reduce the bioavailable levels of VEGF, placental growth factor (PlGF), and TGF-β, resulting in endothelial dysfunction within the maternal circulatory system. This dysfunction can manifest as both increased arterial tone (hypertension) and increased capillary leak (edema/proteinuria/pulmonary congestion). It is unclear what insult prompts the initial increase in sFLT1 and endoglin in some women versus others. One suggestion has been that abnormal trophoblastic invasion of both the maternal decidual arteries with an accompanying abnormal maternal immune response is at the root of this condition. This abnormal placentation is believed to lead to a reduction in placental perfusion and relative placental ischemia. Both sFLT1 and endoglin are

Table 4.1	Risk Factors for Hypertensive Disorders
Risk factor	**Risk ratio**
Nulliparity	3
Age >40	3
African American race	1.5
Family history of PIH	5
Chronic HTN	10
Chronic renal disease	20
Antiphospholipid antibody syndrome	10
Diabetes	2
Twin gestation	4
Angiotensinogen gene T235	
Homozygous	20
Heterozygous	4

HTN = hypertension; PIH = pregnancy-induced hypertension.
Source: ACOG. Hypertension in pregnancy. *Technical Bulletin # 219*, January 1996.

proangiogenic proteins and may represent a placental compensatory response. Recent work has, however, called the implied causality of this hypothesis into question; in early pregnancy, when placental formation is most active, sFLT1 and P1GF levels have failed to reliably predict the occurrence of preeclampsia.

IV. DIAGNOSIS. The classic triad that defines preeclampsia is hypertension, proteinuria, and nondependent edema. At this point, the diagnosis is made exclusively on clinical criteria. The clinical spectrum of preeclampsia ranges from mild to severe. Most patients have mild disease that develops late in the third trimester.

A. **Criteria for the diagnosis of mild preeclampsia**

1. **Hypertension** defined as a blood pressure elevation to 140 mm Hg systolic or 90 mm Hg diastolic over two measurements at least 6 hours apart. Measurements should be taken in the sitting position, and proper cuff size should be ensured.

2. **Proteinuria** defined as at least 300 mg of protein in a 24-hour period.

3. **Nondependent edema** (e.g., facial or upper extremity) is also noted in many but not all cases of preeclampsia.

B. **Criteria for the diagnosis of severe preeclampsia**

1. **Blood pressure** >160 mm Hg systolic or 110 mm Hg diastolic with the diagnostic readings taken twice at least 6 hours apart.

2. **Proteinuria** >5 g per 24-hour collection.

3. **Symptoms suggestive of end-organ dysfunction.** Visual disturbances such as scotomata, diplopia or blindness, persistent severe headache, or epigastric pain.

4. **Pulmonary edema.**

5. **Oliguria** defined as <500 mL of urine per 24-hour collection.

6. **Microangiopathic hemolysis.**

7. **Thrombocytopenia** defined as a platelet count of <100,000.

8. **Hepatocellular dysfunction.** Elevated transaminases.

9. **Intrauterine growth restriction (IUGR) or oligohydramnios.**

C. **HELLP syndrome** (hemolysis, elevated liver enzymes, and low platelets) represents an alternative presentation of preeclampsia associated with disseminated intravascular coagulation (DIC) and reflects systemic end-organ damage. HELLP syndrome often appears without hypertension or proteinuria and may, in fact, have a separate pathologic origin from that of preeclampsia.

V. Complications of preeclampsia result in a **maternal mortality rate** of 3 per 100,000 live births in the United States. Maternal morbidity may include central nervous system complications (e.g., seizures, intracerebral hemorrhage, and blindness), DIC, hepatic failure or rupture, pulmonary edema, and *abruptio placentae* leading to maternal hemorrhage and/or acute renal failure. Fetal mortality markedly increases with rising maternal diastolic blood pressure and proteinuria. Diastolic blood pressures >95 mm Hg are associated with a threefold rise in the fetal death rate. Fetal morbidity may include IUGR, fetal acidemia, and complications from prematurity.

VI. CONSIDERATIONS IN MANAGEMENT

A. **The definitive treatment for preeclampsia is delivery.** However, the severity of disease, dilatation/effacement of the maternal cervix, gestational age at diagnosis, and pulmonary maturity of the fetus all influence obstetric management. Delivery is usually indicated if there is nonreassuring fetal testing in a viable fetus or if the maternal status becomes unstable regardless of either gestational age or fetal maturity.

B. **Delivery should be considered** for all term patients with any degree of preeclampsia. Patients with mild disease and an unfavorable cervix can be closely monitored to await a more favorable cervix.

C. Pregnancies may continue for patients with **preterm gestation and mild preeclampsia**, with close observation as outlined in section VII until 37 weeks' gestation or some other ominous development such as the progression to severe preeclampsia, nonreassuring fetal testing, or maternal instability.

D. **Consideration for delivery should be made in all patients with severe preeclampsia.** Conservative therapy of severe preeclampsia early in gestation has been suggested, with two studies showing that in pregnancies between 28 and 32 weeks, conservative management resulted in a mean prolongation of pregnancy of 2 weeks. However, conservative management of severe preeclampsia may be associated with serious sequelae, such as acute renal failure, DIC, HELLP syndrome, *abruptio placentae*, eclampsia, and intrauterine fetal death. Patients should be counseled that prolongation of pregnancy in the setting of severe preeclampsia is for fetal benefit only as the mother assumes risk to her own well-being. Conservative management should only be undertaken in centers where there is rapid availability of immediate obstetrical and neonatal care.

E. Conservative management entails hospitalization and frequent maternal and fetal surveillance. This should only be undertaken in carefully selected patients after an initial period of observation to ensure stability of the pregnant woman. Women with uncontrolled hypertension, thrombocytopenia, hepatocellular dysfunction, pulmonary edema, compromised renal function, or persistent headache or visual changes are not candidates for conservative management of severe preeclampsia.

F. Although a trial of labor induction is not contraindicated in patients with severe preeclampsia, the success rate is low. The managing team must balance the risks of progression of the disease against the time required to induce labor.

VII. CLINICAL MANAGEMENT OF MILD PREECLAMPSIA

A. Antepartum management. Conservative management of mild preeclampsia generally includes hospitalization with bed rest and close maternal and fetal observation. Outpatient management is an option only for a few carefully selected, well-supported and reliable patients after a period of initial observation to assess maternal and fetal status.

1. **Fetal evaluation**

   a. An initial **ultrasound** should be performed at the time of diagnosis to rule out IUGR and/or oligohydramnios. A **nonstress test** or **biophysical profile** should also be performed.

   b. **Betamethasone** should be administered to accelerate fetal maturity if the fetus is <34 weeks of gestation and no maternal contraindications exist.

   c. If the fetus is appropriately grown with reassuring fetal testing, **testing should be at regular intervals**.

   d. If the estimated fetal weight is <10th percentile or there is oligohydramnios (amniotic fluid index of 5 cm or less), then **testing should be performed at frequent regular intervals** (consider daily) after consideration of delivery.

   e. Any **change in maternal status** should prompt evaluation of fetal status.

   f. **Fetal indications for delivery** include severe fetal growth restriction, nonreassuring fetal testing, and oligohydramnios.

2. **Maternal evaluation**

   a. Women should be **evaluated for signs and symptoms** of preeclampsia and severe preeclampsia.

   b. **Laboratory evaluation** includes hematocrit, platelet count, and quantification of protein excretion in the urine, serum creatinine, transaminases, and uric acid level in addition to prothrombin time/partial thromboplastin time.

   c. **If criteria for mild preeclampsia are met**, laboratory studies should be performed at frequent intervals. For example, at Brigham and Women's Hospital in Boston, women with mild preeclampsia have laboratory testing twice weekly.

   d. **Maternal indications for delivery** include a gestational age ≥37 weeks, thrombocytopenia (<100,000), progressive deterioration in hepatic or renal function, *abruptio placentae*, and persistent severe headaches, visual changes, or epigastric pain.

e. Antihypertensive agents are not routinely given because they have not been shown to improve the outcome in cases of mild preeclampsia.

f. When early delivery is indicated, it is our practice that vaginal delivery is preferred. Cesarean delivery should be reserved for cases when fetal decompensation is suspected, when further fetal evaluation is not possible, or when a rapidly deteriorating maternal condition mandates expeditious delivery (e.g., HELLP with decreasing platelet counts, abruption).

B. Intrapartum management of preeclampsia

1. **Magnesium sulfate** (6 g intravenous [IV] load followed by 2 g/hr infusion), used as seizure prophylaxis, is started when the decision to proceed with delivery is made and is continued for at least 24 hours postpartum or until symptoms are resolving in the mother. Magnesium sulfate has been shown to be the agent of choice for seizure prophylaxis in randomized double-blind comparisons against both placebo and conventional antiepileptics. In patients with a contraindication to magnesium sulfate (e.g., myasthenia gravis, hypocalcemia), it has been our practice to proceed without seizure prophylaxis. Because the kidneys clear magnesium sulfate, urine output should be carefully monitored. Signs and symptoms of maternal toxicity include loss of deep tendon reflexes, somnolence, respiratory depression, cardiac arrhythmia, and, in extreme cases, cardiovascular collapse.

2. **Careful monitoring of fluid balance** is critical because preeclampsia is associated with endothelial dysfunction leading to decreased intravascular volume, pulmonary edema, and oliguria. A serum magnesium level should be considered if reduced renal function is suspected while magnesium sulfate is being administered.

3. **Severe hypertension** may be controlled with agents including hydralazine, labetalol, or nifedipine. Sodium nitroprusside should be avoided before delivery because of potential fetal cyanide toxicity. It is important to avoid large or abrupt reductions in blood pressure because decreased intravascular volume and poor uteroplacental perfusion can lead to acute placental insufficiency and a resulting loss of reassurance regarding fetal well-being.

4. **Continuous electronic fetal monitoring** is recommended given the potential for placental dysfunction in the preeclamptic setting. Monitoring should be established during the initial evaluation, induction of labor, and labor itself. Continuous monitoring is less likely to be useful during intervals of prolonged expectant management. Patterns that suggest fetal compromise include persistent tachycardia, minimal or absent variability, and recurrent late decelerations not responsive to standard resuscitative measures. Reduced fetal heart rate variability may also result from maternal administration of magnesium sulfate.

5. Patients may be safely administered **epidural anesthesia** if the platelet count is >70,000 and there is no evidence of DIC. Consideration should be given for early epidural catheter placement when the platelet count is reasonable and there is concern that it is decreasing. Any anesthesia should be administered by properly trained personnel experienced in the care of women with preeclampsia, given the hemodynamic changes associated with the condition. Adequate preload should be ensured to minimize the risk of hypotension.

6. **Invasive central monitoring** of the mother is rarely indicated, even in the setting of severe preeclampsia.

C. **Postpartum management.** The mother's condition may worsen immediately after delivery. However, signs and symptoms usually begin to resolve within 24 to 48 hours postpartum and completely resolve within 1 to 2 weeks. Some patients, although sufficiently stable for discharge, may require antihypertensive medications for up to 8 weeks. Because postpartum eclamptic seizures generally occur within the first 48 hours and usually within the first 24 hours after delivery, magnesium sulfate prophylaxis is continued for at least 24 hours. Close monitoring of fluid balance is continued. Once a spontaneous maternal diuresis has begun, recovery can be hastened by the administration of oral diuretics.

VIII. MANAGEMENT OF ECLAMPSIA

A. Approximately half of **eclamptic seizures** occur before delivery, 20% occur during delivery, and another 30% occur in the postpartum period. Although there is no clear constellation of symptoms that will accurately predict which patients will have an eclamptic seizure, headache is a frequently reported heralding symptom.

B. **Basic principles of maternal resuscitation** should be followed in the initial management of an eclamptic seizure: airway protection, oxygen, left lateral displacement to prevent uterine compression of vena cava, IV access, and blood pressure control.

C. Magnesium sulfate should be initiated for **prevention of recurrent seizures**. If untreated, 10% of women with eclamptic seizures will have a recurrent seizure.

D. A **transient fetal bradycardia** is usually seen during the seizure followed by a **transient fetal tachycardia** with loss of variability. Ideally, the fetus should be resuscitated *in utero*.

E. **Eclampsia is an indication for delivery but not necessarily an indication for cesarean delivery.** No intervention should be initiated until maternal stability is ensured and the seizure is over. Because of the risk of DIC, coagulation parameters should be assessed and appropriate blood products should be available if necessary.

F. A **neurologic exam** should be performed once the patient recovers from the seizure. If the seizure is atypical or any neurologic deficit persists, **brain imaging** is indicated.

IX. RECURRENCE RISK.

Patients who have a history of preeclampsia are at increased risk for hypertensive disease in a subsequent pregnancy. Recurrence risk is as high as 40% in women with preeclampsia before 32 weeks of gestation, as opposed to 10% or less in women with mild preeclampsia near term. Severe disease and eclampsia are also associated with recurrence. Racial differences exist, with African American women having higher recurrence rates. The recurrence rate for HELLP syndrome is approximately 5%.

X. RISK OF CHRONIC HYPERTENSION.

Preeclampsia may be linked to the development of chronic hypertension later in the mother's life. Women with recurrent preeclampsia, women with early-onset preeclampsia, and multiparas with a diagnosis of preeclampsia (even if not recurrent) are at an increased risk.

XI. INNOVATIONS AND PROPOSED TREATMENTS

A. Several analytic assays based on sFLT1 and PlGF protein levels are currently under evaluation. The ultimate clinical utility of these analyses has yet to be determined.

B. **Reduced maternal 25(OH) vitamin D** levels have recently been associated with an increased risk of preeclampsia. Randomized placebo-controlled trials of vitamin D supplementation are presently ongoing and may yield a widely available means of reducing the risk of preeclampsia.

C. **Low-dose aspirin** has been evaluated as a possible prophylactic. However, no clear benefit has been shown. In fact, there is some suggestion of an increased risk of placental abruption in patients receiving low-dose aspirin.

D. Although earlier studies suggested that **antenatal calcium supplementation** may reduce the incidence of hypertensive disorders of pregnancy, a large National Institutes of Health-sponsored placebo-controlled trial did not show any benefit when given to healthy nulliparous women.

E. Recent enthusiasm for antioxidant therapy has also been dulled after a well-executed trial found vitamin E supplementation during pregnancy to be associated with an increased risk of adverse outcome compared with placebo.

F. The efficacy of **heparin therapy** for the prevention of preeclampsia in women with a genetic thrombophilia is unknown and should only be considered in the setting of a clinical trial.

XII. IMPLICATIONS FOR THE NEWBORN

A. Infants born to mothers with moderate or severe preeclampsia may show evidence of **IUGR** (see Chaps. 1 and 7) and are frequently delivered prematurely. They may tolerate labor poorly and therefore require resuscitation.

B. **Medications used antepartum or intrapartum** may affect the fetus.

    1. **Short-term sequelae of hypermagnesemia**, such as hypotonia and respiratory depression, are sometimes seen. Long-term maternal administration of magnesium sulfate has rarely been associated with neonatal parathyroid abnormalities or other abnormalities of calcium homeostasis (see Chap. 25).

    2. **Antihypertensive medications**, including calcium-channel blockers, may have fetal effects, including hypotension in the infant. Antihypertensive medications and magnesium sulfate generally are not contraindications to breastfeeding.

    3. **Low-dose aspirin therapy** does not appear to increase the incidence of intracranial hemorrhage, asymptomatic bruising, bleeding from circumcision sites, or persistent pulmonary hypertension.

    4. Approximately one-third of infants born to mothers with preeclampsia have **decreased platelet counts at birth**, but the counts generally increase rapidly to normal levels. Approximately 40% to 50% of newborns have neutropenia that generally resolves before 3 days of age. These infants may be at increased risk for neonatal infection.

Suggested Readings

American College of Obstetricians and Gynecologists (ACOG). *ACOG Practice Bulletin 33: Diagnosis and Management of Preeclampsia and Eclampsia.* Washington, DC: American College of Obstetricians and Gynecologists; 2002.

Levine RJ, Maynard SE, Qian C, et al. Circulating angiogenic factors and the risk of preeclampsia. *N Engl J Med* 2004;350:672–683.

Roberts JM. Pregnancy-related hypertension. In: Creasy RK, Resnik R, eds. *Maternal-Fetal Medicine*. 6th ed. Philadelphia: WB Saunders; 2009.

Sibai BM, Mercer BM, Schiff E, et al. Aggressive versus expectant management of severe preeclampsia at 28 to 32 weeks' gestation: a randomized controlled trial. *Am J Obstet Gynecol* 1994;171:818–822.

Sibai BM, Taslimi M, Abdella TN, et al. Maternal and perinatal outcome of conservative management of severe preeclampsia in midtrimester. *Am J Obstet Gynecol* 1985;152:32–37.

5 Resuscitation in the Delivery Room

Steven A. Ringer

I. GENERAL PRINCIPLES. A person skilled in basic neonatal resuscitation, whose primary responsibility is the newly born baby, should be present at every birth. Delivery of all high-risk infants should be ideally attended by personnel who possess the skills required to perform a complete resuscitation.

The highest standard of care requires the following: (i) knowledge of perinatal physiology and principles of resuscitation; (ii) mastery of the technical skills required; and (iii) a clear understanding of the roles of other team members and coordination among team members. This allows anticipation of each person's reactions in a specific instance and helps ensure that care is timely and comprehensive. Completion of the Newborn Resuscitation Program (NRP) of the American Academy of Pediatrics/American Heart Association by every caregiver helps ensure a consistent approach to resuscitations and team-based training. NRP provides an approach to resuscitation that is successful in a very high percentage of cases and aids clinicians in more rapidly identifying those unusual cases in which specialized interventions may be required.

A. Perinatal physiology. Resuscitation efforts at delivery are designed to help the newborn make the respiratory and circulatory transitions that must be accomplished immediately after birth: the lungs expand, fetal lung fluid is cleared, effective air exchange is established, and the right-to-left circulatory shunts terminate. The critical period for these physiologic changes is during the first several breaths, which result in lung expansion and elevation of the partial pressure of oxygen (PO_2) in both the alveoli and the arterial circulation. Elevation of the PO_2 from the fetal level of approximately 25 mm Hg to values of 50 to 70 mm Hg is associated with (i) decrease in pulmonary vascular resistance, (ii) decrease in right-to-left shunting through the ductus arteriosus, (iii) increase in venous return to the left atrium, (iv) rise in left atrial pressure, and (v) cessation of right-to-left shunt through the foramen ovale. The end result is conversion from fetal to transitional to neonatal circulatory pattern. Adequate systemic arterial oxygenation results from perfusion of well-expanded, well-ventilated lungs and adequate circulation.

Conditions at delivery may compromise the fetus's ability to make the necessary transitions. Alterations in tissue perfusion and oxygenation ultimately result in depression of cardiac function, but human fetuses initially respond to hypoxia by becoming apneic. Even a relatively brief period of oxygen deprivation may result in this **primary apnea**. Rapid recovery from this state is generally accomplished with appropriate stimulation and oxygen exposure. If the period of hypoxia continues, the fetus will irregularly gasp and lapse into **secondary apnea**. This state may occur remote from birth or in the peripartum period. Infants born during this period require resuscitation with assisted ventilation and oxygen (see III.D.).

B. Goals of resuscitation are the following:

1. **Minimizing immediate heat loss** by drying and providing warmth, thereby decreasing oxygen consumption by the neonate.

2. **Establishing normal respiration and lung expansion** by clearing the upper airway and using positive-pressure ventilation if necessary.

3. **Increasing arterial PO$_2$** by providing adequate alveolar ventilation. The **routine** use of added oxygen is not warranted, but this therapy may be necessary in some situations.

4. **Supporting adequate cardiac output.**

II. PREPARATION. Anticipation is key to ensuring that adequate preparations have been made for a neonate likely to require resuscitation at birth. It is estimated that as many as 10% of neonates require some assistance at birth for normal transition, while less than 1% require extensive resuscitative measures.

A. Perinatal conditions associated with high-risk deliveries. Ideally, the obstetrician should notify the pediatrician well in advance of the actual birth. The pediatrician may then review the obstetric history and events leading to the high-risk delivery and prepare for the specific problems that may be anticipated. If time permits, the problems should be discussed with the parent(s). The following antepartum and intrapartum events warrant the presence of a resuscitation team at delivery:

1. **Evidence of nonreassuring fetal status**
   a. Category III fetal tracing, including either sinusoidal pattern or absent fetal heart rate variability and any of the following: late decelerations, recurrent variable decelerations or bradycardia.
   b. History of an acute perinatal event (e.g., placental abruption, cord prolapse or abnormal fetal testing, or a scalp pH of 7.20 or less).
   c. History of decreased fetal movement, dimunition in growth, or abnormalites of umbilical vessel Doppler flow studies.

2. **Evidence of fetal disease or potentially serious conditions (see Chap. 1)**
   a. Meconium staining of the amniotic fluid and/or other evidence of possible fetal compromise (see Chap. 35)
   b. Prematurity (<37 weeks), postmaturity (>42 weeks), anticipated low birth weight (<2.0 kg), or high birth weight (>4.5 kg)
   c. Major congenital anomalies diagnosed prenatally
   d. Hydrops fetalis
   e. Multiple gestation (see Chap. 11)

3. **Labor and delivery conditions**
   a. Significant vaginal bleeding
   b. Abnormal fetal presentation
   c. Prolonged or unusual labor
   d. Concern about a possible shoulder dystocia

B. The following conditions do not require a pediatric team to be present, but personnel should be available for assessment and triage:

1. **Neonatal conditions**
   a. Unexpected congenital anomalies
   b. Respiratory distress

    c. Unanticipated neonatal depression, for example, Apgar score of <6 at 5 minutes

  2. Maternal conditions

    a. Signs of maternal infection

       i. Maternal fever

      ii. Membranes ruptured for >24 hours

     iii. Foul-smelling amniotic fluid

     iv. History of sexually transmitted disease

    b. Maternal illness or other conditions

       i. Diabetes mellitus

      ii. Rh or other isoimmunization without evidence of hydrops fetalis

     iii. Chronic hypertension or pregnancy-induced hypertension

     iv. Renal, endocrine, pulmonary, or cardiac disease

      v. Alcohol or other substance abuse

    c. Mode of delivery

    In the absence of other antenatal risk factors, delivery via cesarean section done using regional anesthesia at 37 to 39 weeks' gestation does not increase the likelihood of a baby requiring endotracheal (ET) intubation, compared to vaginal delivery at term.

C. Necessary equipment must be present and operating properly. Each delivery room should be equipped with the following:

  1. Radiant warmer with procedure table or bed. The warmer should be turned on and checked before delivery. For a very low birth weight (VLBW) infant, additional warming techniques should be available, which might include pre-warming the delivery room to 26°C, covering the baby with a plastic wrap or using an exothermic mattress. When used in combination, care should be taken to avoid hyperthermia.

  2. A blended oxygen source (adjustable between 21% and 100%) with adjustable flowmeter and adequate length of tubing. A humidifier and heater may be desirable.

  3. Pulse oximeter available for use when oxygen therapy is anticipated.

  4. Flow-inflating **bag** with adjustable pop-off valve or self-inflating bag with reservoir. The bag must be appropriately sized for neonates (generally about 750 mL) and capable of delivering 100% oxygen.

  5. Face mask(s) of appropriate size for the anticipated infant.

  6. A bulb syringe for suctioning.

  7. Stethoscope with infant- or premature-sized head.

  8. Equipped emergency box or cart

    a. Laryngoscope with no. 0 and no. 1 blades. For extremely low birth weight infants, a no. 00 blade may be preferred.

    b. Extra batteries.

    c. Uniform diameter ET tubes (2.5-, 3.0-, and 3.5-mm internal diameters), two of each.

    d. Drugs, including epinephrine (1:10,000) and NaCl 0.9%. Sodium bicarbonate (0.50 mEq/mL) or other buffers and naloxone are rarely useful.

    e. Umbilical catheterization tray with 3.5 and 5F catheters.

    f. Syringes (1.0, 3.0, 5.0, 10.0, and 20.0 mL), needles (18–25 gauge), T-connectors, and stopcocks.

9. Transport incubator with battery-operated heat source and portable-blended oxygen supply should be available if delivery room is not close to the nursery.

10. The utility of equipment for continuous monitoring of cardiopulmonary status in the delivery room is hampered by difficulty in effectively applying monitor leads. Pulse oximetry can be applied **right** after birth and successfully used to provide information on oxygen saturation and heart rate, and should be available when oxygen use is anticipated or possible.

11. End-tidal CO_2 monitor/indicator to confirm ET tube position after intubation.

D. **Preparation of equipment.** Upon arrival in the delivery room, check that the transport incubator is plugged in and warm, and has a full oxygen tank. The specialist should introduce himself or herself to the obstetrician and anesthesiologist, the mother (if she is awake), and the father (if he is present). While the history or an update is obtained, the following should be done:

1. Ensure that the radiant warmer is on, and that dry, warm blankets are available.

2. Turn on the oxygen source or air–oxygen blend and adjust the flow from 5 to 8 L/minute. Adjust the oxygen concentration to the desired initial level.

3. Test the flow-inflating bag (if used) for pop-off control and adequate flow. Be sure the proper-sized mask is present.

4. Make sure the laryngoscope light is bright and has an appropriate blade (no. 1 for full-term neonates, no. 0 for premature neonates, and no. 00 for extremely low birth weight neonates).

5. Set out an appropriate ET tube for the expected birth weight (3.5 mm for full-term infants, 3.0 mm for premature infants >1,250 g, and 2.5 mm for smaller infants). The NRP recommends a 4.0-mm tube for larger babies, but this is rarely necessary. For all babies, the tube should be 13 cm long. An intubation stylet may be used if the tip is kept at least 0.5 cm from the distal end of the ET tube.

6. If the clinical situation suggests that extensive resuscitation may be needed, the following actions may be required:
   a. Set up an umbilical catheterization tray for venous catheterization.
   b. Draw up 1:10,000 epinephrine and isotonic saline for catheter flush solution and volume replacement.
   c. Check that other potentially necessary drugs are present and ready for administration.

E. **Universal precautions.** Exposure to blood or other body fluids is inevitable in the delivery room. Universal precautions must be practiced by wearing caps, goggles or glasses, gloves, and impervious gowns until the cord is cut and the newborn is dried and wrapped.

III. DURING DELIVERY, the team should be aware of the type and duration of anesthesia, extent of maternal bleeding, and newly recognized problems such as a nuchal cord or meconium in the amniotic fluid.

A. **Immediately following delivery, begin a process of evaluation, decision, and action (resuscitation)**

1. Place the newborn on the warming table.

2. Dry the infant completely and discard the wet linens, including those upon which the infant is lying. Drying should be thorough but gentle; avoid

vigorous rubbing or attempts to clean all blood or vernix from the baby. Make sure the infant is warm. Extremely small infants may require extra warming techniques such as wrapping the body and extremities in a plastic wrap or bag or with the use of an exothermic mattress.

3. Place the infant with head in midline position, with slight neck extension.

4. Suction the mouth, oropharynx, and nares thoroughly with a suction bulb if there is obvious obstruction or if the baby requires positive pressure ventilation. Deep pharyngeal stimulation with a suction catheter may cause arrhythmias that are probably of vagal origin, and this should be avoided. If meconium-stained amniotic fluid is present and the infant is not vigorous, suction the oropharynx and trachea as quickly as possible (see IV.A. and Chap. 35).

B. **Assessment of the need for supplemental oxygen.** In the normal fetal environment, oxygen saturation levels are well below those necessary during extrauterine life. These levels do not completely rise to the normal postnatal range for about 10 minutes after birth, and oxygen saturation levels of 70% to 80% are normal for several minutes. During this time, the baby may appear cyanotic, although clinical assessment of cyanosis has been shown to be an unreliable indicator of actual oxyhemoglobin saturation. However, either insufficient or excessive oxygenation can be harmful to the newborn.

1. **Pulse oximetry.** Several studies have examined the change in oxygen saturation levels in the minutes following birth and have defined percentile ranges for uncompromised babies born at full term. The best-defined data have been obtained using readings made at a "preductal" site (i.e., the right upper extremity) in order to avoid the potentially confounding effect of shunting during the transition to an adult-type circulation. Probes specifically designed for neonates can provide reliable readings within 1 to 2 minutes or less; however, oxygen saturation measurements may be unreliable when cardiac output and skin perfusion are poor. It is recommended that oximetry be available for use in the delivery room so that it will be available when:

   a. Resuscitation can be anticipated, as noted previously.
   b. Positive pressure ventilation is used for more than a few breaths.
   c. Cyanosis is persistent despite interventions.
   d. Supplemental oxygen is administered.

C. **The concentration of oxygen** used to begin resuscitation remains an area of debate. Several trials have shown that survival is improved when resuscitation is initiated with room air compared with 100% oxygen in full-term infants, although there are no studies evaluating other oxygen concentrations. A single study of preterm infants showed that the use of a blended air–oxygen mixture as the initial gas resulted in less hypoxemia or hyperoxemia than did the use of room air or 100% oxygen, but the ideal starting concentration has not been defined. Once oxygen use is started, the concentration should be adjusted so that the measured preductal oxygen saturation value lies within a specified minute-specific reference range (Table 5.1) as advocated by the NRP program. The best available reference is the interquartile range of saturations measured in healthy term babies following vaginal birth at sea level. Different ranges have not been determined for preterm babies or those born via cesarean or vaginal routes.

   Since when using these guidelines the administered oxygen concentration is guided by the measured oxygen saturation, the choice of initial concentration is

Table 5.1	Target Preductal SpO2 during the First 10 Minutes After Birth
1 minute	60%–65%
2 minutes	65%–70%
3 minutes	70%–75%
4 minutes	75%–80%
5 minutes	80%–85%
10 minutes	85%–95%

discretionary, but a uniform approach makes sense. We use **room air** as the initial concentration for term babies, and **60% oxygen** for premature babies less than 32 weeks' gestation.

1. Air should be used if blended oxygen is not available.

2. Oxygen concentration should be increased to 100% if bradycardia (HR< 60 beats per minute [bpm]) does not improve after 90 seconds of resuscitation while employing a lower oxygen concentration.

D. **Sequence of intervention.** While Apgar scores (Table 5.2) are assigned at 1 and 5 minutes, resuscitative efforts should begin during the initial neonatal stabilization period. The NRP recommends that at the time of birth, the baby should be assessed by posing four basic questions: (i) Is it a term gestation? (ii) Is the baby

Table 5.2	Apgar Scoring System		
	Score		
Sign	0	1	2
Heart rate	Absent	<100 bpm	>100 bpm
Respiratory effort	Absent	Slow (irregular)	Good crying
Muscle tone	Limp	Some flexion of extremities	Active motion
Reflex irritability	No response	Grimace	Cough or sneeze
Color	Blue, pale	Pink body, blue extremities	All pink

Source: Adapted from Apgar V. A proposal for a new method of evaluation of the newborn infant. *Curr Res Anesth Analg* 1953;32:260–267.

crying or breathing? (iii) Does the baby have good muscle tone? (iv) Is the baby or amniotic fluid clear of meconium? If the answer to any of these questions is "no," the initial steps of resuscitation should commence. In the newly born infant, essentially all resuscitation problems within the initial postnatal period occur as a result of inadequate respiratory effort or some obstruction to the airway. Therefore, the initial focus should be on ensuring an adequate airway and adequate breathing.

First, assess whether the infant is **breathing spontaneously**. Next, assess whether the **heart rate is >100 bpm**. Finally, evaluate whether the infant's overall color is pink (acrocyanosis is normal) or whether the oxygen saturation level is appropriate (see Table 5.1). If any of these three characteristics is abnormal, take immediate steps to correct the deficiency, and reevaluate every 15 to 30 seconds until all characteristics are present and stable. In this way, adequate support will be given while overly vigorous interventions are avoided when newborns are making adequate progress on their own. This approach will help avoid complications, such as laryngospasm and cardiac arrhythmias, from excessive suctioning or pneumothorax from injudicious bagging. Some interventions are required in specific circumstances.

1. **Infant breathes spontaneously, heart rate is >100 bpm, and color is becoming pink (Apgar score of 8–10).** If measured, oxygen saturation levels during the first several minutes are within or higher than the reference range. This situation is found in over 90% of all term newborns, with a median time to first breath of approximately 10 seconds. Following (or during) warming, drying, positioning, and oropharyngeal suctioning, the infant should be assessed. If respirations, heart rate, and color are normal, the infant should be wrapped and returned to the parents.

   Some newborns do not immediately establish spontaneous respiration but will rapidly respond to tactile stimulation, including vigorous flicking of the soles of the feet or rubbing the back (e.g., cases of **primary apnea**). More vigorous or other techniques of stimulation have no therapeutic value and are potentially harmful. If breathing does not start after **two** attempts at tactile stimulation, the baby should be considered to be in **secondary apnea**, and respiratory support should be initiated. It is better to overdiagnose secondary apnea in this situation than to continue attempts at stimulation that are not successful.

2. **Infant breathes spontaneously, heart rate is >100 bpm, but the overall color appears cyanotic (Apgar score of 5–7).** This situation is not uncommon and may follow primary apnea. A pulse oximeter should be placed on right upper extremity (usually the hand) as soon as possible after birth. If the measured levels are below the range in Table 5.1 at a specific time after birth, blended blow-by oxygen (30%–40%) should be administered at a rate of 5 L/minute by mask or by tubing held approximately 1 cm from the face. If the saturation improves, the oxygen concentration should be adjusted or gradually withdrawn as indicated to maintain saturation levels in the reference range.

   The early initiation of continuous positive airway pressure (CPAP) to a preterm infant who is spontaneously breathing but exhibiting respiratory distress in the delivery room is advocated by some experts. In studies of infants born at less than 29 weeks' gestation, CPAP begun shortly after birth was equally as effective in preventing death or oxygen requirement at 36 weeks postmenstrual age compared with initial intubation and mechanical ventilation. Early CPAP use reduced the need for intubation, mechanical ventilation, and exogenous surfactant administration, but was associated in one study with a higher incidence of pneumothorax. In spontaneously breathing preterm infants with respiratory distress, use of CPAP in the delivery room is a reasonable alternative to intubation and mechanical ventilation. Using a regulated means of administration, such as a T-piece resuscitator or ventilator, is preferable.

3. **The infant is apneic despite tactile stimulation or has a heart rate of <100 bpm despite apparent respiratory effort (Apgar score of 3–4).** This represents **secondary apnea** and requires treatment with bag-and-mask ventilation. When starting this intervention, call for assistance if your team is not already present.

A bag of approximately 750 mL volume should be connected to an air–oxygen blend (initial concentration depending on gestational age as in III.C) at a rate of 5 to 8 L/minute and to a mask of appropriate size. The mask should cover the chin and nose but leave eyes uncovered. After positioning the newborn's head in the midline with slight extension, the initial breath should be delivered at a peak pressure that is adequate to produce appropriate chest rise; often, 20 cm H_2O is effective, but 30 to 40 cm H_2O may be needed in the term infant. This will establish functional residual capacity, and subsequent inflations will be effective at lower inspiratory pressures.

The inspiratory pressures for subsequent breaths should again be chosen to result in adequate chest rise. In infants with normal lungs, this inspiratory pressure is usually no more than 15 to 20 cm H_2O. In infants with known or suspected disease causing decreased pulmonary compliance, continued inspiratory pressures in excess of 20 cm H_2O may be required. If no chest rise can be achieved despite apparently adequate pressure and no evidence of a mechanical obstruction, intubation should be considered. Especially in premature infants, every effort should be made to use the minimal pressures necessary for chest rise and the maintenance of normal oxygen saturation levels. A rate of 40 to 60 breaths per minute should be used, and the infant should be reassessed in 15 to 30 seconds. It is usually preferable to aim for a rate closer to 40 bpm, as many resuscitators deliver less adequate breaths at higher rates. Support should be continued until respirations are spontaneous, and the heart rate is >100 bpm; but effectiveness can also be gauged by improvements in oxygen saturation and tone before spontaneous respirations are established.

Such moderately depressed infants will be acidotic but generally able to correct this respiratory acidosis spontaneously after respiration is established. This process may take up to several hours, but unless the pH remains <7.25, acidosis does not need further treatment.

a. If positive pressure ventilation is continued beyond a few breaths, and especially if the infant is intubated, the use of a T-piece resuscitator (Neopuff Infant Resuscitator [Fisher & Paykel, Inc.]) enhances the ability to provide consistent pressure-regulated breaths. This is a manually triggered, pressure-limited, and manually cycled device that is pneumatically powered by a flowmeter. It offers greater control over manual ventilation by delivering breaths of reproducible size (peak and end-expiratory pressures) and a simplified method to control delivered breath rate.

b. Laryngeal mask airways (LMA) are easy to insert and are effective for ventilating newborns larger than 2,000 g. They should be considered when bag/mask ventilation is not effective and intubation is unsuccessful or no skilled intubator is immediately available. The LMA is not useful for tracheal suctioning and has not been studied as a means of administering intratracheal medications.

4. **The infant is apneic, and the heart rate is below 100 bpm despite 30 seconds of assisted ventilation (Apgar score of 0–2).** If the heart rate is >60, positive-pressure ventilation should be continued and the heart rate rechecked in 30 seconds. It is appropriate to carefully assess the effectiveness of support during this time period using the following steps:
   a. Adequacy of ventilation is the most important and should be assessed by observing chest-wall motion at the cephalad portions of the thorax and listening for equal breath sounds laterally over the right and left hemithoraces at the midaxillary lines. The infant should be ventilated at 40 to 60 breaths per minute using the minimum pressure that will move the chest and produce audible breath sounds. Infants with respiratory distress syndrome, pulmonary hypoplasia, or ascites may require higher pressures. The equipment should be checked, and the presence of a good seal between the mask and the infant's face should be quickly ascertained. At the same time, the position of the infant's head should be checked and returned as needed to midline and slight extension. The airway should be cleared as needed.
   b. Increase the oxygen concentration to 100% for infants of any gestational age if the resuscitation was started using an air–oxygen blend.
      Continue bag-and-mask ventilation and reassess in 15 to 30 seconds. The most important measure of ventilation adequacy is infant response. If, despite good air entry, the heart rate fails to increase and color/oxygen saturation remains poor, intubation should be considered. Air leak (e.g., pneumothorax) should be ruled out (see Chap. 38).
   c. Intubation is absolutely indicated only when a diaphragmatic hernia or similar anomaly is suspected or known to exist. It may be warranted when bag-and-mask ventilation is ineffective, when chest compressions are administered and when an ET tube is needed for emergency administration of drugs, or when the infant requires transportation for more than a short distance after stabilization. Even in these situations, effective ventilation with a bag and mask may be done for long periods, and it is preferred over repeated unsuccessful attempts at intubation or attempts by unsupervised personnel unfamiliar with the procedure.
      Intubation should be accomplished rapidly by a skilled person. If inadequate ventilation was the sole cause of the bradycardia, successful intubation will result in an increase in heart rate to over 100 bpm, and a rapid improvement in oxygen saturation. Detection of expiratory carbon dioxide by a colorimetric detector is an effective means of confirming appropriate tube positioning, especially in the smallest infants.
      The key to successful intubation is to correctly position the infant and laryngoscope and to know the anatomic landmarks. If the baby's chin, sternum, and umbilicus are all lined up in a single plane, and if after insertion into the infant's mouth, the laryngoscope handle and blade are aligned in that plane and held at approximately a 60-degree angle to the baby's chest, only one of four anatomic landmarks will be visible to the intubator: from cephalad to caudad, these include the posterior tongue, the vallecula and epiglottis, the larynx (trachea and vocal cords), or the esophagus. The successful intubator will view the laryngoscope tip and a landmark and should then know whether the landmark being observed is cephalad or caudad to the larynx. The intubator can adjust the position of the blade by several millimeters and locate the vocal cords. The ET tube can then be inserted under direct visualization (see Chap. 66).

d. Circulation. If, after intubation and 30 seconds of ventilation with 100% oxygen, the heart rate remains below 60 bpm, **cardiac massage** should be instituted. The best technique is to stand at the foot of the infant and encircle the chest with both hands, placing the thumbs together over the lower third of the sternum, with the fingers wrapped around and supporting the back. If the infant is intubated, chest compressions can be also given effectively while standing at the head of the bed next to the person performing ventilation, and encircling the chest with the thumbs pointing toward the infant's feet—a configuration that is "upside down" from the first method. Alternatively, one can stand at the side of the infant and compress the lower third of the infant's sternum with the index and third fingers of one hand. In either method, compress the sternum about one-third the diameter of the chest at a rate of 90 times per minute in a ratio of three compressions for each breath. Positive-pressure ventilation should be continued at a rate of 30 breaths per minute, interspersed in the period following every third compression. Determine effectiveness of compressions by palpating the femoral, brachial, or umbilical cord pulse.

Periodically suspend both ventilation and compression as heart rate is assessed, but frequent interruptions of compressions will compromise maintenance of systemic and coronary perfusion. If the rate is >60 bpm, chest compression should be discontinued and ventilation continued until respiration is spontaneous. If no improvement is noted, compression and ventilation should be continued

Infants requiring ventilatory and circulatory support are markedly depressed and require immediate, vigorous resuscitation. Resuscitation may require at least three trained people working together.

e. Medication. If, despite adequate ventilation with 100% oxygen and chest compressions, a heart rate of >60 bpm has not been achieved by 1 to 2 minutes after delivery, medications such as chronotropic and inotropic agents should be given to support the myocardium, to ensure adequate fluid status, and, in some situations, to correct acidosis. (See Table 5.3 for drugs, indications, and dosages.) Medications provide substrate and stimulation for the heart so that it can support circulation of oxygen and nutrients to the brain. For rapid calculations, use 1, 2, or 3 kg as the estimate of birth weight.

   i. The most accessible intravenous (IV) route for neonatal administration of medications is catheterization of the umbilical vein (see Chap. 66), which can be done rapidly and aseptically. Although the saline-filled catheter can be advanced into the inferior vena cava (i.e., 8–10 cm), in 60% to 70% of neonates, the catheter may become wedged in an undesirable or dangerous location (e.g., hepatic, portal, or pulmonary vein). Therefore, insertion of the catheter approximately 2 to 3 cm past the abdominal wall (4–5 cm total in a term neonate), just to the point of easy blood return, is safest before injection of drugs. In this position, the catheter tip will be in or just below the ductus venosus; it is important to flush all medications through the catheter because there is no flow through the vessel after cord separation.

   ii. Drug therapy as an adjunct to oxygen is to support the myocardium and correct acidosis. Continuing bradycardia is an indication for **epinephrine** administration, once effective ventilation has been established. Epinephrine is a powerful adrenergic agonist, and works in both adults and neonates by inducing an intense vasoconstriction and improved

Table 5.3 Neonatal Resuscitation

Drug/therapy	Dose/kg	Weight (kg)	Volume IV (mL)	Volume IT (mL)	Method	Indication
Epinephrine 1:10,000 0.1 mg/mL	0.01–0.03 mg/kg IV 0.03–0.1 mg/kg IT	1 2 3 4	0.2 0.4 0.6 0.8	0.6 1.2 1.8 2.4	Give IV push or IT push. The current IT doses do not require dilution or flushing with saline. **Do not give** into an artery; **do not mix** with bicarbonate; repeat in 5 min PRN	Asystole or severe bradycardia
Volume expanders Normal saline 5% Albumin Whole blood	10 mL/kg	1 2 3 4	10 mL 20 mL 30 mL 40 mL		Give IV over 5–10 min Slower in premature infants	Hypotension because of intravascular volume loss (see Chap. 40)
Naloxone (Narcan) 0.4 mg/mL	0.1–0.2 mg/kg	1 2 3 4	0.25–0.5 0.50–1.0 0.75–1.5 1.0–2.0		Give IV push, IM, SQ, or IT; repeat PRN 3 times if no response, **if material narcotic addiction is suspected, do not give**; do not mix with bicarbonate (see Chap. 12)	Narcotic depression

(continued)

Table 5.3	Neonatal Resuscitation *(Continued)*						
			Volume				
Drug/therapy	Dose/kg	Weight (kg)	IV (mL)	IT (mL)	Method	Indication	
Dopamine	30/60/90 mg/100 mL of solution	—	—		Give as continuous infusion	Hypotension because of poor cardiac output (see Chap. 40)	
Cardioversion/ defibrillation (see Chap. 41)	1–4 J/kg increase 50% each time	—	—		—	Ventricular fibrillation, ventricular tachycardia	
ET tube (see Chap. 66)	—	—	—		Internal diameter (mm)	Distance of tip of ET tube	
		<1,000 g 1,000–2,000 g 2,000–4,000 g >4,000 g			2.5 uncuffed 3.0 uncuffed 3.5 uncuffed 3.5–4.0 uncuffed	7 cm (for nasal 8 cm intubation, 9 cm add 2 cm) 10 cm	
Laryngoscope blades (see Chap. 66)		<2,000 g >2,000 g				0 (straight) 1 (straight)	

IM = intramuscular; IT; = intravenous; SQ = subcutaneous; ET = endotracheal.

coronary (and cerebral) artery perfusion. The recommended dose is extrapolated from the apparently efficacious dose in adults, and is based on both measured responses and empiric experience. The IV dose of 0.1 to 0.3 mL/kg (up to 1.0 mL) of a 1:10,000 epinephrine solution should ideally be given through the umbilical venous catheter and flushed into the central circulation. This dose may be repeated every 3 to 5 minutes if necessary, and there is no apparent benefit to higher doses.

When access to central circulation is difficult or delayed, epinephrine may be delivered through an ET tube for transpulmonary absorption, although a positive effect of this therapy has only been shown in animals at doses much higher than those currently recommended. This route of administration may be considered while IV access is being established, using doses of 0.5 to 1.0 mL/kg of 1:10,000 dilution (0.05–0.1 mg/kg). These larger doses need not be diluted to increase the total volume. If two doses of epinephrine do not produce improvement, additional doses may be given, but one should consider other causes for continuing depression.

iii. **Volume expansion.** If ventilation and oxygenation have been established but blood pressure is still low or the peripheral perfusion is poor, volume expansion may be indicated through the use of normal saline, 5% albumin, packed red blood cells, or whole blood, starting with 10 mL/kg (see IV.B.). Additional indications for volume expansion include evidence of acute bleeding or poor response to resuscitative efforts. Volume expansion should be carried out cautiously in newborns in whom hypotension may be caused by asphyxial myocardial damage rather than hypovolemia. It is important to use the appropriate gestational age– and birth weight–related blood pressure norms to determine volume status (see Chap. 40).

In most situations, there is no value to the administration of bicarbonate or other buffers during immediate resuscitation. Because there are potential risks as well as benefits for all medications (see Table 5.3), drug administration through the umbilical vein should be reserved for those newborns in whom bradycardia persists despite adequate oxygen delivery and ventilation after establishment of an adequate airway. Once an adequate airway has been established, adequate ventilation achieved, and the heart rate exceeds 100 bpm, the infant should be moved to the neonatal intensive care unit (NICU), where physical examination, determination of vital signs, and test results, such as chest radiographic appearance, will more clearly identify needs for specific interventions.

iv. **Reversal of narcotic depression is rarely necessary** during the primary steps of resuscitation and is not recommended. If the mother has received narcotic analgesia within a few hours of delivery, the newborn may manifest respiratory depression because of transplacental passage. The depression usually presents as apnea that persists even after bradycardia and cyanosis have been easily corrected with bag-and-mask ventilation. These infants should be treated with naloxone (0.4 mg/mL), in a dose of 0.25 mL/kg (e.g., 0.1 mg/kg). Naloxone should not be used if the mother is a chronic user of narcotics because of the risk of acute withdrawal in the infant. Respiratory support should be maintained until spontaneous respirations occur.

IV. SPECIAL SITUATIONS

A. Meconium aspiration (see Chap. 35)

1. In the presence of any meconium staining of the amniotic fluid, the obstetrician should quickly assess the infant during the birth process for the presence of secretions or copious amniotic fluid. **Routine suctioning** of all meconium-stained infants is not recommended, but in the presence of significant fluid or secretions, the mouth and pharynx should be aspirated with a bulb syringe after delivery of the head and before breathing begins.

2. The newborn should immediately be assessed to determine whether it is vigorous, as defined by strong respiratory effort, good muscle tone, and a heart rate >100 bpm. Infants who are vigorous should be treated as normal, despite the presence of meconium-stained fluid. If both the obstetric provider and the pediatric team in attendance agree that the infant is vigorous, it is not necessary to take the infant from his or her mother after birth. Infants who are not clearly vigorous should be rapidly intubated and their trachea suctioned for meconium, preferably before the first breath. In many cases, even if the infant has gasped, some meconium may still be removed with direct tracheal suction. Suctioning is accomplished through adapters that allow connection of the ET tube to the suction catheter. The resuscitator should avoid suction techniques that could allow self-contamination with blood or vaginal contents.

3. For infants at risk for meconium aspiration syndrome who show initial respiratory distress, oxygen saturation levels should be monitored and kept in the normal range by administering adequate supplemental oxygen.

B. Shock.

Some newborns present with pallor and shock in the delivery room (see Chaps. 40 and 43). Shock may result from significant intrapartum blood loss because of placental separation, fetal–maternal hemorrhage, avulsion of the umbilical cord from the placenta, vasa or placenta previa, incision through an anterior placenta at cesarean section, twin–twin transfusion, or rupture of an abdominal viscus (liver or spleen) during a difficult delivery. It may also result from vasodilation or loss of vascular tone because of septicemia or hypoxemia and acidosis. These newborns will be pale, tachycardic (over 180 bpm), tachypneic, and hypotensive with poor capillary filling and weak pulses.

After starting respiratory support, immediate transfusion with O-negative packed red blood cells and 5% albumin may be necessary if acute blood loss is the underlying cause. A volume of 20 mL/kg can be given through an umbilical venous catheter. If clinical improvement is not seen, causes of further blood loss should be sought, and more vigorous blood and colloid replacement should be continued. It is important to remember that the hematocrit may be normal immediately after delivery if the blood loss was acute during the intrapartum period.

Except in cases of massive acute blood loss, the emergent use of blood replacement is not necessary and acute stabilization can be achieved with crystalloid solutions. Normal saline is the primary choice of replacement fluid. This allows time to obtain proper products from the blood bank, if blood replacement is subsequently needed.

Except in the most extreme emergency situation where no other therapeutic option exists, the use of autologous blood from the placenta is not recommended.

C. Air leak.

If an infant fails to respond to resuscitation despite apparently effective ventilation, chest compressions, and medications, consider the possibility of air-leak syndromes. Pneumothoraces (unilateral or bilateral) and pneumopericardium should be ruled out by transillumination or diagnostic thoracentesis (see Chap. 38).

D. Prematurity. Premature infants require additional special care in the delivery room, including the use of oxygen–air mixtures and oximetry monitoring, and precautions such as plastic wraps or bags, and/or the use of exothermic mattresses to prevent heat loss because of thinner skin and an increased surface-area-to-body-weight ratio. Apnea secondary to respiratory insufficiency is more likely at lower gestational ages, and support should be provided. Surfactant-deficient lungs are poorly compliant, and higher ventilatory pressures may be needed for the first and subsequent breaths. Depending on the reason for premature birth, perinatal infection is more likely in premature infants, which increases their risk of perinatal depression.

V. APGAR SCORES.

Evaluation and decisions regarding resuscitation measures should be guided by assessment of respiration, heart rate, and color/oxygen saturation. Apgar scores are conventionally assigned after birth and recorded in the newborn's chart. The Apgar score consists of the total points assigned to five objective signs in the newborn. Each sign is evaluated and given a score of 0, 1, or 2. Total scores at 1 and 5 minutes after birth are usually noted. If the 5-minute score is 6 or less, the score is then noted at successive 5-minute intervals until it is >6 (see Table 5.2). A score of 10 indicates an infant in perfect condition; this is quite unusual because most babies have some degree of acrocyanosis. The scoring, if done properly, yields the following information:

A. One-minute Apgar score. This score generally correlates with umbilical cord blood pH and is an index of intrapartum depression. It does not correlate with outcome. Babies with a score of 0 to 4 have been shown to have a significantly lower pH, higher partial pressure of carbon dioxide ($PaCO_2$), and lower buffer base than those with Apgar scores >7. In the VLBW infant, a low Apgar score may not indicate severe depression. As many as 50% of infants with gestational ages of 25 to 26 weeks and Apgar scores of 0 to 3 have a cord pH of >7.25. Therefore, a VLBW infant with a low Apgar score cannot be assumed to be severely depressed. Nonetheless, such infants should be resuscitated actively and will usually respond more promptly and to less invasive measures than newborns whose low Apgar scores reflect acidemia.

B. Apgar scores beyond 1 minute are reflective of the infant's changing condition and the adequacy of resuscitative efforts. Persistence of low Apgar scores indicates need for further therapeutic efforts and usually the severity of the baby's underlying problem. In assessing the adequacy of resuscitation, the most common problem is inadequate pulmonary inflation and ventilation. It is important to verify a good seal with the mask, correct placement of the ET tube, and adequate peak inspiratory pressure applied to the bag if the Apgar score fails to improve as resuscitation proceeds.

The more prolonged the period of severe depression (i.e., Apgar score 3), the more likely is an abnormal long-term neurologic outcome. Nevertheless, many newborns with prolonged depression (>15 minutes) are normal in follow-up. Moreover, most infants with long-term motor abnormalities such as cerebral palsy have not had periods of neonatal depression after birth and have normal Apgar scores (see Chap. 55). Apgar scores were designed to monitor neonatal transition and the effectiveness of resuscitation, and their utility remains essentially limited to this important role. The American Academy of Pediatrics is currently recommending an expanded Apgar score reporting form, which details both the numeric score as well as concurrent resuscitative interventions.

VI. EVOLVING PRACTICES. The practice of neonatal resuscitation continues to evolve with the availability of new devices and enhanced understanding of the best approach to resuscitation.

A. **End-tidal or expiratory CO2 detectors** are already widely used to aid in confirming appropriate ET tube placement in the trachea. These devices may also have utility during bag-and-mask ventilation in helping to identify airway obstruction. Whether they may help ensure that appropriate ventilation is being offered has not yet been determined.

B. **Induced therapeutic hypothermia** is increasingly becoming the standard therapy for infants born at ≥36 weeks' gestation who manifest moderate to severe hypoxic–ischemic encephalopathy. Most protocols include initiation of therapy within 6 hours of birth, but it is currently unknown whether earlier initiation may increase effectiveness, or whether later initiation has any value. The role for passive cooling similarly requires more complete evaluation. Avoidance of maternal or neonatal **hyperthermia** is warranted and may prevent subtle neurologic injury (see Chap. 55).

C. **Withholding or withdrawing resuscitation.** Resuscitation at birth is indicated for those babies likely to have a high rate of survival and a low likelihood of severe morbidity, including those with a gestational age of 25 weeks or greater. In those situations where survival is unlikely or associated morbidity is very high, the wishes of the parents as the best spokespeople for the newborn should guide decisions about initiating resuscitation (see Chap. 19).

If there are no signs of life in an infant after 10 minutes of aggressive resuscitative efforts, with no evidence for other causes of newborn compromise, discontinuation of resuscitation efforts may be appropriate.

Suggested Readings

Burchfield DJ. Medication use in neonatal resuscitation. *Clin Perinatol* 1999;26:683–691.

Davis PG, Tan A, O'Donnell CP, et al. Resuscitation of newborn infants with 100% oxygen or air: a systemic review and meta-analysis. *Lancet* 2004;364:1329–1333.

Dawson JA, Kamlin CO, Wong C, et al. Oxygen saturation and heart rate during delivery room resuscitation of infants <30 weeks' gestation with air or 100% oxygen. *Arch Dis Child Fetal Neonatal Ed* 2009;94:F87–F91.

Kattwinkel J, ed. *Textbook of neonatal resuscitation*. 6th ed. Dallas, TX: American Academy of Pediatrics and American Heart Association; 2011.

Morley CJ, Davis PG, Doyle LW, et al. Nasal CPAP or intubation at birth for very preterm infants. *N Engl J Med* 2008;358:700–708.

Ostrea EM, Odell GB. The influence of bicarbonate administration on blood pH in a "closed system": clinical implications. *J Pediatr* 1972;80:671–680.

Perlman JM, Risser R. Cardiopulmonary resuscitation in the delivery room. Associated clinical events. *Arch Pediatr Adolesc Med* 1995;149:20–25.

Saugstad OD. Resuscitation of newborn infants with room air or oxygen. *Semin Neonatol* 2001;6:233–239.

Saugstad OD, Rootwelt T, Aalen O. Resuscitation of asphyxiated newborn infants with room air or oxygen: an international controlled trial. *Pediatrics* 1998;102:e1.

Vain NE, Szyld EG, Prudent LM, et al. Oropharyngeal and nasopharyngeal suctioning of meconium-stained neonates before delivery of their shoulders: multicentre, randomised controlled trial. *Lancet* 2004;364:597–602.

6 Birth Trauma
Elisa Abdulhayoglu

I. BACKGROUND. Birth injury is defined by the National Vital Statistics Report as "an impairment of the infant's body function or structure due to adverse influences that occurred at birth." Injury may occur antenatally, intrapartum, or during resuscitation and may be avoidable or unavoidable.

A. Incidence. The morbidity rate due to birth trauma is 2.8 per 1,000 live births and varies with the type of injury. The mortality rate in the United States for birth trauma dropped slightly from 2005 to 2006 from 0.6 to 0.5 per 100,000 live births.

B. Risk factors. When fetal size, immaturity, or malpresentation complicates delivery, the normal intrapartum compressions, contortions, and forces can lead to injury in the newborn. Obstetrical instrumentation may increase the mechanical forces, amplifying or inducing a birth injury. Breech presentation carries the greatest risk of injury. However, cesarean delivery without labor does not prevent all birth injuries. The following factors may contribute to an increased risk of birth injury:

1. Primiparity
2. Small maternal stature
3. Maternal pelvic anomalies
4. Prolonged or unusually rapid labor
5. Oligohydramnios
6. Malpresentation of the fetus
7. Use of midforceps or vacuum extraction
8. Versions and extraction
9. Very low birth weight or extreme prematurity
10. Fetal macrosomia or large fetal head
11. Fetal anomalies

C. Evaluation. A newborn at risk for birth injury should have a thorough examination, including a detailed neurologic evaluation. Newborns who require resuscitation after birth should be evaluated, as occult injury may be present. Particular attention should be paid to symmetry of structure and function, cranial nerves, range of motion of individual joints, and integrity of the scalp and skin.

II. TYPES OF BIRTH TRAUMA

A. Head and neck injuries

1. **Injuries associated with intrapartum fetal monitoring.** Placement of an electrode on the fetal scalp or presenting part for fetal heart monitoring occasionally causes superficial abrasions or lacerations. These injuries require minimal local treatment, if any. Facial or ocular trauma may result from a malpositioned electrode. Abscesses rarely form at the electrode site. Hemorrhage is a rare complication of fetal blood sampling.

2. **Extracranial hemorrhage**
   a. **Caput succedaneum**
      i. *Caput succedaneum* is a commonly occurring subcutaneous, extraperiosteal fluid collection that is occasionally hemorrhagic. It has poorly defined margins and can extend over the midline and across suture lines. It typically extends over the presenting portion of the scalp and is usually associated with molding.
      ii. The lesion usually resolves spontaneously without sequelae over the first several days after birth. It rarely causes significant blood loss or jaundice. There are rare reports of scalp necrosis with scarring.
      iii. **Vacuum caput** is a *caput succedaneum* with margins well demarcated by the vacuum cup.
   b. **Cephalohematoma**
      i. A **cephalohematoma** is a subperiosteal collection of blood resulting from rupture of the superficial veins between the skull and periosteum. The lesion is always confined by suture lines. It may occur in as many as 2.5% of all live births. It is more commonly seen in instrumented deliveries, occurring in 1% to 2% of spontaneous vaginal deliveries, 6% to 10% of vacuum-assisted deliveries, and in approximately 4% of forceps-assisted deliveries.
      ii. An extensive cephalohematoma can result in significant hyperbilirubinemia. Hemorrhage is rarely serious enough to necessitate blood transfusion. Infection is also a rare complication and usually occurs in association with septicemia and meningitis. Skull fractures have been associated with 5% of cephalohematomas. A head computed tomography (CT) scan should be obtained if neurologic symptoms are present. Most cephalohematomas resolve within 8 weeks. Occasionally, they calcify and persist for several months or years.
      iii. Management is limited to observation in most cases. Incision and aspiration of a cephalohematoma may introduce infection and is contraindicated. Anemia or hyperbilirubinemia should be treated as needed.
   c. **Subgaleal hematoma**
      i. Subgaleal hematoma is hemorrhage under the aponeurosis of the scalp. It is more often seen after vacuum- or forceps-assisted deliveries.
      ii. Because the subgaleal or subaponeurotic space extends from the orbital ridges to the nape of the neck and laterally to the ears, the hemorrhage can spread across the entire calvarium.
      iii. The initial presentation typically includes pallor, poor tone, and a fluctuant swelling on the scalp. The hematoma may grow slowly or increase rapidly and result in shock. With progressive spread, the ears may be displaced anteriorly and periorbital swelling can occur. Ecchymosis of the scalp may develop. The blood is resorbed slowly, and swelling gradually resolves. The morbidity may be significant in infants with severe hemorrhage who require intensive care for this lesion. The mortality rate can range from 14% to 22%.
      iv. There is no specific therapy. The infant must be observed closely for signs of hypovolemia, and blood volume should be maintained as needed with transfusions. Phototherapy should be provided for hyperbilirubinemia. An investigation for a bleeding disorder should be considered. Surgical drainage should be considered only for unremitting

clinical deterioration. A subgaleal hematoma associated with skin abrasions may become infected; it should be treated with antibiotics and may need drainage.

3. **Intracranial hemorrhage** (see Chap. 54)

4. **Skull fracture**

   a. Skull fractures may be either linear, usually involving the parietal bone, or depressed, involving the parietal or frontal bones. The latter are often associated with forceps use. Occipital bone fractures are most often associated with breech deliveries.

   b. Most infants with linear or depressed skull fractures are asymptomatic unless there is an associated intracranial hemorrhage (e.g., subdural or subarachnoid hemorrhage). Occipital osteodiastasis is a separation of the basal and squamous portions of the occipital bone that often results in cerebellar contusion and significant hemorrhage. It may be a lethal complication in breech deliveries. A linear fracture that is associated with a dural tear may lead to herniation of the meninges and brain, with development of a leptomeningeal cyst.

   c. Uncomplicated linear fractures usually require no therapy. The diagnosis is made by taking a skull x-ray. Head CT scan should be obtained if intracranial injury is suspected. Depressed skull fractures require neurosurgical evaluation. Some may be elevated using closed techniques. Comminuted or large skull fractures associated with neurologic findings need immediate neurosurgical evaluation. If leakage of cerebrospinal fluid from the nares or ears is noted, antibiotic therapy should be started and neurosurgical consultation should be obtained. Follow-up imaging should be performed at 8 to 12 weeks to evaluate possible leptomeningeal cyst formation.

5. **Facial or mandibular fractures**

   a. Facial fractures can be caused by numerous forces, including natural passage through the birth canal, forceps use, or delivery of the head in breech presentation.

   b. Fractures of the mandible, maxilla, and lacrimal bones warrant immediate attention. They may present as facial asymmetry with ecchymoses, edema, and crepitance, or respiratory distress with poor feeding. Untreated fractures can lead to facial deformities, with subsequent malocclusion and mastication difficulties. Treatment should begin promptly because maxillar and lacrimal fractures begin to heal within 7 to 10 days, and mandibular fractures start to repair at 10 to 14 days. Treated fractures usually heal without complication.

   c. Airway patency should be closely monitored. A plastic surgeon or otorhinolaryngologist should be consulted immediately and appropriate radiographic studies obtained. Head CT scan or magnetic resonance imaging (MRI) may be necessary to evaluate for retro-orbital or cribriform plate disruption. Antibiotics should be administered for fractures involving the sinuses or middle ear.

6. **Nasal injuries**

   a. Nasal fracture and dislocation may occur during the birth process. The most frequent nasal injury is dislocation of the nasal cartilage, which may result from pressure applied by the maternal symphysis pubis or sacral promontory. The reported prevalence of dislocation is less than 1%.

   b. Infants with significant nasal trauma may develop respiratory distress. Similar to facial fractures, nasal fractures begin to heal in 7 to 10 days and must be treated promptly. Rapid healing usually occurs once treatment is initiated. If treatment is delayed, deformities are common.

c. A misshapen nose may appear dislocated. To differentiate dislocation from a temporary deformation, compress the tip of the nose. With septal dislocation, the nares collapse and the deviated septum is more apparent. With a misshapen nose, no nasal deviation occurs. Nasal edema from repeated suctioning may mimic partial obstruction. Patency can be assessed with a cotton wisp under the nares. Management involves protection of the airway and otorhinolaryngology consultation.

d. If nasal dislocations are left untreated, there is an increased risk of long-term septal deformity.

7. **Ocular injuries**

a. Retinal and subconjunctival hemorrhages are commonly seen after vaginal delivery. They result from increased venous congestion and pressure during delivery. Malpositioned forceps can result in ocular and periorbital injury, including hyphema, vitreous hemorrhage, lacerations, orbital fracture, lacrimal duct or gland injury, and disruption of Descemet's membrane of the cornea (which can lead to astigmatism and amblyopia). Significant ocular trauma occurs in 0.19% of all deliveries.

b. Retinal hemorrhages usually resolve within 1 to 5 days. Subconjunctival hemorrhages resorb within 1 to 2 weeks. No long-term complications usually occur. For other ocular injuries, prompt diagnosis and treatment are necessary to ensure a good long-term outcome.

c. Management. Prompt ophthalmologic consultation should be obtained.

8. **Ear injuries**

a. Ears are susceptible to injury, particularly with forceps application. More significant injuries occur with fetal malposition. Abrasions, hematomas, and lacerations may develop.

b. Abrasions generally heal well with local care. Hematomas of the pinna may lead to the development of a "cauliflower" ear. Lacerations may result in perichondritis. Temporal bone injury can lead to middle and inner ear complications, such as hemotympanum and ossicular disarticulation.

c. Hematomas of the pinna should be drained to prevent clot organization and development of cauliflower ear. If the cartilage and temporal bone are involved, an otolaryngologist should be consulted. Antibiotic therapy may be required.

9. **Sternocleidomastoid** (see Chap. 58)

a. Sternocleidomastoid (SCM) injury is also referred to as congenital or muscular torticollis. The etiology is uncertain. The most likely cause is a muscle compartment syndrome resulting from intrauterine positioning. Torticollis can also arise during delivery as the muscle is hyperextended and ruptured, with development of a hematoma and subsequent fibrosis and shortening.

b. Torticollis may present at birth with a palpable 1 to 2 cm mass in the SCM region and head tilt to the side of the lesion. More often, it is noted at 1 to 4 weeks of age. Facial asymmetry may be present along with hemihypoplasia on the side of the lesion. Prompt treatment may lessen or correct the torticollis.

c. Other conditions may mimic congenital torticollis and should be ruled out. These include cervical vertebral anomalies, hemangioma, lymphangioma, and teratoma.

d. Treatment is initially conservative. Stretching of the involved muscle should begin promptly and be performed several times per day. Recovery typically occurs within 3 to 4 months in approximately 80% of cases. Surgery is needed if torticollis persists after 6 months of physical therapy.

e. In up to 10% of patients with congenital torticollis, congenital hip dysplasia may be present. A careful hip examination is warranted with further evaluation as indicated.

10. **Pharyngeal injury**

a. Minor submucosal pharyngeal injuries can occur with postpartum bulb suctioning. More serious injury, such as perforation into the mediastinal or pleural cavity, may result from nasogastric or endotracheal tube placement. Affected infants may have copious secretions and difficulty swallowing, and it may be difficult to advance a nasogastric tube.

b. Mild submucosal injuries typically heal without complication. More extensive trauma requires prompt diagnosis and treatment for complete resolution.

c. The diagnosis of a retropharyngeal tear is made radiographically using water-soluble contrast material. Infants are treated with broad-spectrum antibiotics, and oral feedings are withheld for 2 weeks. The contrast study is repeated to confirm healing before feeding is restarted. Infants with pleural effusions may require chest tube placement. Surgical consultation is obtained if the leak persists or if the perforation is large.

B. Cranial nerve, spinal cord, and peripheral nerve injury

1. **Cranial nerve injuries**

a. Facial nerve injury (cranial nerve VII)

i. Injury to the facial nerve is the most common peripheral nerve injury in neonates, occurring in up to 1% of live births. The exact incidence is unknown, as many cases are subtle and resolve readily. The etiology includes compression of the facial nerve by forceps (particularly midforceps), pressure on the nerve secondary to the fetal face lying against the maternal sacral promontory or, rarely, from pressure of a uterine mass (e.g., fibroid).

ii. Facial nerve injury results in asymmetric crying facies.

a) Central facial nerve injury occurs less frequently than peripheral nerve injury. Paralysis is limited to the lower half to two-thirds of the contralateral side, which is smooth with no nasolabial fold present. The corner of the mouth droops. Movement of the forehead and eyelid is unaffected.

b) Peripheral injury involves the entire side of face and is consistent with a lower motor neuron injury. The nasolabial fold is flattened and the mouth droops on the affected side. The infant is unable to wrinkle the forehead and close the eye completely. The tongue is not involved.

c) Peripheral nerve branch injury results in paralysis that is limited to only one group of facial muscles: the forehead, the eyelid, or the mouth.

iii. Differential diagnosis includes Möbius syndrome (nuclear agenesis), intracranial hemorrhage, congenital hypoplasia of the depressor anguli oris muscle, and congenital absence of facial muscles or nerve branches.

iv. The prognosis of acquired facial nerve injury is excellent, with recovery usually complete by 3 weeks. Initial management is directed at prevention of corneal injuries by using artificial tears and protecting the open eye by patching. Electromyography may be helpful to predict recovery or potential residual effects. Full recovery is most likely.

Surgical exploration of the facial nerve should only be performed in infants with complete clinical and electrophysical paralysis, showing no improvement by 5 weeks of age.

b. Recurrent laryngeal nerve injury

   i. Unilateral abductor paralysis may be caused by recurrent laryngeal injury secondary to excessive traction on the fetal head during breech delivery or lateral traction on the head with forceps. The left recurrent laryngeal nerve is involved more often because of its longer course. Bilateral recurrent laryngeal nerve injury can be caused by trauma but is usually due to hypoxia or brain stem hemorrhage.

   ii. A neonate with unilateral abductor paralysis is often asymptomatic at rest, but has hoarseness and inspiratory stridor with crying. Unilateral injury is occasionally associated with hypoglossal nerve injury and presents with difficulty with feedings and secretions. Bilateral paralysis usually results in stridor, severe respiratory distress, and cyanosis.

   iii. Differential diagnosis of symptoms similar to unilateral injury includes congenital laryngeal malformations. Particularly with bilateral paralysis, intrinsic central nervous system (CNS) malformations must be ruled out, including Chiari malformation and hydrocephalus. If there is no history of birth trauma, cardiovascular anomalies and mediastinal masses should be considered.

   iv. The diagnosis can be made using direct or flexible fiberoptic laryngoscopy. A modified barium swallow and speech pathology consultation may be helpful to optimize feeding. Unilateral injury usually resolves by 6 weeks of age without intervention and treatment. Bilateral paralysis has a variable prognosis; tracheostomy may be required.

2. Spinal cord injuries

   a. Vaginal delivery of an infant with a hyperextended head or neck, breech delivery, and severe shoulder dystocia are risk factors for spinal cord injury. However, significant spinal cord injuries are rare with a prevalence rate of 0.14 per 10,000 live births. Injuries include spinal epidural hematomas, vertebral artery injuries, traumatic cervical hematomyelia, spinal artery occlusion, and transection of the cord.

   b. Spinal cord injury presents in four ways:

   i. Some infants with severe high cervical or brain stem injury present as stillborn or in poor condition at birth, with respiratory depression, shock, and hypothermia. Death generally occurs within hours of birth.

   ii. Infants with an upper or midcervical injury present with central respiratory depression. They have lower extremity paralysis, absent deep tendon reflexes and absent sensation in the lower half of the body, urinary retention, and constipation. Bilateral brachial plexus injury may be present.

   iii. Injury at the seventh cervical vertebra or lower may be reversible. However, permanent neurologic complications may result, including muscle atrophy, contractures, bony deformities, and constant micturition.

   iv. Partial spinal injury or spinal artery occlusions may result in subtle neurologic signs and spasticity.

   c. Differential diagnosis includes amyotonia congenita, myelodysplasia associated with spina bifida occulta, spinal cord tumors, and cerebral hypotonia.

d. The prognosis depends on the severity and location of the injury. If a spinal injury is suspected at birth, efforts should focus on resuscitation and prevention of further damage. The head, neck, and spine should be immobilized. Neurology and neurosurgical consultations should be obtained. Careful and repeated examinations are necessary to help predict long-term outcome. Cervical spine radiographs, CT scan, and MRI may be helpful.

3. Cervical nerve root injuries

   a. Phrenic nerve injury (C3, C4, or C5)

      i. Phrenic nerve damage leading to paralysis of the ipsilateral diaphragm may result from a stretch injury due to lateral hyperextension of the neck at birth. Risk factors include breech and difficult forceps deliveries. Injury to the nerve is thought to occur where it crosses the brachial plexus. Therefore, approximately 75% of patients also have brachial plexus injury. Occasionally, chest tube insertion or surgery injures this nerve.

      ii. Respiratory distress and cyanosis are often seen. Some infants present with persistent tachypnea and decreased breath sounds at the lung base. There may be decreased movement of the affected hemithorax. Chest radiographs may show elevation of the affected diaphragm, although this may not be apparent if the infant is on continuous positive airway pressure (CPAP) or mechanical ventilation. If the infant is breathing spontaneously and not on CPAP, an increasing atelectasis may develop. The diagnosis is confirmed by ultrasonography or fluoroscopy that shows paradoxical (upward) movement of the diaphragm with inspiration.

      iii. Differential diagnosis includes cardiac, pulmonary, and other neurologic causes of respiratory distress. These can usually be evaluated by a careful examination and appropriate imaging. Congenital absence of the nerve is rare.

      iv. The initial treatment is supportive. CPAP or mechanical ventilation may be needed, with careful airway care to avoid atelectasis and pneumonia. Most infants recover in 1 to 3 months without permanent sequelae. Diaphragmatic plication is considered in refractory cases. Phrenic nerve pacing is possible for bilateral paralysis.

   b. Brachial plexus injury

      i. The incidence of brachial plexus injury ranges from 0.1% to 0.2% of all births. The cause is excessive traction on the head, neck, and arm during birth. Risk factors include macrosomia, shoulder dystocia, malpresentation, and instrumented deliveries. Injury usually involves the nerve root, especially where the roots come together to form the nerve trunks of the plexus.

      ii. Duchenne-Erb palsy involves the upper trunks (C5, C6, and occasionally C7) and is the most common type of brachial plexus injury, accounting for approximately 90% of cases. Total brachial plexus palsy occurs in some cases and involves all roots from C5 to T1. Klumpke palsy involves C7/C8 to T1 and is the least common.

        a) Duchenne-Erb palsy. The arm is typically adducted and internally rotated at the shoulder. There is extension and pronation at the elbow and flexion of the wrist and fingers in the characteristic "waiter's tip" posture. The deltoid, infraspinatus, biceps, supinator and brachioradialis muscles, and the extensors of the wrist and fingers may be weak or paralyzed. The Moro, biceps, and radial reflexes are absent on the affected side. The grasp reflex is intact. Sensation is variably affected. Diaphragm paralysis occurs in 5% of cases.

b) **Total brachial plexus injury.** Accounts for approximately 10% of all cases. The entire arm is flaccid. All reflexes, including grasp and sensation, are absent. If sympathetic fibers are injured at T1, Horner syndrome may be seen.

c) **Klumpke palsy.** The rarest of the palsies, accounting for <1% of brachial plexus injuries. The lower arm paralysis affects the intrinsic muscles of the hand and the long flexors of the wrist and fingers. The grasp reflex is absent. However, the biceps and radial reflexes are present. There is sensory impairment on the ulnar side of the forearm and hand. Because the first thoracic root is usually injured, its sympathetic fibers are damaged, leading to an ipsilateral Horner syndrome.

iii. **Differential diagnosis** includes a cerebral injury, which usually has other associated CNS symptoms. Injury of the clavicle, upper humerus, and lower cervical spine may mimic a brachial plexus injury.

iv. Radiographs of the shoulder and upper arm should be performed to rule out bony injury. The chest should be carefully examined to detect diaphragm paralysis. Initial treatment is conservative. Physical therapy and passive range of motion exercises prevent contractures. These should be started at 7 to 10 days, when the postinjury neuritis has resolved. "Statue of Liberty" splinting should be avoided, as contractures in the shoulder girdle may develop. Wrist and digit splints may be useful.

v. The prognosis for full recovery varies with the extent of injury. If the nerve roots are intact and not avulsed, the prognosis for full recovery is excellent (>90%). Notable clinical improvement in the first 2 weeks after birth indicates that normal or near-normal function will return. Most infants recover fully by 3 months of age. In those with slow recovery, electromyography and nerve-conduction studies may distinguish an avulsion from a stretch injury. Surgery has most commonly been recommended when there is a lack of biceps function at 3 months of age.

C. Bone injuries

1. **Clavicular fracture** is the most commonly injured bone during delivery, occurring in up to 3% of newborns. Up to 40% of clavicular fractures are not identified until after discharge from the hospital.

   a. These fractures are seen in vertex presentations with shoulder dystocia or in breech deliveries when the arms are extended. Macrosomia is a risk factor.

   b. A greenstick or incomplete fracture may be asymptomatic at birth. The first clinical sign may be a callus at 7 to 10 days of age. Signs of a complete fracture include crepitus, palpable bony irregularity, and spasm of the SCM. The affected arm may have a pseudoparalysis because motion causes pain.

   c. Differential diagnosis includes fracture of the humerus or a brachial plexus palsy.

   d. A **clavicular fracture** is confirmed by chest x-ray. If the arm movement is decreased, the cervical spine, brachial plexus, and humerus should be assessed.

Therapy should be directed at decreasing pain with analgesics. The infant's sleeve should be pinned to the shirt to limit movement until the callus begins to form. Complete healing is expected.

2. **Long bone injuries**

    a. **Humeral fractures** have a prevalence of 0.05 per 1,000 live births.

        i. Humeral fractures typically occur during a difficult delivery of the arms in the breech presentation and/or of the shoulders in vertex. Direct pressure on the humerus may also result in fracture.

        ii. A greenstick fracture may not be noted until the callus forms. The first sign is typically loss of spontaneous arm movement, followed by swelling and pain on passive motion. A complete fracture with displaced fragments presents as an obvious deformity. X-ray confirms the diagnosis.

        iii. Differential diagnosis includes clavicular fracture and brachial plexus injury.

        iv. The prognosis is excellent with complete healing expected. Pain should be treated with analgesics.

           a) A fractured humerus usually requires splinting for 2 weeks. Displaced fractures require closed reduction and casting. Radial nerve injury may be seen.

           b) Epiphyseal displacement occurs when the humeral epiphysis separates at the hypertrophied cartilaginous layer of the growth plate. Severe displacement may result in significant compromise of growth. The diagnosis can be confirmed by ultrasonography because the epiphysis is not ossified at birth. Therapy includes immobilization of the limb for 10 to 14 days.

    b. **Femoral fractures** have a prevalence of 0.13 per 1,000 live births.

        i. Femoral fractures usually follow a breech delivery. Infants with congenital hypotonia are at increased risk.

        ii. Physical examination usually reveals an obvious deformity of the thigh. In some cases, the injury may not be noted for a few days until swelling, decreased movement, or pain with palpation develop. The diagnosis is confirmed by x-ray.

        iii. Complete healing without limb shortening is expected.

           a) Fractures, even if unilateral, should be treated with splinting and immobilization using a spica cast or Pavlik harness.

           b) Femoral epiphyseal separation may be misinterpreted as developmental dysplasia of the hip because the epiphysis is not ossified at birth. Pain and tenderness with palpation are more likely with epiphyseal separation than dislocation. The diagnosis is confirmed by ultrasonography. Therapy includes limb immobilization for 10 to 14 days and analgesics for pain.

D. **Intra-abdominal Injuries.** Intra-abdominal birth trauma is uncommon.

    1. **Hepatic injury**

        a. The liver is the most commonly injured solid organ during birth. Macrosomia, hepatomegaly, and breech presentation are risk factors for hepatic hematoma and/or rupture. The etiology is thought to be a direct pressure on the liver.

        b. Subcapsular hematomas are generally not symptomatic at birth. Nonspecific signs of blood loss such as poor feeding, pallor, tachypnea, tachycardia, and onset of jaundice develop during the first 1 to 3 days after birth. Serial hematocrits may suggest blood loss. Rupture of the hematoma through the capsule results in discoloration of the abdominal wall and circulatory collapse with shock.

c. Differential diagnosis includes trauma to other intra-abdominal organs.

d. Management includes restoration of blood volume, correction of coagulation disturbances, and surgical consultation for probable laparotomy. Early diagnosis and correction of volume loss increase survival.

2. **Splenic injury**

a. Risk factors for splenic injury include macrosomia, breech delivery, and splenomegaly (e.g., congenital syphilis, erythroblastosis fetalis).

b. Signs are similar to hepatic rupture. A mass is sometimes palpable in the left upper quadrant, and the stomach bubble may be displaced medially on an abdominal radiograph.

c. Differential diagnosis includes injury to other abdominal organs.

d. Management includes volume replacement and correction of coagulation disorders. Surgical consultation should be obtained. Expectant management with close observation is appropriate if the bleeding has stopped and the patient has stabilized. If laparotomy is necessary, salvage of the spleen is attempted to minimize the risk of sepsis.

3. **Adrenal hemorrhage**

a. The relatively large size of the adrenal gland at birth may contribute to injury. Risk factors are breech presentation and macrosomia. Ninety percent of adrenal hemorrhages are unilateral; 75% occur on the right.

b. Findings on physical examination depend on the extent of hemorrhage. Classic signs include fever, flank mass, purpura, and pallor. Adrenal insufficiency may present with poor feeding, vomiting, irritability, listlessness, and shock. The diagnosis is made with abdominal ultrasound.

c. Differential diagnosis includes other abdominal trauma. If a flank mass is palpable, neuroblastoma and Wilms tumor should be considered.

d. Treatment includes blood volume replacement. Adrenal insufficiency may require steroid therapy. Extensive bleeding that requires surgical intervention is rare.

E. **Soft tissue injuries**

1. **Petechiae and ecchymoses** are commonly seen in newborns. The birth history, location of lesions, their early appearance without development of new lesions, and the absence of bleeding from other sites help differentiate petechiae and ecchymoses secondary to birth trauma from those caused by a vasculitis or coagulation disorder. If the etiology is uncertain, studies to rule out coagulopathies and infection should be performed. Most petechiae and ecchymoses resolve within 1 week. If bruising is excessive, jaundice and anemia may develop. Treatment is supportive.

2. **Lacerations and abrasions** may be secondary to scalp electrodes and fetal scalp blood sampling or injury during birth. Deep wounds (e.g., scalpel injuries during cesarean section) may require sutures. Infection is a risk, particularly with scalp lesions and an underlying *caput succedaneum* or hematoma. Treatment includes cleansing the wound and close observation.

3. **Subcutaneous fat necrosis** is not usually recognized at birth. It usually presents during the first 2 weeks after birth as sharply demarcated; irregularly shaped; firm; and nonpitting subcutaneous plaques or nodules on the extremities, face, trunk, or buttocks. The injury may be colorless or have a deep red or purple discoloration. Calcification may occur. No treatment is necessary. Lesions typically resolve completely over several weeks to months.

Suggested Readings

Borschel GH, Clarke HM. Obstetrical brachial plexus palsy. *Plast Reconstr Surg* 2009;124(suppl 1):144e–155e.

Doumouchtsis SK, Arulkumaran S. Head trauma after instrumental births. *Clin Perinatol* 2008;35:69–83.

Goetz E. Neonatal spinal cord injury after an uncomplicated vaginal delivery. *Pediatr Neurol* 2010;42:69–71.

Moczygemba CK, Paramsothy P, Meikle S, et al. Route of delivery and neonatal birth trauma. *Am J Obstet Gynecol* 2010;202(4):361.e1–e6.

Rosenberg AA. Traumatic birth injury. *NeoReviews* 2003;4(10):e270–e276.

Uhing MR. Management of birth injuries. *Clin Perinatol* 2005;32:19–38.

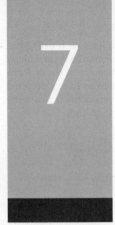

7

The High-Risk Newborn: Anticipation, Evaluation, Management, and Outcome

Vincent C. Smith

I. HIGH-RISK NEWBORNS are often associated with certain maternal, placental, or fetal conditions; when one or more are present, nursery staff should be aware and prepared for possible difficulties. The placenta should be saved after delivery in all cases of high-risk delivery, including cases that involve transfer from the birth hospital, since an elusive diagnosis such as toxoplasmosis may be made on the basis of placental pathology. The following factors are associated with high-risk newborns:

A. Maternal characteristics and associated risk for fetus or neonate

1. **Age at delivery**
   a. **Over 40 years.** Chromosomal abnormalities, macrosomia, intrauterine growth retardation (IUGR), blood loss (abruption or previa).
   b. **Under 16 years.** IUGR, prematurity, child abuse/neglect (mother herself may be abused).

2. **Personal factors**
   a. **Poverty.** Prematurity, IUGR, infection.
   b. **Smoking.** Increased perinatal mortality, IUGR.
   c. **Drug/alcohol use.** IUGR, fetal alcohol syndrome, withdrawal syndrome, sudden infant death syndrome, child abuse/neglect.
   d. **Poor diet.** Mild IUGR to fetal demise in severe malnutrition.
   e. **Trauma (acute, chronic).** Abruptio placentae, fetal demise, prematurity.

3. **Medical conditions**
   a. **Diabetes mellitus.** Stillbirth, macrosomia/birth injury, respiratory distress syndrome (RDS), hypoglycemia, congenital anomalies (see Chap. 2).
   b. **Thyroid disease.** Goiter, hypothyroidism, hyperthyroidism (see Chap. 3).
   c. **Renal disease.** Stillbirth, IUGR, prematurity.
   d. **Urinary tract infection.** Prematurity, sepsis.
   e. **Heart and/or lung disease.** Stillbirth, IUGR, prematurity.
   f. **Hypertension (chronic or pregnancy-related).** Stillbirth, IUGR, prematurity, asphyxia.
   g. **Anemia.** Stillbirth, IUGR, hydrops, prematurity, asphyxia.
   h. **Isoimmunization (red cell antigens).** Stillbirth, hydrops, anemia, jaundice.
   i. **Alloimmunization (platelet antigens).** Stillbirth, bleeding.
   j. **Thrombocytopenia.** Stillbirth, bleeding.

4. **Obstetric history**
   a. **Past history of infant with prematurity, jaundice, RDS, or anomalies.** Same with current pregnancy.
   b. **Maternal medications.** (see Appendices B and C)
   c. **Bleeding in early pregnancy.** Stillbirth, prematurity.
   d. **Hyperthermia.** Fetal demise, fetal anomalies.
   e. **Bleeding in third trimester.** Stillbirth, anemia.
   f. **Premature rupture of membranes.** Infection/sepsis.
   g. **TORCH infections.** (see Chap. 48)
   h. **Trauma.** Fetal demise, prematurity.

B. **Fetal characteristics and associated risk for fetus or neonate**
   1. **Multiple gestation.** IUGR, twin–twin transfusion syndrome, prematurity, birth trauma, asphyxia.
   2. **IUGR.** Fetal demise, congenital anomalies, asphyxia, hypoglycemia, polycythemia.
   3. **Macrosomia.** Congenital anomalies, birth trauma, hypoglycemia.
   4. **Abnormal fetal position/presentation.** Congenital anomalies, birth trauma, hemorrhage.
   5. **Abnormality of fetal heart rate or rhythm.** Congestive heart failure, heart block, hydrops, asphyxia.
   6. **Decreased activity.** Fetal demise, asphyxia.
   7. **Polyhydramnios.** Anencephaly, other central nervous system (CNS) disorders, neuromuscular disorders, problems with swallowing (e.g., agnathia, any mass in the mouth, esophageal atresia), chylothorax, diaphragmatic hernia, omphalocele, gastroschisis, trisomy, tumors, hydrops, isoimmunization, anemia, cardiac failure, intrauterine infection, inability to concentrate urine, large for gestational age, maternal diabetes.
   8. **Oligohydramnios.** Fetal demise, placental insufficiency, IUGR, renal agenesis, pulmonary hypoplasia, deformations, intrapartum distress, postterm delivery.

C. **Conditions of labor and delivery and associated risk for fetus or neonate**
   1. **Preterm delivery.** RDS, other issues of preterm birth (see Chap. 13).
   2. **Postterm delivery (occurring more than 2 weeks after term) (see IV).** Stillbirth, asphyxia, meconium aspiration.
   3. **Maternal fever.** Infection/sepsis.
   4. **Maternal hypotension.** Stillbirth, asphyxia.
   5. **Rapid labor.** Birth trauma, intracranial hemorrhage (ICH), retained fetal lung fluid/transient tachypnea.
   6. **Prolonged labor.** Stillbirth, asphyxia, birth trauma.
   7. **Abnormal presentation.** Birth trauma, asphyxia.
   8. **Uterine tetany.** Asphyxia.
   9. **Meconium-stained amniotic fluid.** Stillbirth, asphyxia, meconium aspiration syndrome, persistent pulmonary hypertension.

10. **Prolapsed cord.** Stillbirth, asphyxia.

11. **Cesarean section.** RDS, retained fetal lung fluid/transient tachypnea, blood loss.

12. **Obstetric analgesia and anesthesia.** Respiratory depression, hypotension, hypothermia.

13. **Placental anomalies**
   a. **Small placenta.** IUGR.
   b. **Large placenta.** Hydrops, maternal diabetes, large infant.
   c. **Torn placenta and/or umbilical vessels.** Blood loss.
   d. **Abnormal attachment of vessels to placenta.** Blood loss.

D. **Immediately evident neonatal conditions and associated risk for fetus or neonate**

1. **Prematurity.** RDS, other sequelae of prematurity.

2. **Low 5-minute Apgar score.** Prolonged transition (especially respiratory).

3. **Low 15-minute Apgar score.** Neurologic damage.

4. **Pallor or shock.** Blood loss.

5. **Foul smell of amniotic fluid or membranes.** Infection.

6. **Small for gestational age (SGA).** (see V.)

7. **Postmaturity syndrome.** (see IV.D.)

II. GESTATIONAL AGE (GA) AND BIRTH WEIGHT CLASSIFICATION. Neonates should be classified by GA, if at all possible, as this is generally more physiologically important than birth weight.

A. **GA classification.**

1. Assessment based on **obstetric information** is covered in Chapter 1. Note that GA estimates by first-trimester ultrasonography are accurate within 4 days.

2. To confirm or supplement obstetric dating, the modified Dubowitz (Ballard) examination for newborns (see Fig. 7.1) may be useful in GA estimation. There are limitations to this method, especially with use of the neuromuscular component in sick newborns.

3. **Infant classification by gestational (postmenstrual) age**
   a. **Preterm.** Less than 37 completed weeks (259 days).
   b. **Late preterm.** A subgroup of infants born at 34 through 36 weeks GA (238–258 days).
   c. **Term.** Thirty-seven to 41 6/7 weeks (260–294 days).
   d. **Postterm.** Forty-two weeks (295 days) or more.

B. **Birth weight classification.** Although there is no universal agreement, the commonly accepted definitions are as follows:

1. **Normal birth weight (NBW).** From 2,500 to 4,000 g.

2. **Low birth weight (LBW).** Less than 2,500 g. Note that, while most LBW infants are preterm, some are term but SGA. LBW infants can be further subclassified as follows:
   a. **Very low birth weight (VLBW).** Less than 1,500 g.
   b. **Extremely low birth weight (ELBW).** Less than 1,000 g.

MATURATIONAL ASSESSMENT OF GESTATIONAL AGE (New Ballard Score)

NAME _____ SEX _____
HOSPITAL NO. _____ BIRTH WEIGHT _____
RACE _____ LENGTH _____
DATE/TIME OF BIRTH _____ HEAD CIRC. _____
DATE/TIME OF EXAM _____ EXAMINER _____
AGE WHEN EXAMINED _____
APGAR SCORE: 1 MINUTE _____ 5 MINUTES _____ 10 MINUTES _____

NEUROMUSCULAR MATURITY

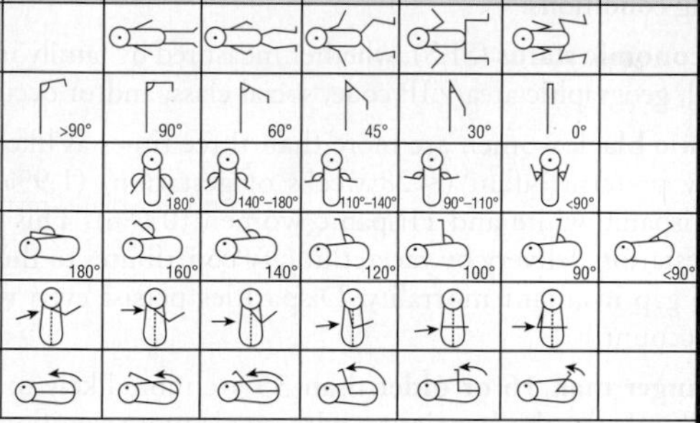

NEUROMUSCULAR MATURITY SIGN	SCORE							RECORD SCORE HERE
	-1	0	1	2	3	4	5	
POSTURE								
SQUARE WINDOW (Wrist)	>90°	90°	60°	45°	30°	0°		
ARM RECOIL		180°	140°–180°	110°–140°	90°–110°	<90°		
POPLITEAL ANGLE	180°	160°	140°	120°	100°	90°	<90°	
SCARF SIGN								
HEEL TO EAR								

TOTAL NEUROMUSCULAR MATURITY SCORE

SCORE
Neuromuscular _____
Physical _____
Total _____

MATURITY RATING

SCORE	WEEKS
-10	20
-5	22
0	24
5	26
10	28
15	30
20	32
25	34
30	36
35	38
40	40
45	42
50	44

GESTATIONAL AGE (weeks)
By dates _____·_____
By ultrasound _____
By exam _____

PHYSICAL MATURITY

PHYSICAL MATURITY SIGN	SCORE							RECORD SCORE HERE
	-1	0	1	2	3	4	5	
SKIN	sticky friable transparent	gelatinous red translucent	smooth pink visible veins	superficial peeling &/or rash, few veins	cracking pale areas rare veins	parchment deep cracking no vessels	leathery cracked wrinkled	
LANUGO	none	sparse	abundant	thinning	bald areas	mostly bald		
PLANTAR SURFACE	heel-toe 40–50 mm: -1 <40 mm: -2	>50 mm no crease	faint red marks	anterior transverse crease only	creases ant. 2/3	creases over entire sole		
BREAST	imperceptible	barely perceptible	flat areola no bud	stippled areola 1–2 mm bud	raised areola 3–4 mm bud	full areola 5–10 mm bud		
EYE / EAR	lids fused loosely: -1 tightly: -2	lids open pinna flat stays folded	sl. curved pinna; soft; slow recoil	well-curved pinna; soft but ready recoil	formed & firm instant recoil	thick cartilage ear shift		
GENITALS (Male)	scrotum flat, smooth	scrotum empty faint rugae	testes in upper canal rare rugae	testes descending few rugae	testes down good rugae	testes pendulous deep rugae		
GENITALS (Female)	clitoris prominent & labia flat	prominent clitoris & small labia minora	prominent clitoris & enlarging minora	majora & minora equally prominent	majora large minora small	majora cover clitoris & minora		

TOTAL PHYSICAL MATURITY SCORE

Figure 7.1. New Ballard score. (From Ballard JL, Khoury JC, Wedig K, et al. New Ballard Score, expanded to include extremely premature infants. *J Pediatr* 1991;119(3):417–423.)

III. PRETERM BIRTH. As noted above, a **preterm neonate** is one whose birth occurs before the end of the 37th week (258th day; i.e., 36 6/7 weeks) following onset of the last menstrual period.

A. **Incidence.** Approximately 12.7% of all births in the United States are preterm. The distribution of this group is gradually shifting to a relatively older gestational age because of a 25% increase in late preterm infants (34 to 36 weeks) since 1990 to current rate of 9.1%.

B. **Etiology** is unknown in most cases. Preterm and/or LBW delivery is associated with the following conditions:

1. **Low socioeconomic status** (SES), whether measured by family income, educational level, geographic area/ZIP code, social class, and/or occupation.

2. **Non-Hispanic black** women are more than three times as likely to deliver an extremely preterm infant (<28 weeks of gestation) (1.9%) compared with non-Hispanic white and Hispanic women (0.6%). This disparity in very short gestation delivery by race/ethnicity contributes to the substantial black–white gap in infant mortality. Disparities persist even when SES is taken into account.

3. **Women younger than 16 or older than 35** are more likely to deliver preterm or LBW infants; the association with age is more significant in whites than in African Americans.

4. **Maternal activity** requiring long periods of standing or substantial amounts of physical stress may be associated with IUGR and prematurity.

5. **Acute or chronic maternal illness** is associated with early delivery, whether spontaneous or, not infrequently, induced.

6. **Multiple-gestation births** frequently deliver preterm (60% of twins and 94% of triplets in the United States in 2005). In such births, higher rate of neonatal mortality is primarily due to prematurity.

7. **Prior poor birth outcome** is the single strongest predictor of poor birth outcome. A preterm first birth is the best predictor of a second preterm birth.

8. **Obstetric factors** such as uterine malformations, uterine trauma, placenta previa, abruptio placentae, hypertensive disorders, preterm cervical shortening, previous cervical surgery, premature rupture of membranes, and chorioamnionitis also contribute to prematurity.

9. **Fetal conditions** such as nonreassuring testing of fetal well-being (see Chap. 1), IUGR, or severe hydrops may require preterm delivery.

10. **Inadvertent early delivery** because of incorrect estimation of GA is increasingly uncommon.

C. **Problems of preterm birth** are related to difficulty in extrauterine adaptation due to immaturity of organ system.

1. **Respiratory.** Preterm infants may experience the following:
   a. Perinatal depression in the delivery room due to poor transition to breathing (see Chaps. 5 and 55).
   b. RDS due to surfactant deficiency and pulmonary immaturity (see Chap. 33).
   c. Apnea due to immaturity in mechanisms controlling breathing (see Chap. 31).

d. Chronic lung disease (CLD) of prematurity formerly called broncho-pulmonary dysplasia (BPD), Wilson-Mikity disease, and chronic pulmonary insufficiency of prematurity (see Chap. 34).

2. **Neurologic.** Preterm infants have a higher risk for neurologic problems, including the following:
   a. Perinatal depression (see Chap. 55).
   b. Intracranial Hemorrhage (ICH) (see Chap. 54).

3. **Cardiovascular.** Preterm infants may present with cardiovascular problems, including the following:
   a. Hypotension
      i. Hypovolemia.
      ii. Cardiac dysfunction.
      iii. Sepsis-induced vasodilation.
   b. Patent ductus arteriosus is common and may lead to pulmonary over-circulation and diastolic hypotension (see Chap. 41).

4. **Hematologic.** Conditions for which preterm infants are at higher risk include the following:
   a. Anemia (see Chap. 45).
   b. Hyperbilirubinemia (see Chap. 26).

5. **Nutritional.** Preterm infants require specific attention to the content, caloric density, volume, and route of feeding (see Chap. 21).

6. **Gastrointestinal.** Premature infants are at increased risk for necrotizing enterocolitis; formula feeding is an additional risk factor; breast milk appears to be protective (see Chap. 27).

7. **Metabolic.** Problems, especially in glucose and calcium metabolism, are more common in preterm infants (see Chaps. 24 and 25).

8. **Renal.** Immature kidneys are characterized by low glomerular filtration rate, as well as an inability to handle water, solute, and acid loads. Therefore, fluid and electrolyte management require close attention (see Chaps. 23 and 28).

9. **Temperature regulation.** Preterm infants are especially susceptible to hypothermia and hyperthermia (see Chap. 15).

10. **Immunologic.** Because of deficiencies in both humoral and cellular response, preterm infants are at greater risk for infection than are term infants.

11. **Ophthalmologic.** Retinopathy of prematurity may develop in the immature retina of infants <32 weeks or with birth weight <1,500 g (see Chap. 64).

D. **Management of the preterm infant** (see Chap. 13).

1. **Immediate postnatal management**
   a. Delivery in an appropriately equipped and staffed hospital is preferable. Risks to the very premature or sick preterm infant are greatly increased by delays in initiating necessary specialized care.
   b. Resuscitation and stabilization require the immediate availability of qualified personnel and equipment. Resuscitation of the newborn at delivery should be in accordance with the American Academy of Pediatrics Neonatal Resuscitation Program (NRP). Anticipation and prevention are always preferred over reaction to problems already present. Adequate oxygen delivery and maintenance of proper temperature are immediate postnatal goals (see Chap. 5).

2. Neonatal management

a. Thermal regulation should be directed toward achieving a neutral thermal zone, that is, environmental temperature sufficient to maintain body temperature, with minimal oxygen consumption. For the small preterm infant, this will require either an overhead radiant warmer (with the advantages of infant accessibility and rapid temperature response) or a closed incubator (with the advantages of diminished insensible water loss) or a combined unit (see Chap. 15).

b. Oxygen therapy and assisted ventilation (see Chap. 29).

c. Patent ductus arteriosus in preterm infants with birth weight >1,000 g often requires only conservative management with fluid restriction and adequate oxygenation. In smaller infants, a prostaglandin antagonist such as indomethacin or ibuprofen may be necessary. In the most symptomatic infants or those for whom medical therapy is either contraindicated or fails to close the ductus, surgical ligation may become necessary (see Chap. 41).

d. Fluid and electrolyte therapy must account for relatively high insensible water loss while maintaining proper hydration and normal glucose and plasma electrolyte concentrations (see Chap. 23).

e. Nutrition may be complicated by the inability of many preterm infants to tolerate enteral feedings, necessitating treatment with parenteral nutrition. Ineffective suck and swallow may necessitate gavage feeding (see Chap. 21).

f. Hyperbilirubinemia, which is inevitable in less mature infants, can usually be managed effectively by careful monitoring of bilirubin levels and early use of phototherapy. In the most severe cases, exchange transfusion may be necessary (see Chap. 26).

g. Infection may be the precipitant of preterm delivery. If an infant displays signs or symptoms that could be attributed to infection, the infant should be carefully evaluated for sepsis (e.g., physical exam, +/− CBC, +/− blood culture). There should be a low threshold for starting broad-spectrum antibiotics (e.g., ampicillin and gentamicin) until sepsis can be ruled out. Consider antistaphylococcal antibiotics for VLBW infants who have undergone multiple procedures or have remained for long periods in the hospital and are at increased risk for nosocomial infection (see Chaps. 48 and 49).

h. Immunizations. Diphtheria, tetanus toxoids, and acellular pertussis (DTaP) vaccine; inactivated poliovirus vaccine (IPV); multivalent pneumococcal conjugate vaccine (PCV); and *Haemophilus influenzae* type b (Hib) vaccine are given in full doses to preterm infants on the basis of their chronologic age (i.e., weeks after birth) and postmenstrual age. Hepatitis B (HepB) vaccine administration for medically stable preterm infants of hepatitis B surface antigen (HBsAg)-negative mothers may be given on a modified schedule. Respiratory syncytial virus (RSV) and influenza prophylaxis should be given as indicated. Special consideration should be given to the rotavirus vaccine (RV) because it is a live oral vaccine that is not given until NICU discharge, with strict limitation on its administration. All Centers for Disease Control and Prevention (CDC) and Advisory Committee on Immunization Practices (ACIP) recommendations can be found at http://www.cdc.gov/vaccines (see Chaps. 48 and 49).

E. **Survival of preterm infants.** For many reasons, survival statistics vary by institution as well as geographic region and country. Figures 7.2 and 7.3 show mortality rates of 56,499 VLBW preterm infants from ~800 hospitals enrolled in the Vermont Oxford Network in 2008. The network maintains data on survival and complications of preterm birth.

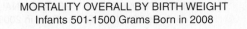

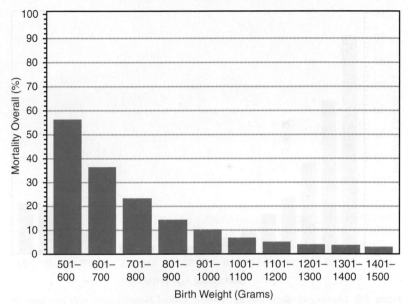

Figure 7.2. Mortality by birth weight. Vermont Oxford Network 2008 with permission of Jeffrey D. Horbar, MD, Editor of 2008 Database Summary. Vermont Oxford Network, 33 Kilburn Street, Burlington, VT 05401. Email: Lynn@vtoxford.org. Website: www.vtoxford.org.

F. **Long-term problems of prematurity.** Preterm infants are vulnerable to a wide spectrum of morbidities. The risk of morbidity and mortality decline markedly with increasing GA.

1. **Developmental disability**

   a. **Major handicaps** (cerebral palsy, mental retardation).

   b. **Sensory impairments** (hearing loss, visual impairment) (see Chaps. 64 and 65).

   c. **Cerebral dysfunction** (language disorders, learning disability, hyperactivity, attention deficits, behavior disorders).

2. **Retinopathy of prematurity** (see Chap. 64).

3. **CLD** (see Chap. 34).

4. **Poor growth.** Preterm infants are at risk for a wide range of growth problems (see Chap. 21). While it is imperative for clinicians to visually assess the size and growth rate of individual infants, there is considerable controversy on which growth charts to use. Traditionally, the Lubchenco and Battaglia growth charts have been popular (see Fig. 7.4). Because these charts are based on an older, nondiverse cohort of infants at a single center using GA estimates before dating by fetal ultrasound was widely practiced, these growth charts have been increasingly questioned regarding their applicability to today's population. The Fenton growth charts use a more recent and diverse cohort of infants who

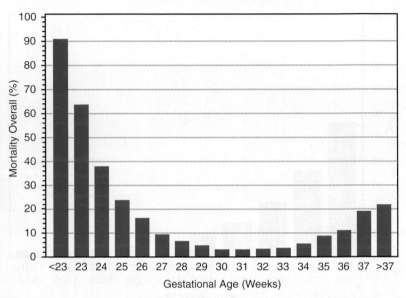

MORTALITY OVERALL BY GESTATIONAL AGE
Infants 501–1500 Grams Born in 2008

Figure 7.3. Mortality by gestational age. Vermont Oxford Network 2008 with permission of Jeffrey D. Horbar, MD, Editor of 2008 Database Summary. Vermont Oxford Network, 33 Kilburn Street, Burlington, VT 05401. Email: Lynn@vtoxford.org. Website: www.vtoxford.org.

had accurate GA assessments, but relies on data that is statistically smoothed between 36 and 46 weeks (see Fig. 7.5). This growth chart may not be appropriate for determining fetal growth in infants older than 36 weeks' gestation. Because extrauterine preterm infants grow at a different rate than their intrauterine fetal counterparts, some argue that a different measure may be needed to assess fetal growth compared to longitudinal preterm infant growth. Thus, there are several approaches to the monitoring of infant growth.

One approach is to assess fetal growth (which is reflected in birth measurement) using one growth chart (Fig. 7.4) while assessing longitudinal growth of preterm infants with the second growth chart (Fig. 7.5). A simpler approach is to use the same growth curve to assess fetal growth (size at birth) and preterm infant longitudinal growth (Fig. 7.5), recognizing that the preterm infants are likely to not achieve the same growth rates as the fetuses of the same postmenstrual age used to generate the growth chart (see Olson reference).

5. **Increased rates of childhood illness and readmission to the hospital.**

IV. POSTTERM INFANTS

A. **Definition.** Approximately 6% (3%–14%) of pregnancies extend beyond 42 weeks of gestation (294 days or more from the first day of the last menstrual period) and are considered postterm. The rate of postterm pregnancies is heavily influenced by local obstetrical practices.

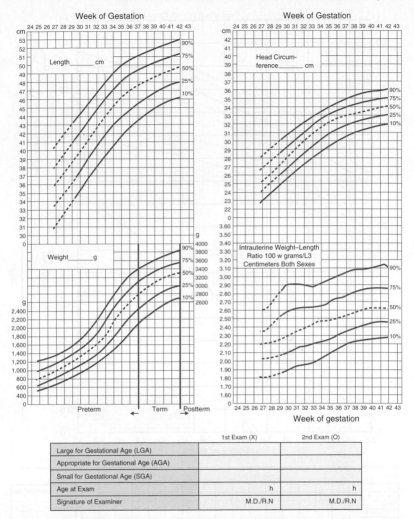

	1st Exam (X)	2nd Exam (O)
Large for Gestational Age (LGA)		
Appropriate for Gestational Age (AGA)		
Small for Gestational Age (SGA)		
Age at Exam	h	h
Signature of Examiner	M.D./R.N	M.D./R.N

Figure 7.4. Intrauterine growth in length and head circumference as estimated from live births at gestational ages from 26 to 42 weeks. (Adapted from Lubchenco LO, Hansman C, Boyd E. Intrauterine growth in length and head circumference as estimated from live births at gestational ages from 26 to 42 weeks. *Pediatrics* 1966;37:403–408; Battaglia FC, Lubchenco LO. A practical classification of newborn infants by weight and gestational age. *J Pediatr* 1967;71:159–163.)

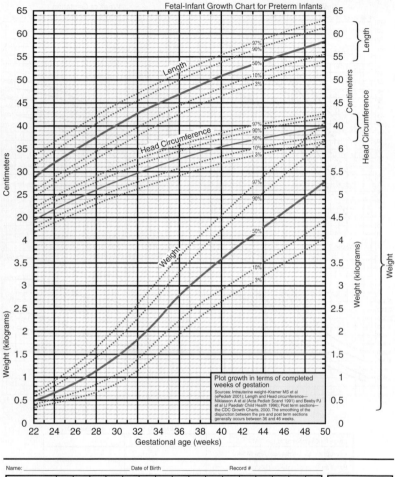

Figure 7.5. Fetal–infant growth chart for preterm infants (weight, head circumference, and length). (Reproduced with permission from Fenton TR; licensee BioMed Central Ltd. This is an Open Access article: Verbatim copying and redistribution of this article are permitted in all media for any purpose, provided this notice is preserved along with the article's original URL. http://www.biomedcentral.com/1471-2431/3/13.)

B. Etiology. Some cases of postterm pregnancy are actually inaccurate dating of the pregnancy. In most cases, the cause of prolonged pregnancy is unknown. There is no association between maternal age or race and the incidence of postterm pregnancy. Risk factors for post-term pregnancies include the following:

1. **Nulliparity**
2. **Previous post-term pregnancy**
3. **Obesity**
4. **Male fetus**
5. **Anencephaly.** An intact fetal pituitary–adrenal axis appears to be necessary for the initiation of labor.
6. **Trisomy 16 and 18**
7. **Seckel syndrome** (bird-headed dwarfism).

C. Morbidities associated with postterm pregnancy include the presence of meconium-stained amniotic fluid, meconium aspiration, oligohydramnios, nonreassuring fetal heart rate tracing in labor, fetal macrosomia, low Apgar scores, and birth injury.

D. Postmaturity syndrome. Postterm infants have begun to lose weight but usually have normal length and head circumference. They may be classified as follows:

1. **Stage 1**
   a. Dry, cracked, peeling, loose, and wrinkled skin.
   b. Malnourished appearance.
   c. Decreased subcutaneous tissue.
   d. Open-eyed and alert.
2. **Stage 2**
   a. All features of stage 1.
   b. Meconium staining of amniotic fluid (MSAF).
   c. Perinatal depression (in some cases).
3. **Stage 3**
   a. The findings in stages 1 and 2.
   b. Meconium staining of cord and nails due to long-term exposure to MSAF.
   c. A higher risk of fetal, intrapartum, or neonatal death.

E. Management

1. **Antepartum management**
   a. Careful estimation of true GA, including ultrasonographic data.
   b. Antepartum assessments by cervical examination and monitoring of fetal well-being (see Chap. 1) should be initiated between 41 and 42 weeks on at least a weekly basis. If fetal testing is not reassuring, delivery is usually indicated. In most instances, a patient is a candidate for induction of labor if the pregnancy is at >41 weeks of gestation and the condition of the cervix is favorable.
2. **Intrapartum management** involves use of fetal monitoring and preparation for possible perinatal depression and meconium aspiration.
3. **Postpartum management**
   a. **Evaluation for other conditions.** Infant conditions more frequently associated with postterm delivery include the following:
      i. Congenital anomalies.
      ii. Perinatal depression.

  iii. Persistent pulmonary hypertension.
  iv. Meconium aspiration syndrome.
  v. Hypoglycemia.
  vi. Hypocalcemia.
  vii. Polycythemia.
 b. Attention to proper nutritional support.

V. INFANTS WHO ARE SGA OR IUGR (see Chap. 1)

A. Definition. Though many use the terms "small for gestational age" (SGA) and "intrauterine growth retardation" (IUGR) interchangeably, they refer to two subtly different populations. SGA describes a neonate whose birth weight or birth crown-heel length is <10th percentile for GA or <2 standard deviations (SD) below the mean for the infant's GA (approximately the 3rd percentile for GA). IUGR describes diminished growth velocity in the fetus as documented by at least two intrauterine growth assessments. Babies who are constitutionally SGA are at overall lower risk compared to those who are IUGR due to some pathologic process. Numerous "normal birth curves" have been defined using studies of large infant populations (see Fig. 7.4); it should be noted that over the past 30 years, birth weight has increased in the general population. The etiology and management of SGA and IUGR fetuses overlaps considerably.

B. SGA/IUGR etiology. Approximately one-third of LBW infants are also SGA/IUGR. There is an association between the following factors and SGA/IUGR infants:

 1. Maternal factors (see Chap. 1) include genetic size; demographic (age at the extremes of reproductive life, race/ethnicity, SES); nulliparity and grand multiparity status; underweight before pregnancy (e.g., malnutrition); uterine anomalies; chronic disease; factors interfering with placental flow and oxygenation (cardiovascular disease, renal disease, hypertension [chronic or pregnancy induced], sickle-cell anemia, pulmonary disease, collagen-vascular disease, diabetes [classes D, E, F, and R], autoimmune diseases, thrombotic disease, postterm delivery, high-altitude environment); exposure to teratogens, including radiation and alcohol; and tobacco or cocaine use.

 2. Placental and umbilical anatomical factors include malformations (e.g., chorioangioma, infarction, circumvallate placenta, placental mosaicism, obliterative vasculopathy of the placental bed, vascular malformations, or velamentous umbilical cord insertion), infarction or focal lesions, abruption, suboptimal implantation site (e.g., low-lying placenta), previa, insufficient uteroplacental perfusion, and single umbilical artery.

 3. Fetal factors include constitutional (normal, "genetically small"), malformations (e.g., abnormalities of CNS and skeletal system), chromosomal abnormality (under 5% of SGA infants; more likely in the presence of malformation), congenital infection (i.e., rubella and cytomegalovirus) (see Chap. 48), and multiple gestation.

C. Management of SGA/IUGR

 1. Pregnancy (see Chap. 1).
  a. Attempt to determine the cause of SGA/IUGR by searching for relevant factors (listed above) by history, laboratory, and ultrasonic examination. Treat any underlying cause (e.g., hypertension) when possible. Chronic fetal

hypoxemia is encountered in about 30% of SGA/IUGR fetuses. Therefore, once the diagnosis is made, changes in obstetrical management may improve outcome.

b. Monitor fetal well-being, including nonstress and oxytocin challenge testing, a biophysical profile, fetal movement counts, amniotic fluid volume evaluation, and serial ultrasonic examinations (see Chap. 1). Doppler evaluation of placental flow may be used to evaluate uteroplacental insufficiency.

c. Consider the issue of fetal lung maturity if early delivery is contemplated (see Chap. 1).

2. **Delivery.** Early delivery is necessary if the risk to the fetus of remaining *in utero* is considered greater than the risks of prematurity.

   a. Generally, indications for delivery are arrest of fetal growth and/or fetal distress, especially in the setting of pulmonary maturity near term.

   b. Acceleration of pulmonary maturity with glucocorticoids administered to the mother should be considered if amniotic fluid analyses suggest pulmonary immaturity, or if delivery is anticipated remote from term.

   c. If there is poor placental blood flow, the fetus may not tolerate labor and may require cesarean delivery.

   d. Infants with extreme SGA/IUGR are at risk for perinatal problems and often require specialized care in the first few days of life. Therefore, if possible, delivery should occur at a center with an NICU or special care nursery. The delivery team should be prepared to manage fetal distress, perinatal depression, meconium aspiration, hypoxia, hypoglycemia, and heat loss.

3. **Postpartum**

   a. If unknown, the etiology of SGA/IUGR should be investigated.

      i. Newborn examination. The infant should be evaluated for signs of any of the previously listed causes of poor fetal growth, especially chromosomal abnormalities, malformations, and congenital infection.

         a) Infants with growth restriction that affects the later part of pregnancy will have a relatively normal head circumference, some reduction in length but a more profound reduction in weight This is thought to be due to the redistribution of fetal blood flow preferentially to vital organs, mainly the brain; hence, the term "head-sparing IUGR." Use of the ponderal index ([cube root of birth weight in grams × 100]/[length in centimeters]) or the weight:length ratio will quantify weight loss. These infants may have little subcutaneous tissue, peeling loose skin, a wasted appearance, and meconium staining. Due to "head-sparing" redistribution of perfusion, the usual physical markers of GA (e.g., vernix, breast buds) may not be reliable.

         b) Infants whose growth restriction began early in pregnancy will have proportionally small head circumference, length, and weight in contrast to IUGR that began late in pregnancy. These infants are sometimes referred to as *symmetrically IUGR* and their ponderal index may be normal. Symmetrical IUGR infants are more likely to have significant intrinsic fetal problems (e.g., chromosomal defects, malformations, and/or congenital infections acquired early in pregnancy).

      ii. **Pathologic examination of the placenta** for infarction or congenital infection may be helpful.

      iii. Generally, **serologic screening** for congenital infection is not indicated unless history or examination suggests infection as a possible cause.

b. SGA infants generally require **more calories per kilogram** than appropriate for gestational age (AGA) infants for "catch-up" growth; term SGA infants will often regulate their intake accordingly.

c. Potential complications related to SGA/IUGR:

    i. Congenital anomalies.

    ii. Perinatal depression.

    iii. Meconium aspiration.

    iv. Pulmonary hemorrhage.

    v. Persistent pulmonary hypertension.

    vi. Hypotension.

    vii. Hypoglycemia from depletion of glycogen stores.

    viii. Hypocalcemia.

    ix. Hypothermia from depletion of subcutaneous fat.

    x. Dyslipidemia.

    xi. Polycythemia.

    xii. Neutropenia.

    xiii. Thrombocytopenia.

    xiv. Acute tubular necrosis/renal insufficiency.

D. Outcomes of SGA/IUGR infants. At the same birth weight, SGA/IUGR infants have a lower risk of neonatal death compared with preterm AGA infants. Compared to AGA infants of the same GA, SGA/IUGR infants have a higher incidence of neonatal morbidity and mortality. In general, SGA/IUGR infants and children (especially those from disadvantaged socioeconomic environments) are at higher risk for poor postnatal growth, neurologic impairment, delayed cognitive development, and poor academic achievement. Finally, some adults who were SGA/IUGR at birth appear to have a higher risk of coronary heart disease, hypertension, non–insulin-dependent diabetes, stroke, obstructive pulmonary disease, renal impairment, decreased reproductive function, as well as other health risks and growth-related psychosocial issues.

E. Management of subsequent pregnancies is important because commonly SGA and IUGR will reoccur. The mother should be cared for by personnel experienced in handling high-risk pregnancies. The health of mother and fetus should be assessed throughout pregnancy with ultrasonography and nonstress tests (see Chap. 1). Early delivery should be considered if fetal growth is poor.

VI. INFANTS WHO ARE LARGE FOR GESTATIONAL AGE (LGA) (see Chap. 1)

A. Definition. As with SGA, there is no uniform definition of LGA, although most reports define it as two standard deviations above the mean for GA or as above the 90th percentile.

B. Etiology

    1. Constitutionally large infants (large parents).

    2. Infants of diabetic mothers (e.g., classes A, B, and C).

    3. Some postterm infants.

    4. Beckwith-Wiedemann and other syndromes.

C. Management

    1. Look for evidence of birth trauma, including brachial plexus injury and perinatal depression (see Chaps. 6 and 55).

2. Allow the infant to feed early, and monitor the blood sugar level. Some LGA infants may develop hypoglycemia secondary to hyperinsulinism (especially infants of diabetic mothers, infants with Beckwith-Wiedemann syndrome, or infants with erythroblastosis (see Chaps. 2 and 24).

3. Consider polycythemia (see Chap. 46).

VII. CORD BLOOD BANKING. The following text is summarized from the American Academy of Pediatrics and American College of Obstetricians and Gynecologists (2007) (see Chap. 42).

A. Prospective parents may seek information regarding umbilical cord blood banking. Balanced and accurate information regarding the advantages and disadvantages of public versus private banking should be provided. Health care providers should dispense the following information:

1. There is clinical potential of hematopoietic stem cells found in cord blood.

2. Where logistically possible, collection and support of umbilical cord blood for public banking is encouraged.

3. The indications for autologous (self) transplantation are limited.

4. Private cord blood banking should be encouraged when there is knowledge of a family member, particularly a full sibling, with a current or potential medical condition (malignant or genetic) that could potentially benefit from cord blood transplantation.

5. Storing cord blood as "biologic insurance" should be discouraged because there is currently no scientific data to support autologous (self) transplantation.

Suggested Readings

American Academy of Pediatrics. *Red Book: 2009 Report of the Committee on Infectious Diseases.* 28th ed. Evanston: American Academy of Pediatrics; 2009.

American Academy of Pediatrics and American College of Obstetricians and Gynecologists. *Guidelines for Perinatal Care.* 6th ed. Elk Grove Village, IL; Washington, DC: American Academy of Pediatrics and American College of Obstetricians and Gynecologists; 2007.

Barker DJ. Early growth and cardiovascular disease. *Arch Dis Child* 1999;80(4):305–307.

Committee on Infectious Diseases. From the American Academy of Pediatrics: policy statements—modified recommendations for use of palivizumab for prevention of respiratory syncytial virus infections. *Pediatrics* 2009;124(6):1694–1701.

Cortese MM, Parashar UD, Centers for Disease Control and Prevention: Prevention of rotavirus gastroenteritis among infants and children: recommendations of the Advisory Committee on Immunization Practices (ACIP). *MMWR Recomm Rep* 2009;58(RR-2):1–25.

Dancis J, O'Connell JR, Holt LE Jr. A grid for recording the weight of premature infants. *J Pediatr* 1948;33(11):570–572.

Doherty L, Norwitz ER. Prolonged pregnancy: when should we intervene? *Curr Opin Obstet Gynecol* 2008;20(6):519–527.

Horbar JD, Badger GJ, Carpenter JH, et al. Trends in mortality and morbidity for very low birth weight infants, 1991–1999. *Pediatrics* 2002;110:143–151.

Lee SK, McMillan DD, Ohlsson A, et al. Variations in practice and outcomes in the Canadian NICU network: 1996–1997. *Pediatrics* 2000;106(5):1070–1079.

Mandruzzato G, Antsaklis A, Botet F, et al. Intrauterine restriction (IUGR). *J Perinat Med* 2008;36(4):277–281.

Martin JA, Hamilton BE, Sutton PD, et al. Births: final data for 2005. *Natl Vital Stat Rep* 2007;56(6):1–103.

McCormick MC, McCarton C, Tonascia J, et al. Early educational intervention for very low birth weight infants: results from the Infant Health and Development Program. *J Pediatr* 1993;123(4):527–533.

Saenger P, Czernichow P, Hughes I, et al. Small for gestational age: short stature and beyond. *Endocr Rev* 2007;28(2):219–251.

Vohr BR, Wright LL, Dusick AM, et al. Neurodevelopmental and functional outcomes of extremely low birth weight infants in the National Institute of Child Health and Human Development Neonatal Research Network, 1993–1994. *Pediatrics* 2000;105(6):1216–1226.

Wiswell TE, Cornish JD, Northam RS. Neonatal polycythemia: frequency of clinical manifestations and other associated findings. *Pediatrics* 1986;78(1):26–30.

8

Assessment of the Newborn History and Physical Examination of the Newborn

Lise Johnson and William D. Cochran

I. **HISTORY.** The family, maternal, pregnancy, perinatal, and social history should be reviewed (Table 8.1).

II. **ROUTINE PHYSICAL EXAMINATION OF THE NEONATE.** Although no statistics are available, the first routine examination probably reveals more abnormalities than any other physical examination. Whenever possible, the examination should be performed in the presence of the parents to encourage them to ask questions regarding their newborn and allow for the shared observation of physical findings both normal and abnormal.

A. **General examination.** At the initial examination, attention should be directed to determine (i) whether any congenital anomalies are present, (ii) whether the infant has made a successful transition from fetal life to air breathing, (iii) to what extent gestation, labor, delivery, analgesics, or anesthetics have affected the neonate, and (iv) whether the infant has any signs of infection or metabolic disease.

1. The infant should be undressed for the examination, ideally in a well-lit room under warming lights to avoid hypothermia, which occurs easily in the neonatal period.

2. Care providers should develop a consistent order to their physical examination, generally beginning with the cardiorespiratory system, which is best assessed when the infant is quiet. If the infant being examined is fussy, a gloved finger to suck on may be offered. The opportunity to perform the eye examination should be seized whenever the infant is noted to be awake and alert.

B. **Vital signs and measurements.** Vital signs should be taken when the infant is quiet, if possible.

1. **Temperature.** Temperature in the neonate is usually measured in the axilla. Rectal temperature can be measured to confirm an abnormal axillary temperature, although they tend to correlate quite closely. Normal axillary temperature is between 36.5° and 37.4°C (97.7° and 99.3°F).

2. **Heart rate.** Normal heart rate in a newborn is between 95 and 160 beats per minute (bpm). Vagal slowing may be noted and appreciated as a reassuring sign. Some infants, particularly those born postdates, may have resting heart rates as low as 80 bpm. Good acceleration with stimulation should be verified

Table 8.1	Important Aspects of Maternal and Perinatal History

FAMILY HISTORY

Inherited diseases (e.g., metabolic disorders, bleeding disorders, hemoglobinopathies, cystic fibrosis, polycystic kidneys, sensorineural hearing loss, genetic disorders or syndromes)

Developmental disorders including autism spectrum disorders

Disorders requiring follow-up screening in family members (e.g., developmental dysplasia of the hip, vesicoureteral reflux, congenital cardiac anomalies, familial arrhythmias)

MATERNAL HISTORY

Age

Gravidity and parity

Infertility treatments required for pregnancy, including source of egg and sperm (donor or parent)

Prior pregnancy outcomes (terminations, spontaneous abortions, fetal demises, neonatal deaths, prematurity, postmaturity, malformations)

Blood type and blood group sensitizations

Chronic maternal illness (e.g., diabetes mellitus, hypertension, renal disease, cardiac disease, thyroid disease, systemic lupus erythematosus, myasthenia gravis)

Infectious disease screening in pregnancy (rubella immunity status; syphilis, gonorrhea, chlamydia, and HIV screening; hepatitis B surface antigen screening, Group B streptococcus (GBS) culture, varicella, cytomegalovirus and toxoplasmosis testing, if performed; purified protein derivative (PPD) status and any past treatments; any recent infections or exposures)

Inherited disorder screening (e.g., hemoglobin electrophoresis, glucose-6-phosphate dehydrogenase (G6PD) deficiency screening, "Jewish panel" screening, cystic fibrosis mutation testing, fragile X testing)

Medications

Tobacco, alcohol, and illegal substance use

Pregnancy complications (e.g., gestational diabetes mellitus, preeclampsia, infections, bleeding, anemia, trauma, surgery, acute illnesses, preterm labor with or without use of tocolytics or glucocorticoids)

FETAL TESTING

First- and/or second-trimester screens for aneuploidy (serum markers and ultrasonographic examination)

Second-trimester (approximately 18 weeks) fetal survey by ultrasound

(continued)

Table 8.1	(Continued)

Genetic testing, including preimplantation, chorionic villus sampling, and amniocentesis genetic screening

Ultrasound monitoring of fetal well-being

Tests of fetal lung maturity

INTRAPARTUM HISTORY

Gestational age at parturition and method of calculation (e.g., ultrasound, artificial insemination or *in vitro* fertilization, last menstrual period)

Presentation

Onset and duration of labor

Timing of rupture of membranes and appearance of amniotic fluid (volume, presence of meconium, blood)

Results of fetal monitoring

Fever

Medications, especially antibiotics, analgesics, anesthetics, and magnesium sulfate

Complications (e.g., excessive blood loss, chorioamnionitis, shoulder dystocia)

Method of delivery

Infant delivery room assessment including Apgar scores and any resuscitation measures required

Placental examination

SOCIAL HISTORY

Cultural background of family

Marital status of mother

Nature of involvement of father of baby

Household members

Custody of prior children

Maternal and paternal occupations

Identified social supports

Current social support service involvement

Past or current history of involvement of child protective agencies

Current or past history of domestic violence

in these infants. A normal blood pressure is reassuring that cardiac output is adequate in the setting of marked sinus bradycardia.

3. **Respiratory rate.** Normal respiratory rate in a newborn is between 30 and 60 breaths per minute. Periodic breathing is common in newborns. Short pauses (usually 5–10 seconds) are considered normal. Apneic spells (defined as 20 seconds or longer) associated with cyanosis and/or bradycardia are not normal in term infants and deserve further evaluation (see Chap. 31).

4. **Blood pressure.** Blood pressure is not routinely measured in otherwise well newborns. When measurement of blood pressure is clinically indicated, care should be taken that the proper neonatal cuff size is chosen and the extremity used is documented in the blood pressure recording. A gradient between upper and lower extremity systolic pressure >10 mm Hg should be considered suspicious for coarctation or other anomalies of the aorta (see Chap. 41).

5. **Pulse oximetry.** Mild cyanosis can be easily overlooked in newborns, particularly those with darker skin pigmentation. The utility of universal pulse oximetry screening in neonates for detection of cyanotic heart disease is a hotly debated issue, mostly due to concern over high false-positive rates. Recent studies have pushed the debate in favor of universal screening. Strategies to lower false-positive rates include performing screening after the first day of life, ensuring staff are properly trained in pulse oximetry measurement, and using later generation pulse oximeters, which are less sensitive to motion artifact. A reasonable criterion meriting further investigation for congenital heart disease is an oxygen saturation <95% in a lower limb after the first day of life.

6. **Measurements.** All newborns should have their weight, length, and head circumference measured shortly after birth. These measurements should be plotted on standard growth curves such that the newborn may be determined to be appropriate for gestational age (AGA), small for gestational age (SGA), or large for gestational age (LGA). SGA or LGA newborns may require further evaluation of both the etiology and sequelae of these conditions (see Chap. 7).

Newborns with extensive molding and/or caput may require a repeat head circumference measurement a few days after birth.

C. **Cardiorespiratory system**

1. **Color.** The healthy newborn should have a reddish pink hue, except for the possible normal cyanosis of the hands and feet (acrocyanosis). Excessive paleness or ruddiness should prompt hematocrit measurement to detect relative anemia (hematocrit <42%) or polycythemia (hematocrit >65%), respectively (see Chaps. 45 and 46).

2. **Respiratory pattern.** The majority of the neonatal respiratory examination may be performed visually without the use of a stethoscope. At rest, a newborn past initial transition should exhibit unlabored breathing without grunting (self-generated positive end-expiratory pressure [PEEP]), nasal flaring (decrease in airway resistance), or intercostal retractions (chest wall stabilization). Significant respiratory disease in the absence of tachypnea is rare unless the infant also has severe central nervous system depression. Rales, decreased breath sounds, decreased or displaced heart sounds, or asymmetry of breath sounds are occasionally found by auscultation in an asymptomatic infant and may reveal occult disease that should be confirmed by chest x-ray (e.g., pulmonary edema, neonatal pneumonia, pneumothorax, pneumomediastinum, dextrocardia).

3. **Heart.** The examiner should observe precordial activity, rate, rhythm, the quality of heart sounds, and the presence or absence of murmurs.

   a. It should be determined whether the heart is on the left or right side of the chest by palpation of the point of maximum impulse (PMI) and auscultation.

   b. Arrhythmias, most often due to premature atrial contractions, are occasionally heard on the routine newborn examination. An electrocardiogram (EKG) with rhythm strip should be obtained to identify the etiology of the arrhythmia and screen for evidence of structural disease.

   c. The heart sounds should be auscultated, with attention paid to the reassuring presence of a split second heart sound (evidence of the presence of two semilunar valves), detection of any gallops (an ominous finding that deserves further evaluation), and detection of ejection clicks, which may indicate pulmonary or aortic valve stenosis or a bicuspid aortic valve.

   d. Murmurs in newborns can be misleading. Systolic murmurs are frequently heard transiently in neonates without significant structural heart disease, particularly as the ductus arteriosus is closing or in those with mild pulmonary branch stenosis. On the other hand, a newborn with serious, hemodynamically significant heart disease may have no murmur. Diastolic murmurs should always be considered abnormal. In an otherwise asymptomatic infant with a persistent or otherwise concerning murmur (e.g., loud, harsh, pansystolic, diastolic), investigation should include an EKG, preductal and postductal oxygen saturation measurement, and four extremity blood pressure measurements. A plain chest x-ray may also be considered. In consultation with a pediatric cardiologist, echocardiogram may also be obtained if readily available. Where echocardiography is not readily available, a hyperoxia test should be obtained to determine the presence of cyanotic heart disease and the potential need for institution of prostaglandin E1 (see Chap. 41).

   e. Femoral pulses should be palpated, although, often, they are weak in the first day or two after birth. Femoral pulses are most easily appreciated if the infant is calm. The following technique may be helpful for locating the femoral pulses: With the infant calm and in a supine position, the examiner uses the palm of his or her hand to extend the knees until the lower extremities lie flat on the bed. The forefingers are gently nestled flat within the femoral grooves of the thighs and then slid upward so that the pads of the fingers may appreciate the femoral pulses usually located just above the groin creases. If there is doubt about the femoral pulses by the time of discharge, the blood pressure in the upper and lower extremities should be measured to investigate the concern for coarctation of the aorta.

D. **Thorax**

   1. The clavicles should be palpated. Crepitus or, less commonly, a "step off" may be appreciated in the presence of a clavicle fracture. Clavicle palpation should always be repeated on the discharge examination because some fractures may be more apparent on the second or third day of life. On follow-up examinations after hospital discharge, a healed clavicle fracture may leave a firm bump on the bone. No special care beyond gentle handling to avoid pain in the first neonatal days is required for clavicle fractures, which generally heal uneventfully and without sequelae. Indeed, many fractured clavicles in the newborn period undoubtedly occur unnoticed.

   2. The thorax should be inspected for shape and symmetry. One or more accessory nipples in the mammary line may be noted occasionally. Tiny periareolar

skin tags that generally dry up and fall off in the first days of life may also be noted. Breast buds due to the influence of maternal hormones can normally be palpated in term newborns. Parents will sometimes need reassurance that the tip of the xiphoid process, which can be quite prominent in the newborn, is also a normal finding.

E. **Abdomen.** The abdominal examination of a newborn differs from that of older infants in that observation can again be used to greater advantage.

1. The anterior abdominal organs (e.g., liver, spleen, bowel) can often be seen through the abdominal wall especially in thin or premature infants. The edge of the liver is occasionally seen, and the intestinal pattern is sometimes visible. Diastasis rectus abdominis is frequently seen in neonates, most evident during crying. Asymmetry due to congenital anomalies or masses is often first appreciated by observation.

2. When palpating the abdomen, start with gentle pressure or stroking, moving from lower to upper quadrants to reveal edges of the liver or spleen. The normal liver edge may extend up to 2.5 cm below the right costal margin. The spleen is usually not palpable. Remember there may be situs inversus.

3. After the abdomen has been gently palpated, deep palpation is possible, not only because of the lack of developed musculature but also because there is no food and little air in the intestine. Kidneys may be palpated and abdominal masses may be appreciated, although the clinically meaningful yield of this portion of the examination may be low in the current age of fetal ultrasonography.

4. The umbilical stump should be inspected. The umbilical vein and one or two umbilical arteries should be identified as well as the amount of Wharton jelly. Discharge, odor, or periumbilical erythema should be noted, if present. Umbilical hernias are frequently seen in neonates and are generally benign and resolve spontaneously.

F. **Genitalia and rectum**

1. **Male**

   a. The **penis** almost invariably has marked phimosis. Stretched penile length under 2.5 cm is abnormal and requires evaluation (see Chap. 61). If present, the degree of hypospadias should be noted, as well as the presence and degree of chordee. Circumcision should be deferred to a urologist whenever hypospadias is identified.

   b. The **scrotum** is often quite large because it is an embryonic analog of the female labia and responds to maternal hormones. Hyperpigmentation of the scrotum should raise suspicion for one of the adrenogenital syndromes (see Chap. 61). The scrotum may also be enlarged due to the presence of a **hydrocele**, which can be identified as a transilluminating mass in either or both sides of the scrotum. Hydroceles are collections of peritoneal fluid in the scrotum due to patency of the processus vaginalis in fetal life. They are common and require no immediate action, although they should be monitored to ensure resolution in the first year of life. The **testes** should be palpated, with the epididymis and vas identified. The testes should be the same size and should not appear blue (a sign of torsion) through the scrotal skin. Normal testicle size in a term newborn ranges from 1.6 cm (length) × 1.0 cm (width) up to 2.9 cm × 1.8 cm. Approximately 2% to 5% of term males will have an undescended testicle at birth, which should be followed for descent in the first months of life.

2. Female

a. The **labia minora** and **labia majora** should be examined. The relative size of the labia majora and labia minora changes over the last weeks of gestation with labia minora receding in prominence as the fetus progresses to term. The labia majora of term newborn girls are frequently reddened and swollen due to the influence of maternal hormones, which are also responsible for a clear or white vaginal discharge in the first days of life. Occasionally, a small amount of blood (pseudomenses) accompanies the discharge after the first few days of life as maternal hormones in the neonate wane.

b. The **vaginal introitus** should be examined and the hymen identified. The finding of an imperforate hymen, which can sometimes be difficult to distinguish from a paraurethral cyst, should prompt referral to a pediatric gynecologist for management. Vaginal tags are commonly noted and their presence is of no clinical significance.

c. The **clitoris**, which recedes in prominence with increasing gestational age, should be noted. Mean clitoral length in term infants ± 1 SD is 4.0 ± 1.24 mm (see Oberfield reference). Clitoral enlargement, particularly when there is accompanying hyperpigmentation, should raise suspicion for androgen excess (see Chap. 61).

3. The anus should be checked carefully for patency, position, and size. Occasionally, a large fistula is mistaken for a normal anus; upon closer examination, it may be noted that the fistula is positioned either anterior or posterior to the usual location of a normal anus.

G. Skin. There are numerous, mostly benign, skin findings commonly seen in newborns (see Chap. 63).

1. Dryness, sometimes accompanied by cracking or peeling of the skin, is common especially in the postmature newborn.

2. Milia, which are inclusion cysts filled with keratinous debris, are tiny, discrete, often solitary, white papules commonly seen on the face and scalp. Milia resolve spontaneously in the first weeks to months of life.

3. Sebaceous hyperplasia appears as tiny yellowish white follicular papules most commonly clustered on the nose. These papules self-resolve in the first weeks of life.

4. Erythema toxicum neonatorum occurs in approximately half of full-term newborns. Classically, the lesions of erythema toxicum are yellowish papules on an erythematous base, prompting the name "flea bite" dermatitis. Presentations may range from a few scattered isolated lesions to extensive, sometimes confluent, areas of pustules or papules with surrounding erythema. When unroofed and scraped, the contents of the papules and pustules will contain many eosinophils on Wright or Giemsa stain. Erythema toxicum most typically appears on the second or third day of life, waxes and wanes for a few days, and resolves within the first week of life.

5. Nevus simplex or salmon patch refers to a frequently seen capillary malformation located on the forehead (typically V shaped), nape of the neck, eyelids, nose, and upper lip. Although most salmon patches on the face ("angel kisses") resolve in the first year or so, those on the nape of the neck ("stork bites") will sometimes persist.

6. Transient pustular melanosis neonatorum (TPMN), most common in darker pigmented infants, consists of 2- to 10-mm fragile, neutrophil-containing pustules that spontaneously break, leaving a collarette of scales and underlying hyperpigmented macules that eventually (weeks to months) fade. Frequently, infants at birth will be found to have the hyperpigmented macules of TPMN with the pustular phase having presumably occurred *in utero*. TPMN may sometimes need to be distinguished from bacterial (usually staph) pustules that are generally larger than TPMN, yield positive cultures and are not associated with the typical hyperpigmented macules.

7. **Dermal melanosis** ("**Mongolian spots**"), commonly seen in darker-skinned and Asian individuals, consists of dermal collections of melanocytes that appear as varying size macules or patches of black, gray, or slate blue skin, most often on the buttocks, although many other locations are also possible. It is prudent to make note of dermal melanosis on the newborn examination so that there is no confusion in the future with traumatic bruises.

8. **Sucking blisters** are occasionally on the hand or forearm of a newborn at birth. They resolve without incident and should not be a cause for concern.

9. The presence of **jaundice** on examination in the first 24 hours of life is not normal and should prompt further evaluation. Some degree of jaundice after the first day of life is common (see Chap. 26).

H. Palpable **lymph nodes** are found in approximately one-third of normal neonates. They are usually under 12 mm in diameter and are often found in the inguinal, the cervical, and, occasionally, the axillary area. Excess lymphadenopathy should prompt further evaluation.

I. **Extremities, joints, and spine** (see Chap. 58).

1. **Extremities.** Anomalies of the digits, such as polydactyly (especially postaxial polydactyly, which is sometimes familial), clinodactyly, or some degree of webbing or syndactyly, are seen relatively frequently. Palmar creases should be examined. Approximately 4% of individuals have a single palmar crease on one hand. Bilateral single palmar creases are less common but need not prompt concern unless associated with other dysmorphic features. Because of fetal positioning, many newborns have forefoot adduction, tibial bowing, or even tibial torsion. Forefoot adduction, also known as metatarsus adductus, will often correct itself within weeks and may be followed expectantly with stretching exercises. Mild degrees of tibial bowing or torsion are also normal. Talipes equinovarus, or clubfoot, always requires orthopedic intervention that should be sought as soon as possible after birth (see Chap. 58).

2. **Joints.** All newborns should be examined for the presence of developmental dysplasia of the hips. Hip "clunks" can be sought by both the Barlow maneuver, which causes posterior dislocation of an unstable hip and the Ortolani maneuver, which causes reduction of the dislocation. Hip "clicks," due to movement of the ligamentum teres in the acetabulum, are much more common than hip "clunks" and not a cause for concern.

3. **Spine.** The infant should be turned over and suspended face down with the examiner's hand supporting the chest. The back, especially the lower lumbar and sacral areas, should be examined. Special care should be taken to look for pilonidal sinus tracts, skin findings, or small soft midline swellings that might indicate a small meningocele or other anomaly (see Chap. 57). Simple, blind-ending midline sacral dimples, a common finding, need no further evaluation

unless they meet high-risk criteria for spinal dysraphism, including being deep, larger than 0.5 cm, are located greater than 2.5 cm from the anal verge, or are associated with other cutaneous markers (see Drolet reference).

J. **Head and neck**

1. **Head**

a. **Scalp.** The scalp should be inspected for cuts, abrasions, or bruises from the birth process. Particular note should be made of puncture wounds from the application of fetal monitor leads as these may occasionally become infected and require further attention. Rarely, cutis aplasia congenita or a nevus sebaceous may also be identified.

b. **Swelling.** Swelling should be noted and identified, distinguishing between **caput succedaneum**, **cephalohematomas**, and **subgaleal hemorrhage**. Caput succedaneum, often boggy in texture, is simply soft tissue swelling from the birth process. Caput is most commonly located occipitally, although may also have a "sausage" shape in the parietal area, may cross suture lines, and most often resolves within a day or two. Cephalohematomas, more common in the setting of an instrumented vaginal birth and most often involving one of the parietal bones, are the result of subperiosteal bleeding and, thus, do not cross suture lines. Cephalohematomas may initially be obscured by overlying caput and become increasingly apparent over the first 3 to 4 days of life. They are typically more tense to palpation than caput and may take weeks to even months to fully resolve. Cephalohematomas are a source of excess bilirubin production, which may contribute to neonatal jaundice. Subgaleal hemorrhages, also associated with vacuum extractions but much rarer in incidence, result from bleeding underneath the aponeurosis of the occipitofrontalis muscle and, classically, result in very loose, soft swelling that may flow freely from the nape of the neck to the forehead. It may even be possible to generate a fluid wave across the swelling from a subgaleal hemorrhage. If a subgaleal hemorrhage is suspected, the newborn should be carefully monitored for possible hemodynamically significant bleeding within the hemorrhage.

c. **Skull bones.** The skull bones (occipital, parietal, and frontal) should be examined and suture lines (sagittal, coronal, lambdoidal, and metopic) should be palpated. Mobility of the sutures will rule out craniosynostosis. Mobility can be appreciated by placing one's thumbs on opposite sides of the suture and then pushing in alternately while feeling for motion. Any molding of the skull bones, which resolves over the first days of life, should be noted. The skull should also be observed for deformational plagiocephaly and, when present, positioning instructions to aid in its resolution should be given. Finally, occasionally craniotabes may be found, with palpation of the skull bones (usually the parietal bones) resulting in an indenting similar to the effect of pressing on a ping-pong ball. Craniotabes generally resolves in a matter of weeks with no further evaluation necessary if an isolated finding.

d. **Fontanelles.** The fontanelles should be palpated. As long as the head circumference is normal and there is motion of the suture lines, one need pay little attention to the size (large or small) of the fontanelles. Very large fontanelles reflect a delay in bone ossification and may be associated with hypothyroidism (see Chap. 3), trisomy syndromes, intrauterine malnutrition, hypophosphatasia, and osteogenesis imperfecta. Fontanelles should be soft, particularly when the infant is in an upright or sitting position. Tense or full fontanelles should raise concern for elevated intracranial pressure due to such causes as meningitis or acute intracranial bleeding.

2. **Eyes**

The eyes should be examined for the presence of scleral hemorrhages, icterus, conjunctival exudate, iris coloring, extraocular muscle movement, and pupillary size, equality, reactivity, and centering. The red reflex should be assessed and cataracts ruled out. Of note, cataracts may cause photophobia resulting in difficulty obtaining cooperation from the infant in maintaining his or her eyes open for the examination. Puffy eyelids sometimes make examination of the eyes impossible. If so, this fact should be noted so that the eyes will be examined upon follow-up.

3. **Ears**

Note the size, shape, position, and presence of auditory canals as well as preauricular sinus, pits, or skin tags.

4. **Nose**

The nose should be inspected, noting any deformation from *in utero* position, patency of the nares, or evidence of septal injury.

5. **Mouth**

The mouth should be inspected for palatal clefts. **Epstein pearls** (small white inclusion cysts clustered about the midline at the juncture of the hard and soft palate) are a frequent and normal finding. Much less common findings include mucoceles of the oral mucosa, a sublingual ranula, alveolar cysts, and natal teeth. The lingual frenulum should also be inspected and any degree of ankyloglossia noted.

6. **Neck**

Because newborns have such short necks, the chin should be lifted to expose the neck for a thorough assessment. The neck should be checked for range of motion, goiter, and thyroglossal and branchial arch sinus tracts.

K. **Neurologic examination.** In approaching the neurologic examination of the neonate, the examiner must be at once humble and ambitious. On the one hand, severe neurologic anomalies may be inapparent on examination in the newborn. In addition, good evidence of the prognostic significance of the neonatal neurologic examination is lacking. On the other hand, with a trained eye, a broad range of clinically relevant observations can be made of the newborn's neurologic system. Categorizing neurobehavioral observations into four systems—autonomic, motor, state, and responsiveness—allows the clinician to capture nuances of a newborn's competence or vulnerability, regulation or dysregulation, maturity or immaturity, as well as identify evidence of neurologic injury or impairment, if present.

1. Examination of the neonatal **autonomic system** includes evaluation of vital sign stability, neurocutaneous stability (pink color vs. mottling or cyanosis), gastrointestinal stability, and the presence or absence of jitteriness or myoclonic jerks. Marked jitteriness should be investigated for etiologies, including hypoglycemia, hypocalcemia, hypomagnesemia, or withdrawal from *in utero* exposure to drugs, including opiates, cocaine, tobacco, or selective serotonin reuptake inhibitors (SSRIs) (see Chap. 12). Sneezes, hiccups, and frequent yawns may also be considered subtle expressions of autonomic stress in the neonate and are very commonly seen in normal term infants. It is worth mention that the majority of the items on the Finnegan Neonatal Abstinence Score are signs and symptoms of autonomic dysregulation.

2. Assessment of the **motor system** begins with noting extremity and axial tone, particularly looking for asymmetries, such as those seen in brachial plexus injuries. An asymmetric grimace during crying may indicate injury to the seventh cranial nerve (especially if accompanied by incomplete ipsilateral eyelid closure) or congenital absence or hypoplasia of the depressor angularis oris muscle, a condition that becomes less noticeable over time. Self-regulatory motor activities such as hand-to-mouth efforts, tucking, bracing, and grasping; or dysregulatory motor activities such as arching, flailing, and hand splaying should also be noted. The motor portion of the neurologic examination is completed by elicitation of the primitive reflexes, including palmar and plantar grasp, Babinski, Moro response, root, suck, galant, tonic neck reflex, stepping, and placing and observation of the quality and quantity of the infant's motor activity.

3. The six behavioral states of the newborn include deep sleep, light sleep, drowsiness, quiet alertness, active alertness (or fussing), and crying. Aspects of the **state system** that can be observed include the clarity of the infant's states, the range of states displayed, the way in which the newborn moves between states, the ability to protect sleep from outside stimulation, and the quality of crying and ability to be consoled.

4. Finally, the newborn's **responsiveness** to the outside world can be observed. The ability to engage socially may be noted, including the ability to fix on and follow a face and voice. Response to inanimate stimuli such as the ability to fix on and follow a small, high contrast object (such as a bright red ball) or respond to a sound such as a bell or rattle can also be observed.

L. **Summary.** All expectant parents dream of the healthy child and worry about the possibility of abnormality or illness in their infant. Whether the newborn examination is performed with the parents or alone in the nursery, the care provider should summarize the findings of the initial assessment for the parents. Most newborns have normal physical examinations and smooth transitions from fetal to extrauterine life; although perhaps mundane knowledge for care providers, this is a source of delight and reassurance to the family of each newborn. When problems or abnormalities are uncovered in the initial newborn assessment, it is of critical importance that they are discussed clearly and sensitively with parents, including any plans for further evaluation, monitoring, or treatment.

Suggested Readings

Brazelton TB, Nugent JK. *Neonatal Behavioral Assessment Scale.* 3rd ed. London: Mac Keith Press; 1995.

Drolet BA. Cutaneous signs of neural tube dysraphism. *Pediatr Clin North Am* 2000;47(4):813–823.

Eichenfeld LF, Frieden IJ, Esterly NB. *Neonatal Dermatology.* 2nd ed. Philadelphia: WB Saunders; 2008.

Mahle WT, Newburger JW, Matherne GP, et al. Role of pulse oximetry in examining newborns for congenital heart disease: a scientific statement from the AHA and AAP. *Pediatrics* 2009; 124(2):823–836.

Mayfield SR, Bhatia J, Nakamura KT, et al. Temperature measurement in term and preterm neonates. *J Pediatr* 1984;104(2):271–275.

Nugent JK, Keefer CH, Minear S, et al. *Understanding Newborn Behavior and Early Relationships: The Newborn Behavioral Observations (NBO) System Handbook.* Baltimore: Paul H. Brookes Publishing Co; 2007.

Oberfield SE, Mondok A, Shahrivar F, et al. Clitoral size in full-term infants. *Am J Perinatol* 1989;6(4):453–454.

Wein AJ, Kavoussi LR, Novick AC, et al. *Campbell-Walsh Urology.* 9th ed. Philadelphia: WB Saunders; 2007.

Suggested Websites

Layton K, Brackbill E. Examination of the newborn. University of Michigan Medical School. 2004. Available at: http://www.med.umich.edu.lrc/newbornexam

Stanford School of Medicine. Newborn Nursery at LPCH: Professional Education. 2010. Available at: http://newborns.stanford.edu/RNMDEducation.html

9 Care of the Well Newborn

Lori A. Sielski and Tiffany M. McKee-Garrett

I. ADMISSION TO THE NEWBORN NURSERY. Healthy newborns should remain in the delivery room with their mother as long as possible to promote immediate initiation of breastfeeding and early bonding (see Chap. 14). Every effort should be made to avoid separation of mother and infant. Family-centered maternity care, in which the nurse cares for the mother and baby together in the mother's room (couplet care), promotes bonding and facilitates teaching.

A. Criteria for admission to the normal newborn nursery or couplet care with the mother vary among hospitals. The minimum requirement typically is a well-appearing infant of at least 35 weeks gestational age, although some nurseries may specify a minimum birth weight, for example, 2 kg.

B. Impeccable **security** in the nursery and mother's room is necessary to protect the safety of families and to prevent the abduction of newborns.

1. Many nurseries use electronic security systems to track newborns.

2. Identification bands with matching numbers are placed on the newborn and mother as soon after birth as possible. Transport of infants between areas should not occur if identification banding has not been done.

3. All staff are required to wear a picture identification (ID) badge, and parents should be instructed to allow the infant to be taken only by someone wearing an ID badge.

II. TRANSITIONAL CARE

A. The transitional period is usually defined as the first 4 to 6 hours after birth. During this period, the infant's pulmonary vascular resistance decreases, blood flow to the lungs is greatly increased, overall oxygenation and perfusion improve, and the ductus arteriosus begins to constrict or close.

B. Interruption of normal transitioning, usually due to complications occurring in the peripartum period, will cause signs of distress in the newborn.

C. Common signs of disordered transitioning are (i) respiratory distress, (ii) poor perfusion with cyanosis or pallor, or (iii) need for supplemental oxygen.

D. Transitional care of the newborn can take place in the mother's room or in the nursery.

1. Infants are evaluated for problems that may require a higher level of care, such as gross malformations and disorders of transition.

2. The infant should be evaluated every 30 to 60 minutes during this period, including assessment of heart rate, respiratory rate, and axillary temperature;

assessment of color and tone; and observation for signs of withdrawal from maternal medications.

3. When disordered transitioning is suspected, a hemodynamically stable infant can be observed closely in the normal nursery setting for a brief period of time. Infants with persistent signs of disordered transitioning require transfer to a higher level of care.

III. ROUTINE CARE

A. Healthy newborns should be with their mothers all or nearly all the time. When possible, physical assessments, administration of medications, routine laboratory tests, and bathing should occur in the mother's room. For family-centered maternity care, nursing ratios should not exceed 1:4 mother–baby couplets.

   1. Upon admission to the nursery, an assessment of gestational age is performed on all infants using the expanded Ballard score (see Chap. 7).

   2. The infant's weight, frontal-occipital circumference (FOC), and length are recorded. On the basis of these measurements, the infant is classified as appropriate for gestational age (AGA), small for gestational age (SGA), or large for gestational age (LGA) (see Chap. 7).

B. The infant's temperature is stabilized with one of three possible modalities:

   1. Skin-to-skin contact with the mother

   2. Open radiant warmer on servo control

   3. Incubator on servo control

C. Universal precautions should be used with all patient contact.

D. The first **bath** is given with warm tap water and nonmedicated soap after an axillary temperature >97.5°F has been recorded.

E. Acceptable practices for **umbilical cord care** include exposure to air, or application of topical antiseptics, such as triple dye, or topical antibiotics, such as bacitracin. The use of topical antiseptics or antibiotics appears to reduce bacterial colonization of the cord, although no single method of cord care has proved to be superior in preventing colonization and disease. Keeping the cord dry promotes earlier detachment of the umbilical stump.

IV. ROUTINE MEDICATIONS

A. All newborns should receive prophylaxis against gonococcal ophthalmia neonatorum within 1 to 2 hours of birth, regardless of the mode of delivery. Prophylaxis is administered as a single ribbon of 0.5% erythromycin ointment or 1% tetracycline ointment bilaterally in the conjunctival sac (see Chap. 49).

B. A single intramuscular dose of 0.5 to 1 mg of vitamin K_1 oxide (phytonadione) should be given to all newborns before 6 hours of age to prevent vitamin K deficiency bleeding (VKDB). Oral vitamin K preparations are **not** recommended because late VKDB (2–12 weeks of age) is best prevented by the administration of parenteral vitamin K (see Chap. 43).

C. Administration of the first dose of preservative-free hepatitis B vaccine is recommended for all infants during the newborn hospitalization, even if the mother is hepatitis B surface antigen (HBsAg) negative (see Chap. 48).

1. Hepatitis B vaccine is administered by 12 hours of age when the maternal HBsAg is positive or unknown. Infants of HBsAg positive mothers also require hepatitis B immune globulin (HBIG) (see Chap. 48).

2. The vaccine is given after parental consent as a single intramuscular injection of 0.5 mL of either Recombivax HB (5 μg) (Merck & Co., Inc., Whitehouse Station, New Jersey) or Engerix-B (10 μg) (GlaxoSmithKline Biologicals, Rixensart, Belgium).

3. Parents must be given a vaccine information statement at the time the vaccine is administered. This is available at www.cdc.gov/nip/publications/vis.

V. SCREENING

A. Prenatal screening test results should be reviewed and documented on the infant's chart at the time of delivery. Maternal prenatal screening tests typically include the following:

1. Blood type, Rh, antibody screen

2. Hemoglobin or hematocrit

3. Rubella antibody

4. HBsAg

5. Serologic test for syphilis (Venereal Disease Research Laboratory [VDRL] or rapid plasma reagin [RPR])

6. Human immunodeficiency virus (HIV)

7. Group B Streptococcus (GBS) culture

8. Gonorrhea and Chlamydia cultures

9. Glucose tolerance test

10. Multiple-marker screening (triple or quadruple screen)

11. Cystic fibrosis carrier testing

B. Cord blood is saved up to 14 to 21 days, depending on blood bank policy.

1. A blood type and direct Coombs (direct antiglobulin test or DAT) should be performed on any infant born to a mother who is Rh negative, has a positive antibody screen, or who has had a previous infant with Coombs-positive hemolytic anemia.

2. A blood type and DAT should be obtained on any infant if jaundice is noted within the first 24 hours of age or there is unexplained hyperbilirubinemia (see Chap. 26).

C. Newborn metabolic screen (see Chap. 60)

1. The American Academy of Pediatrics (AAP), March of Dimes, and American College of Medical Genetics recommend universal newborn screening for specific disorders for which there are demonstrated benefits of early detection and efficacious treatment of the condition being tested.

2. Newborn screening programs are state based. An effort is underway to establish a national consensus on the minimum number and types of disorders that are universally screened. However, all states universally screen for congenital hypothyroidism, phenylketonuria, galactosemia, and hemoglobinopathies. Most states also screen for amino acid, fatty acid, and organic acid disorders, as well as cystic fibrosis and biotinidase deficiency. The National Newborn Screening and Genetics Resource Center (http://genes-r-us.uthscsa.edu/) lists currently screened conditions by state.

   3. Routine collection of the specimen is between 24 and 72 hours of life. In some states, a second screen is routinely performed at 2 weeks of age.

D. Group B streptococcal disease (see Chap. 49)

   1. All newborns should be screened for the risk of perinatally acquired GBS disease as outlined by the Centers for Disease Control and Prevention (http://www.cdc.gov/groupbstrep/guidelines/guidelines.html).

   2. Penicillin is the preferred intrapartum chemotherapeutic agent and ampicillin is an acceptable alternative. Penicillin-allergic mothers should be managed according to the revised management guidelines (see Chap. 49).

   3. Newborns should be managed according to the revised management algorithm (see Chap. 49).

E. Glucose screening

   1. Infants should be fed early and frequently to prevent hypoglycemia.

   2. Infants of diabetic mothers (see Chap. 2) and SGA and LGA infants should be screened for hypoglycemia in the immediate neonatal period (see Chap. 24).

F. Bilirubin screening

   1. Before discharge, all newborns should be screened for the risk of subsequent development of significant hyperbilirubinemia. A predischarge serum or transcutaneous bilirubin measurement combined with risk factor assessment best predicts subsequent hyperbilirubinemia requiring treatment. A total serum bilirubin measurement can be obtained at the time of the newborn metabolic screen. The value should be plotted and interpreted on an hour-specific nomogram (see Chap. 26).

   2. Jaundice during the first 24 hours of life is considered pathologic and warrants a total serum bilirubin level. This result is plotted on an hour-specific nomogram to determine need for phototherapy.

   3. Provide parents with verbal and written information about newborn jaundice.

G. Routine screening for hearing loss in newborns is mandated in most states (see Chap. 65) as outlined by the AAP's Joint Commission on Infant Hearing. Verbal and written documentation of the hearing screen results should be provided to the parents with referral information when needed.

VI. ROUTINE ASSESSMENTS

A. The infant's physician should perform a complete physical examination within 24 hours of birth.

B. Vital signs, including respiratory rate, heart rate, and axillary temperature, are recorded every 8 to 12 hours.

C. Each urine and stool output is recorded in the baby's chart. The first urination should occur by 30 hours of age. The first passage of meconium is expected by

48 hours of age. Delayed urination or stooling is cause for concern and must be investigated.

D. Daily weights are recorded in the infant's chart. Weight loss in excess of 8 to 10% is cause for concern and must be investigated. Excessive weight loss is usually due to insufficient caloric intake and lactation support should be provided (see Chap. 21). If caloric intake is thought to be adequate, organic etiologies should be considered, such as metabolic disorders, infection, or hypothyroidism.

VII. FAMILY AND SOCIAL ISSUES

A. Sibling visitation is encouraged and is an important element of family-centered care. However, siblings with fever, signs of acute respiratory or gastrointestinal illness, or a history of recent exposure to communicable diseases, such as chicken pox, are discouraged from visiting.

B. Social service involvement is helpful in circumstances such as teenaged mothers; lack of, or limited, prenatal care; history of domestic violence; maternal substance abuse; and history of previous involvement with Child Protective Services (CPS) or similar agency.

VIII. FEEDINGS. The frequency, duration, and volume of each feed will depend on whether the infant is breastfeeding or bottle-feeding.

A. The **breast-fed** infant should feed as soon as possible after delivery, preferably in the delivery room, and feed 8 to 12 times per day during the newborn hospitalization. Consultation with a lactation specialist during the postpartum hospitalization is strongly recommended for all breastfeeding mothers (see Chap. 22).

B. Standard 20 cal/oz, iron-containing infant formula is offered to infants for whom breastfeeding is contraindicated or at the request of a mother who desires to bottle-feed. Unless contraindicated by a strong family history, lactose-containing formulas with milk protein (whey and casein) can be given to all newborns.

1. Infants are fed at least every 3 to 4 hours.

2. During the first few days of life, the well newborn should consume at least 0.5 to 1 oz/feed.

3. The frequency and volume of each feed is recorded in the baby's medical record.

IX. NEWBORN CIRCUMCISION

A. The American Academy of Pediatrics (AAP) states that scientific evidence exists that demonstrates potential medical benefits of newborn male circumcision; however, these data are not sufficient to recommend routine neonatal circumcision. Potential benefits are decreased incidence of urinary tract infection in the first year of life; decreased risk for the development of squamous cell carcinoma of the penis; and decreased risk of acquiring sexually transmitted diseases, particularly HIV infection.

B. Informed consent is obtained before performing the procedure. The potential risks and benefits of the procedure are explained to the parents.

1. The overall complication rate for newborn circumcision is approximately 0.5%.

2. The most common complication is bleeding (~0.1%) followed by infection. A family history of bleeding disorders, such as hemophilia or von Willebrand

disease, needs to be explored with the parents when consent is obtained. Appropriate testing to exclude a bleeding disorder must be done before the procedure if the family history is positive.

3. The parents should understand that newborn circumcision is an elective procedure; the decision to have their son circumcised is voluntary and not medically necessary.

4. Contraindications to circumcision in the newborn period include the following:
   a. Sick or unstable clinical status.
   b. Diagnosis of a congenital bleeding disorder. Circumcision can be performed if the infant receives appropriate medical therapy before the procedure (i.e., infusion of factor VIII or IX).
   c. Inconspicuous or "buried" penis.
   d. Anomalies of the penis, including hypospadias, ambiguity, chordee, or micropenis.
   e. Circumcision should be delayed in infants with bilateral cryptorchidism.

C. Adequate analgesia must be provided for neonatal circumcision. Acceptable methods of analgesia are dorsal penile nerve block, subcutaneous ring block, and eutectic mixture of local anesthetics (EMLA) cream: 2.5% prilocaine and 2.5% lidocaine.

D. In addition to analgesia, other methods of comfort are provided to the infant during circumcision.

1. Twenty-four percent sucrose on a pacifier, per nursery protocol, should be given to all infants as an adjunct to analgesia.

2. The infant's upper extremities should be swaddled and the infant placed on a padded circumcision board with restraints on the lower extremities only.

3. Administration of acetaminophen before the procedure is not an effective adjunct to analgesia.

E. Circumcision in the newborn can be performed using one of three different methods:

1. Gomco clamp

2. Mogen clamp

3. Plastibell device

F. Oral or written instructions explaining postcircumcision care should be given to all parents.

X. DISCHARGE PREPARATION

A. Parental education on routine newborn care should be initiated at birth and continued until discharge. Written information in addition to verbal instruction may be helpful, and in some cases, it is mandated. A review of the following newborn issues should be done at discharge:

1. Observation for neonatal jaundice

2. Routine cord and skin care

3. Routine postcircumcision care (when indicated)

4. Back to sleep positioning

5. Subtle signs of infant illness, including fever, irritability, lethargy, or a poor-feeding pattern

6. Adequacy of oral intake, particularly for breast-fed infants (see Chaps. 21 and 22). This includes a minimum of eight feeds per day; at least one wet diaper on the first day, increasing to at least 6 on the 6th day and after; and two stools in a 24-hour period.

7. Appropriate installation and use of an infant car seat.

8. Smoke detectors

9. Lowering of hot water temperature.

10. Avoidance of second-hand smoke.

B. The discharge examination is reviewed in Chapter 8.

C. Discharge readiness

1. Each mother–infant dyad should be evaluated individually to determine the optimal time of discharge.

2. The hospital stay of the mother and her newborn should be long enough to identify early problems and to ensure that the family is able and prepared to care for the infant at home.

3. All efforts should be made to promote the simultaneous discharge of a mother and her infant.

4. The AAP recommends that minimum discharge criteria be met before any term (37–41 weeks) newborn is discharged from the hospital. These criteria include the following:

   a. Unremarkable clinical course and physical examination not revealing any abnormalities that require continued hospitalization.

   b. Normal, stable vital signs in an open crib for at least 12 hours preceding discharge.

   c. Passage of urine and stool spontaneously.

   d. Completion of at least two successful feedings.

   e. Absence of significant bleeding at the circumcision site for at least 2 hours.

   f. Assessment of risk for the subsequent development of significant hyperbilirubinemia.

   g. Adequate evaluation and monitoring for sepsis based on maternal risk factors.

   h. Review of maternal blood and screening tests.

   i. Review and interpretation of infant blood and screening tests.

   j. Assessment of maternal competency to care for her newborn at home.

   k. Administration of initial hepatitis B vaccine.

   l. Completion of hearing and metabolic screens per state regulations.

   m. Assessment of family, environmental, and social risk factors.

   n. Identification of a medical home for continuing medical care.

   o. Definitive follow-up appointments for both the mother and her newborn.

   p. Identification of barriers to adequate follow-up care.

5. **Late-preterm infants** who are 35 to 36 weeks' gestation are often eligible for admission to the normal newborn nursery or couplet care. However, these babies are at greater risk for morbidity and mortality than term infants and are more likely to encounter problems in the neonatal period, such as jaundice, temperature instability, feeding difficulties, and respiratory distress. Late-preterm infants are usually not expected to meet the necessary competencies

for discharge before 48 hours of age. AAP discharge criteria for late-preterm infants are similar to criteria developed for healthy term infants (see number 4 previously) with the following additions:

a. Accurate gestational age has been determined.

b. A physician-directed medical home is identified, and a follow-up visit is arranged within 48 hours of discharge.

c. Demonstration of 24 hours of successful feeding with the ability to coordinate sucking, swallowing, and breathing while feeding.

d. A formal evaluation of breastfeeding has been done and documented in the chart by trained caregivers at least twice daily after birth.

e. A feeding plan has been developed and is understood by the family.

f. Successful completion of a car safety seat test to observe for apnea, bradycardia, or oxygen desaturation, with results documented in the baby's chart.

XI. FOLLOW-UP

A. For newborns discharged less than 48 hours after delivery, outpatient follow-up with a health care professional is preferably within 48 hours of discharge, but no later than 72 hours in most cases. If early follow-up cannot be ensured, early discharge should be deferred.

B. For newborns discharged between 48 and 72 hours of age, outpatient follow-up should be within 2 to 3 days of discharge. Timing should be based on risk for subsequent hyperbilirubinemia, feeding issues, or other concerns.

C. The follow-up visit is designed to perform the following functions:

1. Assess the infant's general state of health, including weight, hydration, and degree of jaundice.

2. Identify any new problems.

3. Perform screening tests in accordance with state regulations.

4. Review adequacy of oral intake and assess elimination patterns.

5. Assess quality of mother–infant bonding.

6. Reinforce parental education.

7. Review results of any outstanding laboratory tests.

8. Provide anticipatory guidance and health care maintenance.

9. Assess parental well-being, including postpartum depression.

Suggested Readings

American Academy of Pediatrics and American College of Obstetricians and Gynecologists. *Guidelines for Perinatal Care*. 6th ed. Elk Grove Village, IL: American Academy of Pediatrics and American College of Obstetricians and Gynecologists; 2007.

American Academy of Pediatrics, Committee on Fetus and Newborn. Hospital stay for healthy term newborns. *Pediatrics.* 2010;125(2):405–409.

Centers for Disease Control and Prevention National Immunization Program (NIP). Available at: http://www.cdc.gov/nip/recs/child-schedule.htm

Centers for Disease Control and Prevention. Recommended childhood and adolescent immunization schedule—United States, 2009. Available at: http://www.immunize .org/acip/

10 Common Genetic Problems in the Newborn

Carlos A. Bacino

I. GENERAL PRINCIPLES

A. Approximately 3% to 4% of newborns are born with a major birth defect and will require genetic evaluation. These birth defects or malformations can be sporadic or associated with other anomalies. Some children may have physical features consistent with a well-known syndrome, while others may have anomalies detected prenatally or postnatally. Other neonatal presentations include some inborn errors of metabolism (acidosis), unexplained seizures, extreme hypotonia, or feeding difficulties. Infants with ambiguous genitalia require a multidisciplinary evaluation involving clinicians from genetics, endocrinology, urology, pediatrics or neonatology, and psychology. A thorough clinical evaluation requires a detailed prenatal history, a family history, and a comprehensive clinical exam, often including anthropometric measurements.

B. Congenital anomalies can be divided into major or minor.

1. **Major malformations** are structural abnormalities that have medical and cosmetic consequence. They may require surgical intervention. Examples include cleft palate and congenital heart disease such as tetralogy of Fallot.

2. **Minor malformations** are anomalies with no medical or cosmetic significance. They may aid in the diagnosis or recognition of a specific syndrome. Most of the minor abnormalities are limited to the head and neck region. Infants with three or more minor malformations are at a high risk for having a major malformation (20%–25%) and/or a syndrome.

C. Major and minor malformations are often part of patterns.

1. A **syndrome** consists of a group of anomalies that are associated due to single or similar etiologies, with known or unknown cause, such as Down syndrome due to trisomy 21.

2. **Associations** are clusters of malformations that occur together more frequently than occur sporadically, such as VACTERL association (vertebral, anal, cardiac, tracheoesophageal fistula, renal, and limbs anomalies, in particular radial ray defects) where at least three anomalies are required for the diagnosis.

3. A **developmental field** defect consists of a group of anomalies resulting from defective development of a related group of cells (developmental field). In this case, the involved embryonic regions are usually spatially related but may not be contiguous in the infant. Holoprosencephaly, affecting the forebrain and face, is an example.

4. **Disruptions** are extrinsic events that occur during normal development. These events can compromise the fetal circulation and result in a major birth defect.

111

An example of a disruption is amniotic bands that may result in amputation of digits or limbs.

5. **Deformations** can occur when physical forces act upon previously formed structures. Examples of deformations include uterine crowding or oligohydramnios that results in plagiocephaly or clubfeet.

II. INCIDENCE.
The Center for Disease Control and Prevention (CDC) monitors rates of birth defects in the United States (http://cdc.gov/ncbddd/bd/). Approximately 1 of 33 children has a major birth defect. Infants with birth defects account for 20% of infant deaths.

III. ETIOLOGY.
The etiology of approximately 50% of birth defects is unknown. Of the remainder, etiology is attributed to 6% to 10% chromosomal, 3% to 7.5% single-gene Mendelian disorders, 20% to 30% multifactorial, and 4% to 5% environmental exposures. The development of more sensitive molecular technology is likely to establish etiology in more cases.

IV. APPROACH TO THE INFANT WITH BIRTH DEFECTS

A. A comprehensive history is an important step in evaluating an infant with a birth defect.

1. **Prenatal**

   a. Chronic maternal illnesses and associated treatment medications, including diabetes (insulin and non-insulin dependent), seizures, hypertension, myotonic dystrophy, phenylketonuria, Graves' disease (see Table 10.1 for prenatal exposures and effects).

   b. Drug exposures should include prescribed drugs, such as antihypertensives (angiotensin-converting-enzyme inhibitors), seizure medications, antineoplastic agents (methotrexate), and illicit drugs (e.g., cocaine). Other drugs that may result in birth defects include misoprostol (to induce abortions). Timing of the exposure is important. Teratogenic agents tend to have their maximum effect during the embryonal period, from the beginning of the fourth to the end of the seventh week postfertilization, with exception of severe forms of holoprosencephaly when exposure may occur around or before 23 days (see Appendix B).

   c. Infections and immunizations.

   d. Social history.

   e. Other exposures may include alcohol; physical agents, such as x-ray and high temperature; chemical agents; and tobacco (see Table 10.1).

   f. Nutritional status.

   g. Fertility issues and use of reproductive assistance (e.g., history of multiple miscarriages, *in vitro* fertilization [IVF], medications to stimulate ovulation). Genetic disorders, such as Beckwith-Wiedemann syndrome, Russell-Silver syndrome, and Angelman syndrome that can be caused by imprinting defects (epigenetic mutations) have been seen in children conceived by assisted reproductive technology using intracytoplasmic sperm injection (ICSI).

   h. Multiple gestations (see Chap. 11).

   i. Results of prenatal studies should be obtained, including ultrasonographic and magnetic resonance imaging (MRI), and chromosome or microarray

Table 10.1	Well-Recognized Human Teratogens
Exposure Type	**Fetal Effect**
Drugs	
Aminopterin/methotrexate	Growth restriction, clefting, syndactyly, skeletal defects, craniosynostosis, dysmorphic features
Retinoic acid	CNS defects, microtia, ID, conotruncal defects: VSD, ASD, TOF
Lithium	Ebstein anomaly
Propylthiouracil, iodine	Hypothyroidism
Warfarin	Skeletal anomalies, stippled epiphyses, nasal hypoplasia
ACE inhibitors	Skull defects, renal hypoplasia/agenesis
Alcohol	Fetal alcohol syndrome or alcohol-related neurodevelopmental disorders
Thalidomide	Limb reduction defects
Valproic acid	Neural tube defects
Phenytoin	Dysmorphic features, nail hypoplasia, cleft lip and palate, ID, growth restriction
Diethylbestrol	Clear cell cervical cancer in female progeny
Cocaine	Vascular disruptions, CNS anomalies
Misoprostol (Cytotec)	Limb malformations, absent digits
Statins (HMG-CoA reductase inhibitor)	Limb defects, CNS abnormalities, congenital heart disease
Maternal conditions	
Maternal phenylketonuria	Microcephaly, intellectual disability
Myasthenia gravis	Neonatal myasthenia
Systemic lupus erythematosus	Cardiac conduction abnormalities
Diabetes	Neural tube defects, sacral agenesis, congenital heart disease, renal anomalies

(continued)

Table 10.1	Well-Recognized Human Teratogens *(Continued)*
Exposure Type	**Fetal Effect**
Other exposures	
Radiation	Miscarriage, growth restriction
Prolonged heat exposure	Microcephaly
Smoking	Growth restriction
Lead	Low birth weight, neurobehavioral and neurologic deficits
Mercury	CNS anomalies, neurobehavioral and neurologic deficits
Infections	
Varicella	Limb scars
Cytomegalovirus	Microcephaly, chorioretinitis, ID
Toxoplasmosis	Microcephaly, brain calcifications, ID
Rubella	Microcephaly, deafness, congenital heart disease, ID

ID = intellectual disability; VSD = ventricular septal defect;
ASD = atrial septal defect; TOF = tetralogy of Fallot;
CNS = central nervous system; ACE = angiotensin converting enzyme

studies done on samples obtained by amniocentesis, chorionic villus sampling (CVS), or percutaneous umbilical blood sampling.

j. Results of first- and second-trimester screening, including triple and quad screens, should be obtained. First-trimester screening combines the use of nuchal translucency with serum levels of pregnancy-associated plasma protein A (PAPP-A) and human chorionic gonadotropin (hCG) measured as free beta subunit (beta hCG) or total hCG. The second-trimester screening includes alpha-fetoprotein (AFP), unconjugated estriol (uE3), free β-hCG for the triple screen, plus inhibin A as part of the quad screen. A low maternal serum AFP (MSAFP) level can be seen in trisomies 21, 18, and 13. A high MSAFP may be a sign of multiple gestation, open neural tube defect, abdominal wall defect, impending fetal death, congenital nephrosis, or epidermolysis bullosa. A high hCG can be seen with trisomy 21, while low hCG may occur with trisomies 18 and 13.

k. Quality and frequency of fetal movements should be documented. Rapid and intense movements could be due to fetal seizures, while decreased movement can be seen with spinal muscular atrophy, Prader-Willi syndrome, and other congenital myopathies.

2. Family history should include the following questions:

   a. Are there any previous children with multiple congenital anomalies?

   b. What is the ethnicity of the parents? Some diseases can be more prevalent in specific populations.

   c. Is there consanguinity or are the parents from the same geographic area? What is the population size of the parents' community? In cases of rare autosomal recessive disorders, the parents may be related.

   d. Is there a history of infertility, multiple miscarriages, multiple congenital anomalies, neonatal deaths, or children with developmental delay? These can be secondary to a balanced chromosome rearrangement in one of the parents but unbalanced in the progeny.

3. Prenatal and perinatal events should be evaluated:

   a. What was the fetal presentation, and how and for how long was the head engaged? Was there fetal crowding, such as might occur with multiple gestation? Are there uterine abnormalities (e.g., septate uterus, myomatosis)? Various deformations, sagittal synostosis, and clubfeet can be caused by fetal constraints.

   b. What was the growth pattern throughout gestation? Was there proportionate or disproportionate growth restriction?

   c. What was the mode of delivery? Was there fetal distress or any events potentially leading to hypoxia?

   d. Placenta appearance: Is there evidence of placental infarcts? Is the umbilical cord normal? Inspection of the cord may reveal severe narrowing, clots, or knots.

4. **Neonatal events**

   a. What were the Apgar scores? Was resuscitation needed? Were intubation and ventilatory assistance needed? Were there severe feeding difficulties necessitating parenteral nutrition or tube feedings? Were there neonatal seizures? Was there hypotonia or hypertonia?

B. **Physical examination**

1. **Anthropometric measurements.** The assessment of growth parameters is extremely valuable to determine growth patterns, such as restriction, overgrowth, disproportion, or microcephaly. In addition, precise measurements of anatomic structures and landmarks can aid the diagnostic evaluation process. Examples are ear length, eye measurements for hypertelorism or hypotelorism (widely or closely spaced eyes), finger length, and internipple distance. Extensive reference tables for many of these measures are available for children of all ages, including premature infants starting from 27 weeks' gestation (Hall et al., 2007).

2. A thorough clinical evaluation is needed to document the presence of dysmorphic features: head shape (e.g., craniosynostosis, trigonocephaly, brachycephaly); ear shape (e.g., microtia, ear pits or tags) and positioning; midface hypoplasia; clefting; micrognathia; short neck; and limb anomalies (e.g., asymmetry, clinodactyly, brachydactyly, polydactyly). A good clinical description can aid the diagnosis as features can be matched to those in a database such as London Dysmorphology Databases or POSSUM web database. Some physical findings can be obscured by aspects of clinical care, such as endotracheal tube

position and taping or intravenous arm board and tape over the limbs. These need to be taken into consideration and the infant should be reexamined when these are no longer present.

3. Ancillary evaluations include a hearing screen that is done typically before discharge from the nursery or NICU and an ophthalmologic evaluation.

C. Laboratory studies

1. Chromosome studies are typically performed on whole blood drawn into sodium heparin tubes. The T lymphocytes in the blood are stimulated with mitogens, cultured for 72 hours, placed on slides, and karyotyped through the help of banding techniques, such as Giemsa trypsin G-banding (GTG). In extremely ill infants, those with immunosuppression, or who have low T-cell counts (as in DiGeorge syndrome), cell growth may be impaired and cell stimulation fails. In this case, a punch skin biopsy may be performed to obtain chromosomes from skin fibroblasts. The disadvantage of using skin fibroblasts is the delay of up to several weeks before a result is available. Chromosome studies can detect up to 5% of abnormalities. Tables 10.2 and 10.4 list the main clinical findings of the most common chromosome aneuploidies.

2. Fluorescent *in situ* hybridization (FISH) studies can be useful for the rapid detection of aneuploidies. These studies are done on unstimulated interphase cells, and the results are typically available in a few hours or overnight. Rapid FISH is used for evaluation in trisomies 13 and 18 and for sex chromosome testing in infants with ambiguous genitalia. More specific studies, such as FISH for SRY (sex-determining region on the Y chromosome), require more time and are done on stimulated metaphase cells.

3. Array comparative genomic hybridization (aCGH), also known as chromosome microarray, is a molecular technique that allows detection of DNA copy number losses (deletions) and copy number gains (duplications, triplications) of small genomic regions, sometimes even at the level of the exons. This study is based on the comparison of a known genome from a normal individual against the test sample and is often done with a matched sex control. Chromosome microarrays can detect 12% to 16% more abnormalities than conventional cytogenetic studies (regular karyotype). Disadvantages of microarray testing include failure to detect inversions, balanced chromosome translocations, and low-level mosaicism. Any loss or gain of genetic material must be confirmed by molecular techniques, such as FISH, polymerase chain reaction (PCR), or multiplex ligation-dependent probe amplification (MLPA). Both parents must be studied after the confirmation to determine if one of them is a carrier and to aid with the interpretation of the finding(s) in case it is a polymorphic variant. Consultation with a cytogeneticist or clinical genetics specialist is essential to interpret abnormal array results. The most common microdeletion syndromes detected in newborns are described in Table 10.3.

4. DNA testing is mainly reserved for single-gene disorders. They are caused by inherited or new mutations and often transmitted in a Mendelian fashion-like autosomal recessive, autosomal dominant, and/or X-linked disorders. Many of them can present in newborns as life-threatening disorders. These include spinal muscular atrophy; congenital adrenal hyperplasia (most commonly due to 21-hydroxylase deficiency); congenital myotonic dystrophy (only when inherited from an affected mother); osteogenesis imperfecta due to type I collagen

Table 10.2	Common Chromosome Anomalies (Aneuploidies)			
	Trisomy 13	Trisomy 18	Trisomy 21	Turner Syndrome
Growth	Growth restriction	Growth restriction	Normal	Mild growth restriction
Craniofacial	Hypotelorism, cleft lip and palate, small malformed ears, colobomas, microphthalmia	Triangular facies, micrognathia, pointy rotated low-set ears	Upslanting palpebral fissures, epicanthal folds, midface hypoplasia, small round ears, tongue thrusting	Frontal prominence, low posterior hairline
Neck	Short		Short, redundant skin	Short, webbed, pterygium, cystic hygroma
Central nervous system	Holoprosencephaly, microcephaly	Microcephaly	Microcephaly	Normal
Neurologic	Hypertonia, seizures, apnea	Hypertonia, apnea	Hypotonia	Normal tone, mild developmental delay
Heart	ASD, VSD	Multiple valvular anomalies	AV canal, VSD, ASD	Aortic coarctation
Abdominal	Multicystic kidneys, horseshoe kidneys, double ureters	Omphalocele, renal anomalies	Duodenal atresia, Hirschsprung disease	Horseshoe kidneys
Limbs	Polydactyly, nail dysplasia	Overlapping fingers, nail hypoplasia, rocker-bottom feet	Brachydactyly, fifth finger clinodactyly, single transverse palmar crease	Hand and feet lymphedema, deep-set nails
Skin	Scalp defects	Decreased subcutaneous tissue	Cutis marmorata	Multiple nevi

AV = atrioventricular; VSD = ventricular septal defect; ASD = atrial septal defect.

Table 10.3 Common Chromosome Microdeletions Ascertained in the Neonatal Period

	Prader-Willi syndrome	DiGeorge syndrome and velocardiofacial syndrome	Williams syndrome	Miller-Dieker syndrome
Chromosomal and genetic defect	15q11q13 deletion 70% UPD 20%–25% Imprinting center defect 5%	22q11.2 deletion	7q11.23 deletion	17p13.3 deletion
Critical gene/s involved	SNRPN	TBX1	ELN (Elastin)	LIS-1
Growth	Normal birth weight. Poor feeding, poor suck	Short stature	Short stature	IUGR
Craniofacial	Bitemporal narrowing, almond-shaped eyes	Prominent tubular nose, small ears, cleft palate, velopharyngeal incompetence (nasal regurgitation)	Supraorbital fullness, stellate pattern of the iris, long philtrum, everted lower lip	Microcephaly, bitemporal hollowing, furrow over mid-forehead, low-set ears
Abdomen		Absent/hypoplastic kidneys	Nephrocalcinosis, renal artery stenosis	Duodenal atresia, omphalocele
Central nervous system	Moderate-to-severe ID	Mild-to-moderate ID	Mild-to-moderate ID	Lissencephaly, agyria, pachygyria, heterotopias, absent corpus callosum, profound ID

Neurologic	Severe hypotonia in the first few weeks of life, poor feeding			Hypertonia, progressive spasticity, decerebrate posture, seizures
Heart	Normal	Conotruncal heart defects: VSD, ASD, tetralogy of Fallot, interrupted aortic arch	Supravalvular aortic stenosis	
Limbs	Small hands and feet	Long digits	Normal	Normal
Skin	Lighter pigmentation than parents (in deletion cases)	Normal	Normal	Normal
Other		T lymphocyte dysfunction: frequent infection	Hypercalcemia	
Natural History	Obesity and hyperphagia after 2–3 years	Normal life span	Normal life span	Death before age 2 years

UPD = uniparental disomy; IUGR = intrauterine growth restriction; VSD = ventricular septal defect; ASD = atrial septal defect; ID = intellectual disability.

Table 10.4 Other Common Chromosome Abnormalities

	Cri-du-chat syndrome	Wolf-Hirschhorn syndrome	1p36.3 Deletion syndrome	Killian /Teschler–Nicola syndrome (Pallister mosaic syndrome)
Chromosomal defect	Deletion of 5p15.2	Deletion of 4p16.3	Deletion of distal short arm of chromosome 1 (1p36.3)	Tetrasomy 12p; mosaicism for isochromosome 12p
Growth	Growth restriction	Growth restriction, FTT	Growth restriction, FTT	Normal or increased weight, later growth deceleration, macrocephaly
Craniofacial	Hypertelorism, round face, low-set ears, epicanthal folds, micrognathia	Hypertelorism, cleft palate, prominent glabella with Greek helmet warrior appearance	Thin horizontal eyebrows, midface hypoplasia, pointy chin, cleft lip/palate, large anterior fontanel	Hypertelorism, sparse hair on lateral frontal region, eyebrows and eyelashes, prominent forehead, chubby cheeks, thick lips, coarse features
Skin		Posterior scalp defects		Linear hyper and hypopigmented skin lesions
Central nervous system	Microcephaly	Microcephaly	Microcephaly	Polymicrogyria
Neurologic	High-pitched characteristic shrill cry (catlike), severe ID	Seizures that may improve with age, hypotonia, severe ID	Moderate-severe MR/absent speech, seizures	Seizures, hypotonia, contractures develop later, profound ID

Heart		Cardiomyopathy	ASD, VSD	
Abdominal	Diaphragmatic hernia, imperforate anus		Malrotation, absent gallbladder	
Limbs	Brachydactyly, broad digits		Clubfeet, hyperconvex nails	Nail hypoplasia
Genitourinary	Hypospadias		Hypospadias, cryptorchidism, absent uterus	
Other	Mosaicism is often found in skin fibroblasts and rarely present in blood chromosomes	Sensorineural hearing loss		
Natural history	Profound ID, no speech, seizures, joint contractures	Moderate to severe ID, seizures in 50% often improve; hearing loss leads to speech delays	Profound ID, major feeding difficulties sometimes require gastrostomy	Severe ID, aggressive behavior, self-mutilation

FTT = failure to thrive; ASD = atrial septal defect; VSD = ventricular septal defect; ID = intellectual disability.

mutations and other rare recessive forms (CRTAP, LEPRE1, PPIB); holoprosencephaly due to mutations in SHH (accounts for 30%–40%), ZIC2, TGIF, SIX3, PTCH1, GLI2; cystic fibrosis due to CFTR mutations and autosomal recessive polycystic kidney disease. A number of inborn errors of metabolism are Mendelian disorders. Other non–life-threatening single-gene disorders that can present in the newborn period include achondroplasia, due to FGFR3 mutations, and nonsyndromic deafness, due to connexin 26 and connexin 30 mutations.

5. **Infection.** TORCH infection may be suspected in children with microcephaly, cataracts, deafness (cytomegalovirus, rubella, toxoplasmosis), and congenital heart disease (rubella). In that case, IgG and IgM antibodies or PCR-based testing should be ordered. Brain imaging studies and fundoscopic exam could reveal brain calcifications and/or chorioretinitis. Parvovirus should be considered in cases of hydrops fetalis. The differential for nonimmune hydrops also includes several rare lysosomal storage disorders (see Chap. 26).

6. **Metabolic testing** for inborn errors of metabolism (IEM) is typically included in newborn screening programs. In most states, mandatory newborn screening is done initially between 24 and 48 hours of age, with a second screen done between 1 and 2 weeks of age. The March of Dimes and the American College of Medical Genetics recommend 29 conditions for testing. Most of these conditions can be managed by medications and/or special diets and treatments in many can be life saving. Additional metabolic studies considered for the diagnosis of IEM include acylcarnitine profile for fatty acid oxidation disorders, urine organic acids for organic acidemias, very long chain fatty acids for peroxisomal disorders (Zellweger syndrome), sterol panel (Smith-Lemli-Opitz syndrome associated with low 7-dehydrocholesterol levels), plasma amino acids for aminoacidopathies (e.g., phenylketonuria, tyrosinemia, nonketotic hyperglycinemia), plasma ammonia, and urine orotic acid (urea cycle disorders). The anion gap should be measured in cases of acidosis; if the anion gap is increased, measure lactic acid in whole plasma from a free-flowing blood sample (ideally arterial), and measure organic acids in urine. It is important to note that many IEM will not manifest symptoms until the infant is receiving milk feedings (see Chap. 60).

D. **Ancillary evaluations**

1. **Imaging studies**

   a. **Ultrasonography:** brain imaging, to detect major malformation and intracranial hemorrhage; abdominal ultrasound exam, to detect major liver and kidney anomalies and presence and position of testicles/ovaries; and echocardiography, to detect heart defects

   b. **Brain MRI,** to delineate brain anatomy in greater detail

   c. Magnetic resonance spectroscopy (MRS) in infants with lactic acidosis, to evaluate for mitochondrial disorders

   d. Magnetic resonance angiography (MRA) in infants with vascular malformations, to rule out further involvement such as arteriovenous fistulas and hemangiomas

   e. **Skeletal survey** in children with IUGR, poor linear growth, especially if disproportionate growth, to evaluate for skeletal dysplasias; if fractures are present, a survey can be valuable to evaluate for osteogenesis imperfecta.

E. Anatomic pathology

1. Muscle biopsy in children with severe hypotonia can be considered in conjunction with nerve biopsy to assess for disorders such as congenital muscular dystrophy, amyoplasia congenita, and hypomyelination syndromes. Sometimes, a muscle biopsy can be postponed until the infant is at least 6 months of age to gather better quality and more complete information.

2. Autopsy studies in stillbirths or infants who died in the neonatal period may provide a diagnosis and help with counseling and recurrence risks. Good documentation should be obtained and radiographs should be considered in addition to pathologic exam.

3. Placental pathology can be useful in infants with growth restriction. A sample of the placenta can also be submitted for genetic studies such as karyotyping.

F. Follow-up

1. Patients with birth defects require close follow-up evaluation after hospital discharge either to aid in the diagnosis or to educate the family. Since approximately 50% of patients born with multiple congenital anomalies have no known diagnosis, the follow-up may reveal new findings that will contribute to the final diagnosis. This will help predict the natural history and allow a proper assessment of the recurrence risk.

2. Infants suspected to be at risk for developmental delay should be referred for therapy services or early childhood intervention programs.

Suggested Readings

GeneTests. Available at: http://www.ncbi.nlm.nih.gov/sites/GeneTests/?db=GeneTests

Hall JG, Allanson JE, Gripp KW, et al. *Handbook of Physical Measurements.* 2nd ed. New York: Oxford University Press; 2007.

Hennekam R, Allanson J, Krantz I. *Gorlin's Syndromes of the Head and Neck.* 5th ed. New York: Oxford University Press; 2010.

Jones KL. *Smith's Recognizable Patterns of Human Malformations.* 6th ed. Philadelphia: Elsevier Saunders; 2006.

Online Mendelian Inheritance in Man. Up-to-date online catalogue of Mendelian genetic disorders and traits with a useful search engine for the identification of syndromes. Available at: http://www.ncbi.nlm.nih.gov/sites/entrez?db=omim

Multiple Births

Yvette R. Johnson

I. CLASSIFICATION

A. **Zygosity.** Monozygotic (MZ) twins originate and develop from a single fertilized egg (zygote) as a result of division of the inner cell mass of the blastocyst. MZ twins are of the same sex and are genetically identical. Dizygotic (DZ) or fraternal twins originate and develop from two separately fertilized eggs. Triplets and higher order pregnancies (quadruplets, quintuplets, sextuplets, septuplets, etc.) can be multizygotic, MZ and identical, or rarely, a combination of both.

B. **Placenta and fetal membranes.** A major portion of the placenta and the fetal membranes originate from the zygote. The placenta consists of two parts: (i) a larger fetal part derived from the villous chorion and (ii) a smaller maternal part derived from the deciduas basalis. The chorionic and amniotic sacs surround the fetus. The chorion begins to form at day 3 after fertilization, and the amnion begins to form between days 6 and 8. The two membranes eventually fuse to form the amniochorionic membrane.

1. MZ twins commonly have one placenta with one chorion and two amnions (**monochorionic diamniotic**) or, rarely, one placenta with one chorion and one amnion (**monochorionic monoamniotic**).

2. If early splitting occurs before the formation of the chorion and amnion (day 0–3), MZ twins can end up having two placentas with two chorions and two amnions (**dichorionic diamniotic**).

3. DZ twins always have two placentas with two chorions and two amnions (dichorionic diamniotic); however, the two placentas and chorions may be fused.

II. EPIDEMIOLOGY

A. **Incidence.** The twin birth rate in 2006 was 32.1 per 1,000 live births and had been stable for the previous 2 years.

1. The rate of MZ twinning has remained relatively constant (3.5 per 1,000 births).

2. The rate of DZ twinning is approximately 1 in 100 births. This rate is influenced by several factors such as ethnicity (1 in 500 Asians, 1 in 125 in whites, and as high as 1 in 20 in African populations) and maternal age. The frequency of DZ twinning has a genetic tendency that is affected by the genotype of the mother and not that of the father. In the United States, approximately two-thirds of twins are DZ.

3. The birth rate of triplet and higher order multiples peaked in 1998 at 194 per 100,000 live births. The rate declined to 153 per 100,000 live births in 2006. The rates for other higher order multiples (quadruplets and higher)

declined by 21% in 2006 compared to peak rates in 1998 (194 per 100,000 live births).

B. Causative factors. Two main factors account for the increase in multiple births over the last 2 decades: (i) increased use of **fertility-enhancing therapies**, including assisted reproductive technologies (ARTs) such as *in vitro* fertilization (IVF), and non-ART therapies such as ovulation-inducing drugs and artificial insemination, and (ii) **older maternal age** at childbearing (peak at 35–39 years), which is associated with an increase in multiples.

III. ETIOLOGY

A. MZ pregnancies result from the splitting of a single egg between day 0 and day 14 postfertilization. The type of placenta that forms depends on the day of embryo splitting.

1. A **dichorionic diamniotic** placenta results when early splitting occurs at day 0 to 3 before chorion formation (which usually occurs about day 3) and before implantation. A **monochorionic diamniotic** placenta results when splitting occurs about day 4 to 7, at which time the blastocyst cavity has developed and the chorion has formed. Amnion formation occurs at day 6 to 8, and splitting of the egg after this time (day 4 to 7) results in a **monochorionic monoamniotic** placenta. At day 14 and thereafter, the primitive streak begins to form, and late splitting of the embryo at this time results in **conjoined twins**.

2. **DZ or multizygous pregnancies** result when more than one dominant follicle has matured during the same menstrual cycle and multiple ovulations occur. Increased levels of follicle-stimulating hormone (FSH) in the mother have been associated with spontaneous DZ twinning. FSH levels increase with advanced maternal age (peak at age 37). A familial tendency toward twinning has also been shown to be associated with increased levels of FSH.

IV. DIAGNOSIS.
Multiple gestational sacs can be detected by ultrasonography as early as 5 weeks and cardiac activity can be detected from more than one fetus at 6 weeks.

A. Placentation. First-trimester ultrasonography can best determine the chorionicity of a multiple gestation; chorionicity is more difficult to determine in the second trimester. From weeks 10 to 14, a fused dichorionic placenta may often be distinguished from a true monochorionic placenta by the presence of an internal dividing membrane or ridge at the placental surface (lambda sign). The dividing septum of a dichorionic placenta appears thicker and includes two amnions and two chorionic layers. In contrast, the dividing septum of a monochorionic placenta consists of two thin amnions. One placenta, same-sex fetuses, and absence of a dividing septum suggest monoamniotic twins, but absence of a dividing septum may also be due to septal disruption. Both conditions have a poor prognosis.

B. Zygosity. Deoxyribonucleic acid (DNA) typing can be used to determine zygosity in same-sex twins. Prenatally, DNA can be obtained by chorionic villus sampling (CVS) or amniocentesis. Postnatally, DNA typing should optimally be performed on umbilical cord tissue, buccal smear, or a skin biopsy specimen rather than blood. There is evidence that DZ twins, even in the absence of vascular connections, can also carry hematopoietic stem cells (HSCs) derived from their twin. HSCs are most likely transferred from one fetus to the other through maternal circulation.

C. **Pathologic examination of the placenta(s)** at birth is important in establishing and verifying chorionicity.

V. PRENATAL SCREENING AND DIAGNOSIS

A. **Zygosity** determines the degree of risk of chromosomal abnormalities in each fetus of a multiple gestation. The risk of aneuploidy in each fetus of an MZ pregnancy is the same as a singleton pregnancy, and except for rare cases of genetic discordancy, both fetuses are affected. In a DZ pregnancy, each twin has an independent risk of aneuploidy; thus, the pregnancy has twice the risk of having a chromosomal abnormality compared with a singleton.

B. **Second-trimester maternal serum screening** for women with multiples is limited because each fetus contributes variable levels of these serum markers. When levels are abnormal, it is difficult to identify which fetus is affected.

C. **First-trimester ultrasonography** to assess for **nuchal translucency** is a more sensitive and specific test to screen for chromosomal abnormalities. A **second-trimester ultrasonography exam** is important in surveying each fetus for **anatomic defects**. **Second-trimester amniocentesis** and **first-trimester CVS** can be safely performed on multiples and are both accurate diagnostic procedures for determining aneuploidy.

VI. MATERNAL COMPLICATIONS

A. **Gestational diabetes** has been shown in some studies to be more common in twin pregnancies.

B. **Spontaneous abortion** occurs in 8% to 36% of multiple pregnancies with reduction to a singleton pregnancy by the end of the first trimester (**"vanishing twin"**). Possible causes include abnormal implantation, early cardiovascular developmental defects, and chromosomal abnormalities. Before fetal viability, the management of the surviving co-twin in a dichorionic pregnancy includes expectant management until term or close to term, in addition to close surveillance for preterm labor, fetal well-being, and fetal growth. The management of a single fetal demise in a monochorionic twin pregnancy is more complicated. The surviving co-twin is at high risk for ischemic multiorgan and neurologic injury that is thought to be secondary to hypotension or thromboembolic events. Fetal imaging by ultrasonography or magnetic resonance imaging (MRI) may be useful in detecting neurologic injury. Termination of pregnancy may be offered as an option when single fetal demise occurs in a previable monochorionic twin pregnancy.

C. **Incompetent cervix** occurs in up to 14% of multiple gestations.

D. **Placental abruption** risk rises as the number of fetuses per pregnancy increases. In a large retrospective cohort study, the incidence of placental abruption was 6.2, 12.2, and 15.6 per 1,000 pregnancies in singletons, twins, and triplets, respectively.

E. **Preterm premature rupture of membranes** complicates 7% to 10% of twin pregnancies compared with 2% to 4% of singleton pregnancies. **Preterm labor and birth** occur in approximately 57% of twin pregnancies and in 76% to 90% of higher order multiple gestations.

F. **Pregnancy-induced hypertension (PIH) and preeclampsia** are 2.5 times more common in multifetal pregnancies compared with singleton pregnancies.

G. **Cesarean delivery.** Approximately 66% of patients with twins and 91% of patients with triplets have cesarean delivery. Breech position of one or more fetuses, cord prolapse, and placental abruption are factors that account for the increased frequency of cesarean deliveries for multiple gestations.

VII. FETAL AND NEONATAL COMPLICATIONS

A. **Prematurity and low birth weight.** The average duration of gestation is shorter in multifetal pregnancies and further shortens as the number of fetuses increases. The mean gestational age at birth is 36, 33, and 29 and one-half weeks, respectively, for twins, triplets, and quadruplets. In developed countries, the incidence of preterm birth in twins was 60.4% in 2006, compared with 11.1% in singletons. Although most of this increased incidence is due to mild prematurity, multifetal pregnancy increases the risk of severe prematurity and very low birth weight (VLBW). The likelihood of a birth weight <1,500 g is 8 and 33 times greater in twins and triplets or higher order multiples, respectively, compared with singletons. In two multicenter surveys, multiples occurred in 21% to 24% of births <1,500 g and in 30% of births <1,000 g.

B. **Intrauterine growth restriction (IUGR).** Fetal growth is independent of the number of fetuses until approximately 30 weeks' gestation, after which growth of multiples gradually falls off compared with singletons. IUGR is defined as an estimated fetal weight (EFW) less than either the third percentile for gestational age or an EFW <10th percentile for gestational age with evidence of fetal compromise. The mechanisms are likely uterine crowding, limitation of placental perfusion, anomalous umbilical cord insertion, infection, fetal anomalies, maternal complications (e.g., maternal hypertension), and monochorionicity. Monochorionic twins are more likely than dichorionic twins to be IUGR and have higher perinatal mortality.

C. **Fetal growth discordance** is typically defined as an intrapair difference in birth weight of more than 20% of the larger twin's weight. It can also be categorized as mild (<15%), moderate (15%–30%), or severe (>30%). Risk factors for discordant growth include monochorionic placentation associated with velamentous cord insertion, placental dysfunction, preeclampsia, antepartum bleeding, twin-to-twin transfusion syndrome (TTTS), fetal infection, and fetal structural and chromosomal abnormalities. The smaller twin has an increased risk of fetal demise, perinatal death, and preterm birth. Five percent to 15% of twins and 30% of triplets have fetal growth discordance that is associated with a sixfold increase in perinatal morbidity and mortality.

D. **Intrauterine fetal demise (IUFD)** refers to fetal demise after 20 weeks' gestation but before delivery and is confirmed by ultrasonographic evidence of absent fetal cardiac activity. The death of one twin, which occurs in 9% of multiple pregnancies, is less common in the second and third trimesters. The risk of IUFD is four to six times greater in MZ pregnancies. Since almost all MZ twins have placental vascular connections with resulting shared circulations, there is a significant risk (20%–40%) of neurologic injury (multicystic encephalomalacia) in the surviving co-twin as a result of associated severe hypotension or thromboembolic events upon death of the co-twin. Because their circulation is not shared, the death of one DZ twin usually has minimal adverse effect on the surviving co-twin. In this case, the co-twin is either completely resorbed if death occurs in the first trimester or is compressed between the amniotic sac of its co-twin and the uterine wall (fetus papyraceous). Other complications involving the surviving co-twin include antepartum stillbirth, preterm birth, placental abruption, and chorioamnionitis.

In the event of a demise of one monochorionic twin, immediate delivery of the surviving co-twin should be considered after fetal viability. However, this does not seem to change the outcome as neurologic injury is thought to occur at the time of the co-twin's death. Disseminated intravascular coagulopathy is a complication seen in 20% to 25% of women who retain a dead fetus for more than 3 weeks. Monitoring of maternal coagulation profiles is recommended and delivery within this time frame should be considered.

E. **Congenital malformations** occur in approximately 6% of twin pregnancies, or 3% of individual twins. The risk in MZ twins is approximately 2.5-fold greater than in DZ twins or singletons. Structural defects specific to MZ twins include (i) early malformations that share a common origin with the twinning process, (ii) vascular disruption syndromes, and (iii) deformations.

1. **Early structural defects** include the following:
   a. Caudal malformations (sirenomelia, sacrococcygeal teratoma)
   b. Urologic malformations (cloacal or bladder exstrophy)
   c. The VATER spectrum (vertebral anomalies, anal atresia, tracheoesophageal fistula, renal agenesis, cardiac defects)
   d. Neural tube defects (anencephaly, encephalocele, or holoprosencephaly)
   e. Defects of laterality (situs inversus, polysplenia, or asplenia)

2. **Vascular disruption syndromes** may occur early or late in gestation.
   a. The presence of large anastomoses between two embryos early in development may cause unequal arterial perfusion resulting in **acardia**. One embryo receives only low-pressure blood flow through the umbilical artery and preferentially perfuses its lower extremities. Profound malformations can result ranging from complete amorphism to severe upper body abnormalities such as anencephaly, holoprosencephaly, rudimentary facial features and limbs, and absent thoracic or abdominal organs. The co-twin is usually well formed. Acardia is rare, occurring in 1% monoamniotic twin pregnancies and affecting 1 in 35,000 to 150,000 births. In acardiac twin pregnancies, the incidence of spontaneous abortion and prematurity is 20% and 60%, respectively. Perinatal mortality in the donor twin is 40%.
   b. Vascular disruptions that occur later in gestation are due to embolic events or the exchange of tissue between twins through placental anastomoses. Late vascular disruptions often occur after the demise of one fetus. Resulting malformations include cutis aplasia, limb interruption, intestinal atresia, gastroschisis, anorchia or gonadal dysgenesis, hemifacial microsomia, Goldenhar syndrome (facio-auriculo-vertebral defects), or Poland sequence. Cranial abnormalities include porencephalic cysts, hydranencephaly, microcephaly, and hydrocephalus.

3. **Deformations** such as clubfoot, dislocated hips, and cranial synostosis are more frequent in multiple pregnancies as a result of overcrowding of the intrauterine environment.

4. **Surveillance.** Twin pregnancies should be evaluated for anomalies by fetal ultrasonography or more invasive procedures if indicated. Congenital anomalies are concordant only in a minority of cases, even in MZ twins. Whether assisted reproductive techniques result in an increased incidence in congenital birth defects is uncertain.

F. **Chromosomal anomalies** occur at a higher frequency in offspring of multiple gestations. **Advanced maternal age** contributes to the increased risk in chromosomal anomalies. The risk in MZ twins is equivalent to that of a singleton. The risk in DZ twins is independent for each fetus, so the risk of chromosomal abnormality in at least one DZ twin is twice that of a singleton fetus.

G. **Conjoined twins** result when incomplete embryonic division occurs late, after day 14 postconception. At this time, differentiation of the chorion and amnion has occurred, and, therefore, conjoined twins are seen only in monochorionic–monoamniotic twins. Conjoined twins are rare and occur in approximately 1 in 50,000 to 100,000 births. The most common sites of fusion are the chest and/or abdomen. Survival is rare when there is cardiac or cerebral fusion. Serial ultrasonography can define the fetal anatomy and help determine management options. Polyhydramnios can affect as many as 50% of cases of conjoined twins and may require amnioreduction. Elective cesarean delivery close to term is recommended, and in cases wherein one twin is not likely to survive, delivery of the co-twin by an *ex utero* intrapartum treatment (EXIT) procedure should be considered. Surgical separation should be performed emergently in the event that one twin dies, and survival of the co-twin in these cases is 30% to 50%. Survival is 80% to 90% in twins that undergo elective separation, which is usually performed at 2 to 4 months of age.

H. **TTTS** occurs only in monochorionic gestations and complicates 10% to 20% of such pregnancies.

1. The **pathophysiology** of TTTS is not completely understood, but placental vascular anastomoses, unequal placental sharing, and abnormal umbilical cord insertions are all necessary for TTTS to occur. Eighty-five percent of monochorionic placentas have vascular connections that include superficial arterial-to-arterial (AA) and venous-to-venous (VV) anastomoses that have bidirectional flow and deep interfetal artery-to-vein (AV) communications with unidirectional flow located in the placental cotyledons that are supplied by one fetus and drained by the other. The number and type of anastomoses impact whether the exchange of blood between the twins is balanced or unbalanced. TTTS results when there is limited bidirectional flow through AA or VV connections. AA connections are thought to be protective, associated with a ninefold reduction in the risk of developing chronic TTTS, while AV anastomoses with unidirectional flow lead to shunting of blood from one twin to the other and are associated with worse perinatal outcome. Ten percent to 20% of monochorionic placentas have sufficient circulatory imbalance to produce TTTS. One fetus (**the donor**) slowly pumps blood into the co-twin's circulation (**the recipient**). Complications in the donor include anemia, hypovolemia and resultant activation of the renin-angiotensin-aldosterone system, growth restriction, brain ischemic lesions, renal hypoperfusion and insufficiency, oligohydramnios ("stuck twin"), lung hypoplasia, limb deformation, and high risk for fetal demise. Complications in the recipient include polycythemia, thrombosis, cerebral emboli, disseminated intravascular coagulation (DIC), polyhydramnios, progressive cardiomyopathy due to volume

overload, and fetal hydrops. Newer evidence suggests that the pathophysiology of TTTS involves changes in the renin-angiotensin system and increased levels of human brain natriuretic peptide (hBNP), atrial natriuretic peptide (ANP), and endothelin-1. Vasoactive mediators produced in the donor are shunted to the recipient resulting in hypertension and contributing to the development of hypertensive cardiomyopathy and hypertensive microangiopathy.

2. Diagnosis is usually made between 17 and 26 weeks' gestation, but the process may occur as early as 13 weeks. Severe cases of TTTS have signs before 20 weeks' gestation and have a mortality rate in at least one fetus of 80% to 100% if left untreated. **Diagnostic criteria** for TTTS include monochorionicity, polyhydramnios in the sac of one twin (the recipient) and oligohydramnios in the sac of the other twin (the donor), umbilical cord size discrepancy, cardiac dysfunction in the polyhydramniotic twin, abnormal umbilical artery and/or ductus venosus velocimetry, and significant growth discordance (>20%). These findings are suggestive of TTTS, although not all are necessary for a diagnosis. Several staging systems have been used to classify disease severity and progression of disease and to provide criteria for escalation of care to a specialty referral center, and a framework to evaluate therapeutic trials. The most commonly used system is the Quintero staging system. Others include the cardiovascular profile system (CVPS), the Children's Hospital of Philadelphia (CHOP) system, and the Cincinnati staging system. The Quintero staging system is based on a series of ultrasonographic findings and does not include fetal echocardiographic findings. The extent to which fetal cardiovascular changes in the recipient twin correlate better with disease severity or predict outcome or disease progression requires further validation. Additional clinical trials are needed to evaluate other physiologic parameters (e.g., cardiac indices or markers of systemic hemodynamic alterations) that will improve prediction of disease severity, progression, and outcome.

3. **Fetal treatment** interventions include serial amnioreduction, microseptostomy of the intertwin membrane, fetoscopic laser photocoagulation, and selective fetoscopic cord coagulation. Amnioreduction for polyhydramnios, initially performed for maternal comfort, was found to improve survival compared to expectant management. Survival in studies of serial amnioreduction ranges from 37% to 83%, with better survival when intervention occurs during early stage disease. Microseptostomy was performed to restore the amniotic fluid dynamics without the need for repeated procedures. However, randomized trials comparing amnioreduction and septostomy showed no survival advantage with either therapy. Microseptostomy has fallen out of favor due to the risk of creating a monoamniotic gestation and umbilical cord entanglement or cord accident. Results from the Eurofoetus trial found that laser photocoagulation improved both perinatal survival and short-term neurologic outcome at 6 months of life compared with serial amnioreduction. The risk of death of both twins and of periventricular leukomalacia (PVL) were also reduced with laser therapy. However, the selection of patients most likely to benefit the best intervention for a particular patient and the optimal timing of intervention remain uncertain. Studies to date suggest that the long-term neurodevelopmental outcome in surviving infants of TTTS (i.e., the incidence of cerebral palsy [CP]) is improved after laser photocoagulation compared to serial amnioreduction. These studies have demonstrated a lower risk of cerebral lesions (PVL, multicystic leukoencephalopathy, intraventricular hemorrhage, hydrocephalus,

and porencephaly) after laser therapy compared to amnioreduction. However, additional studies are needed to compare the long-term neurodevelopmental outcomes of twins after these interventions.

4. **Neonatal management** may include **resuscitation** at birth and need for continued ventilatory and cardiovascular support, rapid establishment of **intravascular access** for volume expansion to treat hypotension, correction of hypoglycemia, red blood cell transfusion to treat anemia, and **partial exchange transfusion** in the recipient to treat significant polycythemia. **Neuroimaging** is performed to detect central nervous system (CNS) injury.

5. **Persistent pulmonary hypertension of the newborn (PPHN).** TTTS is associated with a greater frequency (up to 3%) of PPHN compared to monochorionic twins without TTTS. The association between PPHN and TTTS may result from increased preload, volume overload, polycythemia, increased pulmonary vascular resistance, and increased afterload due to vasoactive substances in the recipient twin. In contrast, the donor twin may also be susceptible due to the presence of IUGR and lower levels of specific amino acids, such as arginine, which, as a nitric oxide precursor, plays a role in decreasing pulmonary vascular resistance after birth (see Chap. 36).

I. **Velamentous cord insertion and vasa previa** occur six to nine times more often in twins than in singletons and even more often in higher order gestations. Probable factors contributing to this higher risk include placental crowding and abnormal blastocyst implantation. All types of placentation can be affected. With velamentous cord insertion, vessels are unprotected by Wharton's jelly and are more prone to compression, thrombosis, or disruption, leading to fetal distress or hemorrhage (see Chap. 43).

J. The perinatal mortality in monochorionic–monoamniotic twins is reported to be approximately 10% to 15%, due primarily to umbilical cord entanglements and compression, congenital anomalies, preterm birth, and IUGR. The period of highest risk for cord accidents is from 26 to 32 weeks.

VIII. OUTCOMES

A. **Neonatal mortality.** Twin birth is associated with an increased risk of neonatal mortality compared to singleton births at all gestational ages; the perinatal mortality rate is increased further in second-born twins compared to first-born twins (26.1 vs. 20.3 per 1,000 live births). The mortality increases threefold and fourfold for triplet and quadruplet births, respectively. As with singleton births, mortality is inversely proportional to gestational age. In addition, the perinatal mortality rate in twin pregnancies peaks again with advancing gestational age, particularly after 37 weeks' gestation; delivery at 37 to 38 weeks is considered optimal timing of twin delivery. Prematurity and low birth weight are the predominating factors that increase the rates of mortality and morbidity for multiple births. Assisted reproduction has contributed to the increased incidence of multifetal pregnancies, and preterm birth is strongly correlated with the number of fetuses. Therefore, techniques that limit the number of reimplanted eggs or transferred embryos or selective reduction of higher order multiples may improve the likelihood of a successful outcome.

B. **Morbidity. Prematurity and growth restriction** are associated with an increased risk of morbidities such as bronchopulmonary dysplasia, necrotizing enterocolitis, retinopathy of prematurity, and intraventricular hemorrhage. These are discussed in more detail elsewhere (see Chaps. 27, 34, 54, and 64).

C. **Long-term morbidity** such as **CP** and other neurologic handicaps affects more twins and multiples than singletons. The risk of CP in multiples compared with singleton gestations is increased from fivefold to tenfold. Twins account for 5% to 10% of all cases of CP in the United States. The prevalence of CP in twins is 7.4%, compared with 1% in singletons. The higher prevalence of CP in twins is primarily observed among larger twins, especially among same-sex pairs; the relative risk of CP in twins ≥2,500 g at birth compared to twins <2,500 g is 6.3 (95% CI 2.0–20.1). Thus, the higher prevalence of CP among twins compared to singleton births is due to a greater frequency of prematurity and low birth weight in twins, as well as a higher prevalence of CP among larger twin pairs. Death of a co-twin is considered an independent risk factor for CP in the surviving twin. Other risk factors for CP in twins include same-sex pairs, monochorionicity, severe birth weight discordance, TTTS, and artificial reproductive technology. Among extremely low birth weight (ELBW) infants, the frequency of CP is not significantly different between singletons and twins. In addition, the frequency of chronic lung disease and IVH are not significantly different between singletons and twins ≤28 weeks' gestation. Twins have a greater risk of learning disabilities even after controlling for CP and low birth weight.

D. **Impact of assisted reproductive technology on outcomes.** In the United States, 18% of twin births result from ART. There have been multiple reports of increased adverse maternal and perinatal outcomes associated with ART. However, the extent to which the disproportionate increased frequency of multiple births (30% twin births with ART vs. 1.5% with non-ART deliveries) following ART contribute to this risk requires further study. Recent population-based studies in the United States demonstrate an increased risk of adverse perinatal outcomes in twin versus singleton ART births and non-ART twins, including prematurity, low birth weight, and VLBW. The rates of cesarean delivery are also increased in ART twins. Studies also demonstrate that adverse long-term neurodevelopmental outcomes are not different among ART compared to non-ART twins or higher order multiples. Although multiple gestation overall is associated with an increased risk of neurodevelopmental abnormalities, this risk is similar in spontaneously conceived and ART multiples and is independent of the type of assisted reproduction. Studies evaluating the increased risk of birth defects among ART births have been inconsistent. However, a number of studies have demonstrated up to a twofold increased risk of congenital anomalies among ART births following either IVF or intracytoplasmic sperm injection (ICSI). Cardiac, urogenital, as well as ocular birth defects have been reported with ART. In addition, rare imprinting disorders have been reported with ART including Beckwith-Wiedemann syndrome (BWS), and Angelman's syndrome. However, larger prospective cohort studies are required to definitively relate these rare conditions to ART.

E. **Economic impact.** Hospital stays for mothers and babies are typically longer for multiple gestations. One study estimated that, compared with singletons, average hospital costs were three and six times higher for twins and triplets, respectively; total family costs were four and 11 times higher, respectively. The increase in multiple births due to the use of ARTs has made an impact on overall medical costs. Thirty-five percent of twins and 75% of triplets resulted from assisted reproduction techniques. In another study, medical costs from induction of IVF pregnancy until the end of the neonatal period for a twin pregnancy were found to be more than five times higher than in a singleton pregnancy.

F. **Social and family impact.** Caring for twins or higher order multiples contributes to increased marital strain, financial stress, parental anxiety, and depression and has a greater influence on the professional and social life of mothers of these infants, particularly first-time mothers, compared with mothers of singletons. However, in one study, IVF twin parents were found to have a lower risk (7.3%) of divorce/separation compared with parents of control twins (13.3%), suggesting that IVF twin parents were able to better cope with the increased stress of twins. Multiples are more likely to have medical complications (i.e., prematurity, congenital defects, IUGR) that result in prolonged hospital stays that contribute further to a family's emotional and financial stress. Social services, lactation support, and assistance from additional caregivers and family members can help parents cope with the increased amount of care required by multiples. Organizations of parents of multiples can provide advice and emotional support that can further help new parents of multiples cope.

Suggested Readings

Chauhan SP, Scardo JA, Hayes E, et al. Twins: prevalence, problems, and preterm birth. *Am J Obstet Gynecol* 2010;203:305–315.

Habli M, Lim FY, Crombleholme T. Twin-to-twin transfusion syndrome: a comprehensive update. *Clin Perinatol* 2009;36:391–416.

Luu TM, Vohr B. Twinning on the brain: the effect on neurodevelopmental outcomes. *Am J Med Genet C Semin Med Genet* 2009;151C:142–147.

12 Maternal Drug Abuse, Exposure, and Withdrawal

Katherine W. Altshul

I. MATERNAL DRUG AND SUBSTANCE USE AND ABUSE. There are many drugs, exposures, and medications that, when taken in pregnancy, can have an adverse impact on the developing fetus and the infant postnatally. These include both illicit drugs as well as prescription medication. The concerns with these prenatal exposures is not only the effect they have on an infant's health and comfort, but also the impact they have on the child's growth, development, and behavior. The most recent National Survey on Drug Use and Health (Substance Abuse and Mental Health Services Administration, www.samhsa.gov), which compares data on drug use among pregnant and nonpregnant women, showed that 4% of pregnant women reported using illicit drugs in a given month compared to 10% of nonpregnant women. However, with the growing drug epidemic in this country, it is important that health care providers have an understanding of how these exposures can affect fetuses and infants.

The most common illicit drugs abused in the United States are cannabinoids, cocaine, heroin, and methamphetamine. There is also a growing epidemic of narcotic abuse and methadone treatment that is having profound impacts on neonates throughout the country. Alcohol and tobacco are also common exposures during pregnancy, despite their known teratogenic effects and the widespread education against their use. Intrauterine exposure to alcohol occurs more often than all the illicit substances listed in the preceding text combined. It is also difficult to tease out the effects of any one of the drugs, as many of them are taken in conjunction with others. Another increasing trend is the use of psychotropic medications taken during pregnancy, most commonly for treatment of maternal depression, anxiety, and bipolar disorder. Many of the medications used to treat these disorders are not recommended in pregnancy, and others, including some of the selective serotonin reuptake inhibitors (SSRIs), are still being studied.

II. DIAGNOSIS OF ILLICIT DRUG USE

A. **Take a comprehensive medical and psychosocial history** including a specific inquiry about maternal drug use as part of every prenatal and newborn evaluation. Accurate information regarding illicit drug use during pregnancy is sometimes difficult to obtain.

1. **Maternal associations with drug abuse**
   a. Poor or no prenatal care
   b. Preterm labor
   c. Placental rupture

This is a revision of the chapter by Sylvia Schechner in the 6th edition.

    d. Precipitous delivery

    e. Frequent demands or requests for large doses of pain medication

2. Signs of maternal drug abuse in the infant

    a. Small for gestational age (SGA)

    b. Microcephaly

    c. Neonatal stroke or any arterial infarction

    d. Any of the symptoms listed in Table 12.1

B. Diagnostic tests. Screen urine if drug withdrawal is a possibility. Urine testing is a quick, noninvasive way to test for drug exposure in the neonate; however, it will only show drug use that occurred within days of delivery. For example, cocaine will remain in the urine up to 3 days after the most recent use, marijuana 7 to 30 days, methamphetamine 3 to 5 days, and opiates (including methadone) 3 to 5 days. Drugs administered during labor may cause difficulty in interpreting urine results.

    Meconium analysis by radioimmunoassay affords a longer view into the drug-use pattern but is an expensive test and results take longer to obtain. Hair analysis of the infant can reveal maternal drug use during the previous 3 months, but hair grows slowly and recent drug use may not be detected. Any negative test does not rule out the possibility of drug exposure, so clinical status is the most important evaluation. Drug screening is also not appropriate in certain situations, and it is important to consider the implications of a positive test result. The following is our statement for testing:

Physician Guidelines for Testing, Reporting, and Care of Neonates Who May Have Been Exposed Prenatally to Controlled Substances
Brigham and Women's Hospital, Boston, MA

1. Testing

    a. Purpose. A positive urine test for controlled substances can serve several purposes: (i) It may help complete a diagnostic workup for an infant with symptoms of drug dependency or withdrawal (e.g., seizures or jitteriness), (ii) it may serve as a marker for an infant at risk for developmental delay, and (iii) it may indicate an at-risk family in need of social services. (A negative test result, however, cannot rule out any of the purposes mentioned earlier.)

    b. Symptomatic infants

        i. Performance of a toxicology screen is strongly recommended for infants with any of the following symptoms: (i) severe intrauterine growth restriction (IUGR), which is defined as a birth weight below the third percentile; (ii) symptoms consistent with neonatal drug dependency; (iii) withdrawal and/or central nervous system (CNS) irritability; and (iv) symptoms consistent with intracranial hemorrhage (ICH) such as focal seizures or paresis. These criteria are intended to serve as guidelines only. The attending physician must decide on a case-by-case basis whether a toxicology screen is indicated, and he or she must order it.

        ii. It is hospital policy not to require a separate specific consent from the parents for a toxicology screen on a symptomatic infant. As testing of symptomatic infants is done to assist in the medical diagnosis and/or treatment of the infant, the general parental consent obtained in the initial admission consent form is sufficient. Parents must be informed by the responsible pediatrician (prior to the test if possible) of the purpose of the toxicology screen. This discussion should be

Table 12.1   Reported Withdrawal Syndromes in Newborns after Maternal Drug Ingestion

Narcotics	Lethargy	Poor state control	Fever	Diaphoresis	Tachycardia	Tachypnea or respiratory distress	Cyanosis	High-pitched or abnormal cry	Altered sleeping	Tremors	Hypotonicity	Hypertonicity	Hyperreflexia	Increased suck	Ineffective suck	Irritability	Jitteriness	Seizures	Nasal congestion	Sneezing/yawning	Ravenous appetite	Vomiting	Excessive regurgitation	Diarrhea	Weight loss	Abdominal distention	Onset	Duration
Codeine			×							×		×	×		×	×	×					×		×			0.5–30 h	4–17 d
Heroin			×	×	×	×		×	×	×		×	×	×		×	×	×	×	×	×	×	×	×	×		1–144 h	7–20 d
Methadone			×	×	×	×		×	×	×		×	×	×		×	×	×	×	×	×	×	×	×	×		1–14 d	20–45 d
Morphine/oxycodone			×	×	×	×		×	×	×		×	×	×		×	×	×	×	×	×	×	×	×	×		1 h–7 d	1–2 wk
Propoxyphene				×	×	×		×		×	×	×		×		×	×	×	×	×	×		×	×	±		3–20 h	56 h–6 d
Pentazocine plus tripelennamine					×	×		×		×		×		×		×	×	×		×		×	×	×		×		
("T's and Blues")						×							×		×	×	×											

Sedatives

	Time	Time
Barbiturates	0.5 h–14 d	11 d–6 mo
Butalbital (Fiorinal, Esgic)	2 d	24 d
Chlordiazepoxide	2 d	37 d
Diazepam	2–6 h	10 d–6 wk
Diphenhydramine	5 d	10 d–5 wk
Ethanol	6–12 d	
Ethchlorvynol (Placidyl) (plus propoxyphene plus diazepam)	24 h	9–10 d
Glutethimide (plus heroin)	8 h	45 d
Hydroxyzine (Vistaril) (600 mg/d plus Pb)	15 min	156 h

Stimulants

	Time	Time
Methamphetamine		5–24 h
Phencyclidine	18–20 h	18 d–2 mo
Cocaine	1–3 d	

(continued)

Table 12.1 Reported Withdrawal Syndromes in Newborns after Maternal Drug Ingestion *(Continued)*

	Lethargy	Poor state control	Fever	Diaphoresis	Tachycardia	Tachypnea or respiratory distress	Cyanosis	High-pitched or abnormal cry	Altered sleeping	Tremors	Hypotonicity	Hypertonicity	Hyperreflexia	Increased suck	Ineffective suck	Irritability	Jitteriness	Seizures	Nasal congestion	Sneezing/yawning	Ravenous appetite	Vomiting	Excessive regurgitation	Diarrhea	Weight loss	Abdominal distention	Onset	Duration
Antidepressants																												
Selective serotonin reuptake inhibitors (SSRIs)	X				X	X	X	X	X	X	X	X	X			X	X	X									12 h–3 d	2–3 wk
Tricyclics antidepressants (TCAs)	X			X	X	X				X	X	X	X		X	X	X	X									5–12 h	96 h–30 d
Antipsychotics																												
Phenothiazines								X		X		X	X	X	X	X	X								X		2 d	>11 d–4 mo

X = symptom usually present; ± = symptom may be present, but not always; Pb = phenobarbital.

documented in the medical record, indicating that the discussion was held and that the parent (mother) assents to the testing. In the event that the parents, when informed, object to the performance of the toxicology screen, the legal office should be contacted for consultation. The results of the test and any follow-up or treatment should also be discussed with the parents. The obstetrician should also be notified of all positive test results.

c. **Asymptomatic infants**

i. When a toxicology screen is to be obtained on an asymptomatic infant, it is the responsibility of the attending physician (or his or her designee) to verbally inform the parent(s) of this plan and its indication. Documentation of this discussion and whether the parent accepted or refused the plan should be made in the infant's medical record. (A separate written consent form signed by the parent is not required.)

ii. Testing of asymptomatic infants is generally indicated in the following circumstances: (i) lack of adequate prenatal care, (ii) past or present parental history or signs of substance abuse, or (iii) abruptio placentae.

These criteria are simply guidelines. It is the responsibility of the attending physician to determine on a case-by-case basis whether testing of an asymptomatic infant may be beneficial.

2. **Referral.** Physicians, nurses, care coordinators, and other patient care employees are required by the State of Massachusetts' Protection and Care of Children Act (commonly known as 51A) to report to the Massachusetts Department of Social Services the cases of suspected child abuse and neglect, including all infants "determined to be physically dependent upon an addictive drug at birth." Reports generated by this hospital are usually filed by the hospital care coordination department. The hospital care coordination department should therefore be notified of all infants with symptoms of physical dependency to an addictive drug so that a 51A report can be filed as legally required.

The hospital care coordination department should also be notified of all asymptomatic infants with a positive toxicology screen and all infants believed to be at risk due to possible parental or family substance abuse. Such cases are not automatically required by law to be reported, and the hospital social worker will conduct a further evaluation to determine whether a potential abuse or negligent situation exists. If such situation is believed to exist, a report will be made. Prior experience indicates that most situations involving an infant with a positive toxicology screen (regardless of whether the infant is asymptomatic) will warrant the filing of a report.

3. **Care and treatment**

a. **Breastfeeding.** Most illicit drugs do not pose a specific risk to the newborn, and the use of them is not in itself a contraindication to breastfeeding. Some drugs may cause undesirable symptoms in the newborn, and the long-term effects of others are not well-studied. Mothers should be counseled about potential and possible risks and recommendations regarding breastfeeding individualized accordingly (see Appendix C).

b. **Screening and treatment for illnesses and disorders associated with drug abuse.** Screening infant–mother pairs for disorders and illnesses related to drug use (particularly HIV) and its associated lifestyle is strongly recommended in cases of known or suspected drug abuse. This includes the following:

   i. Hepatitis B surface antigen status should be known in all women at the time of childbirth. If this information is not readily known, testing should be done to ensure clear establishment of maternal hepatitis B status to allow the administration of hepatitis B vaccine and hepatitis B immune globulin (HBIG) during the effective period. If maternal hepatitis B surface antigen (HBsAg) status is unknown at the time of delivery, hepatitis B vaccine should be administered to the newborn within 12 hours of birth. HBsAg status should be determined as quickly as possible and, if positive, HBIG should be administered as soon as possible but within 7 days of birth at a separate site from the hepatitis B vaccine (see Chap. 48).

  ii. Establishment of the syphilis status of the mother to allow treatment of either or both as necessary. This is particularly important in light of the recent rise in congenital syphilis (see Chap. 51).

 iii. This is an opportune time to explore AIDS and hepatitis C risks with the mother. The discussion may include a recommendation for HIV and/or hepatitis C testing for which specific patient consent is required (see Chap. 48).

A drug-addicted mother is at increased risk for other diseases such as sexually transmitted diseases, tuberculosis, hepatitis B and C, and AIDS, especially if she involves herself in intravenous drug use or prostitution. Approximately 30% of pregnant intravenous drug users are seropositive for HIV (see Chap. 48).

III. NARCOTIC EXPOSURE IN PREGNANCY. Methadone, heroin, and prescribed narcotics are the most common reasons for withdrawal seen in our nurseries. Prescribed narcotics, such as morphine, fentanyl, Percocet, and Dilaudid, are given in pregnancy for management of chronic pain despite their dependence potential.

There has also been a rise in the use of OxyContin in this country since the early 2000s when reports surfaced about the abuse of this opioid. Both its illicit as well as legal use is seen in pregnant women. OxyContin is the extended-release form of oxycodone, an opioid twice as potent as oral morphine. It was originally thought that the extended-release properties would lower the abuse potential. However, when crushed and snorted or injected, the pill rapidly releases oxycodone and has become a powerful drug of abuse. The metabolites of narcotics, including OxyContin, are excreted in the urine and can be detected in the urine opiate and oxycodone screen at minimum levels.

Another narcotic with high abuse potential is heroin, a semisynthetic opioid synthesized from morphine. The high purity of heroin available makes snorting or smoking viable options and has thereby increased heroin consumption compared with years ago when injection was the only option.

Fortunately, with the use of methadone for the treatment of opioid dependence, these addictions can be managed. Small oral doses of methadone act on the same opioid receptors, thereby mitigating opioid withdrawal symptoms. However, this long-acting drug causes similar withdrawal symptoms in neonates, which can sometimes be more severe and prolonged than with exposures to other opioids.

A. Methadone exposure

   1. It can cause withdrawal in 75% to 90% of infants exposed *in utero*. Term infants have more severe abstinence symptoms than preterm infants.

2. The severity of the symptoms correlates with the maternal dose.

3. Maintaining a woman on <20 mg/day of methadone during pregnancy will minimize symptoms in the infant. Higher methadone doses may increase the severity and length of withdrawal. Higher doses have been used in the past few years because better compliance was noted in heroin addicts maintained on methadone doses of >80 mg.

4. Some infants have late withdrawal, which may be of two types:
   a. Symptoms appear shortly after birth, improve, and recur at 2 to 4 weeks.
   b. Symptoms are not seen at birth but develop 2 to 3 weeks later.

5. Effects in the infant exposed to methadone during pregnancy:
   a. Lower birth weight, length, and head circumference
   b. Sleep disturbances
   c. Depressed interactive behavior
   d. Poor self-calming
   e. Tremors
   f. Increased tone
   g. Abstinence-associated seizures
   h. Abnormal pneumograms
   i. Increased incidence of sudden infant death syndrome (SIDS)
   j. Follow-up studies reveal a higher incidence of hyperactivity, learning and behavior disorders, and poor social adjustment. This may be due more to environmental factors than as a consequence of *in utero* methadone exposure.

IV. NARCOTIC WITHDRAWAL IN THE INFANT.
The onset of symptoms for acute narcotic withdrawal varies from shortly after birth to 2 weeks of age, but symptoms usually begin in 24 to 48 hours, depending on the type of drug and when the mother took the last dose. Table 12.1 shows the withdrawal symptoms in newborns.

A. The severity of withdrawal depends on the drugs used. Withdrawal from polydrug use is more severe than that from methadone, which is more severe than that from opiates alone or cocaine alone.

B. **Differential diagnosis.** Consider hypoglycemia, hypocalcemia, hypomagnesemia, sepsis, and meningitis even if the diagnosis of drug-addicted mother is certain.

V. TREATMENT OF INFANT NARCOTIC WITHDRAWAL.
The goal is an infant who is not irritable, has no vomiting or diarrhea, can feed well and sleep between feedings, and yet is not heavily sedated (Fig. 12.1). Never give naloxone (Narcan) to these infants nor to one whose mother was on methadone; it may precipitate immediate withdrawal or seizures.

A. **Symptomatic treatment.** Forty percent need no medication. Symptomatic care includes tight swaddling, holding, rocking, placing in a slightly darkened quiet area, and hypercaloric formula (24 cal/30 mL) as needed.

B. **Medication.** Infants who are unresponsive to symptomatic treatment will need medication. Base the decision to start medication on objective measurement of symptoms recorded on a withdrawal scoring sheet, such as the one shown in Fig. 12.2. A total abstinence score of 8 or higher for three consecutive scorings indicates a need for pharmacologic intervention. Once the infant scores 8 or higher, decrease the scoring interval from 4- to 2-hour intervals. Once the desired effect

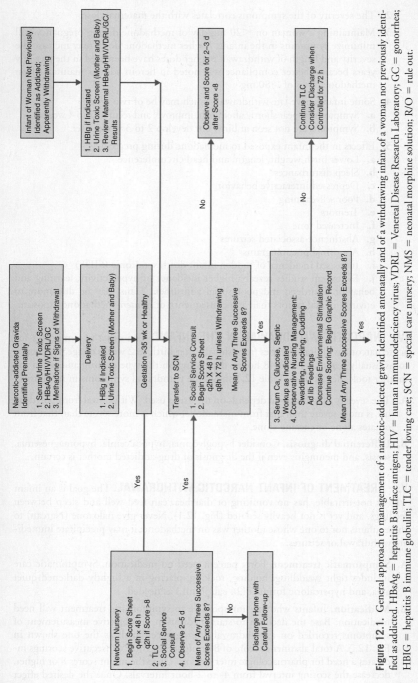

Figure 12.1. General approach to management of a narcotic-addicted gravid identified antenatally and of a withdrawing infant of a woman not previously identified as addicted. HBsAg = hepatitis B surface antigen; HIV = human immunodeficiency virus; VDRL = Venereal Disease Research Laboratory; GC = gonorrhea; HBIG = hepatitis B immune globulin; TLC = tender loving care; SCN = special care nursery; NMS = neonatal morphine solution; R/O = rule out.

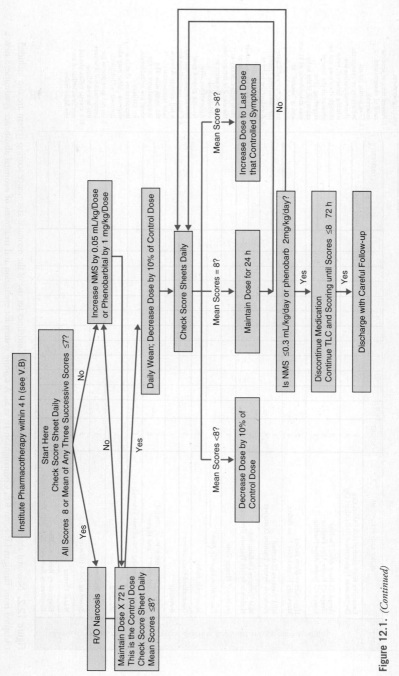

Figure 12.1. (*Continued*)

DATE: _____

SYSTEM	SIGNS AND SYMPTOMS	SCORE	AM	PM	COMMENTS
CENTRAL NERVOUS SYSTEM DISTURBANCES	Excessive High-pitched (OR Other) Cry	2			Daily Weight:
	Continuous High-pitched (OR Other) Cry	3			
	Sleeps <1 Hour After Feeding	3			
	Sleeps <2 Hours After Feeding	2			
	Sleeps <3 Hours After Feeding	1			
	Hyperactive Moro Reflex	2			
	Markedly Hyperactive Moro Reflex	3			
	Mild Tremors Disturbed	1			
	Moderate-Severe Tremors Disturbed	2			
	Mild Tremors Undisturbed	3			
	Moderate-Severe Tremors Undisturbed	4			
	Increased Muscle Tone	2			
	Excoriation (Specify Area): _____	1			
	Myoclonic Jerks	3			
	Generalized Convulsions	5			
METABOLIC/VASOMOTOR/RESPIRATORY DISTURBANCES	Sweating	1			
	Fever <101 (99–100.8° F / 37.2–38.2° C)	1			
	Fever >101 (38.4° C. and Higher)	2			
	Frequent Yawning (>3-4 times/interval)	1			
	Mottling	1			
	Nasal Stuffiness	1			
	Sneezing (>3-4 times/interval)	1			
	Nasal Flaring	2			
	Respiratory Rate >60/Min.	1			
	Respiratory Rate >60/Min. with Retractions	2			

Guidelines for the use of neonatal abstinence scoring system

1. Record time of scoring (end of observation interval).
2. Give points for all behaviors or symptoms observed during the scoring interval, even though they may not be present at the time of recording. (For example, if the baby was diaphoretic at 11 A.M. and is "scored" at noon, when he or she is not, the baby still gets the "sweating" point.)
3. Awaken the baby to test reflexes. Calm before assessing muscle tone, respirations, or Moro reflex. Many of the signs of hunger can appear the same as withdrawal.
4. Count respirations for a full minute. Always take temperature at the same site. The temperatures on the sheet are rectal levels; an axillary temperature that is 2 degrees cooler may also indicate withdrawal.
5. Do not give points for perspiration if it occurs due to swaddling.
6. A startle reflex should not be substituted for the Moro reflex.

Figure 12.2. Neonatal abstinence syndrome assessment and treatment. Guidelines for use of the neonatal abstinence scoring system are also included. (Adapted from Finnigan LP, Kron RE, Connaughton JF, et al. A scoring system for evaluation and treatment of neonatal abstinence syndrome: a new clinical and research tool. In: Morselli PL, Garattini S, Serini F, eds. *Basic and Therapeutic Aspects of Perinatal Pharmacology.* New York: Raven Press; 1975.)

7. Record doses administered (dose/time/initials) on sheet. One hour leeway is acceptable in dosing a fairly stable baby.
8. Record daily weight on graphic sheet.
9. Do not hesitate to get your experienced colleagues' opinions.

GASTROINTESTINAL DISTURBANCES		
Excessive Sucking	1	
Poor Feeding	2	
Regurgitation	2	
Projectile Vomiting	3	
Loose Stools	2	
Watery Stools	3	

TOTAL SCORE

INITIALS OF SCORER

NO.	PHARMACOTHERAPY REGIMEN	STATUS OF PHARMACOTHERAPY	RX	STATUS	DOSE	TIME	STATUS	DOSE	TIME	STATUS	DOSE	TIME	STATUS	DOSE	TIME	STATUS
	TITRATION REGIMENS	Indicate exact dose, time of administration & coded dosing status in the following blocks	#1													
1		Dosing Code	#2													
		Initiation (+)	#3													
2		Maintenance (m)	#4													
		Increase (↑)														
		Decrease (↓)														
		Discontinuation (−)														

	AM PM	AM PM	AM PM	AM PM	AM PM

SEROLOGIC QUANTITATION OF PHARMACOLOGIC AGENTS

Drug Administered:

• BEFORE BIRTH

− AFTER BIRTH

Figure 12.2. (Continued)

has been obtained for 72 hours, slowly taper the dose until it is discontinued. Observe the infant for 2 to 3 days before discharge.

1. **Neonatal morphine solution (NMS).** This solution of morphine sulfate made up in a concentration of 0.4 mg/mL is our treatment of choice for narcotic withdrawal.

   a. It is a pharmacologic replacement.
   b. It controls all symptoms.
   c. It impairs sucking less than other medications do.
   d. It contains few additives.

   However, high doses are often necessary, and withdrawal is slow.

   The previously mentioned dosing for NMS is the equivalent dose of morphine contained in neonatal opium solution (NOS). Because the only diluent is water in NMS, it avoids alcohol, preservatives, or camphor. NMS is made up in the hospital pharmacy. It has greater stability than deodorized tincture of opium (DTO), and if it is prepared properly, there are no problems with overgrowth of mold or microorganisms.

   A dosing scheme for NMS or NOS according to abstinence score is as follows:

Score	NMS or NOS
8–10	0.32 mg (0.8 mL)/kg/d divided q4h
11–13	0.48 mg (1.2 mL)/kg/d divided q4h
14–16	0.64 mg (1.6 mL)/kg/d divided q4h
17 or greater	0.8 mg (2.0 mL)/kg/d divided q4h; increase by 0.4-mL increments until controlled

   Add phenobarbital to control irritability when the NMS or NOS dose is >2 mL/kg/day. Some babies will need medication more often than every 4 hours.

   Once an adequate dose has been found and infant scores have been <8 for 72 hours, wean by 10% of total dose daily. If weaning results in scores >8, restart the last effective dose. Discontinue NMS or NOS when the daily dose is <0.3 mL/kg/day. The infant should be able to tolerate mild symptomatology during reduction. These infants are usually irritable, so all the previously mentioned comfort measures should be continued (see V.A.).

   If the scores are low, make sure that the infant is not overdosed. Effects of overdosage include sleepiness, constipation, poor suck, hypothermia, respiratory depression, apnea, bradycardia, and ultimately profound narcosis with obtundation. If these symptoms occur, stop the medication until the abstinence scores are over 8. Use docusate sodium (Colace) to manage constipation.

2. **Neonatal opium solution (NOS or DTO).** If NMS is not available, use NOS for treatment of narcotic withdrawal. NOS is also called DTO. It is a hydroalcoholic solution containing 10% USP laudanum and is equal to morphine 1.0%. This is diluted 25-fold with sterile water to a concentration and potency equal to that of paregoric (0.4 mg of morphine/mL). The diluted mixture should be called NOS, as suggested in the Neonatal Drug

Withdrawal Statement of the American Academy of Pediatrics (AAP) Committee on Drugs. The NOS dose is the same as that of NMS. This dilution is stable for 2 weeks. Keep the stock solution of tincture of opium in the pharmacy and dilute it there because of the possibility of giving the stronger mixture to the patient in error.

3. **Paregoric.** Paregoric contains opium 0.4%, equivalent to morphine 0.04% (0.4 mg/mL). It also contains anise oil, benzoic acid, camphor, and glycerin in an alcohol base. Dose as for NMS or NOS. Paregoric is readily available and has a long shelf life. Because of the unknown effects of many of the ingredients, we do not use it.

4. **Phenobarbital.** A loading dose of 15 to 20 mg/kg is given. If three consecutive scores are >8, or two consecutive scores are >12, may reload with 10 mg/kg/dose q8–12 h as needed until the cumulative total of all loading doses reaches a maximum of 40 mg/kg. A maintenance dose is given depending on the sum of the total loading doses. It is given q24h.

Cumulative sum of loading doses	Maintenance phenobarbital
20 mg/kg	5 mg/kg/d
30 mg/kg	6.5 mg/kg/d
40 mg/kg	8 mg/kg/d
Phenobarbital can be given orally (PO) or intramuscularly (IM). It is usually given PO.	

a. **Serum levels**
   i. If a cumulative dose of 30 mg/kg or more of phenobarbital has been given, draw a serum level before giving any additional loading doses.
   ii. Draw a serum level before the first maintenance dose to assess initial phenobarbital concentration.
   iii. Draw trough levels weekly.
   iv. Draw serum levels if the infant's scores remain >8 despite appropriate loading doses or repeat scores of <4 with clinical signs of sedation.

   Taper by 10% each day after improvement of symptoms. Phenobarbital is the drug of choice if the infant is thought to be withdrawing from a nonnarcotic drug or from multiple drug use. In narcotic withdrawal, some prefer phenobarbital to NOS to discontinue exposing the developing neonatal brain to narcotics. The possible side effects of phenobarbital include sedation and poor sucking. It does not control the diarrhea that occurs with withdrawal. Using phenobarbital with NMS allows a lower dose of NMS and lessens the side effects.

5. **Morphine and phenobarbital** can be initiated together for infants withdrawing from multiple drugs and may lessen the symptoms compared with single medical therapy.

   Morphine starting dose (0.4 mg/mL) is 0.05 mL/kg q4h, increased by 0.1 mL/kg increments for scores >7. The morphine is reduced by 0.1 mL/kg for scores <5 for 24 hours. Phenobarbital is given in two doses of 10 mg/kg q12h, followed by maintenance therapy of 5 mg/kg/day divided every 12 hours after the last loading dose. Serum phenobarbital levels of 20 to 30 mg/dL are ideal.

Morphine should be withdrawn first and the infant observed for 2 to 3 days off morphine and on phenobarbital alone.

This may allow the discharge of an infant home in the setting of an appropriate environment, with phenobarbital being prescribed. The infant can be allowed to outgrow the dose at home or the dose decreased under the care of the pediatrician. Because of recent literature reporting cognitive impairment and reduced brain mass associated with prenatal or postnatal exposure of humans to antiepileptic therapy, our first choice of drugs in treatment of NAS remains morphine.

Morphine in doses of 0.1 to 0.2 mg/kg can be effective in the emergency treatment of seizures or shock due to acute narcotic withdrawal.

6. **Chlorpromazine** is no longer used by us because of its unacceptable side effects, including tardive dyskinesia. It is useful to control the vomiting and diarrhea that sometimes occur in withdrawal. The dosage is 1.5 to 3 mg/kg/day, administered in four divided doses, initially IM and then PO. Maintain this dose for 2 to 4 days and then taper as tolerated every 2 to 4 days.

7. **Methadone.** Methadone is not routinely used by us for withdrawal from narcotics. Methadone is excreted in breast milk at a very low level. It is now considered safe for methadone-treated mothers to breast-feed if there are no other contraindications. It has a prolonged plasma half-life (24 hours). Doses used are an initial loading dose of 0.1 mg/kg/dose with additional 0.025 mg/kg/doses given every 4 hours until symptoms are controlled. The maximum daily dose is 0.5 mg/kg/day. The maintenance dose is the total methadone dose given over the previous 24 hours divided by 2 and given every 12 hours. Weaning can then be attempted by giving methadone every 12 hours, and then every 24 hours at the last dose used. Once the dose reached is 0.05 mg/kg/day, it could be discontinued. The oral formulation of methadone contains 8% ethanol.

8. **Diazepam (Valium).** We do not recommend diazepam, but it has been used for control of symptoms. Some hospitals use it in doses of 0.1 to 0.3 mg/kg IM until symptoms are controlled, halve the dose, then change to every 12 hours, and lower the dose again. The major side effect is respiratory depression. Breakthrough symptoms, including seizures, respiratory depression, and bradycardia have been seen during use of diazepam. Withdrawal has recurred after termination of therapy. The sodium benzoate included in parenteral diazepam may interfere with the binding of bilirubin to albumin. The manufacturer warns that the safety and efficacy of injectable diazepam have not been established in the newborn (see Appendix A).

9. **Lorazepam (Ativan)** is often used for sedation either alone or with NMS or NOS. The parenteral preparation of lorazepam contains benzyl alcohol and polyethylene glycol. It is given as 0.05 to 0.1 mg/kg IV per dose. When used in conjunction with NOS, it may decrease the amount of NOS needed. Limited data are available about its use in newborns.

Closely monitor fluid and electrolyte intake and losses. Replace as needed.

The narcotic abstinence scoring sheet (Fig. 12.2) will help establish objective criteria for weaning the infant from the medications. Irritability, tremors, and disturbance of sleeping patterns may last for up to 6 months and should not be a reason for continuing medication. For a general approach to management, see Fig. 12.1.

VI. MATERNAL ADDICTION TO DRUGS OTHER THAN NARCOTICS. Infants born to mothers using drugs other than narcotics may be symptomatic.

A. **Cocaine.** Cocaine has a potent anorexic effect and may cause prenatal malnutrition, an increased rate of premature labor, spontaneous abortion, placental abruption, fetal distress, meconium staining, and low Apgar scores. Cocaine increases catecholamines, which can increase uterine contractility and cause maternal hypertension and placental vasoconstriction with diminished uterine blood flow and fetal hypoxia.

1. The following are congenital anomalies associated with cocaine use during pregnancy: cardiac anomalies; genitourinary malformations; intestinal atresias; microcephaly with or without growth retardation; perinatal cerebral infarctions, usually in the distribution of the middle cerebral artery with resultant cystic lesions; early-onset necrotizing enterocolitis; and retinal dysgenesis and retinal coloboma.

2. **Effects in the newborns.** Although cocaine-addicted infants do not show the classic signs of narcotic withdrawal, they demonstrate abnormal sleep patterns, tremors, poor organizational response, inability to be consoled, and transiently abnormal electroencephalograms (EEGs) and visual evoked potentials. Many of these findings are also true of tobacco use, and because many crack cocaine users also smoke cigarettes, it may be difficult to identify which defects are specific to cocaine.

3. **Treatment.** The newborn's withdrawal rarely requires pharmacologic treatment. When the pregnant cocaine abuser also uses other drugs, the neonate may have more severe withdrawal; in this case, we use phenobarbital. If symptomatic treatment is not adequate, use phenobarbital or lorazepam for sedation.

4. **SIDS.** Cocaine-exposed infants appear to be at a three to seven times higher risk for SIDS. This may be due to impaired regulation of respiration and arousal.

5. **Long-term disabilities** such as attention deficits, concentration difficulties, abnormal play patterns, and flat, apathetic moods have been reported. Some believe that the neurologic and cognitive outcomes of cocaine exposure are unclear because standard methods of measuring infant neurologic and behavioral functions are difficult to quantify. It is also difficult to extricate the effects of cocaine use from the effects of lack of prenatal care, polydrug use, smoking, and the increased risks associated with a drug-using lifestyle. Convulsions have been seen both in infants of breastfeeding mothers using cocaine and in infants exposed to passive crack smoke inhalation. Because cocaine and its metabolites can be found in breast milk for up to 60 hours after use, breastfeeding is not recommended.

B. **Ethanol.** Teratogenic studies are confounded by other risk factors, but there is no established safe level of ethanol use in pregnancy. Symmetric growth retardation can occur *in utero*, the extent of which depends on the dose and duration of maternal use and on other factors such as concomitant tobacco or other drug use and overall nutrition. Although alcohol passes freely into breast milk, acetaldehyde—the toxic metabolite of ethanol—does not pass into milk. Therefore, the AAP considers moderate maternal ethanol use to be compatible with breastfeeding.

1. **Fetal alcohol syndrome (FAS)** includes the following features: microcephaly, growth retardation, dysmorphic facial features (such as hypoplastic midface, low nasal bridge, flattened philtrum, thinned upper vermilion, epicanthal fold, shortened palpebral fissure), cardiac problems, hydronephrosis, increased incidence of mental retardation, motor problems, and behavioral issues. Heavy prenatal alcohol exposure with or without physical features of FAS can lead to intelligence quotient (IQ) deficits. As is the case with other syndromes associated with craniofacial anomalies and hearing impairments, speech and language pathologies may also occur in FAS babies.

C. **Tobacco.** Smoking by pregnant women is associated with a higher rate of spontaneous abortions. Placental vascular resistance is increased as a consequence of the effects of nicotine, with resultant chronic ischemia and hypoxia. Nicotine can enter breast milk in relatively low levels and is not well absorbed by the infant's intestinal tract. This does not negate the risks to the infant from passive exposure to smoke.

1. Effects on newborn infants of regular smokers (1 pack per day)
   a. **Such infants** typically weigh 150 to 250 g less than the newborns of nonsmokers. The most pronounced effects of smoking on fetal growth occur after the second trimester. Fetuses may also be at risk by passive exposure.
   b. Increased tremors
   c. Poor auditory responsiveness
   d. Increased tone
   e. No association has been found between maternal smoking during pregnancy and congenital anomalies.
   f. SIDS has been associated, in a dose-response manner, with maternal smoking, possibly secondary to passive exposure to smoke after birth.

D. **Marijuana.** Prenatal use may result in shorter gestation with prolonged or arrested labor. There may be decreased fetal growth but no increase in major or minor morphologic anomalies. No reported adverse effects have been documented with breastfeeding. However, the drug may persist in milk for days after exposure and become concentrated with long-term use. Encourage abstinence if the infant is to be breast-fed. Some have found low Brazelton scores in these neonates and poor McCarthy scores on follow-up.

E. **Methamphetamine.** Methamphetamine, a psychoactive stimulant that increases alertness and energy, is used medically to treat symptoms of attention deficit hyperactivity disorder (ADHD). Its abuse potential lies in the fact that it provides a euphoric rush after being inhaled (smoked), snorted, or injected. It acts in the CNS, activating the catecholamine pathway and causing vasoconstriction, increased heart rate and blood pressure, and decreased appetite. As such, it can have detrimental effects, most notably growth restriction. Withdrawal symptoms from methamphetamines, are difficult to tease out, as the drug is commonly used in conjunction with other drugs such as heroin and cocaine.

F. **Phencyclidine (PCP).** A meta-analysis of 206 infants exposed to PCP prenatally did not show any congenital anomalies. Infants of PCP-abusing mothers are of normal size. Most of the neonatal manifestations of *in utero* exposure center on neurobehavioral effects (irritability, jitteriness, hypertonicity). Because PCP is excreted in breast milk, discourage breastfeeding if the mother uses this drug.

VII.   MATERNAL USE OF PSYCHOTROPIC MEDICATIONS. The use of psychotropic medication during pregnancy has become more common in the past 10 years, especially the SSRIs followed by lithium, antipsychotics, and benzodiazepines. There is growing evidence to show that infants exposed to many of these medications develop irritability, jitteriness, and mild respiratory distress, which are usually transient and self-limited. Women who are on psychotropic medications and become pregnant have to be made aware of the potential risk profiles these medications have for their fetus and infant and decide whether they wish to continue their medications throughout pregnancy. However, the risks to the fetus of a mother with a poorly controlled mood or psychiatric disorder can be harmful to the fetus and infant as well. The risk–benefit ratio of the use of these medications in pregnancy continues to be studied as their prevalence grows. Refer to Appendix B for medications not listed in the following text.

A. SSRI. Long-term developmental outcomes in children exposed to these SSRIs are unknown. Multiple studies have looked at the risk of SSRI use and birth defects. While many studies are inconclusive, there is growing evidence to suggest there is an increased risk of mild cardiac defects with certain medications (reviewed later in this chapter). There also appears to be an increased risk for persistent pulmonary hypertension of the newborn (PPHN) with SSRIs in general, which might partially explain the transient respiratory distress seen in the postnatal period. Another commonly observed outcome is the self-limiting neonatal behavioral syndrome. Infants are irritable with poor sleeping patterns, prolonged crying, and poor feeding, and, although self-limited, it sometimes requires medication as described in the previous sections. Several of the most commonly used SSRIs are indicated in the subsequent text.

It should be noted that we are seeing the use of SSRIs more frequently than tricyclic antidepressant (TCA) medication for the treatment of depression, especially in pregnant women. TCAs are serotonin and/or norepinephrine reuptake inhibitors, and some are also used in the treatment of migraine headaches. Examples of TCAs include medications such as amitriptyline, desipramine, and imipramine. These medications may cause withdrawal symptoms in the neonate similar to those cause by SSRIs (refer to Table 12.1). For a more complete review, please refer to the recommendations of the Committee on the Fetus and Newborn of the AAP on use of psychoactive medications during pregnancy.

1. **Paroxetine hydrochloride (Paxil)** is commonly used to treat depression and anxiety. It readily crosses the placenta, and although it was originally thought that it does not increase teratogenic risk, more recent advisories indicate that infants of women receiving paroxetine in the first trimester had 1.5-fold increased risk of cardiac malformations and a 1.8-fold increased risk of congenital malformations as compared with women receiving other antidepressants. These defects appeared to be mild, such as septal defects (atrial septal defect [ASD], ventricular septal defect [VSD]). The U.S. Food and Drug Administration (FDA) has changed paroxetine's pregnancy category from C to D. Lactation risk is Level II by the FDA.

Levels in breast milk are variable with concentrations higher in foremilk as compared with hind milk. Serum samples of breast-fed infants whose mothers are on Paxil have had minimal amounts of the drug with no untoward resultant symptoms. Therefore, it appears that for healthy full-term infants, there may be no reason to discourage women on Paxil from breastfeeding.

2. **Sertraline (Zoloft).** Mean umbilical cord to maternal serum ratios appear to be significantly lower for sertraline than for fluoxetine (Prozac). It is categorized as pregnancy class C by the FDA.

   A recent study demonstrated detectable serum levels in breastfeeding infants of those mothers who took 100 mg or higher of sertraline. There were no significant adverse sequelae. Lactation risk is categorized as Level II by the FDA.

3. **Fluoxetine (Prozac)** is the SSRI that has been most studied in pregnancy. There does not appear to be an increased risk of fetal loss, major fetal anomalies, or any effect on global IQ or behavioral development. Cases of mild transient respiratory distress, persistent pulmonary hypertension of the newborn, feeding problems, and jitteriness have been reported in women who took fluoxetine late in the third trimester of pregnancy. It is categorized as pregnancy class C by the FDA.

   The level of fluoxetine in breast milk is the highest compared with other SSRIs. This amounted to 10.8% of the weight-adjusted maternal dose. Currently the AAP "considers the effects on the nursing infant unknown, but they may be of concern." For this reason, recommendation might be to consider treating the breastfeeding mother with other SSRIs post delivery, if an SSRI is required. It is classified Level III by the FDA for lactation risk. (See Appendices B and C for information on all these drugs.)

4. **Citalopram (Celexa) and escitalopram oxalate (Lexapro).** Citalopram and its L-isomer escitalopram are emerging as commonly prescribed SSRIs during pregnancy. Their effects on the fetus and infant have been found to be minimal; however, there have been only a few studies with limited sample sizes. Neonatal behavioral syndrome appears to be the common complication in exposed neonates with indications that it may be dose dependent, suggesting that mothers on these medications should be maintained on the lowest effective dose. Both medications are pregnancy class C and lactation Level II by the FDA.

VIII. DISPOSITION. A major issue for infants of a drug-addicted mother is proper disposition and follow-up. Studies show a high incidence of abuse and violence in the lives of drug-abusing women. This, combined with their own drug use and chaotic lifestyles, places them at risk for inadequate parenting. These factors may be more important to the outcome of the child than the drug abuse itself. The health of the mother is significant for the ultimate well-being of the infant.

A. These infants are difficult to care for as they are often irritable, have poor sleeping patterns, and will try the patience of any caregiver. They are at increased risk for child abuse. Infants of HIV-positive mothers should be followed up closely because of their increased risk of AIDS (see Chap. 48).

B. Coordination of plans with social service agencies, drug treatment centers, and the courts, when necessary, is essential for proper follow-up and disposition.

C. Many states require that infants who show signs of withdrawal be reported as battered children.

For mother–infant dyads with SSRI or other psychotropic medication exposure, the risk–benefit ratio of continuing these medications upon discharge must be weighed. The neonatal behavioral syndrome associated with SSRIs is transient, and exposed infants are usually improved by the time of discharge. While limiting their continued exposure is prudent, it is also important to ensure that the mother's depression, anxiety, or other psychiatric illness is well-controlled, thereby enabling her to create a nurturing and safe environment for herself and the infant.

Suggested Readings

Chang G. Substance Use in Pregnancy. *UpToDate*. 2009. Available at: http://www.uptodate .com/online. Accessed April 2010.

Cicero TJ, Inciardi JA, Muñoz A. Trends in abuse of Oxycontin and other opioid analgesics in the United States: 2002–2004. *J Pain* 2005;6(10):662–672.

Fleschler R, Peskin MF. Selective serotonin reuptake inhibitors (SSRIs) in pregnancy: a review. *MCN Am J Matern Child Nurs* 2008;33(6):355–361.

Gomella TL, Cunningham MD, Eyal FG, et al. *Neonatology: Management, Procedures, On-Call Problems, Diseases, and Drugs*. 5th ed. New York: McGraw-Hill; 2004.

Hale TW. *Medications and Mothers' Milk*. 13th ed. Amarillo, TX: Hale Publishing; 2008.

Jansson LM, Velez ML. Infants of drug-dependent mothers. *Pediatr Rev* 2011;32:5–13.

Merlob P, Birk E, Sirota L, et al. Are selective serotonin reuptake inhibitors cardiac teratogens? Echocardiographic screening of newborns with persistent heart murmur. *Birth Defects Res A Clin Mol Teratol* 2009;85(10):837–841.

National Institute on Drug Abuse. Available at: http://www.drugabuse.gov. Accessed April 2010.

Neonatal drug withdrawal. American Academy of Pediatrics Committee on Drugs. *Pediatrics*. 1998;101(6):1079–1088.

Sielski LA. Infants of Mothers with Substance Abuse. *UpToDate*. 2010. Available at: http://www.uptodate.com/online. Accessed April 2010.

Substance Abuse and Mental Health Services Administration. Available at: http://www.samhsa.gov. Accessed April 2010.

Tuccori M, Testi A, Antonioli L, et al. Safety concerns associated with the use of serotonin reuptake inhibitors and other serotonergic/noradrenergic antidepressants during pregnancy: a review. *Clin Ther*. 2009;31(1):1426–1453.

United States National Library of Medicine, National Institutes of Health. Available at: http://www.nlm.nih.gov. Accessed April 2010.

13 Care of the Extremely Low Birth Weight Infant

Steven A. Ringer

I. INTRODUCTION. Extremely low birth weight (ELBW, birth weight <1,000 g) infants are a unique group of patients in the Newborn Intensive Care Unit (NICU). Because these infants are so physiologically immature, they are extremely sensitive to small changes in respiratory management, blood pressure, fluid administration, nutrition, and virtually all other aspects of care. The optimal way to care for these infants ultimately will be established by ongoing research. However, the most effective care based on currently available evidence is best ensured through the implementation of standardized protocols for the care of the ELBW infant within individual NICUs. Our approach is outlined in Table 13.1. Uniformity of approach within an institution and a commitment to provide and evaluate care in a collaborative manner may be the most important aspects of such protocols.

II. PRENATAL CONSIDERATIONS. If possible, extremely premature infants should be delivered in a facility with a high-risk obstetrical service and a Level III NICU. The safety of maternal transport must be weighed against the risks of infant transport (see Chap. 17). Prenatal administration of glucocorticoids to the mother, even if there is no time for a full course, reduces the risk of respiratory distress syndrome (RDS) and other sequelae of prematurity.

A. **Neonatology consultation.** If delivery of an extremely premature infant is threatened, a neonatologist should consult with the parents, with the obstetrician present if possible. A study of ELBWs born in NICUs, participating in the Eunice Kennedy Shriver National Institute of Child Health and Human Development (NICHD) Neonatal Network, determined that survival free from neurodevelopmental disability for infants born between 23 and 25 weeks of gestation was dependent on (i) completed weeks of gestation, (ii) sex, (iii) birth weight, (iv) exposure to antenatal corticosteroids, and (v) singleton or multiple gestation. Using these data, the NICHD developed a web-based tool to estimate the likelihood of survival with and without severe neurosensory disability (http://www .nichd.nih.gov/neonatalestimates). To use the tool, data are entered in each of the five categories (estimated gestational age and birth weight, gender, exposure to antenatal glucocorticoids, and singleton or multiple birth). The tool calculates outcome estimates for survival and survival with moderate or severe disabilities. We find it helpful to use this tool as a guide, tempered by the experience in the individual institution, during antenatal discussions with parents. We generally approach the consultation as follows:

1. **Survival.** To most parents, the impending delivery of an extremely premature infant is frightening, and their initial concern almost always focuses on the

Table 13.1	Elements of a Protocol for Standardizing Care of the Extremely Low Birth Weight (ELBW) Infant

Prenatal consultation

Parental education

Determining parental wishes when viability is questionable

Defining limits of parental choice; need for caregiver–parent teamwork

Delivery room care

Define limits of resuscitative efforts

Respiratory support

Low tidal volume ventilation strategy

Prevention of heat and water loss

Early surfactant therapy

Ventilation strategy

Low tidal volume, short inspiratory time

Avoid hyperoxia and hypocapnia

Early surfactant therapy as indicated

Define indications for high-frequency ventilation

Fluids

Early use of humidified incubators to limit fluid and heat losses

Judicious use of fluid bolus therapy for hypotension

Careful monitoring of fluid and electrolyte status

Use of double-lumen umbilical venous catheters for fluid support

Nutrition

Initiation of parenteral nutrition shortly after birth

Early initiation of trophic feeding with maternal milk

Advancement of feeding density to provide adequate calories for healing and growth

(continued)

Table 13.1	Elements of a Protocol for Standardizing Care of the Extremely Low Birth Weight (ELBW) Infant *(Continued)*

Cardiovascular support

Maintenance of blood pressure within standard range

Use of dopamine for support as indicated

Corticosteroids for unresponsive hypotension

PDA

Avoidance of excess fluid administration

Early medical therapy when hemodynamically significant PDA is present

Surgical ligation after failed medical therapy

Infection control

Scrupulous hand washing, use of bedside alcohol gels

Limiting blood drawing, skin punctures

Protocol for CVL care, acceptable dwell time

Minimal entry into CVLs, no use of fluids prepared in NICU

PDA = patent ductus arteriosus; CVL = central venous line; NICU = Newborn Intensive Care Unit.

likelihood of infant survival. One recent study reported that the survival rate for infants at <23 weeks' gestational age was 0 and at 23, 24, and 25 weeks, the rates were 15%, 55%, and 79%, respectively. Assessments based solely on best obstetrical estimate of gestational age do not allow for the impact of other factors, while those based on birth weight (a more accurately determined parameter), don't fully account for the impact of growth restriction. The use of the NICHD estimator allows the consultant to estimate the impact and interaction between gestational maturity, weight, and the other identified critical factors. While extremely helpful as a starting point, at least two important cautions should be considered in individual cases. First, birth weight has to be estimated for purposes of antenatal discussion, although reliable estimates are often available from ultrasonographic examinations, assuming a technically adequate examination can be performed. If this information is not known, gestational age estimates for appropriate for gestational age (AGA) fetuses can be roughly converted as follows: (i) 600 g = 24 weeks; (ii) 750 g = 25 weeks; (iii) 850 g = 26 weeks; and (iv) 1,000 g = 27 weeks. Second, there may be important additional information in individual cases that will significantly impact prognosis, such as anomalies, infection, chronic growth restriction, or evidence of deteriorating status before birth. Clinical experience should be used to guide interpretation of the impact of such factors.

For antenatal counseling, it may also be important to interpret published data in the light of local results. The best obstetrical estimate of gestational age may vary between institutions, and local practices and capabilities may significantly affect both mortality and morbidity in ELBW infants. Within each institution, practitioners should agree on the gestational age at which an infant has any hope of survival.

In discussions with parents, we attempt to reach a collaborative decision about what course of treatment would be best for their baby. We advocate attempting resuscitation of all newborns who are potentially viable, but recognize that the personal views of parents regarding what might be an acceptable outcome for their child will vary, and thereby impact decisions about offering resuscitation. Currently, we inform them that resuscitation at birth has been technically feasible at gestational age as low as 23 2/7 and 23 5/7 weeks and a birth weight as low as about 500 g, but we recognize that evolving evidence in some centers suggests that this may change in the future. In an individual case, the superimposition of medical problems other than prematurity may make survival extremely unlikely or impossible even at higher gestational ages. In counseling parents, we stress that within these parameters, delivery room resuscitation alone has a high (but not absolute) chance of success, but that this in no way guarantees survival beyond these early minutes. Studies have confirmed our experience that decisions based on the apparent condition at birth are unreliable in terms of viability or long-term outcome. We also note that the initiation of intensive care in no way mandates that it be continued if it is later determined to be futile or very likely to result in a poor long-term outcome. We assure parents that initial resuscitation is always followed by frequent reassessment in the NICU and discussions with them, and that intensive support may be appropriately withdrawn if the degree of immaturity results in no response to therapy, or if a catastrophic and irreversible complication occurs. Parents are counseled that the period of highest vulnerability may last several weeks in infants of lowest gestational ages. Once all these components are discussed, we make a recommendation regarding an approach to initial resuscitation.

If parents disagree with this recommendation, we first attempt to resolve differences by ensuring that they understand the medical information, and we understand their views and concerns, as well as their central role in determining appropriate care for their child. Almost always, a consensus on a plan of care is reached, but if an impasse continues, we seek consultation from the institutional Ethics service (see Chap. 19).

2. **Morbidity.** Care decisions and parental expectations must be based not only on estimates of survival, but on information about likely short- and long-term prognosis. Before delivery, particular attention is paid to the problems that might appear at birth or shortly thereafter. We explain the risk of RDS and the potential need for ventilatory support. In our NICU, all infants of 24 weeks' gestation require some ventilatory support; at 25 to 26 weeks, this proportion drops to 80% to 90%; at 27 to 28 weeks, approximately 50% to 60% of infants require ventilatory support. In our institutions, this usually means mechanical ventilation, but continuous positive airway pressure (CPAP) use beginning at or shortly after birth is an alternative that is being used more

frequently. We also inform parents of the likelihood of infection at birth as well as our plan to screen for it and begin empiric antibiotic therapy while final culture results are pending.

3. During prenatal consultation, we generally avoid giving parents detailed information on every potential sequelae of extreme prematurity because they may be too overwhelmed to process extensive information during this time. We do specifically discuss those problems that are most likely to occur in many ELBW infants or will be screened for during hospitalization. These include apnea of prematurity, intraventricular hemorrhage (IVH), nosocomial sepsis (or evaluations for possible sepsis), and feeding difficulties, as well as long-term sensory disabilities. We make a point of briefly discussing the risks of retinopathy of prematurity and subsequent visual deficits and the need for hearing screening and the potential for hearing loss. These complications are not noted until late in the hospital course, but we find that giving parents some perspective on the entire hospitalization is helpful to them.

4. **Parents' desires.** In most instances, parents are the best surrogate decision makers for their child. We believe that, within each institution, there should be a uniform approach to parental demands for attempting or withholding resuscitation at very low gestational ages. The best practice is to formulate decisions in concert with parents, after providing them with clear, realistic, and factual information about the possibilities for success of therapy and its long-term outcome.

   During the consultation, the neonatologist should try to understand parental wishes about resuscitative efforts and subsequent support, especially when chances for infant survival are slim. When counseling parents around an expected birth at <24 weeks, we specifically offer them the choice of limiting delivery room interventions to those designed to ensure comfort alone if they feel that the prognosis appears too bleak for their child. We encourage them to voice their understanding of the planned approach and their expectations for their soon-to-be-born child. We reassure them that the strength of their wishes does help guide caregivers in determining whether and how long to continue resuscitation attempts. Through this approach, we clarify for parents their role in decision making as well as the limitations of that role. In practice, parents' wishes about resuscitation are central to decision making when the gestational age is <24 6/7 weeks. At 25 weeks and above, in the absence of other factors, we very strongly advocate for attempting resuscitation and make this clear to parents.

III. DELIVERY ROOM CARE. The pediatric team should include an experienced pediatrician or neonatologist, particularly when the fetus is of <26 weeks' gestational age. The approach to resuscitation is similar to that in more mature infants (see Chap. 5). Special attention should be paid to the following:

A. **Warmth and drying.** The ELBW neonate is at particular risk for hypothermia. Conventional practice has been to place the infant under a preheated warmer, quickly dry the baby, and remove the wet toweling. Care should be taken to minimize rubbing so as to limit damage to immature skin. Better temperature control may be achieved with one or more of the following techniques: (i) immediately wrapping the undried baby's body and extremities in plastic wrap or placing them in a plastic bag (we have had most success using a large sheet of plastic and quickly wrapping the baby in a swaddling fashion); (ii) the use of an exothermic mattress;

(iii) ensuring that the delivery room temperature has been set at 26°C. Care must be taken to avoid overheating the baby, especially when more than one of these modalities is employed.

B. **Respiratory support.** Most ELBW infants require some degree of ventilatory support because of pulmonary immaturity and limited respiratory muscle strength. Blended oxygen and air should be available to help avoid prolonged hyperoxia after the initial resuscitation, and it should be used in conjunction with pulse oximetry, using a probe placed on the right upper ("preductal") extremity. Studies have demonstrated that a blend of oxygen and air is preferable over either one alone, but the optimal concentration has not yet been identified; we have chosen to start with 60% oxygen and titrate the concentration based on measured oxygen saturation. We use the saturation targets identified for all babies the first several minutes (see Table 5.1) and, thereafter, adjust the oxygen so as to keep the saturation level the same as that used during NICU care for all babies <32 weeks (a target of 90%–92%, with a range of 85%–93%). If the neonate cries vigorously at birth, we administer blow-by blended oxygen if required on the basis of saturation, and observe the infant for signs of distress.

Many of these infants require bag-and-mask ventilation because of apnea or ineffective respiratory drive. If the infant is breathing spontaneously, albeit with distress, initial respiratory support can be provided by either positive pressure ventilation or CPAP. In studies comparing these modalities, there were no differences in survival or incidence of chronic lung disease. If the infant is not breathing spontaneously, positive pressure ventilation must be started; provision of adequate support will result in or maintain a normal heart rate. Judgment is required regarding ongoing support, depending on the baby's status and local practice patterns. For many babies, support may be maintained using CPAP at 6 to 8 cm H_2O. If positive pressure ventilation is used, moderately high-inflating pressures may be necessary for the initial breaths of an infant whose lungs are deficient in surfactant. Within one or two breaths, the peak pressure should be rapidly lowered to minimize lung injury, with the goal of using the smallest tidal volumes and peak pressure possible while still adequately ventilating the infant. These infants usually require continued respiratory support and do benefit from early application of end-expiratory pressure; our practice is to provide this via endotracheal intubation and ventilation shortly after birth. We employ a T-piece device (Neopuff Infant Resuscitator [Fisher and Paykel]) instead of hand-bagging or face mask CPAP because it ensures adequate and regulated positive end-expiratory pressure and regulated inflation pressures. While commonly practiced in many institutions, administration of exogenous surfactant therapy before the first breath has not yet been proved to be more beneficial than administration after initial stabilization of the infant. Exogenous surfactant may be safely administered in the delivery room once correct endotracheal tube position has been confirmed clinically.

The pediatrician should assess the response to resuscitation and gauge the need for further interventions. If the infant fails to respond, the team should recheck that all supporting measures are being effectively administered. Support for apnea or poor respiratory effort must include intermittent inflating breaths or regulated nasal CPAP. Face mask CPAP alone is not adequate support for an apneic baby, and a failure to respond to this limited intervention does not mean that the infant is too immature to be resuscitated. If, on the other hand, there is no positive response to resuscitation after a reasonable length of time, we consider limiting support to comfort measures alone.

C. **Care after resuscitation.** Immediately after resuscitation, the plastic-wrapped infant should be placed in a prewarmed transport incubator for transfer to the NICU. Within practical limits, we encourage as much interaction between baby and the parents in the delivery room (while in the transport incubator) to enhance the beginning of parent–infant interaction. In the NICU, the infant is moved to an incubator/radiant warmer combination unit (Giraffe Bed, Ohmeda Medical), where a complete assessment is done and treatment initiated. The infant's temperature should be rechecked at this time and closely monitored. As soon as possible, the unit is closed to function as an incubator for continued care. Humidity is maintained at 70% for the first week of life, and 50% to 60% thereafter up to 32 weeks corrected gestation. In addition to reducing insensible fluid losses and thereby simplifying fluid therapy, the use of incubators aids in reducing unnecessary stimulation and noise experienced by the baby.

IV. CARE IN THE INTENSIVE CARE UNIT. Careful attention to detail and frequent monitoring are the basic components of care of the ELBW infant, because critical changes can occur rapidly. Large fluid losses, balances between fluid intake and blood glucose levels, delicate pulmonary status, and the immaturity and increased sensitivity of several organ systems all require close monitoring. Monitoring itself, however, may pose increased risks because each laboratory test requires a significant percentage of the baby's total blood volume, tiny-caliber vessels may be hard to cannulate without several attempts, and limited skin integrity increases susceptibility to injury or infection. Issues in routine care that require special attention in ELBW infants include the following:

A. **Survival.** The first several days after birth, but in particular the first 24 to 48 hours, are the most critical for survival. Infants who require significant respiratory, cardiovascular, and/or fluid support are assessed continuously, and their chances for ongoing survival are evaluated as part of this process. If caregivers and the parents determine that death is imminent, continued treatment is futile, or treatment is likely to result in survival of a child with profound neurologic impairment, we recommend the withdrawal of ventilator and other invasive support and redirection of care to comfort measures and support of the family.

B. **Respiratory support.** Most ELBW infants require initial respiratory support.

1. **Conventional ventilation.** We generally use conventional pressure-limited synchronized intermittent mandatory ventilation (SIMV), usually in a volume guarantee mode, available on the Dräger Babylog ventilator, as our primary mode of mechanical ventilation (see Chap. 29). The lowest possible tidal volume to provide adequate ventilation and oxygenation and a short inspiratory time should be used. Special effort should be made to avoid hyperoxia by targeting oxygen saturations at lower levels than have been traditionally used. Several reports have demonstrated that oxygen saturation limits for babies less than 32 weeks' gestation who require supplemental oxygen should be lower than those used in more mature babies in order to reduce the number of hypoxia–hyperoxia fluctuations and reduce the incidence and severity of retinopathy of prematurity. A recent report found that a target range of 85% to 89% decreased retinopathy but may be associated with an increase in mortality, compared to a range of 90% to 94%. We aim for a target range of 90% to 92%, and set our alarm limits at 85% and 93%. These alarm limits are designed to allow staff a few seconds

to determine if oxygen saturation outside the range will correct without intervention, thereby decreasing the tendency for hypoxia–hyperoxia fluctuations. This can be effectively done while still ensuring that a saturation level that remains, for example, at 86% will be addressed by increasing oxygen concentration, even though the value lies within the alarm limits. It is hypothesized that limiting hyperoxia may also reduce the incidence or severity of chronic lung disease. It is important as well to avoid hypocapnia, although the potential benefit of permissive hypercapnia as a ventilatory strategy remains a subject of debate.

2. **Surfactant therapy** (see Chap. 33). We administer surfactant to infants with RDS who are ventilated with a mean airway pressure of at least 7 cm H_2O and an inspired oxygen concentration (F_1O_2) of 0.3 or higher in the first 2 hours after birth. We give the first dose as soon as possible after birth, preferably within the first hour.

3. **High-frequency oscillatory ventilation (HFOV)** is used in infants who fail to improve after surfactant administration and require conventional ventilation at high peak inspiratory pressures. For infants with an air leak syndrome, especially pulmonary interstitial emphysema (see Chap. 38), high-frequency jet ventilation may be the preferred mode of ventilation.

4. **Vitamin A supplementation.** In many units, infants with birth weight of 1,000 g and less are given 5,000 IU of vitamin A intramuscularly three times a week for the first 4 weeks. This therapy has been shown to result in a small reduction in the incidence of chronic lung disease.

5. **Caffeine citrate** administered within the first 10 days after birth at standard doses (see Appendix A) has been shown to reduce the risk of developing bronchopulmonary dysplasia (BPD).

6. **Nitric oxide** has been shown in one study to reduce the incidence of chronic lung disease when given to infants after the first week of life who continues to require mechanical ventilation. Details regarding the optimal treatment and dosing strategy with this agent remain under investigation.

C. **Fluids and electrolytes** (see Chaps. 23 and 28). Fluid requirements increase tremendously as gestational age decreases <28 weeks, owing to both an increased surface area–body weight ratio and immaturity of the skin. Renal immaturity may result in large losses of fluid and electrolytes that must be replaced. Early use of humidified incubators significantly reduces insensible fluid losses and, therefore, the total administered volume necessary to maintain fluid balance, especially when care interventions are coordinated to ensure that the incubator top is only rarely opened.

1. **Route of administration.** Whenever possible, an umbilical arterial line and a double-lumen umbilical venous line are placed shortly after birth. Arterial lines are maintained for 7 to 10 days and then replaced by peripheral arterial lines if needed. Umbilical venous catheters (UVC) may be used for as long as 7 to 14 days (although we prefer to limit use to 10 days) and are then often replaced by percutaneously inserted central venous catheters (PICC) if continued long-term intravenous (IV) access is required.

2. **Rate of administration.** Table 13.2 presents initial rates of fluid administration for different gestational ages and birth weights when humidified incubators are used. We monitor weight, blood pressure, urine output, and serum

Table 13.2	Fluid Administration Rates for the First 2 Days of Life for Infants on Radiant Warmers*		
Birth weight (g)	Gestational age (wk)	Fluid rate (mL/kg/d)	Frequency of electrolyte testing
500–600	23	110–120	q6h
601–800	24	100–110	q8h
801–1,000	25–26	80–100	q12h

*Rates should be 20%–30% lower when a humidified incubator is used. Urine output and serum electrolytes should be closely monitored to determine the best rates.

electrolyte levels frequently. Fluid rate is adjusted to avoid dehydration or hypernatremia. We generally measure electrolytes before the age of 12 hours (6 hours for infants <800 g) and repeat as often as every 6 hours until the levels are stable. By the second to third day, many infants have a marked diuresis and natriuresis and require continued frequent assessment and adjustment of fluids and electrolytes. Insensible water loss diminishes as the skin thickens and dries over the first few days of life.

3. **Fluid composition.** Initial IV fluids should consist of dextrose solution in a concentration sufficient to maintain serum glucose levels >45 to 50 mg/dL. Often, immature infants do not tolerate dextrose concentrations >10% at high fluid rates, so we generally use dextrose 7.5% or 5% solutions. Usually, a glucose administration rate of 4 to 10 mg/kg/minute is sufficient. If hyperglycemia results, we lower dextrose concentrations but avoid hypo-osmolar solutions (dextrose <5%). If hyperglycemia persists at levels above 180 mg/dL with glycosuria, we begin an insulin infusion at a dose of 0.05 to 0.1 unit/kg/hour and adjust as required (see Chap. 24).

ELBW infants begin losing protein and develop negative nitrogen balance almost immediately after birth. To avoid this, we start parenteral nutrition immediately upon admission to the NICU, using a premixed solution of amino acids and trace elements in dextrose 5% to 7.5%. Multivitamin solutions are not included in this initial parenteral nutrition because of shelf-life issues but are added within 24 hours after delivery. No electrolytes are added to the initial solution other than the small amount of sodium phosphate needed to buffer the amino acids. The solution is designed so that the administration of 60 mL/kg/day (the maximum infusion rate used) provides 2 g of protein/kg/day. Additional fluid needs are met by the solutions described earlier. Customized parenteral nutrition, including lipid infusion, is begun as soon as it is available, generally within the first day.

4. **Skin care.** Immaturity of skin and susceptibility to damage requires close attention to maintenance of skin integrity (see Chap. 63). Topical emollients or petroleum-based products are not used except under extreme situations, but semipermeable coverings (Tegaderm and Vigilon) may be used over areas of skin breakdown.

D. **Cardiovascular support**

1. **Blood pressure.** There is disagreement over acceptable values for blood pressure in extremely premature infants and some suggestions that cerebral perfusion may be adversely affected at levels below a mean blood pressure of 30 mm Hg. In the absence of data demonstrating an impact on long-term neurologic outcome, we accept mean blood pressures of 26 to 28 mm Hg for infants of 24 to 26 weeks' gestational age if the infant appears well perfused and has a stable heart rate. Early hypotension is more commonly due to altered vasoreactivity than hypovolemia, so therapy with fluid boluses is limited to 10 to 20 mL/kg, after which pressor support, initially with dopamine, is begun. Stress dose hydrocortisone (1 mg/kg every 12 hours for two doses) may be useful in infants with hypotension refractory to this strategy (see Chap. 40).

2. **Patent ductus arteriosus (PDA).** The incidence of symptomatic PDA is as high as 70% in infants with a birth weight <1,000 g. The natural timing of presentation has been accelerated by exogenous surfactant therapy, so that a symptomatic PDA now commonly occurs between 24 and 48 hours after birth, manifested by an increasing need for ventilatory support or an increase in oxygen requirement. A murmur may be absent or difficult to hear, and the physical signs of increased pulses or an active precordium may be difficult to discern. Infants with a symptomatic PDA have a higher risk of BPD, but early closure does not decrease this risk. While our practice includes treatment, we have found it prudent to delay indomethacin or ibuprofen therapy until the PDA has been evaluated by echocardiography and demonstrated to be causing a diminution in left ventricular function and distal flow in the descending aorta. Therapy may also be initiated when overt clinical signs of cardiorespiratory compromise are present, and echocardiography is not readily available. Prophylactic treatment with indomethacin has been demonstrated to reduce the incidence and severity of PDA and the need for subsequent ligation. However, it has not been demonstrated to result in a change in long-term neurologic or respiratory outcome. While it has not become routine therapy, many centers continue to use prophylactic indomethacin. Persistent or recurrent confirmed PDA is treated with a second course of indomethacin or ibuprofen. Recurrence of a PDA with a significant left to right shunt after a second treatment course is generally an indication for surgical ligation.

E. **Blood transfusions.** These are often necessary in small infants because of large obligatory phlebotomy losses. Infants who weigh <1,000 g at birth and are moderately or severely ill may receive as many as eight or nine transfusions in the first few weeks of life. Donor exposure can be limited by reducing laboratory testing to the minimum necessary level, employing strict uniform criteria for transfusion and identifying a specific unit of blood for each patient likely to need several transfusions (see Chap. 45). Each such unit can be split to provide as many as eight transfusions for a single patient over a period of 21 days with only a single donor exposure. Erythropoietin therapy in conjunction with adequate iron therapy will result in accelerated erythropoiesis, but it has not been shown to reduce the need for transfusion and is not routinely used in these patients.

F. **Infection and infection control** (see Chap. 49). In general, premature birth is associated with an increased incidence of early-onset sepsis, with an incidence of 1.5% of infants having birth weight <1,500 g. Group B Streptococcus (GBS) remains an important pathogen, but gram-negative organisms now account for most of early-onset sepsis in infants weighing <1,500 g. We almost always screen for infection immediately after birth, and treat with prophylactic antibiotics (ampicillin and gentamicin) pending culture results. ELBW infants are particularly susceptible to nosocomial infections (occurring at >72 hours after birth), and in some reports, as many as one-third of infants weighing <1,000 g at birth have had at least one episode of late-onset sepsis, with wide variations in its incidence between centers. When these infections do occur, almost half are due to coagulase-negative Staphylococcus, 18% due to gram-negative organisms, and 12% due to fungi, although important center differences in pathogens exist. Mortality is higher among infants who develop these late-onset infections, particularly in those with gram-negative infections. Risk factors for late-onset infection include longer duration of mechanical ventilation, umbilical and central venous lines, and parenteral nutrition support.

Several reports have demonstrated that some of these late-onset infections (particularly central line-associated infections) can be prevented by improvements in care practices. Foremost among these is meticulous attention to hand washing. We use alcohol-based gel, containers of which are available at every bedside and prominently in other spots throughout the NICU. We also use periodic anonymous observation to monitor and report on hand hygiene practices before any caregiver–patient contact. In-line suctioning is used in respiratory circuits to minimize disruption, and every effort is made to minimize the duration of mechanical ventilation. We only use parenteral nutrition solutions that have been prepared under laminar flow, and never alter them after preparation. The early introduction of feedings, preferably with human milk, minimizes the need for central lines and provides the benefits of milk-borne immune factors. When central lines are necessary, we have an observer monitor the PICC insertion technique and immediately identify deviation or omission from a standard checklist. Dedicated central line insertion teams are employed in many units and help standardize insertion techniques to reduce the risk of infection. After insertion, attention to scrupulous central line care to avoid line hub bacterial colonization also has been shown to reduce the risk of central line-associated bacterial infection. Laboratory testing is kept to a minimum, and tests clustered whenever possible, to reduce the number of skin punctures and to reduce patient handling. These practices are part of a standardized protocol for skin care for all neonates born with weight of <1,000 g. Ideally, the establishment of a uniform NICU culture that rejects the idea that these infections are inevitable and fosters pride in care and cooperation has helped create an environment of blameless questioning between practitioners.

G. Nutritional support (see Chap. 21)

1. **Initial management.** In all infants who weigh <1,200 g at birth, parenteral nutrition is begun shortly after birth using a standard solution administered at a rate of 60 mL/kg/day (see IV.C.3.), resulting in protein administration of 2 g/kg/day. On subsequent days, customized parenteral solutions are formulated to increase the protein administration rate by 1 g/kg/day up to a maximum of 4 g/kg/day. Parenteral lipids are begun on Day 2 and advanced each day to a maximum of 3 g/kg/day. Enteral feeding is begun as soon as the patient is clinically stable and is not receiving indomethacin or pressor therapy.

2. The safe initiation of enteral feeds begins with the introduction of small trophic amounts of expressed breast milk, donor breast milk, or premature formula (10–20 mL/kg/day), with the goal of priming the gut by inducing local factors necessary for normal function. This amount may be started even in the presence of an umbilical arterial line and are continued for 3 to 4 days without

a change in volume. Feedings of 20 cal/30 mL breast milk or formula are then slowly advanced (10–20 mL/kg/day) while monitoring for signs of feeding intolerance such as abdominal distention, vomiting (which is rare), and increased gastric residuals. It is important but often difficult to differentiate the characteristically poor gastrointestinal motility of ELBW infants from signs of a more serious gastrointestinal disorder such as necrotizing enterocolitis (see Chap. 27). At least two-thirds of our ELBW infants have episodes of feeding intolerance that result in interruption of feeds. Once successful tolerance of feedings is established at 90 to 100 mL/kg/day, caloric density is advanced to 24 cal/30 mL, and then the volume is advanced (see Chap. 21). This eliminates a drop in caloric intake as parenteral nutrition is weaned while feedings advance. Once tolerance of full feedings of 24 cal/30 mL is established, the density of feedings may be advanced by 2 cal/30 mL/day up to a maximum of 30 to 32 cal/30 mL. Protein powder is added to a total protein content of 4 g/kg/day, as this promotes improved somatic and head growth over the first several weeks of life. Many extremely small infants benefit from restriction of total fluids to 130 to 140 mL/kg/day. This minimizes problems with fluid excess while still providing adequate caloric intake.

Suggested Readings

Ballard RA, Truog WE, Cnaan A, et al. Inhaled nitric oxide in preterm infants undergoing mechanical ventilation. *N Engl J Med* 2006;355:343–353.

Horbar JD, Rogowski J, Plsek PE, et al. Collaborative quality improvement for neonatal intensive care. NICQ Project Investigators of the Vermont Oxford Network. *Pediatrics* 2001;107:14–22.

Laughton MM, Simmons MA, Bose CL. Patency of the ductus arteriosus in the premature infant: is it pathologic? Should it be treated? *Curr Opin Pediatr* 2004;16:146–151.

Manley BJ, Dawson JA, Kamlin CO, et al. Clinical assessment of extremely premature infants in the delivery room is a poor predictor of survival. *Pediatrics* 2010;125(3):e559–e564.

Morley CJ, Davis PG, Doyle LW, et al. Nasal CPAP or intubation at birth for very preterm infants. *N Engl J Med* 2008;358:700–708.

Schmidt B, Davis P, Moddemann D, et al. Long-term effects of indomethacin prophylaxis in extremely low birth weight infants. *N Engl J Med* 2001;344(26):1966–1972.

Seri I. Management of hypotension and low systemic blood flow in the very low birth weight neonate during the first postnatal week. *J Perinatol* 2006;26(suppl 1):S8–S13.

Stoll BJ, Hansen N, Fanaroff AA, et al. Late-onset sepsis in very low birth weight neonates: the experience of the NICHD Neonatal Research Network. *Pediatrics* 2002;110:285–291.

SUPPORT Study Group of the Eunice Kennedy Shriver NICHD Neonatal Research Network. Early CPAP versus surfactant in extremely preterm infants. *N Engl J Med* 2010; 362:1970–1979.

SUPPORT Study Group of the Eunice Kennedy Shriver NICHD Neonatal Research Network. Target ranges of oxygen saturation in extremely preterm infants. *N Engl J Med* 2010;362:1959–1969.

Tyson JE, Parikh NA, Langer J, et al. Intensive care for extreme prematurity—moving beyond gestational age. *N Engl J Med* 2008;358(16):1672–1681.

Vohra S, Roberts RS, Zhang B, et al. Heat loss prevention (HeLP) in the delivery room: A randomized controlled trial of polyethylene occlusive skin wrapping in very preterm infants. *J Pediatr* 2004;145(6):750–753.

Wood NS, Marlow N, Costeloe K, et al. Neurologic and developmental disability after extremely preterm birth. EPICure Study Group. *N Engl J Med* 2000;343(6):378–384.

14 Developmentally Supportive Care

Carol Spruill Turnage and Lu-Ann Papile

I. INTRODUCTION. Individualized developmentally supportive care (IDSC) promotes a culture that respects the personhood of preterm and medically fragile term infants and optimizes the care and environment in which health care is delivered to this neurodevelopmentally vulnerable population. Implementing the principles of family-focused IDSC in a neonatal intensive care unit (NICU) environment promotes improved family adaptation and may improve neurodevelopmental outcomes.

Preterm infants have a substantially higher incidence of cognitive, neuromotor, neurosensory, and feeding problems than infants born at full term. Fluctuations in the cerebral circulation that occur in preterm infants even during routine care and smaller than expected brain volumes at 36 to 40 weeks' postmenstrual age (PMA) may contribute to this increased morbidity. Changes in cerebral oxygenation and blood volume measured with near-infrared spectroscopy (NIRS) that occur during diaper changes with elevation of legs and buttocks, during endotracheal tube (ET) suctioning and repositioning, during routine physical assessment, and during standard gavage feedings have been associated with early parenchymal brain abnormalities. IDSC helps to minimize these disturbances.

II. ASSESSMENT. Identification of an infant's stress responses and self-regulating behaviors at rest, as well as during routine care and procedures, is essential in order to create plans of care that support and promote optimal neurodevelopment (Table 14.1). Ideally, an infant's cues are continuously monitored and the care plan is modified as needed to lessen stress and promote stability. Acutely ill term infants have responses to stress and pain similar to those of preterm infants and may not respond as robustly as healthy infants. Their cues are often easier to read than the preterm infant because they have more mature autonomic, motor, and state behaviors.

A. **Stress responses.** Autonomic, motoric, state, organizational behavior and attentional/interactive signs of stress combine to provide a baseline profile of an infant's overall tolerance to various stimuli. Autonomic signs of stress include changes in color, heart rate, and respiratory patterns as well as visceral changes such as gagging, hiccupping, vomiting, and stooling. Motoric signs of stress include facial grimacing, gaping mouth, twitching, hyperextension of limbs, finger splaying, back arching, flailing, and generalized hypertonia or hypotonia. Jerky movements and tremors are associated with the preterm infant's immature neuromotor system. State alterations suggesting stress include rapid state transitions, diffuse sleep states, irritability, and lethargy. Changes in attention or the interactional availability of preterm infants, exhibited by covering eyes/face, gaze aversion, frowning, and hyperalert or panicky facial presentation, represent signs of stress in premature infants.

Table 14.1		Neurobehavioral Organization and Facilitation	
System	Signs of stress	Signs of stability	Interventions
Autonomic			
Respiratory	Tachypnea, pauses, irregular breathing pattern, slow respirations, sighing, or gasping	Smooth, unlabored breathing; regular rate and pattern	Reduce light, noise, and activity at bedside (place pagers/phone on vibrate, lower conversation levels at bedside)
Color	Pale, mottled, red, dusky, or cyanotic	Stable, overall pink color	Use hand containment and pacifier during exams, procedures, or care
			Slowly awaken with soft voice before touch including all procedures, exams, and care unless hearing impaired, use slow movement transitions
Visceral	Several coughs, sneezes, yawns, hiccups, gagging and grunting and straining associated with defecation, spitting up	Visceral stability, smooth digestion, tolerates feeding	Pace feedings by infant's ability and cues in appropriately modified environment
Autonomic-related motor patterns	Tremors, startles, twitches of face and/or body, extremities	Tremors, startles, twitching not observed	Gently reposition while containing extremities close to body if premature
			Avoid sleep disruption

(continued)

Table 14.1	Neurobehavioral Organization and Facilitation *(Continued)*		
System	Signs of stress	Signs of stability	Interventions
			Position appropriately for neuromotor development and comfort; use nesting/boundaries or swaddling as needed to reduce tremors, startles
			Manage pain appropriately
Motor			
Tone	Either hypertonia or hypotonia; limp/flaccid body, extremities and/or face; hyperflexion	Consistent, reliable tone for postmenstrual age (PMA); controlled or more control of movement, activity, and posture	Support rest periods/reduce sleep disruption, minimize stress, contain or swaddle
Posture	Unable to maintain flexed, aligned, comfortable posture	Improved or well-maintained posture; with maturation posture sustainable without supportive aids	Provide boundaries, positioning aids, or swaddling for flexion, containment, alignment, and comfort as appropriate
Level of activity	Frequent squirming, frantic flailing activity or little to no movement	Activity consistent with environment, situation, and PMA	Intervene as needed for pain management, environmental modification, less stimulation; encourage skin-to-skin holding; containment

State		
Sleep	Restless, facial twitching, movement; irregular respirations, fussing, grimacing, whimpers or makes sounds; responsive to environment	Quiet, restful sleep periods; less body/facial movement; little response to environment	Comfortable and age appropriate positioning for sleep with a quiet, dim environment and no interruptions except medical necessity Position with hands to face or mouth or so they can learn to achieve this on their own
Awake	Low level arousal with unfocused eyes; hyperalert expression of worry/panic; cry face or crying; actively avoids eye contact by averting gaze or closing eyes; irritability, prolonged awake periods; difficult to console or inconsolable	Alert, bright, shiny eyes with focused attention on an object or person; robust crying; calms quickly with intervention, consolable in 2–5 minutes	Encourage parent holding as desired either traditional or skin-to-skin May be ready for brief eye contact around 30–32 weeks without displaying stress cues Support awake moments with PMA appropriate activity based on stress and stability data for individual infant

(continued)

Table 14.1	Neurobehavioral Organization and Facilitation *(Continued)*		
System	Signs of stress	Signs of stability	Interventions
Self-regulation			
Motor	Little attempt to flex or tuck body, few attempts to push feet against boundaries, unable to maintain hands to face or mouth, sucking a pacifier may be more stressful than soothing	Strategies for self-regulation include: foot bracing against boundaries or own feet/leg; hands grasped together; hand to mouth or face, grasping blanket or tubes, tucking body/truck; sucking; position changes	Examine using blanket swaddle or nest to support infant regulation by removing only a small part of the body at a time while keeping most of body contained during
			Ask a parent or nurse to provide support during exams, tests, or procedures; swaddle or contain as needed to keep limbs close to body during care or exams and to provide boundaries for grasping or foot bracing
			Position for sleep with hands to face or mouth
			Provide pacifier intermittently when awake and at times other than exams, care, or procedures
			Give older infants something to hold (maybe a finger or blanket)

State	Rapid state transitions, unable to move to drowsy or sleep state when stressed, states are not clear to observers	Transitions smoothly from high arousal states to quiet alert or sleep state; focused attention on an object or person; maintains quiet alert state without stress or with some facilitation	Encourage parenting to support parenting skill; teach parents communication cues and behaviors; model appropriate responses to cues
			Consistently avoid rapid disruption of state behavior (e.g., starting an exam without preparing the baby for the intrusion) by awakening slowly with soft speech or touch, use indirect lighting or shield eyes depending on PMA during exams or care
			Assist return to sleep or quiet alert state after handling
			Provide auditory and facial visual stimulation for quietly alert infants based on cues; premature infants may need to start with only one mode of stimulation initially, adding others based on cues
			Swaddling or containment to facilitate state control or maintenance

Modified from Als H. Toward a synactive theory of development: promise for the assessment and support of infant individuality. *Infant Ment Health J* 1982;3:229–243; Als H. A synactive model of neonatal behavior organization: framework for the assessment of neurobehavioral development in the premature infant and for support of infants and parents in the neonatal intensive care environment. *Phys Occup Ther Pediatr* 1986;6:3–55; Hunter JG. The neonatal intensive care unit. In: Case-Smith J, Allen AS, Pratt PN, eds. *Occupational Therapy for Children.* St. Louis, MO: Mosby; 2001:593; Carrier CT, Walden M, Wilson D. The high-risk newborn and family. In: Hockenberry MJ, ed. *Wong's Nursing Care of Infants and Children.* 7th ed. St. Louis, MO: Mosby; 2003.

B. **Self-regulating behavior.** Preterm infants employ a number of self-consoling behaviors to cope with stress. Self-regulating behaviors include hand or foot bracing, sucking, bringing hands to face, flexed positioning, cooing, and grasping of linens, tubing, or own body parts. Painful procedures may overwhelm an infant's ability to self-console. Infant support during stressful situations requires facilitation by a nurse, physician, or parent.

III. GOALS OF DEVELOPMENTAL SUPPORT.

Developmental support of high-risk infants necessitates attention by caregivers to observable cues (autonomic, motor, and state) and being responsive to these cues. Infant cues provide clues to the type of intervention that may be most effective in decreasing responses to stress and the subsequent physiologic cost. The individual caregiver must learn to recognize and appropriately respond when an infant communicates stress, pain, or the need for attention. A priority of IDSC is for infants to experience auditory, visual, and social input without disrupting autonomic, motor, or state function and integration. Once this objective is achieved, preterm and high-risk neonates can begin to explore their world and relate to their parents during meaningful and reciprocal exchanges.

A. **Supporting autonomic system stability.** Because the autonomic and visceral systems cannot be impacted directly, motor and environmental modifications are used to assist an infant's return to a stable, calm state that supports autonomic stability. Interventions, including swaddling, hand-containment (facilitated tuck), and nesting with boundaries, are efficacious in calming and reducing pain responses. Feedings with anticipatory planning for a quiet, calm environment, swaddling to reduce motor arousal, and letting the infant guide the pace of the feeding are more likely to be successful and elicit less stress behaviors.

B. **Intervening through the motor system.** Support of the motor system is focused on development and function, as well as prevention of acquired positioning deformities or functional limitations. Containment of the motor system or "facilitated tuck" is useful for calming or support during care and/or procedures. Positioning aids are needed when an infant cannot sustain a flexed, aligned posture with midline orientation that is also comfortable. Term infants who cannot maintain age-appropriate posture and/or movement due to neuromuscular disease, congenital anomalies, severity of illness, or medications can develop musculoskeletal problems or loss of skin integrity with improper bedding and support and also need positioning support.

C. **Creating environments that cultivate state organization.** Preterm infants have poor state control with less ability to maintain a state and variable transition between states compared to term infants. Environmental modifications are made to promote quiet, focused attentional states and foster periods of well-defined, restful sleep with regular respirations and little movement. To promote the development of state organization, it is important to avoid activities that cause abrupt state transitions, such as rousing an infant from sleep during repositioning for an examination. Letting an infant know when a caregiver approaches to perform care at the bedside by using soft speech (infant's name), gentle touch, and gradual containment with repositioning can alleviate abrupt state disruption. Staff, parents, and others need to be consistent in their approach.

IV. DEVELOPMENTALLY SUPPORTIVE ENVIRONMENT. By providing a developmentally supportive NICU environment, neonatal caregivers can support neurologic and sensory development and potentially minimize negative outcomes in preterm and medically fragile infants. The acutely ill term infant also requires environmental modifications that reduce stress and promote sleep and recovery. When possible, anticipation of an infant's environmental needs prior to admission is ideal.

A. **Sound.** Increased noise levels in the NICU are associated with physiologic stress and autonomic instability. Intense noise levels at around 55 to 60 dBA and above disrupt sleep and may impact brain development occurring during both active/light sleep and quiet sleep. The development of sleep state organization may also be altered. The American Academy of Pediatrics (AAP) recommends that average NICU sound levels not exceed 50 A-weighted decibels (dBA). An IDSC program includes systematic efforts to manage environmental sound (e.g., low conversational tones, rounding away from the bedside, placing pagers on vibrate mode, care in opening and closing portholes). Baseline sound levels need to be measured along with an evaluation of sources contributing to noise intensity or sudden loud sounds. Random monitoring of sound levels is helpful in sustaining noise abatement.

An important consideration is that the most natural source of sound for the premature and medically fragile infant is mother's voice. If a baby cannot distinguish the maternal voice from ambient noise, auditory development may be altered from the natural evolution that begins in the womb.

B. **Light.** The relationship between ambient light and neurodevelopment is less clear. Reduced illumination (i.e., dark incubator covers and eye patches during phototherapy) is associated with increased autonomic stability in preterm infants and more frequent eye opening among preterm and term infants. An additional developmental benefit of reducing environmental light is a reduction in environmental noise and less handling of infants. Early preterm infants may experience discomfort when exposed to intense light due to very thin eyelids that cannot block light and an immature pupillary reflex that is not apparent until around 30 weeks' PMA. Visual stimulation before 30 to 32 weeks' PMA is often accompanied by stress responses. Protection from light for the early preterm infant can be accomplished with thick, quilted covers that have dark material on the side facing the incubator. Lighting for staff needs to be at levels that allow safe and efficient functioning. During procedures, the infant's eyes need to be protected from direct light using blanket tents or other methods that do not require tactile input. Eye covers can be used but may be another source of tactile stress.

Reduction of light in the NICU does not appear to affect the incidence or progression of retinopathy of prematurity or alter visually evoked potentials measured in early childhood. As these are relatively short-term outcomes, long-term effects of early, atypical lighting and visual stimulation are still unknown.

The AAP Guidelines for Perinatal Care recommends illumination parameters from 10 to 600 lux with separate procedure lighting of not more than 1,000 to 1,500 lux. The AAP also supports the recommendation of the Illuminating Engineering Society and the 2007 Consensus Committee on NICU design that new or renovated NICUs provide ambient lighting of 10 to 20 lux, levels similar to those used in cycled lighting research for the daylight treatment.

Cycled lighting may be beneficial for preterm infants, but the gestational age at which light intensity, day/night pattern, and light duration is safe and beneficial is not known. Preterm infants who have been exposed to cycled lighting at 30 weeks' gestational age and beyond have greater weight gain, earlier oral feeding, and more regulated patterns of rest/activity after discharge than control groups. However, atypical sensory stimulation to one sensory system may adversely affect the function of another sensory system. Until more is understood about light exposure, a conservative approach is best.

V. DEVELOPMENTALLY SUPPORTIVE CARE PRACTICES. Developmental support in the NICU requires collaboration and teamwork to integrate the developmental needs of infants within the context of medical treatment and nursing care. This entails a coordinated, primary team that includes the family and is designed to work in partnership around the infant's state of alertness, sleep cycles, communication cues, medical condition, and family presence. The goal is to maximize rest, minimize stress, and optimize healing and growth in a framework that supports family participation.

A. Positioning. The goals are to facilitate flexed and midline positioning of extremities, stabilize respiratory patterns, and lessen physiologic stress. Interventions include flexion, containment, midline alignment, and comfort. The use of "nesting materials" (e.g., soft blanket rolls, commercially available positioning devices) or swaddling is useful in minimizing the upper/lower extremity abduction, scapular retraction, and cervical hyperextension typical of premature infants. More mature infants with congenital neuromuscular or skeletal disorders may also need positioning support.

Nesting needs to allow sufficient room for the preterm infant to push against boundaries, because the ability to move as a fetus does in the womb allows further development of the neuromotor and skeletal systems.

B. Feeding. Oral feeding is a complex task requiring physiologic maturation, coordination of suck–swallow–breathe mechanics, and development of oral motor skills. Breastfeeding is the preferred method, and breast milk is recommended for both preterm and term infants (see Chap. 22). The transition to bottle from tube feeding requires excellent assessment and judgment on the part of the caregiver. An infant who is successful in learning to nipple and enjoy feeding may be less likely to develop feeding problems after discharge. It is important that the infants learn to feed properly and that family members are able to feed them without using unorthodox techniques at home. Progression to oral feeds is highly contingent upon elements of IDSC and occurs predictably in several phases. Pre–non-nutritive suck (NNS) is characterized by weak suck and instability of motor, autonomic, and state regulation systems; NNS is characterized by more optimal suck patterns and should be encouraged during gavage feeds. Nutritive suck typically begins at approximately 33 weeks' PMA and progresses to full oral intake as autonomic stability and oral motor coordination improve. Strategies to promote successful progression through these phases include identifying and minimizing signs of physiologic stress, environmental modification to promote autonomic stability, feeding in a flexed, midline position, pacing techniques, and use of slow-flow nipples. Considerations for a feeding plan include opportunities to practice, environmental preparation to minimize stressors, and using the infant's feeding readiness cues to start feedings rather than strict adherence to a specific PMA, specific time intervals, and feeding duration. Infants fed using feeding readiness cues experience significantly fewer adverse events during feedings, reach full oral feeding sooner, are discharged earlier, gain the same amount of weight as controls, and demonstrate about three cues per feeding. In addition, experiential feeding, that is feeding frequently during the day without regard for duration, also results in less time to full oral feeding. Leaving a gavage tube in place during initial feeding attempts or repeated insertions may cause discomfort and interfere with feeding progression or generate oral aversion and later feeding disorders. Research is needed to understand more about the risk factors of feeding behavior disorders associated with aversive or repeated noxious stimulation of the oropharynx and gastrointestinal tract.

C. Touch

1. **Hand containment or facilitated tuck** can be provided by parents soon after admission. This technique reduces pain responses during painful and non-painful events. Parents can be taught how to touch their infant in ways that are nurturing and will not create stress.

2. **Kangaroo care** is another technique consistently associated with improved infant outcomes (i.e., fewer respiratory complications, improved weight gain, and temperature regulation) and maternal outcomes (i.e., improved maternal competence and longer breastfeeding duration). Mothers who use kangaroo holding produce a greater volume of breast milk than mothers who hold in the traditional way. Kangaroo care can be initiated as soon as infants are medically stable. Infants are held on their mother's or father's chest wearing only a diaper and are covered with a blanket and hat as needed. A minimum of 1 hour is recommended for kangaroo holding. An NICU protocol for kangaroo holding ensures safety and minimizes an infant's stress response to handling/ positioning. Kangaroo holding impacts several developing sensory systems including tactile (skin), olfactory, and vestibular (rise/fall of chest). A parent is close enough for soft speech to be audible to his or her infant if ambient noise is minimized. The preterm infant's visual capacity is not challenged since eye-to-eye contact is not a necessary component for kangaroo care. Parents can be with their infant earlier in a way that is satisfying for them and supportive for their baby.

D. Team collaboration and consistency of care. Developmental care is not considered additional or "extra" support for an infant that is done only when time allows or in nonemergent situations. The unpredictable nature of care in the NICU can be diminished by consistent caregivers who are familiar with an infant's clinical and behavioral baseline, provide care in a similar manner, respond quickly to cues, and provide relevant information to all members of the infant's team, including the family to create an individualized plan of care. The developmental plan is complementary to the medical plan and uses developmental principles, techniques, and environmental modifications to reduce stressors that challenge an infant's physiologic stability through behavioral instability.

VI. PAIN AND STRESS. Pain assessment and management is a basic right of *all* patients. Evidence-based assessment and practice guidelines facilitate the use of pain management by physicians, nurses, and other practitioners. A streamlined approach using algorithms may enhance utilization at the bedside.

A. Pain. Effective nonpharmacologic interventions incorporate developmental principles such as swaddling, NNS, kangaroo holding, hand containment/facilitated tuck, breastfeeding, and administration of an oral sucrose solution (see Chap. 67). Nonpharmacologic measures are used as an adjunct to pharmacologic treatment of moderate-to-severe pain (see Chap. 67).

B. The AAP and the Canadian Pediatric Society advocate management of both pain and stress. High-stress situations need to be identified and modified to minimize the impact on the ill or preterm neonate. Examples of potential high-stress conditions include delivery room care, transport to NICU, admission process, and diagnostic procedures that often produce pain or discomfort along with stress. During stressful events, developmental support based on infant cues guides the NICU team's care.

VII. PARENT SUPPORT/EDUCATION. Effective IDSC is dependent on implementation of the principles of family-centered care during NICU stay as well as upon transition to home.

A. **In the NICU.** Premature birth and NICU hospitalization negatively impact parent–infant interactions, which, in turn, is associated with long-term adverse developmental sequelae. Individual family-centered interactions (i.e., family-based developmental evaluations, support, and education) have been associated with reduced parent stress and more positive parent–infant interactions. Family-centered NICU policies include welcoming families 24 hours/day, promotion of family participation in infant care, creation of parent advisory boards, implementation of parent support groups, and comfortable rooming-in areas for parents.

B. **Discharge teaching.** Because brain growth and maturation may occur at a slower rate in the extrauterine environment, parents must be prepared for the fact that their baby is not likely to behave as a term baby would, even after he or she has reached 40 weeks' PMA. Many parents report being ill-prepared for discharge from the NICU with respect to recognizing signs of illness, employing effective calming strategies, being aware of typical and delayed development, and using strategies to promote infant development. Teaching that begins well before discharge can help parents be better prepared to assume the primary caregiving role.

C. **Postdischarge family supports.** Parents of premature infants report feeling frightened and alone following discharge from the NICU, even when sent home with services from a visiting nurse and early intervention specialists. Support groups for parents of premature infants designed to provide long-term emotional and educational support are available in many communities. Additionally, magazines, books, and web-based materials related to parenting preterm infants are available. A promising approach to facilitating seamless transition to community-based services includes referral to the federally mandated Early Intervention (EI) program before the infant's discharge and collaboration between NICU and EI professionals to create a developmentally supportive transition plan.

D. **Infant follow-up and EI programs.** The focus of a follow-up program is to prevent or minimize developmental delay through early identification of risk factors and referral to appropriate treatment programs. Close follow-up is paramount to maximizing developmental outcome. Which group of infants is followed and the frequency of follow-up assessments are dependent upon state and medical center resources. Regardless, every center that cares for medically fragile and preterm neonates should have a follow-up program in place.

Suggested Readings

Als H. *Manual for the Naturalistic Observation of Newborn Behavior: Newborn Individualized Developmental Care and Assessment Program.* Boston: Harvard Medical School; 1995.

Kenner C, McGrath JM, eds. *Developmental Care of Newborns and Infants: A Guide for Health Professionals.* St. Louis, MO: Mosby; 2010.

Laadt VL, Woodward BJ, Papile LA. System of risk triage: a conceptual framework to guide referral and developmental intervention decisions in the NICU. *Infants & Young Children* 2007;20(4):336–344.

Turnage-Carrier C. Developmental support. In: Walden M, Verklan T, eds. *Core Curriculum for Neonatal Nursing.* 4th ed. Philadelphia: WB Saunders; 2010:208–232.

Temperature Control
Kimberlee Chatson

I. HEAT PRODUCTION. In adults, thermoregulation is achieved by both metabolic and muscular activity (e.g., shivering). During pregnancy, maternal mechanisms maintain intrauterine temperature. After birth, newborns must adapt to their relatively cold environment by the metabolic production of heat because they are not able to generate an adequate shivering response.

Term newborns have a source for thermogenesis in brown fat, which is highly vascularized and innervated by sympathetic neurons. When these infants face cold stress, norepinephrine levels increase and act in the brown fat tissue to stimulate lipolysis. Most of the free fatty acids (FFAs) are re-esterified or oxidized; both reactions produce heat. Hypoxia or β-adrenergic blockade decreases this response.

II. TEMPERATURE MAINTENANCE

A. Premature infants experience increased mechanisms of heat loss combined with decreased heat production capabilities. These special problems in temperature maintenance put them at a disadvantage compared with term infants; premature infants have the following:

1. A higher ratio of skin surface area to weight
2. Highly permeable skin, which leads to increased transepidermal water loss
3. Decreased subcutaneous fat, with less insulative capacity
4. Less-developed stores of brown fat
5. Decreased glycogen stores
6. The inability to take in enough calories to provide nutrients for thermogenesis and growth
7. Limited oxygen consumption when pulmonary problems exist

B. Cold stress. Premature infants subjected to acute hypothermia respond with peripheral vasoconstriction, causing anaerobic metabolism and metabolic acidosis. This can cause pulmonary vessel constriction, which leads to further hypoxemia, anaerobic metabolism, and acidosis. Hypoxemia further compromises the infant's response to cold. Premature infants are therefore at great risk for hypothermia and its sequelae (i.e., hypoglycemia, metabolic acidosis, increased oxygen consumption). The more common problem facing premature infants is caloric loss from unrecognized chronic cold stress, resulting in excess oxygen consumption and inability to gain weight.

C. Neonatal cold injury occurs in low birth weight infants (LBWs) and term infants with central nervous system (CNS) disorders. It occurs more often in home deliveries, emergency deliveries, and settings where inadequate attention is paid to the thermal environment and heat loss. These infants may have a bright red color because of the failure of oxyhemoglobin to dissociate at low temperature. There may be central pallor or cyanosis. The skin may show edema and sclerema. Core temperature is often <32.2°C (90°F). Signs may include the following: (i) hypotension; (ii) bradycardia; (iii) slow, shallow, irregular respiration; (iv) decreased activity; (v) poor sucking reflex; (vi) decreased response to stimulus; (vii) decreased reflexes; and (viii) abdominal distention or vomiting. Metabolic acidosis, hypoglycemia, hyperkalemia, azotemia, and oliguria are present. Sometimes, there is generalized bleeding, including pulmonary hemorrhage. It is uncertain whether warming should be rapid or slow. Setting the abdominal skin temperature to 1°C higher than the core temperature in a radiant warmer will produce slow rewarming, and setting it to 36.5°C will also result in slow rewarming. If the infant is hypotensive, normal saline (10–20 mL/kg) should be given; sodium bicarbonate is used to correct metabolic acidosis. Infection, bleeding, or injury should be evaluated and treated.

D. Hyperthermia, defined as an elevated core body temperature, may be caused by a relatively hot environment, infection, dehydration, CNS dysfunction, or medications. Placing newborns in sunlight to control bilirubin is hazardous and may be associated with significant hyperthermia.

  If environmental temperature is the cause of hyperthermia, the trunk and extremities are the same temperature and the infant appears vasodilated. In contrast, infants with sepsis are often vasoconstricted, and the extremities are 2°C to 3°C colder than the trunk.

III. MECHANISMS OF HEAT LOSS

A. Radiation. Heat dissipates from the infant to a colder object in the environment.

B. Convection. Heat is lost from the skin to moving air. The amount lost depends on air speed and temperature.

C. Evaporation. The amount of loss depends primarily on air velocity and relative humidity. Wet infants in the delivery room are especially susceptible to evaporative heat loss.

D. Conduction. This is a minor mechanism of heat loss that occurs from the infant to the surface on which he or she lies.

IV. NEUTRAL THERMAL ENVIRONMENTS minimize heat loss. Thermoneutral conditions exist when heat production (measured by oxygen consumption) is minimum and core temperature is within the normal range (Table 15.1).

V. MANAGEMENT TO PREVENT HEAT LOSS

A. Healthy term infant

  1. Standard thermal care guidelines include (i) maintaining the delivery room temperature at 25°C (WHO), (ii) immediately drying the infant (especially the head), (iii) removing wet blankets, and (iv) wrapping the infant in prewarmed blankets. It is also important to prewarm contact surfaces and minimize drafts. A cap is useful in preventing significant heat loss through the scalp, although evidence suggests that only caps made of wool are effective.

Table 15.1	Neutral Thermal Environmental Temperatures	
Age and weight	**Temperature***	
	At start (°C)	**Range (°C)**
0–6 h		
Under 1,200 g	35.0	34.0–35.4
1,200–1,500 g	34.1	33.9–34.4
1,501–2,500 g	33.4	32.8–33.8
Over 2,500 g (and >36 weeks' gestation)	32.9	32.0–33.8
6–12 h		
Under 1,200 g	35.0	34.0–35.4
1,200–1,500 g	34.0	33.5–34.4
1,501–2,500 g	33.1	32.2–33.8
Over 2,500 g (and >36 weeks' gestation)	32.8	31.4–33.8
12–24 h		
Under 1,200 g	34.0	34.0–35.4
1,200–1,500 g	33.8	33.3–34.3
1,501–2,500 g	32.8	31.8–33.8
Over 2,500 g (and >36 weeks' gestation)	32.4	31.0–33.7
24–36 h		
Under 1,200 g	34.0	34.0–35.0
1,200–1,500 g	33.6	33.1–34.2
1,501–2,500 g	32.6	31.6–33.6
Over 2,500 g (and >36 weeks' gestation)	32.1	30.7–33.5

(continued)

Table 15.1	*(Continued)*	
	Temperature*	
Age and weight	**At start (°C)**	**Range (°C)**
36–48 h		
Under 1,200 g	34.0	34.0–35.0
1,200–1,500 g	33.5	33.0–34.1
1,501–2,500 g	32.5	31.4–33.5
Over 2,500 g (and >36 weeks' gestation)	31.9	30.5–33.3
48–72 h		
Under 1,200 g	34.0	34.0–35.0
1,200–1,500 g	33.5	33.0–34.0
1,501–2,500 g	32.3	31.2–33.4
Over 2,500 g (and >36 weeks' gestation)	31.7	30.1–33.2
72–96 h		
Under 1,200 g	34.0	34.0–35.0
1,200–1,500 g	33.5	33.0–34.0
1,501–2,500 g	32.2	31.1–33.2
Over 2,500 g (and >36 weeks' gestation)	31.3	29.8–32.8
4–12 d		
Under 1,500 g	33.5	33.0–34.0
1,501–2,500 g	32.1	31.0–33.2
Over 2,500 g (and >36 weeks' gestation)	—	—
4–5 d	31.0	29.5–32.6

(continued)

Table 15.1	Neutral Thermal Environmental Temperatures *(Continued)*	
Age and weight	**Temperature***	
	At start (°C)	**Range (°C)**
5–6 d	30.9	29.4–32.3
6–8 d	30.6	29.0–32.2
8–10 d	30.3	29.0–31.8
10–12 d	30.1	29.0–31.4
12–14 d		
Under 1,500 g	33.5	32.6–34.0
1,501–2,500 g	32.1	31.0–33.2
Over 2,500 g (and >36 weeks' gestation)	29.8	29.0–30.8
2–3 wk		
Under 1,500 g	33.1	32.2–34.0
1,501–2,500 g	31.7	30.5–33.0
3–4 wk		
Under 1,500 g	32.6	31.6–33.6
1,501–2,500 g	31.4	30.0–32.7
4–5 wk		
Under 1,500 g	32.0	31.2–33.0
1,501–2,500 g	30.9	29.5–35.2
5–6 wk		
Under 1,500 g	31.4	30.6–32.3
1,501–2,500 g	30.4	29.0–31.8

*Generally speaking, the smaller infants in each weight group will require a temperature in the higher portion of the temperature range. Within each time range, the younger infants require the higher temperatures.
Source: Klaus MH, Fanaroff AA. The physical environment. In: *Care of the high risk neonate.* 5th ed. Philadelphia: WB Saunders; 2001.

2. Examination in the delivery room should be done with the infant under a radiant warmer. A skin probe with servo control to keep skin temperature at 36.5°C (97.7°F) should be used for prolonged examinations.

B. Premature infant

1. Standard thermal care guidelines should be utilized. Additional interventions during the first 10 minutes can optimize thermoregulation.

2. External heat sources, including skin-to-skin care and transwarmer mattresses, have demonstrated a reduction in the risk of hypothermia.

3. Barriers to prevent heat loss should also be used in extremely premature infants. These infants should be placed in a polyethylene bag immediately after birth; the wet body is placed in the bag from the neck down. Plastic wraps and plastic caps also have been effective in infants born at less than 29 weeks.

4. A radiant warmer should be used during resuscitation and stabilization. A heated incubator should be used for transport.

5. In the NICU, infants require a thermoneutral environment to minimize energy expenditure; the incubator should be kept at an appropriate temperature on air mode (see Table 15.1) if a skin probe cannot be used due to the potential damage to skin in small premature infants. Alternatively, skin mode or servo control can be set so that the incubator's internal thermostat responds to changes in the infant's skin temperature to ensure a normal temperature despite any environmental fluctuation.

6. Humidification of incubators has been shown to reduce evaporative heat loss and decrease insensible water loss. Risks and concerns for possible bacterial contamination have been addressed in current incubator designs, which include heating devices that elevate the water temperature to a level that destroys most organisms. Notably, the water transforms into a gaseous vapor and not a mist, thus, eliminating the airborne water droplet as a medium for infection.

7. Servocontrolled open warmer beds may be used for very sick infants when access is important. The use of a tent made of plastic wrap or barrier creams such as Aquaphor (or sunflower seed oil in developing countries) prevent both convection heat loss and insensible water loss (see Chap. 23).

8. Double-walled incubators not only limit radiant heat loss but also decrease convective and evaporative losses.

9. Current technology includes the development of hybrid devices such as the Versalet Incuwarmer (Hill-Rom Air-Shields) and the Giraffe Omnibed (Ohmeda Medical). They offer the features of both a traditional radiant warmer bed and an incubator in a single device. This allows for the seamless conversion between modes, which minimizes thermal stress and allows for ready access to the infant for routine and emergency procedures.

10. Premature infants in relatively stable condition can be dressed in clothes and caps and covered with a blanket. This should be done as soon as possible, even if the infant is on a ventilator. Heart rate and respiration should be continuously monitored because the clothing may limit observation.

VI. HAZARDS OF TEMPERATURE CONTROL METHODS

A. **Hyperthermia.** A servocontrolled warmer can generate excess heat, which can cause severe hyperthermia if the probe becomes detached from the infant's skin. Temperature alarms are subject to mechanical failure.

B. **Undetected infections.** Servo control of temperature may mask the hypothermia or hyperthermia associated with infection. A record of both environmental and core temperatures, along with observation for other signs of sepsis, will help detect infections.

C. **Volume depletion.** Radiant warmers can cause increased insensible water loss. Body weight and input and output should be closely monitored in infants cared for on radiant warmers.

Suggested Readings

Cramer K, Wiebe N, Hartling L, et al. Heat loss prevention: a systematic review of occlusive skin wrap for premature neonates. *J Perinatol* 2005;25(12):763–769.

Klaus MH, Fanaroff AA, eds. The physical environment. In: *Care of the high risk neonate.* 5th ed. Philadelphia: WB Saunders; 2001.

McCall EM, Alderdice FA, Halliday HL, et al. Interventions to prevent hypothermia at birth in preterm and/or low birthweight infants. *Cochrane Database Syst Rev* 2010;(3):CD004210.

Sherman TI, Greenspan JS, St Clair N, et al. Optimizing the neonatal thermal environment. *Neonatal Netw* 2006;25(4):251–260.

Sinclair JC. Servo-control for maintaining abdominal skin temperature at 36°C in low-birth-weight infants. *Cochrane Database Syst Rev* 2002;1:CD001074.

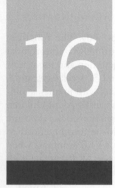

16 Follow-up Care of Very Preterm and Very Low Birth Weight Infants

Jane E. Stewart and Marsha R. Joselow

I. INTRODUCTION. Of the just over four million births per year in this country, 2% or 88,000 are born very preterm, defined as less than 32 weeks' gestational age (GA). Fortunately, the rate of very preterm births appears to have stabilized after a persistent increase over the period from 1990 to 2005; associated with the rising twin and triplet rate presumed to be related to increased use of fertility therapies. With advances in neonatal care, the number of critically ill very preterm infants who survive the neonatal period and are discharged from the NICU has increased; these infants, with their high rate of medical and developmental sequela, have unique follow-up needs that include the utilization of specialized medical and educational resources.

II. MEDICAL CARE ISSUES

A. Respiratory issues (see Chap. 34). Approximately 23% of very low birth weight (VLBW; birth weight <1,500 g) infants and 35% to 45% of extremely low birth weight (ELBW; birth weight <1,000 g) infants develop bronchopulmonary dysplasia (BPD; defined as O_2 dependent at 36 weeks' postmenstrual age). Infants with BPD should be monitored for related morbidities, including acute respiratory exacerbations, upper and lower respiratory infections, reactive airway disease, cardiac problems (e.g., pulmonary hypertension and cor pulmonale), growth failure, and developmental delay. Infants with severe BPD may require treatment with tracheostomy and long-term ventilator support. More commonly, infants with significant BPD require some combination of supplemental oxygen, bronchodilator, steroid, and diuretic therapy.

1. VLBW infants are four times more likely to be rehospitalized during the first year than are higher birth weight infants; up to 60% are rehospitalized at least once by the time they reach school age. Admissions during the first year of life are most commonly for complications of respiratory infections. In a recent study of extremely premature infants, 57% of infants born between 23 to 25 weeks' gestation and 49% of those born between 26 to 28 weeks required rehospitalization in the first 18 months of life. The increased risk of hospitalization persists into early school age; 7% of VLBW children are hospitalized in a given year, compared with 2% of higher birth weight children.

2. **Respiratory syncytial virus (RSV)** is the most important cause of respiratory infection in premature infants, particularly in those with chronic lung disease. To prevent illness caused by RSV, VLBW infants should receive prophylactic

treatment with palivizumab (Synagis) monoclonal antibody. The American Academy of Pediatrics (AAP) recommends treatment during RSV season for at least the first year of life for infants born ≤28 weeks' gestation and for at least the first 6 months of life for those born between 28 and 32 weeks' gestation. Likewise, good hand hygiene by all those in close contact with infants, avoidance of exposure to others with respiratory infections (especially young children during the winter season), and avoidance of passive cigarette smoke exposure to prevent illness caused by respiratory viruses should be recommended to families. The influenza vaccine is also recommended for VLBW infants when they are older than 6 months; until then, care providers in close contact with the infant should strongly consider receiving the influenza vaccine.

3. **Air travel.** In general, air travel is not recommended for infants with BPD because of the increased risk of exposure to infection and because of the lowered cabin pressure resulting in lower oxygen content in the cabin air. If an infant's PaO_2 is ≤80 mm Hg, supplemental oxygen will be needed while flying.

B. **Immunizations.** VLBW infants should receive their routine pediatric immunizations according to the same schedule as term infants, with the exception of Hepatitis B vaccine. Medically stable, thriving infants should receive the Hepatitis B vaccine as early as 30 days of age regardless of gestational age or birth weight. If the baby is ready for discharge to home before 30 days of age, it can be given at the time of discharge to home. Although studies evaluating the long-term immune response to routine immunizations have shown antibody titers to be lower in preterm infants, most achieve titers in the therapeutic range.

C. **Growth.** VLBW infants have a high incidence of feeding and growth problems for multiple reasons. Infants with severe BPD have increased caloric needs for appropriate weight gain. Many of these infants also have abnormal or delayed oral motor development and have oral aversion because of negative oral stimulation during their early life. Growth should be followed carefully on standardized growth curves using the child's age corrected for prematurity for at least the first 2 years of life. Supplemental caloric density is commonly required to optimize growth. Specialized premature infant formulas with increased protein, calcium, and phosphate (either added to human milk or used alone) should be considered in the first 6 to 12 months of life in infants who have borderline growth. ELBW infants commonly demonstrate growth that is close to or below the fifth percentile. However, if their growth runs parallel to the normal curve, they are usually demonstrating a healthy growth pattern. Infants whose growth curve plateaus, or whose growth trajectory falls off, warrant further evaluation to assess caloric intake. If growth failure persists, consultation with a gastroenterologist or endocrinologist to rule out gastrointestinal pathology, such as severe gastroesophageal reflux disease, or endocrinologic problems, such as growth hormone deficiency, should be considered.

Gastrostomy tube placement may be necessary in a small subset of patients with severe feeding problems. Long-term feeding problems are frequent in this population of children and they usually require specialized feeding and oral motor therapy to ultimately wean from gastrostomy tube feedings.

1. **Anemia.** VLBW infants are at risk for iron deficiency anemia and should receive supplemental iron for the first 12 to 15 months of life.

2. **Rickets.** VLBW infants who have had nutritional deficits in calcium, phosphorous, or vitamin D intake are at increased risk for rickets. Infants who are

at highest risk are those treated with long-term parenteral nutrition, furosemide, and those with decreased vitamin D absorption due to fat malabsorption. Infants with rickets diagnosed in the neonatal intensive care unit (NICU) may need continued supplementation of calcium, phosphorous, and vitamin D during the first year of life. All breast fed infants, and those consuming less than 1 Liter per day of formula, should receive 400 IU Vit D supplementation per day for the first year of life.

D. Sensory issues that need follow-up include vision and hearing.

1. Ophthalmologic follow-up (see Chap. 64). Infants with severe retinopathy of prematurity (ROP) are at increased risk for significant vision loss or blindness in the setting of retinal detachment. The risk of severe ROP is highest in the ELBW population in whom the incidence of blindness is 2% to 9%.

In addition to ROP, other ophthalmologic conditions seen in NICU graduates include the following:

a. Refractive errors are more frequent in premature than in term infants. Myopia is the most common problem and may be severe. Hyperopia also occurs more commonly in premature infants. Vision is corrected with eyeglasses.

b. Amblyopia (reduced vision caused by lack of use of one eye during the critical age for visual development) is more frequent in premature infants usually related to strabismus, anisometropia, and bilateral high refractive error (bilateral ametropia). Amblyopia can become permanent if it is not treated before 6 to 10 years of age.

c. Strabismus, or misalignment of the eyes, is more common in premature infants, especially in those with a history of ROP, intracranial hemorrhage, or white matter injury; the most common form is esotropia (crossed eyes), although exotropia (also known as wall-eye) and hypertropia (vertical misalignment of the eyes so that one eye is higher than the other) also occur. Strabismus may be treated with eye patching, atropine drops, corrective lenses, or surgery depending on the cause.

d. Anisometropia, defined as a substantial difference in refractive error between the two eyes, occurs more often in premature than term infants. Because the eyes cannot accommodate (focus) separately, the eye with the higher refractive error can develop amblyopia. Treatment for anisometropia is vision correction with eyeglasses.

In patients who have had severe ROP, including those treated with laser therapy, there is an increased risk of cataracts, glaucoma, late retinal detachment, and visual field deficits.

All VLBW infants should have follow-up with an ophthalmologist who has experience with ophthalmologic problems related to prematurity. This should occur by 8 to 10 months of age and then according to the ophthalmologist's recommendation, usually annually or again at 3 years of age at the latest.

2. Hearing follow-up. Hearing loss occurs in approximately 2% to 11% of VLBW infants. Prematurity increases the risk of both sensorineural and conductive hearing loss. All VLBW infants should be screened both in the neonatal period and again at 1 year of age (earlier if parental concerns are noted or if the infant has additional risk factors for hearing loss) (see Chap. 65). There is also evidence that VLBW infants are at increased risk for auditory dyssynchrony (also called auditory neuropathy) and central auditory processing problems.

E. **Dental problems.** VLBW infants have been noted to have an increased incidence of enamel hypoplasia and discoloration. Long-term oral intubation in the neonatal period may result in palate and alveolar ridge deformation, affecting tooth development. Referral to a pediatric dentist in the first 18 months of life is recommended, as is routine supplemental fluoride.

III. NEURODEVELOPMENTAL OUTCOMES.

Infants with intracranial hemorrhage, in particular parenchymal hemorrhage, or periventricular white matter injury are at increased risk for neuromotor and cognitive delay. Infants with white matter injury are also at increased risk for visuomotor problems, as well as visual field deficits. Among ELBW infants with neonatal complications, including BPD, brain injury (defined on ultrasonographic imaging as intraparenchymal echodensity, periventricular leukomalacia, porencephalic cyst, or grade 3 or 4 intraventricular hemorrhage [IVH]), and severe ROP (threshold or stage 4 or 5 ROP in one or both eyes), 88% had poor neurosensory outcomes at 18 months of age with either cerebral palsy, cognitive delay, severe hearing loss, or bilateral blindness. Infants with cerebellar hemorrhage are at increased risk for abnormal motor development, as well as cognitive, behavioral, functional, and social developmental problems.

A. **Neuromotor problems.** The incidence of cerebral palsy is 7% to 12% in VLBW infants and 11% to 15% in ELBW infants. The most common type of cerebral palsy is spastic diplegia. This correlates with the anatomic location of the corticospinal tracts in the periventricular white matter. VLBW infants are also at risk for other types of abnormal motor development, including motor coordination problems and later problems with motor planning.

1. Both transient and long-term motor problems in infants require assessment and treatment by physical therapists and occupational therapists. These services are usually provided at home through local programs. Infants with sensorineural handicaps require coordination of appropriate clinical services and developmental programs. For older children, consultation with the schools and participation in an educational plan are important.

2. Early diagnosis and referral to a neurologist and orthopedic surgeon will prompt referral for appropriate early intervention services, such as physical and occupational therapy. Some infants with cerebral palsy are candidates for treatment with orthotics or other adaptive equipment. Others with significant spasticity are candidates for treatment with botulinum-A toxin (Botox) injections. In the case of severe spasticity, treatment with baclofen (oral or through an intrathecal catheter with a subcutaneous pump) may be helpful. Older children are candidates for surgical procedures.

B. **Cognitive delay.** Progress is typically assessed by the use of some form of intelligence quotient (IQ) or development quotient (DQ) on an established scale such as the Bayley Scales of Infant Development or the Mullen Scales of Early Learning.

1. VLBW infants tend to have scores somewhat lower on such scales than term infants, but many still fall within the normal range. The percentage of VLBW infants with scores >2 standard deviations below the mean is between 5% and 20% and between 14% and 40% for ELBW infants. Most studies reflect the status of children younger than age 2. Among older children, the percentage of children who are severely affected appears to be the same, but the percentage with school failure or school problems is as high as 50%, with rates of 20%

even among children with average IQ scores. When children were tested at ages 8 to 11, learning disabilities particularly related to visuospatial and visuomotor abilities, written output, and verbal functioning were more common in ELBW infants (without neurologic problems diagnosed) compared to term infants of similar sociodemographic status. More than 50% of ELBW infants require some type of special education assistance compared to <15% of healthy term infants. However, children who were ELBW assessed in the teenage years with measures of self-esteem do not differ from term infants.

2. Referral to **early intervention programs** at the time of discharge from the NICU allows early identification of children with delays and referral for therapy from educational specialists and speech therapists when appropriate. Children with severe language delays may also benefit from referral to special communication programs that utilize adaptive technology to enhance language and communication.

3. **Social development.** Social and communication developmental difficulties are also increasingly a concern in the population of premature infants. Several recent studies have noted prematurity as a risk factor for autism and have noted that in prospective studies of preterm infants at the toddler age, they are more likely to screen positive for autism. These studies are ongoing and the true positive rate for autism will be better understood with further follow-up research.

C. **Emotional and behavioral health**

1. **Sleep problems** are more common in preterm than in term infants. The cause is frequently multifactorial with medical and behavioral components. Parents may benefit from books on sleep training or in more severe cases, referral to a sleep specialist.

2. **Behavior problems.** VLBW children are at increased risk for behavior problems related to hyperactivity and/or attention deficit. The risk factors for behavioral problems also include stress within the family, maternal depression, and smoking. Behavior problems can contribute to school difficulties. In relation to both school problems and other health issues, VLBW children are seen as less socially competent than are normal BW children. Detection of behavioral problems is achieved most commonly using scales developed to elicit parental and teacher concerns. The youngest children for whom such standardized scales are available are 2-year-olds. Management depends on the nature of the problem and the degree of functional disruption. Some problems may be managed with special educational programs; others may involve referral to appropriate psychotherapy services. Screening of NICU mothers for postpartum depression or posttraumatic stress disorder is also recommended; the incidence of depressive symptoms in mothers who have delivered a premature infant is higher and, when identified, provides an opportunity for intervention that will enhance both maternal and child health.

IV. **DEVELOPMENTAL FOLLOW-UP PROGRAMS** support optimization of health outcomes for NICU graduates and provide feedback information for improvement of medical care. Activities can include the following:

A. **Management of sequelae associated with prematurity.** As ever smaller infants survive, the risk of chronic sequelae increases.

B. **Consultative assessment and referral.** Regardless of specific morbidity at the time of discharge, NICU graduates require surveillance for the emergence of a variety of problems that may require referral to and coordination of multiple preventive and rehabilitative services.

C. **Monitoring outcomes.** Information on health problems and use of services by NICU graduates is integral to both the assessment of the effect of services and the counseling of parents regarding an individual child's future.

D. **Program structure**

1. The population requiring follow-up care differs with each NICU and the availability and quality of community resources. Most programs use as criteria some combination of birth weight and specific complications. The criteria must be explicit and well understood by all members of the NICU team, with mechanisms developed for identifying and referring appropriate children.

2. Visits depend on the infant's needs and community resources. Some programs recommend a first visit within a few weeks of discharge to assess the transition to home. If not dictated by acute problems, future visits are scheduled to assess progress in key activities. In the absence of acute care needs, we assess patients routinely at 6-month intervals.

3. Because the focus of follow-up care is enhancement of individual and family function, personnel must have a breadth of expertise, including (i) clinical skill in the management of sequelae of prematurity; (ii) the ability to perform neurologic and cognitive diagnostic assessment; (iii) familiarity with general pediatric problems presenting in premature infants; (iv) the ability to manage children with complex medical, motor, and cognitive problems; and (v) knowledge of the availability of and referral process to community programs.

4. Methods for assessing an individual's progress depend on the need for direct assessment by health professionals and the quality of primary care and early intervention services. A variety of indirect approaches of assessing developmental progress, including parental surveys, exist to provide information identifying children who have delays or other developmental concerns and warrant further assessment and/or intervention. This strategy of initial assessment may be helpful when it is difficult for families to travel the distance back to the medical centers or to reduce program costs. Recommended staff team members and consultants include pediatrician (developmental specialist or neonatologist), neonatology fellows or pediatric residents (for training), pediatric neurologist, physical therapist, psychologist, occupational therapist, dietician, speech and language specialist, and social worker.

5. **Family/parent function and support.** Having a premature infant is often an extremely stressful experience for the parents. Providing specialized care in assessment, supportive counseling, and resources to families caring for the VLBW infant is essential and includes particular attention to issues of postpartum affective conditions and anxiety following the potentially traumatic experience of having a critically ill infant. Provision of specialized behavioral guidance and supportive counseling in addition to facilitating referrals to community providers for additional care should be provided by the team. Addressing the basic needs of families, including health insurance issues, respite, advocating for services in the community, financial resources, and marital stress, are also important.

Suggested Readings

Bhutta AT, Cleves MA, Casey PH, et al. Cognitive and behavioral outcomes of school-aged children who were born preterm: a meta-analysis. *JAMA* 2002;288:728–737.

Delobel-Ayoub M, Arnaud C, White-Koning M, et al. Behavioral problems and cognitive performance at 5 years of age after very preterm birth: the EPIPAGE study. *Pediatrics* 2009;123(6):1485–1492.

Hack M, Fanaroff A. Outcomes of children of extremely low birthweight and gestational age in the 1990s. *Semin Neonatol* 2000;5(2):89–106.

Wilson-Costello D, Friedman H, Minich N, et al. Improved neurodevelopmental outcomes for extremely low birth weight infants in 2000–2002. *Pediatrics* 2007;119(1):37–45.

Wood NS, Costeloe K, et al. The EPICure study: associations and antecedents of neurological and developmental disability at 30 months of age following extremely preterm birth. *Arch Dis Child Fetal Neonatal Ed* 2005;90(2):F134–F140.

17 Neonatal Transport

Caraciolo J. Fernandes

I. INTRODUCTION. Neonatal transport may be defined as the act of moving a neonate from one setting or facility to another to allow the provision of a level of care and/or type of service that is not available at the former. Although neonatal transport typically refers to interfacility transfers of high-risk neonates to tertiary care facilities to allow a higher level of care, the principles pertaining to neonatal transport are equally important for transfer of neonates from the birthing area to special care nurseries within the facility and for transport of infants from tertiary care facilities back to their referral hospitals or sometimes home. Ideally, babies should be delivered and cared for in hospitals adequately equipped and staffed to care for them; thus, high-risk infants should ideally only be born in tertiary care facilities. Careful attention to the history can identify maternal and fetal conditions that suggest a need for infants to be delivered at a hospital capable of providing the appropriate level of care (see Chap. 7). In such instances, maternal transport prior to birth is preferable to having a high-risk neonate be born in a setting that is not equipped to care for it. Unfortunately, not all high-risk infants are identified prior to birth, and infants are delivered in facilities that are not matched to their needs. In this case, prompt contact with the tertiary care facility is essential to allow early and timely involvement of specialists in the care of the infant.

II. INDICATIONS

A. Interhospital transport should be considered if the medical resources or personnel needed for a high-risk infant are not available at the hospital currently providing care. As the birth of high-risk infants cannot always be predicted, all facilities that care for pregnant women and newly born infants should ensure that personnel caring for infants at birth or in the immediate newborn period are proficient in basic neonatal resuscitation and stabilization.

B. Transfer to the regional tertiary neonatal center should be expedited following initial stabilization. Medical personnel from the referring center should contact their affiliated neonatal intensive care unit (NICU) transport service to arrange transfer and to discuss a management plan to optimize patient care before the transport team's arrival at the referring center.

C. **Criteria for neonatal transfer** depend on the capability of the referring hospital as defined by the American Academy of Pediatrics policy statement on levels of neonatal care and as dictated by local and state public health guidelines. Conditions that require transfer to a center that provides neonatal intensive care include the following:

1. Prematurity and/or birth weight <1,500 g

2. Gestational age <32 weeks

3. Respiratory distress requiring ventilatory support (continuous positive airway pressure [CPAP], mechanical ventilation)

4. Hypoxic respiratory failure or persistent pulmonary hypertension

5. Congenital heart disease or cardiac arrhythmias requiring cardiac services

6. Congenital anomalies and/or inborn errors of metabolism

7. Severe hypoxic-ischemic injury

8. Seizures

9. Other conditions requiring neonatology consultation and possible transfer
   a. Severe hyperbilirubinemia that may require exchange transfusion
   b. Infant of diabetic mother
   c. Severe intrauterine growth restriction
   d. Birth weight between 1,500 and 2,000 g and gestational age between 32 and 36 weeks
   e. Procedures unavailable at referring hospital (surgery, extracorporeal membrane oxygenation [ECMO], etc.)

III. ORGANIZATION OF TRANSPORT SERVICES

A. All hospitals with established maternity services and Level I or II neonatal care services should have agreements with regional perinatal centers outlining criteria for perinatal consultations and neonatal transfer.

B. The regional NICU transport team should have an appointed **medical director**. The transport team should follow practice guidelines detailed in easily accessible written protocols and procedures, which should be reviewed on a periodic basis.

C. **Transport teams.** Qualified transport teams should be composed of individuals with pediatric/neonatal critical care experience and training in the needs of infants and children during transport, and who participate in the transport of such patients with sufficient frequency to maintain their expertise. Such teams typically consist of a combination of at least two or three trained personnel and can include one or more of the following: advanced practice nurses, neonatal nurse practitioners, respiratory therapists, and physicians. Senior pediatric residents and subspecialty fellows can provide the physician component for some teams. Skills of the transport team should be assessed periodically, and skills and situational training should be part of routine ongoing education. Each transport team should be supervised by a medical control officer, who may be the attending neonatologist. The medical control officer should be readily available by telephone for consultation to assist in the management of the infant during transport.

Types of transport teams:

1. Unit-based transport teams consist of personnel (nurses, respiratory therapists, neonatal nurse practitioners, etc.) who are involved in routine patient care in the NICU and are deployed when a request for transport is received. If few infants are transported to the NICU, this type of staffing may be most cost-effective; however, this arrangement would lack the experience and expertise of a dedicated transport team.

2. Dedicated transport teams are staffed separately from NICU personnel specifically for the purpose of transport of patients to and from the hospital. These personnel do not have patient assignments, although they may assist NICU staff when they are not on transport. A large volume of transports is necessary to justify a dedicated transport team, which must consist of sufficient personnel for around-the-clock coverage. This arrangement allows dedicated personnel to maintain their skills for safe and efficient transport of patients.

D. **Modes of transport** include ambulance and fixed- (airplane) and rotor-wing (helicopter) aircraft. The type of vehicle chosen will depend on each program's individual needs, specifically the distance of transport anticipated, acuity of patients, and geographic terrain to be covered by the vehicle. Some hospitals own, maintain, and insure their own vehicles, while others contract with commercial vendors for vehicles that can accommodate a transport incubator and appropriate equipment. While the type(s) of vehicle chosen for transport will vary depending on the individual program's needs, the vehicles chosen must be outfitted to conform to standards that ensure safety and efficiency of transport. Vehicles should comply with all local, state, and federal guidelines for air transport and/or ground ambulances. The vehicles should be large enough to allow the transport team to adequately assess and treat patients as needed *en route* to the referral hospital, and should be equipped with appropriate electrical power supply, medical gases (with reserve capacity, in case of a breakdown), and communication systems. All equipment and stretchers should be properly secured. Each mode of transport— ground, fixed wing, and rotor wing—have advantages and disadvantages. **Ground or rotor-wing transport** has the advantage of a rapid response with hospital-to-hospital service for patients up to a distance of 100 to 150 miles or less each way, although a rotor-wing service is more expensive to operate. **Fixed-wing transport** is advisable for transport of patients over greater distances (over 150 miles each way), is moderately expensive to operate, and requires an airport to land and an ambulance at either end of the flight to transport the patient between the airplane and the hospital.

E. **Equipment.** The team should carry with them all equipment, medications, and other supplies that might be needed to stabilize infants at a referring hospital. Teams should use checklists prior to departure to ensure that vital supplies and equipment are not forgotten. Packs especially designed for neonatal transport are commercially available. These packs or other containers should be stocked by members of the transport team, which ensures that they will know where to find required items promptly. The weight of the stocked packs should be documented for air transport (see Tables 17.1–17.3).

F. **Legal issues.** The process of neonatal transport may raise legal issues, which vary among states. Transport teams should periodically review all routine procedures and documentation forms with their hospital legal counsel to ensure compliance with changing laws that govern the transport of infants and accompanying family members (if present). The team should have the ability to contact via telephone appropriate hospital legal counsel as needed.

G. **Malpractice insurance coverage** is required for all team members. The tertiary hospital should decide whether transport is considered as an off-site or extended on-site activity as this can affect the necessary coverage.

Table 17.1	Transport Team Equipment
Transport incubator equipped with ventilators, and monitors for heart rate, vascular pressures, oxygen saturation, and temperature	
Suction device	
Nitric oxide delivery equipment	
Infusion pumps	
Gel-filled mattress	
Adaptors to plug into both hospital and vehicle power	
Airway equipment	
Flow-inflating bag with manometer	
Laryngoscopes with no. 00, 0, and 1 blades	
Magill forceps	
CO_2 detectors	
Instrument tray for chest tubes and vascular catheters	
Stethoscope	
Tanks of oxygen, compressed air, and nitric oxide	
Source of electrical power, heat, and light	

H. **Carrier regulations** vary from state to state and may conflict with transport goals. For example, some states require that an ambulance stop at the scene of an unattended accident to render aid until a second ambulance arrives.

IV. REFERRING HOSPITAL RESPONSIBILITIES

A. **Identify the appropriate tertiary care facility for transfer.** If it is known before birth that the infant will need transfer to a tertiary care facility (e.g., an infant with congenital cyanotic heart disease), both the parents and the appropriate tertiary care facility can be prepared for the transfer. Prompt notification of the referral hospital will allow timely deployment of the transport team and verify that the required services are available. Any risk posed by the patient for communicable diseases must be disclosed to the tertiary center at the time of the request for transfer.

B. **Documentation.** Staff at the referring hospital should complete the administrative forms required for transfer, which include parental consent. A transfer summary should document the care given to the infant at the referring hospital.

Table 17.2	Supplies Used by Transport Teams
Airways
Alcohol swabs
Arm boards
Batteries
Benzoin
Betadine* swabs
Blood culture bottles
Blood pressure cuff
Butterfly needles: 23 and 25 gauge
Chest tubes: 10 and 12 F, and connectors
Chemstrip*
Clipboard with transport data forms, permission forms, progress notes, and booklet for parents
Culture tubes
Endotracheal tubes: 2.5, 3, 3.5, 4 mm
Face masks, term and premature
Feeding tubes: 5 and 8 F
Gauze pads
Gloves, sterile and examination
Heimlich valves
Intravenous tubing
Intravenous catheters: 22 and 24 gauge
Kelly clamp
Lubricating ointment
Monitor leads and transducers
(continued)

Table 17.2	(Continued)
Needles: 18, 20, 26 gauge	
Oxygen tubing	
Pigtail catheters	
Replogle, nasogastric tube	
Scalpel blades, no. 11	
Sterile gowns	
Stopcocks	
Stylus	
Suction catheters: 6, 8, and 10 F and traps	
Suture material (silk 3–0, 4–0, on curved needle)	
Syringes: 1, 3, 10, 50 mL	
Tape	
T-connectors	
Thermometer	
Tubes for blood specimens	
Umbilical catheters: 3.5 and 5 F (double lumen)	
Urine collection bags	
Xeroform* gauze	
*These are trademark items	

The clinician at the referring hospital usually remains the physician of record until the patient leaves the referring hospital with the transport team.

V. TRANSPORT TEAM RESPONSIBILITIES

A. When receiving the initial request for transfer, the transport team should obtain a sufficiently detailed summary from the referring clinician to decide the appropriate team composition and equipment required. Such communication is facilitated by a checklist script such as **SBAR** (**S**ituation, **B**ackground, **A**ssessment, **R**ecommendation) or **ISBARQ** (**I**ntroduction, **S**ituation, **B**ackground, **A**ssessment, **R**ecommendation, **Q**uestions).

Table 17.3	Medications Used on Transport
Adenosine	
Albumin 5%	
Ampicillin	
Atropine	
Calcium	
Calcium gluconate	
Dexamethasone	
Dextrose 50% in water	
Dextrose 10% in water	
Diphenylhydantoin	
Digoxin	
Dobutamine	
Dopamine	
Epinephrine	
Erythromycin eye ointment	
Fentanyl	
Furosemide	
Gentamicin	
Heparin	
Lidocaine	
Midazolam	
Morphine	
Naloxone	
Normal saline	
Pancuronium	
	(continued)

Table 17.3	*(Continued)*
Phenobarbital	
Potassium chloride	
Prostaglandin E_1 (refrigerated)	
Sodium bicarbonate	
Sterile water for injection	
Sucrose oral solution	
Vitamin K_1	

B. The medical control officer or attending neonatologist should discuss the patient's condition, anticipated problems, and potential therapies with team members before departure. Recommendations for management (focused on respiratory, cardiovascular, and metabolic stabilization) should be communicated to staff at the referring hospital for implementation prior to the arrival of the transport team. Interventions concerning airway management and vascular access should be specific, and all recommendations should be documented.

C. Upon arrival at the referring NICU, transport team members should introduce themselves clearly and politely to the referring hospital staff and family members. Appropriate photo identification should be worn. The referring and primary physicians should be identified and their names documented.

D. Transfer of patient information (handoff) should be clear and there should be agreement on when the transport team assumes responsibility for management. The use of checklists for communication (see V.A.) decreases the likelihood of important items being overlooked during handoff.

E. The team should work collegially with the referring hospital staff and be objective in their assessment and stabilization. The referring staff should be included in as much of the care as appropriate.

F. Parents should be given an opportunity to see their infant before the team leaves the referring hospital. While meeting with the family, the team should obtain consent for transfer and other anticipated procedures (including blood transfusion, if indicated), as well as review the team's policy regarding parents traveling with their newborn on transport. Transport teams should have written policies regarding the presence of parents during ground or air transport.

G. Following completion of the transport, the team should call the referring hospital staff with pertinent follow-up of the patient's condition and how he or she tolerated the transport to the tertiary facility.

H. Transport teams should consider an active outreach education program for referring hospital staff that could include conferences, in-service presentations, and case reviews.

VI. MEDICAL MANAGEMENT BEFORE TRANSPORT

A. Medical management of the infant to be transported to a tertiary care facility can be optimized while the transport team is *en route* to the referring hospital. Once the team is deployed, the responsible neonatologist can discuss recommendations for care with the referring hospital staff.

B. The following should be addressed by the referring hospital staff:

1. Establish and maintain a neutral thermal environment.

2. Ensure adequate oxygenation and ventilation.

3. Correct any circulatory deficits, and optimize the blood pressure with inotropic agents, if needed.

4. Ensure adequate blood glucose concentration.

5. Obtain umbilical venous access, if indicated.

6. Obtain umbilical arterial access, if indicated.

7. Obtain appropriate cultures and give first doses of antibiotics, if indicated.

8. Insert a nasogastric tube and decompress the stomach.

9. Obtain initial transport consent from parents.

10. Obtain copies of obstetric and neonatal charts for the transport team.

11. Obtain copies of radiographic and applicable studies for the transport team.

12. Prepare the parents for transport of their infant, and allow them time to visit with their infant.

VII. TRANSPORT BACK TO THE REFERRAL HOSPITAL.

If the infant has been stabilized, most return trips are uneventful. Continuous direct observation of the infant is one of the most important forms of monitoring. The benefit of handling the patient and taking vital signs must be weighed against the possibility of an accidental extubation or thermal loss incurred by opening the transport incubator. In the event of an unexpected clinical deterioration, the transport team may need to contact the medical control officer or neonatologist via wireless phone or radio to discuss the patient's condition and/or plan of care. Ambulance sirens and flashing lights should be used only in rare circumstances as they increase the risk of causing accidents, and have not been shown to save time or reduce mortality.

VIII. ARRIVAL AT THE NICU

A. The team should give the NICU caregivers a succinct and complete summary of the infant's clinical condition and copies of the referring hospital's medical record and radiographic studies. Use of a standardized handoff script will ensure relevant information is not inadvertently omitted.

B. A team member should telephone the parents to let them know that their child has arrived safely.

C. A team member should telephone the referring and primary physicians to inform them of the patient's status and who will be providing further communication.

D. Relevant documentation regarding the transport should be completed and a copy added to the patient's medical record.

E. All transport medications should be immediately restocked, and all equipment checked and prepared for subsequent transports.

F. If an untoward incident occurred during transport, appropriate documentation should be completed and the transport team's medical director should be notified to allow appropriate investigation and debriefing. Quality assurance activities should be performed routinely.

IX. SPECIFIC CONDITIONS AND MANAGEMENT

A. **Premature infants with respiratory distress syndrome** (RDS) who have not responded to early application of continuous positive airway pressure benefit from surfactant administration. Following consultation with the medical control physician, the transport team should administer surfactant and wait at least 30 minutes before moving the newborn to the transport incubator. Weaning of ventilatory support prior to initiation of transport will minimize the likelihood of air leaks and hypocarbia *en route*.

B. **Hypoxic respiratory failure and pulmonary hypertension.** Management should focus on ensuring optimal lung recruitment using ventilatory strategies and surfactant administration and supporting cardiac function and blood pressure. Transport teams should be prepared to institute inhaled nitric oxide at the referring hospital and during transport.

C. **Cardiac disease.** Ideally, a cardiologist at the tertiary care facility should be available to make recommendations for care prior to and during transport of the infant. In infants with suspected ductal-dependent congenital heart disease, prostaglandin E_1 (PGE_1) may be initiated prior to transport. Apnea, fever, and hypotension are common side effects of PGE_1. Endotracheal intubation is usually warranted for transport of an infant requiring PGE_1 infusion.

D. **Surgical conditions.** Special consideration should be given to infants being transported by air (see X.B.).

X. PHYSIOLOGIC CONSIDERATIONS OF AIR TRANSPORTS

A. **Changes in barometric pressure.** As altitude increases, the barometric pressure and partial pressure of oxygen in the air decreases (Table 17.4), which leads to a decrease in alveolar oxygen tension. Even in aircraft with pressurized cabins, because the cabin pressure is usually maintained at a level equal to 8,000 to 10,000 ft above sea level, the FiO_2 delivered to the infant may need to be increased to ensure adequate oxygen delivery. The FiO_2 required to approximate the same oxygen tension that the patient is receiving can be calculated by the formula in Table 17.4. If neonates with severe lung disease are transported by air, the cabin may need to be pressurized to sea level. Ultimately, pulse oximetry and blood gas estimations should be used to guide adjustments in delivered FiO_2 to maintain adequate oxygen saturations.

B. **Gas expansion.** As altitude increases and barometric pressure decreases, gases trapped in closed spaces will expand. This can result in a small pneumothorax or increased gaseous distention of the GI tract causing clinical deterioration in an infant that was stable at sea level. To prevent compromise, pneumothoraces should be drained and the stomach vented with a nasogastric tube before an air transport.

Table 17.4	Barometric Pressure and Partial Pressure of Oxygen with Increasing Altitude					
	Sea level	2,000 ft	4,000 ft	6,000 ft	8,000 ft	10,000 ft
Barometric pressure (torr)	760	706	656	609	565	523
Partial pressure of FiO_2 0.21 (torr)	160	148	138	128	119	110
FiO_2 required $= \dfrac{FiO_2 \times BP_1}{BP_2}$						
FiO_2 = fraction of inspired oxygen patient is currently receiving; BP_1 = current barometric pressure; BP_2 = destination barometric pressure.						

XI. SIMULATION IN TRANSPORT MEDICINE. Transport of critically ill infants involves high-stress situations where it is crucial for the team to work well together to ensure patient and team member safety, enhance efficiencies, and improve patient outcomes. Simulation-based training allows teams to practice working together to enhance their interactions and efficiency in a safe environment.

Suggested Readings

Woodward A, Insoft R, Kleinman M, eds. *Guidelines for Air and Ground Transport of Neonatal and Pediatric Patients.* 3rd ed. Elk Grove Village, IL: American Academy of Pediatrics; 2007.

18 Discharge Planning

Ruth A. Hynes and Theresa M. Andrews

Changes in the health care system in the United States are encouraging earlier discharges and more out of hospital care. This comes at a time when some infants are requiring higher levels of complex care at home. The movement to make the discharge process increasingly family centered and efficient requires careful and organized discharge planning. The optimal safe and successful discharge requires mutual participation between the family and the medical and surgical teams and should begin at admission and follow the continuum of the infants hospital stay.

I. GOALS OF A COMPREHENSIVE DISCHARGE PLAN

A. Is individualized to meet infant and family needs and resources

B. Begins early; planning can begin with a prenatal diagnosis or upon admission to the neonatal intensive care unit (NICU)

C. Includes ongoing daily assessment and clearly identified goals

D. Anticipates potential delays in development and directs care toward prevention and early intervention

E. Promotes multidisciplinary communication as an essential component

F. Is community-based, with early identification of a primary pediatrician and other community resources

G. Promotes access to care and progression through the provider system with minimal fragmentation of care and duplication of services

H. Decreases the possibility of readmission

II. FAMILY ASSESSMENT is a key component of a successful discharge process.

Families are able to build on their strengths if given the opportunity to participate in the care early and be an active participant in the discharge process. Early partnership with the family promotes confidence and decreases stress by enhancing the parents' feeling of control. The ability to provide adequate parent education is vital for the successful transition to home. With early planning, ongoing teaching, and attention to the family's needs and resources, the transition to home can be smooth, even in the most complex cases. The family assessment should address the following questions:

A. Family

1. Who will be the primary caregiver(s) for the infant? How willingly is this responsibility assumed?

2. What is the family structure? Do they have a support system? Does one need to be developed or strengthened?

3. Are there language or learning barriers? Address this early.

4. How do they learn best? The nursing team should maximize the use of educational tools: written materials, visual props, and demonstrations.

5. How do previous or present experiences with the infant's care affect the family's ability to oversee care after discharge?

6. What are the actual as well as perceived complexities of the skills required to care for the infant?

7. What are their coping habits and styles?

8. Do the parents have any medical or psychological concerns that may have an impact on caretaking abilities?

9. What are the cultural beliefs and how might these affect the care of the infant?

10. What are the financial concerns? Will the family's income change? If so, what resources are available to compensate?

11. Are there issues related to the family's living conditions that will be challenging? Families can become overwhelmed by the volume of medical equipment that will be delivered to the home in the days before discharge. Evaluate the home nursery and other spaces for the infant/caregivers and supplies. Have the parent take pictures to evaluate layout options. Discuss supply storage recommendations such as plastic bins on wheels, baskets, and so forth.

B. **Home environment.** If an infant will require in-home respiratory support, make a referral to a durable medical equipment (DME) company. A respiratory therapist (RT) must assess the home to evaluate outlets in the infant's area, measure door openings, inquire about electrical panel location and capacity, and ensure a safe environment.

C. **Stress and coping.** The separation of family and infant, inability to experience a traditional parenting role, and the inclusion of multiple caregivers in daily care can all be stressors to a family. The early establishment of parents as partners and participants in their infant's care helps a family cope with the stress and separation associated with NICU care. The medical team, including the social worker, should assess the family's psychological readiness for a transition to home. Social work can make recommendations for further community psychological supports as needed. It is helpful to keep in mind that while a family is preparing for a child with complex medical needs, they may also be grieving the loss of a traditional experience.

D. **Financial resources.** Social workers and/or resource specialists should assess a family's financial situation early. A preterm delivery or need for complex home care can alter the family's plans for work and child care. Loss of work, income changes, cost of co-payments, and inability to make career moves because of insurance coverage all affect the family's financial stability. Social work can offer secondary insurance resources early if an infant's medical course appears to require a longer than 30 days hospitalization, or if an infant is predicted to have long-term medical needs.

III. SYSTEM ASSESSMENT.

It is important to know how a facility functions, who assumes responsibility for various components of discharge planning, and how communication is carried out. Enough cannot be said about the need for consistency in care providers during the discharge process. Effective relationships with the family, as well as a health care team that is familiar with an infant, will help immensely with concise communication and will enhance an organized discharge process. Identifying payer coverage early promotes timely assessment of contractual requirements.

A. A **physician** or **nurse practitioner** is responsible for daily management of care. In teaching institutions where staff rotates, families may need to adjust to many different providers. For those infants with complex issues, identifying a primary attending physician or practitioner provides the family with more continuity. The team then can coordinate, implement, and evaluate the developed care plan.

B. The infant's **primary nurse and nursing team** follows the family through the NICU stay coordinating, implementing, and evaluating the developed care plan on a daily basis.

C. **Respiratory, physical, and occupational therapists** teach families necessary specific skills and assist in transitioning care to community resources.

D. **Social workers** assess and support the family. Social work should be a part of family and team meetings to help facilitate communication with the family.

E. In the hospital, **case manager/patient care coordinator** gathers the necessary insurance coverage, sets up the homecare systems (i.e., Visiting Nurse Association [VNA], Medical Supply Company, Early Intervention Referral), and blocked hours if approved by the insurance company. The NICU case managers are the key contact in working with services and insurance companies to secure prior authorizations for exceptions to benefits, equipment, and ambulances.

F. The role of a **discharge coordinator or planner** varies by institution. The discharge planner can assist in identifying infants who may be approaching discharge, discuss alternatives to home if necessary, and can work with the medical and nursing teams to ensure that the family receives discharge planning in a timely and organized manner.

G. A **Resource Specialist** can be helpful in finding other financial resources available to families to cover medical costs once the patient is discharged.

H. **Payer resources**, such as health maintenance organizations (HMOs) and third-party payers, often have case managers to assist in the coordination of services. Use of preferred providers may be contractually required. Out-of-hospital case managers can be consulted by the family or by the NICU case manager to help clarify issues of coverage and resource availability.

I. **Interpreters** assist in communication with families when indicated. Any complex discharge updates and teaching should be done with an interpreter when a family is not fluent in English.

IV. INFANT'S READINESS FOR DISCHARGE

A. **Healthy growing preterm infants** are considered ready for discharge when they meet the following criteria:

1. Able to maintain temperature in an open environment

2. Able to take all feedings by bottle or breast without respiratory compromise

3. Demonstrates steady weight gain evidenced by a preterm infant weight gain of 10 to 15 g/kg/day and a term infant weight gain of 20 to 30 g/kg/day

4. Free of apnea or bradycardia for 5 days (see Chap. 31)

5. Able to sleep with head of bed flat without compromising the infant's health and safety. (If reflux is present and compromising infant's health or safety, provide patient with Tucker Wedge & Sling equipment available through Children's Medical Ventures: www.tuckersling.respironics.com)

B. **Infants with specialized needs** require a complex, flexible, ongoing discharge and teaching plan. Medications and special formulas or dietary supplements should be obtained as early as possible to optimize teaching. Some discharge specifics may not be identified until just before discharge. It is important to consider the infant's relative fragility and the complexity of interventions. Include assessment of behavioral and developmental issues, and evaluate parental recognition and response.

C. **Discharge screening.** Complete routine screening tests and immunizations according to individual institutional guidelines (see Table 18.1).

1. **Hearing screening** (see Chap. 65 and Table 18.1).

2. **Eye examinations** (see Chap. 64 and Table 18.1).

3. **Cranial ultrasonography** (see Chap. 54 and Table 18.1) screening for intraventricular hemorrhage and periventricular leukomalacia for all infants who satisfy the following criteria:
   a. Weight <1,500 g or gestational age <32 weeks.
   b. Perform head ultrasonography at day of life 1 to 3, if results alter clinical management, day of life 7 to 10, and then at 1 month of age.

4. **Immunizations.** Administer according to American Academy of Pediatrics' guidelines based on chronologic, not postconceptional, age (http://www.cdc .gov/vaccines and see Chap. 7).

5. **Car seat trial** (see Table 18.1). Infants who fail a car seat test need to be retrialed in a car bed. Car seat testing can be repeated in the community setting 1 month later.

V. PREPARING THE FAMILY FOR DISCHARGE. A well-thought-out plan prepares the family to recognize trouble early and seek medical attention before the health of their infant is compromised. Poor discharge planning has been linked to increased unscheduled health care use and readmissions.

A. **Begin teaching early** to allow the caregivers adequate time to process information, practice skills, and formulate questions. Make teaching protocols detailed and thorough. Include written information for the family to take home to use as references (see Fig. 18.1 and Table 18.2). Standardize information to ensure that every family member receives the same essential information. Create a discharge binder to help organize infant's care and routines. Address necessary medical information, well-baby care, "back to sleep," developmental issues, secondhand smoke, and shaken baby syndrome. Provide cardiopulmonary resuscitation (CPR) education early and possibly repeat closer to discharge date. Include several family members in the learning process so that the parents can get needed support.

B. **Simplify and organize care** by thoroughly reviewing the infant's daily regimen.

Table 18.1	Guidelines for Routine Screening, Testing, Treatment, and Follow-up of Infants Admitted to Neonatal Intensive Care Unit (NICU)

Newborn state screening for metabolic disease (see Chap. 60)

Criteria

- All infants admitted to the NICU

Initial

- Day 3 or discharge (D/C) date (whichever comes first)

Follow-up

- Day 14 or D/C date (whichever comes first)

- Week 6 (if BW <1,500 g)

- Week 10 (if BW <1,500 g)

Head ultrasonography (see Chap. 54)

Criteria

- All infants with GA <32 wk (or any GA at any time if clinically indicated)

Initial

- Day 7–10 (in the case of critically ill infants, when results of an earlier ultrasonography may alter clinical management, an ultrasonography should be performed at the discretion of the clinician)

Follow-up (minimum if no abnormalities noted)

- If no hemorrhage or germinal matrix hemorrhage

  □ If <32 wk: week 4 *and* at 36 wk post menstrual age (or discharge if <36 wk)

- If intraventricular (grade 2+) or intraparenchymal hemorrhage: follow-up at least weekly until stable (more frequently if unstable posthemorrhagic hydrocephalus or clinically indicated)

(continued)

Table 18.1	Guidelines for Routine Screening, Testing, Treatment, and Follow-up of Infants Admitted to Neonatal Intensive Care Unit (NICU) *(Continued)*

Ophthalmologic examination (see Chap. 64)

Criteria

- All infants with BW <1,500 g or GA <32 wk

Initial

- If <27 wk: week 6
- If 27–28 wk: week 5
- If 29–30 wk: week 4
- If 31–32 wk: week 3

Note

- If the infant is transferred to another nursery before 4 wk of age, recommend examination at the receiving hospital

- If the infant is to be discharged home before the first scheduled eye exam, reschedule for before discharge

Follow-up

- Per ophthalmologist (based on initial examination findings)

Audiology screening (see Chap. 65)

Criteria

- All infants to be discharged home from NICU

Timing

- Examine at 34 weeks' gestation or greater

Car seat screening

Criteria

- All infants to be discharged from NICU, born at <37 wk, and all infants with conditions that may compromise respiratory status

(continued)

Table 18.1	**(Continued)**

- Infants who fail the car seat screen should be discharged home in a car bed. The pediatrician generally decides when the infant is ready to travel in a car seat. Some hospitals offer a car seat rechallenge clinic.

Timing

- Screen before discharge home and when off oxygen for at least 24 hours

Hepatitis B vaccination (see Chap. 48)

Criteria

- Infants of mothers with HBsAg negative status

Timing

- Weight >2 kg: before hospital discharge

- Weight <2 kg: one month of age, or at hospital discharge, whichever comes first

- Give dose #2 at least 1 month after dose #1

Social Security

Criteria

- All infants meeting one of the following conditions: (www.socialsecurity.com)

  □ BW <1,200 g

  □ BW 1,200–2,000 g and small for gestational age (SGA)

  □ Any infant with serious handicapping conditions

Timing

- Application completed as early as the first week of life

Follow-up

- Parent notifies social security intake (SSI) office of baby's discharge through form letter

(continued)

Table 18.1	Guidelines for Routine Screening, Testing, Treatment, and Follow-up of Infants Admitted to Neonatal Intensive Care Unit (NICU) *(Continued)*

Infant Follow-Up Program (IFUP)—offered at many hospitals that have a Level III NICU

Criteria

- All infants meeting one of the following conditions:

  □ GA <28 wk

  □ GA <32 wk with one of the following:

    □ IUGR

    □ Maternal age <20

    □ IVH (note grade)

    □ PVL

    □ Surgical NEC

    □ ROP

    □ Psychosocial concerns

Timing

- Referral completed before discharge

Neonatal neurology program

Criteria

- All infants meeting one of the following conditions:

  □ Neurologic disorders (e.g., stroke, intracranial hemorrhage, and neonatal seizures)

  □ Neuromuscular disorders

  □ BW <1,500 g with IVH (or parenchymal hemorrhage) or PVL

Timing

- Referral completed before discharge

(continued)

Table 18.1	*(Continued)*

Early intervention program (EIP)

Criteria

- Infant meeting four or more of the following criteria:

  □ BW <1,200 g

  □ GA <32 wk

  □ NICU admission >5 d

  □ Apgar <5 at 5 min

  □ Intrauterine growth restriction (IUGR) or small for gestational age (SGA) (refer to growth curves)

  □ Hospital stay >25 d

  □ Chronic feeding difficulties

  □ Insecure attachment

  □ Suspected central nervous system abnormality

  □ Maternal age <17 *or* 3 or more births at maternal age <20

  □ Maternal education <10 yr

  □ Parental chronic illness or disability affecting caregiving

  □ Lack of family support

  □ Inadequate food, shelter, and clothing

  □ Open or confirmed protective service investigation ("51-A")

  □ Substance abuse in the home

  □ Domestic violence in the home

Timing

- Referral completed before discharge

ROP = retinopathy of prematurity; IVH = intraventricular hemorrhage; PVL = periventricular leukomalacia; BW = birth weight; GA = gestational age

NEONATAL INTENSIVE CARE UNIT
DISCHARGE INSTRUCTION SHEET

Baby's Caregivers:
Attending Neonatologist at Discharge: _____
Primary Nurse & Team: _____
Social Worker: _____

PARENT INFORMATION

	Reviewed	N/A	RN Signature	Date
NICU parent packet	☐		_____	__/__/__
WIC form	☐	☐	_____	__/__/__
Immunization booklet	☐	☐	_____	__/__/__
Synagis information sheet	☐	☐	_____	__/__/__
Hepatitis B information sheet	☐	☐	_____	__/__/__
Other _____	☐	☐	_____	__/__/__

PREPARATION FOR DISCHARGE

	Reviewed	RN Signature	Date
Feeding: breast milk or formula	☐	_____	__/__/__
Bowel and bladder pattern	☐	_____	__/__/__
Bulb syringe use	☐	_____	__/__/__
Bathing, skin care, cord care	☐	_____	__/__/__
Temperature taking	☐	_____	__/__/__
Circumcision care (if applicable)	☐	_____	__/__/__
CPR instruction	☐	_____	__/__/__
When to call your baby's doctor	☐	_____	__/__/__
Car seat instruction	☐	_____	__/__/__
Car seat screening	☐	_____	__/__/__
Protection from infection	☐	_____	__/__/__
Other _____	☐	_____	__/__/__

DATE OF DISCHARGE: __/__/__

Discharge Measurements: RN Signature Date
Weight _____ gms (____ lbs ____ oz) _____ __/__/__
Length ____ cm (____ in) _____ __/__/__
Head Circumference ____ cm (____ in) _____ __/__/__

STATE NEWBORN SCREENING: Most recent test: __/__/__

NEWBORN HEARING SCREEN: ☐Pass ☐Refer (see follow-up care)

ADDITIONAL NOTES:

BABY'S FOLLOW UP CARE

Primary Pediatric Provider: ☐N/A
Name: _____
Telephone: _____
Appt. Date: __/__/__ Time: _____

Early Intervention: ☐N/A
Center Name/Town: _____
Initial Contact: __/__/__ Date Confirmed: __/__/__

Visiting Nurse: ☐N/A
Center Name/Town: _____
Telephone: _____
Date Contacted: __/__/__ ☐ referral faxed

Infant Follow-up Program: (617) 667-1330 ☐N/A
(<1500g–see criteria on referral sheet)
Date Contacted: __/__/__ ☐ referral faxed

Neonatal Neurology Program: (617) 355-6388 ☐N/A
Children's Hospital
(see criteria on referral sheet)
Date Contacted: __/__/__

Lactation Consultant: ☐N/A
Name: _____
Telephone: _____

Ophthalmologist: ☐N/A
Name: _____
Telephone: _____
Date: __/__/__ Time: _____
☐ Recommended Follow-up at 8 months

Follow-up Hearing Screen: ☐N/A
Date: __/__/__ Time: _____
Location:
☐ Children's Hospital - Fegan 11 (617) 355-6461
☐ Children's Hospital - Lexington (781) 672-2000
☐ HVMA - Kenmore (617) 421-8888
☐ Other: _____ ( ) ___-____

Other:

Medication/Feeding Additives	Reason	Amount to give	When to give	How to give
☐ Check medroom for stored breastmilk				

This information has been reviewed with me, and my questions have been answered. I authorize the NICU staff to provide necessary information from my child's medical record to the above named providers/services.

_____ ☐ Copy given to parent _____ __/__/__
Parent Signature   RN Signature   Date

MC0104   Revised 5/00   White - Medical Record   Yellow - Parent

Note: This is a general guideline, and it does not represent a professional standard of care governing providers' obligations to patients. Care is revised to meet individual patient needs.

©Beth Israel Deaconess Medical Center

Figure 18.1. Newborn discharge instruction sheet. (Adapted from Beth Israel Deaconess Medical Center.)

C. Teach clustering of care to help organize the daily routine for the parent and patient.

D. Evaluate the medication schedule and change times to fit into the parent/patient's home schedule. Eliminate unnecessary medications and make any needed changes prior to discharge. Have prescriptions written and filled at least 2 to 3 days prior to discharge. Some medications may not be commercially prepared and must be compounded by a specialty pharmacy. Review medications early with a hospital pharmacist, as finding a compounding pharmacy and allowing for the time for a

Table 18.2	Additional Discharge Instruction Sheet

Community Resources

- **Poison Control Center**...(800) 222–1222
- **Parents Helping Parents**...(800) 632–8188
- **National Domestic Violence Hotline (24 h)**............................(800) 799–SAFE
- **Alcohol and Drug Addiction Resource Center**.........................(800) 448–3000
- **Mother of Twins Association**.......................................(248) 231–4480

Breastfeeding

- **La Leche**..(800)–LaLeche

Guidelines for when parents should call their baby's doctor

Any sudden changes in baby's usual patterns of behavior:

- Increased sleepiness
- Increased irritability
- Poor feeding

Any of the following:

- Breathing difficulty
- Blueness around lips, mouth, or eyes
- Fever (by rectal temperature) over 100°F or (under the arm) over 99.6°F or low temperature (rectal) under 97°F
- Vomiting or diarrhea
- Dry diaper for >12 h
- No bowel movement for >4 d
- Black or bright red color in stool

medication to be mixed can be time consuming. Once prescription is filled, ask the family to bring in the filled bottle and practice drawing up the medication before going home.

E. **Evaluate feeding schedule** to allow adequate sleeping time for parents while ensuring sufficient caloric intake for the infant. Establish whether or not the formula and additives are covered by insurance. Some formulas are not carried by all pharmacies and may need to be specially ordered. Ordering formulas through a store or pharmacy can take a day or two. The nutritionist can teach families how to mix calorie-enriched formula or breast milk. The case manager/discharge coordinator can obtain the paper work necessary for insurance approval of specialized formulas.

F. **Approaching readiness for discharge.** Do not leave the bulk of teaching for the final week. Provide transitional programs for parents. Schedule blocks of hands-on care with each parent, either individually or together. Prior to discharge, encourage the parents to spend the night with their infant in order to assess their readiness for discharge. This maximizes parental competence and confidence and helps strengthen the parent–infant bond. Ideally, the day of discharge is a stress-free day with almost all details wrapped up and teaching complete.

VI. PREPARING HOME SERVICES FOR THE INFANT'S DISCHARGE

A. **Home care services** are becoming more widely available; however, their ability to provide specialized pediatric or neonatal services is variable. Consult the NICU case manager to assess the infant's home care needs, review insurance, and make community referrals.

B. **Home Nursing Care**
   1. **Visiting nurse associations** provide home visits for reinforcement of teaching, health and psychosocial assessments, and short-term treatments or nursing care.
   2. **Private duty nursing or block nursing** may be provided to infants who are discharged home with high acuity, such as with a tracheostomy. Case management should be consulted as soon as it is known that an infant with complex medical needs will be discharged to home. The case manager will make referrals to have an infants care reviewed to determine the allotment of hours. This level of in-home care will require secondary insurance.

C. **Notify emergency care providers,** including community hospital emergency departments and local emergency medical technicians (EMT) or first responders of the child's condition, medical needs, and possible problems. This will optimize appropriate emergency response. Helping the family to prepare a succinct summary of the infant's medical conditions, and current medications can be extremely useful. An electronic copy is preferable so that the information can be updated easily.

D. **Local utility companies,** such as telephone, electricity, fuel, and public works for snow removal, should be notified in writing of the child's presence in the home so they will assign priority resumption of services if there is an interruption.

E. **Supplies and equipment**
   1. Order **equipment** well before discharge to ensure availability and time for teaching.
   2. **Supplies, medications, and special formulas** or dietary supplements should also be specified and ordered as early as possible. Many preparations vary in the community; obtaining and using these items during hands-on teaching in the NICU increase the family's familiarity and promote safe administration.

VII. FOLLOW-UP CARE. Infants with special needs may require many different services and providers to meet all of their needs.

A. **Primary care** is usually provided through a pediatrician, family practitioner, or nurse practitioner. Ongoing communication between NICU staff and the primary care provider begins long before discharge. This maintains continuity and facilitates appropriate medical care after discharge. A family should make a pediatrician appointment for 1 to 3 days after discharge, preferably not on the same day as a visiting nurse appointment, if applicable.

B. **Follow-up appointments** are sometimes needed for a variety of clinics. Consider assisting the family to make this initial set of appointments to help ease an already complex discharge process. Identify which services will be managing what issues so that it is clear to families. For example, will the nutritionist or the pediatrician adjust the formula as a patient grows?

C. **Infant follow-up programs** affiliated with many Level III nurseries offer multidisciplinary services, including developmental assessments, hearing and visual screening, physical therapy assessments, and referrals to community-based providers and support groups (see Chap. 16).

D. **Early intervention programs** are community-based and offer multidisciplinary services for children from birth to age 3. Children deemed at biologic, environmental, or emotional risk are eligible. Programs are partially federally funded and are offered on a sliding scale. They provide multidisciplinary services, including physical therapy, occupational therapy, speech and feeding therapy, early childhood education, social services, and parental support groups. Services may be home based or center based. For further detailed criteria, see Table 18.1.

VIII. COMMUNICATION WITH COMMUNITY PROVIDERS is essential for a smooth transition to home. A verbal conversation before discharge promptly followed up with the written summary (Table 18.3) and copies of hospital studies will allow for optimal communication. A discharge summary may also need to be sent to follow-up programs. VNA and EIP's will require a patient care referral form to be sent by the day of discharge.

IX. ALTERNATIVES TO HOME DISCHARGE may be temporary or permanent. Integrating the child into the home may be difficult because of medical needs or family situation. Decisions regarding alternative placement may be painful for the family and therefore require extra support. Alternatives vary widely from community to community.

A. **Inpatient pediatric ward or Level II nurseries** may be options for the baby who is stable but needs a less intense level of hospital care before going home. Pediatric wards may have a place for parents to room in, and community hospitals may be closer to home. Both options can offer more opportunities for families to be together to participate in care and have more time to learn.

B. **Pediatric rehabilitation hospitals** can be used for the high-risk infant who requires ongoing but less-acute hospital care.

C. **Pediatric nursing homes** provide extended care at a skilled level.

Table 18.3	Neonatal Intensive Care Unit (NICU) Discharge/Interim Summary Dictation Guideline/Discharge Summary Content

NICU Discharge/Interim Summary Dictation Guideline

1. Name of dictator (spell name)

2. Name of attending physician (spell name)

3. Patient's name (spell name)

4. Service ("neonatology")

5. Patient MR#

6. Date of birth and gender of patient

7. Date of admission

8. Date of discharge. If interim summary, state "interim date."

9. History

    a. If interim summary, specify dates covered and author/date of prior summary.

    b. Include reason for admission, birth weight, and gestational age.

    c. Maternal history—including prenatal labs, pregnancy, labor, and birth history.

10. Physical examination on admission

    a. Include weight, head circumference, and length with percentile.

11. Summary of hospital course by systems (concise). Include pertinent lab results

    a. Respiratory – Surfactant if given, maximum level of support. Days on ventilation, continuous positive airway pressure (CPAP), supplemental oxygen. If apnea, report how patient was treated, when treatment ended, and when condition resolved (levels if still on therapy).

    b. Cardiovascular – Diagnoses/therapies in summary form. Echo/electrocardiogram (ECG) results

    c. Fluids, electrolytes, nutrition – Brief feeding history. Include recent weight, length, and head circumference.

    d. Gastrointestinal (GI) – Pertinent diagnoses and treatment. Maximum bilirubin and therapy used.

(continued)

Table 18.3	*(Continued)*

e. Hematology – Patient blood type, brief transfusion summary, recent hematocrit (Hct).
f. Infectious disease – Cultures, antibiotic courses.
g. Neurology – Describe ultrasonographic findings.
h. Sensory
i. Audiology – Hearing screening results. (If baby didn't pass or testing was not performed, indicated date/location of follow-up test or recommend test before discharge.)
ii. Psychosocial – Social work involved with family. Follow-up will be provided by (name of agency/social worker and telephone number).
12. Condition at discharge.
13. Discharge disposition (e.g., home, Level II, Level III, chronic care)
14. Name of primary pediatrician (spell name). Phone # and Fax #.
15. Care/recommendations (quick summary for those assuming care of the infant).
a. Feeds at discharge *(if transitional formula, e.g., Neosure, recommend until 6 to 9 months corrected age)*
b. Medications
c. Car seat screening
d. State newborn screening status
e. Immunizations received
f. Immunizations recommended
i. Synagis (www.synagis.com).
ii. Influenza immunization should be considered annually in the fall for all infants once they reach 6 mo of age. Before this age (and for the first 24 mo of the child's life), immunization against influenza is recommended for household contacts and out-of-home caregivers.
g. Follow-up appointments scheduled/recommended
16. Discharge diagnoses list

D. Medical foster care places the special-needs infant in a home setting with specially trained caregivers. The ultimate goal is to place the infant back with the family.

E. Hospice care may be institutional or home based. It focuses on maximizing the quality of life when cure is not expected.

Suggested Readings

American Academy of Pediatrics. Changing concepts of sudden infant death syndrome: implications for infant sleeping environment and sleep position. *Pediatrics* 2000;105:650–656.

Discenza D. NICU parents' top ten worries at discharge. *Neonatal Netw.* 2009;28(3):202–203.

Griffin T, Abraham M. Transition to home from the newborn intensive care unit: applying the principles of family-centered care to the discharge process. *J Perinat Neonatal Nurs* 2006;20(3):243–249.

Hansen A, Puder M. *Manual of Neonatal Surgical Intensive Care.* 2nd ed. Shelton: People's Medical Publishing House; 2009;612–628.

Hummel P, Cronin J. Home care of the high-risk infant. *Adv Neonatal Care* 2004;4(6):354–364.

Mills MM, Sims DC, Jacob J. Implementation and case-study results of potentially better practices to improve the discharge process in the neonatal intensive care unit. *Pediatrics.* 2006;118(suppl 2):S124–S133.

Scherf RF, Reid KW. Going home: what NICU nurses need to know about home care. *Neonatal Netw* 2006;25(6):421–425.

Section on Ophthalmology American Academy of Pediatrics, American Academy of Ophthalmology, American Association for Pediatric Ophthalmology and Strabismus. Screening examination of premature infants for retinopathy of prematurity. *Pediatrics* 2006;117(2):572–576.

Smith VC, Young S, Pursley DM, et al. Are families prepared for discharge from the NICU? *J Perinatol* 2009;29(9):623–629.

Decision Making and Ethical Dilemmas

Frank X. Placencia

I. BACKGROUND. The practice of neonatology necessitates decision making in all aspects of care. Most neonatologists feel comfortable making routine clinical decisions regarding management of pulmonary or cardiac function, infection, nutrition, and neurodevelopmental care. On the other hand, clinical situations with ethical implications are more difficult for professionals and families. These include decisions regarding instituting, withholding, or withdrawing life-sustaining therapy in patients with irreversible or terminal conditions such as extreme immaturity, severe hypoxic–ischemic encephalopathy, certain congenital anomalies, or other conditions that are refractory to the best available treatments.

A. The **ethical principles** that must be considered in the decision-making process in the neonatal intensive care unit (NICU) include beneficence, nonmaleficence, respect for autonomy, justice, and other principles associated with the physician–patient relationship. Other principles that must be considered include:

1. Treatment decisions must be based on the infant's best interests, free from considerations of race, ethnicity, ability to pay, or other influences. The American Academy of Pediatrics (AAP), the judicial system, and various bioethicists have all embraced some form of this standard, although their interpretations have differed.

2. The infant's parents serve as the legal and moral fiduciaries (or advocates) for their child. The relationship of parents to children is that of responsibility, not rights. Because infants are incapable of making decisions for themselves, the parents become their surrogate decision makers. Therefore, the parents are owed respect for autonomy in making decisions for their infants as long as their decisions do not conflict with the best interests of their child.

3. The physician serves as a fiduciary who acts in the best interest of the patient, using the most current evidence-based medical information. In this role as infant advocate, the physician oversees the responses (decisions) of his or her patient's parents. It is the responsibility of the physician to involve the court system when he or she perceives that the infant's interests are inappropriately threatened by the parents' decision.

B. There is considerable debate on how to define the "best interests" of the infant. The most controversial issue is whether the primary focus should be the preservation of life (the vitalist approach) or to maintaining a particular quality of life (the nonvitalist approach). This debate enters into difficult decisions more frequently as it becomes technically possible to sustain smaller and sicker infants. Staff and parents often struggle with identifying the medical and moral choices and with making decisions based on those choices. These choices, including the understanding of what defines a fulfilling or adequate quality of life, vary substantially among families and professionals.

C. Parental consent versus parental permission. The 1995 AAP Committee on Bioethics policy statement "Informed Consent, Parental Permission, and Assent in Pediatric Practice" embraced the concept of parental permission. Parental permission, like informed consent, requires that parents be informed of the various treatment options, as well as their risks and benefits, and allows them to make decisions in cooperation with the physician. It differs from informed consent in that it is derived from the obligation shared by the parents and physicians to make decisions in the best interest of the infant, thereby enabling the physician to proceed with a treatment plan without parental permission if doing so is clearly in the best interests of the infant.

II. DEVELOPING A PROCESS FOR ETHICAL DECISION MAKING. An ethically sound, well-defined, and rigorous process for making decisions in ethically challenging cases is key to avoiding unwanted intervention by a state agency or court. An NICU should define the decision-making process and identify the individuals (nursing staff, primary medical team, subspecialists, social services, ethicists, hospital legal counsel) that may need to participate in that process. Developing this process allows for healthy discussions among NICU personnel that incorporate ethical knowledge and values at a time and place distant from a specific patient. Ideally, this preparation will ease the stress when an actual decision needs to be made.

A. **Develop an educational program to prepare the NICU caregivers to** address difficult decisions regarding patient care. Focus on process (who, when, where) as well as on substance (how). Identifying areas of frequent consensus and disagreement within an NICU and outlining a general approach to those situations can provide helpful guidance. The educational program should be available for NICU staff and discussed during the orientation of new personnel. The hospital ethics committee can serve as an educational resource for personnel regarding how to deal with ethical decision making.

B. **Part of the educational program could be to identify common ethical situations** (e.g., extreme prematurity, multiple congenital anomalies, severe asphyxia) that might produce conflict and have a series of multidisciplinary discussions about these models. These conversations should include a review of the common underlying ethical principles likely to be in conflict and illuminate common areas of agreement or disagreement. These discussions help develop a consensus on group values, promote a tolerance for individual differences, and establish trust and respect among professionals. The overall goal is to better prepare caregivers when actual situations arise.

C. **Define and support the role of the parents** who should be seen as the primary decision makers for their infant unless they have indicated otherwise. The parents' desired decision making should be explored with them in open and honest discussions. The ethical and legal presumption is that they will make decisions that are in the best interests of their child (best interests standard) and within the context of accepted legal and social boundaries. If the health care providers believe that the parental choice is not in the child's best interest, then they have an obligation as the infant advocate to override the parental decision. Although every effort must be made to align the views of the parents and medical team, in cases of continued disagreement by the parents with the course chosen by the physician to be in the best interests of their infant, the hospital ethics committee, hospital legal counsel, and social services should be consulted, and the court system may need to be involved. In this situation, the physician should continue to serve as the infant's advocate.

D. **Develop consensus among the primary clinical team** and consultants prior to meeting with the parents. Team meetings prior to family meetings provide the opportunity for caregivers to clarify the dilemmas and options that will be offered to the family and, hopefully, to reach a consensus regarding recommendations. It also allows the team to establish who will communicate with the family to help maintain consistency during the discussion of complicated medical and ethical issues.

In large practices, a diverse array of opinions is common. Establishing a forum in which the primary team may solicit the opinions of other staff members on the medical and ethical questions specific to the case serves multiple purposes: (i) identification of alternative treatment options; (ii) identification of staff members (physicians, nurses, etc.) comfortable with pursuing a course of action that current members may not be; (iii) creation of consensus within the group on a specific course of action that can be presented to the hospital ethics committee if need be.

E. **Identify available resources.** Determine the roles of social service, chaplain, hospital attorney, and the hospital ethics committee. Although a general knowledge of existing hospital policies on common situations such as "do not attempt resuscitate" orders or withdrawal of life support should be included in the multidisciplinary discussions mentioned previously, the NICU should identify one or two key resource people who are easily accessible. These professionals should be familiar with hospital policies, the ethics codes of the hospital as well as those of national organizations such as the AAP or the American Medical Association, and applicable federal and state laws. This key resource person is often a member of the hospital ethics committee who can be available without pursuing a formal ethics consult.

F. **Base decisions on the most accurate, up-to-date medical information.** Good ethics begins with good facts. Take the time to accumulate the relevant data. Consultation services are likely to provide valuable input. Be consistent in asking the same appropriate questions in each clinical setting. The answers to these questions may vary from case to case, but the questions regarding the ethical principles must always be asked. Be wary of setting certainty as a goal, as it is almost never achievable in the NICU. Instead, a reasonable degree of medical certainty is often more achievable. As the weight of a decision's consequences increases, so does the rigor of the requirement for a reasonable degree of certainty and the importance of parental involvement in the decision-making process.

G. **People of good conscience can disagree.** Individual caregivers must feel free to remove themselves from patient care if their ethical sense conflicts with the decision of the primary team and parents. This conflict should be handled with the director of nursing or medical director of the NICU. Parents and caregivers must be able to appeal decisions to an individual such as the NICU medical director or to the hospital's ethics committee. No system will provide absolute certainty that the "right" decision will always be made. However, a system that is inclusive, systematic, and built on an approach that establishes a procedure for handling these difficult issues is most likely to produce acceptable decisions.

III. EXTREMELY PREMATURE INFANTS. Nearly all NICUs have struggled with decisions about infants at the threshold of viability and the question of "how small is too small." The practice of resuscitating extremely preterm infants presents difficult medical and ethical challenges. Current technology allows some of these infants to survive, but with a great risk of substantial handicap. Parents may ask that neonatologists pursue aggressive therapies despite poor prognoses. Neonatologists are concerned that instituting those therapies may not be the most appropriate course of action. The AAP statement on perinatal care at the threshold of viability stresses several key areas: (i) parents must receive adequate and current information about potential infant survival and short- and long-term outcomes; (ii) physicians are obligated to be aware of the most current national and local survival data; and (iii) parental choice should be respected as much as possible with joint decision making by both the parents and the physicians as the standard. As more experience is gained with these very difficult situations, further debate and discussion are likely to lead to greater consensus in this area. Guidelines for resuscitation by gestational age or birth weight are intentionally vague. In making these decisions and recommendations, clinicians should take into account the specifics of each pregnancy as well as the local outcomes data (see NICHD Neonatal Research Network (NRN): Extremely Preterm Birth Outcome Data at http://www.nichd.nih.gov/about/org/cdbpm/pp/prog_epbo/epbo_case.cfr site can also be accessed through www.aap.org/sections/perinatal: Pediatricians–Useful Links–NICHD Preemie Outcome Calculator).

IV. THE DECISION TO REDIRECT LIFE-SUSTAINING TREATMENT TO COMFORT MEASURES. One of the most difficult issues is deciding when to withhold or withdraw life-sustaining therapies. Philosophies and approaches vary among caregivers and NICUs. The AAP statement on noninitiation or withdrawal of intensive care for high-risk newborns stresses several key areas: (i) decisions about noninitiation or withdrawal of intensive care should be made by the health care team in collaboration with the parents, who must be well informed about the condition and prognosis of their infant; (ii) parents should be active participants in the decision-making process; (iii) compassionate comfort care should be provided to all infants, including those for whom intensive care is not provided; (iv) it is appropriate to provide intensive care when it is thought to be of benefit to the infant, and not when it is thought to be harmful, of no benefit, or futile.

One model to consider emphasizes an objective interdisciplinary approach to determine the best course of action.

A. The goal of the process is to identify the action that is in the **baby's best interest.** The interests of others, including family and caregivers, are of less priority than are the baby's.

B. Decision making should be guided by data. Caregivers should explore every reasonable avenue to maximize collection of data relevant to the ethical question at hand. Information about alternative therapies and prognosis should be sought. The objective data are evaluated in the context of the primary team's meetings. Subspecialty consultations should be obtained when indicated and included in the primary team's deliberations. Often, these consultations may add extra input to assist in the questions that the primary team is trying to address. It is important that these consultants' input be reviewed with the primary team before discussing such findings with the parents.

C. As the decision to withhold or withdraw life-sustaining medical treatment becomes the focus, the team discusses the best data available, their implications, and their degree of certainty. The goal should be to build a **consensus** regarding the best plan of care for the baby and/or recommendations for the parents. Sometimes there will be strong scientific support for a particular option. In other instances, the best course of action must be estimated. During this time, it is especially important to actively seek feedback from the parents regarding their thoughts, feelings, and understanding of the clinical situation. It should be emphasized that different caregivers reach the consensus at different rates and times. It may be the nursing caregivers who understand and accept the futility of a patient's condition long before the physicians and parents or vice versa. Supporting each participant through this process is important until all understand and accept the consensus and can then readily agree upon a decision.

D. **The parents' role as surrogate decision makers is respected.** This starts with communication that is completely transparent. The primary care team should meet at least daily with the parents to discuss the baby's progress, current status, plan of care, and to summarize the team's medical and ethical discussions. Parental views are always considered; they are most likely to influence decisions when it remains unclear which option (e.g., continuing vs. discontinuing life-sustaining treatment) is in the child's best interest. Parents are not expected to evaluate clinical data in isolation. Even in instances of medical uncertainty, the primary team objectively assesses what is known as well as what remains uncertain about the infant's condition and/or prognosis. The team should also provide the parents with their best assessment and recommendation. In the face of true medical uncertainty, parental wishes should be supported in deference to those of the primary medical team.

E. There is an agreement among ethical and legal scholars that no important distinction exists between **withholding or withdrawing life-sustaining treatments**. Therefore, a therapeutic trial of life-sustaining treatment is acceptable, and parents and staff should not feel remorse in withdrawing those treatments if they no longer, or never did, improve the infant's condition and, therefore, serve his or her best interests. Not using this approach of starting therapy and stopping therapy that is nonbeneficial may result in one of two adverse outcomes: (i) nonbeneficial, possibly even harmful, treatment may be continued longer than necessary; and (ii) some infants who might benefit from treatment may be excluded if it is feared that treatment would needlessly prolong the lives of a greater number of infants whose condition would not respond. The President's Commission on Medical Ethics argues that withdrawal of life-sustaining treatment after having shown no efficacy may be more justifiable than presuming futility and thus withholding treatment. This approach supports the concept of a "trial of intensive care" wherein the staff and family agree to start life-sustaining treatment and to discontinue it if it becomes clear that continued treatment is no longer in the infant's best interest.

The 1984 amendment to the Child Abuse and Prevention and Treatment Act (CAPTA) defines treatment as *not* medically indicated if the infant is irreversibly comatose, if it would merely prolong dying, not be effective in ameliorating or correcting all of the life-threatening conditions, if it would be futile in terms of survival, or if it would be virtually futile in terms of survival and be inhumane. These conditions both protect the rights of children to treatment despite underlying conditions or potential handicaps and support the importance of quality-of-life determinations in the provision of care. Substantial conflict can arise if the caregivers and parents disagree about the goals of care. An NICU must be prepared for these circumstances.

F. The **hospital ethics committee** is helpful when the primary team is unable to reach consensus or disagrees with the parents' wishes. In our experience, consultation with the ethics committee helps encourage communication among all involved parties and improve collaborative decision making. The ethics committee can often ease tensions between parents and caregivers, allowing for a resolution to the dilemma.

Suggested Readings

American Academy of Pediatrics Committee on Fetus and Newborn, Bell EF. Noninitiation or withdrawal of intensive care for high-risk newborns. *Pediatrics* 2007;119(2):401–403.

Batton DG; Committee on Fetus and Newborn. Clinical report—Antenatal counseling regarding resuscitation at an extremely low gestational age. *Pediatrics* 2009;124(1):422–427.

Informed consent, parental permission, and assent in pediatric practice. Committee on Bioethics, American Academy of Pediatrics. *Pediatrics* 1995;95(2):314–317.

President's Commission for the Study of Ethical Problems in Medicine and Biomedical and Behavioral Research. *Deciding to Forego Life-Sustaining Treatment: A Report on the Ethical, Medical, and Legal Issues in Treatment Decisions.* Washington, DC: U.S. G.P.O.; 1983.

Pub L No. 98-457, the Amendment to Child Abuse Prevention and Treatment Act (CAPTA).

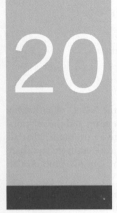

20 Management of Neonatal End-of-Life Care and Bereavement Follow-up

Caryn E. Douma

I. INTRODUCTION. Providing compassionate, family-centered, end-of-life care in the neonatal intensive care unit (NICU) environment is challenging for caregivers. The care team must balance the medical needs of the infant with those of the parents and family. Parents are profoundly affected by the compassion and treatment they receive from health care providers during end-of-life care. Although the death of a baby is a devastating event, the knowledge and skill of the multidisciplinary team can greatly influence the ability of the parents to effectively cope with their loss.

Despite advances in neonatal care, more children die in the perinatal and neonatal period than in any other time in childhood. The majority of neonatal deaths in the United States are due to congenital malformations and disorders related to short gestation and low birth weight.

For many families, a lethal or life-limiting condition may be diagnosed early in the pregnancy, thus the opportunity to begin the decision-making process occurs prior to admission to the NICU. Perinatal hospice is an alternative to termination of pregnancy and provides a structured approach for the parents and the care team when developing a plan to create the best possible outcome for the baby and family.

II. FAMILY-CENTERED END-OF-LIFE CARE PRINCIPLES AND DOMAINS. The provision of quality end-of-life care is a process that allows for clear and consistent communication delivered by a compassionate multidisciplinary team within a framework of shared decision making. Providing physical and emotional support and follow-up care enables the parents to begin the healing process as they return home.

End-of-life domains comprise family-centered care in the intensive care unit. These domains provide guidance and process measures to assess and provide quality of care at the end of life.

A. Patient- and family-centered decision making

B. Communication among the multidisciplinary team members and between the team and the parents and families

C. Spiritual support of families

D. Emotional and practical support of families

E. Symptom management and comfort care

F. Continuity of care

G. Emotional and organizational support for health care workers

III. COORDINATION OF CARE

A. Communication and collaboration. Family support in the NICU relies heavily on communication between the family and the health care team and the relationship among the members of the care team. A collaborative care model that allows physicians, nurses, and other team members to work cooperatively and share decisions, while respecting each professional's unique contribution, promotes an environment where the best care can be delivered.

1. Care provided at the end of life is an extension of the relationship already in place between the care providers and the infant and family. Staff can facilitate this relationship in the following ways:

   a. Communicate with families through frequent meetings with the primary team

   b. Include the obstetrical care team and other consultants when appropriate

   c. Encourage sibling visitation and extended family support

   d. Encourage incorporation of cultural and spiritual customs

   e. Provide an environment that allows parents to develop a relationship with their infant, visiting and holding as often as medically appropriate

2. Parents want to be given information in a clear, concise manner and value honesty and transparency.

3. Clear recommendations about the goals of care (life support vs. comfort care) from the health care team are appropriate and may relieve parents of some of the burden of decision making in the end-of-life context.

4. Most neonatal deaths occur following a decision to remove life-sustaining treatment.

5. Prior to meeting with the family to discuss redirection of care from treatment to comfort, it is important for the multidisciplinary team to agree on goals of care and identify the needs of the patient and family.

6. Address conflicts within the team early in the process, utilizing available professional supports, such as ethical or spiritual consultants.

7. It is essential for the team to reach agreement prior to meeting with the family.

8. One spokesperson (usually the attending physician) is recommended to maintain continuity of communication.

B. Patient- and family-centered decision making

1. Most parents want to be involved in the decision to transition care from treatment to comfort, yet not all are able to participate or want to feel responsible for the final decision. They rely on the care team to interpret the information and deliver the choices in a compassionate, sensitive manner that incorporates their individual needs and desired level of involvement.

2. The parents need to feel supported regardless of the decision that is made.

3. The quality of the relationship and the communication style of the team members can influence the ability of the parents to understand the information presented and to reach consensus with the heath care team.

4. Shared decision making involves the support and participation of the entire team.

5. Meet with the family in a private, quiet area and allow ample time for the family to understand the information presented and the recommendations of the team.

   a. Provide a medical translator if needed.

   b. Refer to the baby by name.

   c. Ask the parents how they feel and how they perceive the situation.

   d. Once the decision has been made to redirect care away from supporting life to comfort measures, develop a specific plan with the family that involves a description of how life-sustaining support will be withdrawn and determine their desired level of participation.

C. Withdrawing life-sustaining treatment

1. Once a decision has been made to withdraw life-sustaining treatment and provide comfort care, the family should be provided an environment that is quiet, private, and will accommodate everyone the family wishes to include.

2. Staffing should be arranged so that one nurse and one physician will be readily available to the family at all times.

3. Allow parents ample time to create memories and become a family. Allow them to hold, photograph, bathe, and dress their infant before, during, or after withdrawing mechanical ventilation or other life support.

4. Discuss the entire process with parents, including endotracheal tube removal and pain control. Gently describe how the infant will look and the measures that the staff will take to provide the infant with a comfortable, pain-free death. Let them know that death will not always occur immediately.

5. Arrange for baptism and spiritual support if desired; incorporate spiritual and cultural customs into the plan of care if desired.

6. The goal of comfort care is to provide a pain-free comfortable death. Anticipate medications that may be required, leaving intravenous access in place. Discontinue muscle relaxation before extubation. The goal of medication use should be to ensure that the infant is as comfortable as possible.

7. When the infant is extubated, discontinue all unnecessary intravenous catheters and equipment.

8. Allow parents to hold their infant for as long as they desire after withdrawing life support. The nurse and attending physician should be nearby to assist the family and assess heart rate and comfort of the infant.

9. When the family has a surviving multiple, it is important that the care team acknowledge the difficulty that this will present both at the time of death and during the grieving process.

10. Autopsy should be discussed before or after death at the discretion of the attending physician.

11. Create a memory box including crib cards, photographs, clothing, a lock of hair, footprints, handprints, and any other mementos accumulated during the infant's life. Keep them in a designated place if the family does not desire to see or keep them at the time of death. Parents often change their minds later and are grateful that these items have been retained.

12. Be sure that photographs of the infant have been taken. Parents of multiples will often want a photograph of their children together or a family picture. It is helpful for the NICU to have a digital camera and printer available. Now I Lay Me Down To Sleep (NILMDTS) is an organization that utilizes volunteer professional photographers and is available in many communities.

D. Emotional and organizational support for staff

1. A debriefing meeting for all members of the health care team after a baby's death provides an opportunity for those involved with the death to share their thoughts and emotions, if desired. Chaplains and social workers are often good resources for staff support and are usually considered a part of the care team.

2. Reviewing the events surrounding the death helps to identify what went well and opportunities for improvement.

3. Institutional support may include paid funeral leave, counseling, and remembrance ceremonies.

4. Recognizing and addressing staff response to grief in the workplace is a necessary part of providing end-of-life care.

5. Many institutions have developed formal programs to support staff working with dying patients. Programs often include support groups, counseling, writing workshops, and other interventions. Creating rituals around the time of death and providing time to reflect before returning to care for patients can be helpful.

IV. BEREAVEMENT FOLLOW-UP

A. General principles. Bereavement follow-up provides continuing support to families as they return home to continue the grieving process. Some families may not wish any contact with the team after they return home and others may desire more frequent meetings or calls. Prior to leaving the hospital, it is important for a member of the team to review the follow-up support that will be provided. A bereavement packet with literature and a summary of hospital specific programs are useful to provide the family with grief resources and contact information. Most programs include follow-up calls and cards within the first week and again between four and six weeks after the death of the infant. A follow-up meeting with the team allows the family the opportunity to review the events that surrounded the death, including the autopsy results if appropriate. In addition to providing support to the family, the meeting allows the team to assess the need for further support and provide referrals that might include support groups or counseling.

B. Hospital care

1. A designated team member or bereavement coordinator should review the program and bereavement materials with the parents or a family member. Often, a family support person is best able to absorb this information and communicate to the parents at the appropriate time.

2. Briefly describe the normal grieving process and what to expect in the following days and weeks.

3. Lactation support should be offered if appropriate and a plan made for lactation suppression and follow-up.

4. Provide assistance in making burial or cremation arrangements.

5. The family's obstetrician, pediatrician, and other community supports should be notified of the infant's death.

6. A representative from the primary team or appropriately trained designee should assume responsibility for coordinating bereavement follow-up. This person will be responsible for arranging and documenting the follow-up process.

7. Provide assistance to the family as they leave the hospital without their child. If possible, arrange for prepaid valet parking or an escort to the door.

C. Follow-up after discharge

1. Contact the family within the first week to provide an opportunity for questions and offer support. The designated follow-up coordinator usually takes responsibility for placing the call and documentation. Other members of the care team may wish to maintain contact if they developed a close relationship with the family. It is important to discuss specific follow-up details with the family prior to discharge home.

2. Parents appreciate receiving a sympathy card, signed by members of the primary team sent to their home within the first few weeks, and communication at selected intervals.

3. Schedule a follow-up meeting with the family approximately 4 to 6 weeks after the infant's death. Timing will depend on availability of autopsy results and parental preference. In some cases, the family will not want to return to the hospital or continue contact. The coordinator will make sure this is documented and arrange for the family to be followed through a primary care provider or other community agency. Follow-up calls can still be made if the family consents.

4. Meetings should include a review of events surrounding the infant's death, results of the autopsy or other studies, and implications for future pregnancies.

5. Assessment should be made to determine the coping ability of the family as they continue with the grieving process and referrals made to appropriate professionals or agencies including bereavement support groups if needed.

6. Send a card and initiate a phone call around the 1-year anniversary of the infant's death. This can be a difficult time for the family. Many families develop their own rituals to celebrate the life of their child during this time. Contact from members of their care team is greatly appreciated.

7. Plan for future meetings if the family desires.

Suggested Readings

Abe N, Catlin A, Mihara D. End of life in the NICU: a study of ventilator withdrawal. *Am J Matern Child Nurs* 2001;26(3):141–146.

Clarke EB, Curtis JR, Luce JM, et al. Quality indicators for end-of-life care in the intensive care unit. *Crit Care Med* 2003;31(9):2255–2262.

Gale G, Brooks A. Implementing a palliative care protocol in a newborn intensive care unit. *Adv Neonatal Care* 2006;6(1):37–53.

Munson D, Leuthner SR. Palliative care for the family carrying a fetus with a life-limiting diagnosis. *Pediatr Clin N Am* 2007;54(5):787–798.

21 Nutrition

Deirdre M. Ellard and Diane M. Anderson

Following birth, term infants rapidly adapt from a relatively constant intrauterine supply of nutrients to intermittent feedings of milk. Preterm infants, however, are at increased risk for potential nutritional compromise. These infants are born with limited nutrient reserves, immature metabolic pathways, and increased nutrient demands. In addition, medical and surgical conditions commonly associated with prematurity have the potential to alter nutrient requirements and complicate adequate nutrient delivery. As survival for these high-risk newborns continues to improve, current data suggest that early, aggressive nutrition intervention is advantageous.

I. GROWTH

A. Fetal body composition changes throughout gestation, with accretion of most nutrients occurring primarily in the late second and throughout the third trimester. Term infants will normally have sufficient glycogen and fat stores to meet energy requirements during the relative starvation of the first day after birth. In contrast, preterm infants will rapidly deplete their limited nutrient reserves, becoming both hypoglycemic and catabolic unless appropriate nutritional therapy is provided. In practice, it is generally assumed that the severity of nutrient insufficiency is inversely related to gestational age at birth and birth weight.

B. Postnatal growth varies from intrauterine growth in that it begins with a period of weight loss, primarily through the loss of extracellular fluid. The typical loss of 5% to 10% of birth weight for a full-term infant may increase to as much as 15% of birth weight in infants born preterm. The nadir in weight loss usually occurs by 4 to 6 days of life, with birth weight being regained by 14 to 21 days of life in most preterm infants. Currently, there is no widely accepted measure of neonatal growth that captures both the weight loss and subsequent gain characteristic of this period. Goals in practice are to limit the degree and duration of initial weight loss in preterm infants and to facilitate regain of birth weight within 7 to 14 days of life.

C. After achieving birth weight, intrauterine growth and nutrient accretion rate data are widely accepted as reference standards for assessing growth and nutrient requirements. Goals of 10 to 20 g/kg/day weight gain (15–20 g/kg/day for infants <1,500 g), approximately 1 cm/week in length, and 0.5 to 1 cm/week in head circumference are used. Although these goals are not initially attainable in most preterm infants, replicating growth of the fetus at the same gestational age remains an appropriate goal as recommended by the American Academy of Pediatrics (AAP).

D. Serial measurements of weight, head circumference, and length plotted on growth curves provide valuable information in the nutritional assessment of the preterm infant. Historically, the Lubchenco intrauterine growth curves (1966) have been widely used because the chart is based on a reasonable sample size, provides curves to monitor weight, length, and head circumference, and is easy to use and interpret. Of late, the Fenton (2003) fetal-infant chart has been more frequently utilized. The chart is based on a larger number of infants from a wider geographic location and reflects infants born more recently. With the Fenton chart, the premature infant's growth can be monitored for a longer period of time, from 22 to 50 weeks postmenstrual age (PMA). Most recently, the Olsen (2010) growth curves have become available (Figure 21.1A–D). These newer growth charts are drawn from a large, contemporary, racially diverse US sample. Gender-specific weight, length, and head circumference curves are provided. Postnatal growth curves are also available. Postnatal growth curves follow the same infants over time (i.e., longitudinal growth curves), and are available from a number of single–neonatal intensive care unit (NICU) studies and from the National Institute for Child Health and Human Development (NICHD) multicenter study (2000). These curves, however, show **actual**, not ideal, growth. Although these curves provide interesting information by allowing comparison of the growth of infants in one NICU to those in another, they do not indicate if either group of infants is growing adequately. Intrauterine growth remains the gold standard for comparison.

E. When an infant is in full-term corrected gestational age, the Centers for Disease Control and Prevention (CDC) recommends the World Health Organization (WHO) Child Growth Standards 2006 be used for monitoring of growth. Infants should be plotted by corrected age and followed for catch-up growth. The charts can be downloaded from www.cdc.gov/growthcharts/who_charts.htm.

II. NUTRIENT RECOMMENDATIONS

A. Sources for nutrient recommendations for preterm infants include the American Academy of Pediatrics Committee on Nutrition (AAP-CON), the European Society for Paediatric Gastroenterology, Hepatology, and Nutrition Committee on Nutrition (ESPGHAN-CON), and the Reasonable Ranges of Nutrient Intakes published by Tsang and colleagues (Table 21.1). These recommendations are based on (i) intrauterine accretion rate data, (ii) the nutrient content of human milk, (iii) the assumed decreased nutrient stores and higher nutritional needs in preterm infants, and (iv) the available data on biochemical measures reflecting adequate intake. However, due to the limitations of the currently available data, the goals for nutrient intake for preterm infants are considered to be recommendations only.

B. **Fluid** (see Chaps. 13 and 23). The initial step in nutritional support is to determine an infant's fluid requirement, which is dependent on gestational age, postnatal age, and environmental conditions. Generally, baseline fluid needs are inversely related to gestational age at birth and birth weight. During the first week of life, very low birth weight (VLBW) infants are known to experience increased water loss because of the immaturity of their skin, which has a higher water content and increased permeability, and the immaturity of their renal function with a decreased ability to concentrate urine. Environmental factors, such as radiant warmers and phototherapy versus humidified incubators, also impact insensible losses and may affect fluid requirements. Conversely, restriction of fluid intake may be necessary to assist with the prevention and/or treatment of patent ductus arteriosus, renal insufficiency, and bronchopulmonary dysplasia (BPD). Fluid

Intrauterine Growth Curves

Name _____

Record # _____

FEMALES

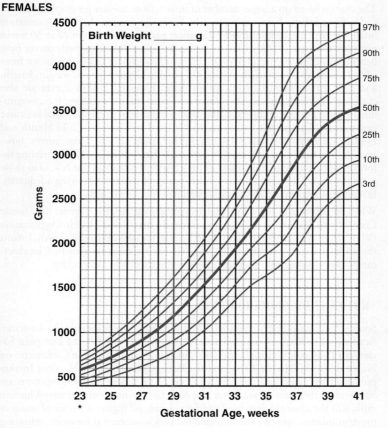

Birth Weight _____ g

BIRTH SIZE ASSESSMENT:

Date of Birth: / / (wks GA)	Select One
Large-for-gestational age (LGA) >90th percentile	☐
Appropriate-for-gestational age (AGA) 10–90th percentile	☐
Small-for-gestational age (SGA) <10th percentile	☐

* 3rd and 97th percentile on all curves for 23 weeks should be interpreted cautiously given the small sample size.

Figure 21.1. Intrauterine growth curves for males and females. Reproduced with permission from Olsen IE, Groveman S, Lawson ML, et al. New intrauterine growth curves based on United States data. *Pediatrics* 2010;125:e214–e224. Copyright 2010 by the American Academy of Pediatrics. Data source: Pediatrix Medical Group.

Page 2

Name _____

Record # _____

FEMALES

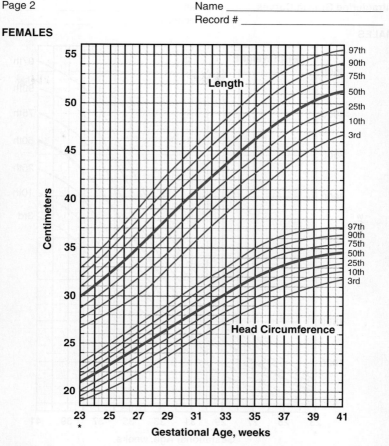

Date																		
GA (wks)																		
WT (g)																		
L (cm)																		
HC (cm)																		

* 3rd and 97th percentile on all curves for 23 weeks should be interpreted cautiously given the small sample size.

Figure 21.1. *(Continued)*

Intrauterine Growth Curves

Name _____

Record # _____

MALES

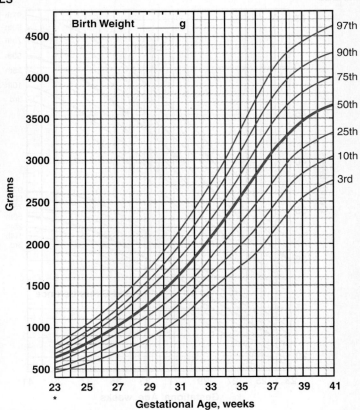

BIRTH SIZE ASSESSMENT:

Date of Birth: / / (wks GA)	Select One
Large-for-gestational age (LGA) >90th percentile	☐
Appropriate-for-gestational age (AGA) 10–90th percentile	☐
Small-for-gestational age (SGA) <10th percentile	☐

* 3rd and 97th percentile on all curves for 23 weeks should be interpreted cautiously given the small sample size.

Figure 21.1. *(Continued)*

Page 2   Name _____

    Record # _____

MALES

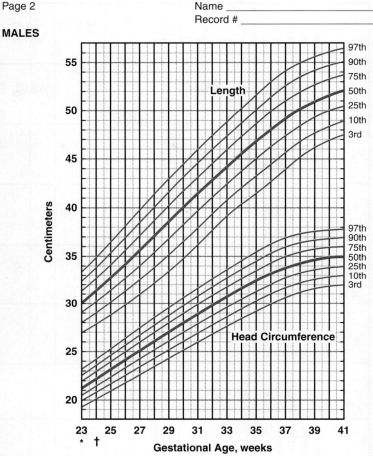

Date																
GA (wks)																
WT (g)																
L (cm)																
HC (cm)																

* 3rd and 97th percentile on all curves for 23 weeks should be interpreted cautiously given the small sample size.

† Male head circumference curve at 24 weeks all percentiles should be interpreted cautiously as the distribution of data is skewed left.

Figure 21.1. *(Continued)*

Table 21.1 Comparison of Enteral Intake Recommendations and Selected Feeding Regimens* for the Preterm Infant

Nutrient	Unit	Enteral intake recommendations for growing, stable preterm infants (2, 8)	Mature human milk‡	Mature human milk plus 4 packets Enfamil HMF/dL	Mature human milk plus 4 vials Enfamil HMF acidified liquid	Mature human milk plus 4 packets Similac HMF/dL	Mature human milk plus Prolact +4	24 kcal/oz Enfamil Premature w/ Iron	24 kcal/oz Similac Special Care w/ Iron
Protein‡‡	g/kg/day		1.6	3.2	4	3	3	3.6	3.6
ELBW infants	g/kg/day	3.8–4.4							
VLBW infants	g/kg/day	3.4–4.2							
Carbohydrate	g/kg/day		10.8	11.4	9.7	13.5	11.4	13.4	12.6
ELBW infants	g/kg/day	9–20							
VLBW infants	g/kg/day	7–17							
Fat	g/kg/day		5.9	7.4	7.7	6.4	7.4	6.2	6.6
ELBW infants	g/kg/day	6.2–8.4							
VLBW infants	g/kg/day	5.3–7.2							
Docosahexaenoic acid	mg/kg/day				≥15			20.7	17.1

	Units								
ELBW infants	mg/kg/day	≥21							
VLBW infants	mg/kg/day	≥18							
Arachidonic acid	mg/kg/day							42	26.9
ELBW infants	mg/kg/day	≥28							
VLBW infants	mg/kg/day	≥24							
Vitamin A	IU/kg/day	700–1,500	338	1,763	1,731	1,268	360	1,515	1,521
Vitamin D	IU/day	150–400‡‡‡	3	228	237	183	42	292.5	183
Vitamin E	IU/kg/day	6–12	0.6	7.5	7.5	5.4	1	7.7	4.8
Vitamin K	mcg/kg/day	8–10	0.3	6.9	7.4	12.8	0.2	9.8	14.6
Thiamine	mcg/kg/day	180–240	32	257	257	381	31.5	243	304.5
Riboflavin	mcg/kg/day	250–360	52	382	373	677	64.5	360	754.5
Vitamin B_6	mcg/kg/day	150–210	30.6	203	200	347	24	183	304.5
Vitamin B_{12}	mcg/kg/day	0.3	0.07	0.3	1	1	0.06	0.3	0.67
Niacin	mg/kg/day	3.6–4.8	0.2	4.7	4.8	5.6	0.26	4.8	6.1

(continued)

Table 21.1		Comparison of Enteral Intake Recommendations and Selected Feeding Regimens* for the Preterm Infant *(Continued)*							
Nutrient	Unit	Enteral intake recommendations for growing, stable preterm infants (2, 8)	Mature human milk‡	Mature human milk plus 4 packets Enfamil HMF/dL	Mature human milk plus 4 vials Enfamil HMF acidified liquid	Mature human milk plus 4 packets Similac HMF/dL	Mature human milk plus Prolact +4	24 kcal/oz Enfamil Premature w/ Iron	24 kcal/oz Similac Special Care w/ Iron
Folate	mcg/kg/day	25–50	7.2	44.7	44.4	41.7	13.5	48	45
Pantothenic acid	mg/kg/day	1.2–1.7	0.27	1.4	1.4	2.5	0.33	1.5	2.3
Biotin	mcg/kg/day	3.6–6	0.6	4.7	4.7	39.6	0.75	4.8	45
Vitamin C	mg/kg/day	18–24	6.1	24	24	43.5	4.5	24.3	45
Choline	mg/kg/day	14.4–28	14.3			17.2	12	24.3	12
Inositol	mg/kg/day	32–81	22.5			28.5	18	54	48
Taurine	mg/kg/day	4.5–9						7.3	
Carnitine	mg/kg/day	~2.9						2.9	
Calcium	mg/kg/day	100–220	42	177	180	217.5	210	201	219

		60–140	21.4	96.3	97	121.9	121.5	100.5	121.5
Phosphorus	mg/kg/day	60–140	21.4	96.3	97	121.9	121.5	100.5	121.5
Magnesium	mg/kg/day	7.9–15	5.2	6.7	6.6	15.6	11.9	11	14.6
Iron	mg/kg/day	2–4	0.04	2.2	2.2	0.6	0.15	2.2	2.2
Zinc	mcg/kg/day	1,000–3,000	183	1,263	1,352	1,683	960	1,830	1,830
Manganese	mcg/kg/day	0.7–7.5	1	16	13	11.8	19.5	7.7	15
Copper	mcg/kg/day	120–150	37.8	103.8	107	292.8	121.5	145.5	304.5
Iodine	mcg/kg/day	10–60	16.3				13.5	30	7.5
Selenium	mcg/kg/day	1.3–4.5	2.3			3		3.5	2.3
Sodium	mEq/kg/day	3–5	1.2	2.2	2.5	2.2	3.3	3.1	2.3
Potassium	mEq/kg/day	2–3	2	3.1	3.1	4.4	3	3.1	4
Chloride	mEq/kg/day	3–7	1.8	2.3	2.5	3.4	3	3.1	2.9

HMF = Human Milk Fortifier
*Calculated intakes of human milk feedings and formulas are based on an intake of 150 mL/kg/day.
‡ Denotes milk of mothers of preterm infants post the first 21 days of lactation.
‡‡ The AAP suggests the estimated requirements based on the fetal accretion rate of protein are 3.5 to 4 g/kg/day.
‡‡‡ Aim for 400 IU/day.

requirements in the first weeks of life are, therefore, continually reassessed, as the transition is made from fetal to neonatal life and at least daily afterward.

C. **Energy.** Estimates suggest that preterm infants in a thermoneutral environment require approximately 40 to 60 kcal/kg/day for maintenance of body weight, assuming adequate protein is provided. Additional calories are needed for growth, with the smallest neonates tending to demonstrate the greatest need, as their rate of growth is highest (Table 21.2). The AAP recommends 105 to 130 kcal/kg/day. Practice generally strives for energy intakes of 110 to 130 kcal/kg/day. Infants with severe and/or prolonged illness frequently require a range of 130 to 150 kcal/kg/day. Lesser intakes (90–120 kcal/kg/day) may sustain intrauterine growth rates if energy expenditure is minimal or if parenteral nutrition (PN) is used.

III. PN

A. **Nutrient goals.** Our initial goal for PN is to provide adequate calories and amino acids to prevent negative energy and nitrogen balance. Goals thereafter include the promotion of appropriate weight gain and growth, while awaiting the attainment of adequate enteral intake.

B. **Indications for initiating PN**

PN is started the first postnatal day for infants who are <1,500 g birth weight. Infants for whom significant enteral intake is not anticipated by 5 days of age or those with cardiac disease requiring calcium supplementation may also be considered for PN.

Table 21.2	Estimation of Energy Requirement of the Low Birth Weight Infant*
	Average estimation, kcal/kg/day
Energy expended	40–60
Resting metabolic rate	40–50†
Activity	0–5†
Thermoregulation	0–5†
Synthesis	15‡
Energy stored	20–30‡
Energy excreted	15
Energy intake	90–120

*From: American Academy of Pediatrics, Committee on Nutrition (AAP-CON). *Pediatric Nutrition Handbook*. 6th ed. Elk Grove Village, IL: American Academy of Pediatrics; 2009.
† Energy for maintenance.
‡ Energy cost of growth.

C. Peripheral versus central PN

1. Parenteral solutions may be infused through peripheral veins or a central vein, accessed from the antecubital and saphenous veins, respectively. Historically, the AAP has recommended that peripheral solutions maintain an osmolarity between 300 and 900 mOsm/L. Because of this limitation, peripheral solutions often cannot adequately support growth in extremely low birth weight (ELBW) infants. Central PN not only allows for the use of more hypertonic solutions but also incurs greater risks, particularly catheter-related sepsis.

2. Central PN is considered to be warranted under the following conditions:
   a. Nutritional needs exceed the capabilities of peripheral PN
   b. An extended period (e.g., >7 days) of inability to take enteral feedings, such as in infants with necrotizing enterocolitis (NEC) and in some postoperative infants
   c. Imminent lack of peripheral venous access

D. Carbohydrate. Dextrose (D-glucose) is the carbohydrate source in intravenous (IV) solutions (see Chap. 24).

1. The caloric value of dextrose is 3.4 kcal/g.

2. Because dextrose contributes to the osmolarity of a solution, it is generally recommended that the concentration administered through peripheral veins be limited to ≤12.5% dextrose. Higher concentrations of dextrose may be used for central venous infusions in circumstances when fluid volume is severely restricted. Infants receiving extracorporeal membrane oxygenation (ECMO) therapy may require up to 40% dextrose.

3. Dextrose infusions are typically referred to in terms of the milligrams of glucose per kilogram per minute (mg/kg/min) delivered, which expresses the total glucose load and accounts for infusion rate, dextrose concentration, and patient weight (Figure 21.2).

4. The initial glucose requirement for term infants is defined as the amount that is necessary to avoid hypoglycemia. In general, this may be achieved with initial infusion rates of approximately 4 mg/kg/minute.

5. Preterm infants usually require higher rates of glucose, as they have a higher brain-to-body weight ratio and higher total energy needs. Initial infusion rates of 4 to 8 mg/kg/minute may be required to maintain euglycemia.

6. Initial rates may be advanced, as tolerated, by 1 to 2 mg/kg/minute daily to a maximum of 11 to 12 mg/kg/minute. This may be accomplished by increasing dextrose concentration, by increasing infusion rate, or by a combination of both. Infusion rates above 11 to 12 mg/kg/minute may exceed the infant's oxidative capacity and are generally not recommended, as this may cause the excess glucose to be converted to fat, particularly in the liver. This conversion may also increase oxygen consumption, energy expenditure, and CO_2 production.

7. The quantity of dextrose that an infant can tolerate will vary with gestational and postnatal age. Signs of glucose intolerance include hyperglycemia and secondary glucosuria with osmotic diuresis.

E. Protein. Crystalline amino acid solutions provide the nitrogen source in PN.

1. The caloric value of amino acids is 4 kcal/g.

2. Three pediatric amino acid formulations are commercially available in the United States: TrophAmine (B. Braun), Aminosyn-PF (Hospira), and PremaSol

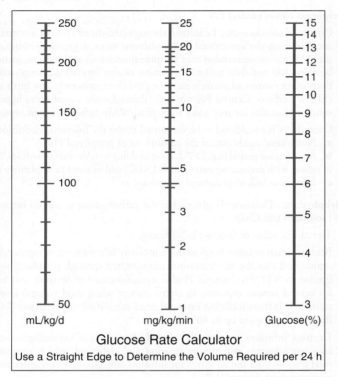

Figure 21.2. Interconversion of glucose infusion units. From Klaus MH, Faranoff AA, eds. *Care of the High-Risk Neonate.* 2nd ed. Philadelphia: WB Saunders, 1979:430.

(Baxter). In theory, these products are better adapted to the needs of newborns than are standard adult formulations, as they have been modified for improved tolerance and contain conditionally essential amino acids. However, the optimal amino acid composition for neonatal PN has not yet been defined, and there are no products currently available that are specifically designed for preterm infants.

3. It has been demonstrated that VLBW infants who do not receive amino acids in the first postnatal days catabolize body protein at a rate of at least 1 g/kg/day. Studies investigating the use of early amino acids have consistently shown a reversal of this catabolism without adverse metabolic consequences. Current recommendations support the infusion of amino acids in a dose of 2 g/kg/day beginning in the first 24 hours after birth.

4. Infants with a birth weight <1,250 g are provided with 2 to 2.4 g/kg/day beginning immediately after birth. Infants with a birth weight between 1,250 and 1,500 g are initiated on 2 g/kg/day within the first 24 hours of life. Infants >1,500 g are only initiated on 2 g/kg/day if indicated, depending on their size, clinical condition, and estimated time to achieve significant enteral volumes.

5. Protein infusion rates are generally advanced to a target of 3.5 g/kg/day for premature infants and up to 3 g/kg/day for the term neonates.

F. **Lipid.** Soybean oil, or a combination of soybean and safflower oil, provides the fat source for IV fat emulsions.

1. The caloric value of 20% lipid emulsions is 2 kcal/mL (approximately 10 kcal/g). The use of 20% emulsions is preferred over 10% because the higher ratio of phospholipids to triglyceride in the 10% emulsion interferes with plasma triglyceride clearance. Twenty percent emulsions also provide a more concentrated source of calories. For these reasons, only 20% lipid emulsions are used.

2. Current data suggest that preterm infants are at risk for essential fatty acid (EFA) deficiency within 72 hours after birth if an exogenous fat source is not delivered. This deficiency state can be avoided by the administration of 0.5 to 1 g/kg/day of lipid emulsion. Therefore, infants weighing <1,500 g at birth are provided with approximately 1 to 2 g/kg/day within the first 24 to 48 hours after birth. This rate is advanced by approximately 1 g/kg/day, as tolerated, to a target of 3 g/kg/day.

3. Tolerance also correlates with hourly infusion rate, and no benefit to a rest period has been identified. Therefore, lipid emulsions are infused over 24 hours for optimal clearance. However, due to sepsis risk factors, syringes may be changed every 12 hours.

G. **Electrolytes**

1. Sodium and potassium concentrations are adjusted daily based on individual requirements (see Chap. 23). Maintenance requirements are estimated at approximately 2 to 4 mEq/kg.

2. Increasing the proportion of anions provided as acetate aids in the treatment of metabolic acidosis in VLBW infants.

H. **Vitamins.** The current vitamin formulations (MVI Pediatric, Hospira, INFU-VITE Pediatric, Baxter) do not maintain blood levels of all vitamins within an acceptable range for preterm infants. However, there are no products currently available that are specifically designed for preterm infants. Table 21.3 provides guidelines for the use of the available formulations for term and preterm infants. For infants less than 2,500 g, the AAP suggests a dose of 40% of the MVI Pediatric (INFUVITE Pediatric) 5 mL vial/kg/day. This guideline may be met by adding 1.5 mL MVI Pediatric/100 mL PN and administered at a rate of approximately 140 mL/kg. For infants 2,500 g or greater, the AAP suggests the 5 mL MVI Pediatric (INFUVITE Pediatric) per day. Vitamin A is the most difficult to provide in adequate amounts to the VLBW infant without providing excess amounts of the other vitamins, as it is subject to losses through photodegradation and absorption to plastic tubing and solution-containing bags. B vitamins may also be affected by photodegradation. This is of particular concern with long-term PN use and, for this reason, consideration should be given to shielding the PN-containing plastic bags and tubing from light.

I. **Minerals.** The amount of calcium and phosphorus that can be administered through IV is limited by the precipitation of calcium phosphate. Unfortunately, the variables that determine calcium and phosphate compatibility in PN are

Table 21.3	Suggested Intakes of Parenteral Vitamins in Infants			
	Estimated needs		2 mL of a 5 mL single-dose vial MVI Pediatric (Hospira), INFUVITE Pediatric (Baxter)	1.5 mL MVI Pediatric (Hospira), INFUVITE Pediatric (Baxter) per 100 mL PN administered at a rate of 140 mL/kg/day[†]
Vitamins	Term infants (≥2.5 kg) (dose/day)	Preterm infants (≤2.5 kg)*		
Lipid soluble				
A (mcg)[‡]	700	280	280	294
D (IU)[‡]	400	160	160	168
E (mg)[‡]	7	2.8	2.8	2.9
K (mcg)	200	80	80	84
Water soluble				
Thiamine (mg)	1.2	0.48	0.48	0.5
Riboflavin (mg)	1.4	0.56	0.56	0.59
Niacin (mg)	17	6.8	6.8	7.1
Pantothenate (mg)	5	2	2	2.1
Pyridoxine (mg)	1	0.4	0.4	0.42
Biotin (mcg)	20	8	8	8.4
Vitamin B_{12} (mcg)	1	0.4	0.4	0.42
Ascorbic acid (mg)	80	32	32	34
Folic acid (mcg)	140	56	56	59

* Dose/kg of body weight per day for preterm infants, not to exceed daily dose for term (>2.5 kg) infants.
† Assumes 140 mL/kg is the maximum PN administration rate.
‡ 700 mcg retinol equivalent = 2,300 IU; 7 mg alpha-tocopherol = 7 IU; 10 mcg vitamin D = 400 IU.

complex and what constitutes maximal safe concentrations is controversial. The aluminum content of these preparations should also be considered.

1. Calcium to phosphorus ratios of approximately 1.3:1 to 1.7:1 by weight (1:1–1.3:1 molar) are suggested. However, despite efforts to optimize mineral intake, preterm infants receiving prolonged PN remain at increased risk for metabolic bone disease (see Chap. 59).

2. 3-in-1 PN solutions are not used (dextrose, amino acid, and lipid mixed in single bag) for the following reasons:

   a. The pH of lipid emulsions is more basic and increases the pH of the total solution, which decreases the solubility of calcium and phosphorus and limits the amount of these minerals in the solution.

   b. If the calcium and phosphorus in a 3-in-1 solution did precipitate, it would be difficult to detect, as the solution is already cloudy.

   c. 3-in-1 solutions require either a larger micron filter or no filter, which may pose a greater sepsis risk.

J. Trace elements

1. Currently, 0.2 mL/dL of NeoTrace and 1.5 mcg/dL of selenium are added, beginning in the first days of PN. However, when PN is supplementing enteral nutrition or limited to <2 weeks, only zinc may be needed.

2. As copper and manganese are excreted in bile, these trace elements are routinely reduced or omitted if impaired biliary excretion and/or cholestatic liver disease is present.

K. General PN procedures

1. If possible, the continuity of a central line should not be broken for blood drawing or blood transfusion because of the risk of infection.

2. Most medications are not given in PN solutions. If necessary, the PN catheter may be flushed with saline solution and a medication then infused in a compatible IV solution. Refer to the table in Appendix A for guidelines for parenteral nutrition (dextrose and amino acid solution) and intravenous lipid and medication compatibility.

3. Heparin is added to all central lines at a concentration of 0.5 unit/mL of solution.

L. Metabolic monitoring for infants receiving PN. Infants receiving PN are typically monitored according to the schedule indicated in Table 21.4.

M. Potential complications associated with PN

1. Cholestasis (see Chap. 26) may be seen and is more often transient than progressive. Experimentally, even short-term PN can reduce bile flow and bile salt formation.

   a. Risk factors include:

      i. Prematurity

      ii. Duration of PN administration

      iii. Duration of fasting (lack of enteral feeding also produces bile inspissation and cholestasis)

      iv. Infection

      v. Narcotic administration

   b. Recommended management:

      i. Attempt enteral feeding. Even minimal enteral feedings may stimulate bile secretion.

Table 21.4	Schedule for Metabolic Monitoring of Infants Receiving Parenteral Nutrition
Measurement	**Frequency of measurement**
Blood	
Glucose, electrolytes, including total carbon dioxide or pH	Daily until stable, then as clinically indicated
Blood urea nitrogen, creatinine, calcium, phosphorus, magnesium, total and direct bilirubin, triglycerides	Weekly to every 14 days, as clinically indicated
ALT, AST, alkaline phosphatase	As clinically indicated
Urine	
Total volume	Daily

ALT = alanine aminotransferase; AST = aspartate aminotransferase.

    ii. Avoid excess nutrition with PN.

    iii. Provision of a mixed fuel source may be helpful.

    iv. Research is ongoing regarding the use of an omega-3 fatty acid lipid emulsion for the prevention and/or treatment of cholestasis (see Chap. 26).

  2. Metabolic bone disease (see Chap. 59). The use of earlier enteral feedings and central PN, with higher calcium and phosphorus ratios, has reduced the incidence of metabolic bone disease. However, this continues to be seen with the prolonged use of PN in place of enteral nutrition or the feeding of enteral formulations designed for the term infant.

  3. Metabolic abnormalities. Azotemia, hyperammonemia, and hyperchloremic metabolic acidosis have become uncommon since introduction of the current crystalline amino acid solutions. These complications may occur, however, with amino acid intakes exceeding 4 g/kg/day.

  4. Metabolic abnormalities related to lipid emulsions

    a. Hyperlipidemia/hypertriglyceridemia. The incidence tends to be inversely related to gestational age at birth and postnatal age. A short-term decrease in the lipid infusion rate usually is sufficient to normalize serum lipid levels. The AAP suggests serum triglyceride concentrations be maintained below 200 mg/dL.

    b. Indirect hyperbilirubinemia. Because free fatty acids can theoretically displace bilirubin from albumin binding sites, the use of lipid emulsions during periods of neonatal hyperbilirubinemia has been questioned. Research, however, suggests that infusion of lipids, at rates up to 3 g/kg/day, is unlikely to displace bilirubin. However, during periods of extreme hyperbilirubinemia (e.g., requiring exchange transfusion), rates <3 g/kg/day are typically provided.

c. Sepsis has been associated with decreased lipoprotein lipase activity and impaired triglyceride clearance. Therefore, during a sepsis episode, it may be necessary to temporarily reduce and/or limit the lipid infusion to avoid hypertriglyceridemia.

d. The potential adverse effects of lipid emulsions on pulmonary function, the risk of bronchopulmonary dysplasia (BPD), and impaired immune function remain subjects of debate. Because of the concern about toxic products of lipid peroxidation, protecting lipid emulsions from both ambient and phototherapy lights should also be considered.

N. Other additives

1. **Carnitine** facilitates the transport of long-chain fatty acids into the mitochondria for oxidation. However, this nutrient is not routinely added to PN solutions. Preterm infants who receive prolonged, unsupplemented PN are at risk for carnitine deficiency due to their limited reserves and inadequate rates of carnitine synthesis. Infants who are able to tolerate enteral nutrition receive a source of carnitine via human milk and/or carnitine-containing infant formula. However, for infants requiring prolonged (e.g., >2–4 weeks) PN, a parenteral source of carnitine may be provided at an initial dose of approximately 10 to 20 mg/kg/day until enteral nutrition can be established.

2. **Cysteine** is not a component of current crystalline amino acid solutions, as it is unstable over time and will form a precipitate. Cysteine is ordinarily synthesized from methionine and provides a substrate for taurine. However, this may be considered an essential amino acid for preterm infants due to low activity of the enzyme hepatic cystathionase, which converts methionine to cysteine. Supplementation with L-cysteine hydrochloride lowers the pH of the PN solution and may necessitate the use of additional acetate to prevent acidosis. However, the lower pH also enhances the solubility of calcium and phosphorus and allows for improved mineral intake. Cysteine is routinely supplemented in PN at a rate of approximately 30 to 40 mg/g protein.

3. **Glutamine** is an important fuel for intestinal epithelial cells and lymphocytes; however, due to its instability, it is presently not a component of crystalline amino acid solutions. Studies to date have not proven its addition to PN as helpful for the neonate.

4. **Insulin** is not routinely added to PN. Its use must be weighed against the risk of wide swings in blood glucose levels, as well as the concerns surrounding the overall effects of the increased uptake of glucose. When hyperglycemia is severe or persistent, an insulin infusion may be useful (see Chap. 24).

5. **Vitamin A** is important for normal growth and differentiation of epithelial tissue, particularly the development and maintenance of pulmonary epithelial tissue. ELBW infants are known to have low vitamin A stores at birth, minimal enteral intake for the first several weeks after birth, reduced enteral absorption of vitamin A, and unreliable parenteral delivery. Studies have suggested that vitamin A supplementation can reduce the risk of BPD. At present, infants weighing <1,000 g at birth are supplemented with 5,000 IU vitamin A intramuscularly three times per week for the first 4 weeks of life, beginning in the first 72 hours of life (see Chap. 34).

IV. ENTERAL NUTRITION

A. Early enteral feeding

1. The structural and functional integrity of the gastrointestinal (GI) tract is dependent upon the provision of enteral nutrition. Withholding enteral feeding after birth places the infant at risk for all the complications associated with luminal starvation, including mucosal thinning, flattening of the villi, and bacterial translocation. **Minimal enteral nutrition** (also referred to as "gut priming" or "trophic feedings") may be described as the nonnutritive use of very small volumes of human milk or formula for the intended purpose of preservation of gut maturation rather than nutrient delivery. Definitive conclusions cannot be drawn as to what constitutes the optimal volume for minimal enteral nutrition.

2. **Benefits associated with minimal enteral nutrition include:**
   a. Improved levels of gut hormones
   b. Less feeding intolerance
   c. Earlier progression to full enteral feedings
   d. Improved weight gain
   e. Improved calcium and phosphorus retention
   f. Fewer days on PN

3. **The following are guidelines for the use of gut priming in preterm infants:**
   a. Begin as soon after birth as possible, ideally by postnatal day 2 to 3.
   b. Use full-strength colostrum/preterm maternal milk or pasteurized donor human milk (PDHM). In instances where the supply of maternal milk is insufficient for 100% gut priming volume, and PDHM has been declined or is unavailable, full-strength 20 kcal/oz preterm formula may be used. Gut priming may be administered as a fixed dose (i.e., 0.5 mL every 4 hours, regardless of birth weight or gestational age). Alternatively, a low volume per kilogram may be delivered (i.e., 10–20 mL/kg/day divided into 8 aliquots).
   c. Gut priming is not used in infants with severe hemodynamic instability, suspected or confirmed NEC, evidence of ileus, or clinical signs of intestinal pathology. Infants who are undergoing medical treatment for patent ductus arteriosus may receive gut priming, pending the discretion of the care term.
   d. Controlled trials of gut priming with umbilical arterial catheters (UACs) in place have not shown an increased incidence of NEC. Therefore, the presence of a UAC is not considered a contraindication to minimal enteral nutrition. However, the clinical condition accompanying the prolonged use of a UAC may serve as a contraindication.

B. Preterm infants

1. **Fortified human milk.** Human milk provides the gold standard for feeding term infants. Although there is no such gold standard for preterm infants, the use of human milk offers many nutritional and nonnutritional advantages for the premature infant. Feeding tolerance is improved with more rapid advancement of feedings. The incidence of sepsis and NEC is decreased. Earlier discharge is facilitated by better feeding tolerance and less illness. Therefore, the use of fortified human milk is considered the preferred feeding for preterm infants.
   a. Preterm human milk contains higher amounts of protein, sodium, chloride, and magnesium than term milk. However, the levels of these nutrients

remain below preterm recommendations, the differences only persist for approximately the first 21 days of lactation, and composition is known to vary.

b. For these reasons, human milk for preterm infants is routinely supplemented with human milk fortifier (HMF). Recently only powdered, bovine milk–based HMF has been available in the United States. A liquid human milk–based HMF has now become available. The addition of bovine milk–based HMF to human milk (see Table 21.1) increases energy, protein, vitamin, and mineral contents to levels more appropriate for preterm infants. The human milk–based fortifier increases energy, protein, and mineral intake. However, as vitamin content of the feeding is not appreciably increased with the use of this product, a multivitamin and iron supplement is typically administered daily.

c. When powdered, bovine milk–based HMF is used, the addition of HMF is considered (at 2–4 kcal/oz) at approximately 100 mL/kg of human milk for infants born weighing <1,500 g. For larger neonates, HMF is considered at full-volume feedings.

d. In instances when the liquid human milk–based HMF is employed, the addition of this HMF may be considered at approximately 60 mL/kg of human milk for those infants born weighing <1,250 g.

e. When 100% maternal milk is unavailable in our units, PDHM is offered to infants who are considered to be at highest risk for feeding intolerance and NEC. Most typically, this includes VLBW newborns and/or those born at <30 weeks' gestation. Consent is obtained from the parent or guardian prior to administering PDHM. Maternal milk is preferentially fed, as available, with PDHM being used, as needed, to reach goal volumes. PDHM is typically offered until 100% maternal milk is achieved or an established endpoint has been reached. This endpoint may be full-volume feedings for a certain period of time (i.e., full feeds for 48 hours), or until a goal weight or PMA has been reached (i.e., 34 weeks' PMA). Once at this previously established endpoint, the infant is slowly transitioned off of PDHM by gradually adding in formula feedings. This process usually occurs over several days.

f. When human milk is fed through continuous infusion, incomplete delivery of nutrients may occur; in particular, the nonhomogenized fat and nutrients in the HMF may cling to the tubing. Small, frequent bolus feedings may result in improved nutrient delivery and absorption compared with continuous feedings.

g. Our protocols for the collection and storage of human milk are outlined in Chapter 22.

2. **Preterm formulas** (see Tables 21.1 and 21.6) are designed to meet the nutritional and physiologic needs of preterm infants and have some common features:

a. Whey-predominant, taurine-supplemented protein source, which is better tolerated and produces a more normal plasma amino acid profile than casein-predominant protein

b. Carbohydrate mixtures of 40% to 50% lactose and 50% to 60% glucose polymers to compensate for preterm infants' relative lactase deficiency

c. Fat mixtures containing approximately 50% medium-chain triglycerides (MCTs) to compensate for limited pancreatic lipase secretion and small bile acid pools, as well as 50% long-chain triglycerides to provide a source of EFAs

d. Higher concentrations of protein, vitamins, minerals, and electrolytes to meet the increased needs associated with rapid growth and limited fluid tolerance

Table 21.5	Tube Feeding Guidelines*,†,‡,§	
Birth weight (g)	**Initial rate (mL/kg/day)**	**Volume increase (mL/kg every 12 hours)**
<1,000	10	10
1,001–1,250	10–20	10
1,251–1,500	20–30	10–15
1,501–1,800	30	15
1,801–2,500	30–40	15–20

* The initial volume should be administered for at least 24 hours prior to advancement.
† The cited guidelines should be individualized based on the infant's clinical status/ history of present illness.
‡ Once feeding volume has reached approximately 80 mL/kg/day, infants weighing <1,250 g should be considered for feeding intervals of every 2 hours or every 3 hours, as opposed to every 4 hours.
‡ Once feeding volume has reached approximately 100 mL/kg/day, consider advancing to 22 kcal/oz or 24 kcal/oz for all infants weighing <1,500 g.
‡ Consider advancing feeding volume more rapidly than the prescribed guidelines once tolerance of >100 mL/kg/day is established, but do not exceed increments of 15 mL/kg every 12 hours in most infants weighing <1,500 g.
§ The recommended volume goal for feedings is 140–160 mL/kg/day. These guidelines do not apply to infants capable of *ad libitum* feedings.

3. **Feeding advancement.** When attempting to determine how best to advance a preterm infant to full enteral nutrition, there is very limited data to support any one method as optimal. The following guidelines reflect current practice:
   a. Use full-strength, 20 kcal/oz human milk or preterm formula and advance feeding volume according to the guidelines in Table 21.5 for any infant being fed by tube feedings.
   b. As previously discussed, for human milk–fed infants, the caloric density may be advanced by 2 to 4 kcal/oz at 100 mL/kg of volume with powdered, bovine milk–based HMF. When the liquid human milk–based fortifier is used, this may be added at 60 mL/kg/day of human milk. For those VLBW infants receiving 20 kcal/oz premature infant formula, the caloric density may be advanced from 20 to 24 kcal/oz at 100 mL/kg. Volume, at the new caloric density, is typically maintained for approximately 24 hours before the advancement schedule is resumed.
   c. As enteral volumes are increased, the rate of any IV fluid is reduced accordingly so that the total daily fluid volume remains the same. Enteral nutrients are taken into account when administering any supplemental PN.

C. **Term infants**
   1. **Human milk** is considered the preferred feeding choice for term infants.
   2. **Term formulas.** The AAP provides specific guidelines for the composition of infant formulas so that term infant formulas approximate human milk in general composition. Table 21.6 describes the composition of commonly available formulas, many of which are derived from modified cow's milk.

Table 21.6 Nutrient Composition of Human Milk and Select Infant Formula

	kcal/30 mL	Protein (g/dL)	Fat (g/dL)	DHA (mg/dL)	ARA (mg/dL)	Carbohydrate* (g/dL)	Electrolytes (mEq/dL)			Minerals (mg/dL)			Vitamins (IU/dL)			Folic acid (mcg/dL)	Osmolality (mOsmol/ kg H₂O)	PRSL (mOsmol/L)
							Na	K	Cl	Ca	P	Fe†	A	D	E			
Mature human milk (composition varies)	20	1	3.9			7.2	0.8	1.4	1.2	28	14	0.03	225	2	0.4	4.8	286	97.6
Formula (manufacturer††)																		
Preterm formulas																		
Enfamil Premature (Mead Johnson)	20	2	3.4	11.5	23	7.4	1.7	1.7	1.7	112	56	1.22	850	162	4.3	27	240	181
Enfamil Premature (Mead Johnson)	24	2.4	4.1	13.8	28	8.9	2	2	2.1	134	67	1.46	1,010	195	5.1	32	300	220
Enfamil Premature High Protein (Mead Johnson)	24	2.8	4.1	13.6	27.2	8.4	2	2	2	132	66	1.44	1,000	192	5	32	300	241
Similac Special Care (Abbott)	20	2	3.7	9.2	14.7	7	1.3	2.2	1.6	122	68	1.22	845	101	2.7	25	235	188.2
Similac Special Care (Abbott)	24	2.4	4.4	11	17.6	8.4	1.5	2.7	1.9	146	81	1.46	1,014	122	3.3	30	280	225.8
Similac Special Care High Protein (Abbott)	24	2.68	4.4	11	17.6	8.1	1.5	2.7	1.9	146	81	1.46	1,014	122	3.3	30	280	240
Similac Special Care (Abbott)	30	3	6.7	14	22.1	7.8	1.9	3.4	2.3	183	101	1.8	1,268	152	4.1	37.5	325	282.3

(continued)

Table 21.6 Nutrient Composition of Human Milk and Select Infant Formula (Continued)

	kcal/30 mL	Protein (g/dL)	Fat (g/dL)	DHA (mg/dL)	ARA (mg/dL)	Carbohydrate* (g/dL)	Electrolytes (mEq/dL) Na	K	Cl	Minerals (mg/dL) Ca	P	Fe†	Vitamins (IU/dL) A	D	E	Folic acid (mcg/dL)	Osmolality (mOsmol/ kg H₂O)	PRSL (mOsmol/L)
Nutrient-enriched postdischarge formulas																		
Enfamil EnfaCare (Mead Johnson)	22	2.1	3.9	12.6	25	7.7	1.1	2	1.6	89	49	1.33	330	52	3	19.2	Liquid 250 Powder 310	Liquid 181 Powder 184
Similac Expert Care NeoSure (Abbott)	22	2.1	4.1	10.4	16.4	7.5	1.1	2.7	1.6	78	46	1.34	342	52	2.7	18.6	250	187.4
Standard cow's milk–based formula																		
Enfamil PREMIUM Newborn (Mead Johnson)	20	1.4	3.6	11.5	23	7.6	0.8	1.9	1.2	53	29	1.22	200	51	1.35	10.8	300	129
Enfamil PREMIUM (Mead Johnson)	20	1.4	3.6	11.5	23	7.6	0.8	1.9	1.2	53	29	1.22	200	41	1.36	10.9	300	129
Enfamil LIPIL (Mead Johnson)	24	1.7	4.3	13.8	28	8.8	1	2.3	1.4	63	35	1.46	240	49	1.62	13	NA	156
Similac Advance (Abbott)	20	1.4	3.6	5.4	14.6	7.6	0.7	1.8	1.2	53	28	1.2	203	41	1	10	310	126.7
Similac Expert Care (Abbott)	24	2.2	4.3			8.5	1.2	2.7	1.9	72	56	1.5	242	48	1.2	12	280	201

Specialized formulas

Formula																		
Similac Expert Care Alimentum (Abbott)	20	1.9	3.7	5.6	14.9	6.9	1.3	2	1.6	71	51	1.2	203	30	2	10	370	171.3
Elecare with DHA/ARA (Abbott)	20	2.1	3.3	5.4	14.9	7.2	1.3	2.6	1.1	78	57	1	185	28	1.4	20	350	187
Nutramigen LIPIL (Mead Johnson)	20	1.9	3.6	11.5	23	7	1.4	1.9	1.6	64	35	1.22	200	34	1.35	10.8	Liquid 320 Powder 300	168
Nutramigen w/ Enflora LGG Powder (Mead Johnson)	20	1.9	3.6	11.5	23	7	1.4	1.9	1.6	64	35	1.22	200	34	1.35	10.8	300	168
Nutramigen AA (powder) (Mead Johnson)	20	1.9	3.6	11.5	23	7	1.4	1.9	1.6	64	35	1.22	200	34	1.35	10.8	350	168
Pregestimil LIPIL (Mead Johnson)	20	1.9	3.8	11.5	23	6.9	1.4	1.9	1.6	64	35	1.22	260 (Liquid) 240 (Powder)	34 34	2.7 2.7	10.8	Liquid 290 Powder 320	168
Pregestimil LIPIL (liquid) (Mead Johnson)	24	2.3	4.5	13.7	27.5	8.3	1.7	2.3	2	76	42	1.5	308	41	3.2	13	340	200
Neocate Infant w/ DHA/ARA (Nutricia)	20	2.1	3	5.75	10.14	7.8	1.1	2.7	1.5	83	62	1.2	274	40	0.8	6.8	375	192
Enfaport (Mead Johnson)	20	2.4	3.7	11.5	23	6.9	0.9	2	1.7	64	35	1.22	240	34	2.7	10.8	170	193.4

(continued)

Table 21.6   Nutrient Composition of Human Milk and Select Infant Formula (Continued)

	kcal/30 mL	Protein (g/dL)	Fat (g/dL)	DHA (mg/dL)	ARA (mg/dL)	Carbohydrate* (g/dL)	Electrolytes (mEq/dL)			Minerals (mg/dL)			Vitamins (IU/dL)			Folic acid (mcg/dL)	Osmolality (mOsmol/ kg H₂O)	PRSL (mOsmol/L)
							Na	K	Cl	Ca	P	Fe†	A	D	E			
Monogen (Nutricia)	20	1.8	1.9			10.8	1.4	1.5	1	41	32	0.67	172	42	0.7	7.5		151
Enfamil A.R. (Mead Johnson)	20	1.7	3.4	11.5	23	7.4	1.2	1.9	1.4	53	36	1.22	200	41	1.35	10.8	Liquid 240 Powder 230	Liquid 151 Powder 153
Similac Sensitive for Spit Up (Abbott)	20	1.4	3.7	5.5	14.6	7.2	0.9	1.9	1.2	57	38	1.22	203	41	2	10.1	180	134.7
Similac PM 60/40 (Abbott)	20	1.5	3.8			6.9	0.7	1.4	1.1	38	19	0.5	203	41	1	10.1	280	124.1
Similac Isomil Advance (Abbott)	20	1.7	3.7	5.5	14.7	7	1.3	1.9	1.2	71	51	1.22	203	41	1	10.1	200	154.5
Prosobee (Mead Johnson)	20	1.7	3.6	11.5	23	7.2	1	2.1	1.5	71	47	1.22	200	41	1.35	10.8	Liquid 170 Powder 180	156

DHA = docosahexaenoic acid; ARA = arachidonic acid; Ca = calcium; P = phosphorus; Fe = iron; Na = sodium; K = potassium; Cl = chloride; NA = not analyzed.

*See text for types of carbohydrates used in formulas.

†In instances where high and low Fe formulations are available, the iron fortified value appears.

††Additional product information and nutrient composition data may be found at the following websites: www.meadjohnson.com, www.abbott.com, www.nutricia-na.com

D. Specialized formulas have been designed for a variety of congenital and neonatal disorders, including milk protein allergy, malabsorption syndromes, and several inborn errors of metabolism. Indications for the most commonly used of these specialized formulas are briefly reviewed in Table 21.7, whereas composition is outlined in Table 21.6. However, it is important to note that **these formulas were not designed to meet the special nutritional needs of preterm infants**. Preterm infants who are fed these formulas require close nutritional assessment and monitoring for potential protein, mineral, and multivitamin supplementation.

E. Caloric-enhanced feedings. Many ill and preterm infants require increased energy/nutrient intakes in order to achieve optimal rates of growth.

1. As previously discussed, for preterm infants, when using bovine milk–based HMF, the caloric density of human milk is first increased by concentrating feedings to 24 kcal/oz. If needed, infant formula powder, MCT or corn oil and/or Polycose, may then be added in increments of 2 to 3 kcal/oz (typically not to exceed a maximum caloric density of 30 kcal/oz). Adjustments should be made gradually with feeding tolerance assessed after each change. If the mother's milk production is greater than her infant's intake, the use of hindmilk may be employed to enhance caloric intake. However, this should not replace the use of HMF. The provision of energy and protein is preferred over just energy. Growth is enhanced with the intake of protein. Powdered infant formula may be used, as there is not a sterile, liquid, nutritionally adequate supplement to retain the volume of human milk provided. The formula powder is not sterile and does present the risk of *Cronobacter* spp. contamination. Fat modulars may be added to the feeding as a bolus or as mixed with the feeding. However, fat mixed with the feeding is subject to adherence to the storage container over time.

2. For infants receiving the liquid human milk–based HMF, the fortifiers designed to make 26 to 30 kcal/oz milk may be used. The energy and protein content of the milk will be increased.

3. Protein supplementation, with a whey protein modular, may be considered for VLBW infants in order to increase the protein content to approximately 4 g/kg/day as needed.

4. Formula-fed, fluid-restricted preterm infants may be switched to a 26 to 30 kcal/oz premature infant formula once they are tolerating appropriate volumes of 24 kcal/oz feedings.

5. Human milk–fed term infants requiring caloric enhancement may also utilize infant formula powder, MCT or corn oil and/or Polycose, added in increments of 2 to 3 kcal/oz (typically not to exceed a maximum caloric density of 30 kcal/oz). As with preterm infants, adjustments should be made gradually with feeding tolerance assessed after each change. Hindmilk may also be used.

6. For term infants receiving standard formula, the formula density may be increased as needed by the use of standard formula powder, and/or modulars, or formula concentrate diluted to a more calorically dense feeding. The overall nutrient composition of these feedings should be considered.

7. The previously mentioned supplements are further described in Table 21.8.

8. Growth patterns of infants receiving these supplements are monitored closely and the nutritional care plan is adjusted accordingly.

Table 21.7	Indications for Use of Infant Formulas	
Clinical condition	Suggested type of infant formula	Rationale
Allergy to cow's milk protein or soy protein	Extensively hydrolyzed protein or free amino acids	Impaired digestion/utilization of intact protein
Bronchopulmonary dysplasia	High energy, nutrient dense	Increased energy requirement, fluid restriction
Biliary atresia	Semielemental, containing reduced LCT (~45%), with supplemented MCT (~55%)	Impaired intraluminal digestion and absorption of long-chain fats
Chylothorax (persistent)	Significantly reduced LCT (~15%), with supplemented MCT (~84%)	Decreased lymphatic absorption of fats
Congestive heart failure	High-energy formula	Lower fluid and sodium intake; increased energy requirement
Cystic fibrosis	Semielemental formula, containing reduced LCT (~45%), with supplemented MCT (~55%) or standard formula with pancreatic enzyme supplementation	Impaired intraluminal digestion and absorption of long-chain fats
Galactosemia	Soy protein–based formula	Lactose free
Gastroesophageal reflux	Standard formula, Enfamil A.R.	Consider small, frequent feedings
Hepatic insufficiency	Semielemental formula, containing reduced LCT (~45%), with supplemented MCT (~55%)	Impaired intraluminal digestion and absorption of long-chain fats
Lactose intolerance	Low lactose formula	Impaired digestion or utilization of lactose
Lymphatic anomalies	Significantly reduced LCT (~15%), with supplemented MCT (~84%)	Impaired absorption of long-chain fats

(continued)

Table 21.7	*(Continued)*	
Clinical condition	**Suggested type of infant formula**	**Rationale**
Necrotizing enterocolitis	Preterm formula or semielemental formula, if indicated	Impaired digestion
Renal insufficiency	Standard formula	
	Similac PM 60/40	Low phosphate content, low renal solute load

LCT = long-chain triglyceride; MCT = medium-chain triglyceride.

F. Feeding method. These should be individualized based on gestational age, clinical condition, and feeding tolerance.

    1. Nasogastric/orogastric feedings. Nasogastric tube feedings are utilized more frequently, as orogastric tubes tend to be more difficult to secure.

      a. Candidates

        i. Infants <34 weeks' gestation, as most do not yet have the ability to coordinate suck–swallow–breathe patterns.

        ii. Infants with impaired suck/swallow coordination due to conditions such as encephalopathy, hypotonia, and maxillofacial abnormalities.

      b. Bolus versus continuous. Studies may be found in support of either method and, in practice, both are utilized. Feedings are usually initiated as

Table 21.8	Oral Dietary Supplements Available for Use in Infants		
Nutrient	**Product**	**Source**	**Energy content**
Fat	MCT oil (Novartis)	Medium-chain triglycerides	8.3 kcal/g 7.7 kcal/mL
	Microlipid (Novartis)	Long-chain triglycerides	4.5 kcal/mL
	Corn oil	Long-chain triglycerides	8.6 kcal/g 8 kcal/mL
Carbohydrate	Polycose (Abbott)	Glucose polymers	3.8 kcal/g 8 kcal/tsp (powder)
Protein	Beneprotein (Nestle)	Whey protein isolates	3.6 kcal/g 5.5 kcal/tsp

MCT = medium-chain triglyceride.

bolus, divided every 3 to 4 hours. If difficulties with feeding tolerance occur, the amount of time over which a feeding is given may be lengthened by delivery via a syringe pump for 30 to 120 minutes.

2. **Transpyloric feedings**
   a. **Candidates.** There are only a few indications for transpyloric feedings.
      i. Infants intolerant to nasogastric/orogastric feedings
      ii. Infants at increased risk for aspiration
      iii. Severe gastric retention or regurgitation
      iv. Anatomic abnormalities of the GI tract such as microgastria
   b. **Other considerations**
      i. Transpyloric feedings should be delivered continuously, as the small intestine does not have the same capacity for expansion as does the stomach.
      ii. There is an increased risk of fat malabsorption, as lingual and gastric lipase secretions are bypassed.
      iii. These tubes are routinely placed under guided fluoroscopy.

3. **Transition to breast/bottle feedings** is a gradual process. Infants who are approximately 33 to 34 weeks' gestation, who have coordinated suck–swallow–breathe patterns and respiratory rates <60 per minute, are appropriate candidates for introducing breast/bottle feedings.

4. **Gastrostomy feedings**
   a. **Candidates**
      i. Infants with neurologic impairment and/or those who are unable to take sufficient volumes through breast/bottle feeding to maintain adequate growth/hydration status

G. **Iron.** The AAP recommends that growing preterm infants receive a source of iron, provided at 2 to 4 mg/kg/day, after 2 weeks of age. The AAP further suggests that preterm infants on iron-fortified preterm formula do not need additional iron. The Summary of Reasonable Nutrient Intakes continues to recommend 2 to 4 mg/kg/day for VLBW and ELBW infants. It has been suggested that greater than 2 mg/kg/day may be needed when adjusted for noncompensated phlebotomy losses and the number of days during which the infant does not receive iron due to feeding intolerance or illness. Iron supplementation is recommended until the infant is 12 months of age. Iron-fortified formulas and iron-fortified HMF provide approximately 2.2 mg/kg/day when delivered at a rate of 150 mL/kg/day. Low-iron formulas are not recommended for use.

1. **Vitamin E** is an important antioxidant that acts to prevent fatty acid peroxidation in the cell membrane. The recommendation for preterm infants is 6 to 12 IU vitamin E/kg/day. Preterm infants are not initiated on iron supplements until they are tolerating full enteral volumes of 24 kcal/oz feedings, which provides vitamin E at the low to midrange of the recommendations. An additional vitamin E supplement would be required to meet the upper end of the recommendation.

H. **Other nutrients**

1. **Glutamine.** As with parenteral glutamine supplementation, there are presently no recommendations for enteral glutamine supplementation in preterm infants.

2. **Long-chain polyunsaturated fatty acids (LCPUFAs).** The inclusion of LCPUFAs, specifically docosahexaenoic acid (DHA) and arachidonic acid (ARA),

in infant formulas has been the subject of much debate. These LCPUFAs are derivatives of the EFAs, linoleic acid, and alpha-linolenic acid, and they are important in cognitive development and visual acuity. Human milk contains these LCPUFAs but, until recently, standard infant formula did not. Controlled trials investigating the effects of LCPUFA-supplemented formula on cognitive development in preterm infants have been inconclusive. The effects on visual acuity have more consistently suggested an advantage. Furthermore, no adverse effects were noted.

V. SPECIAL CONSIDERATIONS

A. **Gastroesophageal reflux (GER).** Episodes of GER, as monitored by esophageal pH probes, are common in both preterm and full-term infants. The majority of infants, however, do not exhibit clinical compromise from GER.

1. **Introduction of enteral feeds.** Emesis can be associated during the introduction and advancement of enteral feeds in preterm infants. These episodes are most commonly related to intestinal dysmotility secondary to prematurity and will respond to modifications of the feeding regimen.

   a. Temporary reductions in the feeding volume, lengthening the duration of the feeding (sometimes to the point of using continuous feeding), removal of nutritional additives, and temporary cessation of enteral feeds are all possible strategies depending upon the clinical course of the infant.

   b. Rarely, specialized formulas are used when all other feeding modifications have been tried without improvement. In general, these formulas should only be used for short periods of time with close nutritional monitoring.

   c. Infants who have repeated episodes of symptomatic emesis that prevent achievement of full-volume enteral feeds may require evaluation for anatomic problems such as malrotation or Hirschsprung disease. In general, radiographic studies are not undertaken unless feeding problems have persisted for 2 or more weeks, or unless bilious emesis occurs (see Chap. 62).

2. **Established feeds.** Preterm infants on full-volume enteral feeds will have occasional episodes of symptomatic emesis. If these episodes do not compromise the respiratory status or growth of the infant, no intervention is required other than continued close monitoring of the infant. If symptomatic emesis is associated with respiratory compromise, repeated apnea, or growth restriction, therapeutic maneuvers are indicated.

   a. Positioning. Reposition the infant to elevate the head and upper body, in either a prone or a right-side-down position.

   b. Feeding intervals. Shortening the interval between feeds to give a smaller volume during each feed may sometimes improve signs of GER. Infants fed by gavage may have the duration of the feed increased.

   c. Metoclopramide. Infants who remain clinically compromised from GER after positioning and feeding interval changes can have a therapeutic trial of metoclopramide. The metoclopramide should be discontinued after 1 week if there is no improvement in clinical status (see Appendix A).

3. **Apnea.** Studies using pH probes and esophageal manometry have not shown an association between GER and apnea episodes. Treatment with promotility agents should not be used for uncomplicated apnea of prematurity (see Chap. 31).

B. NEC (see Chap. 27). Nutritional support of the patient with NEC focuses around providing complete PN during the acute phase of the disease, followed by gradual introduction of enteral nutrition after the patient has stabilized and the gut has been allowed to heal.

1. **PN.** For at least 2 weeks after the initial diagnosis of NEC, the patient is kept nothing by mouth (NPO) and receives total PN. The goals for PN were delineated previously in Section III.

2. **Initiation of feedings.** If the patient is clinically stable after a minimum 2 weeks of bowel rest, feeds are generally introduced at approximately 10 to 20 mL/kg/day, preferably with maternal milk or PDHM, although a standard formula appropriate for the gestational age of the patient may also be used (i.e., preterm formula for the typical NICU infant). More specialized formulas containing elemental proteins are rarely indicated.

3. **Feeding advancement.** If low volume feedings (10–20 mL/kg/day) are tolerated for 24 to 48 hours, gradual advancement is continued at approximately 10 mL/kg every 12 to 24 hours for the next 2 to 3 days. If this advancement is tolerated, further advancement proceeds according to the guidelines in Table 21.5. Supplemental PN is continued until enteral feeds are providing approximately 100 to 120 mL/kg/day volume.

4. **Feeding intolerance.** Signs of feeding intolerance include emesis, large gastric residuals, abdominal distension, and increased numbers of apnea episodes. Reduction of feeding volume or cessation of feeding is usually indicated. If these clinical signs prevent attainment of full-volume enteral feeds despite several attempts to advance feeds, radiographic contrast studies may be indicated to rule out intestinal strictures. This type of evaluation would typically take place after 1 to 2 weeks of attempting to achieve full-volume enteral feeds.

5. **Enterostomies.** If one or more enterostomies are created as a result of surgical therapy for NEC, it may be difficult to achieve full nutritional intake by enteral feeds. Depending on the length and function of the upper intestinal tract, increasing feeding volume or nutritional density may result in problems with malabsorption, dumping syndrome, and poor growth.

   a. Refeeding. Output from the proximal intestinal enterostomy can be refed into the distal portion(s) of the intestine through the mucous fistula(s). This may improve the absorption of both fluid and nutrients.

   b. PN support. If growth targets cannot be achieved using enteral feeds, continued use of supplemental PN may be indicated depending on the patient's overall status and liver function. Enteral feeding should be continued at the highest rate and nutritional density tolerated, and supplemental PN should be given to achieve the nutritional goals and growth outcomes as previously outlined.

C. BPD. Preterm infants who have BPD have increased caloric requirements due to their increased metabolic expenditure, and at the same time have a lower tolerance for excess fluid intake (see Chap. 34).

1. **Fluid restriction.** Total fluid intake is typically restricted from the usual 150 mL/kg/day to 140 mL/kg/day. In cases of severe BPD, further restriction to 130 mL/kg/day may be required. Careful monitoring is required when fluid restrictions are implemented to ensure adequate caloric and micronutrient intake. Growth parameters must also be monitored so that continued growth is not compromised.

2. **Caloric density.** Infants with BPD will commonly require up to 30 kcal/oz feeds in order to achieve the desired growth targets.

VI. NUTRITIONAL CONSIDERATIONS IN DISCHARGE PLANNING. Recent

data describing postnatal growth in the United States suggest that a significant number of VLBW and ELBW infants continue to have catch-up growth requirements at the time of discharge from the hospital. However, there is a paucity of data regarding what to feed the preterm infant after discharge.

A. **Human milk.** The use of human milk and efforts to transition to full breastfeeding in former preterm infants who continue to require enhanced caloric density feedings, poses a unique challenge. Individualized care plans are indicated in order to support the transition to full breastfeeding while continuing to allow for optimal rates of growth. Usually, this is accomplished by a combination of a specified number of nursing sessions per day, supplemented by feedings of calorically enhanced breast milk or nursing on demand supplemented by several feeds per day of nutrient-enriched postdischarge formula. Growth rate data obtained in the hospital are typically forwarded to infant follow-up clinics and the private pediatrician for VLBW and ELBW infants.

B. **Formula choices**

1. **Nutrient-enriched postdischarge formulas.** The AAP suggests a recent meta-analysis of randomized controlled trials concluded that these formulas have limited benefits at best for growth and development up to 18 months after term compared with standard infant formulas. In some of the trials, infants on standard formula increased their volume of intake, therefore, mostly compensating for any additional nutrients from the postdischarge formulas. The ESPGHAN has suggested that preterm infants who demonstrate subnormal weight for age at discharge should be fed with fortified human milk or special formula fortified with high contents of protein, minerals, and trace elements, as well as LCPUFAs until at least 40 weeks' PMA, but possibly for another 3 months thereafter. In practice, preterm infants are considered to be appropriate candidates for the use of these formulas, either as an additive to human milk or as a sole formula choice, once they are >2,000 g and 35 weeks' corrected gestational age. However, the length of time after discharge these formulas should be continued remains unclear.

2. **Term formulas** may also be utilized; however, careful monitoring of growth after discharge should continue.

C. **Vitamin supplementation**

1. The AAP recommends 400 IU vitamin D per day for all infants. Unless they are consuming at least 1,000 mL/day of vitamin D–fortified formula, they will not meet this goal. The American Academy of Breastfeeding Medicine suggests up to 400 IU vitamin D per day for the NICU graduate. In practice, preterm infants who are >2,000 g and 35 weeks' corrected gestational age, and human milk–fed, are supplemented daily with 1 mL pediatric MVI without iron, with ferrous sulfate drops administered separately.

2. Preterm infants who are >2,000 g and 35 weeks' corrected gestational age, and fed a combination of human milk and formula, are supplemented with 0.5 to 1 mL vitamin D drops to a goal vitamin D intake of 400 IU per day. Ferrous sulfate drops should be administered separately, as needed.

3. Preterm infants who are >2,000 g and 35 weeks' corrected gestational age, and formula fed, are supplemented with 0.5 mL (400 units/mL) vitamin D drops, up to a goal intake of 400 IU vitamin D per day. Ferrous sulfate drops are administered separately, if needed.

4. Term infants, who are exclusively human milk–fed, are supplemented daily with 1 mL (400 units/mL) vitamin D drops once feedings have been established.

5. Term infants, who are formula-fed, may be supplemented daily with 0.5 mL vitamin D drops to a goal intake of 400 IU per day once feedings have been established.

6. Iron supplementation guidelines for preterm infants are recommended as previously described.

Suggested Readings

Agostoni C, Buonocore G, Carnielli VP, et al. Enteral nutrient supply for preterm infants: commentary from the European Society for Paediatric Gastroenterology, Hepatology, and Nutrition Committee on Nutrition. *J Pediatr Gastroenterol Nutr* 2010;50:85–91.

American Academy of Pediatrics, Committee on Nutrition (AAP-CON). *Pediatric Nutrition Handbook*, 6th ed. Elk Grove Village, IL: American Academy of Pediatrics, 2009.

Ehrenkranz RA, Younes N, Lemons JA, et al. Longitudinal growth of hospitalized very low birth weight infants. *Pediatrics* 1999;104(2 Pt 1):280–289.

Fenton TR. A new growth chart for preterm babies: Babson and Benda's chart updated with recent data and a new format. *BMC Pediatr* 2003;3:13. Chart may be downloaded from: http://members.shaw.ca/growthchart.

Lubchenco LO, Hansman C, Boyd E. Intrauterine growth in length and head circumference as estimated from live births at gestational ages from 26–42 weeks. *Pediatrics* 1966;37:403–408.

Martinez JA, Ballew MP. Infant formulas. *Pediatr Rev.* 2011;32(5):179–189.

Olsen IE, Groveman S, Lawson ML, et al. New intrauterine growth curves based on United States data. *Pediatrics* 2010;125:e214–e224. Chart may be downloaded from: http://www.nursing.upenn.edu/media/infantgrowthcurves/Documents/Olsen-NewIU GrowthCurves_2010permission.pdf.

Tsang RC, Uauy R, Koletzko B, et al, eds. *Nutritional Needs of the Premature Infant: Scientific Basis and Practical Guidelines*. 3rd ed. Baltimore: Lippincott Williams & Wilkins, 2005.

"Use of World Health Organization and CDC growth charts for children aged 0–59 months in the United States". *MMWR Recomm Rep* 2010;59(RR-9):1–15. Available at: http://www.cdc.gov/mmwr/pdf/rr/rr5909.pdf.

World Health Organization Child Growth Standards. Birth to 24 months: boys head circumference-for-age and weight-for-length percentiles. *Centers for Disease Control and Prevention.* November 1, 2009. Available at: http://www.cdc.gov/growthcharts/data/who/GrChrt_Boys_24HdCirc-L4W_rev90910.pdf.

World Health Organization Child Growth Standards. Birth to 24 months: boys length-for-age and weight-for-age percentiles. *Centers for Disease Control and Prevention.* November 1, 2009. Available at: http://www.cdc.gov/growthcharts/data/who/GrChrt_Boys _24LW_9210.pdf.

World Health Organization Child Growth Standards. Birth to 24 months: Girls head circumference-for-age and weight-for-length percentiles. *Centers for Disease Control and Prevention.* November 1, 2009. Available at: http://www.cdc.gov/growthcharts/data/who/GrChrt_Girls_24HdCirc-L4W_9210.pdf.

World Health Organization Child Growth Standards. Birth to 24 months: Girls length-for-age and weight-for-age percentiles. *Centers for Disease Control and Prevention.* November 1, 2009. Available at: http://www.cdc.gov/growthcharts/data/who/GrChrt_Girls_24LW_9210.pdf.

22 Breastfeeding
Nancy Hurst

I. RATIONALE FOR BREASTFEEDING.

Breastfeeding enhances maternal involvement, interaction, and bonding; provides species-specific nutrients to support normal infant growth; provides nonnutrient growth factors, immune factors, hormones, and other bioactive components that can act as biological signals; and can decrease the incidence and severity of infectious diseases, enhance neurodevelopment, decrease the incidence of childhood obesity and some chronic illnesses, and decrease the incidence and severity of atopic disease. Breastfeeding is beneficial for the mother's health because it increases maternal metabolism; has maternal contraceptive effects with exclusive, frequent breastfeeding; is associated with decreased incidence of maternal premenopausal breast cancer and osteoporosis; and imparts community benefits by decreasing health care costs and economic savings related to commercial infant formula expenses.

II. RECOMMENDATIONS ON BREASTFEEDING FOR HEALTHY TERM INFANTS INCLUDE THE FOLLOWING GENERAL PRINCIPLES

A. Exclusive breastfeeding for the first 6 months

B. When direct breastfeeding is not possible, expressed breast milk should be provided

C. Place infants skin to skin with their mothers immediately after birth and encourage frequent feedings (8–12 feeds/24-hour period)

D. Supplements (i.e., water or formula) should not be given unless medically indicated

E. Breastfeeding should be well established before pacifiers are used

F. Complementary foods should be introduced around 6 months with continued breastfeeding up to and beyond the first year

G. Oral vitamin D drops (400 IU/daily) should be given to the infant beginning within the first few days of age

H. Supplemental fluoride should not be provided during the first 6 months of age

III. MANAGEMENT AND SUPPORT ARE NEEDED FOR SUCCESSFUL BREASTFEEDING

A. **Early postpartum period.** Prior to hospital discharge, all mothers should receive:

1. Breastfeeding assessment by a lactation and/or nurse specialist

2. General breastfeeding information about:
   a. Basic positioning of infant to allow correct infant attachment at the breast
   b. Minimum anticipated feeding frequency (eight times/24-hour period)
   c. Expected physiologically appropriate small colostrum intakes (about 15–20 mL in first 24 hours).

    d. Infant signs of hunger and adequacy of milk intake

    e. Common breast conditions experienced during early breastfeeding and basic management strategies

    f. Proper referral sources when indicated

B. All breastfeeding infants should be seen by a pediatrician or other health care provider at 3 to 5 days of age to ensure that the infant has stopped losing weight and lost no more than 8 to 10% birth weight; has yellow, seedy stools (approximately 3/d)—no more meconium stools; and has at least six wet diapers per day.

    1. At 3 to 5 days postdelivery, the mother should experience some breast fullness, and notice some dripping of milk from opposite breast during breastfeeding; demonstrate ability to latch infant to breast; understand infant signs of hunger and satiety; understand expectations and treatment of minor breast/nipple conditions.

    2. Expect a return to birth weight by 12 to 14 days of age and a continued rate of growth of at least ½ ounce per day during the first month.

    3. If infant growth is inadequate, after ruling out any underlying health conditions in the infant, breastfeeding assessment should include adequacy of infant attachment to the breast; presence or absence of signs of normal lactogenesis (i.e., breast fullness, leaking); and maternal history of conditions (i.e., endocrine, breast surgery) that may affect lactation.

      a. The ability of infant to transfer milk at breast can be measured by weighing the infant before and after feeding using the following guidelines:

        i. Weighing the diapered infant before and immediately after the feeding (without changing the diaper)

        ii. 1 g infant weight gain equals 1 mL milk intake

    4. If milk transfer is inadequate, supplementation (preferably with expressed breast milk) may be indicated.

    5. Instructing the mother to express her milk with a mechanical breast pump following feeding will allow additional breast stimulation to increase milk production.

IV. MANAGEMENT OF BREASTFEEDING PROBLEMS

A. Sore, tender nipples. Most mothers will experience some degree of nipple soreness most likely a result of hormonal changes and increased friction caused by the infant's sucking action. A common description of this soreness includes an intense onset at the initial latch-on with a rapid subsiding of discomfort as milk flow increases. Nipple tenderness should diminish during the first few weeks until no discomfort is experienced during breastfeeding. Purified lanolin and/or expressed breast milk applied sparingly to the nipples following feedings may hasten this process.

B. Traumatized, painful nipples (may include bleeding, blisters, cracks). Nipple discomfort associated with breastfeeding that does not follow the scenario described previously requires immediate attention to determine cause and develop appropriate treatment modalities. Possible causes include ineffective, poor latch-on to breast; improper infant sucking technique; removing infant from breast without first breaking suction; and underlying nipple condition or infection (i.e., yeast, eczema). Management includes (i) assessment of infant positioning and latch-on with correction of improper techniques. Ensure that mother can duplicate positioning technique and experiences relief with adjusted latch-on. (ii) Diagnose any underlying nipple condition and prescribe appropriate treatment. (iii) In cases of severely traumatized nipples, temporary cessation of breastfeeding may be indicated to allow for healing. It is important to instruct the mother to maintain lactation with mechanical/hand expression until direct breastfeeding is resumed.

C. **Engorgement** is a severe form of increased breast fullness that usually presents on day 3 to 5 postpartum signaling the onset of copious milk production. Engorgement may be caused by inadequate and/or infrequent breast stimulation resulting in swollen, hard breasts that are warm to the touch. The infant may have difficulty latching on to the breast until the engorgement is resolved. Treatment includes (i) application of warm, moist heat to the breast alternating with cold compresses to relieve edema of the breast tissue; (ii) gentle hand expression of milk to soften areola to facilitate infant attachment to the breast; (iii) gentle massage of the breast during feeding and/or milk expression; (iv) mild analgesic (acetaminophen) or anti-inflammatory (naproxen) for pain relief and/or reduction of inflammation.

D. **Plugged ducts** usually present as a palpable lump or area of the breast that does not soften during a feeding or pumping session. It may be the result of an ill-fitting bra; tight, constricting clothing; or a missed or delayed feeding/pumping. Treatment includes (i) frequent feedings/pumpings beginning with the affected breast; (ii) application of moist heat and breast massage before and during feeding; (iii) positioning infant during feeding to locate the chin toward the affected area to allow for maximum application of suction pressure to facilitate breast emptying.

E. **Mastitis** is an inflammatory and/or infectious breast condition—usually affecting only one breast. Signs and symptoms include rapid onset of fatigue, body aches, headache, fever, and tender, reddened breast area. Treatment includes (i) immediate bed rest concurrent with continued breastfeeding on affected and unaffected breasts; (ii) frequent and efficient milk removal—using an electric breast pump when necessary (it is not necessary to discard expressed breast milk); (iii) appropriate antibiotics for a sufficient period (10–14 days); (iv) comfort measures to relieve breast discomfort and general malaise (i.e., analgesics, moist heat/massage to breast).

V. SPECIAL SITUATIONS.
Certain conditions in the infant, mother, or both may indicate specific strategies that require a delay and/or modification of the normal breastfeeding relationship. Whenever breastfeeding is delayed or suspended for a period of time, frequent breast emptying with an electric breast pump is recommended to ensure maintenance of lactation.

A. **Infant conditions.** Hyperbilirubinemia is not a contraindication to breastfeeding. Special attention should be given to ensuring infant is breastfeeding effectively in order to enhance gut motility and facilitate bilirubin excretion. In rare instances of severe hyperbilirubinemia, breastfeeding may be interrupted temporarily for a short period of time.

    1. **Congenital anomalies** may require special management.

        a. Craniofacial anomalies (i.e., cleft lip/palate, Pierre-Robin) present challenges to the infant's ability to latch effectively to the breast. Modified positioning and special devices (i.e., obturator, nipple shield) may be utilized to achieve an effective latch.

        b. Cardiac or respiratory conditions may require fluid restriction and special attention to pacing of feeds to minimize fatigue during feeding.

c. Restrictive lingual frenulum (ankyloglossia/tongue-tie) may interfere with the infant's ability to effectively breast-feed. The inability of the infant to extend the tongue over the lower gum line and lift the tongue to compress the underlying breast tissue may compromise effective milk transfer. Frenulotomy is often the treatment of choice.

2. Premature infants receive profound benefits from breastfeeding and the receipt of mother's own milk. Mothers should be encouraged to express their milk (see breast milk collection and storage in the subsequent text)—even if they do not plan on direct breastfeeding—in order to provide their infant with the special nutritional and nonnutritional human milk components.

Although mother's own milk imparts the greatest benefit to preterm and high-risk infants, pasteurized donor breast milk may be an alternative when mother's own milk is not available. When considering donor milk feeding, the product should be obtained from milk banks that adhere to the guidelines established by the Human Milk Banking Association of North America (HMBANA). These guidelines ensure safe handling and maintain the maximum amount of active human milk components. We obtain parental informed consent prior to using donor milk.

a. Special attention should be given to late preterm and near-term infants (35–37 weeks' gestation) who are often discharged from the hospital before they are breastfeeding effectively. Management should include (i) mechanical milk expression concurrent with breastfeeding until the infant is breastfeeding effectively; (ii) systematic assessment (and documentation) of breastfeeding by a trained observer; (iii) weighing the infant before and after breastfeeding to evaluate adequacy of milk intake and determine need for supplementation.

b. For premature infants less than 35 weeks, mothers should be encouraged to practice early and frequent skin-to-skin holding and suckling at the emptied breast to facilitate early nipple stimulation to enhance milk volume and enable infant oral feeding assessment.

B. Maternal conditions

1. Endocrine diseases have the potential to affect lactation and milk production.
a. Women with diabetes should be encouraged to breast-feed, and many find an improvement in their glucose metabolism during lactation. Early, close monitoring to ensure the establishment of lactation and adequacy of infant growth are recommended due to a well-documented delay (1–2 days) in the secretory phase of lactogenesis.
b. Thyroid disease does not preclude breastfeeding, although without proper treatment of the underlying thyroid condition, poor milk production (hypothyroidism) or maternal loss of weight, agitation, and heart palpitations (hyperthyroidism) may negatively affect lactation. With proper pharmacologic treatment, the ability to lactate does not appear to be affected.
c. Gestational ovarian theca lutein cysts and retained placental fragments are conditions that delay the secretory phase of lactogenesis.

2. Women with a history of breast or chest surgery should be able to breast-feed successfully. Prenatal assessment should include documenting the type of procedure (i.e., augmentation, reduction mammoplasty) and surgical approach (i.e., submammary, periareolar, free nipple transplantation) utilized in order to evaluate the level of follow-up indicated in the early postpartum period to monitor the progress of breastfeeding and adequacy of milk production and infant growth.

VI. CARE AND HANDLING OF EXPRESSED BREAST MILK.

When possible, direct breastfeeding provides the greatest benefit for mother and infant, especially in terms of provision of specific human milk components and maternal–infant interaction. However, when direct breastfeeding is not possible, expressed breast milk should be encouraged with special attention to milk expression and storage techniques. Mothers separated from their infants immediately following delivery due to infant prematurity or illness must initiate lactation by mechanical milk expression. Milk expression and storage techniques can affect the composition and bacterial content of mother's own milk.

A. **Breast milk expression and collection.** Recommendations for initiation and maintenance of mechanical milk expression for pump-dependent mothers of hospitalized infants include (i) breast stimulation with a hospital-grade electric breast pump combined with hand expression/breast massage initiated within the first few hours following delivery; (ii) frequent pumping/hand expression (8–10 times daily) during the first 2 weeks following birth theoretically stimulates mammary alveolar growth and maximizes potential milk yield; (iii) pumping 10 to 15 minutes per session during the first few days until the onset of increased milk flow at which time pumping time per session can be modified to continue 1 to 2 minutes beyond a steady milk flow; (iv) a target daily milk volume of 800 to 1,000 mL at the end of the second week following delivery is optimal.

B. **Guidelines for breast milk collection** include (i) instructing the mother to wash hands and scrub under fingernails prior to each milk expression; (ii) all milk collection equipment coming in contact with the breast and breast milk should be thoroughly cleaned prior to and following each use; (iii) sterilizing milk collection equipment once a day; (iv) collect milk in sterile glass or hard plastic containers—plastic bags are not recommended for milk storage for preterm infants; (v) label each milk container with infant's identifying information, date, and time of milk expression.

C. **Guidelines for breast milk storage** include (i) use fresh, unrefrigerated milk within 4 hours of milk expression; (ii) refrigerate milk immediately following expression when the infant will be fed within 72 hours; (iii) freeze milk when infant is not being fed, or the mother is unable to deliver the milk to the hospital within 24 hours of expression; (iv) in the event that frozen milk partially thaws, either complete thawing process and feed the milk or refreeze.

VII. CONTRAINDICATIONS AND CONDITIONS *NOT* CONTRAINDICATED TO BREASTFEEDING

There are a few contraindications to breastfeeding or expressed breast milk feeding. Maternal health conditions should be evaluated and appropriate treatments prescribed in order to support continued breastfeeding and/or minimal interruption of feeding when possible. Most maternal medications enter breast milk to some degree; however, with few exceptions, the concentrations of most are relatively low and the dose delivered to the infant often subclinical (see Appendix C).

A. Contraindications to breastfeeding

1. An infant with **galactosemia** will be unable to breast-feed or receive breast milk.

2. A mother with **active untreated tuberculosis** will be isolated from her newborn for initial treatment. She can express her milk to initiate and maintain

her milk volume during this period, and once it is deemed safe for her to have contact with her infant, she can begin breastfeeding.

3. The Centers for Disease Control and Prevention recommends that **women who test positive for HIV in the United States** should avoid breastfeeding.

4. **Some maternal medications** are contraindicated during breastfeeding. Clinicians should maintain reliable resources for information on the transfer of drugs into human milk (see Appendix C).

B. Conditions that are **not** contraindications to breastfeeding

1. Mothers who are hepatitis B surface antigen positive. Infants should receive hepatitis B immune globulin and hepatitis B vaccine to eliminate risk of transmission.

2. Although hepatitis C virus has been found in breast milk, transmission through breastfeeding has not been shown (see Chap. 48).

3. In full-term infants, the benefits of breastfeeding appear to outweigh the risk of transmission from cytomegalovirus (CMV)-positive mothers. The extremely preterm infant is at increased risk for perinatal CMV acquisition. Frozen milk or pasteurization may reduce the risk of transmission in human milk.

4. Mothers who are febrile

5. Mothers exposed to low-level environmental chemical agents

6. Although tobacco smoking is not contraindicated, mothers should be advised to avoid smoking in the home and make every effort to stop smoking while breastfeeding.

7. Alcohol use should be avoided because it is concentrated in milk and it can inhibit short-term milk production. Although an occasional, small alcoholic drink is acceptable, breastfeeding should be avoided for 2 hours after the drink.

Suggested Readings

American Academy of Pediatrics. Breastfeeding and the use of human milk. *Pediatrics* 2005;115(2):496–506.

Hale T. *Medications and Mother's Milk*. 14th ed. Amarillo, TX: Pharmasoft Medical Publishing, 2010.

Hurst NM, Meier PP. Breastfeeding the preterm infant. In: Riordan J, Wambach K, eds. *Breastfeeding and Human Lactation*. 4th ed. Boston, MA: Jones & Bartlett, 2010:425–470.

Lawrence RA. *Breastfeeding: A Guide for the Medical Profession*. 6th ed. St. Louis, MO: Mosby, 2005.

Suggested Websites

The Academy of Breastfeeding Medicine, http://www.bfmed.org

Baby Friendly Hospital Initiative in the United States, http://www.babyfriendlyusa.org

Human Milk Banking Association of North America, http://www.hmbana.org

International Lactation Consultant Association, http://www.ilca.org

La Leche League International, http://www.llli.org

LactMed—drugs and lactation database, http://toxnet.nlm.nih.gov/cgi-bin/sis/htmlgen?LACT

Wellstart International, http://www.wellstart.org

23 Fluid and Electrolyte Management
Elizabeth G. Doherty

Careful fluid and electrolyte management in term and preterm infants is an essential component of neonatal care. Developmental changes in body composition in conjunction with functional changes in skin, renal, and neuroendocrine systems account for the fluid balance challenges faced by neonatologists on a daily basis. Fluid management requires the understanding of several physiologic principles.

I. DISTRIBUTION OF BODY WATER

A. **General principles.** Transition from fetal to newborn life is associated with major changes in water and electrolyte homeostatic control. Before birth, the fetus has constant supply of water and electrolytes from the mother across the placenta. After birth, the newborn assumes responsibility for its own fluid and electrolyte homeostasis. The body composition of the fetus changes during gestation with a smaller proportion of body weight being composed of water as gestation progresses.

B. **Definitions**

1. Total body water (TBW) = intracellular fluid (ICF) + extracellular fluid (ECF) (see Fig. 23.1)

2. ECF is composed of intravascular and interstitial fluid.

3. Insensible water loss (IWL) = fluid intake − urine output + weight change

C. **Perinatal changes in TBW.** A proportion of diuresis in both term and preterm infants during the first days of life should be regarded as physiologic. This diuresis results in a weight loss of 5% to 10% in term infants and up to 15% in preterm infants. At lower gestational ages, ECF accounts for a greater proportion of birth weight (Fig. 23.1). Therefore, very low birth weight (VLBW) infants must lose a greater percentage of birth weight to maintain ECF proportions equivalent to those of term infants. Larger weight loss is possibly beneficial to the preterm infant, as administration of excessive fluid and sodium (Na) may increase risk of chronic lung disease (CLD) and patent ductus arteriosus (PDA).

D. **Sources of water loss**

1. **Renal losses.** Renal function matures with increasing gestational age (GA). Immature Na and water homeostasis is common in the preterm infant. Contributing factors leading to varying urinary water and electrolyte losses include the following:

   a. Decreased glomerular filtration rate (GFR)
   b. Reduced proximal and distal tubule Na reabsorption
   c. Decreased capacity to concentrate or dilute urine
   d. Decreased bicarbonate, potassium (K), and hydrogen ion secretion

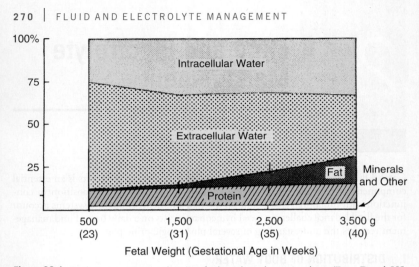

Figure 23.1. Body composition in relation to fetal weight and gestational age. (From Dweck HS. Feeding the prematurely born infant. Fluids, calories, and methods of feeding during the period of extrauterine growth retardation. *Clin Perinatol* 1975;2:183–202. Data from Widdowson EM. Growth and composition of the fetus and newborn. In: Assali NS, ed. *Biology of Gestation*, Vol. 2. New York: Academic Press, 1968).

    2. **Extra renal losses.** In VLBW infants, IWL can exceed 150 mL/kg/day, owing to increased environmental and body temperatures, skin breakdown, radiant warmers, phototherapy, and extreme prematurity (see Table 23.1). Respiratory water loss increases with decreasing GA and with increasing respiratory rate; in intubated infants, inadequate humidification of the inspired gas may lead to increased IWL. Other fluid losses that should be replaced if amount is deemed significant include stool (diarrhea or ostomy drainage), cerebrospinal fluid (from ventriculotomy or serial lumbar punctures), and nasogastric tube or thoracostomy tube drainage.

    Incubators for newborn infants are being designed to improve maintenance of warmth and humidity and may lead to decreased IWL (e.g., the Giraffe isolette).

Table 23.1	Insensible Water Loss (IWL)*
Birth weight (g)	**IWL (mL/kg/day)**
750–1,000	82
1,001–1,250	56
1,251–1,500	46
>1,501	26

*Values represent mean IWL for infants in incubators during the first week of life. IWL is increased by phototherapy (up to 40%), radiant warmers (up to 50%), and fever. IWL is decreased by the use of humidified gas with respirators and heat shields in incubators (Bell et al., 1980; Fanaroff et al., 1972; and Okken et al., 1979).

II. ASSESSMENT OF FLUID AND ELECTROLYTE STATUS

A. History

1. **Maternal.** The newborn's fluid and electrolyte status partially reflects maternal hydration status and drug administration. Excessive use of oxytocin, diuretics, or hyponatremic intravenous (IV) fluid can lead to maternal and fetal hyponatremia. Antenatal steroids may increase skin maturation, subsequently decreasing IWL and the risk of hyperkalemia.

2. **Fetal/perinatal.** The presence of oligohydramnios may be associated with congenital renal dysfunction, including renal agenesis, polycystic kidney disease, or posterior urethral valves. Severe *in utero* hypoxemia or birth asphyxia may lead to acute tubular necrosis.

B. Physical examination

1. **Change in body weight.** Acute changes in an infant's weight generally reflect a change in TBW. The compartment affected will depend on the gestational age and clinical course of the infant. For example, long-term use of paralytic agents and peritonitis may lead to increased interstitial fluid volume and body weight but decreased intravascular volume. Therefore, weight should be measured at least daily.

2. **Skin and mucosal manifestations.** Altered skin turgor, sunken anterior fontanelle, and dry mucous membranes are not sensitive indicators of fluid or electrolyte balance.

3. **Cardiovascular.** Tachycardia can result from ECF excess (e.g., heart failure) or hypovolemia. Capillary refill time can be delayed with reduced cardiac output or peripheral vasoconstriction, and hepatomegaly can occur with increased ECF volume. Blood pressure changes occur late in the sequence of responses to reduced cardiac output.

C. Laboratory studies

1. **Serum electrolytes and plasma osmolarity** reflect the composition and tonicity of the ECF. Frequent monitoring, every 4 to 6 hours, should be done in the extremely low birth weight (ELBW) infants during the first few days of life owing to high IWL.

2. **Fluid balance** with input and output measurements should be monitored. Normal urine output is 1 to 3 mL/kg/hour. With ECF depletion (dehydration), urine output may fall to <1 mL/kg/hour. However, in neonates with immature renal function, urine output may not decrease despite ECF volume depletion.

3. **Urine electrolytes and specific gravity (SG)** can reflect renal capacity to concentrate or dilute urine and reabsorb or excrete Na. Increases in SG can occur when the infant is receiving decreased fluids, has decreased urine output, or is spilling glucose. Neither urine electrolytes nor SG is very helpful when infant is on diuretics.

4. **Fractional excretion of Na (FENa)** reflects the balance between glomerular filtration and tubular reabsorption of Na.

   FENa = (urine Na × plasma creatinine)/(plasma Na × urine creatinine) × 100

   ■ Level of <1% indicates prerenal factors reducing renal blood flow.
   ■ Level of 2.5% occurs with acute renal failure (ARF).
   ■ Level of >2.5% is frequently seen in infants of <32 weeks' gestation.

5. **Blood urea nitrogen (BUN) and serum creatinine (Cr)** values provide indirect information about ECF volume and GFR. Values in the early postnatal period reflect placental clearance.

6. **Arterial pH, carbon dioxide tension (Pco$_2$), and Na bicarbonate** determinations can provide indirect evidence of intravascular volume depletion because poor tissue perfusion leads to high anion gap metabolic acidosis (lactic acidosis).

III. MANAGEMENT OF FLUIDS AND ELECTROLYTES.

The goal of early management is to allow initial ECF loss over the first 5 to 6 days as reflected by weight loss, while maintaining normal tonicity and intravascular volume as reflected by blood pressure, heart rate, urine output, serum electrolyte levels, and pH. Subsequent fluid management should maintain water and electrolyte balance including requirements for body growth.

A. **The term infant.** Body weight decreases by 3% to 5% over the first 5 to 6 days. Subsequently, fluids should be adjusted so that changes in body weight are consistent with caloric intake. Clinical status should be monitored for maldistribution of water (e.g., edema). Na supplementation is not usually required in the first 24 hours unless ECF expansion is necessary. Small-for-gestational-age term infants may require early Na supplementation to maintain adequate ECF volume.

B. **The premature infant.** Allow a 5% to 15% weight loss over the first 5 to 6 days. Table 23.2 summarizes initial fluid therapy. Then, adjust fluids to maintain stable weight until an anabolic state is achieved and growth occurs. Frequently assess response to fluid and electrolyte therapy during the first 2 days of life. **Physical examination, urine output, SG, and serum electrolyte determinations may be required initially as frequent as every 6 to 8 hours in infants <1,000 g** (see VIII.A.).

Water loss through skin and urine may exceed 200 mL/kg/day, which can represent up to **one-third of TBW**. IV Na supplementation is not required for the first 24 hours unless ECF volume loss exceeds 5% of body weight per day (see Chap. 13). If ECF volume expansion is necessary, **normal saline (NS) is preferred over 5% albumin solutions** in order to reduce risk of CLD.

Table 23.2	Initial Fluid Therapy*			
		Fluid rate (mL/kg/day)		
Birth weight (kg)	Dextrose (g/100 mL)	<24 h	24–48 h	>48 h
<1	5–10	100–150†	120–150	140–190
1–1.5	10	80–100	100–120	120–160
>1.5	10	60–80	80–120	120–160

*Infants in humidified incubators. Infants under radiant warmers usually require higher initial fluid rates.
†Very low birth weight (VLBW) infants frequently require even higher initial rates of fluid administration, and frequent reassessment of serum electrolytes, urine output, and body weight.

IV. APPROACH TO DISORDERS OF NA AND WATER BALANCE. Abnormalities

can be grouped into disorders of **tonicity** or **ECF volume**. The conceptual approach to disorders of tonicity (e.g., hyponatremia) depends on whether the newborn exhibits normal ECF (euvolemia), ECF depletion (dehydration), or ECF excess (edema).

A. Isonatremic disorders

1. Dehydration

a. Predisposing factors frequently involve equivalent losses of Na and water (through thoracostomy, nasogastric, or ventriculostomy drainage) or third-space losses that accompany peritonitis, gastroschisis, or omphalocele. Renal Na and water losses in the VLBW infant can lead to hypovolemia despite normal body tonicity.

b. Diagnosis. Dehydration is usually manifested by weight loss, decreased urine output, and increased urine SG. However, infants of <32 weeks' gestation may not demonstrate oliguria in response to hypovolemia. Poor skin turgor, tachycardia, hypotension, metabolic acidosis, and increasing BUN may coexist. A low FENa (<1%) is usually seen in infants of >32 weeks' gestational age (see II.C.4.).

c. Therapy. Administer Na and water to first correct deficits and then adjust to equal maintenance needs plus ongoing losses. Acute isonatremic dehydration may require IV infusion of 10 mL/kg of NS if acute weight loss is >10% of body weight with signs of poor cardiac output.

2. Edema

a. Predisposing factors include excessive isotonic fluid administration, heart failure, sepsis, and neuromuscular paralysis.

b. Diagnosis. Clinical signs include periorbital and extremity edema, increased weight, and hepatomegaly.

c. Therapy includes **Na restriction** (to decrease total body Na) and water restriction (depending on electrolyte response).

B. Hyponatremic disorders (see Table 23.3). Consider **factitious hyponatremia**

due to hyperlipidemia or **hypoosmolar hyponatremia** due to osmotic agents. True hypoosmolar hyponatremia can then be evaluated.

1. Hyponatremia due to ECF volume depletion

a. Predisposing factors include diuretic use, osmotic diuresis (glycosuria), VLBW with renal water and Na wasting, adrenal or renal tubular salt-losing disorders, gastrointestinal losses (vomiting, diarrhea), and third-space losses of ECF (skin sloughing, early necrotizing enterocolitis [NEC]).

b. Diagnosis. Decreased weight, poor skin turgor, tachycardia, rising BUN, and metabolic acidosis are frequently observed. If renal function is mature, the newborn may develop decreased urine output, increased urine SG, and a low FENa.

c. Therapy. If possible, reduce ongoing Na loss. Administer Na and water to replace deficits and then adjust to match maintenance needs plus ongoing losses.

2. Hyponatremia with normal ECF volume

a. Predisposing factors include excess fluid administration and the syndrome of inappropriate antidiuretic hormone (SIADH) secretion. Factors that cause SIADH include pain, opiate administration, intraventricular hemorrhage (IVH), asphyxia, meningitis, pneumothorax, and positive-pressure ventilation.

b. Diagnosis of SIADH. Weight gain usually occurs without edema. Excessive fluid administration without SIADH results in low urine SG and high urine

Table 23.3	Hyponatremic Disorders	
Clinical diagnosis	Etiology	Therapy
Factitious hyponatremia	Hyperlipidemia	
Hypertonic hyponatremia	Mannitol	
	Hyperglycemia	
ECF volume normal	Syndrome of inappropriate antidiuretic hormone (SIADH)	Restrict water intake
	Pain	
	Opiates	
	Excess intravenous fluids	
ECF volume deficit	Diuretics	Increase Na intake
	Late-onset hyponatremia of prematurity	
	Congenital adrenal hyperplasia	
	Severe glomerulotubular imbalance (immaturity)	
	Renal tubular acidosis	
	Gastrointestinal losses	
	Necrotizing enterocolitis (third-space loss)	
ECF volume excess	Heart failure	Restrict water intake
	Neuromuscular blockade (e.g., pancuronium)	
	Sepsis	
ECF = extracellular fluid.		

output. In contrast, SIADH leads to **decreased urine output** and **increased urine osmolarity**. Urinary Na excretion in infants with SIADH varies widely and reflects Na intake. The diagnosis of SIADH presumes no volume-related stimulus to antidiuretic hormone (ADH) release, such as reduced cardiac output or abnormal renal, adrenal, or thyroid function.

   c. Therapy. Water restriction is therapeutic unless (i) serum Na concentration is less than approximately 120 mEq/L or (ii) neurologic signs such as obtundation or seizure activity develop. In these instances, **furosemide** 1 mg/kg IV q6h can be initiated while replacing urinary Na excretion with **hypertonic NaCl (3%) (1–3 mL/kg initial dose).** This strategy leads to loss of free water with no net change in total body Na. Fluid restriction alone can be utilized once serum Na concentration is >120 mEq/L and neurologic signs abate.

  3. Hyponatremia due to ECF volume excess
    a. Predisposing factors include sepsis with decreased cardiac output, late NEC, heart failure, abnormal lymphatic drainage, and neuromuscular paralysis.
    b. Diagnosis. Weight increase with edema is observed. Decreasing urine output, increasing BUN and urine SG, and a low FENa are often present in infants with mature renal function.
    c. Therapy. Treat the underlying disorder and **restrict water** to alleviate hypotonicity. Na restriction and improving cardiac output may be beneficial.

C. Hypernatremic disorders

  1. Hypernatremia with normal or deficient ECF volume
    a. Predisposing factors include increased renal and IWL in VLBW infants. Skin sloughing can accelerate water loss. ADH deficiency secondary to IVH can occasionally exacerbate renal water loss.
    b. Diagnosis. Weight loss, tachycardia and hypotension, metabolic acidosis, decreasing urine output, and increasing urine SG may occur. Urine may be dilute if the newborn exhibits central or nephrogenic diabetes insipidus.
    c. Therapy. Increase **free water administration** to reduce serum Na no faster than 1 mEq/kg/hour. If signs of ECF depletion or excess develop, adjust Na intake. **Hypernatremia does not necessarily imply excess total body Na.** For example, **in the VLBW infant, hypernatremia in the first 24 hours of life is almost always due to free water deficits** (see VIII.A.1.).

  2. Hypernatremia with ECF volume excess
    a. Predisposing factors include excessive isotonic or hypertonic fluid administration, especially in the face of reduced cardiac output.
    b. Diagnosis. Weight gain associated with edema is observed. The infant may exhibit normal heart rate, blood pressure, and urine output and SG, but an elevated FENa.
    c. Therapy. Restrict Na administration.

V. OLIGURIA exists if urine flow is <1 mL/kg/hour. Although delayed micturition in a healthy infant is not of concern until 24 hours after birth, urine output in a critically ill infant should be assessed by 8 to 12 hours of life, using urethral catheterization if indicated. Diminished urine output may reflect abnormal prerenal, renal parenchymal, or postrenal factors (see Table 23.4). The most common causes of neonatal ARF are asphyxia, sepsis, and severe respiratory illness. It is important to exclude other potentially treatable etiologies (see Chap. 28). In VLBW infants, oliguria may be normal in the first 24 hours of life (see VIII.A.1.).

A. History and physical examination. Screen the maternal and infant history for maternal diabetes (renal vein thrombosis), birth asphyxia (acute tubular necrosis), and oligohydramnios (Potter syndrome). Force of the infant's urinary stream (posterior urethral valves), rate and nature of fluid administration and urine

Table 23.4	Etiologies of Oliguria	
Prerenal	Renal parenchymal	Postrenal
Decreased inotropy	Acute tubular necrosis	Posterior urethral valves
	Ischemia (hypoxia, hypovolemia)	
Decreased preload	Disseminated intravascular coagulation	
	Renal artery or vein thrombosis	Neuropathic bladder
Increased peripheral resistance	Nephrotoxin	
	Congenital malformation	Prune belly syndrome
	Polycystic disease	
	Agenesis	
	Dysplasia	Uric acid nephropathy

output, and nephrotoxic drug use (aminoglycosides, indomethacin, furosemide) should be evaluated. **Physical examination** should determine blood pressure and ECF volume status; evidence of cardiac disease, abdominal masses, or ascites; and the presence of any congenital anomalies associated with renal abnormalities (e.g., Potter syndrome, epispadias).

B. Diagnosis

1. **Initial laboratory examination** should include urinalysis, BUN, Cr, and FENa determinations. These aid in diagnosis and provide baseline values for further management.

2. **Fluid challenge**, consisting of a total of 20 mL/kg of NS, is administered as two infusions at 10 mL/kg/hour if no suspicion of structural heart disease or heart failure exists. Decreased cardiac output not responsive to ECF expansion may require the institution of inotropic or chronotropic pressor agents. Dopamine at a dose of 1 to 5 µg/kg/minute may increase renal blood flow and a dose of 2 to 15 µg/kg/minute may increase total cardiac output. These effects may augment GFR and urine output (see Chap. 40).

3. **If no response to fluid challenge occurs,** one may induce diuresis with **furosemide** 2 mg/kg IV.

4. Patients who are unresponsive to increased cardiac output and diuresis should be evaluated with an **abdominal ultrasonography** to define renal, urethral, and bladder anatomy. IV pyelography, renal scanning, angiography, or cystourethrography may be required (see Chap. 28).

C. Management. Prenatal oliguria should respond to increased cardiac output. **Postrenal** obstruction requires urologic consultation, with possible urinary diversion and surgical correction. If parenchymal **ARF** is suspected, minimize excessive ECF expansion and electrolyte abnormalities. If possible, eliminate reversible causes of declining GFR, such as nephrotoxic drug use.

1. **Monitor** daily weight, input and output, and BUN, Cr, and serum electrolytes.

2. **Fluid restriction.** Replace insensible fluid loss plus urine output. **Withhold K supplementation** unless hypokalemia develops. Replace urinary Na losses unless edema develops.

3. **Adjust dosage and frequency of drugs** eliminated by renal excretion. Monitor serum drug concentrations to guide drug dosing intervals.

4. **Peritoneal or hemodialysis** may be indicated in patients whose GFR progressively declines causing complications related to ECF volume or electrolyte abnormalities (see Chap. 28).

VI. METABOLIC ACID–BASE DISORDERS

A. Normal acid–base physiology. Metabolic acidosis results from excessive loss of buffer or from an increase of volatile or nonvolatile acid in the extracellular space. Normal sources of acid production include the metabolism of amino acids containing sulfur and phosphate, as well as hydrogen ion released from bone mineralization. Intravascular buffers include bicarbonate, phosphate, and intracellular hemoglobin. Maintenance of normal pH depends on excretion of volatile acid (e.g., carbonic acid) from the lungs, skeletal exchange of cations for hydrogen, and renal regeneration and reclamation of bicarbonate. Kidneys contribute to maintenance of acid–base balance by reabsorbing the filtered load of bicarbonate, secreting hydrogen ions as titratable acidity (e.g., H_2PO_4), and excreting ammonium ions.

B. Metabolic acidosis (see Chap. 60)

1. **Anion gap.** Metabolic acidosis can result from accumulation of acid or loss of buffering equivalents. Anion gap determination will suggest mechanism. Na, Cl, and bicarbonate are the primary ions of the extracellular space and exist in approximately electroneutral balance. The **anion gap,** calculated as the difference between the Na concentration and sum of the Cl and bicarbonate concentrations, reflects the unaccounted for anion composition of the ECF. An increased anion gap indicates an accumulation of organic acid, whereas a normal anion gap indicates a loss of buffer equivalents. Normal values for the neonatal anion gap are from 5 to 15 mEq/L and vary directly with serum albumin concentration.

2. **Metabolic acidosis associated with an increased anion gap (>15 mEq/L).** Disorders (see Table 23.5) include renal failure, inborn errors of metabolism, lactic acidosis, late metabolic acidosis, and toxin exposure. Lactic acidosis results from diminished tissue perfusion and resultant anaerobic metabolism in infants with asphyxia or severe cardiorespiratory disease. Late metabolic acidosis typically occurs during the second or third week of life in premature infants who ingest high casein-containing formulas. Metabolism of sulfur-containing amino acids in casein and increased hydrogen ion release due to the rapid mineralization of bone cause an increased acid load. Subsequently, inadequate hydrogen ion excretion by the premature kidney results in acidosis.

Table 23.5	Metabolic Acidosis
Increased anion gap (>15 mEq/L)	**Normal anion gap (<15 mEq/L)**
Acute renal failure	Renal bicarbonate loss
Inborn errors of metabolism	Renal tubular acidosis
Lactic acidosis	Acetazolamide
Late metabolic acidosis	Renal dysplasia
Toxins (e.g., benzyl alcohol)	Gastrointestinal bicarbonate loss
	Diarrhea
	Cholestyramine
	Small-bowel drainage
	Dilutional acidosis
	Hyperalimentation acidosis

3. **Metabolic acidosis associated with a normal anion gap (<15 mEq/L)** results from buffer loss through the renal or gastrointestinal systems (Table 23.5). Premature infants <32 weeks' gestation frequently manifest a proximal or distal renal tubular acidosis (RTA). Urine pH persistently >7 in an infant with metabolic acidosis suggests a distal RTA. Urinary pH <5 documents normal distal tubule hydrogen ion secretion but proximal tubular bicarbonate resorption could still be inadequate (proximal RTA). IV Na bicarbonate infusion in infants with proximal RTA will result in a urinary pH >7 before attaining a normal serum bicarbonate concentration (22–24 mEq/L).

4. **Therapy.** Whenever possible, **treat the underlying cause**. Lactic acidosis due to low cardiac output or due to decreased peripheral oxygen delivery should be treated with specific measures. The use of a low-casein formula may alleviate late metabolic acidosis. Treat normal anion gap metabolic acidosis by decreasing the rate of bicarbonate loss (e.g., decreased small bowel drainage) or providing buffer equivalents. **IV Na bicarbonate or Na acetate** (which is compatible with Ca salts) is most commonly used to treat arterial pH <7.25. Oral buffer supplements can include citric acid (Bicitra) or Na citrate (1–3 mEq/kg/day). Estimate bicarbonate deficit from the following formula:
Deficit = 0.4 × body weight × (desired bicarbonate − actual bicarbonate)
The premature infant's acid–base status can change rapidly, and frequent monitoring is warranted. The infant's ability to tolerate an increased Na load and to metabolize acetate is an important variable that influences acid–base status during treatment.

C. **Metabolic alkalosis.** The etiology of metabolic alkalosis can be clarified by determining urinary Cl concentration. Alkalosis accompanied by ECF depletion is

Table 23.6	Metabolic Alkalosis
Low urinary Cl (<10 mEq/L)	**High urinary Cl (>20 mEq/L)**
Diuretic therapy (late)	Barters syndrome with mineralocorticoid excess
Acute correction of chronically compensated respiratory acidosis	Alkali administration
Nasogastric suction	Massive blood product transfusion
Vomiting	Diuretic therapy (early)
Secretory diarrhea	Hypokalemia
Cl = chloride.	

associated with decreased urinary Cl, whereas states of mineralocorticoid excess are usually associated with increased urinary Cl (see Table 23.6). Treat the underlying disorder.

VII. DISORDERS OF K BALANCE.
K is the fundamental intracellular cation. Serum K concentrations do not necessarily reflect total body K because extracellular and intracellular K distribution also depends on the pH of body compartments. **An increase of 0.1 pH unit in serum results in approximately a 0.6 mEq/L fall in serum K concentration due to an intracellular shift of K ions.** Total body K is regulated by balancing K intake (normally 1–2 mEq/kg/day) and excretion through urine and the gastrointestinal tract.

A. **Hypokalemia** can lead to arrhythmias, ileus, renal concentrating defects, and obtundation in the newborn.
   1. **Predisposing factors** include nasogastric or ileostomy drainage, chronic diuretic use, and renal tubular defects.
   2. **Diagnosis.** Obtain serum and urine electrolytes, pH, and an electrocardiogram (ECG) to detect possible conduction defects (prolonged QT interval and U waves).
   3. **Therapy.** Reduce renal or gastrointestinal losses of K. Gradually increase intake of K as needed.

B. **Hyperkalemia.** The normal serum K level in a nonhemolyzed blood specimen at normal pH is 3.5 to 5.5 mEq/L; symptomatic hyperkalemia may begin at a serum K level >6 mEq/L.
   1. **Predisposing factors.** Hyperkalemia can occur unexpectedly in any patient but should be **anticipated** and **screened** for in the following scenarios:
      a. Increased K release secondary to tissue destruction, trauma, cephalhematoma, hypothermia, bleeding, intravascular or extravascular hemolysis, asphyxia/ischemia, and IVH.
      b. Decreased K clearance due to renal failure, oliguria, hyponatremia, and congenital adrenal hyperplasia.

c. Miscellaneous associations, including dehydration, birth weight <1,500 g (see VIII.A.2.), blood transfusion, inadvertent excess (KCl) administration, CLD with KCl supplementation, and exchange transfusion.

d. Up to 50% of VLBW infants born before 25 weeks' gestation manifest serum K levels >6 mEq/L in the first 48 hours of life (see VIII.A.2.). **The most common cause of sudden unexpected hyperkalemia in the neonatal intensive care unit (NICU) is medication error.**

2. **Diagnosis.** Obtain serum and urine electrolytes, serum pH, and Ca concentrations. The hyperkalemic infant may be asymptomatic or may present with a spectrum of signs, including bradyarrhythmias or tachyarrhythmias, cardiovascular instability or collapse. The ECG findings progress with increasing serum K from peaked T waves (increased rate of repolarization), flattened P waves and increasing PR interval (suppression of atrial conductivity), to QRS widening and slurring (conduction delay in ventricular conduction tissue, as well as in the myocardium itself), and finally, supraventricular/ventricular tachycardia, bradycardia, or ventricular fibrillation. The ECG findings may be the first indication of hyperkalemia (see Chap. 41).

Once hyperkalemia is diagnosed, remove all sources of exogenous K (change all IV solutions and analyze for K content, check all feedings for K content), rehydrate the patient if necessary, and eliminate arrhythmia-promoting factors. The pharmacologic therapy of neonatal hyperkalemia consists of three components:

a. Goal 1: Stabilization of conducting tissues. This can be accomplished by Na or Ca ion administration. **Ca gluconate (10%) given carefully at 1 to 2 mL/kg IV (over 0.5–1 hour)** may be the most useful in the NICU. Treatment with hypertonic NaCl solution is not done routinely. However, if the patient is both hyperkalemic and hyponatremic, NS infusion may be beneficial. Use of antiarrhythmic agents such as lidocaine and bretylium should be considered for refractory ventricular tachycardia (see Chap. 41).

b. Goal 2: Dilution and intracellular shifting of K. Increased serum K in the setting of dehydration should respond to fluid resuscitation. Alkalemia will promote intracellular K-for-hydrogen-ion exchange. **Na bicarbonate 1 to 2 mEq/kg/hour IV** may be used, although the resultant pH change may not be sufficient to markedly shift K ions. Na treatment as described in goal 1 may be effective. **In order to reduce risk of IVH, avoid rapid Na bicarbonate administration, especially in infants born before 34 weeks' gestation and younger than 3 days.** Respiratory alkalosis may be produced in an intubated infant by hyperventilation, although the risk of hypocarbia-diminishing cerebral perfusion may make this option more suited to emergency situations. Theoretically, every 0.1 pH unit increase leads to a decrease of 0.6 mEq/L in serum K.

Insulin enhances intracellular K uptake by direct stimulation of the membrane-bound Na–K ATPase. Insulin infusion with concomitant glucose administration to maintain normal blood glucose concentration is relatively safe, as long as serum or blood glucose levels are frequently monitored. **This therapy may begin with a bolus of insulin and glucose (0.05 unit/kg of human regular insulin with 2 mL/kg of dextrose 10% in water [D10W]) followed by continuous infusion of D10W at 2 to 4 mL/kg/hour and human regular insulin (10 units/100 mL) at 1 mL/kg/hour.** To minimize the effect of binding to IV tubing, insulin diluted in D10W may be flushed through the tubing. Adjustments in infusion rate of either glucose or insulin in response to hyperglycemia or hypoglycemia may be simplified if the two solutions are prepared individually (see Chap. 24).

β-2-Adrenergic stimulation enhances K uptake, probably through stimulation of the Na–K ATPase. The immaturity of the β-receptor response in preterm infants may contribute to nonoliguric hyperkalemia in these patients (see VIII.A.2.). To date, β stimulation is not primary therapy for hyperkalemia in the pediatric population. However, if cardiac dysfunction and hypotension are present, use of dopamine or other adrenergic agents could, through β-2 stimulation, lower serum K.

c. Goal 3: Enhanced K excretion. Diuretic therapy (e.g., **furosemide 1 mg/kg IV**) may increase K excretion by increasing flow and Na delivery to the distal tubules. In the clinical setting of inadequate urine output and reversible renal disease (e.g., indomethacin-induced oliguria), **peritoneal dialysis** and **double volume exchange transfusion** are potentially life-saving options. Peritoneal dialysis can be successful in infants weighing <1,000 g and should be considered if the patient's clinical status and etiology of hyperkalemia suggest a reasonable chance for good long-term outcome. **Use fresh whole blood (<24 hours old) or deglycerolized red blood cells reconstituted with fresh-frozen plasma for double volume exchange transfusion.** Aged, banked blood may have K levels as high as 10 to 12 mEq/L; aged, washed, packed red blood cells will have low K levels (see Chap. 42).

Enhanced K excretion using cation-exchange resins, such as Na or Ca polystyrene sulfonate, has been studied primarily in adults. The resins can be administered orally per gavage (PG) or rectally. A study involving uremic and control rats demonstrated that Na polystyrene sulfonate (Kayexalate) administered by rectum with sorbitol was toxic to the colon, but rectal administration after suspension in distilled water produced only mild mucosal erythema in 10% of animals. Another possible complication of resins is bowel obstruction secondary to bezoar or plug formation.

The reported experience with resin use in neonates covers those born at 25 to 40 weeks' gestation. **PG administration of Kayexalate is not recommended in preterm infants because they are prone to hypomotility and are at risk for NEC. Rectal administration of Kayexalate (1 g/kg at 0.5 g/mL of NS) with a minimum retention time of 30 minutes should be effective in lowering serum K levels by approximately 1 mEq/L. The enema should be inserted 1 to 3 cm using a thin silastic feeding tube.** Published evidence supports the efficacy of this treatment in infants. Kayexalate prepared in water or NS (eliminating sorbitol as a solubilizing agent) and delivered rectally should be a therapeutic agent with an acceptable risk–benefit ratio.

The clinical condition, ECG, and actual serum K level all affect the choice of therapy for hyperkalemia. Figure 23.2 contains guidelines for treatment of hyperkalemia.

VIII. COMMON CLINICAL SITUATIONS

A. **VLBW infant**

1. **VLBW infants undergo three phases of fluid and electrolyte homeostasis:** prediuretic (first day of life), diuretic (second to third day of life), and postdiuretic (fourth to fifth day of life). Marked diuresis can occur during the diuretic phase leading to **hypernatremia** and the need for frequent serum

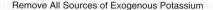

Remove All Sources of Exogenous Potassium

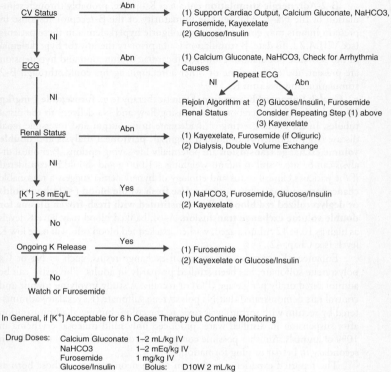

In General, if [K⁺] Acceptable for 6 h Cease Therapy but Continue Monitoring

Drug Doses:

Calcium Gluconate	1–2 mL/kg IV	
NaHCO3	1–2 mEq/kg IV	
Furosemide	1 mg/kg IV	
Glucose/Insulin	Bolus:	D10W 2 mL/kg
		Humulin 0.05 U/kg
	Infusion:	D10W 2–4 mL/kg/h
		Humulin, 10 U/100 mL D10W or 5% albumin, 1 mL/kg/h
Kayexelate	1 g/kg PR, Used Cautiously in the Setting of an Immature Ischemic GI Tract	

Figure 23.2. Treatment of hyperkalemia (CV = cardiovascular; Nl = normal; Abn = abnormal; ECG = electrocardiogram; GI = gastrointestinal). For a given algorithm outcome proceed by administering the entire set of treatments labeled (1). If unsuccessful in lowering [K⁺] or improving clinical condition, proceed to the next set of treatments, for example, (2) and then (3).

electrolyte determinations (q6–8h) and increased rates of parenteral fluid administration. Increased free water loss through skin and dopamine-associated natriuresis (due to increased GFR) can further complicate management. Hypernatremia often occurs despite a total body Na deficit. Lack of a brisk diuretic phase has been associated with increased CLD incidence.

In addition, **impaired glucose tolerance** can lead to hyperglycemia, requiring reduced rates of parenteral glucose infusion (see Chap. 24). This combination frequently leads to administration of reduced dextrose concentrations (<5%) in parenteral solutions. Avoid the infusion of parenteral solutions containing <200 mOsmol/L (i.e., D3W), to minimize local osmotic hemolysis and thereby reduce renal K load.

2. **VLBW infants often develop a nonoliguric hyperkalemia** in the first few days of life. This is caused by a relatively low GFR combined with an intracellular to extracellular K shift due to decreased Na–K ATPase activity. Postnatal glucocorticoid use may further inhibit Na–K ATPase activity. Insulin infusion to treat hyperkalemia may be necessary but elevates the risk of iatrogenic hypoglycemia. Treatment with Kayexalate (see VII.B.2.c.) can occasionally be beneficial in infants born before 32 weeks' gestation despite the obligate Na load and potential irritation of bowel mucosa by rectal administration. Na restriction can reduce the risk of CLD.

3. **Late-onset hyponatremia of prematurity** often occurs 6 to 8 weeks postnatally in the growing premature infant. Failure of the immature renal tubules to reabsorb filtered Na in a rapidly growing infant often causes this condition. Other contributing factors include the low Na content in breast milk and diuretic therapy for CLD. Infants at risk should be monitored with periodic electrolytes measurements and if affected, treated with simple Na supplementation (start with 2 mEq/kg/day).

B. **Severe CLD** (see Chap. 34). CLD requiring **diuretic** therapy often leads to **hypokalemic, hypochloremic metabolic alkalosis.** Affected infants frequently have a chronic respiratory acidosis with partial metabolic compensation. Subsequently, vigorous diuresis can lead to total body K and ECF volume depletion, causing a superimposed metabolic alkalosis. If the alkalosis is severe, alkalemia (pH >7.45) can supervene and result in central hypoventilation. If possible, gradually reduce urinary Na and K loss by reducing the diuretic dose, and/or increase K intake by administration of KCl (starting at 1 mEq/kg/day). Rarely, administration of ammonium chloride (0.5 mEq/kg) is required to treat the metabolic alkalosis. Long-term use of loop diuretics such as furosemide promotes excessive urinary Ca losses and nephrocalcinosis. Urinary Ca losses may be reduced through concomitant thiazide diuretic therapy (see Chap. 34).

Suggested Readings

Baumgart S. What's new from this millennium in fluids and electrolyte management for the VLBW and ELBW prematures. *J Neonatal-Perinatal Med* 2009;2:1–9.

Baumgart S, Costarino AT. Water and electrolyte metabolism of the micropremie. *Clin Perinatol* 2000;27(1):131–146.

Bell EF, Gray JC, Weinstein MR, et al. The effects of thermal environment on heat balance and insensible water loss in low-birth-weight infants. *J Pediatr* 1980;96:452–459.

Bhatia J. Fluid and electrolyte management in the very low birth weight neonate. *J Perinatol* 2006;26(Suppl 1):S19–S21.

Costarino AT Jr, Gruskay JA, Corcoran L, et al. Sodium restriction versus daily maintenance replacement in very low birth weight premature neonates: a randomized, blind therapeutic trial. *J Pediatr* 1992;120:99–106.

Fanaroff AA, Wald M, Gruber HS, et al. Insensible water loss in low birth weight infants. *Pediatrics* 1972;50(2):236–245.

Lorenz JM, Kleinman LI, Ahmed G, et al. Phases of fluid and electrolyte homeostasis in the extremely low birth weight infant. *Pediatrics* 1995;96(3 Pt 1):484–489.

Lorenz JM, Kleinman LI, Kotagal UR, et al. Water balance in very low-birth-weight infants: relationship to water and sodium intake and effect on outcome. *J Pediatr* 1982;101(3):423–432.

Shaffer SG, Kilbride HW, Hayen LK, et al. Hyperkalemia in very low birth weight infants. *J Pediatr* 1992;121(2):275–279.

24 Hypoglycemia and Hyperglycemia

Richard E. Wilker

Hypoglycemia is historically one of the most common metabolic problems seen in both the newborn nursery and neonatal intensive care unit (NICU), but confirming a diagnosis of clinically significant hypoglycemia requires that one interpret the blood glucose value within the clinical context. The definition of hypoglycemia as well as its clinical significance and management remain controversial. Blood glucose levels in the first hours of life are typically lower than normal values of older children or adults. In healthy babies, the blood glucose level can often be maintained in the appropriate range by initiating feeding soon after birth. Most cases of neonatal hypoglycemia are transient, respond readily to treatment, and are associated with an excellent prognosis. Persistent hypoglycemia is more likely to be associated with abnormal endocrine conditions, including hyperinsulinemia, as well as possible neurologic sequelae, but it is not possible to validly quantify the effects of neonatal hypoglycemia on subsequent neurodevelopment.

Persistent **hyperglycemia** is very rarely seen in the newborn nursery, but frequently occurs in very low birth weight (VLBW) babies in the NICU.

I. HYPOGLYCEMIA. Glucose provides the fetus with approximately 60% to 70% of its energy needs. Almost all fetal glucose derives from the maternal circulation by the process of transplacental-facilitated diffusion that maintains fetal glucose levels at approximately two-thirds of maternal levels. The severing of the umbilical cord at birth abruptly interrupts the source of glucose, and to maintain adequate glucose levels, the newborn must rapidly respond by glycogenolysis of hepatic stores, inducing gluconeogenesis, and utilizing exogenous nutrients from feeding. During this normal transition, newborn glucose levels fall to a low point in the first 1 to 2 hours of life, and then increase and stabilize at mean levels of 65 to 70 mg/dL by the age of 3 to 4 hours.

A. Incidence. The reported incidence of hypoglycemia varies with its definition, but it has been estimated to occur in up to 16% of large-for-gestational-age (LGA) infants and 15% of small-for-gestational-age (SGA) infants. Since blood glucose levels change markedly within the first hours of life, it is necessary to know the baby's exact age in order to interpret the glucose level.

B. Definition. The continued lack of a rational evidence-based definition of neonatal hypoglycemia has hampered the discussion of its incidence, effects, and treatment goals.

1. Historical Definitions

   a. Previous epidemiologic definitions that resulted in the acceptance of repeated glucose levels in the range of 20 to 30 mg/dL are no longer considered valid.

   b. Using a clinical definition (*Whipple's triad*) that required demonstrating symptoms in association with low glucose levels and resolution when the levels were restored to the normal range is also problematic since the development of clinical signs or symptoms may be a late manifestation of hypoglycemia. One of the goals of current management is to anticipate and attempt to prevent symptomatic hypoglycemia rather than react to it.

2. **Operational threshold.** In 2000, Cornblath recommended the use of an "*operational threshold*" for blood sugar management in newborn infants. The operational threshold is an indication for action and is not diagnostic of disease or abnormality.

   Cornblath's description of operational thresholds suggested glucose levels at which intervention should be considered based on clinical experience and analysis of the available evidence. Some important features of operational thresholds are listed subsequently:

   a. Lower than therapeutic goal

   b. Dependent on clinical state and age

   c. Do not define normal or abnormal

   d. Provide margin of safety

   e. Operational thresholds as suggested by Cornblath et al.

      i. Healthy full-term infant

         a) <24 hours of age—30 to 35 mg/dL may be acceptable at one time, but threshold is raised to 45 mg/dL if it persists after feeding or if it recurs in first 24 hours.

         b) After 24 hours, threshold should be increased to 45 to 50 mg/dL.

      ii. Infant with abnormal signs or symptoms—45 mg/dL.

      iii. Asymptomatic infants with risk factors for low blood sugar—36 mg/dL. Close surveillance is required and intervention is needed if plasma glucose remains below this level, does not increase after feeding, or if abnormal clinical signs are seen.

      iv. For any baby, if glucose levels are <20 to 25 mg/dL, IV glucose is needed to raise the plasma glucose to >45 mg/dL.

3. The significance of a given glucose level depends on the method of measurement, the infant's gestational age, chronological age, and other risk factors.

4. The absence of overt symptoms at low glucose levels does not rule out central nervous system (CNS) injury. There is no evidence indicating that the premature or young infant is protected from the effects of inadequate glucose delivery to the CNS.

5. There is no single value below which brain injury definitely occurs.

6. Within the first hours of life, normal asymptomatic babies may have a transient glucose level in the 30s (mg/dL) that will increase either spontaneously or in response to feeding. These babies have an excellent prognosis.

7. A glucose level less than 40 mg/dL at any time in any newborn requires a prompt follow-up glucose measurement to document normal values. If the value has not increased, an intervention is needed.

8. On the basis of developmental, neuroanatomic, metabolic, and clinical studies, our goal is to maintain the glucose value above 45 mg/dL in the first day, and more than 50 mg/dL thereafter.

C. Knowledge gaps. A report from the Eunice Kennedy Shriver National Institute of Child Health and Human Development workshop on neonatal hypoglycemia in 2009 identified the following knowledge gaps:

1. The complex nature and maturational features of global and regional brain energy use remain to be studied in human neonates.

2. There is no evidence-based study to identify any specific plasma glucose concentration (or range of glucose values) to define pathologic "hypoglycemia." Research studies are needed to fulfill this basic gap in knowledge and to help demonstrate the relationship between plasma glucose concentrations during the neonatal period and later neurologic outcomes.

3. There is great inconsistency in the sources and sampling methods of blood (capillary, venous, arterial) and the methods used for subsequent analysis, including processing techniques, thus affecting "normal" values on the basis of existing literature.

   There are no noninvasive methods for measuring concentrations of glucose and other energy substrates (intermittently or continuously); the existing minimally invasive methods need further refinement for their utility.

   The role of neuroimaging and electroencephalogram (EEG) studies in the management and prediction of hypoglycemia-related neuronal injuries remains to be determined.

D. Etiology

1. **Hyperinsulinemic hypoglycemia** is recognized as a major cause of persistent recurrent hypoglycemia in newborns, and it may be associated with an increased risk of brain injury since it not only decreases serum glucose levels but also prevents the brain from utilizing secondary fuel sources by suppressing fatty acid release and ketone body synthesis. Some cases of hyperinsulinemic hypoglycemia are transient and resolve over the course of several days, while others require more aggressive and prolonged treatment.

   a. Historically, the most common example of hyperinsulinism is the infant of diabetic mothers (see Chap. 2).

   b. Congenital genetic. Hyperinsulinism is seen in mutations of genes encoding the pancreatic beta cell ATP-sensitive potassium channel, such as ABCC8 and KCNJ11, which encode for sulfonylurea receptor (SUR1) and Kir6.2. Elevated insulin levels are also associated with loss of function mutations in HNF4A gene. Additional mutations continue to be identified.

   c. Secondary to other conditions
      i. Birth asphyxia
      ii. Developmental syndromes such as Beckwith-Wiedemann syndrome (macrosomia, mild microcephaly, omphalocele, macroglossia, hypoglycemia, and visceromegaly)
      iii. Congenital disorders of glycosylation and other metabolic conditions
      iv. Erythroblastosis (hyperplastic islets of Langerhans) (see Chap. 26)
      v. Maternal tocolytic therapy with beta-sympathomimetic agents (terbutaline)
      vi. Malpositioned umbilical artery catheter used to infuse glucose in high concentration into the celiac and superior mesenteric arteries T11 to 12, stimulating insulin release from the pancreas
      vii. Abrupt cessation of high glucose infusion

    viii. After exchange transfusion with blood containing high glucose concentration

    ix. Insulin-producing tumors (nesidioblastosis, islet cell adenoma, or islet cell dysmaturity)

2. **Large-for-gestational-age infants.** Current prenatal obstetric care includes testing women for glucose intolerance, and the number of undiagnosed infants of gestational diabetic mothers has decreased. The incidence of hypoglycemia in this heterogeneous population is not accurately known, but this group continues to be considered at high risk for hypoglycemia and warrants routine screening.

3. **Decreased production/stores**

    a. Prematurity

    b. Intrauterine growth restriction (IUGR)

    c. Inadequate caloric intake

    d. Delayed onset of feeding

4. **Increased utilization and/or decreased production.** Any baby with one of the following conditions should be evaluated for hypoglycemia; parenteral glucose may be necessary for the management of these infants.

    a. Perinatal stress

        i. Sepsis

        ii. Shock

        iii. Asphyxia

        iv. Hypothermia (increased utilization)

        v. Respiratory distress

        vi. Postresuscitation

    b. S/p exchange transfusion with heparinized blood that has a low glucose level in the absence of a glucose infusion; reactive hypoglycemia after exchange with relatively hyperglycemic citrate-phosphate-dextrose (CPD) blood.

    c. Defects in carbohydrate metabolism (see Chap. 60)

        i. Glycogen storage disease

        ii. Fructose intolerance

        iii. Galactosemia

    d. Endocrine deficiency

        i. Adrenal insufficiency

        ii. Hypothalamic deficiency

        iii. Congenital hypopituitarism

        iv. Glucagon deficiency

        v. Epinephrine deficiency

    e. Defects in amino acid metabolism (see Chap. 60)

        i. Maple syrup urine disease

        ii. Propionic acidemia

        iii. Methylmalonic acidemia

        iv. Tyrosinemia

        v. Glutaric acidemia type II

        vi. Ethylmalonic adipic aciduria

    f. Polycythemia. Hypoglycemia may be due to higher glucose utilization by the increased mass of red blood cells. The decreased amount of serum per drop of blood may cause a reading consistent with hypoglycemia on whole blood measurements, but may yield a normal glucose level on laboratory analysis of serum (see Chap. 46).

g. **Maternal therapy with beta-blockers (e.g., labetalol or propranolol).** Possible mechanisms include the following:

i. Prevention of sympathetic stimulation of glycogenolysis

ii. Prevention of recovery from insulin-induced decreases in free fatty acids and glycerol

iii. Inhibition of epinephrine-induced increases in free fatty acids and lactate after exercise

E. **Diagnosis**

1. **Symptoms that have been attributed to hypoglycemia are nonspecific.**

   a. Tremors, jitteriness, or irritability

   b. Seizures, coma

   c. Lethargy, apathy, and limpness

   d. Poor feeding, vomiting

   e. Apnea

   f. Weak or high-pitched cry

   g. Cyanosis

   h. Many infants may have no symptoms

2. **Screening.** Serial blood glucose levels should be routinely measured in infants who have risk factors for hypoglycemia, and in infants who have symptoms that could be due to hypoglycemia (see I.D. and I.E.1.).

   a. We start screening babies with risk factors at 30 to 60 minutes of life. In many cases, low glucose levels in the first hour will increase spontaneously or in response to feeding. The length of time to continue screening depends on the glucose levels measured and the etiology of hypoglycemia.

   i. Infants of diabetic mothers usually develop hypoglycemia in the first hours of life and should have frequent early measurements of blood glucose level (see Chap. 2).

   ii. Preterm and SGA infants should have blood glucose measurements within 30 to 60 minutes of birth and continuing during the first 3 to 4 postnatal days. Late preterm infants are at risk for hypoglycemia due to their decreased energy stores, immature enzyme systems for gluconeogenesis, and decreased oral intake.

   iii. Infants with erythroblastosis fetalis should routinely be screened for hypoglycemia after birth because of hyperinsulinism, and it is important to monitor for reactive hypoglycemia after exchange transfusion due to the high sugar content of banked blood.

   iv. Infants with symptoms should be evaluated for hypoglycemia when the symptoms are present.

3. **Reagent strips with reflectance meter.** Although in widespread use as a screening tool, reagent strips are of unproven reliability in documenting hypoglycemia in neonates.

   a. Reagent strips measure whole blood glucose, which is 15% lower than plasma levels.

   b. Reagent strips are subject to false-positive and false-negative results as a screen for hypoglycemia, even when used with a reflectance meter.

   c. A valid confirmatory laboratory glucose determination is required before one can diagnose hypoglycemia.

   d. If a reagent strip reveals a concentration of less than 45 mg/dL, treatment should not be delayed while one is awaiting confirmation of hypoglycemia by laboratory analysis. If an infant has either symptoms that could be due to hypoglycemia and/or a low glucose level as measured by a reagent strip, treatment should be initiated immediately after the confirmatory blood sample is obtained.

4. New point of care devices are available to allow for the accurate and rapid determination of glucose levels on small volume samples, but we do not use them for routine screening.

5. **Laboratory diagnosis**
   a. The laboratory sample must be obtained and analyzed promptly to avoid the measurement being falsely lowered by glycolysis. The glucose level can fall 18 mg/dL per hour in a blood sample that awaits analysis.

6. **Additional evaluation for persistent hypoglycemia.** Most hypoglycemia will resolve in 2 to 3 days. A requirement of more than 8 to 10 mg of glucose per kilogram per minute suggests increased utilization due to hyperinsulinism (Figure 24.1). This condition is usually transient, but if it persists, endocrine evaluation may be necessary to specifically evaluate for hyperinsulinism or other rare causes of hypoglycemia as listed in I.D. Many evaluations are not productive because they are done too early in the course of a transient

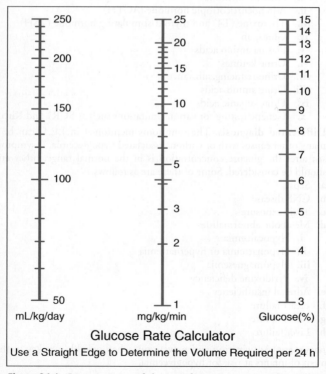

Glucose Rate Calculator

Use a Straight Edge to Determine the Volume Required per 24 h

Figure 24.1. Interconversion of glucose infusion units. From Klaus MH, Faranoff AA, eds. *Care of the High-Risk Neonate.* 2nd ed. Philadelphia: WB Saunders, 1979:430.

hypoglycemic state or the samples to determine hormone levels are drawn when the glucose level is normal.

    a. Critical lab sample. Diagnosing hyperinsulinemia requires measuring an insulin level that is inappropriately high for a simultaneous serum glucose. Evaluation requires drawing blood for insulin, cortisol, and amino acids at a time when the glucose level is less than 40 mg/dL. The typical critical lab sample includes the following:

        i. Glucose

        ii. Insulin

        iii. Cortisol. Cortisol levels can be used to screen for the integrity of the hypothalamic-pituitary-adrenal axis.

        iv. Beta-hydroxybutyrate and free fatty acid levels. Measurement of plasma beta-hydroxybutyrate and free fatty acid levels can be useful, because decreased levels of these substances can indicate excessive insulin action even if insulin levels are not significantly elevated.

    b. If the insulin level is normal for the blood glucose level, consider additional testing as indicated subsequently to evaluate for other causes of persistent hypoglycemia such as defects in carbohydrate metabolism (see I.D.4.c.), endocrine deficiency (see I.C.4.d.), and defects in amino acid metabolism (see I.D.4.e.).

        i. Growth hormone

        ii. Adrenocorticotropic hormone (ACTH)

        iii. Thyroxine (T4) and thyroid-stimulating hormone (TSH)

        iv. Glucagon

        v. Plasma amino acids

        vi. Urine ketones

        vii. Urine-reducing substance

        viii. Urine amino acids

        ix. Urine organic acids

        x. Genetic testing for various mutations such as SUR1 and Kir6.2

    7. Differential diagnosis. The symptoms mentioned in I.E.1. can be due to many other causes with or without associated hypoglycemia. If symptoms persist after the glucose concentration is in the normal range, other etiologies should be considered. Some of these are as follows:

    a. Sepsis

    b. CNS disease

    c. Toxic exposure

    d. Metabolic abnormalities

        i. Hypocalcemia

        ii. Hyponatremia or hypernatremia

        iii. Hypomagnesemia

        iv. Pyridoxine deficiency

    e. Adrenal insufficiency

    f. Heart failure

    g. Renal failure

    h. Liver failure

F. Management. Anticipation and prevention, when possible, are key to the management of infants at risk for hypoglycemia.

    1. Well infants who are at risk for hypoglycemia (see I.D.) should have serial blood glucose levels measured. *Infants of diabetic mothers* should have glucose measured and should be treated according to the protocol in Chapter 2.

2. Other *asymptomatic* well full-term infants who are at risk for hypoglycemia should have blood glucose measured in the first 1 to 2 hours of life. As soon after birth as their condition allows, they should be nursed or given formula per the mother's preference. This feeding should be repeated every 2 to 3 hours.

3. *The interval between measurements of glucose levels requires clinical judgment.* If the glucose concentration is as low as 20 to 25 mg/dL, the baby should be treated with intravenous (IV) glucose with a goal of maintaining the glucose greater than 45 mg/dL in the first 24 hours, and greater than 50 mg/dL thereafter.

4. **Feeding.** Some asymptomatic infants with early glucose levels in the 30s (mg/dL) will respond to feeding (breast or bottle). A follow-up blood glucose should be measured 1 hour after the start of the feeding. If the glucose level does not rise, more aggressive therapy may be needed. Feeding of glucose water is not recommended. The early introduction of milk feeding is preferable and will often result in raising glucose levels to normal, maintaining normal stable levels, and avoiding problems with rebound hypoglycemia. We sometimes find it useful to add calories to feedings in infants who feed well but have marginal glucose levels.

5. **Breastfeeding.** Babies who are breast-fed have lower glucose levels but higher ketone body levels than those who are formula-fed. The use of alternate fuels may be an adaptive mechanism during the first days of life as the maternal milk supply and the baby's feeding ability both increase. Early breastfeeding enhances gluconeogenesis and increases the production of gluconeogenic precursors. Some infants will have difficulty in adapting to breastfeeding, and symptomatic hypoglycemia has been reported to develop in breast-fed babies after hospital discharge. Late preterm infants will sometimes have a delay in achieving adequate oral feeding volumes and should have glucose levels measured. It is important to document that breast-fed babies are latching on and appear to be sucking milk, but there is no need to routinely monitor glucose levels in healthy full-term breast-fed babies who do not have additional risk factors.

6. **IV therapy**
   a. **Indications**
      i. Inability to tolerate oral feeding
      ii. Symptoms
      iii. Oral feedings do not maintain normal glucose levels
      iv. Glucose levels less than 25 mg/dL
   b. **Urgent treatment**
      i. 200 mg/kg of glucose over 1 minute, to be followed by continuing therapy discussed subsequently
      ii. This initial treatment is equivalent to 2 mL/kg of dextrose 10% in water (10% D/W) infused intravenously
   c. **Continuing therapy**
      i. Infusion of glucose at a rate of 6 to 8 mg of glucose/kg per minute
      ii. 10% D/W at a rate of 86.4 mL/kg per day or 3.6 mL/kg per hour gives 6 mg/kg per minute of glucose. Glucose infusion rate (GIR) may be calculated using the following formula:

$$\text{(GIR) in mg/kg/min} = \frac{\text{dextrose\% concentration} \times \text{mL/kg/day}}{144}$$

For example, in an infant receiving 10% D/W at 80 mL/kg/day, the GIR would be $\frac{10 \times 80}{144} = 5.6$ mg/kg/min

See Figure 24.1.

Many hospitals now have computerized provider order entry systems that automatically calculate the GIR.

   iii. Recheck glucose level 20 to 30 minutes after IV bolus, and then hourly until stable, to determine if additional therapy is needed.

   iv. Additional bolus infusions of 2 mL/kg of 10% D/W may be needed

   v. If glucose is stable and in acceptable range, feedings may be continued and the glucose infusion tapered as permitted by glucose measurements prior to feeding.

 d. For most infants, IV 10% D/W at daily maintenance rates will provide adequate glucose. The required concentration of dextrose in the IV fluids will depend on the daily water requirement. It is suggested that calculation of both glucose intake (i.e., milligrams of glucose per kilogram per minute) and water requirements be done each day, or more frequently, if glucose levels are unstable. For example, on the first day, the fluid requirement is generally about 80 mL/kg per day, or 0.055 mL/kg per minute; therefore, 10% D/W provides about 5.6 mg of glucose per kilogram per minute, and 15% D/W at 80 mL/kg per day, provides 8.25 mg of glucose per kilogram per minute.

 e. Some infants with hyperinsulinism and infants with IUGR will require 12 to 15 mg of dextrose per kilogram per minute (often as 15% or 20% D/W).

 f. The concentration of glucose and the rate of infusion are increased as necessary to maintain a normal blood glucose level. A central venous catheter may be necessary to give adequate glucose (15% to 20% D/W) in an acceptable fluid volume. After glucose levels have been stable in the normal range, it is appropriate to taper the GIR and concentration while monitoring glucose levels before feeding. IV fluids should be weaned slowly while feedings are advanced.

7. Consider adding **hydrocortisone**, 5 mg/kg per day intravenously in two divided doses, if it is difficult to maintain the infant's glucose levels in the normal range despite receiving more than 12 to 15 mg of glucose per kilogram per minute. Hydrocortisone reduces peripheral glucose utilization, increases gluconeogenesis, and increases the effects of glucagon. The hydrocortisone will usually result in stable and adequate glucose levels, and it can then be rapidly tapered over the course of a few days. Before administering hydrocortisone, it is important that a cortisol level be drawn and sent to the laboratory.

8. **Diazoxide** (5–8 mg/kg/day in divided doses every 8–12 hours) may be given orally for infants who are persistently hyperinsulinemic. This drug inhibits insulin release by acting as a specific adenosine triphosphate (ATP)-sensitive potassium channel agonist in normal pancreatic beta cells and decreases insulin release. It can take up to 5 days for a positive effect to be seen.

9. **Octreotide** (5–20 mcg/kg/day subcutaneously or intravenously divided every 6–8 hours). A long-acting somatostatin analog that inhibits insulin secretion, it can be used when diazoxide does not successfully control the glucose level. Tachyphylaxis can develop.

10. **Glucagon** (0.025 to 0.2 mg/kg intramuscularly, subcutaneously, or intravenously, maximum 1.0 mg) is rarely used. It may be given to hypoglycemic infants with good glycogen stores, but it is only a temporizing measure to mobilize glucose for

2 to 3 hours in an emergency until IV glucose can be given. The glucose level will often fall after the effects of glucagon have worn off, and it remains important to obtain IV access to adequately treat these babies. For infants of diabetic mothers, the dose is 0.3 mg/kg (maximum dose is 1.0 mg) (see Chap. 2).

11. If medical treatment does not control the blood glucose level, consider an 18F-fluoro-L-DOPA PET scan to identify focal lesions in the pancreas and consider surgical treatment by subtotal pancreatectomy. Referral to a subspecialty center with experience in these procedures should be considered if a genetic defect of glucose control is suspected or confirmed.

G. Long-term follow-up and evaluation

MRI scans. Babies with hypoglycemia have been reported to exhibit a typical pattern of CNS injury particularly in the parieto-occipital cortex and subcortical white matter. Recent studies report more widespread and varied patterns of injury, as well as diffusion-weighted imaging changes that are seen within 6 days of the insult. It is often difficult clinically to separate isolated hypoglycemia from hypoxic ischemic encephalopathy plus hypoglycemia. Some clinicians believe that it is useful to obtain an MRI scan on babies with symptomatic hypoglycemia, but the report of the National Institute of Child Health and Human Development workshop on knowledge gaps regarding neonatal hypoglycemia stated that the role of neuroimaging in assessing babies with symptomatic hypoglycemia remains to be determined. Babies who have had symptomatic hypoglycemia should have close follow-up of their neurodevelopmental status.

II. HYPERGLYCEMIA

is usually defined as a whole-blood glucose level higher than 125 mg/dL or plasma glucose values higher than 145 mg/dL. This problem is commonly encountered in low birth weight (LBW) premature infants receiving parenteral glucose but is also seen in other infants who are sick. There are usually not any specific symptoms associated with neonatal hyperglycemia, but the major clinical problems associated with hyperglycemia are hyperosmolarity and osmotic diuresis. Osmolarity of more than 300 mOsm/L usually leads to osmotic diuresis (each 18 mg/dL rise in blood glucose concentration increases serum osmolarity 1 mOsm/L). Subsequent dehydration may occur rapidly in small premature infants with large insensible fluid losses.

The hyperosmolar state, an increase of 25 to 40 mOsm or a glucose level of more than 450 to 720 mg/dL, can cause water to move from the intracellular compartment to the extracellular compartment. The resultant contraction of the intracellular volume of the brain may be a cause of intracranial hemorrhage.

Although rarely seen in the first months of life, diabetes mellitus can present with severe clinical symptoms, including polyuria, dehydration, and ketoacidosis that require prompt treatment. The genetic basis of neonatal diabetes is beginning to be understood and has implications for its treatment (see subsequent discussion).

A. Etiology

1. **Exogenous parenteral glucose** administration of more than 4 to 5 mg/kg/min of glucose in preterm infants weighing less than 1,000 g may be associated with hyperglycemia.

2. **Drugs.** The most common association is with steroids. Other drugs associated with hyperglycemia are caffeine, theophylline, phenytoin, and diazoxide.

3. **Extremely low birth weight (ELBW) infants** (<1,000 g), possibly due to variable insulin response, to persistent endogenous hepatic glucose production despite significant elevations in plasma insulin, or to insulin resistance that may in part be due to immature glycogenolysis enzyme systems. ELBW infants sometimes must be administered fluids in excess of 200 mL/kg per day, and a minimum glucose concentration of dextrose 5% must be used to avoid infusing a hypotonic solution. When this amount of fluid is administered, the infant is presented with a large glucose load. Modifications to the physical environment (i.e., humidified incubators, see Chaps. 13, 15, and 23) that decrease free water loss help limit the amount of IV fluid needed to treat these babies.

4. **Lipid infusion.** Free fatty acids are associated with increased glucose levels.

5. **Sepsis,** possibly due to depressed insulin release, cytokines, or endotoxin, resulting in decreased glucose utilization. Stress hormones such as cortisol and catecholamines are elevated in sepsis. In an infant who has normal glucose levels and then becomes hyperglycemic without an excess glucose load, sepsis should be the prime consideration.

6. **"Stressed" premature infants** requiring mechanical ventilation or other painful procedures have persistent endogenous glucose production due to catecholamines and other "stress hormones." Insulin levels are usually appropriate for the glucose level.

7. **Hypoxia,** possibly due to increased glucose production in the absence of a change in peripheral utilization.

8. **Surgical procedures.** Hyperglycemia in this setting is possibly due to the secretion of epinephrine, glucocorticoids, and glucagon as well as excess administration of glucose-containing IV fluids.

9. **Neonatal diabetes mellitus.** In this rare disorder, infants present with significant hyperglycemia that requires insulin treatment in the first months of life. They characteristically are SGA term infants, with no gender predilection, and a third have a family history of diabetes mellitus. They present with marked glycosuria, hyperglycemia (240 to 2,300 mg/dL), polyuria, severe dehydration, acidosis, mild or absent ketonuria, reduced subcutaneous fat, and failure to thrive. Insulin values are either absolutely or relatively low for the corresponding blood glucose elevation. Approximately half of the infants have a transient need for insulin treatment and are at risk for recurrence of diabetes in the second or third decade. Many of the patients with permanent diabetes have mutations involving regulation of the ATP-sensitive potassium channels of the pancreatic beta cells. Activating mutations of either the KCNJ11 gene that encodes the Kir6.2 subunit or the ABCC8 gene that encodes the SUR1 have been implicated in the cause of neonatal diabetes. Repeated plasma insulin values are necessary to distinguish transient from permanent diabetes mellitus. Molecular genetic diagnosis can help distinguish the infants with transient diabetes from those with permanent diabetes, and it can also be important for determining which babies are likely to respond to treatment with sulfonylureas.

10. **Diabetes due to pancreatic lesions** such as pancreatic aplasia, or hypoplastic or absent pancreatic beta cells is usually seen in SGA infants who may have other congenital defects. They usually present soon after birth and survival has been rare.

11. **Transient hyperglycemia associated with ingestion of hyperosmolar formula.** Clinical presentation may mimic transient neonatal diabetes with glycosuria, hyperglycemia, and dehydration. A history of inappropriate formula dilution is key. Treatment consists of rehydration, discontinuation of the hyperosmolar formula, and appropriate instructions for mixing concentrated or powder formula.

12. **Hepatic glucose production** can persist despite normal or elevated glucose levels.

13. **Immature development of glucose transport proteins**, such as GLUT-4.

B. **Treatment.** The primary goal is prevention and early detection of hyperglycemia by carefully adjusting GIRs, and frequent monitoring of blood glucose levels and urine for glycosuria. If present, evaluation and possible intervention are indicated.

1. Measure glucose levels in premature infants or infants with abnormal symptoms.

2. ELBW premature infants (<1,000 g) should start with a GIR of at least 4 to 6 mg/kg/min. Glucose levels and fluid balance need to be followed closely to provide data for adjusting the concentration and/or the rate of glucose infusion. Hypotonic fluids (dextrose solutions with concentrations under 5%) should be avoided.

3. As appropriate, decrease the GIR and closely follow the blood glucose levels.

4. Begin parenteral nutrition as soon as possible in LBW infants. Some amino acids promote insulin secretion.

5. Feed if condition allows; feeding can promote the secretion of hormones that promote insulin secretion.

6. Many small infants will initially be unable to tolerate a certain glucose load (e.g., 6 mg/kg per minute) but will eventually develop tolerance if they are presented with just enough glucose to keep their glucose level high yet not enough to cause glycosuria.

7. Exogenous insulin therapy has been used when glucose values exceed 250 mg/dL despite efforts to lower the amount of glucose delivered or when prolonged restriction of parenterally administered glucose would substantially decrease the required total caloric intake. Neonates may be extremely sensitive to the effects of insulin. It is desirable to decrease the glucose level gradually to avoid rapid fluid shifts. Very small doses of insulin are used and the actual amount delivered may be difficult to determine because some of the insulin is adsorbed on the plastic surfaces of the IV tubing. Unlike in adult ICUs where insulin and tight glucose control has been shown to increase survival, the routine use of insulin is not recommended in the NICU.

   a. **Insulin infusion**

      i. One standard dilution is 15 units regular human insulin (0.15 mL) added to 150 mL normal saline for a concentration of 0.1 unit/mL.

      ii. Prior to starting the infusion, purge the IV tubing with a minimum of twice the volume of the connecting tubing using the insulin-containing solution to saturate the plastic binding sites.

      iii. Bolus insulin infusion
         a) Dose 0.05 to 0.1 unit/kg every 4 to 6 hours prn
         b) Infuse over 15 minutes via syringe pump
         c) Monitor glucose every 30 minutes to 1 hour

d) If glucose remains >200 mg/dL after three doses, consider continuous infusion of insulin

iv. Continuous insulin infusion

a) Rate of infusion is 0.01 to 0.2 unit/kg per hour. (Usual starting dose is 0.05 unit/kg/hr)

$$\text{Flow rate (mL/hr)} = \frac{\text{dose (units/kg/hr)} \times \text{weight (kg)}}{\text{concentration (units/mL)}}$$

For example:
Ordered dose: 0.05 unit/kg/hr and infant weighs 600 g (0.6 kg)
0.05 unit/kg/hr × 0.6 kg = 0.03 unit/hr
Concentration is 0.5 unit/mL

Infusion rate is: $\dfrac{0.03 \text{ unit/hr}}{0.5 \text{ mL}} = 0.06 \text{ mL/hr}$

b) Check glucose levels every 30 minutes until stable to adjust the infusion rate.

c) If glucose remains > 180 mg/dL, titrate in increments of 0.01 unit/kg/hr.

d) If hypoglycemia occurs, discontinue insulin infusion and administer IV bolus of 10% D/W at 2 mL/kg × 1 dose.

e) Monitor potassium level.

f) Monitor for rebound hyperglycemia.

b. Subcutaneous insulin lispro

i. This is rarely used except in neonatal diabetes. A typical dose is 0.03 unit/kg as needed for glucose >200 mg/dL.

ii. Do not administer more frequently than every 3 hours to avoid hypoglycemia.

iii. Rotate administration sites.

iv. Monitor glucose level frequently.

v. Monitor electrolytes including potassium level every 6 hours initially.

vi. Insulin lispro has a rapid onset of action (15–30 minutes) and peak effect is 30 minutes to 2 ½ hours.

c. Oral sulfonylureas have been used in the long-term management of babies with Kir6.2 and SUR1 defects.

Suggested Readings

Beardsall K, Vanhaesebrouck S, Ogilvy-Stuart AL, et al. Early insulin therapy in very low birth weight infants. *N Engl J Med* 2008;359:1873–1884.

Burns CM, Rutherford MA, Boardman JP, et al. Patterns of cerebral injury and neurodevelopmental outcomes after symptomatic neonatal hypoglycemia. *Pediatrics* 2008;122:65–74.

Cornblath M, Hawdon JM, Williams AF, et al. Controversies regarding definition of neonatal hypoglycemia: suggested operational thresholds. *Pediatrics* 2000;105:1141–1145.

De León DD, Stanley CA. Mechanisms of disease: advances in diagnosis and treatment of hyperinsulinism in neonates. *Nat Clin Pract* 2007;3:57–68.

Hay WW, Raju TN, Higgins RD, et al. Knowledge gaps and research needs for understanding and treating neonatal hypoglycemia: workshop report from Eunice Kennedy Shriver National Institute of Child Health and Human Development. *J Pediatr* 2009;155:612–617.

Kapoor RR, Flanagan SE, James C, et al. Hyperinsulinaemic hypoglycaemia. *Arch Dis Child* 2008;94:450–457.

Tam EW, Widjaja E, Blaser SI, et al. Occipital lobe injury and cortical visual outcomes after neonatal hypoglycemia. *Pediatrics* 2008;122:507–512.

25 Abnormalities of Serum Calcium and Magnesium

Steven A. Abrams

I. HYPOCALCEMIA

A. General principles

1. **Definition.** Neonatal hypocalcemia is defined as a total serum calcium concentration of <7 mg/dL or an ionized calcium concentration of <4 mg/dL (1 mmol/L). In very low birth weight (VLBW) infants, ionized calcium values of 0.8 to 1 mmol/L are common and not usually associated with clinical symptoms. In larger infants and in infants of >32 weeks' gestation, symptoms may more readily occur with an ionized calcium concentration of <1 mmol/L.

2. **Pathophysiology**

   a. Calcium ions (Ca^{2+}) in cellular and extracellular fluid (ECF) are essential for many biochemical processes. Significant aberrations of serum calcium concentrations are frequently observed in the neonatal period.

      i. **Hormonal regulation of calcium homeostasis.** Regulation of serum and ECF-ionized calcium concentration within a narrow range is critical for blood coagulation, neuromuscular excitability, cell membrane integrity and function, and cellular enzymatic and secretory activity. The principal calcitropic or calcium-regulating hormones are parathyroid hormone (PTH) and 1,25-dihydroxyvitamin D (1,25[OH]$_2$D), also referred to as *calcitriol*.

      ii. When the ECF-ionized calcium level declines, parathyroid cells secrete PTH. PTH mobilizes calcium from bone, increases calcium resorption in the renal tubule, and stimulates renal production of 1,25(OH)$_2$D. PTH secretion causes the serum calcium level to rise and the serum phosphorus level either to be maintained or to fall.

      iii. Vitamin D is synthesized from provitamin D in the skin after exposure to sunlight and is also ingested in the diet. Vitamin D is transported to the liver, where it is converted to 25(OH)D (the major storage form of the hormone). This is transported to the kidney, where it is converted to the biologically active hormone 1,25(OH)$_2$D (calcitriol). Calcitriol increases intestinal calcium and phosphate absorption and mobilizes calcium and phosphate from bone.

3. **Etiology**

   a. **Prematurity.** Preterm infants are capable of mounting a PTH response to hypocalcemia, but target organ responsiveness to PTH may be diminished.

   b. Infants of diabetic mothers (IDMs) have a 25% to 50% incidence of hypocalcemia if maternal control is poor. Hypercalcitoninemia, hypoparathyroidism, abnormal vitamin D metabolism, and hyperphosphatemia have all been implicated, but the etiology remains uncertain (see Chap. 2).

c. Severe neonatal birth depression is frequently associated with hypocalcemia and hyperphosphatemia. Decreased calcium intake and increased endogenous phosphate load are likely the causes.

d. Congenital. Parathyroids may be absent in DiGeorge sequence (hypoplasia or absence of the third and fourth branchial pouch structures) as an isolated defect in the development of the parathyroid glands or as part of the Kenny-Caffey syndrome.

e. Pseudohypoparathyroidism. Maternal hyperparathyroidism.

f. Magnesium deficiency (including inborn error of intestinal magnesium transport) impairs PTH secretion.

g. Vitamin D deficiency (rarely a cause in the first weeks of life).

h. Alkalosis and bicarbonate therapy.

i. Rapid infusion of citrate-buffered blood (exchange transfusion) chelates ionized calcium.

j. Shock or sepsis.

k. Phototherapy may be associated with hypocalcemia by decreasing melatonin secretion and increasing uptake of calcium into the bone.

l. For late-onset hypocalcemia, high phosphate intakes lead to excess phosphorus and decreased serum calcium.

B. Diagnosis

1. Clinical presentation

a. Hypocalcemia increases both cellular permeability to sodium ions and cell membrane excitability. The signs are usually nonspecific: apnea, seizures, jitteriness, increased extensor tone, clonus, hyperreflexia, and stridor (laryngospasm).

b. Early-onset hypocalcemia in preterm newborns is often asymptomatic but may show apnea, seizures, or abnormalities of cardiac function.

c. Late-onset syndromes, in contrast, may present as hypocalcemic seizures. Often, they must be differentiated from other causes of newborn seizures, including "fifth-day" fits.

2. History

a. For late-onset presentation, mothers may report partial breastfeeding. Abnormal movements and lethargy may precede obvious seizure activity. Rarely, use of goat's milk or whole milk of cow may be reported. Symptoms are usually described beginning from the third to fifth days of life.

3. Physical examination

a. General physical findings associated with seizure disorder in the newborn may be present in some cases. Usually, there are no apparent physical findings.

4. Laboratory studies

a. There are three definable fractions of calcium in serum: (i) ionized calcium (~50% of serum total calcium); (ii) calcium bound to serum proteins, principally albumin (~40%); and (iii) calcium complexed to serum anions, mostly phosphates, citrate, and sulfates (~10%). Ionized calcium is the only biologically available form of calcium.

b. Assessment of calcium status using ionized calcium is preferred, especially in the first week of life. Correction nomograms, used to convert total calcium into ionized calcium, are not reliable.

c. Calcium concentration reported as milligrams per deciliter can be converted to molar units by dividing by 4 (e.g., 10 mg/dL converts to 2.5 mmol/L).

d. Postnatal changes in serum calcium concentrations: At birth, the umbilical serum calcium level is elevated (10–11 mg/dL). In healthy term babies, calcium concentrations decline for the first 24 to 48 hours; the nadir is usually 7.5 to 8.5 mg/dL. Thereafter, calcium concentrations progressively rise to the mean values observed in older children and adults.

e. Although an association with vitamin D deficiency is uncommon, an assessment of both maternal and neonatal serum 25(OH)D level may be warranted. Values <10 to 12 ng/dL are suggestive of severe deficiency that may be associated with clinical symptoms in some, but probably not most infants.

5. **Monitoring**

   a. Suggested schedule for monitoring calcium levels in infants, such as VLBW, IDM, and birth depression, who are at risk for developing hypocalcemia are as follows:

   i. Ionized calcium at 12, 24, and 48 hours of life.

   ii. Total serum phosphorus and total serum magnesium for infants with hypocalcemia.

   iii. Other lab tests, including serum concentrations of PTH, 25(OH)D, and 1,25(OH)₂D are not usually needed unless neonatal hypocalcemia does not readily resolve with calcium therapy. It is extremely rare that 1,25(OH)₂D is ever measured in neonates.

   iv. A prolonged electrocardiographic QTc interval is a traditional indicator that is typically not clinically useful in the newborn period.

6. **Imaging**

   a. Absence of a thymic shadow on a chest radiograph and the presence of conotruncal cardiac abnormalities may suggest a diagnosis of 22q11.2 deletion syndrome, also known as *CATCH22* or *DiGeorge sequence*.

C. **Treatment**

1. **Medications**

   a. Therapy with calcium is usually adequate for most cases. In some cases (see the following text), concurrent therapy with magnesium is indicated.

   b. Rapid intravenous infusion of calcium can cause a sudden elevation of serum calcium level, leading to bradycardia or other dysrhythmias. Intravenous calcium should only be "pushed" for treatment of hypocalcemic crisis (e.g., seizures) and done with careful cardiovascular monitoring.

   c. Infusion by means of the umbilical vein may result in hepatic necrosis if the catheter is lodged in a branch of the portal vein.

   d. Rapid infusion by means of the umbilical artery can cause arterial spasms and, at least experimentally, intestinal necrosis and thus, is generally not indicated.

   e. Intravenous calcium solutions are incompatible with sodium bicarbonate since calcium carbonate will precipitate.

   f. Extravasation of calcium solutions into subcutaneous tissues can cause severe necrosis and subcutaneous calcifications.

   g. Calcium preparations. Calcium gluconate 10% solution is preferred for intravenous use. Calcium glubionate syrup (Neo-Calglucon) is a convenient oral preparation. However, the high sugar content and osmolality may cause gastrointestinal irritation or diarrhea.

   i. If the ionized calcium level drops to 1 mmol/L or less (>1,500 g) or 0.8 mmol/L or less (<1,500 g), a continuous intravenous calcium infusion may be commenced. For infants with early hypocalcemia, this may be done using total parenteral nutrition (TPN). For use without other TPN components, a dose of 40 to 50 mg/kg/day of elemental calcium is typical.

ii. It may be desirable to prevent the onset of hypocalcemia for newborns who exhibit cardiovascular compromise (e.g., severe respiratory distress syndrome, asphyxia, septic shock, and persistent pulmonary hypertension of the newborn). Use a continuous calcium infusion, preferably by means of a central catheter, to maintain an ionized calcium of 1 to 1.4 mmol/L (<1,500 g) or 1.2 to 1.5 mmol/L (>1,500 g).

iii. Emergency calcium therapy (for active seizures or profound cardiac failure thought to be associated with severe hypocalcemia) consists of 100 to 200 mg/kg of 10% calcium gluconate (9–18 mg of elemental calcium/kg) by intravenous infusion over 10 to 15 minutes.

h. Monitor heart rate and rhythm and the infusion site throughout the infusion.

i. Repeat the dose in 10 minutes if there is no clinical response.

j. Following the initial dose(s), maintenance calcium should be given through continuous intravenous infusion.

k. Hypocalcemia associated with hyperphosphatemia presenting after day of life (DOL) #3.

i. The goal of initial therapy is to reduce renal phosphate load while increasing calcium intake. Reduce phosphate intake by feeding the infant human milk or a low-phosphorus formula (Similac PM 60/40 is most widely used, but other relatively low-mineral formulas, including Nestle Good Start, may be used).

ii. Avoid the use of preterm formulas, lactose-free or other special formulas, or transitional formulas. These have high levels of phosphorus or may be more limited in calcium bioavailability.

iii. Increase the oral calcium intake using supplements (e.g., 20–40 mg/kg/day of elemental calcium added to Similac PM 60/40). Phosphate binders are generally not necessary and may not be safe for use, especially in premature infants.

iv. Gradually wean calcium supplements over 2 to 4 weeks. Monitor serum calcium and phosphorus levels one to two times weekly.

v. The use of vitamin D or active vitamin D ($1,25[OH]_2D$) in this circumstance is controversial and not usually necessary. If a serum 25(OH)D level was obtained and is <10 to 12 ng/mL, then 1,000 IU of vitamin D should be given daily and the value rechecked in 14 to 21 days. Rarely should higher doses of vitamin D be given to neonates.

l. **Rare defects in vitamin D metabolism** are treated with vitamin D analogs, for example, dihydrotachysterol (Hytakerol) and calcitriol (Rocaltrol). The rapid onset of action and short half-life of these drugs lessen the risk of rebound hypercalcemia.

II. HYPERCALCEMIA

A. General principles

1. Definition

a. Neonatal hypercalcemia (serum total calcium level >11 mg/dL, serum ionized calcium level >1.45 mmol/L) may be asymptomatic and discovered incidentally during routine screening. Alternatively, the presentation of severe hypercalcemia (>16 mg/dL or ionized calcium >1.8 mmol/L) can require immediate medical intervention. Very mild hypercalcemia (serum calcium 11–12 mg/dL) is common and does not require any intervention at all.

2. **Etiology**

   a. Imbalance in intake or use of calcium.

   b. Clinical adjustment of TPN by removing the phosphorus (due to, for example, concern about excess sodium or potassium intake) can rapidly lead to hypercalcemia, especially in VLBW infants. This commonly leads to ionized calcium values from 1.45 to 1.6 mmol/L.

   c. Extreme prematurity. Moderate to extreme hypercalcemia is not uncommon in infants <700 g birth weight on usual TPN. Values up to 2.2 mmol/L of ionized calcium occur. This is likely due to inability to utilize calcium in these infants and may or may not be associated with high serum phosphorus.

   d. Hyperparathyroidism

      i. Congenital hyperparathyroidism associated with maternal hypoparathyroidism usually resolves over several weeks.

      ii. Neonatal severe primary hyperparathyroidism (NSPHP). The parathyroids are refractory to regulation by calcium, producing marked hypercalcemia (frequently 15–30 mg/dL).

      iii. Self-limited secondary hyperparathyroidism associated with neonatal renal tubular acidosis.

   e. **Hyperthyroidism.** Thyroid hormone stimulates bone resorption and bone turnover.

   f. Hypophosphatasia, an autosomal recessive bone dysplasia, produces severe bone demineralization and fractures.

   g. Increased intestinal absorption of calcium.

   h. Hypervitaminosis D may result from excessive vitamin D ingestion by the mother (during pregnancy) or the neonate. Since vitamin D is extensively stored in fat, intoxication may persist for weeks to months (see Chap. 21).

   i. Decreased renal calcium clearance.

   j. Familial hypocalciuric hypercalcemia, a clinically benign autosomal dominant disorder, can present in the neonatal period. The gene mutation is on chromosome 3q21–24.

   k. Idiopathic neonatal/infantile hypercalcemia occurs in the constellation of Williams syndrome (hypercalcemia, supravalvular aortic stenosis or other cardiac anomalies, "elfin" facies, psychomotor retardation) and in a familial pattern lacking the Williams phenotype. Increased calcium absorption has been demonstrated; increased vitamin D sensitivity and impaired calcitonin secretion are proposed as possible mechanisms.

   l. Subcutaneous fat necrosis is a sequela of trauma or asphyxia. Only the more generalized necrosis seen in asphyxia is associated with significant hypercalcemia. Granulomatous (macrophage) inflammation of the necrotic lesions may be a source of unregulated $1,25(OH)_2D_3$ synthesis.

   m. Acute renal failure, usually during the diuretic or recovery phase.

B. **Diagnosis**

1. **Clinical presentation**

   a. Hyperparathyroidism includes hypotonia, encephalopathy, poor feeding, vomiting, constipation, polyuria, hepatosplenomegaly, anemia, and extraskeletal calcifications, including nephrocalcinosis.

   b. Milder hypercalcemia may present as feeding difficulties or poor linear growth.

2. History

a. Maternal/family history of hypercalcemia or hypocalcemia, parathyroid disorders, and nephrocalcinosis

b. Family history of hypercalcemia or familial hypocalciuric hypercalcemia

c. Manipulations of TPN

3. Physical examination

a. Small for dates (hyperparathyroidism, Williams syndrome).

b. Craniotabes, fractures (hyperparathyroidism), or characteristic bone dysplasia (hypophosphatasia).

c. "Elfin" facies (Williams syndrome).

d. Cardiac murmur (supravalvular aortic stenosis and peripheral pulmonic stenosis associated with Williams syndrome).

e. Indurated, bluish-red lesions (subcutaneous fat necrosis).

f. Evidence of hyperthyroidism.

4. Laboratory evaluation

a. The clinical history, serum and urine mineral levels of phosphorus, and the urinary calcium: creatinine ratio (U_{Ca}/U_{Cr}) should suggest a likely diagnosis.

    i. A very elevated serum calcium level (>16 mg/dL) usually indicates primary hyperparathyroidism or, in VLBW infants, phosphate depletion or the inability to utilize calcium for bone formation.

    ii. Low serum phosphorus level indicates phosphate depletion, hyperparathyroidism, or familial hypocalciuric hypercalcemia.

    iii. Very low U_{Ca}/U_{Cr} suggests familial hypocalciuric hypercalcemia.

b. Specific serum hormone levels (PTH, 25[OH]D) may confirm the diagnostic impression in cases where obvious manipulations of diet/TPN are not apparent. Measurement of $1,25(OH)_2D$ is rarely indicated unless hypercalcemia persists in infants >1,000 g with no other apparent etiology.

c. A very low level of serum alkaline phosphatase activity suggests hypophosphatasia (confirmed by increased urinary phosphoethanolamine level).

d. Radiography of hand/wrist may suggest hyperparathyroidism (demineralization, subperiosteal resorption) or hypervitaminosis D (submetaphyseal rarefaction).

C. Treatment

1. Emergency medical treatment (symptomatic or calcium >16 mg/dL, ionized Ca >1.8 mmol/L).

a. Volume expansion with isotonic saline solution. Hydration and sodium promote urinary calcium excretion. If cardiac function is normal, infuse normal saline solution (10–20 mL/kg) over 15 to 30 minutes.

b. Furosemide (1 mg/kg intravenously) induces calciuria.

2. Inorganic phosphate may lower serum calcium levels in hypophosphatemic patients by inhibiting bone resorption and promoting bone mineral accretion.

a. Glucocorticoids are effective in hypervitaminosis A and D and subcutaneous fat necrosis by inhibiting both bone resorption and intestinal calcium absorption; they are ineffective in hyperparathyroidism.

b. Low-calcium, low-vitamin D diets are an effective adjunctive therapy for subcutaneous fat necrosis and Williams syndrome.

c. Calcitonin is a potent inhibitor of bone resorption. The antihypercalcemic effect is transient but may be prolonged if glucocorticoids are used concomitantly. There is little reported experience in neonates.

d. Parathyroidectomy with autologous reimplantation may be indicated for severe persistent neonatal hyperparathyroidism.

III. DISORDERS OF MAGNESIUM: HYPOMAGNESEMIA AND HYPERMAGNESEMIA

A. Etiology

1. Hypermagnesemia is usually due to an exogenous magnesium load exceeding renal excretion capacity.
   a. Magnesium sulfate therapy for maternal preeclampsia or preterm labor.
   b. Administration of magnesium-containing antacids to the newborn.
   c. Excessive magnesium in parenteral nutrition.
   d. Hypomagnesemia is uncommon but is often seen with late onset hypocalcemia.

B. Diagnosis

1. Elevated serum magnesium level (>3 mg/dL) suggests hypermagnesemia although symptoms are uncommon with serum values <4 to 5 mg/dL. Low serum magnesium level of <1.6 mg/dL suggests hypomagnesemia.

2. Severe hypermagnesemic symptoms are unusual in neonates with serum magnesium level <6 mg/dL. The common curariform effects include apnea, respiratory depression, lethargy, hypotonia, hyporeflexia, poor suck, decreased intestinal motility, and delayed passage of meconium.

3. Hypomagnesemia is usually seen along with hypocalcemia in the newborn. Hypomagnesemia symptoms can also include apnea and poor motor tone.

C. Treatment

1. Hypocalcemia seizures with concurrent hypomagnesemia should include treatment for the hypomagnesemia.
   a. The preferred preparation for treatment is magnesium sulfate. The 50% solution contains 500 mg or 4 mEq/mL.
   b. Correct severe hypomagnesemia (<1.6 mg/dL) with 50 to 100 mg/kg of magnesium sulfate intravenously given over 1 to 2 hours. When administering intravenously, infuse slowly and monitor heart rate. The dose may be repeated after 12 hours. Obtain serum magnesium levels before each dose.

2. Often, the only intervention necessary for hypermagnesemia is removal of the source of exogenous magnesium.

3. Exchange transfusion, peritoneal dialysis, and hemodialysis are not used in the newborn period.

4. For hypermagnesemic babies, begin feedings only after suck and intestinal motility are established. Rarely, respiratory support may be needed.

Suggested Readings

De Marini S, Mimouni FB, Tsang RC, et al. Disorders of calcium, phosphorus, and magnesium metabolism. In: Fanaroff AA, Mouton RJ, eds. *Neonatal–perinatal medicine*, 6th ed. St. Louis: Mosby, 1997.

Tsang RC. Calcium, phosphorus, and magnesium metabolism. In: Polin RA, Fox WW, eds. *Fetal and Neonatal Physiology*, 2nd ed. Philadelphia: WB Saunders 1992.

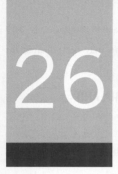

26 Neonatal Hyperbilirubinemia

Mary Lucia P. Gregory, Camilia R. Martin, and John P. Cloherty

I. BACKGROUND. The normal adult serum bilirubin level is <1 mg/dL. Adults appear jaundiced when the serum bilirubin level is >2 mg/dL, and newborns appear jaundiced when it is >7 mg/dL. Approximately 85% of all term newborns and most premature infants develop clinical jaundice. Also, 6.1% of well term newborns have a maximal serum bilirubin level >12.9 mg/dL. A serum bilirubin level >15 mg/dL is found in 3% of normal term babies. **Physical examination is not a reliable measure of serum bilirubin.**

A. **Source of bilirubin.** Bilirubin is derived from the breakdown of heme-containing proteins in the reticuloendothelial system. The normal newborn produces 6 to 10 mg of bilirubin/kg/day, as opposed to the production of 3 to 4 mg/kg/day in the adult.

1. The major heme-containing protein is **red blood cell (RBC) hemoglobin**. Hemoglobin released from senescent RBCs in the reticuloendothelial system is the source of 75% of all bilirubin production. One gram of hemoglobin produces 34 mg of bilirubin. Accelerated release of hemoglobin from RBCs is the cause of hyperbilirubinemia in isoimmunization (e.g., Rh and ABO incompatibility), erythrocyte biochemical abnormalities (e.g., glucose-6-phosphate dehydrogenase [G6PD] and pyruvate kinase deficiencies), abnormal erythrocyte morphology (e.g., hereditary spherocytosis [HS]), sequestered blood (e.g., bruising and cephalohematoma), and polycythemia.

2. The other 25% of bilirubin is called **early-labeled bilirubin**. It is derived from hemoglobin released by ineffective erythropoiesis in the bone marrow, from other heme-containing proteins in tissues (e.g., myoglobin, cytochromes, catalase, and peroxidase), and from free heme.

B. **Bilirubin metabolism.** The heme ring from heme-containing proteins is oxidized in reticuloendothelial cells to **biliverdin** by the microsomal enzyme heme oxygenase. This reaction releases **carbon monoxide (CO)** (excreted from the lung) and **iron** (reutilized). Biliverdin is then reduced to bilirubin by the enzyme **biliverdin reductase**. Catabolism of 1 mol of hemoglobin produces 1 mol each of CO and bilirubin. Increased bilirubin production, as measured by CO excretion rates, accounts for the higher bilirubin levels seen in Asian, Native American, and Greek infants.

1. **Transport.** Bilirubin is nonpolar, insoluble in water, and is transported to liver cells bound to serum **albumin**. Bilirubin bound to albumin does not usually enter the central nervous system (CNS) and is thought to be nontoxic. Displacement of bilirubin from albumin by drugs, such as the sulfonamides, or by free fatty acids (FFAs) at high molar ratios of FFA:albumin, may increase bilirubin toxicity (see Table 26.1).

Table 26.1	Drugs That Cause Significant Displacement of Bilirubin from Albumin *In vitro*
Sulfonamides	
Moxalactam	
Ticarcillin, azlocillin, carbenicillin	
Ceftriaxone; cefotetan; cefmetazole, cefonicid	
Fusidic acid	
Radiographic contrast media for cholangiography (sodium iodipamide, sodium ipodate, iopanoic acid, meglumine loglycamate)	
Benzyl alcohol (preservative), benzoate	
Aspirin	
Ibuprofen	
Aminophylline	
Diatrizoate	
Apazone	
Tolbutamide	
Rapid infusions of albumin preservatives (sodium caprylate and N-acetyltryptophan)	
Rapid infusions of ampicillin	
Long-chain FFAs at high molar ratios of FFA:albumin	

FFA = free fatty acid.
Sources: From Roth P, Polin RA. Controversial topics in kernicterus. *Clin Perinatol* 1988;15:965–990 and Robertson A, Karp W, Broderson R. Bilirubin displacing effect of drugs used in neonatology. *Acta Paediatr Scand* 1991;80:1119–1127.

2. **Uptake.** Nonpolar, fat-soluble bilirubin (dissociated from albumin) crosses the hepatocyte plasma membrane and is bound mainly to cytoplasmic **ligandin** (Y protein) for transport to the smooth endoplasmic reticulum. Phenobarbital increases the concentration of ligandin.

3. **Conjugation.** Unconjugated (indirect) bilirubin (UCB) is converted to water-soluble conjugated (direct) bilirubin (CB) in the smooth endoplasmic reticulum by **uridine diphosphogluconurate glucuronosyltransferase (UGT).**

This enzyme is inducible by phenobarbital and catalyzes the formation of bilirubin monoglucuronide. The monoglucuronide may be further conjugated to bilirubin diglucuronide. Both monoglucuronide and diglucuronide forms of CB are able to be excreted into the bile canaliculi against a concentration gradient.

Inherited deficiencies and polymorphisms of the conjugating enzyme gene can cause severe hyperbilirubinemia in neonates. **Bilirubin uridine diphosphogluconurate glucuronosyltransferase gene (UGT1A1) polymorphisms** have been described, which diminish the expression of the UGT enzyme. The **TATA box mutation** is the most common mutation found and is implicated in Gilbert syndrome in the Western population. Instead of the usual six (TA) repeats in the promoter region, there is an extra two-base pair (TA) repeat resulting in seven (TA) repeats ([TA]7TAA). The estimated allele frequency among whites is 0.33 to 0.4, and among Asians, it is 0.15. Alone, this mutation may not result in significant neonatal hyperbilirubinemia; however, with other risk factors for hyperbilirubinemia present (G6PD deficiency, ABO incompatibility, HS, and breast milk jaundice), the presence of this mutation may confer a significant risk for neonatal hyperbilirubinemia. The **211G → A (G71R)** mutation occurs with increased frequency among the Japanese population, and the presence of this mutation alone (homozygote or heterozygote) can result in reduced enzyme activity and neonatal hyperbilirubinemia. This mutation is also the most common mutation in Japanese patients with Gilbert syndrome. The G71R mutation has not been found in the white population. Other mutations have been described, such as **1456T → G** and the **CAT box mutation** (CCAAT → GTGCT); however, less is known about these mutations and their role in hyperbilirubinemia in the newborn. The population differences in allele frequencies likely account for some of the racial and ethnic variation seen in the development of jaundice.

4. **Excretion.** CB in the biliary tree enters the gastrointestinal (GI) tract and is then eliminated in the stool, which contains large amounts of bilirubin. CB is not normally resorbed from the bowel unless it is converted back to UCB by the intestinal enzyme **β-glucuronidase**. Resorption of bilirubin from the GI tract and delivery back to the liver for reconjugation is called **enterohepatic circulation**. Intestinal bacteria can prevent enterohepatic circulation of bilirubin by converting CB to **urobilinoids**, which are not substrates for β-glucuronidase. Pathologic conditions leading to increased enterohepatic circulation include decreased enteral intake, intestinal atresias, meconium ileus, and Hirschsprung disease.

5. **Fetal bilirubin metabolism.** Most UCB formed by the fetus is cleared by the placenta into the maternal circulation. Formation of CB is limited in the fetus because of decreased fetal hepatic blood flow, decreased hepatic ligandin, and decreased UGT activity. The small amount of CB excreted into the fetal gut is usually hydrolyzed by β-glucuronidase and resorbed. Bilirubin is normally found in amniotic fluid by 12 weeks' gestation and is usually gone by 37 weeks' gestation. Increased amniotic fluid bilirubin is found in hemolytic disease of the newborn and in fetal intestinal obstruction below the bile ducts.

II. PHYSIOLOGIC HYPERBILIRUBINEMIA. The serum UCB level of most newborn infants rises to >2 mg/dL in the first week of life. This level usually rises in

full-term infants to a peak of 6 to 8 mg/dL by 3 to 5 days of age and then falls. A rise to 12 mg/dL is in the physiologic range. In premature infants, the peak may be 10 to 12 mg/dL on the fifth day of life, possibly rising >15 mg/dL without any specific abnormality of bilirubin metabolism. Levels <2 mg/dL may not be seen until 1 month of age in both full term and premature infants. This "normal jaundice" is attributed to the following mechanisms:

A. **Increased bilirubin production due to:**

1. Increased RBC volume per kilogram and decreased RBC survival (90 days versus 120 days) in infants compared with adults.

2. Increased ineffective erythropoiesis and increased turnover of nonhemoglobin heme proteins.

B. Increased enterohepatic circulation caused by high levels of intestinal β-glucuronidase, preponderance of bilirubin monoglucuronide rather than diglucuronide, decreased intestinal bacteria, and decreased gut motility with poor evacuation of bilirubin-laden meconium.

C. **Defective uptake** of bilirubin from plasma caused by decreased ligandin and binding of ligandin by other anions.

D. **Defective conjugation** due to decreased UGT activity.

E. **Decreased hepatic excretion** of bilirubin.

III. NONPHYSIOLOGIC HYPERBILIRUBINEMIA.

Nonphysiologic jaundice may not be easy to distinguish from physiologic jaundice. The following situations suggest nonphysiologic hyperbilirubinemia and require evaluation (see Fig. 26.1 and Table 26.2):

A. **General conditions** (see Tables 26.2 and 26.4)

1. Onset of jaundice before 24 hours of age.

2. Any elevation of serum bilirubin that requires phototherapy (see Figs. 26.2 and 26.4 and VI.D.).

3. A rise in serum bilirubin levels of >0.2 mg/dL/hour.

4. Signs of underlying illness in any infant (vomiting, lethargy, poor feeding, excessive weight loss, apnea, tachypnea, or temperature instability).

5. Jaundice persisting after 8 days in a term infant or after 14 days in a premature infant.

B. **History**

1. A family history of jaundice, anemia, splenectomy, or early gallbladder disease suggests hereditary hemolytic anemia (e.g., spherocytosis, G6PD deficiency).

2. A family history of liver disease may suggest galactosemia, α1-antitrypsin deficiency, tyrosinosis, hypermethioninemia, Gilbert disease, Crigler-Najjar syndrome types I and II, or cystic fibrosis.

3. Ethnic or geographic origin associated with hyperbilirubinemia (East Asian, Greek, and American Indian) (see I.B.3. for potential genetic influences).

4. A sibling with jaundice or anemia may suggest blood group incompatibility, breast milk jaundice, or Lucey-Driscoll syndrome.

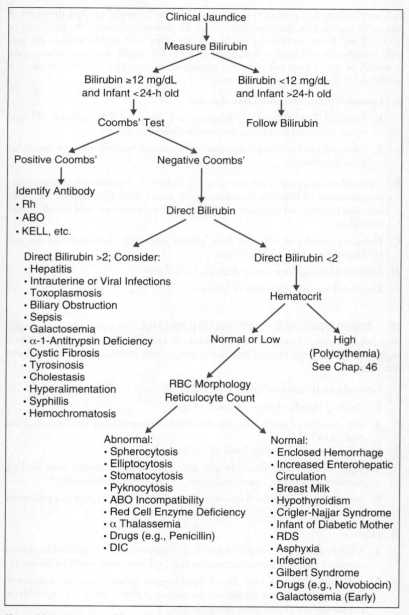

Clinical Jaundice
↓
Measure Bilirubin

Bilirubin ≥12 mg/dL and Infant <24-h old → Coombs' Test

Bilirubin <12 mg/dL and Infant >24-h old → Follow Bilirubin

Positive Coombs' → Identify Antibody
• Rh
• ABO
• KELL, etc.

Negative Coombs' → Direct Bilirubin

Direct Bilirubin >2; Consider:
• Hepatitis
• Intrauterine or Viral Infections
• Toxoplasmosis
• Biliary Obstruction
• Sepsis
• Galactosemia
• α-1-Antitrypsin Deficiency
• Cystic Fibrosis
• Tyrosinosis
• Cholestasis
• Hyperalimentation
• Syphillis
• Hemochromatosis

Direct Bilirubin <2 → Hematocrit

Normal or Low → RBC Morphology Reticulocyte Count

High (Polycythemia) See Chap. 46

Abnormal:
• Spherocytosis
• Elliptocytosis
• Stomatocytosis
• Pyknocytosis
• ABO Incompatibility
• Red Cell Enzyme Deficiency
• α Thalassemia
• Drugs (e.g., Penicillin)
• DIC

Normal:
• Enclosed Hemorrhage
• Increased Enterohepatic Circulation
• Breast Milk
• Hypothyroidism
• Crigler-Najjar Syndrome
• Infant of Diabetic Mother
• RDS
• Asphyxia
• Infection
• Gilbert Syndrome
• Drugs (e.g., Novobiocin)
• Galactosemia (Early)

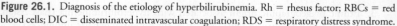

Figure 26.1. Diagnosis of the etiology of hyperbilirubinemia. Rh = rhesus factor; RBCs = red blood cells; DIC = disseminated intravascular coagulation; RDS = respiratory distress syndrome.

Table 26.2 Causes of Neonatal Hyperbilirubinemia

Overproduction	Undersecretion	Mixed	Uncertain mechanism
Fetomaternal blood group incompatibility (e.g., Rh, ABO)	**Metabolic and endocrine conditions**	Sepsis	Chinese, Japanese, Korean, and American Indian infants (see polymorphism discussion, section I.B.3.)
Hereditary spherocytosis (MCHC >36.0 g/dL), eliptocytosis, somatocytosis	Galactosemia	Intrauterine infections	Breast milk jaundice
Nonspherocytic hemolytic anemias	Familial nonhemolytic jaundice types 1 and 2 (Crigler-Najjar syndrome)	Toxoplasmosis	
G6PD deficiency and drugs	Gilbert disease	Rubella	
Pyruvate-kinase deficiency	Hypothyroidism	CID	
Other red cell enzyme deficiencies	Tyrosinosis	Herpes simplex	
α Thalassemia	Hypermethioninemia	Syphilis	
δ–β Thalassemia	Drugs and hormones	Hepatitis	
Acquired hemolysis due to vitamin K, nitrofurantonin, sulfonamides, antimalarials, penicillin, oxytocin, bupivacaine, or infection	Novobiocin	Respiratory distress syndrome	
	Pregnanediol	Hypoxia-ischemia	
	Lucey-Driscoll syndrome	Infant of diabetic mother	
	Infants of diabetic mothers	Severe erythroblastosis fetalis	
Extravascular blood	Prematurity		
Petechiae	Hypopituitarism and anencephaly		
Hematomas	**Obstructive disorders**		
Pulmonary, cerebral, or occult hemorrhage	Biliary atresia*		
	Dubin-Johnson and Rotor syndrome*		
	Choledochal cyst*		

(continued)

Table 26.2 Causes of Neonatal Hyperbilirubinemia *(Continued)*

Overproduction	Undersecretion	Mixed	Uncertain mechanism
Polycythemia	Cystic fibrosis (inspissated bile)*		
Fetomaternal or fetofetal transfusion	Tumor* or band* (extrinsic obstruction)		
Delayed clamping of the umbilical cord	α1-antitrypsin deficiency*		
Increased enterohepatic circulation	Parenteral nutrition		
Pyloric stenosis*			
Intestinal atresia or stenosis, including annular pancreas			
Hirschsprung disease			
Meconium ileus and/or meconium plug syndrome			
Fasting or hypoperistalsis from other causes			
Drug-induced paralytic ileus (hexamethonium)			
Swallowed blood			

MCHC = mean corpuscular hemoglobin concentration; G6PD = glucose-6-phosphate dehydrogenase; CID = cytomegalovirus inclusion disease, as in TORCH (toxoplasmosis, other, rubella, cytomegalovirus, herpes simplex).

* Jaundice may not be seen in the neonatal period.

Source: Modified from Odell GB, Poland RL, Nostrea E Jr. Neonatal hyperbilirubinemia. In: Klaus MH, Fanaroff A, eds. *Care of the High-Risk Neonate.* Philadelphia: WB Saunders, 1973, Chapter 11.

Table 26.3	Timing of Follow-up
Infant discharged	**Should be seen by age**
Before age 24 h	72 h
Between 24 and 47.9 h	96 h
Between 48 and 72 h	120 h

For some newborns discharged before 48 h, two follow-up visits may be required, the first visit between 24 and 72 h and the second between 72 and 120 h. Clinical judgment should be used in determining follow-up. Earlier or more frequent follow-up should be provided for those who have risk factors for hyperbilirubinemia (Table 26.4), whereas those discharged with few or no risk factors can be seen after longer intervals.
Source: Reprinted with permission from the American Academy of Pediatrics Subcommittee on Hyperbilirubinemia. Management of hyperbilirubinemia in the newborn infant 35 or more weeks of gestation. *Pediatrics* 2004;114:297–316.

5. Maternal illness during pregnancy may suggest congenital viral infection or toxoplasmosis. Infants of diabetic mothers tend to develop hyperbilirubinemia (see Chap. 2).

6. Maternal drugs may interfere with bilirubin binding to albumin, making bilirubin toxic at relatively low levels (sulfonamides) or may cause hemolysis in a G6PD-deficient infant (sulfonamides, nitrofurantoin, antimalarials).

7. The labor and delivery history may show trauma associated with extravascular bleeding and hemolysis. Oxytocin use may be associated with neonatal hyperbilirubinemia, although this is controversial. Infants with hypoxic-ischemic

Table 26.4	Important Risk Factors for Severe Hyperbilirubinemia
Predischarge TSB or TcB measurement in high-risk or high-intermediate zone	
Lower gestational age	
Exclusive breastfeeding, especially if it is not going well and infant has excessive weight loss	
Jaundice in the first 24 hours of age	
Isoimmune or other hemolytic disease	
Previous sibling with jaundice	
Cephalohematoma or significant bruising	
East Asian race	

Source: Maisels MJ, Bhutani VK, Bogen D, et al. Hyperbilirubinemia in the newborn infant ≥35 weeks' gestation: an update with clarifications. *Pediatrics* 2009;124:1193–1198.

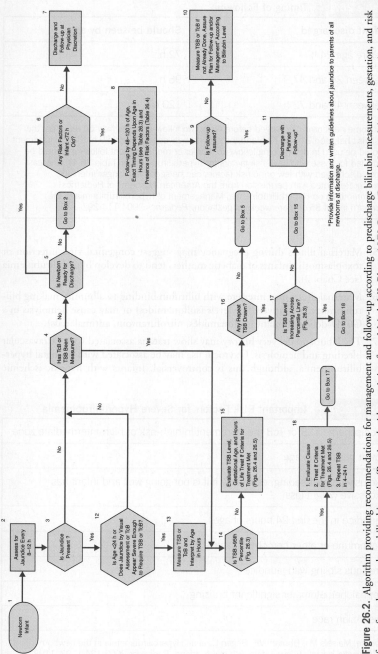

Figure 26.2. Algorithm providing recommendations for management and follow-up according to predischarge bilirubin measurements, gestation, and risk factors for subsequent hyperbilirubinemia. (Reprinted with permission from Maisels MJ, Bhutani VK, Bogen D, et al. Hyperbilirubinemia in the newborn infant ≥35 weeks' gestation: an update with clarifications. *Pediatrics* 2009;123:1193–1198.)

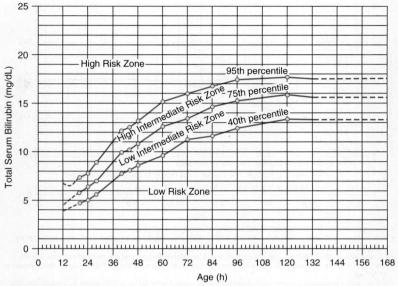

Risk designation of term and near-term well newborns based on their hour-specific serum bilirubin values. The high-risk zone is designated by the 95th percentile track. The intermediate-risk zone is subdivided to upper- and lower-risk zones by the 75th percentile track. The low-risk zone has been electively and statistically defined by the 40th percentile track. (Dotted extensions are based on <300 TSB values/epoch). This study is based on heel stick venous bilirubins and lower bilirubins.

Figure 26.3. Hour-specific bilirubin nomogram. G6PD = glucose-6-phosphate dehydrogenase; TSB = total serum bilirubin. (Reprinted with permission from Bhutani VK, Johnson L, Sivieri EM. Predictive ability of a predischarge hour-specific serum bilirubin for subsequent significant hyperbilirubinemia in healthy term and near-term newborns. *Pediatrics* 1999;103:6–14.)

injuries may have elevated bilirubin levels; causes include inability of the liver to process bilirubin and intracranial hemorrhage. Delayed cord clamping may be associated with neonatal polycythemia and increased bilirubin load.

8. The infant's history may show delayed or infrequent stooling, which can be caused by poor caloric intake or intestinal obstruction and lead to increased enterohepatic circulation of bilirubin. Poor caloric intake may also decrease bilirubin uptake by the liver. Vomiting can be due to sepsis, pyloric stenosis, or galactosemia.

9. **Breastfeeding.** A distinction is made between breast milk jaundice, in which jaundice is thought to be due to factors in breast milk, and breastfeeding jaundice, typically seen when breastfeeding is not going well and intake is inadequate.
   a. Breastfeeding jaundice. Infants who are breast-fed have higher bilirubin levels after day 3 of life compared to formula-fed infants. The differences in the levels of bilirubin are usually not clinically significant. The incidence of peak bilirubin levels >12 mg/dL in breast-fed term infants is 12% to 13%. The main factor thought to be responsible for breastfeeding jaundice is a decreased intake of milk that leads to slower bilirubin elimination and increased enterohepatic circulation.

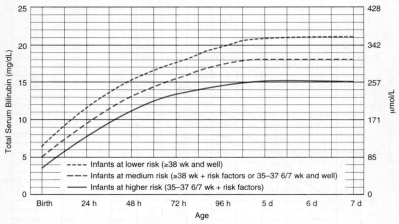

Figure 26.4. Guidelines for phototherapy in hospitalized infants of 35 or more weeks' gestation. TSB = total serum bilirubin. (Reprinted with permission from the American Academy of Pediatrics Subcommittee on Hyperbilirubinemia. Management of hyperbilirubinemia in the newborn infant 35 or more weeks of gestation. *Pediatrics* 2004;114:297–316.)

> **b. Breast milk jaundice** is of late onset and has an incidence in term infants of 2% to 4%. By day 4, instead of the usual fall in the serum bilirubin level, the bilirubin level continues to rise and may reach 20 to 30 mg/dL by 14 days of age if no treatment is instituted. If breastfeeding is continued, the levels will stay elevated and then fall slowly at 2 weeks of age, returning to normal by 4 to 12 weeks of age. If breastfeeding is stopped, the bilirubin level will fall rapidly in 48 hours. If nursing is then resumed, the bilirubin may rise for 2 to 4 mg/dL but usually will not reach the previous high level. These infants show good weight gain, have normal liver function test (LFT) results, and show no evidence of hemolysis. Mothers with infants who have breast milk jaundice syndrome have a recurrence rate of 70% in future pregnancies (see I.B.3. for potential genetic influences). The mechanism of true breast milk jaundice is unknown but is thought to be due to an unidentified factor (or factors) in breast milk interfering with bilirubin metabolism. Additionally, compared with formula-fed infants, breast-fed infants are more likely to have increased enterohepatic circulation because they ingest the β-glucuronidase present in breast milk, they are slower to be colonized with intestinal bacteria that convert CB to urobilinoids, and they excrete less stool.

C. The physical examination. Jaundice is detected by blanching the skin with finger pressure to observe the color of the skin and subcutaneous tissues. Jaundice progresses in a cephalocaudal direction. The highest bilirubin levels are typically associated with jaundice below the knees and in the hands, although there is substantial overlap of serum bilirubin levels associated with jaundice progression. **Visual inspection is not a reliable indicator of serum bilirubin levels.**

Jaundiced infants should be examined for the following physical findings:

1. **Prematurity. Gestational age is an important predictor of risk for hyperbilirubinemia; this should be evaluated and documented for each newborn.**

2. **Small-for-gestational-age (SGA),** which may be associated with polycythemia and *in utero* infections.

3. **Microcephaly,** which may be associated with *in utero* infections.

4. **Extravascular blood** bruising, cephalohematoma, or other enclosed hemorrhage.

5. **Pallor** associated with hemolytic anemia or extravascular blood loss.

6. **Petechiae** associated with congenital infection, sepsis, or erythroblastosis.

7. **Hepatosplenomegaly** associated with hemolytic anemia, congenital infection, or liver disease.

8. **Omphalitis.**

9. **Chorioretinitis** associated with congenital infection.

10. Evidence of **hypothyroidism** (see Chap. 3).

D. Prediction of hyperbilirubinemia that may require treatment in otherwise healthy infants ≥35 weeks' gestation

1. Visual inspection is **not** a reliable measure of serum bilirubin level.

2. A **screening total serum bilirubin (TSB)** collected predischarge from the newborn nursery at the time of the metabolic screen and plotted on an hour-specific bilirubin nomogram (Fig. 26.3) is helpful in identifying infants at increased risk for developing hyperbilirubinemia that requires treatment.

3. Alternatively, **transcutaneous bilirubin (TcB)** measurement using multiple wavelength analysis (versus two-wavelength method) can reliably estimate serum bilirubin levels independent of skin pigmentation, postnatal age, and weight of infant. Similar to TSB, TcB can be used as a screening tool to identify infants at high risk for severe hyperbilirubinemia by plotting obtained values on an hour-specific bilirubin nomogram. Despite advancements in transcutaneous technology, extrapolation to serum bilirubin levels from TcB should continue to be done with caution. We check TcB in all well term infants prior to discharge from the hospital.

TcB is a screening tool and can underestimate the TSB. Several options are recommended to avoid missing a high TSB. These include checking TSB if (i) TcB exceeds the 70th percentile of the TSB level recommended for phototherapy (Fig. 26.4), (ii) TcB exceeds the 75th percentile on the Bhutani nomogram (Fig. 26.3), or (iii) at follow-up after discharge, the TcB is >13 mg/dL. Our practical approach is to send a TSB simultaneously with the state metabolic screen if the TcB is >8, so that it is available for the discharging physician to evaluate.

It is important to note that TcB monitoring is unreliable after phototherapy has begun due to bleaching of the skin with treatment. However, TcB checked on skin that is unexposed to the phototherapy (e.g., under the eye shield) correlates with or overestimates TSB. TcB as a screening tool has the potential to reduce the number of invasive blood tests performed in newborns and reduce related health care costs.

4. **End-tidal carbon monoxide (ETCOc)** does not improve the sensitivity or specificity of predicting nonphysiologic hyperbilirubinemia over TSB or TcB alone. Although it may offer insight to the underlying pathologic process contributing to the hyperbilirubinemia (hemolysis versus conjugation defects), it is not commercially available at this time in the United States.

E. **Clinical tests** (Figs. 26.1 and 26.2). The following tests are indicated when TSB is above the 95th percentile for age in hours at or near the threshold for initiation of phototherapy treatment.

1. **Blood type, Rh, and antibody screen of the mother** should have been done during pregnancy, and the antibody screen repeated at delivery.

2. **Blood type, Rh, and direct Coombs test of the infant** to test for isoimmune hemolytic disease. Infants of women who are Rh negative should have a blood type, Rh, and Coombs test performed at birth. Routine blood typing and Coombs testing of all infants born to O Rh-positive mothers to determine whether there is risk for ABO incompatibility is unnecessary. Such testing is reserved for infants with clinically significant hyperbilirubinemia, those in whom follow-up is difficult, or those whose skin pigmentation is such that jaundice may not be easily recognized. Blood typing and Coombs testing should be considered for infants who are discharged early, especially if the mother is type O (see Chap. 9).

3. **Peripheral smear for RBC morphology and reticulocyte count** to detect causes of Coombs-negative hemolytic disease (e.g., spherocytosis). HS occurs in about 1 per 2,000 births and may be missed if family history alone is used for screening, as many cases are *de novo* and in infants of Japanese ancestry may be autosomal recessive. In one report, a mean corpuscular hemoglobin concentration (MCHC) of ≥36.0 g/dL has an 82% sensitivity and a 98% specificity for diagnosing HS.

4. **Hematocrit** will detect polycythemia or suggest blood loss from occult hemorrhage.

5. Identification of **antibody on infant's RBCs** (if result of direct Coombs test is positive).

6. **Direct bilirubin** should be measured when bilirubin levels are at or above the 95th percentile or when the phototherapy threshold is approaching. Direct bilirubin should also be measured when jaundice persists beyond the first 2 weeks of life or whenever there are signs of cholestasis (light-colored stools and bilirubin in urine). If elevated, a urinalysis and a urine culture should be obtained. Check state newborn screen for hypothyroidism and galactosemia. Check urine for reducing substances.

7. In prolonged jaundice, tests for liver disease, congenital infection, sepsis, metabolic defects, or hypothyroidism are indicated. Total parenteral nutrition (PN) is a well-recognized cause of prolonged direct hyperbilirubinemia.

8. **A G6PD screen** may be helpful, especially in male infants of African, Asian, southern European, and Mediterranean or Middle Eastern descent. The incidence of G6PD deficiency among African Americans males is 11% to 13%, comprising the most affected subpopulation in America. Affected infants are at increased risk for hyperbilirubinemia. A combination of genetic and environmental risk factors will determine the individual infant's risk of neonatal hyperbilirubinemia (see I.B.3. for potential genetic influences). Screening the

parents for G6PD deficiency is also helpful in making the diagnosis. Infants who had G6PD deficiency and were discharged early have been reported with severe hyperbilirubinemia and significant sequelae.

IV. DIAGNOSIS OF NEONATAL HYPERBILIRUBINEMIA (TABLE 26.2 AND FIG. 26.1).

V. BILIRUBIN TOXICITY. The level of bilirubin associated with toxicity in healthy term or preterm infants is uncertain and appears to vary among infants and in different clinical circumstances.

A. Bilirubin enters the brain as free (unbound) bilirubin or as bilirubin bound to albumin in the presence of a disrupted blood–brain barrier. It is estimated that 8.5 mg of bilirubin will bind tightly to 1 g of albumin (molar ratio of 1), although this binding capacity is less in small and sick premature infants. FFAs and certain drugs (Table 26.1) interfere with bilirubin binding to albumin, although acidosis affects bilirubin solubility and its deposition into brain tissue. Factors that disrupt the blood–brain barrier include hyperosmolarity, asphyxia, and hypercarbia; the barrier may be more permeable in premature infants.

B. **Kernicterus** is a pathologic diagnosis and refers to **yellow staining** of the brain by bilirubin together with evidence of **neuronal injury**. Grossly, bilirubin staining is most commonly seen in the basal ganglia, various cranial nerve nuclei, other brainstem nuclei, cerebellar nuclei, hippocampus, and anterior horn cells of the spinal cord. Microscopically, there is necrosis, neuronal loss, and gliosis. Abnormal signal intensity may be seen on brain magnetic resonance (MR) imaging, and a metabolic signature on MR spectroscopy is being investigated. The term **kernicterus** in the clinical setting should be used to denote the *chronic* and *permanent sequelae* of bilirubin toxicity.

C. **Acute bilirubin encephalopathy** is the clinical manifestation of bilirubin toxicity seen in the neonatal period. The clinical presentation of acute bilirubin encephalopathy can be divided into three phases:

1. **Early phase.** Hypotonia, lethargy, high-pitched cry, and poor suck.

2. **Intermediate phase.** Hypertonia of extensor muscles (with opisthotonus, rigidity, oculogyric crisis, and retrocollis), irritability, fever, and seizures. Many infants die in this phase. All infants who survive this phase develop chronic bilirubin encephalopathy (clinical diagnosis of kernicterus).

3. **Advanced phase.** Pronounced opisthotonus (although hypotonia replaces hypertonia after approximately 1 week of age), shrill cry, apnea, seizures, coma, and death.

D. **Chronic bilirubin encephalopathy** (kernicterus) is marked by athetosis, complete or partial sensorineural deafness (auditory neuropathy), limitation of upward gaze, dental dysplasia, and sometimes, intellectual deficits.

E. **Bilirubin toxicity and hemolytic disease.** There is general agreement that in Rh hemolytic disease, there is a direct association between marked elevations of bilirubin and signs of bilirubin encephalopathy with kernicterus at autopsy. Studies and clinical experience have shown that in full-term infants with hemolytic disease, if the total bilirubin level is kept <20 mg/dL, bilirubin encephalopathy is unlikely to occur. Theoretically, this should apply to other causes of isoimmune hemolytic disease, such as ABO incompatibility, and to hereditary hemolytic processes, such as HS, pyruvate kinase deficiency, or G6PD deficiency.

F. **Bilirubin toxicity and the healthy full-term infant.** In contrast to infants with hemolytic disease, there is little evidence showing adverse neurologic outcome in healthy term neonates with bilirubin levels <25 to 30 mg/dL. A large prospective cohort study failed to demonstrate a clinically significant association between bilirubin levels >20 mg/dL and neurologic abnormality, long-term hearing loss, or intelligence quotient (IQ) deficits. However, an increase in minor motor abnormalities of unclear significance was detected in those with serum bilirubin levels >20 mg/dL. Hyperbilirubinemia in term infants has been associated with abnormalities in brainstem auditory-evoked responses (BAERs), cry characteristics, and neurobehavioral measures. However, these changes disappear when bilirubin levels fall and there are no measurable long-term sequelae. Kernicterus has been reported in jaundiced healthy, full-term, breast-fed infants. **All predictive values for bilirubin toxicity are based on heel stick values.**

G. **Bilirubin toxicity and the low birth weight infant.** Initial early studies of babies of 1,250 to 2,500 g and 28 to 36 weeks' gestational age showed no relation between neurologic damage and bilirubin levels >18 to 20 mg/dL. Later studies, however, began to report "kernicterus" at autopsy or neurodevelopmental abnormalities at follow-up in premature infants <1,250 g who had bilirubin levels previously thought to be safe (e.g., <10–20 mg/dL). Because kernicterus in preterm infants is now considered uncommon, hindsight suggests that this so-called "low bilirubin kernicterus" was largely due to factors other than bilirubin alone. For example, unrecognized intracranial hemorrhage, inadvertent exposure to drugs that displace bilirubin from albumin, or the use of solutions (e.g., benzyl alcohol) that can alter the blood–brain barrier may have accounted for developmental handicaps or kernicterus in infants with low levels of serum bilirubin. In addition, premature infants are more likely to suffer from anoxia, hypercarbia, and sepsis, which open the blood–brain barrier and lead to enhanced bilirubin deposition in neural tissue. Finally, the pathologic changes seen in postmortem preterm infant brains have been more consistent with nonspecific damage than with true kernicterus. Therefore, bilirubin toxicity in low birth weight infants may not be a function of bilirubin levels *per se* but of their overall clinical status.

VI. MANAGEMENT OF UNCONJUGATED HYPERBILIRUBINEMIA. Given the uncertainty of determining what levels of bilirubin are toxic, these are general clinical guidelines only and should be modified in any sick infant with acidosis, hypercapnia, hypoxemia, asphyxia, sepsis, hypoalbuminemia (<2.5 mg/dL), or signs of bilirubin encephalopathy. When evaluating need for phototherapy or exchange transfusion, total bilirubin level should be used. Direct bilirubin is not subtracted from the total, except possibly if it constitutes >50% of total bilirubin.

A. **General principles.** Management of unconjugated hyperbilirubinemia is clearly tied to the etiology. Early identification of known causes of nonphysiologic hyperbilirubinemia (see III.B., C., and D.) should prompt close observation for development of jaundice, appropriate laboratory investigation, and timely intervention. Any medication (Table 26.1) or clinical factor that may interfere with bilirubin metabolism, bilirubin binding to albumin, or the integrity of the blood–brain barrier should be discontinued or corrected. Infants who are receiving inadequate feedings, or who have decreased urine and stool output, need increased feedings both in volume and in calories to reduce the enterohepatic circulation of bilirubin. Infants with hypothyroidism need adequate replacement of the thyroid hormone. If levels of bilirubin are so high that the infant is at risk for kernicterus, bilirubin may be removed mechanically by exchange transfusion, or its excretion increased by alternative pathways using phototherapy.

B. Infants with hemolytic disease (see XII. and XIII.)

1. In Rh disease, we start intensive phototherapy immediately. An exchange transfusion is performed if the bilirubin level is predicted to reach 20 mg/dL (see Figs. 26.5A and B).

2. High-dose intravenous immune globulin (IVIG) (500–1,000 mg/kg IV given over 2–4 hours) has been used to reduce bilirubin levels in infants with isoimmune hemolytic disease. The mechanism is unknown, but the immune globulin is thought to act by occupying the Fc receptors of reticuloendothelial cells, thereby preventing them from taking up and lysing antibody-coated RBCs. We give IVIG in cases of A–O or B–O incompatability if phototherapy is not effective in lowering TSB, and the TSB is approaching the level for exchange transfusion.

3. In ABO hemolytic disease, TSB levels for initiation of intensive phototherapy or exchange transfusion follow the medium or high risk line, depending on gestational age (see Figs. 26.4 and 26.6). Our approach has been more conservative: We start intensive phototherapy if the bilirubin level exceeds 10 mg/dL at 12 hours, 12 mg/dL at 18 hours, 14 mg/dL at 24 hours, or 15 mg/dL at any time and perform an exchange transfusion if the bilirubin reaches 20 mg/dL.

4. In hemolytic disease of other causes, we treat as if it were Rh disease (see Tables 26.5–26.7).

C. Healthy late-preterm and term infants (Figs. 26.2, 26.3, 26.4, and 26.6). The American Academy of Pediatrics (AAP) practice guideline for the treatment of unconjugated hyperbilirubinemia in healthy, newborn infants at 35 weeks' gestation and greater rests on three general principles to reduce the occurrence of severe hyperbilirubinemia while also reducing unintended harm: universal systematic assessment before discharge, close follow-up, and prompt intervention when indicated.

1. In our nurseries, we use either universal TcB (see III.D.) measurements or TSB levels sampled at the time of the metabolic screen. These bilirubin measurements are plotted on an hour-specific bilirubin nomogram to identify infants at risk for significant hyperbilirubinemia.

2. Most healthy, late-preterm and term infants are discharged home by 24 to 48 hours of age; therefore, parents should be informed about neonatal jaundice before discharge from the hospital. **Arrangements should be made for follow-up by a clinician within 1 or 2 days of discharge. This is especially true if the infant is <38 weeks' gestation, is the first child, is breastfeeding, or has any other risk factors for hyperbilirubinemia.**

3. In healthy, late-preterm and term infants who are jaundiced, we follow the guidelines published by the AAP (Fig. 26.2).

4. In **breast-fed infants** with hyperbilirubinemia, preventive measures are the best approach and include encouragement of frequent nursing (at least every 3 hours) and, if necessary, supplementation with expressed breast milk or formula (***not*** with water or dextrose water) (see III.B.9.).

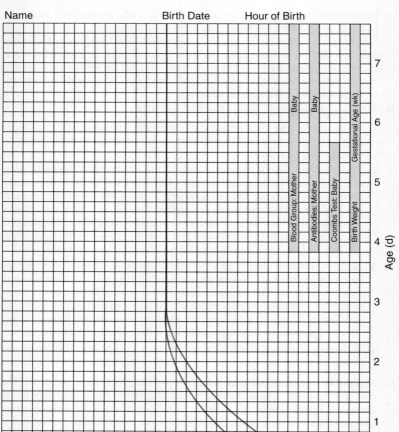

Name   Birth Date   Hour of Birth

A   Serum Bilirubin (mg/dL) in Term Infants

Figure 26.5. Serum bilirubin levels plotted against age in term infants (**A**) and premature infants (**B**) with erythroblastosis. Infants with levels plotting below the bottom line require no action, those with levels between the two lines should receive phototherapy, and those with levels above the top line should undergo exchange transfusion.

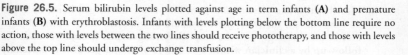

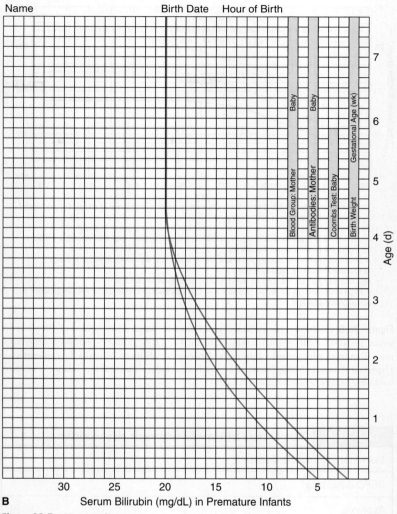

B   Serum Bilirubin (mg/dL) in Premature Infants

Figure 26.5. *(Continued)*

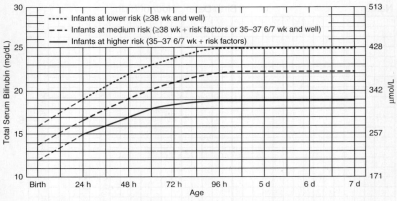

- The dashed lines for the first 24 h indicate uncertainty due to a wide range of clinical circumstances and a range of responses to phototherapy.
- Immediate exchange transfusion is recommended if infant shows signs of acute bilirubin encephalopathy (hypertonia, arching, retrocollis, opisthotonos, fever, high pitched cry) or if TSB is ≥5 mg/dL (85 μmol/L) above these lines.
- Risk factors–isoimmune hemolytic disease, G6PD deficiency, asphyxia, significant lethargy, temperature instability, sepsis, acidosis.
- Use total bilirubin. Do not subtract direct reacting or conjugated bilirubin.
- If infant is well and 35–37 6/7 wk (medium risk) can individualize TSB levels for exchange based on actual gestational age.

Figure 26.6 Guidelines for exchange transfusion in hospitalized infants of 35 or more weeks' gestation. TSB = total serum bilirubin; G6PD = glucose-6-phosphate dehydrogenase. (Reprinted with permission from the American Academy of Pediatrics Subcommittee on Hyperbilirubinemia. Management of hyperbilirubinemia in the newborn infant 35 or more weeks of gestation. *Pediatrics* 2004;114:297–316.)

Table 26.5	Risk Factors for Hyperbilirubinemia Neurotoxicity
Isoimmune hemolytic disease	
G6PD deficiency	
Asphyxia	
Sepsis	
Acidosis	
Albumin less than 3.0 mg/dL	

Source: Maisels MJ, Bhutani VK, Bogen D, et al. Hyperbilirubinemia in the newborn infant ≥35 weeks' gestation: an update with clarifications. *Pediatrics* 2009;124:1193–1198.

Table 26.6	Other Antigens Involved in Hemolytic Diseases of the Newborn	
Antigen	**Alternative symbol or name**	**Blood group system**
Co^a	—	Colton
Di^b	—	Diego
Ge	—	Gerbich
Hy	Holley	—
Jr	—	—
Js^b	Matthews, K:7	Kell
K	Cellano, K:2	Kell
Kp^b	Rautenberg, K:4	Kell
Lan	Langereis	—
Lu^b	—	Lutheran
LW	Landsteinder-Wiener	—
P, P1, P^k	Tj^a	P
U	—	MNSs
Yt^a	—	Cartwright

5. Guidelines for phototherapy and exchange transfusion are identical for breast-fed and formula-fed infants. However, in **breast-fed infants**, a decision is often made whether to interrupt breastfeeding. In a randomized controlled trial of breast-fed infants with bilirubin levels of at least 17 mg/dL, 3% of those who switched to formula and received phototherapy reached bilirubin levels >20 mg/dL compared with 14% of those who continued nursing while they were receiving phototherapy. In infants not receiving phototherapy, 19% of those who switched to formula reached bilirubin levels >20 mg/dL compared with 24% of those who simply continued nursing. No infant in any group had a bilirubin >23 mg/dL, and none required exchange transfusion. However, interrupting breastfeeding entirely may not be necessary. In a later prospective trial, breast-fed infants who continued to breastfeed and were supplemented with formula had a comparable response to treatment to infants who stopped breastfeeding and were fed with formula alone.

In general, **our current practice** is that if the bilirubin reaches a level that requires phototherapy, we start phototherapy and have the mother continue to breastfeed or pump and feed the breast milk. Fiberoptic blankets can be used when phototherapy is discontinued for feeding. If there is inadequate breast milk, or the infant has excessive weight loss or hypovolemia, or the

Table 26.7	Infrequent Antigens Implicated in Hemolytic Diseases of the Newborn	
Antigen	**Alternative symbol or name**	**Blood group system**
Be^a	Berrens	Rh
Bi	Biles	—
By	Batty	—
C^w	Rh:8	Rh
C^x	Rh:9	Rh
Di^a*	—	Diego
Evans	—	Rh
E^w	Rh:11	Rh
Far	See Kam	—
Ga	Gambino	—
Go^a	Gonzales	Rh
Good	—	—
Heibel	—	—
Hil	Hill	MNSs Mi sub+
Ht^a	Hunt	—
Hut	Hutchinson	MNSs Mi sub
Js^a	Sutter	Kell
Kam (Far)	Kamhuber	—
Kp^a	Penney	Kell
Mit	Mitchell	—
Mt^a	Martin	MNSs#
Mull	Lu:9	Lutheran
Mur	Murrell	MNSs Mi sub
		(continued)

Table 26.7	(Continued)	
Antigen	**Alternative symbol or name**	**Blood group system**
Rd	Radin	—
Re^a	Reid	—
R^N	Rh:32	Rh
Vw (Gr)	Verweyst (Graydon)	MNSs Mi sub
Wi^a	Wright	—
Zd	—	—

*This may not be a complete list. Any antigen that the father has and the mother does not have and that induces an immunoglobulin G (IgG) response in the mother may cause sensitization.

bilirubin level is not declining, supplementation with formula is instituted. The mother requires much support through this process and is encouraged to resume breastfeeding as soon as possible.

D. Premature infants. No consensus guidelines exist for phototherapy and exchange transfusion in low birth weight infants. A large randomized controlled trial of aggressive versus conservative phototherapy in extremely low birth weight (ELBW) infants performed by the National Institute of Child Health and Human Development (NICHD) Neonatal Research Network showed a significant decrease in neurodevelopmental impairment, especially profound impairment, at 18 to 20 months corrected age with aggressive phototherapy. However, in the 501 to 750 g birth weight category, aggressive phototherapy was associated with a 5% increase in mortality. No evidence is available in preterm infants of moderate birth weight.

Our current practice for treating jaundiced premature infants is as follows:

1. **Infants <1,000 g.** Phototherapy is started within 24 hours, and exchange transfusion is performed at levels of 10 to 12 mg/dL.

2. **Infants 1,000 to 1,500 g.** Phototherapy at bilirubin levels of 7 to 9 mg/dL and exchange transfusion at levels of 12 to 15 mg/dL.

3. **Infants 1,500 to 2,000 g.** Phototherapy at bilirubin levels of 10 to 12 mg/dL and exchange transfusion at levels of 15 to 18 mg/dL.

4. **Infants 2,000 to 2,500 g.** Phototherapy at bilirubin levels of 13 to 15 mg/dL and exchange transfusion at levels of 18 to 20 mg/dL.

VII. PHOTOTHERAPY. Although bilirubin absorbs visible light with wavelengths of approximately 400 to 500 nm, the most effective lights for phototherapy are those with high energy output near the maximum absorption peak of bilirubin (450–460 nm). Special blue lamps with a peak output at 425 to 475 nm are the most efficient for phototherapy. Cool white lamps with a principal peak at 550 to 600 nm and a range of 380 to 700 nm are usually adequate for treatment. Fiberoptic phototherapy (phototherapy blankets) has been shown to reduce bilirubin levels, although less effectively for term infants, likely due to limited skin exposure.

A. Photochemical reactions. When bilirubin absorbs light, three types of photochemical reactions occur.

1. Photoisomerization occurs in the extravascular space of the skin. The natural isomer of UCB (4Z,15Z) is rapidly converted to a less toxic polar isomer (4Z,15E) that diffuses into the blood and is excreted into the bile without conjugation. However, excretion is slow, and the photoisomer is readily converted back to UCB, which is resorbed from the gut if the baby is not having stools. After approximately 12 hours of phototherapy, the photoisomers make up approximately 20% of total bilirubin. Standard tests do not distinguish between naturally occurring bilirubin and the photoisomer, so bilirubin levels may not change much although the phototherapy has made the bilirubin present less toxic. Photoisomerization occurs at low-dose phototherapy (6 μW/cm^2/nm) with no significant benefit from doubling the irradiance.

2. Structural isomerization is the intramolecular cyclization of bilirubin to **lumirubin.** Lumirubin makes up 2% to 6% of serum concentration of bilirubin during phototherapy and is rapidly excreted in the bile and urine without conjugation. Unlike photoisomerization, the conversion of bilirubin to lumirubin is irreversible, and it cannot be reabsorbed. It is the most important pathway for the lowering of serum bilirubin levels and is strongly related to the dose of phototherapy used in the range of 6 to 12 μW/cm^2/nm.

3. The slow process of **photo-oxidation** converts bilirubin to small polar products that are excreted in the urine. It is the least important reaction for lowering bilirubin levels.

B. Indications for phototherapy

1. Phototherapy should be used when the level of bilirubin may be hazardous to the infant if it were to increase, although it has not reached levels requiring exchange transfusion (see VI.).

2. Prophylactic phototherapy may be indicated in special circumstances, such as with ELBW infants or with severely bruised infants, when the TSB is anticipated to increase rapidly. In hemolytic disease of the newborn, phototherapy is started immediately while the rise in the serum bilirubin level is plotted (Figs. 26.5 and 26.6) and during the wait for exchange transfusion.

3. Phototherapy is usually contraindicated in infants with direct hyperbilirubinemia caused by liver disease or obstructive jaundice, because indirect bilirubin levels are not usually high in these conditions and because phototherapy may lead to the **"bronze baby" syndrome**. If both direct and indirect bilirubin are high, exchange transfusion is probably safer than phototherapy because it is not known whether the bronze pigment is toxic.

C. Technique of phototherapy. Effective phototherapy depends on the light spectrum, irradiance (energy output), distance from the infant (closer maximizes irradiance), and the extent of skin area exposure. Conventional phototherapy should deliver spectral irradiance at the infant's level of 8 to 10 μW/cm^2/nm, 430 to 490 nm, when positioned 20 cm above the infant; intensive phototherapy delivers at least 30 $\mu W/cm^2/nm$ at that spectrum. All devices should be used according to the manufacturers' instructions to avoid overheating.

1. We have found that **light banks** with alternating special blue (narrow-spectrum) and daylight fluorescent lights are effective and do not make the baby appear cyanotic. In infants with severe hyperbilirubinemia, we use neoBLUE phototherapy lights (Natus, 1501 Industrial Park, San Carlos, CA 94070, www. natus.com), which deliver the irradiance needed for intensive phototherapy and do not cause overheating. Bulbs should be changed at intervals specified by the manufacturer. Our practice is to change all the bulbs every 3 months because this approximates the correct number of hours of use in our unit.

2. For infants under radiant warmers, we place infants on fiberoptic blankets and/or use **spot phototherapy** overhead with quartz halide white light having output in the blue spectrum.

3. **Fiberoptic blankets** with light output in the blue-green spectrum have proved very useful in our unit, not only for single phototherapy, but also for delivering **"double phototherapy"** in which the infant lies on a fiberoptic blanket with phototherapy lights overhead.

4. Infants under phototherapy lights are kept naked except for eye patches and a diaper used as a diaper to ensure light exposure to the greatest skin surface area. We use eyecovers called *Biliband* (Natus, 1501 Industrial Park, San Carlos, CA 94070, www.natus.com). The infants are turned every 2 hours. Care should be taken to ensure that the eye patches do not occlude the nares, as asphyxia and apnea can result.

5. If an incubator is used, there should be a 5- to 8-cm space between it and the lamp cover to prevent overheating.

6. The infants' temperature should be carefully monitored and servo-controlled.

7. Infants should be weighed daily (small infants are weighed twice each day). Between 10% and 20% extra fluid over the usual requirements is given to compensate for the increased insensible water loss in infants in open cribs or warmers who are receiving phototherapy. Infants also have increased fluid losses caused by increased stooling (see Chap. 23).

8. Skin color is not a guide to TSB levels in infants undergoing phototherapy; consequently, we typically monitor bilirubin level every 12 to 24 hours, depending on the bilirubin level, rate of rise or decline, and gestational and postnatal age.

9. Once a satisfactory decline in bilirubin levels has occurred (e.g., exchange transfusion has been averted), we interrupt phototherapy for feedings and brief parental visits.

10. **Phototherapy is stopped** when it is believed that the level is low enough to eliminate concern about the toxic effects of bilirubin, when the risk factors for toxic levels of bilirubin are gone, and when the baby is old enough to handle the bilirubin load. In general, we stop phototherapy started during the birth hospitalization when the TSB is less than the level at which phototherapy was started. A bilirubin level is usually checked 12 to 24 hours after phototherapy is stopped in babies who had hemolytic disease and in preterm infants. In a recent study of infants with nonhemolytic hyperbilirubinemia, phototherapy was discontinued at mean bilirubin levels of 13 ± 0.7 mg/dL in term and 10.7 ± 1.2

mg/dL in preterm infants. Rebound bilirubin levels 12 to 15 hours later averaged a rise of <1 mg/dL, and no infant required reinstitution of phototherapy.

11. **Home phototherapy** is effective, cheaper than hospital phototherapy, and easy to implement with the use of fiberoptic blankets. It may not have the same irradiance as the hospital phototherapy. Most candidates for home phototherapy are breast-fed infants, whose bilirubin problems can be resolved with a brief interruption of breastfeeding and increased fluid intake. Constant supervision is required, and attention to all the other details of phototherapy, such as temperature control and fluid intake, are also required. The AAP recommends the use of home phototherapy only for infants with bilirubin levels in the "phototherapy optional" range (Fig. 26.4).

12. It is contraindicated to put jaundiced infants under direct sunlight, as sunburn or hyperthermia may result.

D. Side effects of phototherapy

1. **Insensible water loss** is increased in infants undergoing phototherapy, especially those under radiant warmers. The increase may be as much as 40% for term and 80% to 190% in premature infants. Incubators with servo-controlled warmers decrease this water loss. Extra fluid must be given to make up for these losses (see Chap. 23).

2. **Redistribution of blood flow.** In **term** infants, left ventricular output and renal blood flow velocity decrease, whereas left pulmonary artery and cerebral blood flow velocity increase. All velocities return to baseline after discontinuation of phototherapy. In the **preterm** infant, cerebral blood flow velocity also increases and renal vascular resistance increases with a reduction of renal blood flow velocity. In ventilated preterm infants, the changes in blood flow velocities do not return to baseline even after discontinuation of phototherapy. In addition, in preterm infants under conventional phototherapy, it has been shown that the usual postprandial increase in superior mesenteric blood flow is blunted. Fiberoptic phototherapy did not seem to affect the postprandial response. Although the changes in cerebral, renal, and superior mesenteric artery blood flow with phototherapy treatment in preterm infants is of potential concern, no detrimental clinical effects due to these changes have been determined.

3. **Watery diarrhea and increased fecal water loss** may occur. The diarrhea may be caused by increased bile salts and UCB in the bowel.

4. **Low calcium** levels have been described in preterm infants under phototherapy.

5. **Retinal damage** has been described in animals whose eyes have been exposed to phototherapy lamps. The eyes should be shielded with eye patches. Follow-up studies of infants whose eyes have been adequately shielded show normal vision and electroretinography.

6. **Tanning** of the skin of black infants. Erythema and increased skin blood flow may also be seen.

7. **"Bronze baby" syndrome** (see VII.B.3.).

8. **Mutations, sister chromatid exchange, and DNA strand breaks** have been described in cell culture.

9. **Tryptophan is reduced in amino acid solutions** exposed to phototherapy. Methionine and histidine are also reduced in these solutions if multivitamins

are added. The effects on outcome or of shielding these solutions with aluminum foil on the lines and bottles are unknown.

10. **No significant long-term developmental differences** have been found in infants treated with phototherapy compared with controls.

11. Phototherapy upsets **maternal–infant interactions** and, therefore, should be used only with adequate thought and explanation.

VIII. EXCHANGE TRANSFUSION

A. **Mechanisms.** Exchange transfusion removes partially hemolyzed and antibody-coated RBCs, as well as unattached antibodies, and replaces them with donor RBCs, lacking the sensitizing antigen. As bilirubin is removed from the plasma, extravascular bilirubin will rapidly equilibrate and bind to the albumin in the exchanged blood. Within half an hour after the exchange, bilirubin levels return to 60% of preexchange levels, representing the rapid influx of bilirubin into the vascular space. Further increases in postexchange bilirubin levels are due to hemolysis of antibody-coated RBCs sequestered in bone marrow or spleen, from senescent donor RBCs, and from early-labeled bilirubin.

B. **Indications for exchange transfusion**

1. When phototherapy fails to prevent a rise in bilirubin to toxic levels (see VI. and Figs. 26.2–26.5).

2. To correct anemia and improve heart failure in hydropic infants with hemolytic disease.

3. To stop hemolysis and bilirubin production by removing antibody and sensitized RBCs.

4. Figure 26.5 shows the natural history of bilirubin rise in infants with Rh sensitization without phototherapy. In hemolytic disease, immediate exchange transfusion is usually indicated if:
   a. The cord bilirubin level is >4.5 mg/dL and the cord hemoglobin level is under 11 g/dL.
   b. The bilirubin level is rising >1 mg/dL/hour despite phototherapy.
   c. The hemoglobin level is between 11 and 13 g/dL, and the bilirubin level is rising >0.5 mg/dL/hour despite phototherapy.
   d. The bilirubin level is 20 mg/dL, or it appears that it will reach 20 mg/dL at the rate it is rising (Figs. 26.5 and 26.6).
   e. There is progression of anemia in the face of adequate control of bilirubin by other methods (e.g., phototherapy).

5. Repeat exchanges are done for the same indications as the initial exchange. All infants should be under intensive phototherapy while decisions regarding exchange transfusion are being made.

C. **Blood for exchange transfusion**

1. We use fresh (<7 days old), irradiated, and reconstituted whole blood (hematocrit 45–50%) made from packed red blood cells (PRBCs) and fresh frozen plasma collected in citrate-phosphate-dextrose (CPD). Cooperation

with the obstetrician and the blood bank is essential in preparing for the birth of an infant requiring exchange transfusion (see Chap. 42).

2. **In Rh hemolytic disease**, if blood is prepared before delivery, it should be type O Rh-negative, cross-matched against the mother. If the blood is obtained after delivery, it also may be cross-matched against the infant.

3. **In ABO incompatibility**, the blood should be type O Rh-negative or Rh-compatible with the mother and infant, be cross-matched against the mother and infant, and have a low titer of naturally occurring anti-A or anti-B antibodies. Usually, type O cells are used with AB plasma to ensure that no anti-A or anti-B antibodies are present.

4. In other isoimmune hemolytic disease, the blood should not contain the sensitizing antigen and should be cross-matched against the mother.

5. In nonimmune hyperbilirubinemia, blood is typed and cross-matched against the plasma and red cells of the infant.

6. Exchange transfusion usually involves double the volume of the infant's blood and is known as a two-volume exchange. If the infant's blood volume is 80 mL/kg, then a two-volume exchange transfusion uses 160 mL/kg of blood. This replaces 87% of the infant's blood volume with new blood.

D. Technique of exchange transfusion

1. Exchange transfusion is done with the infant under a servo-controlled radiant warmer and cardiac, blood pressure, and oxygen saturation monitoring in place. Equipment and personnel for resuscitation must be readily available, and an intravenous line should be in place for the administration of glucose and medication. The infant's arms and legs should be restrained.

2. An assistant should be assigned to the infant to record volumes of blood, observe the infant, and check vital signs.

3. Measurement of potassium and pH of the blood for exchange may be indicated if the blood is >7 days old or if metabolic abnormalities are noted following exchange transfusion.

4. The blood should be warmed to 37°C.

5. Sterile technique should be used. Old, dried umbilical cords can be softened with saline-soaked gauze to facilitate locating the vein and inserting the catheter. If an umbilical line is placed in an infant more than 1 or 2 days of age, or if there was a break in sterile technique, we treat with oxacillin and gentamicin for 2 to 3 days.

6. We do most exchanges by the **push–pull technique** through the umbilical vein inserted only as far as required to permit free blood exchange. A catheter in the heart may cause arrhythmias (see Chap. 66).

7. **Isovolumetric** exchange transfusion (simultaneously pulling blood out of the umbilical artery and pushing new blood in the umbilical vein) may be tolerated better in small, sick, or hydropic infants.

8. If it is not possible to insert the catheter in the umbilical vein, exchange transfusion can be accomplished through a central venous catheter placed through the antecubital fossa or into the femoral vein through the saphenous vein.

9. In the push–pull method, blood is removed in aliquots that are tolerated by the infant. This usually is **5 mL** for infants <1,500 g, **10 mL** for infants

1,500 to 2,500 g, **15 mL** for infants 2,500 to 3,500 g, and **20 mL** for infants >3,500 g. The rate of exchange and aliquot size have little effect on the efficiency of bilirubin removal, but smaller aliquots and a slower rate place less stress on the cardiovascular system. The recommended time for the exchange transfusion is 1 hour.

10. The blood should be gently mixed after every deciliter of exchange to prevent the settling of RBCs and the transfusion of anemic blood at the end of the exchange.

11. After exchange transfusion, phototherapy is continued and bilirubin levels are measured every 4 hours.

12. When the exchange transfusion is finished, a silk purse-string suture should be placed around the vein; the tails of the suture material should be left. This localization of the vein will facilitate the next exchange transfusion, if needed.

13. When the catheter is removed, the tie around the cord should be tightened snugly for approximately 1 hour. It is important to remember to loosen the tie after 1 hour to avoid necrosis of the skin.

E. **Complications of exchange transfusions**

1. **Hypocalcemia and hypomagnesemia.** The citrate in CPD blood binds ionic calcium and magnesium. Hypocalcemia associated with exchange transfusion may produce cardiac and other effects (see Chap. 25). We usually do not give extra calcium unless the electrocardiogram (ECG) and clinical assessment suggest hypocalcemia. The fall in magnesium associated with exchange transfusion has not been associated with clinical problems.

2. **Hypoglycemia.** The glucose concentration of CPD blood is approximately 300 mg/dL and may stimulate insulin secretion and cause hypoglycemia 1 to 2 hours after an exchange. Blood glucose is monitored for several hours after exchange and the infant should have an intravenous line containing glucose (see Chap. 24).

3. **Acid–base balance.** Citrate in CPD blood is metabolized to alkali by the healthy liver and may result in a late metabolic alkalosis. If the baby is very ill and unable to metabolize citrate, the citrate may produce significant acidosis.

4. **Hyperkalemia.** Potassium levels may be greatly elevated in stored PRBCs, but washing the cells before reconstitution with fresh frozen plasma removes this excess potassium. Washing by some methods (IBM cell washer) may cause hypokalemia. If blood is >7 days old, we check the potassium level before using it (see Chap. 23).

5. **Cardiovascular.** Perforation of vessels, embolization (with air or clots), vasospasm, thrombosis, infarction, arrhythmias, volume overload, and arrest.

6. **Bleeding.** Thrombocytopenia, deficient clotting factors (see Chap. 43).

7. **Infections.** Bacteremia, hepatitis, cytomegalovirus (CMV), human immunodeficiency virus (HIV) (acquired immune deficiency syndrome [AIDS]), West Nile virus, and malaria (see Chaps. 48 and 49).

8. **Hemolysis.** Hemoglobinemia, hemoglobinuria, and hyperkalemia caused by overheating of the blood have been reported. Massive hemolysis, intravascular sickling, and death have occurred from the use of hemoglobin sickle cell (SC) donor blood.

9. **Graft-versus-host disease.** This is prevented by using **irradiated blood**. Before blood was routinely irradiated for newborns, a syndrome of transient maculopapular rash, eosinophilia, lymphopenia, and thrombocytopenia without other signs of immunodeficiency was described in infants receiving multiple exchange transfusions. This did not usually progress to graft-versus-host disease.

10. **Miscellaneous.** Hypothermia, hyperthermia, and possibly necrotizing enterocolitis.

IX. NO LONGER USED OR INVESTIGATIONAL THERAPIES. The following therapies have been tested but are not in routine use:

A. **Increasing bilirubin conjugation. Phenobarbital** induces microsomal enzymes, increases bilirubin conjugation and excretion, and increases bile flow. It is useful in treating the indirect hyperbilirubinemia of Crigler-Najjar syndrome type II (but not type I). Phenobarbital, given antenatally to the mother, is effective in lowering bilirubin levels in erythroblastotic infants, but concerns about toxicity prevent its routine use in pregnant women in the United States. Phenobarbital does not augment the effects of phototherapy. We do not use phenobarbital to treat neonatal hyperbilirubinemia.

B. **Decreasing enterohepatic circulation.** In breast-fed and formula-fed infants with bilirubins >15 mg/dL, oral agar significantly increases the efficiency and shortens the duration of phototherapy. In fact, oral agar alone was as effective as phototherapy in lowering bilirubin levels. Although oral agar may prove to be an economical therapy for hyperbilirubinemia, this has not been adopted widely and has not been used in our nurseries.

C. **Inhibiting bilirubin production.** Metalloprotoporphyrins (e.g., tin and zinc protoporphyrins) are competitive inhibitors of heme oxygenase, the first enzyme in converting heme to bilirubin. They have been used to treat hyperbilirubinemia in Coombs-positive ABO incompatibility and in Crigler-Najjar type I patients. In addition, a single dose of tin mesoporphyrin given shortly after birth substantially reduced the incidence of hyperbilirubinemia and the duration of phototherapy in Greek preterm (30–36 weeks) infants. A follow-up study by the same research group demonstrated that a single dose of Sn-mesoporphyrin in G6PD-deficient newborns significantly reduced bilirubin levels and eliminated the need for phototherapy. These agents are still experimental and are not in routine use.

X. DIRECT OR CONJUGATED HYPERBILIRUBINEMIA is due to failure to excrete CB from the hepatocyte into the duodenum. It is manifested by a CB level >2 mL/dL or a CB level >15% of the total bilirubin level. It may be associated with hepatomegaly, splenomegaly, pale stools, and dark urine. CB is found in the urine, UCB is not. The preferred term to describe it is **cholestasis**, which includes retention of CB, bile acids, and other components of bile.

A. **Differential diagnosis**

1. **Liver cell injury (normal bile ducts)**
   a. **Toxic.** Prolonged use of PN (generally greater than 2 weeks) in low birth weight infants is a major cause of elevated CB in the neonatal intensive care unit (NICU). It appears to be related to the parenteral use of lipid. Sepsis and ischemic necrosis may also cause cholestasis.

b. Infection. Viral: hepatitis (B, C), giant cell neonatal hepatitis, rubella, CMV, herpes, Epstein-Barr virus, coxsackievirus, adenovirus, echoviruses 14 and 19. Bacterial: syphilis, *Escherichia coli*, group B β-hemolytic streptococcus, listeria, tuberculosis, staphylococcus. Parasitic: toxoplasma.

c. Metabolic. α1-antitrypsin deficiency, cystic fibrosis, galactosemia, tyrosinemia, hypermethionemia, fructosemia, storage diseases (Gaucher, Niemann-Pick, glycogenosis type IV, Wolmans), Rotor syndrome, Dubin-Johnson syndrome, Byler disease, Zellweger syndrome, idiopathic cirrhosis, porphyria, hemochromatosis, trisomy 18.

2. **Excessive bilirubin load (inspissated bile syndrome)** may be seen in any severe hemolytic disease but especially in infants with erythroblastosis fetalis who have been treated with intrauterine transfusion. In addition, a self-limited cholestatic jaundice is frequently seen in infants supported on extracorporeal membrane oxygenation (ECMO) (see Chap. 39). The cholestasis may last as long as 9 weeks and is thought to be secondary to hemolysis during ECMO.

3. **Bile flow obstruction (biliary atresia, extrahepatic or intrahepatic).** The extrahepatic type may be isolated or associated with a choledochal cyst, trisomy 13 or 18, or polysplenia. The intrahepatic type may be associated with the Alagille syndrome, intrahepatic atresia with lymphedema (Aagenaes syndrome), nonsyndromic paucity of intrahepatic bile ducts, coprostanic acidemia, choledochal cyst, bile duct stenosis, rupture of bile duct, lymph node enlargement, hemangiomas, tumors, pancreatic cyst, inspissated bile syndrome, and cystic fibrosis. Genetic testing is available for the diagnosis of Alagille syndrome.

4. In the NICU, the most common causes of elevated CB, in decreasing order of frequency, are PN, idiopathic hepatitis, biliary atresia, α1-antitrypsin deficiency, intrauterine infection, choledochal cyst, galactosemia, and increased bilirubin load from hemolytic disease.

B. **Diagnostic tests and management**

1. Evaluate for hepatomegaly, splenomegaly, petechiae, chorioretinitis, and microcephaly.

2. Evaluate liver damage and function by measurement of serum glutamic oxaloacetic transaminase (SGOT) level, serum glutamic pyruvic transaminase (SGPT) level, alkaline phosphatase level, prothrombin time (PT), partial thromboplastin time (PTT), and serum albumin level.

3. Establish enteral feeds so that PN can be stopped. If PN is the cause, the liver dysfunction will usually resolve.

4. Test for bacterial, viral, and intrauterine infections (see Chaps. 48, 49, and 51).

5. Serum analysis for α1-antitrypsin deficiency.

6. Serum and urine amino acids determinations (see Chap. 60).

7. Urinalysis for glucose and reducing substances (see Chap. 60).

8. If known causes are ruled out, the problem is to differentiate idiopathic neonatal hepatitis from bile duct abnormalities, such as intrahepatic biliary atresia or hypoplasia, choledochal cyst, bile plug syndrome, extrahepatic biliary atresia, hypoplasia, or total biliary atresia.

   a. Abdominal ultrasound should be done to rule out a choledochal cyst or mass.

   b. We use a hepatobiliary scan with technetium ^{99m}Tc–diisopropyliminodiacetic acid (DISIDA) as the next step to visualize the biliary tree.

c. ^{131}I–rose bengal fecal excretion test may be useful if the ^{99m}Tc-DISIDA scan is not available.

d. A nasoduodenal tube can be passed and fluid collected in 2-hour aliquots for 24 hours. If there is no bile, treat with phenobarbital, 5 mg/kg/day for 7 days, and repeat the duodenal fluid collection.

e. If the duodenal fluid collections, scans, and ultrasonography suggest no extrahepatic obstruction, the child may be observed with careful follow-up.

f. If the ultrasonography scans or fluid collections suggest extrahepatic obstruction disease, the baby will need an exploratory laparotomy, cholangiogram, and open liver biopsy to enable a definite diagnosis.

g. If the diagnosis of extrahepatic obstruction disease cannot be ruled out, the baby must have the studies outlined, because surgical therapy for choledochal cyst is curative if done early, and hepatoportoenterostomy has better results if done early.

h. Most cholestasis in the NICU is due to prolonged exposure to PN. After ruling out other causes (sepsis, metabolic disorders, ultrasound for choledochal cyst, and the presence of a gallbladder), we institute the following:

    i. Enteral feedings, even at "trophic" volumes of 10 mL/kg/day should be initiated as soon as can be safely done.

    ii. Once enteral feedings are restarted, infants with persistently elevated direct bilirubin and LFTs should receive fat-soluble vitamin supplements (A, D, E, and K).

    iii. Patients on PN should have LFTs checked regularly (once a week); and if the direct bilirubin, alanine aminotransferase (ALT), and gamma-glutamyltransferase (GGT) begin to rise, the PN should be adjusted. Decrease mineral content to minimize toxic effects of mineral accumulation. Copper and manganese, which are excreted in the bile, should be eliminated from or reduced in the PN (see Chap. 21). Cycle PN, on for 18 to 20 hours, off for 4 to 6 hours (run dextrose solution when PN is off).

    iv. Phenobarbital should not be used to treat cholestasis in this patient population.

    v. We obtain a gastroenterology/liver consultation and consider use of ursodiol (Actigall) in infants who tolerate enteral feeding.

    vi. We use parenteral fish oil (Omegaven 10% fish oil emulsions—Fresenius Kabi, Homburg, Germany) on an investigational protocol in infants with PN-associated liver disease. Intralipid is discontinued and replaced with Omegaven at a dose of 1 g/kg/day. Extra calories are given as glucose. So far, more than 100 patients with PN-associated liver disease mostly related to severe short gut syndromes have been treated with Omegaven at Children's Hospital Boston with encouraging results. Parenteral fish oil is not approved for use in the United States; use requires application to the US Food and Drug Administration (FDA) for compassionate use and purchase through an international pharmacy in Germany.

XI. HYDROPS is a term used to describe generalized subcutaneous edema in the fetus or neonate. It is usually accompanied by ascites and often by pleural and/or pericardial effusions. Hydrops fetalis is discussed here, because in the past, hemolytic disease of the newborn was the major cause of both fetal and neonatal hydrops.

However, because of the decline in Rh sensitization, nonimmune conditions are now the major causes of hydrops in the United States.

A. Etiology. The pathogenesis of hydrops includes anemia, cardiac failure, decreased colloid oncotic pressure (hypoalbuminemia), increased capillary permeability, asphyxia, and placental perfusion abnormalities. There is a general, but not a constant relation between the degree of anemia, the serum albumin level, and the presence of hydrops. There is no correlation between the severity of hydrops and the blood volume of the infant. Most hydropic infants have normal blood volume (80 mg/kg).

1. **Hematologic** due to chronic *in utero* anemia (10% of cases). Isoimmune hemolytic disease (e.g., Rh incompatibility), homozygous α- thalassemia, homozygous G6PD deficiency, chronic fetomaternal hemorrhage, twin-to-twin transfusion, hemorrhage, thrombosis, bone marrow failure (chloramphenicol, maternal parvovirus infection), bone marrow replacement (Gaucher disease), leukemia.

2. **Cardiovascular** due to heart failure (20% of cases) (see Chap. 41).
   a. Rhythm disturbances. Heart block, supraventricular tachycardia, atrial flutter.
   b. Major cardiac disease. Hypoplastic left heart, Ebstein anomaly, truncus arteriosus, myocarditis (coxsackie virus), endocardial fibroelastosis, cardiac neoplasm (rhabdomyoma), cardiac thrombosis, arteriovenous malformations, premature closure of foramen ovale, generalized arterial calcification, premature restructure of the foramen ovale.

3. **Renal** (5% of cases). Nephrosis, renal vein thrombosis, renal hypoplasia, urinary obstruction.

4. **Infection** (8% of cases). Syphilis, rubella, CMV, congenital hepatitis, herpes virus, adenovirus, toxoplasmosis, leptospirosis, Chagas disease, parvovirus (see Chaps. 48, 50, and 51).

5. **Pulmonary** (5% of cases). Congenital chylothorax, diaphragmatic hernia, pulmonary lymphangiectasia, cystic adenomatoid malformations, intrathoracic mass.

6. **Placenta or cord** (rare cause). Chorangioma, umbilical vein thrombosis, arteriovenous malformation, chorionic vein thrombosis, true knot in umbilical cord, cord compression, choriocarcinoma.

7. **Maternal conditions** (5% of cases). Toxemia, diabetes, thyrotoxicosis.

8. **GI** (5% of cases). Meconium peritonitis, *in utero* volvulus, atresia.

9. **Chromosomal** (10% of cases). Turner syndrome; aneuploidy, including trisomy 13, 18, 21; triploidy.

10. **Miscellaneous** (10% of cases). Wilms tumor, angioma, teratoma, neuroblastoma, CNS malformations, amniotic band syndrome, lysosomal storage disorders, glycogen storage disease type II, Gaucher disease, GM1 gangliosidosis, Niemann-Pick disease, congenital myotonic dystrophy, skeletal abnormalities (osteogenesis imperfecta, achondrogenesis, hypophosphatasia, thanatophoric dwarf, arthrogryposis), Noonan syndrome, acardia, absent ductus venosus, renal venous thrombosis, cystic hygroma.

11. **Unknown** (20% of cases).

B. **Diagnosis.** A pregnant woman with polyhydramnios, severe anemia, toxemia, or isoimmune disease should undergo ultrasonic examination of the fetus. If the fetus is hydropic, a careful search by ultrasonography and real-time fetal echocardiography may reveal the cause and guide fetal treatment. The accumulation of pericardial or ascitic fluid may be the first sign of impending hydrops in an Rh-sensitized fetus. Investigations should be carried out for the causes of fetal hydrops mentioned in XI.A. The usual investigation includes the following:

1. **Maternal** blood type and Coombs test, red cell antibody titers, complete blood count (CBC) and RBC indices, hemoglobin electrophoresis, Kleihauer-Betke stain of maternal blood for fetal red cells, tests for syphilis, studies for viral infection, and toxoplasmosis (see Chaps. 48, 50, and 51), sedimentation rate, and lupus tests.

2. **Fetal** echocardiography for cardiac abnormalities and ultrasonography for other structural lesions.

3. **Amniocentesis** for karyotype, metabolic studies, fetoprotein, cultures, and polymerase chain reaction (PCR) for viral infections and restriction endonucleases as indicated.

4. **Doppler** ultrasonographic measurements of peak velocity of blood flow in the fetal middle cerebral artery have good correlation with fetal anemia.

5. **Fetal blood sampling—percutaneous umbilical blood sampling (PUBS)** (see Chap. 1). Karyotype, CBC, hemoglobin electrophoresis, cultures and PCR, DNA studies, and albumin.

6. **Neonatal.** Following delivery, many of the same studies may be carried out on the infant. A CBC, blood typing, and Coombs test; ultrasonographic studies of the head, heart, and abdomen; and a search for the causes listed in XI.A should be done. Examination of pleural and/or ascitic fluid, LFTs, urinalysis, viral titers, chromosomes, placental examination, and x-rays may be indicated. If the infant is stillborn or dies, a detailed autopsy should be performed.

C. **Management**

1. A hydropic fetus is at great risk for intrauterine death. A decision must be made about intrauterine treatment if possible, for example, fetal transfusion in isoimmune hemolytic anemia (see Chap. 1) or maternal digitalis therapy for supraventricular tachycardia (see Chap. 41). If fetal treatment is not possible, the fetus must be evaluated for the relative possibility of intrauterine death versus the risks of premature delivery. If premature delivery is planned, pulmonary maturity should be induced with steroids if it is not present (see Chap. 33). Intrauterine paracentesis or thoracentesis just before delivery may facilitate subsequent newborn resuscitation.

2. Resuscitation of the hydropic infant is complex and requires advance preparation whenever feasible. Intubation can be extremely difficult with massive edema of the head, neck, and oropharynx and should be done by a skilled operator immediately after birth. (A fiberoptic laryngoscope may facilitate placement of the endotracheal tube.) A second individual should provide rapid relief of hydrostatic pressure on the diaphragm and lungs by paracentesis and/or thoracentesis with an 18- to 20-gauge angiocatheter attached to a three-way stopcock and syringe. After entry into the chest or abdominal cavity, the needle is withdrawn so that the plastic catheter can remain without fear of

laceration. Pericardiocentesis may also be required if there is electromechanical dissociation due to cardiac tamponade.

3. Ventilator management can be complicated by pulmonary hypoplasia, barotrauma, pulmonary edema, or reaccumulation of ascites and/or pleural fluid. If repeated thoracenteses cannot control hydrothorax, chest tube drainage may be indicated. Judicious use of diuretics (e.g., furosemide) is often helpful in reducing pulmonary edema. Arterial access is needed to monitor blood gases and acid–base balance.

4. Because hydropic infants have enormous quantities of extravascular salt and water, fluid intake is based on an estimate of the infant's "dry weight" (e.g., 50th percentile for gestational age). Free water and salt are kept at a minimum (e.g., 40–60 mL/kg/day as dextrose water) until edema is resolved. Monitoring the electrolyte composition of serum, urine, ascites fluid, and/or pleural fluid and careful measurement of intake, output, and weight are essential for guiding therapy. Normoglycemia is achieved by providing glucose at a rate of 4 to 8 mg/kg/minute. Unless cardiovascular and/or renal function is compromised, edema will eventually resolve, and salt and water intake can then be normalized.

5. If the hematocrit is <30%, a partial exchange transfusion with 50 to 80 mL/kg PRBCs (hematocrit 70%) should be performed to raise the hematocrit and increase oxygen-carrying capacity. If the problem is Rh isoimmunization, the blood should be type O Rh-negative. We often use O Rh-negative cells and AB serum prepared before delivery and cross-matched against the mother. An isovolumetric exchange (simultaneous removal of blood from the umbilical artery while blood is transfused in the umbilical vein at 2 to 4 mL/kg/minute) may be better tolerated in infants with compromised cardiovascular systems.

6. Inotropic support (e.g., dopamine) may be required to improve cardiac output. Central venous and arterial lines are needed for monitoring pressures. Most hydropic infants are normovolemic, but manipulation of the blood volume may be indicated after measurement of arterial and venous pressures and after correction of acidosis and asphyxia. If a low serum albumin level is contributing to hydrops, fresh frozen plasma may help. Care must be taken not to volume overload an already failing heart; infusions of colloid may need to be followed by a diuretic.

7. Hyperbilirubinemia should be treated as in VI.

8. Many infants with hydrops will survive if aggressive neonatal care is provided.

XII. ISOIMMUNE HEMOLYTIC DISEASE OF THE NEWBORN

A. **Etiology.** Maternal exposure (through blood transfusion, fetomaternal hemorrhage, amniocentesis, or abortion) to foreign antigens on fetal RBCs causes the production and transplacental passage of specific maternal immunoglobulin G (IgG) antibodies directed against the fetal antigens, resulting in the immune destruction of fetal RBCs. The usual antigen involved prenatally is the Rh(D) antigen, and postnatally, the A and B antigens. The frequency of the Rh antigen varies worldwide by region (http://anthro.palomar.edu/vary/vary_3.htm). A positive Coombs test result in an infant should prompt identification of the antibody. If the antibody is not Rh (D), anti-A or anti-B, or known from antibody screening tests, then it should be identified by testing the mother's serum against a panel of red cell antigens or the father's red cells. This may have implications for subsequent pregnancies. Since the dramatic decline in Rh hemolytic disease with the use of Rho(D) immune globulin, maternal antibody against A or B antigens (ABO incompatibility) is now the most common cause of isoimmune hemolytic disease. In addition, other relatively uncommon antigens (Kell, Duffy, E, C, and c) now account for a greater proportion of cases of isoimmune hemolytic anemia (Tables 26.5–26.7). The **Lewis antigen** is a commonly found antigen, but this antigen does not cause hemolytic disease of the newborn. Most Lewis antibodies are of the immunoglobulin M (IgM) class (which do not cross the placenta), and the Lewis antigen is poorly developed and expressed on the fetal and/or neonatal erythrocytes.

B. Neonatal management. About half of the infants with a positive Coombs test result with Rh hemolytic disease will have minimum hemolysis and hyperbilirubinemia (cord bilirubin level <4 mg/dL and hemoglobin level >14 g/dL). These infants may require no treatment or only phototherapy. One-fourth of infants with Rh hemolytic disease present with anemia (hemoglobin level less than 14 g/dL) and hyperbilirubinemia (cord bilirubin greater than 4 mg/dL). They have increased nucleated red cells and reticulocytes on blood smear. These infants may have thrombocytopenia and a very elevated white blood cell count. They have an enlarged liver and spleen and require early exchange transfusion and phototherapy (see VI.B., VII., and VIII.). Figure 26.6 and Tables 26.5–26.7 can be used in deciding what treatment to use. Infants with isoimmune hemolytic anemia may develop an exaggerated physiologic anemia at 12 weeks of age, requiring blood transfusion. Erythropoietin is currently being evaluated for use in preventing late anemia. High-dose intravenous immune γ-globulin therapy 500 to 1,000 mg/kg IV is used for hemolytic disease (see VI.B.2.).

D. Prevention. Eliminating exposure of women to foreign red cell antigens will prevent immune hemolytic disease of the newborn. Avoiding unnecessary transfusions and medical procedures that carry the risk of transplacental passage of blood will help decrease sensitization. Rh hemolytic disease is now being prevented by the administration of **Rho(D) immune globulin** to unsensitized Rh-negative mothers. This is usually done at 28 weeks' gestation and again within 72 hours after delivery. Other indications for Rho(D) immune globulin (or for using larger doses) are prophylaxis following abortion, amniocentesis, chorionic villus sampling, and transplacental hemorrhage. ABO incompatibility between mother and fetus protects against sensitization of an Rh-negative mother, probably because maternal antibodies eliminate fetal RBCs from the maternal circulation before they can encounter antibody-forming lymphocytes.

XIII. ABO HEMOLYTIC DISEASE OF THE NEWBORN. Since the introduction of Rh immune globulin, ABO incompatibility has been the most common cause of hemolytic disease of the newborn in the United States.

A. Etiology. The cause is the reaction of maternal anti-A or anti-B antibodies to the A or B antigen on the RBCs of the fetus or newborn. It is usually seen only in type A or B infants born to type O mothers because these mothers make anti-A or anti-B antibodies of the IgG class, which cross the placenta, whereas mothers of type A or B usually make anti-A or anti-B antibodies of the IgM class, which do not cross the placenta. The combination of a type O mother and a type A or type B infant occurs in 15% of pregnancies in the United States. Only one-fifth of infants with this blood group setup (or 3% of all infants) will develop significant jaundice. Some bacterial vaccines, such as tetanus toxoid and pneumococcal vaccine, had A and B substance in the culture media and were associated with significant hemolysis in type A or type B neonates born to type O mothers who were given these vaccines. New preparations of the vaccine are said to be free of these A and B substances.

B. **Clinical presentation.** The typical presentation is a type O mother with a type A or type B infant who becomes jaundiced in the first 24 hours of life. Approximately 50% of the cases occur in firstborn infants. There is no predictable pattern of recurrence in subsequent infants. **Most ABO-incompatible infants have anti-A or anti-B antibody on their RBCs, yet only a small number have significant ABO hemolytic disease of the newborn.** Infants may have a low concentration of antibody on their red cells; consequently, their antibody will not be demonstrated by elution techniques or by a positive direct antiglobulin test (Coombs test). As the antibody concentration increases, the antibody can be demonstrated first by elution techniques and then by the Coombs test. Although all ABO-incompatible infants have some degree of hemolysis, significant hemolysis is usually associated only with a positive direct Coombs test result on the infant's red cells. If there are other causes of neonatal jaundice, ABO incompatibility will add to the bilirubin production. In infants with significant ABO incompatibility, there will be many spherocytes on the blood smear and an elevated reticulocyte count. RBCs from infants with ABO incompatibility may have increased osmotic fragility and autohemolysis, as in HS. The autohemolysis is not corrected by glucose, as in HS. The family history, long-term course, and MCHC will usually help with the diagnosis of HS (see III.E.3.).

C. **Management.** Most infants with ABO incompatibility do not develop significant jaundice. Approximately 10% of these infants with a positive direct Coombs test will need phototherapy. See sections III.E.2. and VI.B. above for evaluation and management.

Suggested Readings

American Academy of Pediatrics Subcommittee on Hyperbilirubinemia. Management of hyperbilirubinemia in the newborn infant 35 or more weeks of gestation. *Pediatrics* 2004;114:297–316.

Fallon EM, Le HD, Puder M. Prevention of parenteral nutrition-associated liver disease: role of omega-3 fish oil. *Curr Opin Organ Transplant* 2010;15(3):334–340.

Maisels MJ, Bhutani VK, Bogen D, et al. Hyperbilirubinemia in the newborn infant ≥ 35 weeks' gestation: an update with clarifications. *Pediatrics* 2009;124:1193–1198.

Maisels MJ, McDonagh AF. Phototherapy for neonatal jaundice. *N Eng J Med* 2008;358: 920–928.

Necrotizing Enterocolitis

Muralidhar H. Premkumar

I. BACKGROUND. NECROTIZING ENTEROCOLITIS (NEC) is the most common gastrointestinal (GI) emergency of the neonate. Its pathogenesis is complex and multifactorial, and etiology unclear. In spite of the advances in neonatology over the last few decades, the mortality and morbidity secondary to NEC remains high. Current clinical practice is directed mainly toward prompt, early diagnosis and institution of proper intensive care management.

A. **Epidemiology.** NEC is the most common serious surgical disorder among infants in a neonatal intensive care unit (NICU) and is a significant cause of neonatal morbidity and mortality.

1. The **incidence** of NEC varies from center to center and from year to year within centers. There are endemic and epidemic occurrences. An estimated 0.3 to 2.4 cases occur in every 1,000 live births. In most centers, NEC occurs in 2% to 5% of all NICU admissions and 5% to 10% of very low birth weight (VLBW) infants. If VLBW infants who die early are excluded and only infants who have been fed included, the incidence is approximately 15%.

2. Sex, race, geography, climate, and season do not appear to play any determining role in the incidence or course of NEC.

3. **Prematurity** is the single greatest risk factor. Decreasing gestational age is associated with an increased risk of NEC. The mean gestational age of infants with NEC is 30 to 32 weeks, and the infants generally are weight appropriate for gestational age. Approximately 10% of infants with NEC are full term. The postnatal age at onset is inversely related to birth weight and gestational age, with a mean age at onset of 12 days.

4. Enteral feeding is perhaps the next greatest risk factor. More than 90% of infants have been fed before the onset of this disease. In the extremely premature infants, the risk is least with infants who are exclusively breast-fed, and any kind of exposure to bovine milk–based products may increase the risk of NEC.

5. Similar to the effect on the lungs, antenatal steroids have been shown to improve the maturity of the GI tract. Randomized controlled trials performed even before the widespread use of antenatal steroids have shown reduced incidence of NEC among the infants treated with antenatal steroids.

6. Infants exposed to cocaine have a 2.5 times increased risk of developing NEC. The vasoconstrictive and hemodynamic properties of cocaine may promote intestinal ischemia (see Chap. 12).

7. The overall **mortality** is 9% to 28% regardless of surgical or medical intervention. The mortality for infants weighing <1,500 g can be as high as 45%; for those weighing <750 g, it may be much higher. The introduction of standardized therapeutic protocols with criteria for medical management and surgical

intervention, a high index of suspicion for the disease, and general improvements in neonatal intensive care have decreased the mortality rate. Infants exposed to cocaine who develop NEC have a significantly higher incidence of massive gangrene, perforation, and mortality than do infants not exposed.

8. Case-controlled epidemiologic studies have revealed that almost all previously described risk factors for NEC, including maternal disorders (e.g., toxemia), the infant's course (e.g., asphyxia, patent ductus arteriosus [PDA]), and the type of management (e.g., umbilical artery catheterization [UAC]), simply describe a population of high-risk neonates. Apart from prematurity, exposure to artificial formula feeds, and cocaine exposure, no maternal or neonatal factors are known to increase the risk of NEC. This suggests that immaturity of the GI tract is the greatest risk factor.

9. Although NEC is primarily a disease of preterm infants, term infants also are rarely affected. The incidence of NEC in term infants is 1 in 20,000 live births. Some authors believe that NEC in term infants is a different disease process compared to that in preterm infants, displaying a more definite association with splanchnic hypoperfusion. Those term infants in whom NEC develops commonly have other risk factors such as congenital heart disease, polycythemia, sepsis, hypotension, and asphyxia.

B. Pathogenesis

1. The pathogenesis of NEC is not well defined. NEC is a multifactorial disease resulting from complex interactions between immaturity, mucosal injury secondary to a variety of factors (including ischemia, luminal substrate, and infection), and poor host work response to injury.

2. The concept of a **hypoxic or hemodynamic insult**, resulting in splanchnic vasoconstriction and reduced mesenteric flow, inducing bowel mucosal hypoxia, and rendering the intestine susceptible to injury, has long been considered a contributing factor in the pathogenesis of NEC. The pathologic findings of NEC resemble those seen in older individuals with gut vascular compromise. However, in a significant number of cases, no hypoxic or ischemic problems can be identified, and the temporal sequence of events does not support an ischemic event alone.

3. **Enteral feedings** have been implicated in the pathogenesis of NEC, as almost all babies who develop NEC have been fed. Factors that have been considered include osmolality of formula, the lack of immunoprotective factors in formula, and the timing, volume, and rate of feeding. Breast milk has been shown to have protective factors. Although breast milk alone does not prevent development of NEC in extremely premature infants, exclusive human milk diet in contrast to a combination of mother's milk and bovine-based products has shown to reduce the rates of NEC and surgical NEC. Some case control studies suggest judicious introduction of feedings and avoidance of large day-to-day volume increases may lower the incidence of NEC. However, the rate of daily feeding increment that may protect infants from developing NEC has not been identified, and the mechanism by which larger volumes may predispose to the development of NEC is not known. It has been shown that adoption of standardized feeding regimen, dictating the advance of feedings in the VLBW population, and strict adherence to it reduce the risk of NEC by up to 87% despite heterogeneity of the feeding regimens used.

4. The **microbiologic flora** involved in NEC is not unique but represents the predominant bowel organisms present in the infant at the time of onset.

Various bacterial and viral agents have been reported in the microbial picture that is sometimes associated with NEC, especially with epidemic NEC, but none has yet been proved to be causal. Most often, it simply represents the gut flora translocating the compromised gut barrier. Release of endotoxin and cytokines by proliferation of colonizing bacteria, and bacterial fermentation with gaseous distension, may play a role as well. Presence of bacteria is likely important in the pathogenesis of NEC, since antenatal intestinal ischemia when the gut is in a sterile environment results in stenosis and not NEC.

5. Evidence supports a critical role for inflammatory mediators. **Platelet activating factor** (PAF), endotoxin lipopolysaccharide (LPS), tumor necrosis factor *a* (TNF-*a*), interleukins, and nitric oxide are some of the inflammatory mediators that have been suspected to have a role in the pathophysiology of NEC. Both animal studies and samples from human infants demonstrate the association of elevated levels of PAF in infants with NEC compared with those without. In animal models, exogenous administration of PAF mimics NEC-like injury and PAF antagonists limit such injury. The discovery of the roles of several inflammatory mediators points to the multifactorial etiology of the disease and underlines the fact that not one but several strategies are necessary for the prevention of NEC. Improved understanding of the role inflammation and pro-inflammatory mediators play in the development of NEC is needed before devising strategies to either limit or prevent this inflammatory cascade.

6. **Histopathologic examination** of tissue after surgery or autopsy shows that the terminal ileum and ascending colon are the most frequently involved areas, but in the most severe cases, the entire bowel may be involved. This localization has implications for long-term sequelae (see IV.). The pathologic lesions consist of coagulation necrosis, bacterial overgrowth, inflammation, and reparative changes.

7. Use of **H2 blockers** have been implicated in a higher risk of NEC in extremely low birth weight (ELBW) infants, suggesting that an acidic GI environment may be protective.

8. Several studies have suggested a temporal association of packed red blood cell (PRBC) transfusions with the onset of NEC. Hypothesized mechanisms include T cell activation, immune-mediated hemolysis, and splanchnic vasoconstriction associated with the transfusion. However, a consistent description of risk factors such as gestation, severity of anemia, or the stability of the infant prior to the transfusion is lacking, thereby making it difficult to institute evidence-based transfusion guidelines.

II. DIAGNOSIS. Early diagnosis of NEC may be an important factor in determining outcome. This is accomplished by a high index of suspicion and careful clinical observation for signs in infants at risk.

A. **Clinical characteristics.** There is a broad spectrum of disease manifestations. The clinical features of NEC can be divided into systemic and abdominal signs. Most infants have a combination of both, although abdominal signs usually predominate.

1. **Systemic signs.** Respiratory distress, apnea and/or bradycardia, lethargy, temperature instability, irritability, poor feeding, hypotension (shock), decreased peripheral perfusion, acidosis, oliguria, or bleeding diathesis.

2. **Abdominal (enteric) signs.** Abdominal distension or tenderness, gastric aspirates (feeding residuals), vomiting (of bile, blood, or both), ileus (decreased or

absent bowel sounds), bloody stools, abdominal wall erythema or induration, persistent localized abdominal mass, or ascites.

3. The **course of the disease** varies among infants. Most frequently, it will appear (i) as a fulminant, rapidly progressive presentation of signs consistent with intestinal necrosis and sepsis or (ii) as a slow, paroxysmal presentation of abdominal distension, ileus, and possible infection. The latter course will vary with the rapidity of therapeutic intervention and require consistent monitoring and anticipatory evaluation (see III.).

B. **Laboratory features.** The diagnosis is suspected from clinical presentation but must be confirmed by diagnostic radiographs, surgery, or autopsy. No laboratory tests are specific for NEC; nevertheless, some tests are valuable in confirming diagnostic impressions.

1. **Radiology studies.** The abdominal radiograph will often reveal an abnormal gas pattern consistent with ileus. Both anteroposterior (AP) and cross-table lateral or left lateral decubitus views should be included. These films may reveal bowel wall edema, a fixed position loop on serial studies, the appearance of a mass, pneumatosis intestinalis (the radiologic hallmark used to confirm the diagnosis), portal or hepatic venous air, pneumobilia, or pneumoperitoneum taking the appearance of gas under the diaphragm. Isolated intestinal perforation (IP) may present with pneumoperitoneum without other clinical signs.

2. **Blood and serum studies.** Thrombocytopenia, persistent metabolic acidosis, and severe refractory hyponatremia constitute the most common triad of signs. Serial measurements of C-reactive protein (CRP) may also be helpful in the diagnosis and assessment of response to therapy of severe NEC. Blood cultures may reveal bacteremia with a pathogenic organism.

3. **Analysis of stool** for blood has been used to detect infants with NEC based on changes in intestinal integrity. Although grossly bloody stools may be an indication of NEC, occult hematochezia does not correlate well with NEC, and routine testing of stool for occult blood is not recommended.

C. **Bell staging criteria** with the Walsh and Kleigman modification allow for uniformity of diagnosis across centers. Bell staging is not a continuum; babies may present with advanced NEC without earlier signs or symptoms.

1. **Stage I** (suspect) clinical signs and symptoms, including abdominal signs and nondiagnostic radiographs

2. **Stage II** (definite) clinical signs and symptoms, pneumatosis intestinalis, and portal venous gas on radiograph
   a. Mildly ill
   b. Moderately ill with systemic toxicity

3. **Stage III** (advanced) clinical signs and symptoms, pneumatosis intestinalis on radiograph, and critically ill
   a. Impending IP
   b. Proven IP

D. **Differential diagnosis**

1. **Pneumonia and sepsis** are common and frequently associated with an intestinal ileus. The abdominal tenderness characteristic of NEC will be absent in infants with ileus not due to NEC.

2. **Surgical abdominal catastrophes** include malrotation with obstruction (complete or intermittent), malrotation with midgut volvulus, intussusception, ulcer, gastric perforation, and mesenteric vessel thrombosis. The clinical presentation of these disorders may overlap with that of NEC. Occasionally, the diagnosis is made only at the time of exploratory laparotomy (see Chap. 62).

3. **Isolated IP** is a distinct clinical entity that occurs in approximately 2% of ELBW infants. It often presents as asymptomatic pneumoperitoneum, although other clinical and laboratory abnormalities may be present. IP tends to occur at an earlier postnatal age than NEC and is not associated with feeding. The risk of IP is increased with early glucocorticoid exposure and indomethacin treatment for PDA. Concurrent treatment with glucocorticoids and indomethacin increases the risk of IP.

4. **Infectious enterocolitis** is rare in this population but must be considered if diarrhea is present. *Campylobacter* species have been associated with bloody diarrhea in the newborn. These infants lack any other systemic or enteric signs of NEC.

5. Severe forms of **inherited metabolic disease** (e.g., galactosemia with *Escherichia coli* sepsis) may lead to profound acidosis, shock, and vomiting and may initially overlap with some signs of NEC.

6. Severe **allergic colitis** can present with abdominal distension and bloody stools. Usually these infants are well appearing and have normal abdominal radiographs and laboratory studies.

7. **Feeding intolerance** is a common but ill-defined problem in premature infants. Despite adequate GI function *in utero*, some premature infants will have periods of gastric residuals and abdominal distension associated with advancing feedings. The differentiation of this problem from NEC can be difficult. Cautious evaluation by withholding enteral feedings and administering parenteral nutrition (PN) and antibiotics for 48 to 72 hours may be indicated until this benign disorder can be distinguished from NEC. Serial monitoring of CRP can sometimes help in distinguishing this from NEC.

E. **Additional diagnostic considerations**

1. Since the early abdominal signs may be nonspecific, at present, **a high index of suspicion** is the most reliable approach to early diagnosis. Attempts at identifying biomarkers that might allow early identification of an infant with NEC have been largely unsuccessful. The entire picture of history, physical examination, and laboratory features must be considered in the context of the particular infant's course. Isolated signs or laboratory values often indicate the need for a careful differential diagnosis, despite the obvious concern over NEC.

2. **Diarrhea** is an uncommon presentation of NEC in the absence of bloody stools. This sign should point away from NEC.

3. **Radiographic findings** can often be subtle and confusing. For example, perforation of an abdominal viscus will not always cause pneumoperitoneum, and conversely, pneumoperitoneum does not necessarily indicate abdominal perforation from NEC. Serial review of the radiographs with a pediatric radiologist is indicated to assist in interpretation and to plan for further appropriate studies.

III. MANAGEMENT

A. Immediate medical management (Table 27.1). Treatment should begin promptly when a diagnosis of NEC is suspected. Therapy is based on intensive care measures and the anticipation of potential problems.

1. Respiratory function. Rapid assessment of ventilatory status (physical examination, arterial blood gases) should be made, and supplemental oxygen and mechanical ventilatory support should be provided as needed.

Table 27.1	Management of Necrotizing Enterocolitis	
Bell staging criteria	**Diagnosis**	**Management (usual attention to respiratory, cardiovascular, and hematologic resuscitation presumed)**
Stage I (suspect)	Clinical signs and symptoms Nondiagnostic radiograph	NPO with IV fluids Nasogastric drainage CBC, lytes, abdominal radiograph q6–8 h × 48 h Blood culture Stool heme test and Clinitest Ampicillin and gentamicin × 48 hours
Stage II (definite)	Clinical signs and symptoms Pneumatosis intestinalis on radiograph	NPO with parenteral nutrition (by CVL once sepsis ruled out) Nasogastric drainage CBC, lytes, abdominal radiograph (AP and lateral) q6–8 h × 48–72 h, then prn Blood culture Stool heme test and Clinitest Ampicillin, gentamicin, and clindamycin × 14 days Surgical consultation
Stage III (advanced)	Clinical signs and symptoms	NPO with parenteral nutrition (by CVL once sepsis ruled out)
	Critically ill	Nasogastric drainage
	Pneumatosis intestinalis or pneumo-peritoneum on radiograph	CBC, lytes, abdominal radiograph (AP and lateral) q6–8 h × 48–72 h, then prn Stool heme test and Clinitest Ampicillin, gentamicin, and clindamycin × 14 days Surgical consultation with intervention, if indicated: Resection with enterostomy or primary anastomosis In selected cases (usually <1,000 g and unstable), bedside drainage under local anesthesia

AP = anteroposterior; CBC = complete blood count, CVL = central venous line; NPO = nothing by mouth; prn = as needed.

2. **Cardiovascular function.** Assessment of circulatory status (physical examination, blood pressure) should be made, and circulatory support provided as needed. Volume in the form of normal saline, fresh frozen plasma, or packed red cells (dose 10 mL/kg) may be used if circulatory volume is compromised. Pharmacologic support may be necessary; in this case, we use low doses of dopamine (3–5 μ/kg per minute) to optimize the effect on splanchnic and renal blood flow; however, higher doses may be necessary to ensure adequate blood pressure and tissue perfusion. Impending circulatory collapse will often be reflected by poor perfusion and oxygenation, although arterial blood pressure may be maintained. Intra-arterial blood pressure monitoring is often necessary, but the proximity of the umbilical arteries to the mesenteric circulation precludes the use of these vessels. In fact, any umbilical artery catheter should be promptly removed and peripheral artery catheters alternatively used if needed. Further monitoring of central venous pressure (CVP) may become necessary if additional pharmacologic support of the circulation or failing myocardium is needed (see Chap. 40).

3. **Metabolic function.** Metabolic acidosis will generally respond to volume expansion. Sodium bicarbonate should be reserved for severe metabolic acidosis (dose 1–2 mEq/kg). The blood pH and lactate level should be monitored; in addition, serum electrolyte levels, blood glucose, and liver function should be measured.

4. **Nutrition.** All GI feedings are discontinued, and the bowel is decompressed by suctioning through a nasogastric or orogastric tube. PN is given through a peripheral vein as soon as possible, with the aim of providing 90 to 110 cal/kg per day once amino acid solutions and Intralipid are both tolerated. A central venous catheter is almost always necessary to provide adequate calories in the VLBW infant. We wait to place a central catheter for this purpose until the blood cultures are negative, during which time adaptation to peripheral PN can take place (see Chap. 21).

5. **Infectious disease.** Blood, urine, stool, and cerebrospinal fluid (CSF) specimens are obtained, examined carefully for indications of infection, and sent for culture and sensitivities. We routinely begin broad-spectrum antibiotics as soon as possible, utilizing ampicillin, gentamicin, and clindamycin to cover most enteric flora. Piperacillin-tazobactam (Zosyn) has recently been used due to its broad spectrum and the ability to be used as a single agent. With changing antibiotic sensitivities, one must be aware of the predominant local NICU flora, the organisms associated with NEC and their resistance patterns, and adjust antibiotic coverage accordingly. Antibiotic therapy is adjusted on the basis of culture results, but only 10% to 40% of blood cultures will be positive, necessitating continued broad-spectrum coverage in most cases. In infants requiring surgery, peritoneal fluid cultures may also help target appropriate antibiotic treatment. Treatment is generally maintained for 14 days. There is no evidence to support the use of enteral antibiotics.

6. **Hematologic aspects.** Analysis of the complete blood count and differential, with examination of the blood smear, is always indicated. We use platelet transfusions to correct severe thrombocytopenia and PRBCs to maintain the hematocrit above 35%. The prothrombin time, partial thromboplastin time, fibrinogen, and platelet count should be evaluated for evidence of disseminated intravascular coagulation. Fresh frozen plasma is used to treat coagulation problems (see Chap. 42).

7. **Renal function.** Oliguria often accompanies the initial hypotension and hypoperfusion of NEC; measurement of urine output is essential. In addition, serum blood urea nitrogen (BUN), creatinine, and serum electrolyte levels should be monitored. Impending renal failure from acute tubular necrosis, coagulative necrosis, or vascular accident must be anticipated, and fluid therapy adjusted accordingly (see Chap. 28).

8. **Neurologic function.** Evaluation of the infant's condition may be difficult given the degree of illness, but one must be alert to the problems of associated meningitis and intraventricular hemorrhage. Seizures may occur secondary to either meningitis, intraventricular hemorrhage (IVH), or from the metabolic perturbations associated with NEC. These complications must be anticipated and promptly recognized and treated.

9. **GI function.** Physical examination and serial (every 6–8 hours during the first 2–3 days) radiographs are used to assess ongoing GI damage. Unless perforation occurs or full-thickness necrosis precipitates severe peritonitis, management remains medical. The evaluation for surgical intervention, however, is an important and complex management issue (see III.B.).

10. **Family support.** Any family of an infant in the NICU may be overwhelmed by the crisis. Infants with NEC present a particular challenge because the disease often causes sudden deterioration for "no apparent reason." Furthermore, the impending possibility of surgical intervention and the high mortality and uncertain prognosis make this situation most difficult for parents. Careful anticipatory sharing of information must be utilized by the staff to establish a trusting alliance with the family.

B. **Surgical intervention (see Chap. 62)**

1. **Prompt early consultation** should be obtained with a pediatric surgeon. This will allow the surgeon to become familiar with the infant and will provide an additional evaluation by another skilled individual. If a pediatric surgeon is not available, the infant should be transferred to a site where one is.

2. **GI perforation** is a generally agreed-upon indication for surgical intervention. Unfortunately, there is no reliable or absolute indicator of imminent perforation; therefore, frequent monitoring is necessary. Perforation occurs in 20% to 30% of patients, usually 12 to 48 hours after the onset of NEC, although it can occur later. In some cases, the absence of pneumoperitoneum on the abdominal radiograph can delay the diagnosis, and paracentesis may aid in establishing the diagnosis. In general, an infant with increasing abdominal distension, an abdominal mass, a worsening clinical picture despite medical management, or a persistent fixed loop on serial radiographs may have a perforation and may require operative intervention.

3. **Full-thickness necrosis of the GI tract** may require surgical intervention, although this diagnosis is difficult to establish in the absence of perforation. In most cases, the infant with bowel necrosis will have signs of peritonitis, such as ascites, abdominal mass, abdominal wall erythema, induration, persistent thrombocytopenia, progressive shock from third-space losses, or refractory metabolic acidosis. Paracentesis may help to identify these patients before perforation occurs.

4. The mainstay of **surgical treatment** is resection with enterostomy, although resection with primary reanastomosis is sometimes used in selected cases. At surgery, the goal is to excise necrotic bowel while preserving as much bowel

length as possible. Peritoneal fluid is examined for signs of infection and sent for culture, necrotic bowel is resected and sent for pathologic confirmation, and viable bowel ends are exteriorized as stomas. All sites of diseased bowel are noted, whether or not removal is indicated. If there is extensive involvement, a "second look" operation may be done within 24 to 48 hours to determine whether any areas that appeared necrotic are actually viable. The length and areas of removed bowel are recorded. If large areas are resected, the length and position of the remaining bowel are noted, as this will affect the long-term outcome. In approximately 14% of infants with this condition, NEC totalis (bowel necrosis from duodenum to rectum) is found. In these cases, mortality is almost certain.

5. In ELBW infants (<1,000 g) and extremely unstable infants, **peritoneal drainage** under local anesthesia may be a management option. In many cases, this temporizes laparotomy until the infant is more stable, and in some cases, no further operative procedure is required. A recent multicenter cohort study comparing laparotomy versus peritoneal drainage in NEC with perforation showed no significant differences in survival or need for long-term total PN between the two procedures. However, some studies have suggested worse long-term neurodevelopmental outcome in infants with NEC treated with peritoneal drains alone, perhaps representing the infants who were too sick to undergo laparotomy. Optimal surgical therapy still remains controversial.

C. **Long-term management.** Once the infant has been stabilized and effectively treated, feedings can be reintroduced. We generally begin this process after 2 weeks of treatment by stopping gastric decompression. If infants can tolerate their own secretions, feedings are begun very slowly while parenteral alimentation is gradually tapered. No conclusive data are available on the best method or type of feeding, but breast milk may be better tolerated and is preferred. The occurrence of strictures may complicate feeding plans. The incidence of recurrent NEC is 4% and appears to be independent of type of management. Recurrent disease should be treated as before and will generally respond similarly. If surgical intervention was required and an ileostomy or colostomy was created, intestinal reanastomosis can be electively undertaken after an adequate period of healing. If an infant tolerates enteral feedings, reanastomosis may be performed after a period of growth at home. However, earlier surgical intervention may be indicated in infants who cannot be advanced to full-volume or strength feedings because of malabsorption and intestinal dumping. Before reanastomosis, a contrast study of the distal bowel is obtained to establish the presence of a stricture that can be resected at the time of ostomy closure.

IV. **PROGNOSIS.** Few detailed and accurate studies are available on prognosis. In uncomplicated cases of NEC, the long-term prognosis may be comparable with that of other low birth weight infants; however, those with stage IIB and stage III NEC have a higher incidence of mortality (of over 50%), growth delay (delay in growth of head circumference is of most concern), and poor neurodevelopmental outcome. NEC requiring surgical intervention may have more serious sequelae, including mortality secondary to infection, respiratory failure, PN-associated hepatic disease (see Chap. 26), rickets, and significant developmental delay.

A. **Sequelae** of NEC can be directly related to the disease process or to the long-term NICU management often necessary to treat it. GI sequelae include strictures, enteric fistulas, short bowel syndrome, malabsorption and chronic diarrhea, dumping syndromes related to loss of terminal ileum and ileocecal valve, fluid and electrolyte losses with rapid dehydration, and hepatitis or cholestasis related to long-term PN. Strictures occur in 25% to 35% of patients with or without surgery and are most common in the large bowel. However, not all strictures are clinically significant, and may not preclude advancement to full feeding volumes. Short bowel syndrome occurs in approximately 10% to 20% following surgical treatment. Metabolic sequelae include failure to thrive, metabolic bone disease, and problems related to central nervous system (CNS) function in the VLBW infant. Studies have shown that infants with NEC are at a higher risk of impaired neurodevelopmental outcome.

B. Prevention of NEC is the ultimate goal. Unfortunately, this can best be accomplished only by preventing premature birth. If prematurity cannot be avoided, several preventive strategies may be of benefit.

1. **Induction of GI maturation.** The incidence of NEC is significantly reduced after prenatal steroid therapy.

2. **Exclusive feeding of human milk–based diet.** Premature infants who are fed exclusively with expressed human milk are at decreased risk for developing NEC. Mothers should be strongly encouraged to provide expressed milk for their premature babies when able; the role of donor human milk has not been adequately studied.

3. **Optimization of enteral feedings** (see Chap. 21). Because of the lack of adequately sized randomized trials in ELBW infants, currently there is not enough evidence to support either early versus delayed feedings, or an optimum rate of advancement of feedings. However, from the available evidence, it is clear that adoption and strict adherence to a particular standardized feeding regimen significantly reduces the risk of NEC; therefore, individual NICUs should agree on a feeding regimen and monitor adherence.

4. **Enterally fed probiotics** are a promising new approach to the prevention of NEC. Probiotics fed to preterm infants may help to normalize intestinal microflora colonization. A recent meta-analysis has shown reduced incidence of NEC by over 50% in infants fed probiotics (e.g., *Lactobacillus GG, Bifidobacterium breve, Saccharomyces boulardii, Lactobacillus acidophilus*) compared with controls. Until further evidence is available to help determine the most effective probiotic(s), their optimum dosage, and long and short-term safety, the use of probiotics in the prevention and treatment of NEC should be confined to carefully monitored trials.

Suggested Readings

Deshpande G, Rao S, Patole S, Bulsara M. Updated meta-analysis of probiotics for preventing necrotizing enterocolitis in preterm neonates. *Pediatrics* 2010;125(5):921–930.

Patole S, de Klerk N. Impact of standardised feeding regimens on incidence of neonatal necrotising enterocolitis: a systematic review and meta-analysis of observational studies. *Arch Dis Child Fetal Neonatal Ed* 2005;90(2):F147–F151.

Sullivan S, Schanler RJ, Kim JH, et al. An exclusively human milk-based diet is associated with a lower rate of necrotizing enterocolitis than a diet of human milk and bovine milk-based products. *J Pediatr* 2010;156(4):562–567.e1.

28 Renal Conditions
David J. Askenazi and Stuart L. Goldstein

Renal problems in the neonate may be the result of specific inherited developmental abnormalities or the result of acquired events either in the prenatal or postnatal period. For this reason, evaluation includes a detailed review of the history (family history, gestational history, and the neonatal events) as well as a review of the presenting clinical features and relevant laboratory/radiologic findings. An understanding of the developmental process and the differences in renal physiology in the neonatal period compared to that at later ages is necessary for evaluation.

I. RENAL EMBRYOGENESIS AND FUNCTIONAL DEVELOPMENT

A. Embryology

1. Three paired renal systems develop from the nephrogenic ridge of the mesoderm.

2. The first two systems, the **pronephros** and the **mesonephros**, have limited function in the human being and are transient. The mesonephric tubules and duct form the efferent ductules of the epididymis, the vas deferens, the ejaculatory ducts, and the seminal vesicles in men. In women, they result in the vestigial epoophoron and the paroophoron.

3. The **metanephros** is the third and final excretory system and appears in the fifth week of gestation. The metanephros is made up of two different cell types. These differentiate into the **pelvicalyceal** system, which is well delineated by the 13th or 14th week, and the **nephrons,** which continue to form up to the 34th week of gestation to a final complement of 1 million nephrons per kidney. Urine is produced by the 12th week.

4. Parallel development of the lower urinary tract occurs with opening of the mesonephric duct to the allantois and cloaca at 5 weeks gestation. Shortly thereafter, at 6 weeks, the urorectal fold forms as a septum dividing the gastrointestinal (GI) tract (posterior compartment) from the anterior genitourinary (GU) compartment—the urogenital sinus. At 7 weeks, separate vesicoureteral openings form and the allantois degenerates to a cord that becomes the urachus and the upper bladder, although the trigone develops from the Wolffian duct remnant. Müllerian system development produces a ureterovaginal cord, which in women becomes the vaginal vestibule, vagina, and uterine cervix. In men, müllerian system regression leads to the prostatic urethra.

5. Disruption of normal renal development may lead to renal malformations, such as renal agenesis, renal hypoplasia, renal ectopy, renal dysplasia, and cystic disease.

B. Functional development.
At birth, the kidney replaces the placenta as the major homeostatic organ, maintaining fluid and electrolyte balance and removing harmful waste products. This transition occurs with changes in renal blood flow (RBF),

glomerular filtration rate (GFR), and tubular functions. The level of renal function relates more closely to the postnatal age than to the gestational age at birth.

1. **RBF** remains low in the fetus, accounting for only 2% to 3% of cardiac output. At birth, RBF rapidly increases to 15% to 18% of cardiac output because of (i) a decrease in renal vascular resistance, which is proportionally greater in the kidney compared to other organs; (ii) an increase in systemic blood pressure; and (iii) an increase in inner to outer cortical blood flow.

2. **Glomerular filtration** begins soon after the first nephrons are formed and GFR increases in parallel with body and kidney growth (approximately 1 mL/min/kg of body weight). Once all the glomeruli are formed by 34 weeks' gestation, the GFR continues to increase until birth because of decreases in renal vascular resistance. GFR is less well autoregulated in the neonate. It is controlled by maintenance of glomerular capillary pressure by the greater vasoconstrictive effect of angiotensin II at the efferent then afferent arteriole where the effect is attenuated by concurrent prostaglandin-induced vasodilatation.

   GFR at birth is lower in the most premature and after birth rises dependent on the degree of prematurity. In term babies, GFR rises quickly, doubling by 2 weeks of age and reaching adult levels by 1 year of age and similar values are eventually reached by premature infants (Table 28.5).

3. **Tubular function**
   a. Sodium (Na^+) handling. The ability to reabsorb Na^+ is developed by 24 weeks' gestation. However, tubular resorption of Na^+ is low until 34 weeks gestation. This is important when evaluating the infant for prerenal azotemia, as they will be unable to reabsorb sodium maximally and thus will have elevated fractional excretion of sodium (FeNa; see Table 28.1). Very premature infants cannot conserve Na^+ even when Na^+ balance is negative. Hence, premature infants below 34 weeks' gestation receiving formula or breast milk without Na^+ supplementation can develop hyponatremia. After 34 weeks' gestation, Na^+ reabsorption becomes more efficient, so that 99% of filtered Na^+

Table 28.1	Commonly Used Equations and Formulas
$CrCl \ (mL/min/1.73 \ m^2) = K \times Length \ (cm)/P_{Cr}$	
$CrCl \ (mL/min/1.73 \ m^2) = U_{Cr} \times U_{vol} \times 1.73/P_{Cr} \times BSA$	
$FeNa = 100 \times (U_{Na^+} \times P_{Cr})/(P_{Na^+} \times U_{Cr})$	
$TRP = 100 \times (1 - ((U_P \times P_{Cr})/(P_P \times U_{Cr})))$	
Calculated $P_{osm} \geq 2 \times plasma \ [Na^+] + [glucose]/18 + BUN/2.8$	
Plasma anion gap $= [Na^+] - [Cl^-] - [HCO_3^-]$	
BSA = body surface area; CrCl = creatinine clearance; FeNa = fractional excretion of sodium; P_{Cr} = plasma creatinine; P_{osm} = plasma osmolarity; P_{Na} = plasma sodium; TRP = tubular reabsorption of phosphorus; U_{Cr} = urinary creatinine; U_{vol} = urinary volume per minute.	

can be reabsorbed, resulting in an FeNa of <1% if challenged with renal hypoperfusion. Full-term neonates can retain Na^+ when in negative Na^+ balance but, like premature infants, are also limited in their ability to excrete a Na^+ load because of their low GFR.

b. Water handling. The newborn infant has a limited ability to concentrate urine due to limited urea concentration within the interstitium because of low protein intake and anabolic growth. The resulting decreased osmolality of the interstitium leads to a decreased capacity to reabsorb water and concentrating ability of the neonatal kidney. The maximal urine osmolality is 500 mOsm/L in premature infants and 800 mOsm/L in term infants. Although this is of little consequence in infants receiving appropriate amounts of water with hypotonic feeding, it can become clinically relevant in infants receiving high osmotic loads. In contrast, both premature and full-term infants can dilute their urine with a minimal urine osmolality of 25 to 35 mOsm/L. Their low GFR, however, limits their ability to handle water loads.

c. Potassium (K^+) handling. The limited ability of premature infants to excrete large K^+ loads is related to decreased distal tubular K^+ secretion, a result of decreased aldosterone sensitivity, low $Na^+ - K^+$ adenosine triphosphatase (ATPase) activity, and low GFR.

d. Acid and bicarbonate handling are limited by a low serum bicarbonate threshold in the proximal tubule (14–16 mEq/L in premature infants, 18–21 mEq/L in full-term infants), which improves as maturation of $Na^+ - K^+$ ATPase and Na^+–H transporter occurs. In addition, the production of ammonia in the distal tubule and proximal tubular glutamine synthesis are decreased. The lower rate of phosphate excretion limits the generation of titratable acid, further limiting their ability to eliminate an acid load. Very low birth weight infants can develop mild metabolic acidosis during the second to fourth week after birth that may require administration of additional sodium bicarbonate.

e. Calcium and phosphorous handling in the neonate is characterized by a pattern of increased phosphate retention associated with growth. The intake and filtered load of phosphate, parathyroid hormone (PTH), and growth factors modulate phosphate transport. The higher phosphate level and higher rate of phosphate reabsorption are not explained by a low GFR or tubular unresponsiveness to extrarenal factors (PTH, vitamin D). More likely, there is a developmental mechanism that favors renal conservation of phosphate, in part, due to growth hormone effects, as well as a growth-related Na^+-dependent phosphate transporter, so that a positive phosphate balance for growth is maintained. Tubular reabsorption of phosphate (TRP) is also altered by gestational age, increasing from 85% at 28 weeks to 93% at 34 weeks and 98% by 40 weeks.

Calcium levels in the fetus and cord blood are higher than those in the neonate. Calcium levels fall in the first 24 hours, but low levels of PTH persist. This relative hypoparathyroidism in the first few days after birth may be the result of this physiologic response to hypercalcemia in the normal fetus. Although plasma Ca^+ values <8 mg/dL in premature infants are common, they are usually asymptomatic, because the ionized calcium level is usually normal. Factors that favor this normal ionized Ca^+ fraction include lower serum albumin and the relative metabolic acidosis in the neonate.

Urinary calcium excretion is lower in premature infants and correlates with gestational age. At term, calcium excretion rises and persists until approximately 96 months of age. The urine calcium excretion in premature infants varies directly with $Na+$ intake, urinary $Na+$ excretion, and inversely with plasma Ca^2+. Neonatal stress and therapies such as aggressive fluid use or furosemide administration increase Ca^2+ excretion, aggravating the tendency to hypocalcemia.

4. Fetal urine contribution to amniotic fluid volume is minimal (10 mL/hour) in the first half of gestation but increases significantly to an average of 50 mL/hour and is a necessary contribution to pulmonary development. Oligohydramnios or polyhydramnios may reflect dysfunction of the developing kidney.

II. CLINICAL ASSESSMENT OF RENAL FUNCTION.

Assessment of renal function is based on the patient's history, physical examination, and appropriate laboratory and radiologic tests.

A. History

1. Prenatal history includes any maternal illness, drug use, or exposure to known and potential teratogens.

a. Maternal use of ACE-inhibitors, angiotensin receptor blockers, or indomethacin decreases glomerular capillary pressure and GFR and has been associated with neonatal renal failure.

b. Oligohydramnios may indicate a decrease in fetal urine production. It may be associated with renal agenesis, renal dysplasia, polycystic kidney disease, or severe obstruction of the urinary tract system. It most often is a sign of poor fetal perfusion due to placental insufficiency as seen in preeclampsia or maternal vascular disease or premature rupture of membranes (see Chaps. 2 and 4).

Polyhydramnios is seen in pregnancies complicated by maternal diabetes (see Chap. 2) and in fetal anomalies such as esophageal atresia (see Chap. 62) or anencephaly (see Chap. 57). It also may be a result of renal tubular dysfunction with inability to fully concentrate urine.

c. Elevated serum/amniotic fluid α-fetoprotein and enlarged placenta are associated with congenital nephrotic syndrome.

2. Family history. The risk of renal disease is increased if there is a family history of urinary tract anomalies, polycystic kidney disease, consanguinity, or inherited renal tubular disorders. Familial diseases (congenital nephrotic syndrome, autosomal recessive polycystic kidney disease [ARPKD], hydronephrosis, dysplasia) may be recognized *in utero* or remain asymptomatic until later life.

3. Delivery history. Fetal distress, perinatal asphyxia, sepsis, and volume loss may lead to ischemic or anoxic injury.

4. Micturition. Seventeen percent of newborns void in the delivery room, approximately 90% void by 24 hours, and 99% void by 48 hours. The rate of urine formation ranges from 0.5 to 5.0 mL/kg/hour at all gestational ages. The most common cause of delayed or decreased urine production is inadequate perfusion of the kidneys; however, delay in micturition may be due to intrinsic renal abnormalities or obstruction of the urinary tract.

B. Physical examination. Careful examination will detect abdominal masses in 0.8% of neonates. Most of these masses are either renal in origin or related to the GU system. It is important to consider in the differential diagnosis whether the mass is unilateral or bilateral (see Table 28.2). Edema may be present in infants

Table 28.2	Abdominal Masses in the Neonate (see Chap. 62)
Type of mass	**Total percentage**
Renal	55
Hydronephrosis	
Multicystic dysplastic kidney	
Polycystic kidney disease	
Mesoblastic nephroma	
Renal ectopia	
Renal vein thrombosis	
Nephroblastomatosis	
Wilms tumor	
Genital	15
Hydrometrocolpos	
Ovarian cyst	
Gastrointestinal	20

Source: From Pinto E, Guignard JP. Renal masses in the neonate. *Biol Neonate* 1995;68(3):175–184.

with congenital nephrotic syndrome (due to low oncotic pressure) or from fluid overload if input exceeds output. Tubular defects and use of diuretics can cause salt and water losses, which can lead to dehydration.

Many congenital syndromes may affect the kidneys; thus, a thorough evaluation is necessary in those presenting with congenital renal anomalies. Findings associated with congenital renal anomalies include low-set ears, ambiguous genitalia, anal atresia, abdominal wall defect, vertebral anomalies, aniridia, meningomyelocele, tethered cord, pneumothorax, pulmonary hypoplasia, hemihypertrophy, persistent urachus, hypospadias, and cryptorchidism among others (see Table 28.3). Spontaneous pneumothorax may occur in those who have pulmonary hypoplasia associated with renal abnormalities.

C. Laboratory evaluation. Renal function tests must be interpreted in relation to gestational and postnatal age (see Tables 28.4 and 28.5).

1. Urinalysis reflects the developmental stages of renal physiology.

   a. Specific gravity. Full-term infants have a limited concentrating ability with a maximum specific gravity of 1.021 to 1.025.

Table 28.3	Congenital Syndromes with Renal Components (see Chap. 10)	
Dysmorphic disorders, sequences, and associations	General features	Renal abnormalities
Oligohydramnios sequence (Potter syndrome)	Altered facies, pulmonary hypoplasia, abnormal limb and head position	Renal agenesis, severe bilateral obstruction, severe bilateral dysplasia, autosomal recessive polycystic kidney disease
VATER and VACTERL syndrome	Vertebral anomalies, anal atresia, tracheo-esophageal fistula, radial dysplasia, cardiac and limb defects	Renal agenesis, renal dysplasia, renal ectopia
MURCS association and Rokitansky sequence	Failure of parameso-nephric ducts, vaginal and uterus hypoplasia/atresia, cervicothoracic somite dysplasia	Renal hypoplasia/agenesis, renal ectopia, double ureters
Prune belly	Hypoplasia of abdominal muscle, cryptorchidism	Megaureters, hydro-nephrosis, dysplastic kidneys, atonic bladder
Spina bifida	Meningomyelocele	Neurogenic bladder, vesicoureteral reflux, hydronephrosis, double ureter, horseshoe kidney
Caudal dysplasia sequence (caudal regression syndrome)	Sacral (and lumbar) hypoplasia, disruption of the distal spinal cord	Neurogenic bladder, vesicoureteral reflux, hydronephrosis, renal agenesis
Anal atresia (high imperforate anus)	Rectovaginal, rectovesical, or recto-urethral fistula tethered to the spinal cord	Renal agenesis, renal dysplasia
Hemihypertrophy	Hemihypertrophy	Wilms tumor, hypospadias
Aniridia	Aniridia, cryptorchidism	Wilms tumor
		(continued)

Table 28.3	Congenital Syndromes with Renal Components *(Continued)*	
Dysmorphic disorders, sequences, and associations	**General features**	**Renal abnormalities**
Drash syndrome	Ambiguous genitalia	Mesangial sclerosis, Wilms tumor
Small deformed or low-set ears		Renal agenesis/ dysplasia
Autosomal recessive		
Cerebrohepatorenal syndrome (Zellweger syndrome)	Hepatomegaly, glaucoma, brain anomalies, chondrodystrophy	Cortical renal cysts
Jeune syndrome (asphyxiating thoracic dystrophy)	Small thoracic cage, short ribs, abnormal costochondral junctions, pulmonary hypoplasia	Cystic tubular dysplasia, glomerulosclerosis, hydronephrosis, horseshoe kidneys
Meckel-Gruber syndrome (dysencephalia splanchnocystica)	Encephalocele, microcephaly, polydactyly, cryptorchidism, cardiac anomalies, liver disease	Polycystic/dysplastic kidneys
Johanson-Blizzard syndrome	Hypoplastic alae nasi, hypothyroidism, deafness, imperforate anus, cryptorchidism	Hydronephrosis, caliectasis
Schinzel-Giedion syndrome	Short limbs, abnormal facies, bone abnormalities, hypospadias	Hydronephrosis, megaureter
Short rib-polydactyly syndrome	Short horizontal ribs, pulmonary hypoplasia, polysyndactyly, bone and cardiac defects, ambiguous genitalia	Glomerular and tubular cysts
Bardet-Biedl syndrome	Obesity, retinal pigmentation, polydactyly	Interstitial nephritis
		(continued)

Table 28.3	*(Continued)*	
Dysmorphic disorders, sequences, and associations	**General features**	**Renal abnormalities**
Autosomal dominant		
Tuberous sclerosis	Fibrous-angiomatous lesions, hypopigmented macules, intracranial calcifications, seizures, bone lesions	Polycystic kidneys, renal angiomyolipoma
Melnick-Fraser syndrome (branchio-oto-renal [BOR] syndrome)	Preauricular pits, branchial clefts, deafness	Renal dysplasia, duplicated ureters
Nail-patella syndrome (hereditary osteo-onychodysplasia)	Hypoplastic nails, hypoplastic or absent patella, other bone anomalies	Proteinuria, nephrotic syndrome
Townes syndrome	Thumb, auricular and anal anomalies	Various renal abnormalities
X-Linked		
Oculocerebrorenal syndrome (Lowe syndrome)	Cataracts, rickets, mental retardation	Fanconi syndrome
Oral-facial-digital (OFD) syndrome type I	Oral clefts, hypoplastic alae nasi, digital asymmetry (X-linked, lethal in men)	Renal microcysts
Trisomy 21 (Down syndrome)	Abnormal facies, brachycephaly, congenital heart disease	Cystic dysplastic kidney and other renal abnormalities
XO syndrome (Turner syndrome)	Small stature, congenital heart disease, amenorrhea	Horseshoe kidney, duplications and malrotations of the urinary collecting system
Trisomy 13 (Patau syndrome)	Abnormal facies, cleft lip and palate, congenital heart disease	Cystic dysplastic kidneys and other renal anomalies

(continued)

Table 28.3	**Congenital Syndromes with Renal Components** *(Continued)*	
Dysmorphic disorders, sequences, and associations	**General features**	**Renal abnormalities**
Trisomy 18 (Edwards syndrome)	Abnormal facies, abnormal ears, overlapping digits, congenital heart disease	Cystic dysplastic kidneys, horseshoe kidney, or duplication
XXY, XXX syndrome (Triploidy syndrome)	Abnormal facies, cardiac defects, hypospadias and cryptorchidism in men, syndactyly	Various renal abnormalities
Partial trisomy 10q	Abnormal facies, microcephaly, limb and cardiac abnormalities	Various renal abnormalities

b. Protein excretion varies with gestational age. Urinary protein excretion is higher in premature infants and decreases progressively with postnatal age. In normal full-term infants, protein excretion is minimal after the second week of life.

c. Glycosuria is commonly present in premature infants of <34 weeks' gestation. The tubular resorption of glucose is <93% in infants born before 34 weeks' gestation compared with 99% in infants born after 34 weeks' gestation. Glucose excretion rates are highest in infants born before 28 weeks' gestation.

d. Hematuria is abnormal and may indicate intrinsic renal damage or result from a bleeding or clotting abnormality (see III.G.).

e. The sediment examination will usually demonstrate multiple epithelial cells (thought to be urethral mucosal cells) for the first 24 to 48 hours. In infants with asphyxia, there is an increase in epithelial cells and transient microscopic hematuria with leukocytes is common. Further investigation is necessary if these sediment findings persist. Hyaline and fine granular casts are common in dehydration or hypotension. Uric acid crystals are common in dehydration states and concentrated urine samples. They may be seen as pink or reddish brown diaper staining (particularly with the newer absorptive diapers).

2. Method of collection

a. Suprapubic aspiration is the most reliable method to obtain an uncontaminated sample collection for urine culture. Ultrasound guidance will improve chance of success.

b. Bladder catheterization is used if an infant has failed to pass urine by 36 to 48 hours and is not hypovolemic (see III.B.), if precise determination of urine volume is needed, or to optimize urine drainage if functional or anatomic obstruction is suspected.

c. Bag collections are adequate for most studies such as determinations of specific gravity, pH, electrolytes, protein, glucose, and sediment but not urine culture. It is the preferred method for detecting red blood cells in the urine.

Table 28.4	Normal Urinary and Renal Values in Term and Preterm Infants			
	Preterm infants <34 wk	Term infants at birth	Term infants 2 wk	Term infants 8 wk
GFR (mL/min/1.73 m^2)	13–58	15–60	63–80	
Bicarbonate threshold (mEq/L)	14–18	21	21.5	
TRP (%)	>85%	>95%		
Protein excretion (mg/m^2/24 h) (mean ± 1 SD)	60 ± 96	31 ± 44		
Maximal concentration ability (mOsmol/L)	500	800	900	1,200
Maximal diluting ability (mOsmol/L)	25–30	25–30	25–30	25–30
Specific gravity	1.002–1.015	1.002–1.020	1.002–1.025	1.002–1.030
Dipstick				
pH	5.0–8.0	4.5–8.0	4.5–8.0	4.5–8.0
Proteins	Neg to ++	Neg to +	Neg	Neg
Glucose	Neg to ++	Neg	Neg	Neg
Blood	Neg	Neg	Neg	Neg
Leukocytes	Neg	Neg	Neg	Neg
Neg = negative.				

    d. Diaper urine specimens are reliable for estimation of pH and qualitative determination of the presence of glucose, protein, and blood.

  3. Evaluation of renal function

    a. Serum creatinine at birth reflects maternal renal function. In healthy term infants, serum creatinine levels fall from 0.8 mg/dL at birth to 0.5 mg/dL at 5 to 7 days and reach a stable level of 0.3 to 0.4 mg/dL by 9 days. Premature infants' serum creatinine may rise transiently for the first few days and then will reduce slowly over weeks to months, depending on the level of prematurity (Fig. 28.1). The rate of decrease in serum creatinine in the first few weeks is slower in younger gestational age infants with lower GFR (Table 28.5).

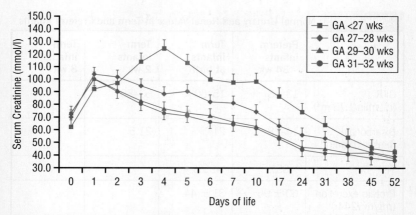

Figure 28.1 Serum creatinine concentration (mmol/l) (mean and standard error) in neonates vary by gestational age. (Adapted from Gallini et al. *Pediatric Nephrology* 2000.)

b. Blood urea nitrogen (BUN) is a useful indicator of renal function. However, BUN can be elevated as a result of increased production of urea nitrogen in hypercatabolic states, sequestered blood, tissue breakdown, steroid use, hemoconcentration, or increased protein intake.

c. GFR can be measured by clearance studies of either exogenous substances (inulin, Cr-EDTA [chromium ethylene diamine tetra-acetic acid], sodium iothalamate) or endogenous substances such as creatinine (see Table 28.6). Practical considerations, such as frequent blood sampling, urine collection, or infusion of an exogenous substance, limit their use and are used only for research purposes. GFR can be estimated from serum creatinine and body length (Table 28.1), although this equation must be used with caution as it was

Table 28.5	Normal Serum Creatinine Values in Term and Preterm Infants (Mean ± SD)			
Age (d)	<28 wk	28–32 wk	32–37 wk	>37 wk
3	1.05 ± 0.27	0.88 ± 0.25	0.78 ± 0.22	0.75 ± 0.2
7	0.95 ± 0.36	0.94 ± 0.37	0.77 ± 0.48	0.56 ± 0.4
14	0.81 ± 0.26	0.78 ± 0.36	0.62 ± 0.4	0.43 ± 0.25
28	0.66 ± 0.28	0.59 ± 0.38	0.40 ± 0.28	0.34 ± 0.2

Source: From Rudd PT, Hughes EA, Placzek MM, et al. Reference ranges for plasma creatinine during the first month of life. *Arch Dis Child* 1983;58(3):212–215; van den Anker JN, de Groot R, Broerse HM, et al. Assessment of glomerular filtration rate in preterm infants by serum creatinine: comparison with inulin clearance. *Pediatrics* 1995;96(6):1156–1158.

Table 28.6	Inulin Clearance GFR in Healthy Premature Infants
Age	mL/min/1.73 m^2
1–3 days	14.0 ± 5
1–7 days	18.7 ± 5.5
4–8 days	44.3 ± 9.3
3–13 days	47.8 ± 10.7
1.5–4 mo	67.4 ± 16.6
8 years	103 ± 12

designed using the Jaffe method to detect serum creatinine, and it is strictly an estimate with significant predictive variability in determining true GFR.

d. Measurement of serum and urine electrolytes is used to guide fluid and electrolyte management and in assessing renal tubular function. One must consider serum values and clinical context in order to interpret urine electrolyte measurements (see Chap. 23).

D. Radiological studies

1. **Ultrasonography** is the initial imaging study to delineate renal parenchymal architecture. Color Doppler flow techniques can estimate RBF but have significant intra-operator variability. The length of the kidneys in millimeters is approximately the gestational age in weeks. The renal cortex has echogenicity similar to that of the liver or spleen in the neonate, in contrast to the hypoechoic renal cortex seen in adults and older children. In addition, the medullary pyramids in the neonate are much more hypoechoic than the cortex and hence are more prominent in appearance.

2. **Voiding cystourethrography (VCUG),** with fluoroscopy, is an excellent method to determine vesicoureteral reflux (VUR), bladder anatomy, and define lower urinary tract anatomy such as in posterior urethral valves. Radionuclide cystography is often used to evaluate VUR because of its lower radiation dose. However, VCUG produces better static imaging for anatomical defects and is preferred for the initial evaluation of obstructive uropathy.

3. **Radionuclide scintigraphy** is useful in demonstrating the position and relative function of the kidneys. Isotopes such as ^{99m}Tc-diethylenetriamine pentaacetic acid (DTPA) or ^{99m}Tc-mercaptoacetyltriglycine (MAG 3) are handled by glomerular filtration and can be used to assess RBF and renal function. In conjunction with intravenously administered furosemide, it can help differentiate obstructive from nonobstructive hydronephrosis. Isotopes that bind to the renal tubules, such as ^{99m}Tc-dimercaptosuccinic acid (DMSA), produce static images of the renal cortex. This may be helpful for assessing acute pyelonephritis and renal scarring from renal artery emboli or renal vascular disorders and for quantifying the amount of renal cortex in patients with renal dysplasia and hypoplasia.

III. COMMON CLINICAL RENAL PROBLEMS

A. **Prenatal ultrasonography.** Routine maternal ultrasonographic screening detects an incidence of fetal GU abnormalities of 0.3% to 0.5%.

1. The most common finding is **hydronephrosis**, reported in >80% of the cases. Approximately 75% of these are confirmed postnatally.

   a. Initial management of a newborn with prenatally identified hydronephrosis depends on the clinical condition of the patient and the suspected nature of the lesion.

   b. Unilateral hydronephrosis is more common and is not associated with systemic or pulmonary complications if the contralateral kidney is normal. Postnatal ultrasonographic confirmation may be carried out electively at approximately 2 to 4 weeks of life, depending on severity. It is important not to perform the ultrasonographic examination in the first few days after birth, when hydronephrosis may not be detected because of physiologic dehydration.

   c. Bilateral hydronephrosis is more worrisome, especially if oligohydramnios or pulmonary disease is present. In the male infant, postnatal evaluation (VCUG and ultrasonography) should be performed within the first day to determine the etiology (posterior urethral valves [PUV], ureteropelvic junction [UPJ] obstruction, ureterovesical junction (UVJ) obstruction, Prune-Belly syndrome, or VUR). With postbladder obstruction such as PUV, ultrasonography will often demonstrate a trabeculated and thickened bladder wall.

2. Routine prenatal ultrasonography has increased the diagnosis of multicystic dysplastic kidney (MCDK), especially with unilateral involvement. A MCDK is one in which no functional parenchyma is present and a lobulated "ball of grapes" like structure is present. Infants with unilateral MCDK are usually asymptomatic, and the affected kidney has no renal function as demonstrated by DMSA renal scan. There is general agreement that surgical removal is indicated in cases with associated hypertension or infection, or with respiratory compromise secondary to abdominal compression by the abnormal kidney. Although surgical removal had been suggested to decrease the potential of renal cell carcinoma, there is no evidence that surgical removal of asymptomatic MCDK improves long-term outcomes. In asymptomatic patients, medical observation is the current practice, and surgical removal is reserved only if symptoms develop.

3. Renal abnormalities may be associated with other congenital anomalies, including neural tube defects, congenital heart lesions, intestinal obstructive lesions, abdominal wall defects, central nervous system (CNS) or spinal abnormalities, and urological abnormalities of the lower urinary tract.

B. **Acute kidney injury (AKI), previously termed acute renal failure,** may be secondary to prerenal azotemia, intrinsic (tubular, glomerular, or interstitial disease), or postrenal disorders (obstructive) (see Table 28.7). **Prerenal azotemia** occurs when the kidney becomes underperfused. The most common causes of prerenal azotemia are loss of effective blood volume, relative loss of intravascular volume from increased capillary leak, poor cardiac output, medications, and intra-abdominal compartment syndrome. These conditions can lead to intrinsic renal tubular damage if not corrected expeditiously. **Intrinsic AKI** implies direct damage to the glomeruli, interstitia, or tubules. In neonates, tubular injury is most commonly caused by prolonged or severe ischemia, nephrotoxins, or sepsis. Glomerular and primary interstitial injury is very rare in neonates. It results from

Table 28.7	Causes of Acute Kidney Injury in the Neonatal Period
A. Prerenal	
1. Reduced effective circulatory volume	
a. Hemorrhage	
b. Dehydration	
c. Sepsis	
d. Necrotizing enterocolitis	
e. Congenital heart disease	
f. Hypoalbuminemia	
2. Increased renal vascular resistance	
a. Polycythemia	
b. Indomethacin	
c. Adrenergic drugs	
3. Hypoxia/asphyxia	
B. Intrinsic or renal parenchymal	
1. Sustained hypoperfusion leading to acute tubular necrosis	
2. Congenital anomalies	
a. Agenesis	
b. Hypoplasia/dysplasia	
c. Polycystic kidney disease	
3. Thromboembolic disease	
a. Bilateral renal vein thrombosis	
b. Bilateral renal arterial thrombosis	
4. Nephrotoxins	
a. Aminoglycosides	
b. Radiographic contrast media	
c. Maternal use of captopril or indomethacin	

(continued)

Table 28.7	Causes of Acute Kidney Injury in the Neonatal Period *(Continued)*
C. Obstructive	
1. Urethral obstruction	
a. Posterior urethral valves	
b. Stricture	
c. Prune belly syndrome	
2. Ureterocele	
3. Ureteropelvic/ureterovesical obstruction	
4. Extrinsic tumors	
5. Neurogenic bladder	
6. Megacystis or megaureter syndrome	

obstruction to urinary flow in both kidneys. In boys, the most common lesion is PUV; however, acquired obstruction (from masses, stones, or fungal balls) can also occur. Renal function may be abnormal even after correction of the obstruction.

1. **Evaluation to determine the underlying etiology of rising creatinine or decreased urine output is critical to AKI management.**
   a. Evaluate history for oligohydramnios, perinatal asphyxia, bleeding disorders, polycythemia, thrombocytosis, thrombocytopenia, sepsis, or maternal drug use. Evaluate for the presence of nephrotoxic medication.
   b. Place an indwelling urinary catheter.
   c. Evaluate for signs and symptoms of intravascular depletion (tachycardia, sunken fontanelle, poor skin turgor, dry mucous membranes). Laboratory evaluation can help determine the underlying etiology. Table 28.8 lists laboratory tests

Table 28.8	Renal Failure Indices in the Oliguric Neonate	
Indices	**Prerenal failure**	**Intrinsic renal failure**
Urine sodium (mEq/L)	10–50	30–90
Urine/plasma creatinine	29.2 ± 1.6	9.7 ± 3.6
FENa*	0.9 ± 0.6	4.3 ± 2.2

*Fractional excretion of sodium defined in Chapter 23.
Source: Modified from Mathew OP, Jones AS, James E, et al. Neonatal renal failure: usefulness of diagnostic indices. *Pediatrics* 1980;65(1):57–60.

that are helpful in differentiating prerenal azotemia from intrinsic and obstructive causes. Test samples should be obtained before fluid challenge if possible.

d. If edema is present, evaluation to determine whether intravascular volume is depleted (in hypoalbuminemia, for example) or elevated is helpful in determining the etiology and plan of action.

e. A fluid challenge with normal saline 10 to 20 mL/kg over 30 minutes not only can replete intravascular volume, but also can help to determine if intravascular depletion is present. Evaluation for cardiac failure is imperative prior to aggressive fluid resuscitation for renal failure.

f. Renal ultrasonogram should be performed to rule out bladder obstruction and to assess for congenital anomalies of the kidney and urinary tract.

2. Management of those who develop AKI should focus on treating the underlying etiology, avoiding further injury, and addressing consequences of decreased renal function.

   a. As mentioned, response to fluid challenge not only provides information about the underlying cause of AKI, but also serves as the beginning of the management plan. Close evaluation of the cause of the intravascular volume depletion should be sought, and appropriate fluid management should be given. Intravenous albumin should be considered for those with low serum albumin.

   b. Avoidance of nephrotoxic medications to prevent further insult and dose adjustment of concurrent medications based on estimated renal function are necessary.

   c. Furosemide may be given to correct fluid overload but has not been shown to prevent AKI. Low- or "renal-dose" dopamine has NOT been shown to prevent AKI.

   d. If blood pressure is low in relation to vascular congestion and/or abdominal pressures, consider increasing blood pressure with inotropes to increase glomerular filtration (see Chap. 40).

3. **Management of complications**

   a. Hyperkalemia. Discontinue or minimize potassium (K^+) intake. Low-K^+ formula such as Similac PM 60/40 or K^+-free IV solution is used. Treatment of hyperkalemia ($K^+ > 6$ mEq/L) is as follows (see Chap. 23):

   i. Sodium polystyrene sulfonate (Kayexalate) is administered rectally in a dose of 1 to 1.5 g/kg (dissolved in normal saline at 0.5 g/mL saline) or orally in a dose of 1 g/kg (dissolved in dextrose 10% in water) as needed to decrease serum K^+ levels. The enema tube, a thin Silastic feeding tube, is inserted 1 to 3 cm. If possible, we avoid using Kayexalate in low birth weight infants because of the risk of intestinal perforation. Kayexalate of 1 g/kg removes 1 mEq/L of potassium.

   ii. Calcium is given as 1 to 2 mL/kg of calcium gluconate 10% over 2 to 4 minutes for cardioprotection. The electrocardiogram (ECG) is monitored.

   iii. Sodium bicarbonate will shift K into the cells and can temporarily lower serum K^+. 1 mEq/kg given intravenously over 5 to 10 minutes, will decrease serum K+ by 1 mEq/L.

   iv. Glucose and insulin will also shift K^+ into cells to temporarily lower serum K^+ levels. Begin with a bolus of regular human insulin (0.05 units/kg) and dextrose 10% in water (2 mL/kg) followed by a continuous infusion of dextrose 10% in water at 2 to 4 mL/kg/hour and human regular insulin (10 units/100 mL) at 1 mL/kg/hour. Monitor blood glucose level frequently. Maintain a ratio of 1 or 2 units of insulin to 4 g of glucose.

   v. Furosemide can be given for kaliuresis as well as natiuresis if volume expansion is present. A trial of 1 mg/kg intermittently is given.

vi. **Dialysis** is considered when hyperkalemia cannot be controlled with medical therapy. Although hemodialysis (HD) is the most efficient way to remove K^+, peritoneal dialysis (PD) or continuous venovenous hemoperfusion (CVVH) can be used.

b. **Fluid management** is based on the patient's fluid status and determination of ongoing losses. Unless dehydration or polyuric states are present, volume should be limited to replacement of insensible losses and urine output (see Chap. 23). The inability to adequately prescribe nutrition due to fluid restriction and/or significant fluid overload are indication for dialysis.

c. **Sodium** (Na^+) is restricted and Na^+ concentration is monitored, accounting for fluid balance. Hyponatremia is usually secondary to excess free water. Close monitoring of electrolytes especially sodium is needed during diuretic therapy or with dialysis.

d. **Phosphorus** is restricted by using a low-phosphorus formula (e.g., Similac PM 60/40). Oral calcium carbonate can be used as a phosphate-binding agent.

e. **Calcium** supplementation is given if ionized calcium is decreased or the patient is symptomatic. In infants with chronic renal failure, 1,25-dihydroxyvitamin D or its analog is given to maximize Ca^{2+} absorption and prevent renal osteodystrophy (see Chap. 25).

f. **Metabolic acidosis** is usually mild, unless there is (i) significant tubular dysfunction with decreased ability to reabsorb bicarbonate, or (ii) increased lactate production due to decreased perfusion due to heart failure or volume loss from hemorrhage (see I.B.1.). Consider using sodium bicarbonate or sodium citrate to correct severe metabolic acidosis.

g. **Nutrition** is critical to the growing newborn. Infants who can take oral feeding are given a low-phosphate and low-potassium formula with a low renal solute load (e.g., Similac PM 60/40). Caloric density can be progressively increased to a maximum of 50 kcal/oz with glucose polymers (Polycose) and oil. Adequate protein for neonates with otherwise normal renal function should be provided unless they are on continuous hemodialysis or peritoneal dialysis. As these therapies can cause protein losses of 1 to 1.5 g/kg/day, additional supplementation is necessary.

h. **Hypertension** (see III.D.2.).

i. **Dialysis** is indicated when conservative management has been unsuccessful in correcting severe fluid overload, hyperkalemia, acidosis, and uremia. Inadequate nutrition because of severe fluid restriction in the anuric infant is a relative indication for dialysis. Because the technical aspects and the supportive care are specialized and demanding, this procedure must be performed in centers where the staff have experience with dialysis in infants and neonates.

C. Congenital anomalies of the kidney and urinary tract (CAKUT) may become apparent with prenatal ultrasound, discovered at birth, or present later in life. Common lesions are hydronephrosis, dysplastic kidneys (with or without cysts), multicystic dysplastic kidney (MCDK), and obstruction of the urinary system either at the level of the UPJ, UVJ, or by valves at the urethra (PUV). Besides CAKUT anomalies, ARPKD, which is associated with liver fibrosis, is another cause of renal failure in neonates. Autosomal dominant polycystic kidney disease (ADPKD) is more common in the general population, but does not generally present until later in life. Differential diagnosis includes other renal masses (Table 28.2). The severity of renal impairment in these diseases varies from extreme oligohydramnios and *in utero* compromise to late presentation in adulthood. Ultimately, the prognosis depends on the severity of the anomaly, whether the contralateral kidney is viable and on extrarenal organ dysfunction. In the newborn course, the degree of pulmonary hypoplasia will dictate the likelihood of viability.

D. Blood pressure in the newborn is related to weight and gestational age. Blood pressure rises with postnatal age, 1 to 2 mm Hg/day during the first week and 1 mm Hg/week during the next 6 weeks in both the preterm and full-term infant.

1. Normative values of blood pressure for full-term infants and premature infants are shown in Tables 28.9 to 28.11.

2. **Hypertension** is defined as persistent blood pressure >2 standard deviations above the mean. The clinical signs and symptoms, which may be absent or nonspecific, include cardiorespiratory abnormalities such as tachypnea, cardiomegaly, heart failure; neurologic findings such as irritability, lethargy, or seizure; failure to thrive; or GI difficulties.

3. Neonatal hypertension has many causes (see Table 28.12). The three most common causes of hypertension in newborns are secondary to bronchopulmonary dysplasia, umbilical artery thrombus emboli, and coarctation of the aorta. History and physical examination, a review of fluid status, medications, location of arterial thrombus, and weak distal pulses, may provide clues about the underlying etiology. Renin-mediated hypertension and fluid overload may both contribute to renal causes of hypertension. Urinalysis, renal function studies, serum electrolyte levels, and renal ultrasonographic examination should also be obtained. Color Doppler flow studies may detect aortic or renal vascular thrombosis, although this test is not reliable with the possibility of both false positives and false negatives. A DMSA renal scan may detect segmental renal arterial infarctions. Plasma renin levels are difficult to interpret. Echocardiogram is indicated if coarctation is suspected and can determine if left ventricular hypertrophy has occurred from sustained hypertension.

Table 28.9	Normal Longitudinal Blood Pressure in Full-term Infants (mm Hg)			
	Boys		Girls	
Age	Systolic	Diastolic	Systolic	Diastolic
1st d	67 ± 7	37 ± 7	68 ± 8	38 ± 7
4th d	76 ± 8	44 ± 9	75 ± 8	45 ± 8
1 mo	84 ± 10	46 ± 9	82 ± 9	46 ± 10
3 mo	92 ± 11	55 ± 10	89 ± 11	54 ± 10
6 mo	96 ± 9	58 ± 10	92 ± 10	56 ± 10

Source: From Gemelli M, Manganaro R, Mamì C, et al. Longitudinal study of blood pressure during the 1st year of life. *Eur J Pediatr* 1990;149(5):318–320.

Table 28.10	Systolic and Diastolic Blood Pressure Ranges in Infants of 500–2,000 Grams Birth Weight at 3–6 h of Life	
Birth weight (g)	Systolic (mm Hg)	Diastolic (mm Hg)
501–750	50–62	26–36
751–1,000	48–59	23–36
1,001–1,250	49–61	26–35
1,251–1,500	46–56	23–33
1,501–1,750	46–58	23–33
1,751–2,000	48–61	24–35

Source: From Hegyi T, Carbone MT, Anwar M, et al. Blood pressure ranges in premature infants. I. The first hours of life. *J Pediatr* 1994;124(4):627–633.

4. Management is directed at correcting the underlying cause whenever possible. Antihypertensive therapy (see Table 28.13) is administered for sustained hypertension not related to volume overload or medications. Hydralazine is most commonly used. Captopril is often used if hypertension persists.

E. **Renal vascular thrombosis**

1. **Renal artery thrombosis (RAT)** is often related to the use of indwelling umbilical artery catheters, which can obstruct or emit an embolus into the renal artery. Other rare causes include congenital hypercoagulable states and severe hypotension. While the management is controversial, potential options include surgical thrombectomy, thrombolytic agents, and conservative medical care, including antihypertensive therapy. The surgical renal salvage rate is no better than medical

Table 28.11	Mean Arterial Blood Pressure (MAP) in Infants of 500–1,500 Grams Birth Weight		
	MAP ± SD (mm Hg)		
Birth weight (g)	Day 3	Day 17	Day 31
501–750	38 ± 8	44 ± 8	46 ± 11
751–1,000	43 ± 9	45 ± 7	47 ± 9
1,001–1,250	43 ± 8	46 ± 9	48 ± 8
1,251–1,500	45 ± 8	47 ± 8	47 ± 9

Source: From Klaus MH, Fanaroff AA, eds. *Care of the High-risk Neonate.* Philadelphia: WB Saunders, 1993, p. 497.

Table 28.12	Causes of Hypertension in the Neonate

A. Vascular

   1. Renal artery thrombosis

   2. Renal vein thrombosis

   3. Coarctation of the aorta

   4. Renal artery stenosis

   5. Idiopathic arterial calcification

B. Renal

   1. Obstructive uropathy

   2. Polycystic kidney disease

   3. Renal insufficiency

   4. Renal tumor

   5. Wilms tumor

   6. Glomerulonephritis

   7. Pyelonephritis

C. Endocrine

   1. Congenital adrenal hypoplasia

   2. Primary hyperaldosteronism

   3. Hyperthyroidism

D. Neurologic

   1. Increased intracranial pressure

   2. Cushing's disease

   3. Neural crest tumor

   4. Cerebral angioma

   5. Drug withdrawal

E. Pulmonary

   1. Bronchopulmonary dysplasia

(continued)

Table 28.12	Causes of Hypertension in the Neonate *(Continued)*
F. Drugs	
1. Corticosteroids	
2. Theophylline	
3. Adrenergic agents	
4. Phenylephrine	
G. Other	
1. Fluid/electrolyte overload	
2. Abdominal surgery	
3. Associated with extracorporeal membrane oxygenation (ECMO)	

management and carries a considerable mortality rate of 33%. Patients with unilateral RAT who received conservative medical treatment are usually normotensive by 2 years of age, no longer receiving antihypertensive medications, and have normal creatinine clearance, although some have unilateral renal atrophy with compensatory contralateral hypertrophy. There have been reports of long-term complications with hypertension and/or proteinuria and progression to renal failure in adolescence (see Chap. 44).

2. **Renal vein thrombosis (RVT)** has the predisposing conditions of hyperosmolarity, polycythemia, hypovolemia, and hypercoagulable states and is therefore often associated with infant of diabetic mothers, or use of umbilical venous catheters. Cases of intrauterine renal venous thrombosis have been described and present with calcification of the clot in the inferior vena cava (IVC). The classic clinical findings include gross hematuria often with clots, enlarged kidneys, hypertension, and thrombocytopenia. Other symptoms include vomiting, shock, lower extremity edema, and abdominal distention. The diagnosis of RVT is confirmed by ultrasonography, which typically shows an enlarged kidney with diffuse homogenous hyperechogenicity; Doppler flow studies may detect thrombi in the IVC or renal vein leading to absent renal flow. The differential diagnosis includes renal masses or hemolytic uremic syndrome.

The management of RVT is also controversial. Initial therapy should focus on the maintenance of circulation, fluid, and electrolyte balance while examining for underlying predisposing clinical conditions. Assessment of the coagulation status includes platelet count, prothrombin time (PT), partial thromboplastin time (PTT), fibrinogen, and fibrin split products. Thorough evaluation for hypercoaguable states is necessary as over 50% of infants with RVT have at least one defect (see Chap. 44).

No consensus exists on the use of heparin. If there is unilateral involvement without evidence of disseminated intravascular coagulation (DIC), conservative management is warranted. If there is bilateral involvement and

Table 28.13	Antihypertensive Agents for the Newborn (See Appendix A for Specific Dosing Recommendations)	
	Dose	Comment
Diuretics		
Furosemide	0.5–1.0 mg/kg/dose IV, IM, PO	May cause hyponatremia, hypokalemia, hypercalciuria
Chlorothiazide	20–40 mg/kg/d PO; divided q12h 2–8 mg/kg/day IV divided q12h	May cause hyponatremia, hypokalemia, hypochloremia
Vasodilators		
Hydralazine	1–8 mg/kg/day; divided q 6–8 h	May cause tachycardia
Calcium channel blockers		
Nifedipine	0.2 mg/kg/dose	Onset in 15–30 minutes; lasts 4-8 hours
Nicardipine	Start at 0.5 mcg/kg/min and titrate to effect (max 4–5 mcg/kg/min)	Onset within minutes—titrate every 5–10 minutes
Isradipine	0.1–0.2 mg/kg/dose PO	Onset in 15–30 minutes; lasts 4–8 hours
Amlodipine	0.1–0.4 mg/kg/day PO divided q12h	Onset 3 hours; time to peak 6–12 hours duration 12–24 hours
Basal receptor antagonist		
Propranolol	0.5–5.0 mg/kg/d PO; divided q 6–8 h	May cause bronchospasm
α/β-receptor antagonist		
Labetalol	0.5–1.0 mg/kg/dose IV, q 4–6 h	Limited use in neonates
ACE inhibitor		
Captopril	0.15–2.0 mg/kg/d PO, divided q 8–12 h	May cause oliguria hyperkalemia, renal failure
Enalapril	5–10 μg/kg/dose IV, 8–24 h	May cause oliguria, hyperkalemia, renal failure
ACE = angiotensin-converting enzyme.		

evidence of DIC, more aggressive therapy is indicated since the infant is at risk for complete loss of kidney function. Heparin therapy should be initiated with an initial bolus of 50 to 100 units/kg followed by continuous infusion at 25 to 50 units/kg to maintain PTT of 1.5 times normal. Antithrombin III (AT III) activity should be reassessed before heparin therapy is instituted as AT III is required for the anticoagulant action of heparin. Recently, low-molecular-weight heparin has been used both as initial treatment for thrombosis and as prophylactic therapy after recannulization of the occluded vessel. In the treatment of patients with thrombosis, dosages of 200 to 300 anti-Fxa U/kg are reported to reach a therapeutic level of 0.5 to 1.0 anti-Fxa U/mL. Reported dosages range from 45 to 100 anti-Fxa U/kg to reach prophylactic levels of 0.2 to 0.4 anti-Fxa U/mL.

Thrombolytic therapy with streptokinase and urokinase have been used in both RAT and RVT, with variable success but are no longer commercially available. There is limited experience with the use of thromboplastin activator (TPA). This is used in low dose (0.02–0.03 mg/kg) if there is evidence of bleeding, and titrated to PTT value of 1.5 times normal. Plasma infusion may be necessary to provide thromboplastin activation. Protamine and e-caproic acid should be present at the bedside because significant bleeding can occur. Surgical intervention should be considered if there has been an indwelling umbilical vein catheter, the thrombosis is bilateral, and involves the main renal veins leading to renal failure. This type of thrombosis is likely to have started in the IVC rather than intrarenal and hence is more likely amenable to surgical attention (see Chap. 44).

F. **Proteinuria** in small quantities during the first weeks of life is frequently found. After the first week, persistent proteinuria >250 mg/m^2/day should be investigated (Table 28.4).

1. In general, **mild proteinuria** reflects a vascular or tubular injury to the kidney, or the inability of the immature tubules to reabsorb protein. Administration of large amounts of colloid can exceed the reabsorptive capacity of the neonatal renal tubules and may result in mild proteinuria.

2. **Massive proteinuria** (>1.5 g/m^2/day), hypoalbuminemia with serum albumin levels <2.5 g/dL, and edema are all components of congenital nephrotic syndrome. Prenatal clues to the diagnosis include elevated maternal/amniotic α-fetoprotein levels and enlarged placenta. Children with severe forms of congenital nephrotic syndrome require daily intravenous albumin and Lasix for fluid removal, high caloric diets, replacement of thyroid, iron and vitamins due to excess losses of binding proteins and ultimately require bilateral nephrectomies and renal transplantation. They are at high risk for infections and thrombosis due to immunoglobulin losses and loss of anticoagulant proteins.

3. No specific treatment is required for mild proteinuria. Treat the underlying disease and monitor the proteinuria until resolved.

4. Glomerular disease is rare and usually associated with congenital nephrotic syndrome if presentation is in the nursery.

G. **Hematuria** is defined as >5 red blood cells (RBCs) per high-power field. It is uncommon in newborns and should always be investigated.

1. Hematuria has many causes (see Table 28.14), including hemorrhagic disease of the newborn if vitamin K supplementation has not been given. The differential diagnosis for hematuria includes urate staining of the diaper, myoglobinuria,

Table 28.14	Etiology of Hematuria in the Newborn
Acute tubular necrosis	
Cortical necrosis	
Vascular diseases	
Renal vein thrombosis	
Renal artery thrombosis	
Bleeding and clotting disorders (including hemorrhagic disease of newborn)	
Disseminated intravascular coagulation	
Severe thrombocytopenia	
Clotting factors deficiency	
Urological anomalies	
Urinary tract infection	
Glomerular diseases (see III.F.4.)	
Tumors	
Wilms tumor	
Neuroblastoma	
Angiomas	
Nephrocalcinosis	
Trauma	
Suprapubic bladder aspiration	
Urethral catheterization	

or hemoglobinuria. A negative dipstick with benign sediment suggests urates, whereas a positive dipstick with negative sediment for RBCs indicates the presence of globin pigments. Vaginal bleeding ("pseudomenses") in girls or a severe diaper rash is also a possible cause of blood in the diaper or positive dipstick for heme.

2. Evaluation of neonatal hematuria depends on the clinical situation. Depending on the clinical situation, one may consider performing includes the following tests: urinalysis with examination of the sediment, urine culture, ultrasonography of the upper and lower urinary tract, evaluation of renal function (serum creatinine and BUN), and coagulation studies.

H. Urinary Tract Infection (UTI)

1. Infections of the urinary tract in newborns can result in asymptomatic bacteriuria or can lead to pyelonephritis and/or sepsis. A urine culture should be obtained from every infant with fever, poor weight gain, poor feeding, unexplained prolonged jaundice, or any clinical signs of sepsis. A UTI is uncommon in the first 48 hours of life.

2. The diagnosis is confirmed by positive urine culture obtained by suprapubic bladder aspiration or catheterized specimen with a colony count exceeding 1,000 colonies per millimeter. A blood culture should also be obtained, even from asymptomatic infant with UTI. Although most newborns with UTIs have leukocytes in the urine, an infection can be present in the absence of leukocyturia.

3. *Escherichia coli* accounts for approximately 75% of the infections. The remainder are caused by other gram-negative bacilli (Klebsiella, Enterobacter, Proteus) and by gram-positive cocci (Enterococci, *Staphylococcus epidermidis*, *Staphylococcus aureus*).

4. Evaluation of the urinary tract by ultrasonography is required to rule out obstructive uropathy, severe reflux, or neurogenic bladder with inability to empty the bladder. Adequate drainage or relief of obstruction is necessary for antibiotic control of the infection. VCUG is needed to detect reflux and define lower tract abnormalities. VUR occurs in 40% of neonates with UTIs and predominates slightly in boys. Inadequate therapy, particularly in the presence of urological abnormalities, could lead to renal scarring with potential development of hypertension and loss of renal function.

5. The initial treatment is antibiotics, usually a combination of ampicillin and gentamicin, given parenterally. The final choice of antibiotic is based on the sensitivity of the cultured organism. Treatment is continued for 10 to 14 days, and amoxicillin prophylaxis (20 mg/kg/day) is administered until a VCUG is performed. If VUR is present, prophylactic treatment should be considered. For later onset infections (>7 days) in hospitalized infants, some experts would suggest using vancomycin rather than ampicillin to cover the possibility of hospital acquired organisms until definitive culture results are available.

I. Tubular disorders

1. **Fanconi syndrome** is a group of disorders with generalized dysfunction of the proximal tubule resulting in excessive urinary losses of amino acids, glucose, phosphate, and bicarbonate. The glomerular function is usually normal.

   a. **Clinical and laboratory findings** include the following:

      i. Hypophosphatemia due to the excessive urinary loss of phosphate. In these patients, the tubular reabsorption of phosphate (TRP) is abnormally low. Rickets and osteoporosis are secondary to hypophosphatemia and can appear in the neonatal period.

      ii. Metabolic acidosis is secondary to bicarbonate wasting (proximal renal tubular acidosis [RTA]).

      iii. Aminoaciduria and glycosuria do not result in significant clinical signs or symptoms.

      iv. These infants are often polyuric and therefore at risk for dehydration.

      v. Hypokalemia, due to increased excretion by the distal tubule to compensate for the increased sodium reabsorption, is also frequent and sometimes profound.

b. Etiology. The primary form of Fanconi syndrome is rare in the neonatal period and is a diagnosis of exclusion. Although familial cases (mainly autosomal dominant) have been reported, it is generally sporadic. Most secondary forms of the syndrome in the neonatal period are related to inborn errors of metabolism, including cystinosis, hereditary tyrosinemia, hereditary fructose intolerance, galactosemia, glycogenosis, Lowe syndrome (oculocerebrorenal syndrome), and mitochondrial disorders. Cases associated with heavy metal toxicity have also been described.

2. **RTA** is defined as metabolic acidosis resulting from the inability of the kidney to excrete hydrogen ions or to reabsorb bicarbonate. Poor growth may result from RTA.

   a. Distal RTA (type I) is caused by a defect in the secretion of hydrogen ions by the distal tubule. The urine cannot be acidified below 6 pH. It is frequently associated with hypercalciuria. Nephrocalcinosis (NC) is common later in life. In the neonatal period, distal RTA may be primary, due to a genetic defect, or secondary to several disorders.

   b. Proximal RTA (type II) is a defect in the proximal tubule with reduced bicarbonate reabsorption leading to bicarbonate wasting. Serum bicarbonate concentration falls until the abnormally low threshold for bicarbonate reabsorption is reached in the proximal tubule (generally <16 mEq/L). Once this threshold has been reached, no significant amount of bicarbonate reaches the distal tubule, and the urine can be acidified at that level. Proximal RTA can occur as an isolated defect or in association with Fanconi syndrome (see III.I.1.).

   c. Hyperkalemic RTA (type IV) is a result of a combined impaired ability of the distal tubule to excrete hydrogen ions and potassium. In the neonatal period, this disorder is seen in infants with aldosterone deficiency, adrenogenital syndrome, reduced tubular responsiveness to aldosterone, or associated obstructive uropathies.

   d. The treatment of RTA is based on correction of the acidosis with alkaline therapy. Bicitra or sodium citrate, 2 to 3 mEq/kg/day in divided doses, is usually sufficient to treat type I and type IV RTA. The treatment of proximal RTA requires larger doses sometimes as high as 10 mEq/kg/day bicarbonate. In secondary forms of RTA, the treatment of the primary cause often results in the resolution of the RTA.

J. **Nephrocalcinosis** is detected by renal ultrasound examinations.

1. NC is generally associated with a hypercalciuric state. Drugs that are associated with NC and increased urinary calcium excretion include loop diuretics such as furosemide, methylxanthines, glucocorticoids, and vitamin D in pharmacologic doses. In addition, hyperoxaluria, often associated with parenteral nutrition, and hyperphosphaturia facilitate the deposition of calcium crystals in the kidney.

2. Renal stones and NC secondary to primary hyperoxaluria/oxalosis, RTA, or UTIs are rare in newborns.

3. Few follow-up studies of NC in premature infants are available. In general, renal function is not significantly impaired, and 75% of cases resolve spontaneously often within the first year of life as demonstrated by ultrasonography but resolution may take up to 5 to 7 years. However, significant tubular dysfunction at 1 to 2 years of age has been reported.

4. It is unclear whether NC requires a specific treatment. If possible, drugs that cause hypercalciuria should be discontinued. Change to or addition of thiazide diuretics and supplemental magnesium in patients with bronchopulmonary dysplasia, with a need for long-term diuretic therapy may be helpful. Monitoring of urinary calcium excretion (urine calcium:creatinine ratio) helps in determining response to therapy.

K. Cystic disease of the kidney may result from abnormalities in development, such as multicystic dysplasia, or from genetically induced diseases. The principal differential diagnosis of bilateral cystic kidney disease in the newborn includes **ARPKD**, the infantile form of **ADPKD**, and glomerulocystic kidney disease.

1. In ARPKD, the genetic defect has been mapped to chromosome 6p21, which encodes a novel protein product named fibrocystin or polyductin. In infants with ARPKD, the kidneys appear markedly enlarged and hyperechogenic by ultrasonography, with a typical "snowstorm" appearance with concurrent liver fibrosis and/or dilated bile ducts. In contrast, macroscopic cysts are usually detected in cases of ADPKD and glomerulocystic disease, and the liver is spared. The clinical findings of ARPKD are variable and include bilateral smooth enlarged kidneys, varying degrees of renal insufficiency, which usually progresses to renal failure over time and severe renin-mediated hypertension. Infants with more severe involvement may have oligohydramnios with pulmonary hypoplasia and Potter syndrome, but those patients who survive the neonatal period can be carried to renal transplantation in later childhood or adolescence. ARPKD is always associated with liver involvement, which may progress to liver failure requiring transplantation in adolescence.

2. In ADPKD, an abnormal gene, PKD1, has been identified and located on the short arm of chromosome 16, and a second gene, PKD2, located on the long arm of chromosome 4. These two genes account for most of the ADPKD patients. Clinical manifestations include bilateral renal masses that are usually less symmetrical than in ARPKD.

3. Other hereditary syndromes that can manifest as renal cystic disease include tuberous sclerosis, von Hippel-Lindau disease, Jeune syndrome or asphyxiating thoracic dystrophy, oral-facial-digital syndrome type 1, brachymesomelia-renal syndrome, and trisomy 9, 13, and 18.

L. The decision for **circumcision** is based primarily on cultural or ethnic background. Data on risk of UTIs, penile cancer, and protection from sexually transmitted diseases in circumcised and uncircumcised men are insufficient to recommend routine circumcisions. Medical indications for circumcision include recurrent urinary tract infection, urinary retention due to adhesions of the foreskin or to tight phimosis. Circumcision should be avoided in cases of hypospadias, ambiguous genitalia, and bleeding disorders (see Chap. 9).

M. Renal tumors are rare in the neonatal period. These include mesoblastic nephroma and nephroblastomatosis. The differential diagnosis includes other causes of renal masses (Table 28.2).

Suggested Readings

Andreoli SP. Acute renal failure in the newborn. *Semin Perinatol* 2004;28:112.

Bailie MD, ed. Renal function and disease. *Clin Perinatol* 1992;19(1):91–92.

Chevalier RL. Perinatal obstructive nephropathy. *Semin Perinatol* 2004;28:124.

Guignard JP, Drukker A. Clinical neonatal nephrology. In: Barratt TM, Avner ED, Harmon WE, eds. *Pediatric Nephrology*. Philadelphia: Lippincott Williams & Wilkins, 1999.

Mesrobian HG. Urologic problems of the neonate: an update. *Clin Perinatol* 2007;34:667.

Moghal NE, Embleton ND. Management of acute renal failure in the newborn. *Semin Fetal Neonatal Med* 2006;11(3):207–213.

29 Mechanical Ventilation
Eric C. Eichenwald

I. GENERAL PRINCIPLES. Mechanical ventilation is an invasive life support procedure with many effects on the cardiopulmonary system. The goal is to optimize both gas exchange and clinical status at minimum fractional concentration of inspired oxygen (FiO_2) and ventilator pressures/tidal volume. The ventilator strategy employed to accomplish this goal depends, in part, on the infant's disease process. In addition, recent advances in technology have brought more options for ventilatory therapy of newborns.

II. TYPES OF VENTILATORY SUPPORT

A. Continuous positive airway pressure (CPAP)

1. **CPAP is usually administered by means of a ventilator or stand-alone CPAP delivery system.** Any system used to deliver CPAP should allow continuous monitoring of the delivered pressure, and be equipped with safety alarms to indicate when the pressure is above or below the desired level. Alternatively, CPAP may be delivered by a simplified system providing blended oxygen flowing past the infant's airway, with the end of the tubing submerged in 0.25% acetic acid in sterile water solution to the desired depth to generate pressure ("bubble CPAP"). Stand-alone variable flow CPAP devices, in which expiratory resistance is decreased via a "fluidic flip" of flow at the nosepiece during expiration, are also available.

2. **General characteristics.** A continuous flow of heated, humidified gas is circulated past the infant's airway, typically at a set pressure of 3 to 8 cm H_2O, maintaining an elevated end-expiratory lung volume while the infant breathes spontaneously. The air–oxygen mixture and airway pressure can be adjusted. Variable flow CPAP systems may decrease the work of breathing and improve lung recruitment in infants on CPAP, but have not been shown to be clearly superior to conventional means of delivery. CPAP is usually delivered by means of nasal prongs, nasopharyngeal tube, or nasal mask. Endotracheal CPAP should not be used, because the high resistance of the endotracheal tube increases the work of breathing, especially in small infants. Positive-pressure hoods and continuous-mask CPAP are not recommended.

3. **Advantages**
   a. CPAP is less invasive than mechanical ventilation and causes less lung injury.
   b. When used early in infants with respiratory distress syndrome (RDS), CPAP can help prevent alveolar and airway collapse, and thereby reduce the need for mechanical ventilation.
   c. Use of immediate CPAP in the delivery room for immature infants ≥25 weeks' gestation decreases the need for mechanical ventilation and administration

of surfactant, although trials comparing initial CPAP and mechanical ventilation show similar rates of bronchopulmonary dysplasia (BPD).

    d. CPAP decreases the frequency of obstructive and mixed apneic spells in some infants.

  4. Disadvantages

    a. CPAP is not effective in patients with apnea or inadequate respiratory drive.

    b. CPAP provides inadequate respiratory support in the face of severely abnormal pulmonary compliance and resistance.

    c. Maintaining nasal or nasopharyngeal CPAP in large, active infants may be technically difficult.

    d. Infants on CPAP frequently swallow air, leading to gastric distension and elevation of the diaphragm, necessitating decompression by a gastric tube.

  5. Indications (see III.A.)

B. Pressure-limited, time-cycled, continuous flow ventilators are used most frequently in newborns with respiratory failure.

  1. General characteristics. A continuous flow of heated and humidified gas is circulated past the infant's airway; the gas is a mixture of air, blended with oxygen to maintain the desired oxygen saturation level. Peak inspiratory pressure (PI or PIP), positive end-expiratory pressure (PEEP), and respiratory timing (rate and duration of inspiration and expiration) are selected.

  2. Advantages

    a. The continuous flow of fresh gas allows the infant to make spontaneous respiratory efforts between ventilator breaths (intermittent mandatory ventilation [IMV]).

    b. Good control is maintained over respiratory pressures.

    c. Inspiratory and expiratory time can be independently controlled.

    d. The system is relatively simple and inexpensive.

  3. Disadvantages

    a. Tidal volume (VT) is poorly controlled.

    b. The system does not respond to changes in respiratory system compliance.

    c. Spontaneously breathing infants, who breathe out of phase with too many IMV breaths ("bucking" or "fighting" the ventilator), may receive inadequate ventilation and are at increased risk for air leak.

C. Synchronized and patient-triggered (assist/control or pressure support) ventilators are adaptations of conventional pressure-limited ventilators used for newborns and are currently the "gold standard" for mechanical ventilation of newborns.

  1. General characteristics. These ventilators combine the features of pressure-limited, time-cycled, continuous flow ventilators with an airway pressure, airflow, or respiratory movement sensor. By measuring inspiratory flow or movement, these ventilators deliver intermittent positive-pressure breaths at a fixed rate, in synchrony with the baby's inspiratory efforts ("synchronized IMV," or synchronized intermittent mandatory ventilation [SIMV]). During apnea, SIMV ventilators continue to deliver the set IMV rate. In patient-triggered ventilation, a positive pressure breath is delivered with every inspiratory effort. As a result, the ventilator delivers more frequent positive pressure breaths, usually allowing a decrease in the inspiratory pressure (PIP) needed for adequate gas exchange. During apnea, the ventilator in patient-triggered mode delivers an operator-selected IMV ("control") rate. In some ventilators, synchronized IMV breaths can be supplemented by pressure-supported breaths in the spontaneously breathing infant. Ventilators equipped with a flow sensor can also be used to monitor delivered V_T continuously by integration of the flow signal.

2. **Advantages**

   a. Synchronizing the delivery of positive pressure breaths with the infant's inspiratory effort reduces the phenomenon of breathing out of phase with IMV breaths ("fighting" the ventilator). This may decrease the need for sedative medications, and aid in weaning mechanically ventilated infants.

   b. Pronounced asynchrony with ventilator breaths, during conventional IMV, has been associated with the development of air leak and intraventricular hemorrhage. Whether the use of SIMV or assist/control ventilation reduces these complications is not known.

3. **Disadvantages**

   a. Under certain conditions, the ventilators may inappropriately trigger a breath because of signal artifacts, or fail to trigger because of problems with the sensor.

   b. Limited data are available comparing patient-triggered ventilation to other modes of ventilation in newborns. Pressure support ventilation may not be appropriate for small premature infants with irregular respiratory patterns and frequent apnea because of the potential for significant variability in ventilation. However, some data suggest that use of patient-triggered modes of ventilation in premature infants may decrease markers of lung inflammation and facilitate earlier extubation, when used as the initial mode of mechanical ventilator support.

4. **Indications.** SIMV can be used when a conventional pressure-limited ventilator is indicated. If available, it is the preferable mode of ventilator therapy in infants who are breathing spontaneously while on IMV. The indications for assist/control and pressure support ventilation have not been established, although many neonatal intensive care units (NICUs) use these modes as initial ventilator support because of perceived advantages of using lower peak inspired pressure and smaller V_Ts.

D. **Volume-cycled ventilators** are rarely used in newborn infants, although recent advances in technology have renewed interest in this mode of ventilation in selected situations. Only volume-cycled ventilators specifically designed for newborns should be used.

1. **General characteristics.** Volume-cycled ventilators are similar to pressure-limited ventilators, except that the operator selects the volume delivered rather than the PIP. "Volume guarantee" is a mode of pressure-limited SIMV, in which the ventilator targets an operator-chosen V_T (usually 4–6 mL/kg) during mechanically delivered breaths. Volume guarantee allows rapid response of the ventilator pressures to changing lung compliance, and may be particularly useful in infants with RDS who receive surfactant therapy.

2. **Advantages.** The pressure automatically varies with respiratory system compliance to deliver the selected V_T, theoretically minimizing variability in minute ventilation.

3. **Disadvantages**

    a. The system is complicated and requires more skill to operate.

    b. Because VTs in infants are small, most of the VTs selected are lost in the ventilator circuit or from air leaks around uncuffed endotracheal tubes. Some ventilators compensate for these losses by targeting expired rather than inspired VTs.

4. **Indications.** Volume-cycled ventilators may be useful if lung compliance is rapidly changing, as would be seen in infants receiving surfactant therapy.

E. **High-frequency ventilation** (HFV) is an important adjunct to conventional mechanical ventilation in newborns. The recommended uses and the ventilatory strategies employed with HFV continue to evolve with clinical experience. Three types of high-frequency ventilators are approved for use in newborns: a high-frequency oscillator (HFO), a high-frequency flow interrupter (HFFI), and a high-frequency jet (HFJ) ventilator.

    1. **General characteristics.** Available high-frequency ventilators are similar despite considerable differences in design. All are capable of delivering extremely rapid rates (300–1,500 breaths/minute, 5–25 Hz; 1 Hz = 60 breaths/minute), with VTs equal to or smaller than anatomic dead space. These ventilators apply continuous distending pressure to maintain an elevated lung volume; small VTs are superimposed at a rapid rate. HFJ ventilators are paired with a conventional pressure-limited device, which is used to deliver intermittent "sigh" breaths to help prevent atelectasis. "Sigh" breaths are not used with HFO ventilation. Expiration is passive (i.e., dependent on chest wall and lung recoil) with HFFI and HFJ machines, while expiration is active with HFO. The mechanisms of gas exchange are incompletely understood.

    2. **Advantages**

        a. **HFV** can achieve adequate ventilation while avoiding the large swings in lung volume required by conventional ventilators and associated with lung injury. Because of this, HFV may be useful in pulmonary air leak syndromes (pulmonary interstitial emphysema [PIE], pneumothorax), or in infants failing conventional mechanical ventilation.

        b. **HFV** allows the use of a high mean airway pressure (MAP) for alveolar recruitment and resultant improvement in ventilation–perfusion ($\dot{V}/\dot{Q}$) matching. This may be advantageous in infants with severe respiratory failure requiring high MAP to maintain adequate oxygenation on a conventional mechanical ventilator.

    3. **Disadvantages.** Despite theoretical advantages of HFV, no significant benefit of this method has been demonstrated in routine clinical use over more conventional ventilators. Only one rigorously controlled study found a small reduction in BPD in infants at high risk treated with high-frequency oscillatory ventilation (HFOV) as the primary mode of ventilation. This experience is likely not generally applicable, however, as other studies have shown no difference. These ventilators are more complex and expensive, and there is less long-term clinical experience. The initial studies with HFO suggested an increased risk of significant intraventricular hemorrhage, although this complication has not been observed in recent clinical trials. Studies comparing the different types of high-frequency ventilators are unavailable; therefore, the relative advantages or disadvantages of HFO, HFFI, and HFJ, if any, are not characterized.

4. **Indications.** HFV is primarily used as a rescue therapy for infants failing conventional ventilation. Both HFJ and HFO ventilators have been shown to be superior to conventional ventilation in infants with air leak syndromes, especially PIE. Because of the potential for complications and equivalence to conventional ventilation in the incidence of BPD, we do not use high-frequency ventilation as the primary mode of ventilatory support in infants.

F. **Negative pressure.** These infant versions of the adult "iron lung" are rarely used, because nursing access is limited by the negative-pressure cylinder and because the neck seal makes them feasible only for large babies. Their use is restricted to older infants with neuromuscular problems who can therefore be ventilated without an endotracheal tube.

III. INDICATIONS FOR RESPIRATORY SUPPORT

A. **Indications** for CPAP in the preterm infant with RDS include the following:

1. Recently delivered premature infant with minimal respiratory distress and low supplemental oxygen requirement (to prevent atelectasis)

2. Respiratory distress and requirement of FiO_2 above 0.30 by hood

3. FiO_2 above 0.40 by hood

4. Initial stabilization in the delivery room for spontaneously breathing, extremely premature infants (25–28 weeks' gestation)

5. Initial management of premature infants with moderately severe respiratory distress

6. Clinically significant retractions and/or distress after recent extubation

7. In general, infants with RDS who require FiO_2 above 0.35 to 0.40 on CPAP should be intubated, ventilated, and given surfactant replacement therapy. In some NICUs, intubation for surfactant therapy in infants with RDS is followed by immediate extubation to CPAP. We generally use mechanical ventilation for all infants who are given surfactant.

8. After extubation to facilitate maintenance of lung volume

B. **Relative indications for mechanical ventilation** in any infant include the following:

1. Frequent intermittent apnea unresponsive to drug therapy

2. Early treatment when use of mechanical ventilation is anticipated because of deteriorating gas exchange

3. Relieving "increased work of breathing" in an infant with signs of moderate-to-severe respiratory distress

4. Administration of surfactant therapy in infants with RDS

C. **Absolute indications for mechanical ventilation**

1. Prolonged apnea

2. PaO_2 below 50 mm Hg, or FiO_2 above 0.80. This indication may not apply to the infant with cyanotic congenital heart disease.

3. $PaCO_2$ above 60 to 65 mm Hg with persistent acidemia

4. General anesthesia

IV. HOW VENTILATOR CHANGES AFFECT BLOOD GASES

A. Oxygenation (see Table 29.1)

1. **FiO₂.** The goal is to maintain adequate tissue oxygen delivery. Generally, this can be accomplished by achieving a PaO_2 of 50 to 70 mm Hg and results in a hemoglobin saturation of 88% to 95% (see Fig. 29.1). Increasing inspired oxygen is the simplest and most direct means of improving oxygenation. In premature infants, the risk of retinopathy and pulmonary oxygen toxicity argue for minimizing PaO_2. For infants with other conditions, the optimum PaO_2 may be higher. Direct pulmonary oxygen toxicity begins to occur at FiO_2 values greater than 0.60 to 0.70.

Table 29.1	Ventilator Manipulations to Increase Oxygenation	
Parameter	**Advantage**	**Disadvantage**
↑ FiO₂	Minimizes barotrauma	Fails to affect V̇/Q̇ matching
	Easily administered	Direct toxicity, especially >0.6
↑ PIP	Improves V̇/Q̇	Lung injury: air leak, BPD
↑ PEEP	Maintains FRC/prevents collapse	Shifts to stiffer part of compliance curve
	Splints obstructed airways	May impede venous return
		Increases expiratory work and CO₂
		Increases dead space
↑ Tɪ	Increases MAP	Results in slower rates; may need to increase PIP
	"Critical opening time"	Lower minute ventilation for given PIP—PEEP combination
↑ Flow	Square wave—maximizes MAP	Greater shear force, more lung injury
		Greater resistance at greater flows
↑ Rate	Increases MAP while using lower PIP	Inadvertent PEEP with high rates or long time constant

↑ = increase; BPD = bronchopulmonary dysplasia; FiO₂ = fractional concentration of inspired oxygen; FRC = functional residual capacity; PIP = inspiratory pressure; Tɪ = inspiratory time; MAP = mean airway pressure; PEEP = positive end-expiratory pressure; V̇/Q̇ = ventilation–perfusion ratio.
Increase in any setting (except FiO₂) results in higher mean airway pressure (MAP).

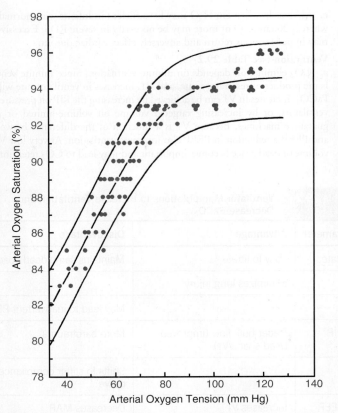

Figure 29.1. Comparison of paired measurements of oxygen saturation by pulse oximetry and of oxygen tension by indwelling umbilical artery oxygen electrode. The lines represent ±2 standard deviations. (Modified from Wasunna A, Whitelaw AG. Pulse oximetry in preterm infants. *Arch Dis Child* 1987;62[9]:957.)

2. **Mean Airway Pressure (MAP)**

   a. MAP is the average area under the curve of the pressure waveform. Many ventilators now display MAP or can be equipped with a device to do so; it may also be calculated using the following equation: MAP = ([PIP − PEEP][TI / TI + TE) + PEEP. MAP is increased by increases in PEEP, PIP, TI, rate, and flow rate. All these changes lead to higher PaO_2, but each has different effects on $PaCO_2$. For a given rise in MAP, increasing PEEP gives the greatest improvement in PaO_2. Other ways to raise MAP are to increase PIP and prolong TI.

   b. Optimum MAP results from a balance between optimizing PaO_2, minimizing direct oxygen toxicity, minimizing barotrauma and volutrauma, achieving adequate ventilation, and minimizing adverse cardiovascular effects. Ventilator-induced lung injury is probably most closely related to peak-to-peak swings in lung volume, although changes in airway pressure are also implicated.

  c. MAP as low as 5 cm H_2O may be sufficient in infants with normal lungs, whereas 20 cm H_2O or more may be necessary in severe RDS. Excessive MAP may impede venous return and adversely affect cardiac output.

3. Ventilation (see Table 29.2)

  a. CO_2 elimination depends on minute ventilation. Since minute ventilation is the product of respiratory rate, and V_T, increases in ventilator rate will lower $PaCO_2$. Increases in V_T can be achieved by increasing the PIP on pressure-cycled ventilators, or by increasing targeted volume on volume-limited or volume guarantee machines. Because V_T is a function of the difference between PIP and PEEP, a reduction in PEEP also improves ventilation. At very low V_Ts, the volume of dead space becomes important and may lead to CO_2 retention.

Table 29.2	Ventilator Manipulations to Increase Ventilation and Decrease $PaCO_2$	
Parameter	**Advantage**	**Disadvantage**
↑ Rate	Easy to titrate	Maintains same dead space/V_T
	Minimizes lung injury	
		May lead to inadvertent PEEP
↑ PIP	Better bulk flow (improved dead space/V_T)	More barotrauma
		Shifts to stiffer compliance curve
↓ PEEP	Increases V_T	Decreases MAP
	Decreases dead space	Decreases oxygenation; may result in alveolar collapse
	Shifts to steeper part of compliance curve	Decreases splinting of obstructed/closed airways
↑ Flow	Permits shorter T_I, longer T_E	More barotrauma
↑ T_E	Allows longer time for passive expiration in face of prolonged time constant	Shortens T_I
		Decreases MAP
		Decreases oxygenation
T_E = expiratory time; FiO_2 = fractional concentration of inspired oxygen; T_I = inspiratory time; MAP = mean airway pressure; $PaCO_2$ = partial pressure of carbon dioxide, arterial; PIP = peak inspiratory pressure; PEEP = positive end-expiratory pressure; ↓ = decrease; ↑ = increase.		

b. Optimal $PaCO_2$ varies according to disease state. For very immature infants or infants with air leak, a $PaCO_2$ of 50 to 60 mm Hg may be tolerated to minimize ventilator-induced lung injury, provided pH can be maintained >7.20 to 7.25.

V. DISEASE STATES

A. **Effects of diseases.** Respiratory failure can result from numerous illnesses through a variety of pathophysiologic mechanisms. Optimal ventilatory strategy must take into account the pathophysiology, expected time course, and particular vulnerabilities of the patient.

B. **Pulmonary mechanics** influence the ventilator strategy selected.

1. **Compliance is the stiffness** or distensibility of the lung and chest wall; that is, the change in volume (ΔV) produced by a change in pressure (ΔP), or $\Delta V/\Delta P$. It is decreased with surfactant deficiency, excess lung water, and lung fibrosis. It is also decreased when the lungs are hyperexpanded.

2. **Resistance is the impediment** to airflow due to friction between gas and airways (airway resistance) and between tissues of the lungs and chest wall (viscous tissue resistance). Almost half of airway resistance is in the upper airways, including the endotracheal tube when in use. Resistance is high in diseases characterized by airway obstruction, such as meconium aspiration and BPD. Resistance can change rapidly if, for example, secretions partially occlude the endotracheal tube.

3. **Time constant** is the product of compliance and resistance. This is a measure of the time it takes to equilibrate pressure between the proximal airway and the alveoli. Expiratory time constants are somewhat longer than inspiratory ones. When time constants are long, as in meconium aspiration, care must be taken to set ventilator inspiratory times and rates that permit adequate inspiration to deliver the required V_T and adequate expiration to avoid inadvertent PEEP.

4. **Functional residual capacity (FRC)** is a measure of the volume of the lungs at end expiration. FRC is decreased in diseases that permit alveolar collapse, particularly surfactant deficiency.

5. **$\dot{V}/\dot{Q}$ matching.** Diseases that reduce alveolar surface area (through atelectasis, inflammatory exudates, or obstruction) permit intrapulmonary shunting of desaturated blood. The opposite occurs in persistent pulmonary hypertension when extrapulmonary shunting diverts blood flow away from the ventilated lung. Both mechanisms result in systemic recirculation of desaturated blood.

6. **Work of breathing** is especially important in the smallest infants and those with chronic lung disease whose high airway resistance, decreased lung compliance, compliant chest wall, and weak musculature may overwhelm their metabolic energy requirements and impede growth.

C. **Specific disease states.** Several of the more common neonatal disease processes are described in the subsequent text and are presented in Table 29.3, along with the optimal ventilatory strategies. Before initiating ventilatory support, clinicians must evaluate for mechanical causes of distress, including pneumothorax or airway obstruction.

1. **RDS (see Chap. 33)**
   a. Pathophysiology. RDS is caused by surfactant deficiency, which results in a severe decrease in compliance (stiff lung). This causes diffuse alveolar collapse with $\dot{V}/\dot{Q}$ mismatching and increased work of breathing.

Table 29.3		Neonatal Pulmonary Physiology by Disease State				
Disease	Compliance mL/cm H_2O	Resistance cm $H_2O/mL/s$	Time constant (s)	FRC (mL/kg)	$\dot{V}/\dot{Q}$ matching	Work
Normal term	4–6	20–40	0.25	30	—	—
RDS	↓↓	—	↓↓	↓	↓/↓↓	↑
Meconium aspiration	—/↓	↑↑	↑	↑/↑↑	↓↓	↑
BPD	↑/↓	↑↑	↑	↑↑	↓↓/↓	↑↑
Air leak	↓↓	—/↑	—/↑	↑↑	↓/↓↓	↑↑
VLBW apnea	↓	—	↓↓	—/↓	↓/—	—/↑

BPD = bronchopulmonary dysplasia; FRC = functional residual capacity; RDS = respiratory distress syndrome; $\dot{V}/\dot{Q}$ = ventilation–perfusion ratio; VLBW = very low birth weight; ↓ = decrease; / = either/or; ↓ = decrease; ↑ = increase; — = little or no change.

b. Surfactant replacement. Early initiation of CPAP, usually starting in the delivery room, may avoid the need for mechanical ventilation and surfactant therapy in some infants, even at very early gestational ages. Alternatively, some recommend intubation and initiation of mechanical ventilation early in the course of RDS in order to provide surfactant therapy promptly. Surfactant therapy modifies the distinctive time course of escalation, plateau, and weaning in classic RDS. Ventilatory strategy should anticipate the increased risk of pneumothorax as compliance increases and time constants lengthen, especially with the rapid improvement that can be seen after surfactant administration. In all approaches, a $PaCO_2$ value higher than the physiologic value is acceptable to minimize ventilator-induced lung injury.

c. Ventilator strategy

    i. CPAP. In mild to moderately affected infants who may not require intubation and surfactant administration, CPAP is used very early in the disease course to prevent further atelectasis. CPAP is initiated at 5 to 6 cm H_2O, and increased to a maximum of 7 to 8 cm H_2O. The risk of pneumothorax may be increased at higher levels of CPAP pressure. CPAP is titrated by clinical assessment of retractions and respiratory rate and by observation of O_2 saturation. Alternatively, in infants with more severe RDS, consideration may be given to intubation for surfactant administration, a short period of mechanical ventilation, and followed by CPAP as gas exchange improves.

    ii. Mechanical ventilation is used when $\dot{V}/\dot{Q}$ mismatching is so severe that increased FiO_2 and CPAP are inadequate to maintain gas exchange, or in infants who tire from the increased work of breathing.

Data suggest that a ventilator strategy that avoids large changes in V_T may reduce ventilator-induced lung injury. The objective of all strategies of assisted ventilation in the infant with RDS should be to provide the lowest level of ventilatory support possible to support adequate oxygenation and ventilation while attempting to reduce acute and chronic lung injury secondary to barotrauma/volutrauma and oxygen toxicity. Our preferred approach is to maintain the appropriate MAP with a T_I initially set at 0.3 second, and rate of approximately 20 to 40 breaths/minute. Rarely, a longer T_I is required to provide adequate oxygenation. This ventilatory approach requires a moderate PIP to provide adequate minute ventilation and to maintain alveolar recruitment.

iii. **PIP and PEEP.** PIP, applied to recruit alveoli, is initially estimated by visible chest excursion and is usually 20 to 25 cm H_2O. PEEP is usually set at 4 to 6 cm H_2O. Higher PEEP may interfere with cardiac output, and should be avoided in acute RDS.

iv. **Flow.** Flow rates of 7 to 12 L/minute are needed to provide a relatively square pressure waveform. Higher flows may be required at very high PIP (>35 cm H_2O).

v. **Rates** are generally set initially at 20 to 40 breaths/minute, and adjusted according to blood gas results.

vi. When using volume-controlled or volume-guarantee modes, the V_T targets are usually 4 to 6 mL/kg (expired volume).

vii. **Weaning.** When the patient improves, FiO_2 and PIP are weaned first, alternating with rate, in response to assessment of chest excursion, oxygen saturation, and blood gas results. In patient-triggered modes, the back-up rate of the ventilator is usually not changed, and progressive decreases in PIP are used to wean the ventilator. In volume-guarantee ventilation, the PIP will decrease automatically in response to improved compliance; weaning may be accomplished by decreasing the targeted level of V_T. Extubation is usually successful when ventilator rates are <20 to 25 breaths/minute, or PIP is below 16 to 18 cm H_2O. Caffeine citrate may be used to facilitate spontaneous breathing before extubation and may increase the success rate of extubation in very low birth weight infants.

viii. **Advantages and disadvantages.** This ventilatory strategy maximizes alveolar recruitment, but with a potential for greater lung injury secondary to higher PIP and volutrauma secondary to higher V_T.

ix. **Alternative ventilator strategies.** An alternative approach to mechanical ventilation in RDS relies on high rates to maintain MAP while reducing PIP and V_T to minimize lung injury. Rates of 60 to 80 breaths/minute are used, with T_I as low as 0.2 second. Inadvertent PEEP is not encountered, because the time constant in RDS may be as short as 0.05 second. PIP is set as low as 12 to 18 cm H_2O, with PEEP of 4 to 5 cm H_2O. Initial settings are based on auscultation of good breath sounds and are increased as needed to maintain adequate minute ventilation and oxygenation. In general, pressure is weaned first, while the rate remains high, or by 10% drops in rate alternating with pressure, as tolerated. This ventilator strategy may minimize barotrauma due to lower PIP and V_T, with the disadvantage of less alveolar recruitment and consequent need for higher FiO_2 to maintain adequate oxygen saturation.

High-frequency ventilation may be initiated if conventional ventilation fails to maintain adequate gas exchange at acceptable settings. High-frequency ventilation should be used only by clinicians familiar with its use. We consider the use of HFV when the MAP required for adequate gas exchange exceeds 10 to 11 cm H_2O in small infants, and 12 cm H_2O in larger infants, or if air leak occurs. Strategies differ depending on whether HFJ, HFO, or HFFI is used. We prefer HFOV over other available HFV because of its ease of use and applicability in a wide range of pulmonary diseases and infant weights.

a) **HFJ ventilation.** HFJ requires a special adapter for a standard endotracheal tube to allow connection to the jet port of the ventilator.

1) **PIP and PEEP.** Peak pressures on the jet ventilator are initially set approximately 20% lower than on those being used with conventional ventilation, and adjusted to provide adequate chest vibration assessed clinically and by blood gas determinations. PIP, PEEP, and FiO_2 are adjusted as needed to maintain oxygenation. CO_2 elimination is dependent on the pressure difference (PIP − PEEP). Because of the lower peak pressures required to ventilate, PEEP may be increased to 8 to 10 cm H_2O if needed to improve oxygenation.

2) **Rate.** The frequency is usually set at 420 breaths/minute, with an inspiratory jet valve on-time of 0.02 second.

3) **Conventional ventilator settings.** Once the HFJ is properly adjusted, the conventional ventilator rate is decreased to 2 to 10 breaths/minute to help maintain alveolar recruitment, with PIP set at 2 to 3 cm H_2O lower than the jet PIP. In air leak syndromes, it may be advantageous to provide no sigh breaths from the conventional ventilator as long as the PEEP is set high enough to maintain lung volume.

4) **Weaning** from HFJ ventilation is accomplished by decreasing the jet PIP in response to blood gas determinations and the FiO_2. PEEP is weaned as tolerated if pressures higher than 4 to 5 cm H_2O are used. Frequency and jet valve on-time are generally not adjusted.

5) **Similar strategies** outlined for the HFJ apply in use of the HFFI.

b) **HFOV.** With HFO, operator-selected parameters include MAP, frequency, and piston amplitude.

1) **MAP.** In RDS, the initial MAP selected is usually 2 to 5 cm H_2O higher than that being used on the conventional ventilator to enhance alveolar recruitment. MAP used with HFO is titrated to O_2 requirement and to provide adequate lung expansion on chest x-ray. Care must be exercised to avoid lung hyperinflation, which might adversely affect oxygen delivery by reducing cardiac output.

2) **Frequency is usually set at 10 to 15 Hz.** Inspiratory time is set at 33%.

3) **Amplitude.** Changes in piston amplitude primarily affect ventilation. It is set to provide adequate chest vibration, assessed clinically and by blood gas determinations.

4) **Flow rates** of 8 to 15 L/minute are usually adequate.

5) **Weaning.** In general, FiO_2 is weaned first, followed by MAP in decrements of 1 to 2 cm H_2O once the FiO_2 falls below 0.6. Piston amplitude is adjusted by frequent assessment of chest vibration and blood gas determinations. Frequency is usually not adjusted unless adequate oxygenation or ventilation cannot otherwise be achieved. In contrast to conventional mechanical ventilation, decreasing the frequency of breaths in HFOV will improve ventilation because of effects on delivered VT. In both HFJ and HFO, we usually wean to extubation after transfer back to conventional ventilation, although infants can be extubated directly from HFV.

2. **Meconium aspiration syndrome (MAS) (see Chap. 35)**

   a. Pathophysiology. MAS results from aspiration of meconium-stained amniotic fluid. The severity of the syndrome is related to the associated asphyxial insult and the amount of fluid aspirated. The aspirated meconium causes acute airway obstruction, markedly increased airway resistance, scattered atelectasis with $\dot{V}/\dot{Q}$ mismatching, and hyperexpansion due to obstructive ball-valve effects. The obstructive phase is followed by an inflammatory phase 12 to 24 hours later, which results in further alveolar involvement. Aspiration of other fluids (such as blood or amniotic fluid) has similar but milder effects.

   b. Ventilator strategy. Because of the ball-valve effects, the application of positive pressure may result in pneumothorax or other air leak, so initiating mechanical ventilation requires careful consideration of the risks and benefits. Low levels of PEEP (4–5 cm H_2O) are helpful in splinting open partially obstructed airways and equalizing $\dot{V}/\dot{Q}$ matching. Higher levels may lead to hyperinflation. If airway resistance is high and compliance is normal, a slow-rate, moderate-pressure strategy is needed. If pneumonitis is more prominent, more rapid rates can be used. Sedation or muscle relaxation may be used to minimize the risks of air leak in severe MAS, because of the high transpulmonary pressures these large infants can generate when "fighting" the ventilator and the ball-valve hyperexpansion caused by their disease. Use of patient-triggered ventilation may be helpful in some infants and avoid the need for muscle relaxation. Weaning may be rapid if the illness is primarily related to airway obstruction, or prolonged if complicated by lung injury and severe inflammation. Due to secondary surfactant inactivation, the use of surfactant therapy may improve lung compliance and oxygenation, and should be considered in more severe cases of MAS.

   High-frequency ventilation has also been successfully used in infants with MAS who are failing conventional ventilation or who have air leak. The strategies are similar to those described in the preceding text. During HFO, slower frequencies (8–10 Hz) may be useful to improve oxygenation in severe cases.

3. **BPD (see Chap. 34)**

   a. Pathophysiology. BPD results from injury to the alveoli and airways. Bleb formation may lead to poor recoil. Fibrosis and excess lung water may cause stiffer compliance. Airways may be narrowed and fibrotic or hyperreactive. The upper airways may be overdistended and conduct airflow poorly. BPD is marked by shifting focal atelectasis, hyperinflation with $\dot{V}/\dot{Q}$ mismatch, chronic and acute increases in airway resistance, and a significant increase in the work of breathing.

b. Ventilator strategy. The optimal strategy is to wean infants off the ventilator as soon as possible to prevent further mechanical injury and oxygen toxicity. If this is not feasible, ventilator settings should be minimized to permit tissue repair and long-term growth. Rates less than about 20 breaths/minute should generally be avoided to prevent increased work of breathing, but longer Ti (0.4–0.5 second) may be used to maintain FRC. Some centers use SIMV in combination with pressure support ventilation in severe cases to improve work of breathing and ventilation. Higher PIPs are sometimes required (20–30 cm H_2O) because of the stiff lungs, although the high resistance prevents transfer of most of this to the alveoli. Oxygenation should be maintained (saturations of 90%–92%), but higher $PaCO_2$ values can be permitted (55–65 mm Hg), provided the pH is acceptable. Acute decompensations can result from bronchospasm and interstitial fluid accumulation. These must be treated with adjustment of PIP, bronchodilators, and diuretics. Acute BPD "spells" in which oxygenation and airway resistance worsen rapidly are usually due to larger airway collapse, and may be treated successfully with higher PEEP (7–8 cm H_2O). Frequent rapid desaturations secondary to acute decreases in FRC with crying or infant movement respond to changes in FiO_2, but may also be partially ameliorated by using higher PEEP. Weaning is a slow and difficult process, decreasing rate by 1 to 2 breaths/minute or 1 cm H_2O decrements in PIP every day when tolerated. Fortunately, with improved medical and ventilatory care of these infants, it is rare for infants with BPD to require tracheostomy for chronic ventilation.

4. **Air leak (see Chap. 38)**

a. Pathophysiology. Pneumothorax and PIE are the two most common air leak syndromes. Pneumothorax results when air ruptures into the pleural space. In PIE, the interstitial air substantially reduces tissue compliance as well as recoil. In addition, peribronchial and perivascular air may compress the airways and vascular supply, causing "air block."

b. Ventilator strategy. Since air is driven into the interstitium throughout the ventilatory cycle, the primary goal is to reduce MAP through any of its components (PIP, Ti, or PEEP) and to rely on increased FiO_2 to provide oxygenation. This strategy holds for all air leak syndromes. If dropping the MAP is not tolerated, other techniques may be tried. Because the time constants for interstitial air are much longer than those for the alveoli, we sometimes use very rapid conventional rates (up to 60 breaths/minute), which may preferentially ventilate the alveoli.

High-frequency ventilation is an important alternative therapy for severe air leak and, if available, may be the ventilatory treatment of choice. HFV strategies for air leak differ from those used in diffuse alveolar disease. As described for conventional ventilation, the ventilatory goal in air leak syndromes is to decrease MAP, relying on FiO_2 to provide oxygenation. With HFJ and HFFI, PEEP is maintained at lower levels (4–6 cm H_2O), and few to no-sigh breaths are provided. With HFO, the MAP initially used is the same as that being used on the conventional ventilator, and the frequency set at 15 Hz. While weaning, MAP is decreased progressively, tolerating higher FiO_2 in the attempt to limit the MAP exposure.

5. Apnea (see Chap. 31)

    a. Pathophysiology. Occasionally, apnea is severe enough to warrant ventilator support, even in the absence of pulmonary disease. This may result from apnea of prematurity, during or following general anesthesia, or from neuromuscular paralysis.

    b. Ventilator strategy. For infants completely dependent on the ventilator, the goal should be to provide "physiologic" ventilation using moderate PEEP (3–4 cm H_2O), low gas flow, and normal rates (30–40 breaths/minute), with PIP adjusted to prevent hyperventilation (10–18 cm H_2O). Prolonged Tı is unnecessary. For infants requiring a ventilator because of intermittent but prolonged apnea, low rates (12–15 breaths/minute) may be sufficient.

VI. ADJUNCTS TO MECHANICAL VENTILATION

A. Sedation (see chart on intubation sedation guidelines, and Chap. 67) can be used when agitation or distress is associated with excessive lability of oxygenation and hypoxemia. Although this problem is more common in the neonate receiving long-term ventilation, acutely ill newborns may occasionally benefit from sedation. Morphine (0.05–0.1 mg/kg) or fentanyl (1–3 μg/kg) can be used but may cause neurologic depression. Prolonged use may lead to dependence. Lorazepam (0.05–0.1 mg/kg/dose given every 4–6 hours) or midazolam (0.05–0.1 mg/kg/dose given every 2–4 hours) has been used in more mature infants and in more chronic situations. In preterm infants, nonpharmacologic methods, such as limiting environmental light and noise and providing behavioral supports may help decrease agitation and limit the need for sedative medications. As discussed, synchronized IMV or patient-triggered ventilation may also help diminish agitation and ventilatory lability.

B. Muscle relaxation with pancuronium bromide (0.1 mg/kg/dose, repeated as needed) or vecuronium (0.1 mg/kg/dose) is rarely used, but may be indicated in some infants who continue to breathe out of phase with the ventilator after attempts at finding appropriate settings and sedation have failed. Although unequivocal data are not available, gas exchange may be improved in some infants following muscle relaxation. Prolonged muscle relaxation leads to fluid retention and may result in deterioration in compliance. Sedation is routinely administered to infants receiving muscle relaxants.

C. Blood gas monitoring (see Chap. 30). All infants receiving mechanical ventilation require continuous monitoring of oxygen saturation and intermittent blood gas measurements.

VII. COMPLICATIONS AND SEQUELAE. As a complex and invasive technology, mechanical ventilation can result in numerous adverse outcomes, both iatrogenic and unavoidable.

A. Lung injury and oxygen toxicity

    1. BPD is related to increased airway pressure and changes in lung volume, although oxygen toxicity, anatomic and physiologic immaturity, and individual susceptibility also contribute.

2. **Air leak** is directly related to increased airway pressure. Risk is increased at MAPs in excess of 14 cm H_2O.

B. **Mechanical**

1. Obstruction of endotracheal tubes may result in hypoxemia and respiratory acidosis.

2. Equipment malfunction, particularly disconnection, is not uncommon and requires functioning alarm systems and vigilance.

C. **Complications of invasive monitoring**

1. Peripheral arterial occlusion with infarction (see Chap. 44)

2. Aortic thrombosis from umbilical arterial catheters, occasionally leading to renal impairment and hypertension

3. Emboli from flushed catheters, particularly to the lower extremities, the splanchnic bed, or even the brain

D. **Anatomic**

1. Subglottic stenosis from prolonged intubation; risk increases with multiple reintubations

2. Palatal grooves from prolonged orotracheal intubation

3. Vocal cord damage

Suggested Reading

Goldsmith J, Karotkin E. *Assisted Ventilation of the Neonate.* 5th ed. Philadelphia, PA: Saunders-Elsevier, 2010.

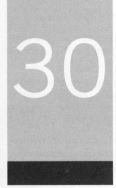

30

Blood Gas and Pulmonary Function Monitoring

James M. Adams

I. **GENERAL PRINCIPLES.** Blood gas monitoring in neonatal critical care units allows (i) assessment of pulmonary gas exchange; (ii) determination of hemoglobin oxygen saturation and arterial oxygen content; and (iii) evaluation, although limited, of adequacy of tissue oxygen delivery. Both invasive and noninvasive techniques are used in the clinical setting.

II. **OXYGEN USE AND MONITORING.** In emergency situations, sufficient oxygen to abolish cyanosis should be administered. Oxygen monitoring with pulse oximetry should be initiated as soon as possible, and the concentration of oxygen should be adjusted to maintain saturation values within a targeted range. An oxygen blender and pulse oximeter should be used whenever supplemental oxygen is administered. Monitoring of oxygen use is necessary to reduce both hypoxic injury to tissues and to minimize oxidative injury to the lungs or the immature retina of the premature infant.

A. **Arterial blood gas measurements.** Arterial PO_2 and PCO_2 are direct indicators of efficiency of pulmonary gas exchange in babies with acute lung disease. Arterial oxygen tension (PaO_2), measured under steady state conditions from an indwelling catheter, is the "gold standard" for oxygen monitoring.

1. **Usual values.** Most sources consider 50 to 80 mm Hg to be an acceptable target range for newborn PaO_2. Premature infants who require respiratory support may exhibit wide swings in PaO_2 values. In such circumstances, a single blood gas value may not accurately reflect the overall trend of oxygenation.

2. **Sampling.** To minimize sampling and dilutional artifacts, arterial blood gas samples should be collected in dry heparin syringes that are commercially available for this purpose. Most blood gas analyzers allow determination of blood gas values, as well as other whole blood parameters, on 0.2 to 0.3 mL samples. Samples should be analyzed within 15 minutes or preserved on ice if sent to a remote laboratory site. Blood gas sampling by percutaneous puncture is utilized when the need for measurement is infrequent or an indwelling catheter is not available. However, the discomfort of the puncture may result in agitation and a fall in PaO_2, such that the value obtained underestimates the true steady state value.

B. **Capillary blood gas determination.** This technique requires extensive warming of the extremity, free-flowing puncture, and strictly anaerobic collection. Under these conditions, capillary sampling may be useful for determination of pH and

PCO_2. Proper collection techniques are often difficult to guarantee in the clinical setting however, and capillary sampling should not be used for determination of PaO_2.

C. **Continuous blood gas analysis** via an indwelling catheter has been advocated to provide rapid, real-time data and reduce the volume of blood required for repeated blood gas measurements. However, because of technical limitations, a role for these devices in neonatal intensive care has not been established.

D. **Noninvasive oxygen monitoring** provides real-time trend data that are particularly useful in babies exhibiting frequent swings in PaO_2 and oxygen saturation. Noninvasive devices also may reduce the frequency of blood gas sampling in some patients.

1. **Pulse oximetry** is the primary tool for noninvasive oxygen monitoring in neonates. Pulse oximeters provide continuous measurement of hemoglobin oxygen saturation (SpO_2) with a high level of accuracy ($\pm 3\%$) when compared to control values measured by co-oximetry, at least down to the range of 70%.

a. **General characteristics.** Oximeters depend upon different absorption characteristics of oxygenated versus reduced hemoglobin for various wavelengths of light. Differences in transmission of two (usually red and near infrared) or more wavelengths through tissues with pulsatile blood flow are measured. Using the measured values, the proportion of oxygenated and reduced hemoglobin is calculated and displayed as percent saturation.

b. **Disadvantages.** Pulse oximetry does not measure the PaO_2 and, thus, is insensitive in detecting hyperoxemia. Due to the shape of the oxyhemoglobin dissociation curve, if SpO_2 is >95%, PaO_2 is unpredictable. Under such conditions, PaO_2 may well be greater than 100 mm Hg. Patient movement and the low amplitude pulse wave of small premature infants may introduce artifacts that result in false episodes of desaturation, although software modifications have reduced this problem. Other potential sources of artifact include inappropriate sensor placement, presence of high intensity light (some phototherapy devices), fetal hemoglobin values >50%, and presence of carboxyhemoglobin or methemoglobin.

c. **Targeted saturation values.** The optimal range of oxygen saturation, especially for preterm infants, is uncertain. In the Surfactant, Positive Pressure, and Oxygenation Randomized Trial (SUPPORT), infants born at 24 to 27 weeks' gestation were randomly assigned to target oxygen saturation ranges of 85% to 89% or 91% to 95%. The rate of severe retinopathy (ROP) or death (the primary outcome) was not different between the groups. Death before discharge was more frequent in the lower saturation group, although ROP occurred less often in survivors. In older studies that targeted oxygen saturation values in preterm infants after the immediate newborn period (supplemental therapeutic oxygen for prethreshold retinopathy of prematurity [STOP-ROP], benefits of oxygen saturation targeting [BOOST]), SpO_2 values >95% in preterm infants receiving supplemental oxygen were associated with increased need for prolonged supplemental oxygen. For infants who require supplemental oxygen, one approach is to target SpO_2 in the 88% to 92% range for infants less than 30 weeks' gestation or 1,250 g (set monitor alarm limits 85%–95%). For infants 30 weeks' gestation or more, or when infants reach 30 weeks' postmenstrual age, target SpO_2 from 88% to 95% (set alarm limits 85%–97%). If these targets are maintained, arterial PO_2 rarely will exceed 90 mm Hg.

2. **Transcutaneous oxygen monitoring** ($PtcO_2$) can be useful in management of acute cardiopulmonary disease during the first 2 weeks of life or if arterial catheterization is not possible. However, this technique has been largely supplanted in the neonatal intensive care unit (NICU) environment by pulse oximetry.

III. ASSESSMENT OF PULMONARY VENTILATION.

Assessment of alveolar ventilation is accomplished by direct or noninvasive measurement of PCO_2. Low values should be avoided because of the association with lung injury due to excessive volume distension of the immature lung. A strategy of "permissive hypercarbia" in mechanically ventilated infants generally tolerates PCO_2 values in the range of 50 to 65 mm Hg.

A. **Blood gas determination.** As is the case with oxygen monitoring, a $PaCO_2$ value obtained at steady state from an indwelling arterial catheter provides the most accurate indicator of alveolar ventilation. Lack of a catheter, however, limits the availability of this sampling for many patients. Blood obtained by percutaneous arterial puncture is an alternative but may not reflect steady state values because of artifacts introduced by pain and agitation.

1. **Venous blood** from a central catheter also may be useful in certain circumstances. If alveolar ventilation and circulatory function are normal, venous PCO_2 usually exceeds arterial values by 5 to 6 mm Hg. However, if significant hypoventilation or circulatory dysfunction is present, this relationship is unpredictable.

2. **Capillary blood gases.** PCO_2 and pH values obtained from properly collected capillary blood samples can closely reflect arterial values. The extremity must be warmed and a free-flowing blood sample collected under strictly anaerobic conditions without squeezing the extremity. In smaller premature infants, these conditions are difficult to achieve.

B. **Transcutaneous CO_2 monitoring.** Most current transcutaneous oxygen monitor sensors also include a transcutaneous CO_2 electrode. Accurate $PtcCO_2$ values, however, are more difficult to obtain than values for transcutaneous oxygen tension. Tissue diffusion rates and temperature coefficients for CO_2 are different than those for oxygen. Gas calibration of the electrode is required and a calibration factor must be built into the algorithm. Transcutaneous CO_2 tension exceeds that of arterial blood by a mean of 4 mm Hg, but this gradient may more than double in the presence of hypercapnia. The need for a high level of user attention and expertise has severely limited the use of this technique.

C. **Capnography.** The utility of end-tidal CO_2 measurements in neonates is limited by several factors. Mechanical ventilation typically occurs at relatively rapid rates compared to adult strategies, and most ventilator circuits deliver a continuous fresh flow of gas throughout the respiratory cycle. This limits the ability to obtain a true end-expiratory plateau. Also, arterial–alveolar CO_2 gradients are elevated in babies with serious primary lung disease because of maldistribution of ventilation (mean 6–10 mm Hg). Resulting end-tidal measurements, thus, may significantly underestimate arterial PCO_2 values in neonates with parenchymal lung disease. However, the technique may be useful for trend monitoring in babies with more uniform distribution of ventilation.

1. **Endotracheal intubation monitoring.** The Neonatal Resuscitation Program recommends the use of an exhaled CO_2 detector (colorimetric device or capnograph) to confirm correct tube placement during endotracheal intubation.

2. **Monitoring during anesthesia.** The Standards for Basic Anesthetic Monitoring of the American Society of Anesthesiologists specifies the use of continuous end-tidal CO_2 monitoring during general anesthesia with endotracheal tube or laryngeal mask airway. This monitoring is performed during intraoperative care, including that of neonates, using capnography, capnometry, or mass spectroscopy.

IV. PULMONARY GRAPHICS MONITORING. Several devices are marketed for bedside pulmonary function testing in infants and young children. Likewise, most newer generation ventilators graphically display a variety of measured or calculated parameters. Despite the added cost and increasing availability of these modalities, evidence of beneficial effect on neonatal outcomes is lacking. Several techniques have been advocated in limited studies.

A. **Measurement of tidal volume.** Tidal volume measurements may be used to assist in manual adjustment of ventilator settings. Alternatively, such measurements may form the basis for software-automated ventilator adjustments designed to maintain a defined range of delivered tidal volume ("volume guarantee") or consistent tidal volume delivery employing minimal peak airway pressure ("pressure-regulated volume control"). However, technical issues may limit efficacy of these modalities. Marked variations in measured tidal volume exist among devices from different manufacturers. Although newer modes of ventilation may improve consistency of delivered tidal volume, a significant proportion of values still remain outside the target range. Reasons for these discrepancies include differences in site of measurements in ventilator systems, variations in tubing system compliance, and use of differing strategies to compensate for endotracheal tube leaks. In addition, some software algorithms average adjustments in tidal volume over several breaths. Despite these shortcomings, tidal volume measurements employing the same device consistently over time may provide clinically useful information during chronic mechanical ventilation and may be helpful with weaning following surfactant treatment where rapid changes in lung compliance and delivered tidal volume are of significant concern (see Chap. 29, Mechanical Ventilation).

B. **Flow-volume loops.** The use of positive end-expiratory pressure (PEEP) is an important tool in management of infants with congenital or acquired bronchomalacia (a common complication of severe bronchopulmonary dysplasia [BPD]). Limited case studies have reported the use of real-time flow-volume loop tracings to guide in determination of optimal PEEP to oppose airway collapse. However, indices that quantitate the flow–volume relationship have not been validated in young infants. Because of rapid breathing, onset of inspiration often occurs before end-expiratory closure of the loop is achieved. As a result, "normal" tracings are difficult to obtain and clinical application of this technique in small infants is limited.

Suggested Readings

Askie L, Henderson-Smart D, Irwig L, et al. Oxygen-saturation targets and outcomes in extremely preterm infants (BOOST trial). *N Engl J Med* 2003;349:959–967.

The STOP-ROP Multicenter Study Group. Supplemental therapeutic oxygen for prethreshold retinopathy of prematurity (STOP-ROP), a randomized, controlled trial. I: primary outcomes. *Pediatrics* 2000;105:295–310.

SUPPORT Study Group of the Eunice Kennedy Shriver NICHD Neonatal Research Network. Target ranges of oxygen saturation in extremely preterm infants. *N Engl J Med* 2010;362:1959–1969.

Apnea

Ann R. Stark

I. BACKGROUND

A. Definition. Apnea is defined as the cessation of airflow. Apnea is pathologic (an apneic spell) when absent airflow is prolonged (usually 20 seconds or more) or accompanied by bradycardia (heart rate <100 beats/minute) or hypoxemia that is detected clinically (cyanosis) or by oxygen saturation monitoring. Bradycardia and desaturation are usually present after 20 seconds of apnea, although they typically occur more rapidly in the small premature infant. As the spell continues, pallor and hypotonia are seen, and infants may be unresponsive to tactile stimulation. The level or duration of bradycardia or desaturation that may increase the risk of neurodevelopmental impairment is not known.

B. Classification of apnea is based on whether absent airflow is accompanied by continued inspiratory efforts and upper airway obstruction. Most spells are central or mixed apnea.

1. Central apnea occurs when inspiratory efforts are absent.

2. Obstructive apnea occurs when inspiratory efforts persist in the presence of airway obstruction.

3. Mixed apnea occurs when airway obstruction with inspiratory efforts precedes or follows central apnea.

C. Incidence. Apneic spells occur frequently in premature infants. The incidence of apnea increases with decreasing gestational age. Essentially, all infants <28 weeks' gestational age have apnea. As many as 25% of all premature infants who weigh <1,800 g (~34 weeks' gestational age) have at least one apneic episode.

1. **Onset.** Apneic spells generally begin at 1 or 2 days after birth; if they do not occur during the first 7 days, they are unlikely to occur later.

2. **Duration.** Apneic spells persist for variable periods postnatally and usually cease by 37 weeks' gestational age. In infants born before 28 weeks' gestation, however, spells often persist beyond term postmenstrual age. In a study in which infants were monitored at home, significant apnea and/or bradycardia were recorded up to 43 weeks' postmenstrual age in 20% of preterm infants who were free of spells for at least 5 days before discharge, and in 33% of those who had spells observed during that period. The clinical significance of these events is uncertain.

3. **Term infants.** Apneic spells occurring in infants at or near term are always abnormal and are nearly always associated with serious, identifiable causes, such as birth asphyxia, intracranial hemorrhage, seizures, or depression from medication. Failure to breathe at birth in the absence of drug depression or asphyxia is generally caused by irreversible structural abnormalities of the central nervous system (CNS).

II. PATHOGENESIS. Several mechanisms have been proposed to explain apnea in premature infants, although those responsible for this disorder are unknown. Many clinical conditions have also been associated with apneic spells, and some may be causative.

A. **Developmental immaturity of central respiratory drive** is a likely contributing factor because apneic spells occur more frequently in immature infants.

1. The occurrence of apnea may correlate with brain stem neural function. The frequency of apnea decreases over a period in which brain stem conduction time of the auditory evoked response shortens as gestational age increases.

2. Breathing in infants is strongly influenced by sleep state. Active or rapid eye movement (REM) sleep is marked by irregularity of tidal volume and respiratory frequency. REM sleep predominates in preterm infants, and apneic spells occur more frequently in this state than in quiet sleep.

B. **Chemoreceptor response**

1. In preterm infants, hypoxia results in transient hyperventilation, followed by hypoventilation and sometimes apnea, in contrast to the response in adults. In addition, hypoxia makes the premature infant less responsive to increased levels of carbon dioxide. This suggests that immaturity of peripheral chemoreceptors may be involved in the pathogenesis of apnea. Although most infants do not appear to be hypoxemic before the onset of apnea, hypoxemia might play a role in prolonging the spell.

2. The ventilatory response to increased carbon dioxide is decreased in preterm infants with apnea compared with a matched group without apnea and is also decreased compared to term infants or adults. This suggests the possible contribution of immature central chemoreceptors to the pathogenesis of apnea.

C. **Reflexes.** Active reflexes invoked by stimulation of the posterior pharynx, lung inflation, fluid in the larynx, or chest wall distortion can precipitate apnea in infants. These reflexes may be involved in the apnea that is sometimes associated, for example, with vigorous use of suction catheters in the pharynx or with fluid in the upper airway during feeding.

D. **Respiratory muscles.** Ineffective ventilation may result from impaired coordination of the inspiratory muscles (diaphragm and intercostal muscles) and the muscles of the upper airway (larynx and pharynx).

1. Airway obstruction contributes to mixed and obstructive apneic spells. The site of this obstruction is usually the upper pharynx, which is vulnerable because of poor muscle tone, especially in REM sleep. Passive neck flexion, pressure on the lower rim of a face mask, and submental pressure (all encountered during nursery procedures) can obstruct the airway in infants and lead to apnea, especially in a small premature infant. Spontaneously occurring airway obstruction is seen more frequently when preterm infants assume a position of neck flexion.

2. Nasal obstruction can lead to apnea, especially in preterm infants who usually do not switch to oral breathing after nasal occlusion.

E. **Gastroesophageal reflux** is common in preterm infants. However, no association has been demonstrated between apnea of prematurity and gastroesophageal reflux.

F. Many **inhibitory neurotransmitters** are thought to play a role in the pathogenesis of apnea.

III. MONITORING AND EVALUATION. All infants <35 weeks' gestational age should be monitored for apneic spells for at least the first week after birth because of the risk of apneic spells in this group. Monitoring should continue until no significant apneic episode has been detected for at least 5 days. Because impedance apnea monitors may not distinguish respiratory efforts during airway obstruction from normal breaths, heart rate should be monitored in addition to, or instead of, respiration. Pulse oximetry should be monitored to detect episodes of desaturation. Even with careful monitoring, some prolonged spells of apnea and bradycardia may not be recognized.

A. When a monitor alarm sounds, one should remember to respond to the infant, not the monitor, checking for bradycardia, cyanosis, and airway obstruction.

B. Most apneic spells in premature infants respond to tactile stimulation. Infants who fail to respond to stimulation should be ventilated during the spell with bag and mask, generally starting with a fractional concentration of inspired oxygen (FiO_2) equal to the FiO_2 used before the spell to avoid marked elevations in arterial oxygen tension (PO_2).

C. After the first apneic spell, the infant should be evaluated for a possible underlying cause (Table 31.1); if a cause is identified, specific treatment can then be

Table 31.1   Evaluation of an Infant with Apnea

Potential cause	Associated history of signs	Evaluation
Infection	Feeding intolerance, lethargy, temperature instability	Complete blood count, cultures, if appropriate
Impaired oxygenation	Desaturation, tachypnea, respiratory distress	Continuous oxygen saturation monitoring, arterial blood gas measurement, chest x-ray examination
Metabolic disorders	Jitteriness, poor feeding, lethargy, CNS depression, irritability	Glucose, calcium, electrolytes
Drugs	CNS depression, hypotonia, maternal history	Magnesium, screen for toxic substances in urine
Temperature instability	Lethargy	Monitor temperature of patient and environment
Intracranial pathology	Abnormal neurologic examination, seizures	Cranial ultrasonographic examination

CNS = central nervous system.

initiated. One should be particularly alert to the possibility of a precipitating cause in infants who are more than 34 weeks' gestational age. Evaluation should include a history and physical examination, arterial blood gas measurement with continuous oxygen saturation monitoring, complete blood count, and measurement of blood glucose, calcium, and electrolyte levels.

IV. TREATMENT. When apneic spells are repeated and prolonged (i.e., more than two to three times per hour) or when they require frequent bag-and-mask ventilation, treatment should be initiated.

A. **General measures**

1. **Specific therapy** should be directed at an underlying cause, if one is identified.

2. The optimal range of oxygen saturation for preterm infants is not certain. However, supplemental oxygen should be provided if needed to maintain values in the targeted range (see Chap. 30, Section II.D.1.c. Targeted saturation values).

3. **Care should be taken** to avoid reflexes that may trigger apnea. Suctioning of the pharynx should be done carefully, and oral feedings should be avoided.

4. **Positions of extreme flexion** or extension of the neck should be avoided to reduce the likelihood of airway obstruction. Prone positioning stabilizes the chest wall and may reduce apnea.

B. **Nasal continuous positive airway pressure** (CPAP) at moderate levels (4–6 cm H_2O) can reduce the number of mixed and obstructive apneic spells. It is especially useful in infants <32 to 34 weeks' gestational age and those with residual lung disease. Nasal intermittent positive pressure ventilation (NIPPV) may reduce extubation failure due to apnea following mechanical ventilation, but more evidence is needed.

C. **Treatment with caffeine, a methylxanthine,** markedly reduces the number of apneic spells and the need for mechanical ventilation. Mechanisms by which methylxanthines may decrease apnea include (i) respiratory center stimulation; (ii) antagonism of adenosine, a neurotransmitter that can cause respiratory depression; and (iii) improvement of diaphragmatic contractility.

In the Caffeine for Apnea of Prematurity (CAP) study, survival without neurodevelopmental disability at 18 to 21 months of age, the primary outcome, was improved in infants 500 to 1,250 g birth weight treated early with caffeine compared to placebo. Caffeine treatment also reduced the rate of bronchopulmonary dysplasia. We therefore begin caffeine citrate treatment in all infants less than 1,250 g birth weight soon after birth and continue until it is deemed no longer necessary to treat apnea. In preterm infants more than 1,250 g birth weight who require mechanical ventilation, we begin caffeine treatment prior to extubation. In other infants with apnea of prematurity, we begin caffeine to treat frequent and/or severe apnea.

1. We use a loading dose of 20 mg/kg of caffeine citrate (10 mg/kg caffeine base) orally or intravenously over 30 minutes, followed by maintenance doses of 5 to 8 mg/kg (2.5–5 mg/kg caffeine base) in one daily dose beginning 24 hours after the loading dose.

   a. If apnea continues, we give an additional dose of 10 mg/kg caffeine citrate and increase the maintenance dose by 20%.

   b. Caffeine serum levels of 5 to 20 μg/mL are considered therapeutic. We do not routinely measure serum drug concentration because of the wide therapeutic index and the lack of an established dose–response relationship.

c. Caffeine is generally discontinued at 34 to 36 weeks' postmenstrual age if no apneic spells have occurred for 5 to 7 days. As noted previously, apnea in infants born at less than 28 weeks' gestation frequently persists beyond this postmenstrual age and caffeine is continued until the spells resolve. The effect of caffeine likely remains for approximately 1 week after it has been discontinued. We continue monitoring until no apnea has been detected for at least 5 days after that period.

2. Additional long-term benefits or risks of caffeine therapy are uncertain. In the CAP trial, weight gain was less during the first 3 weeks after randomization in infants treated with caffeine, but not at 4 and 6 weeks, and head circumference was similar in the two groups during the 6-week observation period. Mean percentiles for growth parameters were similar at 18 to 21 months corrected age.

3. Most reports of side effects of methylxanthines in newborns are based on experience with theophylline. Caffeine appears to be less toxic than theophylline and is well tolerated.

4. We do not use doxapram, a respiratory stimulant that may reduce apnea if methylxanthine therapy has failed.

D. Whether blood transfusion reduces the frequency of apneic spells in some infants is controversial. We consider a transfusion of packed red blood cells (PRBCs) if the hematocrit is <25% and the infant has episodes of apnea and bradycardia that are frequent or severe while continuing treatment with caffeine (see Chap. 45).

E. Mechanical ventilation may be required if the other interventions are unsuccessful.

V. PERSISTENT APNEA.
In some infants, especially those born at <28 weeks' gestation, apneic spells may persist at 37 to 40 weeks' postmenstrual age, when the infant may be otherwise ready for discharge home. There is no consensus on the appropriate management of these infants, but efforts are directed at reducing the risk of apneic spells so that the child can be cared for at home.

A. Recordings of impedance pneumography and electrocardiograms (ECGs) for 12 to 24 hours ("pneumograms") can be used to document the occurrence of apnea and bradycardia during that time period, but they do not predict the risk of sudden infant death syndrome (SIDS).

B. Continued use of caffeine may be helpful in infants whose spells recur when the drug is discontinued. Attempts to withdraw the drug can be made at intervals of approximately 2 months while the child is closely monitored.

C. Some infants are cared for with cardiorespiratory monitoring at home, although few data are available on its effectiveness. Extensive psychosocial support must be provided for the parents, who should be skilled in cardiopulmonary resuscitation (CPR) and in the use of the monitor. Routine home monitoring of asymptomatic preterm infants is not indicated.

VI. STRATEGIES TO PREVENT SIDS.
Although the peak incidence of SIDS occurs after the newborn period, parents frequently express concern about their child's risk. Although SIDS occurs more frequently in premature or low birth weight infants, a history of apnea of prematurity does not increase this risk.

We encourage strategies that may reduce the risk of SIDS.

A. **Sleeping position.** Prone sleeping position increases the risk of SIDS, and sleeping on the back reduces the risk. In general, babies should be placed to sleep on their back on a firm surface. The exceptions include preterm infants with respiratory disease, infants with symptomatic gastroesophageal reflux, and infants with craniofacial abnormalities or evidence of upper airway obstruction. For these infants, soft bedding should be avoided. The American Academy of Pediatrics (AAP) recommends a sleeping environment that is separate from but near the mother. Use of a pacifier during sleep also appears to reduce the risk of SIDS.

B. **Smoking.** Infants exposed to maternal smoking during pregnancy and postnatally have a higher risk of SIDS. Smoking should be avoided by parents, and infants should not be exposed to smoke.

C. **Overheating.** Infants exposed to excessively high room temperatures or overheating from excess wrapping have an increased risk of SIDS. Caregivers should avoid practices that result in overheating.

D. **Breastfeeding.** Infants who were never breast-fed have a higher risk of SIDS than do breast-fed infants. We encourage breastfeeding for many reasons (see Chap. 22).

Suggested Readings

Kinney HC, Thach BT. The sudden infant death syndrome. *N Engl J Med* 2009;361:795–805.

32 Transient Tachypnea of the Newborn
Kirsten A. Kienstra

I. DEFINITION. Transient tachypnea of the newborn (TTN), first described by Avery and coworkers in 1966, results from delayed clearance of fetal lung fluid. As the name implies, it is usually a benign, self-limited process. It generally affects infants born at late preterm or term gestation. The disorder is characterized by tachypnea with signs of mild respiratory distress, including retractions and cyanosis; decreased oxygen saturation is usually alleviated by supplemental oxygen with FiO_2 <0.04.

II. PATHOPHYSIOLOGY. To accommodate the transition to breathing air at birth, the lungs must switch from a secretory mode, which provides the fetal lung fluid required for normal lung growth and development *in utero*, to an absorptive mode. This transition is thought to be facilitated by changes in the maternal–fetal hormonal milieu, including a surge in glucocorticoids and catecholamines, associated with physiologic events near the end of pregnancy and during spontaneous labor. Amiloride-sensitive sodium channels expressed in the apical membrane of the alveolar epithelium play an important role in lung fluid clearance. Adrenergic stimulation and other changes near birth lead to passive transport of sodium through the epithelial sodium channels, followed by transport into the interstitium via basolateral Na^+/K^+-ATPase, and passive movement of chloride and water through paracellular and intracellular pathways. Interstitial lung fluid pools in perivascular cuffs of tissue and in the interlobar fissures and is then cleared into pulmonary capillaries and lung lymphatics. Disruption or delay in clearance of fetal lung fluid results in the transient pulmonary edema that characterizes TTN. Compression of the compliant airways by fluid accumulated in the interstitium can lead to airway obstruction, air trapping, and ventilation-perfusion mismatch. Because infants usually recover, a precise pathologic definition is lacking.

III. EPIDEMIOLOGY. Risk factors for TTN include birth by cesarean section with or without labor, precipitous birth, and preterm birth. These have been attributed to delayed or abnormal fetal lung fluid clearance due to the absence of the hormonal changes that accompany spontaneous labor. For infants delivered by elective cesarean section, the presence of labor and the gestational age at delivery impact the risk of respiratory complications, with some degree of protection provided by onset of labor and term gestation. Delivery at lower gestational ages, including late preterm birth, increases the risk of TTN. Diagnosis at earlier gestations is complicated by the presence of other comorbidities such as respiratory distress syndrome (RDS). Other risk factors include male gender and family history of asthma (especially the mother). The mechanism underlying the gender- and asthma-associated risks is unclear but may be related to altered sensitivity to catecholamines that play a role in lung fluid clearance. Genetic polymorphisms in β-adrenergic receptors in alveolar type II cells have been associated with TTN and may influence lung fluid clearance by regulating epithelial sodium channel expression. Macrosomia, maternal diabetes, and multiple gestations also increase the risk of TTN. The associations between TTN and other obstetric factors such as excessive maternal sedation, prolonged labor, and volume of maternal intravenous fluids have been less consistent.

IV. CLINICAL PRESENTATION. Affected term or late preterm infants usually present within the first 6 hours of life with tachypnea; respiratory rates are typically 60 to 120 breaths per minute. The tachypnea may be associated with mild to moderate respiratory distress with retractions, grunting, nasal flaring, and/or mild cyanosis that usually responds to supplemental oxygen at <0.40 FiO_2. Respiratory failure and mechanical ventilation are rare. Infants may have an increased anteroposterior diameter of the chest (barrel-shaped) due to hyperinflation, which may also push down the liver and spleen, making them palpable. Auscultation usually reveals good air entry, and crackles may or may not be appreciated. Signs of TTN usually persist for 12 to 24 hours in cases of mild disease but can last up to 72 hours in more severe cases.

V. DIFFERENTIAL DIAGNOSIS. The diagnosis of TTN requires the exclusion of other potential etiologies for mild to moderate respiratory distress presenting in the first 6 hours of age. The differential diagnosis includes pneumonia/sepsis, RDS, pulmonary hypertension, meconium aspiration, cyanotic congenital heart disease, congenital malformations (e.g., congenital diaphragmatic hernia, cystic adenomatoid malformations), central nervous system (CNS) insults (subarachnoid hemorrhage, hypoxic-ischemic encephalopathy) causing central hyperventilation, pneumothorax, polycythemia, and metabolic acidosis.

VI. EVALUATION

A. **History and physical examination.** A careful history identifies elements such as prematurity, infectious risk factors, meconium, or perinatal depression that may aid in directing the evaluation. Similarly, findings on physical examination such as cardiac or neurologic abnormalities may lead to a more targeted investigation.

B. **Radiographic evaluation.** The chest radiograph of an infant with TTN is consistent with retained fetal lung fluid, with characteristic prominent perihilar streaking (*sunburst pattern*) due to engorgement of periarterial lymphatics that participate in the clearance of alveolar fluid. Coarse, fluffy densities may reflect alveolar edema. Hyperaeration with widening of intercostal spaces, mild cardiomegaly, widened and fluid-filled interlobar fissure, and mild pleural effusions may also be observed. The radiographic findings in TTN usually improve by 12 to 18 hours and resolve by 48 to 72 hours. This rapid resolution helps distinguish the process from pneumonia and meconium aspiration. The chest radiograph can also be used to exclude other diagnoses such as pneumothorax, RDS, and congenital malformations. Of note, the presence of increased pulmonary vascularity in the absence of cardiomegaly may represent total anomalous pulmonary venous return.

C. **Laboratory evaluation.** A complete blood count (CBC) and appropriate cultures can provide information concerning possible pneumonia or sepsis. If risk factors or laboratory data suggest infection, or if respiratory distress does not improve, broad-spectrum antibiotics should be initiated. An arterial blood gas may be used to determine the extent of hypoxemia and adequacy of ventilation. Infants with TTN may have mild hypoxemia and mild respiratory acidosis that typically resolve over 24 hours. With persistent or severe hypoxemia, a cardiac evaluation should be considered. Respiratory alkalosis may reflect central hyperventilation due to CNS pathology.

VII. TREATMENT.
Treatment is mainly supportive with provision of supplemental oxygen, as needed. More severe cases may respond to continuous positive airway pressure (CPAP) to improve lung recruitment. Infants often undergo an evaluation for infection and are treated with antibiotics for 24 to 48 hours until blood cultures are negative. If tachypnea persists and is associated with increased work of breathing, gavage feedings or intravenous fluids may be needed. Strategies aimed to facilitate lung fluid absorption have not shown clinical efficacy. Oral furosemide has not been shown to improve the duration of tachypnea or length of hospitalization. In a study based on the hypothesis that infants with TTN have relatively low levels of catecholamines that facilitate fetal lung fluid absorption, treatment with racemic epinephrine did not change the rate of resolution of tachypnea compared to placebo.

VIII. COMPLICATIONS.
Although TTN is a self-limited process, supportive therapy may be accompanied by complications. CPAP is associated with increased risk of air leak. Delayed initiation of oral feeds may interfere with parental bonding and establishment of breastfeeding, and may prolong hospitalization.

IX. PROGNOSIS.
By definition, TTN is a self-limited process with no risk of recurrence and the prognosis is excellent. Generally, there are no significant long-term residual effects. However, there is an increasing body of literature describing a possible link between TTN and reactive airway disease; the correlation remains to be confirmed.

Suggested Readings

Guglani L, Lakshminrusimha S, Ryan RM. Transient tachypnea of the newborn. *Pediatr Rev* 2008;29:e59–e65.

Tutdibi E, Gries K, Bucheler N, et al. Impact of labor on outcomes in transient tachypnea of the newborn. *Pediatrics* 2010;125:e577–e583.

33 Respiratory Distress Syndrome

Kushal Y. Bhakta

The primary cause of respiratory distress syndrome (RDS), formerly known as hyaline membrane disease, is inadequate pulmonary surfactant. Preterm birth is the most common etiologic factor. The manifestations of the disease are caused by the resultant diffuse alveolar atelectasis, edema, and cell injury. Subsequently, serum proteins that inhibit surfactant function leak into the alveoli. The increased water content, immature mechanisms for clearance of lung liquid, lack of alveolar-capillary apposition, and low surface area for gas exchange typical of the immature lung also contribute to the disease. Prenatal diagnosis to identify infants at risk, prevention of the disease by antenatal administration of glucocorticoids, improvements in perinatal and neonatal care, advances in respiratory support, and surfactant replacement therapy have reduced mortality from RDS. However, RDS remains an important contributing cause of neonatal mortality and morbidity, especially among the most immature infants.

I. IDENTIFICATION

A. Perinatal risk factors

1. **Factors** that affect the state of lung development at birth include prematurity, maternal diabetes, and genetic factors (white race, history of RDS in siblings, male sex). Thoracic malformations that cause lung hypoplasia, such as diaphragmatic hernia, may also increase the risk of surfactant deficiency. Genetic disorders of surfactant production and metabolism include surfactant protein B and surfactant protein C gene mutations, and mutations of the ABCA3 gene, whose product is an adenosine triphosphate (ATP)-binding cassette transporter localized to the lamellar bodies of alveolar type II cells. These rare disorders cause a severe RDS-like picture, often in term infants, and are usually fatal without lung transplantation.

2. **Factors** that may acutely impair surfactant production, release, or function include perinatal asphyxia in premature infants and cesarean section without labor. Infants delivered before labor starts do not benefit from the adrenergic and steroid hormones released during labor, which increase surfactant production and release. As a result, RDS may be seen in late preterm or early term infants delivered by elective cesarean section.

B. Prenatal prediction

1. **Assessment** of fetal lung maturity (FLM). Prenatal prediction of lung maturity can be made by testing amniotic fluid obtained by amniocentesis.

   a. The lecithin/sphingomyelin (L/S) ratio is performed by thin-layer chromatography. Specific techniques vary among laboratories and may affect the results. In general, the risk of RDS is very low if the L/S ratio is >2. Exceptions to the prediction of pulmonary maturity with an L/S ratio >2 are infants of diabetic mothers (IDMs), infants with erythroblastosis fetalis, and infants who have suffered intrapartum asphyxia. Possible exceptions are intrauterine growth restriction (IUGR), abruptio placentae, preeclampsia, and hydrops fetalis. Contaminants, such as blood and meconium, affect the interpretation of results.

b. The TDx-FLM II measures the surfactant to albumin ratio using fluorescent polarization technology. A value of >55 mg surfactant/g albumin correlates with lung maturity; the predictive capacity of the test may improve if gestational age–specific threshold values are used. Contamination with blood or meconium may interfere with interpretation of this test.

c. Lamellar body counts in the amniotic fluid have also been used as a rapid and inexpensive test to determine FLM. Lamellar bodies are "packages" of phospholipids produced by type II alveolar cells and are present in amniotic fluid in increasing numbers with advancing gestational age. A value of >50,000 lamellar bodies/microliter predicts lung maturity. Lamellar bodies can also be assessed indirectly by measuring optical density of amniotic fluid.

d. The presence of phosphatidylglycerol (PG) can also be used to determine FLM, but PG appears late in the maturation process of the lung. An advantage to this test is that it is not affected by contamination with blood or meconium. The major disadvantage is that its sensitivity is low, and thus can give a false-negative result when other tests indicate lung maturity.

e. Foam stability index (FSI) predicts FLM based on the formation of a stable foam when amniotic fluid is shaken with ethanol in a test tube. Blood and meconium contamination interfere with interpretation of this test; interpretation may also vary among users.

2. **Antenatal** corticosteroid therapy should be given to pregnant women 24 to 34 weeks' gestation with intact membranes or with preterm rupture of the membranes (ROM) without chorioamnionitis who are at high risk for preterm delivery within the next 7 days. The efficacy of treatment at gestational ages earlier than 24 weeks is uncertain; however, administration below this age may be reasonable depending upon clinical circumstances. This strategy induces surfactant production and accelerates maturation of the lungs and other fetal tissues, resulting in a substantial reduction of RDS, intraventricular hemorrhage (IVH), necrotizing enterocolitis (NEC), and perinatal mortality. A full course consists of two doses of betamethasone (12 mg IM) separated by a 24-hour interval, or four doses of dexamethasone (6 mg IM) at 12-hour intervals, although incomplete courses may improve outcome. Contraindications to treatment include chorioamnionitis or other indications for immediate delivery. Most studies suggest that betamethasone may be preferable because of potential neurotoxicity of dexamethasone. However, the only randomized trial (Betacode trial) comparing both drugs found no difference in most outcomes, except that the rate of IVH and brain lesions was higher in infants exposed to betamethasone.

C. **Postnatal diagnosis.** A premature infant with RDS has clinical signs shortly after birth. These include tachypnea, retractions, flaring of the nasal alae, grunting, and cyanosis. The classic radiographic appearance is of low-volume lungs with a diffuse reticulogranular pattern and air bronchograms.

II. MANAGEMENT. The keys to the management of infants with RDS are (i) to prevent hypoxemia and acidosis (this allows normal tissue metabolism, optimizes surfactant production, and prevents right-to-left shunting); (ii) to optimize fluid management (avoiding hypovolemia and shock, on the one hand, and edema, particularly pulmonary edema, on the other); (iii) to reduce metabolic demands; (iv) to prevent worsening atelectasis and pulmonary edema; (v) to minimize oxidant lung injury; and (vi) to minimize lung injury caused by mechanical ventilation.

A. **Oxygen**

1. **Delivery of oxygen** should be sufficient to meet target saturation values, although the range of optimal oxygenation is uncertain. For infants who require supplemental oxygen, one approach is to target SpO_2 in the 88% to 92% range for infants less than 30 weeks' gestation or 1,250 g (set monitor alarm limits 85%–95%). For infants 30 weeks' gestation or more, or when infants reach 30 weeks' postmenstrual age, target SpO_2 from 88% to 95% (set alarm limits 85%–97%). If these targets are maintained, arterial PO_2 rarely will exceed 90 mm Hg. (see Chap. 30, Section II.D.1.c. Targeted saturation values). Higher than necessary fractional concentration of inspired oxygen (FiO_2) levels should be avoided because of the danger of potentiating the development of lung injury and retinopathy of prematurity. The oxygen is warmed, humidified, and delivered through an air-oxygen blender that allows precise control over the oxygen concentration. For infants with acute RDS, oxygen is ordered by concentration to be delivered to the infant's airway, not by flow, and oxygen concentration is checked at least hourly. It should be titrated to the targeted oxygen saturation, which should be monitored continuously. When hand ventilation is required during suctioning of the airway, during insertion of an endotracheal tube, or during an apneic spell, the oxygen concentration should be similar to that before bagging to avoid hyperoxia and should be adjusted in response to continuous monitoring.

2. **Blood gas monitoring** (see Chap. 30). During the acute stages of illness, frequent sampling may be required to maintain arterial blood gases within appropriate ranges. Arterial blood gases (arterial oxygen tension [PaO_2], arterial carbon dioxide tension [$PaCO_2$], and pH) should be measured 30 minutes after changes in respiratory therapy, such as alteration in the FiO_2 or ventilator settings. We use indwelling arterial catheters for this purpose. To monitor trends in oxygenation continuously, we use pulse oximeters. In more stable infants, capillary blood from warmed heels may be adequate for monitoring $PaCO_2$ and pH.

B. **Continuous positive airway pressure**

1. **Indications.** We begin continuous positive airway pressure (CPAP) therapy as soon as possible after birth in infants with RDS, including those at extremely low gestational age (see Chap. 29). Although both the CPAP or Intubation at Birth (COIN) and Surfactant, Positive Pressure, and Oxygenation Randomized Trial (SUPPORT) trials found that the rate of death or bronchopulmonary dysplasia (BPD) was not different between groups that received early CPAP or surfactant treatment, infants in the nasal CPAP group required less mechanical ventilation. The rate of pneumothorax was higher in the CPAP infants in the COIN trial, but not in SUPPORT trial. In infants with RDS, CPAP appears to help prevent atelectasis, thereby minimizing lung injury and preserving the functional properties of surfactant, and allowing reduction of oxygen concentration as the

PaO_2 rises. Infants who fail early nasal CPAP and require intubation are typically extremely immature or those with severe respiratory distress, who require FiO_2 higher than 0.4 or 0.5 to maintain the targeted oxygen saturation, and have $PaCO_2$ greater than 55 to 60 mm Hg. Infants with RDS who require intubation and mechanical ventilation should be treated with surfactant.

If CPAP enables the infant to inspire on a more compliant portion of the pressure–volume curve, $PaCO_2$ may fall. However, minute ventilation may decrease on CPAP, particularly if the distending pressure is too great. We obtain a chest radiograph before or soon after starting CPAP to confirm the diagnosis of RDS and to exclude disorders in which this type of therapy should be approached with caution, such as air leak.

2. Methods of administering CPAP. We usually begin CPAP through nasal prongs using a continuous-flow ventilator. We generally start at a pressure of 5 to 7 cm H_2O, using a flow high enough to avoid rebreathing (5–10 L/minute), then adjust the pressure in increments of 1 to 2 cm H_2O to a maximum of 8 cm H_2O, observing the baby's respiratory rate and effort and monitoring oxygen saturation. An orogastric tube is placed to decompress swallowed air. Simpler CPAP delivery devices utilizing tubing submerged in sterile water to deliver the desired distending pressure ("bubble" CPAP) can also be used and may have some benefits over a continuous-flow ventilator. Variable flow CPAP devices that reduce the work of breathing, especially during expiration, are available, although significant long-term clinical benefits have not been observed with their use.

3. Problems encountered with CPAP
a. CPAP may interfere with venous return to the heart and thereby decrease cardiac output. Positive pressure may be transmitted to the pulmonary vascular bed, raising pulmonary vascular resistance and thereby promoting right-to-left shunting. The risk of these phenomena increases as RDS resolves and lung compliance improves. In this circumstance, reduction of the CPAP may improve oxygenation.
b. Hypercarbia may indicate that CPAP is too high and tidal volume is reduced.
c. The use of nasal prongs may be unsuccessful if crying or mouth opening prevents adequate transmission of pressure or if the infant's abdomen becomes distended despite insertion of an orogastric tube. In these situations, endotracheal intubation may be necessary.

4. Weaning. As the infant improves, we reduce the FiO_2 in decrements of 0.05 to maintain the targeted oxygen saturation. Generally, when FiO_2 is <0.30, CPAP can be reduced to 5 cm H_2O, monitoring oxygen saturation. Physical examination will provide evidence of respiratory effort during weaning, and chest radiographs may help estimate lung volume. Lowering of the distending pressure should be attempted with caution if lung volume appears low and alveolar atelectasis persists. We generally discontinue CPAP if there is no distress and if the FiO_2 remains <0.3.

C. Surfactant replacement is one of the best-studied therapies in neonates. It has been shown in numerous clinical trials to be successful in ameliorating RDS. These trials have examined the effects of surfactant preparations delivered through the endotracheal tube either within minutes of birth (prophylactic treatment) or after the symptoms and signs of RDS are present (selective or "rescue" treatment). Surfactants of human, bovine, or porcine origin and synthetic preparations have been studied. In general, these studies have shown improvement in oxygenation and decreased need for ventilator support lasting hours to days after treatment and, in many of the larger studies, decreased incidence of air leaks and death. Beractant (Survanta, a bovine lung extract), calfactant (Infasurf, a calf lung extract), and poractant alfa (Curosurf, a porcine lung extract) are available in the United States (Table 33.1).

1. **Timing.** Prophylactic treatment of surfactant deficiency, before lung injury occurs, results in better distribution and less lung injury than supplementation once respiratory failure is severe. "Early rescue" (before 2 hours of age) is preferable to delayed treatment, although whether prophylactic treatment is better than early treatment is uncertain. However, early intubation and surfactant administration must be balanced against the application of nasal CPAP, which may reduce the need for subsequent mechanical ventilation.

2. **The response to surfactant therapy** varies among infants. The causes of this variability include timing of treatment and patient factors such as other concurrent illnesses and degree of lung immaturity. Delayed resuscitation, insufficient lung inflation, improper ventilator strategies, and excessive fluid administration may negate the benefits of surfactant therapy. The combined use of antenatal corticosteroids and postnatal surfactant when indicated improves neonatal outcome more than postnatal surfactant therapy alone.

   In infants with established RDS, repeated surfactant treatment results in greater improvement in oxygenation and ventilation, decreased risk of pneumothorax, and a trend toward improved survival when compared to single-dose therapy. However, there is no clear benefit to more than four doses of beractant or calfactant or three doses of poractant alfa. Whether all infants should be given additional doses or only those who meet certain criteria for severity of illness at the recommended intervals for retreatment is not known. We generally re-treat infants who still require mechanical ventilation with mean airway pressures above 7 cm H_2O and FiO_2 over 0.30 up to the maximum number of doses, although most infants require only one or two doses.

3. **Administration.** See Table 33.1 for dosing information, source, and phospholipid and protein concentration for beractant (Survanta), calfactant (Infasurf), and poractant alfa (Curosurf). Specific instructions about administration of these preparations vary slightly and are available on the package insert. Surfactant is administered during brief disconnection from the ventilator, in two or four divided doses depending on the product, through an end-hole catheter that is just slightly longer than that of the endotracheal tube; alternatively, an adapter can be used with closed suction devices so that ventilation is not interrupted. Desaturation, bradycardia, and apnea are frequent adverse effects. Administration should be adjusted according to the infant's tolerance. Apnea commonly occurs at slow ventilation rates, so the rate should be at least 30 breaths per minute during administration. In addition, infants may respond rapidly and need careful adjustment of ventilator settings to prevent hypotension or pneumothorax secondary to sudden improvement in compliance. Others become transiently hypoxemic during treatment and require additional oxygen.

4. **Complications.** Pulmonary hemorrhage is an infrequent adverse event after surfactant therapy. It most commonly occurs in extremely low birth weight (ELBW) infants, in males, and in infants who have clinical evidence of patent ductus arteriosus (PDA) (see Chap. 37, Pulmonary Hemorrhage).

   Surfactant treatment has not consistently reduced the incidence of IVH, NEC, and retinopathy of prematurity. Although these disorders tend to be

Table 33.1 Dosing Information, Source, and Phospholipid and Protein Concentration for Beractant (Survanta), Calfactant (Infasurf), and Poractant Alfa (Curosurf)

Trade name	Active ingredient	Source	Dosing	Phospholipid concentration	Protein concentration
Survanta	Beractant	Bovine lung extract	• 4 mL/kg (100 mg/kg phospholipid) divided into four quarter doses through endotracheal tube. Prophylaxis: give within 15 minutes of birth in infants at risk for surfactant deficiency. Rescue therapy: give when diagnosis of surfactant deficiency is made • Can use up to four doses, given no more frequently than every 6 hours	25 mg/mL	<1 mg/mL (SP-B and SP-C; does not contain SP-A)
Infasurf	Calfactant	Calf lung lavage fluid	• 3 mL/kg (105 mg/kg phospholipid) through endotracheal tube for prophylaxis or rescue therapy • Can use up to three doses, given 12 hours apart	35 mg/mL	0.7 mg/mL (SP-B and SP-C; does not contain SP-A)
Curosurf	Poractant alfa	Porcine lung extract	• Initial dose: 2.5 mL/kg through endotracheal tube (200 mg/kg phospholipid) • Can use up to two subsequent doses of 1.25 mL/kg administered 12 hours apart (maximum volume 5 mL/kg)	76 mg/mL	1 mg/mL (SP-B and SP-C; does not contain SP-A)

References: Survanta package insert, Abbott Nutrition, Columbus, OH; Infasurf package insert, ONY, Inc., Amherst, NY; Curosurf package insert, Chiesi Farmaceutici, S.p.A., Parma, Italy.

associated with severe RDS, they are primarily caused by immaturity of other organs. Likewise, most studies have not demonstrated a reduced incidence of BPD, particularly in the smallest infants who are at the highest risk. However, the reduction in mortality attributable to surfactant therapy has not typically been associated with a large increase in rates of BPD, suggesting that surfactant therapy prevents BPD in some infants. No significant difference has been shown in infants treated with surfactant versus placebo with regard to both neurodevelopmental outcomes and physical growth.

D. Mechanical ventilation (see Chap. 29)

1. **The initiation of ventilator therapy** is influenced by the decision to administer surfactant (see II.C.). The goals, once mechanical ventilation is initiated, are to limit tidal volume without losing lung volume or promoting atelectasis and to wean to extubation as soon as possible. Indications to start ventilation are a respiratory acidosis with a $PaCO_2$ >55 mm Hg or rapidly rising, a PaO_2 <50 mm Hg or oxygen saturation <90% with an FiO_2 above 0.50, or severe apnea. The actual levels of PaO_2 and $PaCO_2$ necessitating intervention depend on the course of the disease and the gestational age of the infant. For example, a high $PaCO_2$ early in the course of RDS will generally indicate the need for ventilator support, while the same $PaCO_2$ when the infant is recovering might be managed, after careful evaluation, by observation and repeated sampling before any intervention is made.

2. **Ventilators.** A continuous-flow, pressure-limited, time-cycled ventilator is useful for ventilating newborns because pressure waveforms, inspiratory and expiratory duration, and pressure can be varied independently and because the flow of gas permits unobstructed spontaneous breathing. Synchronized intermittent mechanical ventilation (SIMV), which synchronizes with the infant's own respiratory effort, is preferred (see Chap. 29). Other modes of pressure-limited ventilation including assist-control, pressure support, and volume-guarantee are used as well, although clinical benefits have not been shown with these newer modes.

   High-frequency oscillatory ventilation (HFOV) may be useful to minimize lung injury in very small and/or sick infants who require high peak inspiratory pressures and oxygen concentration to maintain adequate gas exchange and to manage infants in whom air leak syndromes complicate RDS.

   a. Initial settings. We generally start mechanical ventilation with a peak inspiratory pressure of 20 to 25 cm H_2O, positive end-expiratory pressure (PEEP) of 5 to 6 cm H_2O, frequency of 25 to 30 breaths per minute, inspiratory duration of 0.3 to 0.4 seconds, and the previously required FiO_2 (usually 0.50–1). Because of the short lung time constant in early RDS, faster rates (40–60 breaths per minute) with a shorter inspiratory time (0.2 seconds) may also be used. It is useful to ventilate the infant first by hand; a flow-inflating bag and manometer can be helpful to determine the actual pressures required. The infant should be observed for color, chest motion, and respiratory effort, and the examiner should listen for breath sounds and observe changes in oxygen saturation. Adjustments in ventilator settings may be required on the basis of these observations or arterial blood gas results.

   b. Adjustments (see Chap. 29). $PaCO_2$ should be maintained in the range of 45 to 55 mm Hg. Acidosis may exacerbate RDS. Therefore, if relative hypercapnia is accepted to minimize lung injury, metabolic acidosis should be minimized. Rising $PaCO_2$ levels may indicate the onset of complications, including atelectasis, air leak, or symptomatic PDA. PaO_2 usually rises in response to increases in FiO_2 or mean airway pressure. Some infants have pulmonary hypertension resulting in right-to-left shunting through fetal pathways; in these infants, interventions to reduce pulmonary vascular resistance may improve oxygenation (see Chap. 36). More commonly, premature infants remain hypoxemic because of shunting through atelectatic lung and respond to measures that improve lung recruitment, including HFOV.

3. **Care of the infant receiving ventilator therapy** includes scrupulous attention to vital signs and clinical condition. FiO_2 and ventilator settings must be checked frequently. Oxygen saturation should be monitored continuously. Blood gas levels should be checked at least every 4 to 6 hours during the acute illness, or more frequently if the infant's condition is changing rapidly, and 30 minutes following changes in ventilator settings. Airway secretions may require periodic suctioning, preferably using closed (in-line) suction devices.

4. **Danger signs**
   a. If an infant receiving mechanical ventilation deteriorates, the following should be suspected:
      i. Blocked or dislodged endotracheal tube
      ii. Malfunctioning ventilator
      iii. Air leak
   b. Remedial action. The infant should be removed from the ventilator and hand ventilated with a bag that is immediately available at the bedside. An appropriate suction catheter is passed to determine patency of the tube, and the tube position is checked by auscultation of breath sounds or by laryngoscopy. If there is any doubt, the tube should be removed and the infant should be ventilated by bag and mask pending replacement of the tube. The ventilator should be checked to ensure that FiO_2 settings are appropriate. The baby's chest is auscultated and transilluminated to check for pneumothorax (see Chap. 38). If pneumothorax is suspected, chest radiographs should be obtained, but if the infant's condition is critical, immediate aspiration by needle is both diagnostic and therapeutic. Hypotension secondary to hemorrhage, capillary leak, or myocardial dysfunction also can complicate RDS and should be treated by blood volume expansion or pressors or both. Pneumopericardium and pulmonary hemorrhage or IVH can also cause a sudden deterioration. Immediate attention to treatable conditions is appropriate.

5. **Weaning.** As the infant shows signs of improvement, weaning from the ventilator should be attempted. Specific steps to reduce inspiratory pressure, PEEP, rate, and FiO_2 depend on the infant's blood gases, physical examination, and responses.
   a. The settings at which mechanical ventilation can be successfully discontinued will vary with the size, condition, respiratory drive, and individual pulmonary mechanics of the infant. Infants weighing <2 kg are usually best weaned to ventilator rates of approximately 20 breaths per minute and then extubated if they are stable on FiO_2 <0.30 and peak inspiratory pressure <18 cm H_2O. Larger infants may tolerate extubation from higher settings. We generally use nasal CPAP to stabilize lung volumes after extubation, especially in smaller infants.

b. Failure to wean may result from a number of causes, of which the following is a partial list.

   i. Pulmonary edema may be present owing to capillary leak during acute stages of the illness or may develop secondary to patency of the ductus arteriosus. However, diuretic treatment in the acute phase of RDS is not helpful.

   ii. Recovery of the lung from RDS is not uniform, and segmental or lobar atelectasis, edema, or interstitial emphysema may delay weaning.

   iii. As the infant's lungs become more compliant, the inspiratory and expiratory times may have to be increased to allow optimal inflation and deflation of the lungs.

   iv. Other reasons include onset of BPD or of apnea of prematurity. We routinely start caffeine soon after birth in infants with birth weight <1,250 g. We begin caffeine therapy before extubation in infants <30 weeks' gestation who have not previously been treated to improve respiratory drive and prevent apnea (see Chap. 31). Glottic or subglottic edema resulting in obstruction may respond to inhaled racemic epinephrine; a brief course of systemic glucocorticoids may rarely be needed.

E. Supportive therapy

 1. Temperature (see Chap. 15). Temperature control is crucial in all low birth weight (LBW) infants, especially in those with respiratory disease. If the infant's temperature is too high or low, metabolic demands increase considerably. If oxygen uptake is limited by RDS, the increased demand cannot be met. An incubator or a radiant warmer must be used to maintain a neutral thermal environment for the infant.

 2. Fluids and nutrition (see Chaps. 21 and 23)

   a. Infants with RDS initially require intravascular administration of fluids. We generally start fluid therapy at 60 to 80 mL/kg/day, using dextrose 10% in water. Very low birth weight (VLBW) infants in whom poor glucose tolerance and large transcutaneous losses are expected are usually started at 100 to 120 mL/kg/day. ELBW infants may be started as high as 120 to 140 mL/kg/day with a lower glucose concentration, although use of humidified incubators decreases insensible losses and resultant fluid requirements. Phototherapy, skin trauma, and radiant warmers increase insensible losses. Excessive fluid administration may cause pulmonary edema and increases the risk of a symptomatic PDA. The key to fluid management is careful monitoring of serum electrolytes and body weight and frequent adjustments in fluids as indicated. Fluid retention is common in infants with RDS. However, extremely immature infants often lack renal concentration efficiency and have enormous evaporative losses if not placed in humidified incubators.

   b. By the second day, we usually add sodium (2 mEq/kg/day), potassium (1 mEq/kg/day), and calcium (100–200 mg/kg/day) to the fluids. If it seems unlikely that adequate enteral nutrition will be achieved within several days, total parenteral nutrition should be started by the first day after birth.

   c. In most infants with RDS, spontaneous diuresis occurs on the second to fourth day, preceding improvement in pulmonary function. Diuresis and improvement in pulmonary compliance occur much sooner in surfactant-treated infants, often within hours. If diuresis and improvement in lung disease do not occur by 1 to 2 weeks of age, this may indicate the onset of BPD (see Chap. 34). The routine use of diuretics in the treatment of RDS is discouraged, as there are no data to show improvement in any outcome measures, and these medications have potential side effects.

3. **Circulation is assessed** by monitoring the heart rate, blood pressure, and peripheral perfusion. Judicious use of blood or a volume expander (normal saline) may be necessary, and pressors may be used to support the circulation. In general, we attempt to limit crystalloid administration (attempting to avoid both capillary leak of fluid into inflamed lung parenchyma and the excessive administration of sodium from repeated bolus infusions of saline). We often use dopamine (starting at 5 μg/kg/minute) to maintain adequate blood pressure and cardiac output, ensure improved tissue perfusion and urine output, and avoid metabolic acidosis. After the first 12 to 24 hours, hypotension and poor perfusion can also result from a large left-to-right shunt through a PDA, so careful assessment is warranted. The volume of blood drawn should be monitored and, in VLBW infants who are sick with RDS, generally should be replaced by packed red blood cell (PRBC) transfusion when the hematocrit falls below 35% to 40% (see Chaps. 40, 41, and 45).

4. **Possible infection.** Because pneumonia or sepsis (classically with Group B *Streptococcus*) can duplicate the clinical signs and radiographic appearance of RDS, we obtain blood cultures and complete blood counts with differential from all infants with RDS considered to be at risk for infection and treat with broad-spectrum antibiotics (ampicillin and gentamicin); these are typically discontinued when the blood culture is negative for 48 hours unless infection is strongly suspected.

F. **Acute complications**

1. **Air leak** (see Chap. 38). Pneumothorax, pneumomediastinum, pneumopericardium, or interstitial emphysema should be suspected when an infant with RDS deteriorates, typically with hypotension, apnea, bradycardia, or persistent acidosis.

2. **Infection** (see Chap. 49) may accompany RDS and may present in a variety of ways. Also, instrumentation, such as catheters or respiratory equipment, provides access for organisms to invade the immunologically immature preterm infant. Whenever there is suspicion of infection, appropriate cultures should be obtained and antibiotics administered promptly.

3. **Intracranial hemorrhage** (see Chap. 54). Infants with severe RDS are at increased risk for intracranial hemorrhage and should be monitored with cranial ultrasound examinations.

4. **PDA** (see Chap. 41) frequently complicates RDS. PDA typically presents as pulmonary vascular pressures begin to fall. Increasing left-to-right shunt may cause heart failure, manifested by respiratory decompensation and cardiomegaly. The systemic consequences of the shunt may include low mean blood pressure, metabolic acidosis, decreased urine output, and worsening jaundice due to impaired organ perfusion. We consider treatment of infants, especially those weighing <1,500 g, with intravenous indomethacin or ibuprofen if they develop signs of a symptomatic PDA, such as a systolic or continuous murmur, hyperdynamic precordium, bounding pulses, or widened pulse pressure, and have respiratory decompensation or are unable to be weaned from

mechanical ventilation. We usually confirm the diagnosis of PDA by cardiac echo. We consider surgical ligation for infants in whom medical treatment is contraindicated (e.g., those with renal failure or NEC) or those in whom two courses of medical treatment have failed. In infants who are improving steadily despite signs of PDA and who have no evidence of heart failure, mild fluid restriction and time may result in closure.

G. **Long-term complications** include BPD (see Chap. 34) and other complications of prematurity, including neurodevelopmental impairment and retinopathy of prematurity. The risk of these complications increases with decreasing birth weight and gestational age.

Suggested Readings

Morley CJ, Davis PG, Doyle LW, et al. Nasal CPAP or intubation at birth for very preterm infants. *N Engl J Med* 2008;358:700–708.

SUPPORT Study Group of the Eunice Kennedy Shriver NICHD Neonatal Research Network, Carlo WA, Finer NN, et al. Target ranges of oxygen saturation in extremely preterm infants. *N Engl J Med* 2010;362:1959–1969.

SUPPORT Study Group of the Eunice Kennedy Shriver NICHD Neonatal Research Network, Finer NN, Carlo WA, et al. Early CPAP versus surfactant in extremely preterm infants. *N Engl J Med* 2010;362:1970–1979.

34 Bronchopulmonary Dysplasia/Chronic Lung Disease

Richard B. Parad

I. DEFINITION. A National Institutes of Health (NIH) conference proposed definitions for bronchopulmonary dysplasia (BPD), also known as *chronic lung disease* (CLD) of prematurity, which is a more general term. For infants born at <32 weeks' gestation who remain in oxygen for the first 28 days at 36 weeks' postmenstrual age (PMA), mild BPD is defined as no supplemental O_2 requirement; moderate BPD is a requirement of supplemental O_2 $<30\%$; and severe BPD is a requirement of $\geq30\%$ O_2 and/or continuous positive airway pressure (CPAP) or ventilator support. For infants born at ≥32 weeks, BPD is defined as a supplemental O_2 requirement for the first 28 days with severity level based on O_2 requirement at 56 days. A physiologic definition of BPD has been proposed based on SaO_2 during a room air challenge performed at 36 weeks (or 56 days for infants >32 weeks) or before hospital discharge, with persistent SaO_2 $<90\%$, the cutoff at which supplemental O_2 is required. Lung parenchyma usually appears abnormal on chest radiographs. This definition can apply to term babies with meconium aspiration syndrome, pneumonia, and certain cardiac and gastrointestinal (GI) anomalies who require chronic ventilatory support. BPD is associated with the development of chronic respiratory morbidity (CRM).

II. EPIDEMIOLOGY. Approximately 15,000 new cases of BPD occur in the United States each year. Infants $<1,250$ g birth weight are most susceptible to developing this condition. Differences in populations (race/ethnicity/socioeconomic status); clinical practices; and definitions account for a wide variation in the rate reported among centers. The relative risk is decreased in African Americans and females. Of infants with birth weight $<1,000$ g, gestational age <32 weeks, and alive at 36 weeks' PMA, 44% who require O_2 at 36 weeks' PMA develop CRM (defined as a requirement for pulmonary medications at 18 months corrected age), while 29% without O_2 requirement at 36 weeks' PMA also develop CRM.

III. PATHOGENESIS

A. **Acute lung injury** is caused by the combination of O_2 toxicity, barotrauma, and volutrauma from mechanical ventilation. Cellular and interstitial injury results in the release of proinflammatory cytokines (interleukin 1β [IL-1β], IL-6, IL-8, tumor necrosis factor-α [TNF-α]) that cause secondary changes in alveolar permeability and recruit inflammatory cells into interstitial and alveolar spaces; further injury from proteases, oxidants, and additional chemokines, and chemoattractants cause ongoing inflammatory cell recruitment and leakage of water and protein.

Airway and vascular tone may be altered. Alveolar development is interrupted, and parenchyma is destroyed, leading to emphysematous changes. Sloughed cells and accumulated secretions not cleared adequately by the damaged mucociliary transport system cause inhomogeneous peripheral airway obstruction that leads to alternating areas of collapse and hyperinflation and proximal airway dilation. Bombesin-like protein, a proinflammatory peptide produced by neuroendocrine cells, is elevated in the urine of infants who subsequently develop BPD. Historically, "old" BPD, as originally reported by Northway in 1967, was described in infants with a mean gestational age of 33 weeks and a birth weight of 2,000 g. Pathology of nonsurvivors showed a predominance of small airway injury, fibrosis, and emphysema. In the postsurfactant therapy era, "new" BPD now predominates, affecting a different population of preterm infants, with a mean gestational age under 28 weeks and birth weight under 1,000 g. For this group, the most significant pathologic finding in nonsurvivors is decreased alveolarization.

B. **In the chronic phase of lung injury,** the interstitium may be altered by fibrosis and cellular hyperplasia that results from excessive release of growth factors and cytokines, leading to insufficient repair. Interstitial fluid clearance is disrupted, resulting in pulmonary fluid retention. Airways develop increased muscularization and hyperreactivity. The physiologic effects are decreased lung compliance, increased airway resistance, and impaired gas exchange with resulting ventilation–perfusion mismatching and air trapping.

C. **Factors that may contribute to the development of BPD include the following:**

1. **Immature lung substrate.** The lung is most susceptible before alveolar septation begins. Injury at this stage may lead to an arrest of alveolarization.

2. **Inadequate activity** of the antioxidant enzymes superoxide dismutase, catalase, glutathione peroxidase, and/or deficiency of free radical sinks such as vitamin E, glutathione, and ceruloplasmin may predispose the lung to O_2 toxicity. Similarly, inadequate antiprotease protection may predispose the lung to injury from the unchecked proteases released by recruited inflammatory cells.

3. **Excessive early intravenous fluid administration,** perhaps by contributing to pulmonary edema.

4. **Persistent left-to-right shunt through the patent ductus arteriosus (PDA).** Although prophylactic PDA ligation or administration of indomethacin or ibuprofen does not prevent BPD, persistent left-to-right shunt and late PDA closure appear associated with increased BPD risk. However, surgical PDA closure is also associated with increased BPD risk.

5. **Intrauterine or perinatal infection,** with cytokine release, may contribute to the etiology of BPD or may modify its course. *Ureaplasma urealyticum* has been associated with BPD in premature infants, although it remains unclear whether this relationship is causal. Intrauterine *Chlamydia trachomatis* and other viral infections have been similarly implicated.

6. **Familial airway hyperreactivity** is found more commonly in the setting of preterm labor, which confounds the increased risk estimate of both premature and BPD affected infants.

7. **Increased inositol clearance may** lead to diminished plasma inositol levels and decreased surfactant synthesis or impaired surfactant metabolism.

8. **An increase in vasopressin** and a decrease in atrial natriuretic peptide release may alter pulmonary and systemic fluid balance in the setting of obstructive lung disease.

IV. CLINICAL PRESENTATION

A. **Physical examination** typically reveals tachypnea, retractions, and rales on auscultation.

B. **Arterial blood gas** (ABG) analysis shows hypoxemia and hypercarbia with eventual metabolic compensation for the respiratory acidosis.

C. **The chest radiograph appearance** changes as the disease progresses. In early descriptions of BPD, stage I had the same appearance as respiratory distress syndrome (RDS); stage II showed diffuse haziness with increased density and normal-to-low lung volumes; stage III demonstrated streaky densities with bubbly lucencies and early hyperinflation; and stage IV showed hyperinflation with larger hyperlucent areas interspersed with thicker, streaky densities. Not all infants progressed to stage IV, and some transitioned directly from stage I to stage III. Radiographic abnormalities often persisted into childhood. *New BPD* is often associated with stage II changes that may evolve if the condition progresses.

D. **Cardiac evaluation.** Nonpulmonary causes of respiratory failure should be excluded. Electrocardiogram (ECG) can show persistent or progressive right ventricular hypertrophy if *cor pulmonale* develops. Left ventricular hypertrophy may develop with systemic hypertension. Two-dimensional echocardiography may be useful in excluding left-to-right shunts (see Chap. 41) and pulmonary hypertension (see Chap. 36). Biventricular failure is unusual when good oxygenation is maintained, and the development of pulmonary hypertension is avoided.

E. **Infant pulmonary function testing (iPFT).** Increased respiratory system resistance (Rrs) and decreased dynamic compliance (Crs) have been the hallmarks of BPD. In the first year of life, iPFTs reveal decreased forced expiratory flow rate, increased functional residual capacity (FRC), increased residual volume (RV), and increased RV/total lung capacity ratio and bronchodilator responsiveness, with an overall pattern of mild-to-moderate airflow obstruction, air trapping, and increased airway reactivity.

F. **Pathologic changes are detectable** in severe cases by the first few days after birth. By the end of the first week, necrotizing bronchiolitis, obstruction of small airway lumens by debris and edema, and areas of peribronchial and interstitial fibrosis are present. Emphysematous changes and significant impairment in alveolar development result in diminished surface area for gas exchange. Changes in both large airways (glandular hyperplasia) and small airways (smooth muscle hyperplasia) likely form the histologic basis for reactive airway disease. Pulmonary vascular changes associated with pulmonary hypertension may be seen. Arrest of alveolarization is more significant at lower gestational ages.

V. INPATIENT TREATMENT. The goals of treatment during the neonatal intensive care unit (NICU) course are to minimize further lung injury (barotrauma and volutrauma, O_2 toxicity, inflammation), maximize nutrition, and diminish O_2 consumption.

A. **Mechanical ventilation**

1. **Acute phase.** Ventilator adjustments are made to minimize airway pressures and tidal volumes (generally 3–5 ml/kg/breath) while providing adequate gas exchange (see Chap. 30). It is possible that use of patient-controlled ventilator techniques such as patient-triggered breaths, pressure-supported spontaneous

breaths, and volume-targeted patient-triggered breaths may lower BPD risk, although recent trials have not clearly demonstrated this advantage, and some identified increased rates of pneumothorax and mortality. Early use of nasal intermittent positive pressure ventilation (NIPPV) may be more effective than standard nasal CPAP in avoiding need for intubation and surfactant therapy, and NIPPV may also decrease extubation failure rate, although appropriately powered trials are needed.

In most circumstances, we avoid hyperventilation (keeping arterial carbon dioxide tension [$PaCO_2$] at >55 mm Hg, with pH >7.25) and maintain oxygen saturation (SaO_2) at 90% to 95% or lower and arterial oxygen tension (PaO_2) 60 to 80 mm Hg. We do not routinely use high-frequency oscillatory ventilation because most available evidence suggests that this technique does not prevent BPD in high-risk infants. Early CPAP, with avoidance of mechanical ventilation, and earlier transition from mechanical ventilation to CPAP are management strategies that may be associated with decreased BPD risk.

2. **Chronic phase.** Once baseline ventilator settings are established with an $PaCO_2$ not higher than 65 mm Hg, we maintain the ventilator rate without weaning until a pattern of steady weight gain is established.

B. **Supplemental oxygen** is supplied to maintain the PaO_2 >55 mm Hg. The SaO_2 should be correlated with PaO_2 in each infant. Several studies published prior to 2007 that evaluated the impact of limiting O_2 exposure on retinopathy of prematurity (ROP) risk noted that BPD risk was lower in the groups with lower oximeter saturation ranges. Based on these findings and on other cohort studies, we set oximeter alarm limits at 85% to 93% for infants <32 weeks' gestation, and then relax the range to 87% to 97% at 32 weeks' PMA and older. Of caution, the SUPPORT trial (2010) of low (85%–89%) versus high (91%–95%) SaO_2 in infants <28 weeks' gestation revealed a higher mortality rate and no reduction in BPD rate in the low SaO_2 group, although severe ROP was less frequent in survivors.

When <30% O_2 concentration is required by hood, we supply O_2 by nasal cannula. If adequate SaO_2 cannot be maintained on <1 L/min of flow, we restore hood O_2. We use a flowmeter that is accurate at low rates, and gradually decrease the flow of 100% O_2 while maintaining the appropriate SaO_2. Alternatively, flow can be decreased to the lowest marking on the flowmeter, as tolerated, and then O_2 concentration can be decreased. Estimates of the actual concentration of O_2 delivered to the lungs by nasal cannula at different flows of 100% O_2 have been generated by hypopharyngeal measurements (see Fig. 34.1). SaO_2 should remain >90% during sleep, feedings, and active periods before supplemental O_2 is discontinued.

C. **Surfactant replacement therapy** decreases the combined outcome of CLD or death at 28 days of age, although it has made little or no impact on the overall incidence of CLD. Meta-analyses suggest that the incidence is decreased in larger premature infants but is higher in smaller premature infants who would have died without surfactant therapy (see Chap. 33). Late surfactant exhaustion may contribute to the development of BPD; an ongoing trial is testing late surfactant dosing in infants with decompensation or persistent requirement for mechanical ventilation.

D. **PDA.** We consider treatment of a hemodynamically significant PDA in infants who have respiratory decompensation or cannot be weaned from mechanical ventilation (see Chap. 41).

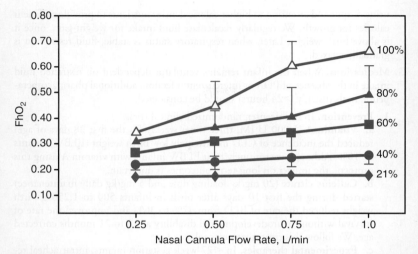

Figure 34.1. Approximate conversion from nasal cannula flow FiO$_2$ to hypopharyngeal FiO$_2$ (FhO$_2$). FiO$_2$, fraction of inspired O$_2$. (From Vain NE, Prudent LM, Stevens DP, et al. Regulation of oxygen concentration delivered to infants through nasal cannulas. *Am J Dis Child* 1989;143(12):1459–1460. By permission.)

E. Monitoring (see Chap. 30)

1. **ABG analysis** is used to monitor gas exchange and confirm noninvasive monitoring values.

2. **We use continuous pulse oximetry** for long-term monitoring of infants with CLD, set oximeter alarm limits at 85% to 93% for infants <32 weeks' gestation and adjust the range to 87% to 97% at 32 weeks' PMA. The long-term goal is to keep the PaO$_2$ ≥55 mm Hg and avoid hyperoxemia.

3. **Capillary blood gas** (CBG) values are useful to monitor pH and pCO$_2$. Because pH and pCO$_2$ sometimes vary from central values, we compare them with ABG values. If CBG and ABG values are similar, we monitor stable ventilator-dependent infants with pulse oximetry and one or two CBG analyses per day initially or less often if clinical condition is unchanged. Less frequent CBG measurements are obtained for patients receiving O$_2$ by nasal cannula.

4. **Transcutaneous pCO$_2$ monitors** have undergone recent technical improvements so that they require less frequent calibration and operate at lower temperatures (minimizing skin injury). They may be useful to monitor pCO$_2$ trends, which allow more real-time ventilator adjustment to both minimize barotrauma and respond earlier to decompensations.

5. **Pulmonary function testing** is used in some centers to document functional responses to trials of bronchodilators and diuretics (see V.G.1–4.).

F. Fluid management. Initial fluid intake is limited to the minimum required. Early on, we provide intake adequate to maintain urine output at least 1 mL/kg/hour and serum sodium concentration of 140 to 145 mEq/L. In the chronic phase, we may limit fluids to as low as 130 mL/kg/day with monitoring for adequate urine output and attention to higher caloric density nutrients to provide sufficient calories for growth. We regularly recalculate fluid intake for weight gain, once it is above birth weight. Later, when respiratory status is stable, fluid restriction is gradually relaxed.

G. **Medications.** When the infant remains ventilator dependent on restricted fluid intake in the absence of PDA or intercurrent infection, additional pharmacotherapeutic trials (usually >24 hours) should be considered.

1. **Prevention.** In multicenter, randomized clinical trials:

   a. Vitamin A (5,000 U IM, three times weekly for the first 28 days of age) reduced the incidence of CLD in extremely low birth weight (ELBW) infants by 10%. Although we routinely treat ELBW infants with vitamin A using this protocol, the impact on long-term outcomes is uncertain.

   b. Caffeine citrate (20 mg/kg loading dose and 5 mg/kg daily maintenance) started during the first 10 days after birth in infants 500 to 1,250 g birth weight reduced the rate of BPD from 47% to 36% and improved the rate of survival without neurodevelopmental disability at 18 to 21 months corrected age. We follow this treatment protocol.

   c. Experimental therapies. In <27-week gestation infants, intratracheal recombinant human Cu/Zn superoxide dismutase administered intratracheally every 48 hours while intubated resulted in an approximately 50% reduction in use of asthma medications, emergency room visits, and hospitalizations in the first year of life. Recombinant human Clara cell protein 10, a natural innate anti-inflammatory protein abundant in the lung, is also undergoing evaluation for intratracheal administration for prophylaxis against CRM. These treatments remain investigational.

   d. Azithromycin may decrease the risk of developing BPD in infants with documented *Ureaplasma* colonization or infection.

   e. Inhaled nitric oxide (iNO). In animal models of BPD, iNO may act to relax airway and pulmonary vascular tone and diminish lung inflammation. Several multicenter clinical trials assessed the potential efficacy of iNO in attenuating or preventing BPD using different treatment regimens. One trial found that BPD was reduced in infants >1,000 g although not for the overall group; the other found overall benefit that was limited to those treated at 7 to 14 days. Because benefit is unclear and both safety and long-term impact have not been established, an NIH consensus panel recommended that use of iNO to prevent or treat BPD is not supported by available evidence.

2. **Diuretics** are used to treat pulmonary fluid retention. Diuretics indirectly attenuate symptoms of respiratory distress and result in decreased Rrs and increased Crs; gas exchange is variably affected. An acute clinical response may be seen within 1 hour, although maximal effect may not be achieved until 1 week of therapy. The clinical improvement is likely due to decreased lung water content, with decreased interstitial and peribronchial fluid resulting in less resistance and better compliance. The mechanisms of action may be due to either diuresis or nondiuretic effects. Diuretics have not been shown to improve clinical outcomes such as duration of ventilator dependence, hospital length of stay, or long-term outcome.

   a. Furosemide is used initially at a dose of 0.5 to 1.0 mg/kg intravenously one to two times daily. The dose may be given at the time of blood transfusions if these have been associated with increased pulmonary fluid and respiratory distress. Immature infants are at increased risk for toxicity from larger or more frequent doses because of the prolonged drug half-life. Side effects include hypercalciuria, nephrocalcinosis, ototoxicity, electrolyte imbalance, and nephrolithiasis.

b. Chlorothiazide. If a trial of furosemide suggests clinical improvement, we prefer treatment with chlorothiazide (20–40 mg/kg/day orally, divided BID) to avoid furosemide toxicities. Chlorothiazide decreases calcium excretion and, if used in combination with furosemide, may minimize calcium loss and reverse nephrocalcinosis due to furosemide. The combination may allow for the use of a lower furosemide dose.

3. **Bronchodilators.** Acute obstructive episodes or chronically increased resistance may be related to increased airway tone or bronchospasm and may respond to bronchodilator therapy. Infants with developing CLD may benefit as early as the second week of age.

   a. Administration of nebulized β-adrenergic agonists (BAAs) results in decreased Rrs and increased Crs. Tachycardia is the major limiting side effect. Newer agents have increased β2 specificity with less β1 toxicity. We use an albuterol metered-dose inhaler (MDI) with a spacer device (1 puff) or nebulized 0.5% solution (5 mg/mL) 0.02 to 0.04 mL/kg (up to 0.1 mL total in 2 mL of normal saline solution) every 6 to 8 hours. In ventilated infants, for efficiency, our preference is an MDI with a spacer device placed in line with the ventilator near the endotracheal tube.

   b. Muscarinic agents. MDI (1 puff) or nebulized (25 mg/kg/dose) ipratropium bromide increases Crs and decreases Rrs. Combination MDI containing both BAAs and muscarinic agents may provide a synergistic effect, but this has not been studied in preterm infants.

   c. Caffeine citrate is used for the treatment of apnea in most infants with BPD. Although not well studied, infants treated with caffeine for apnea may have improved Crs.

4. **Postnatal corticosteroids.** In early trials, treatment with glucocorticoids (usually dexamethasone) in infants, who remained ventilator dependent for 2 to 3 weeks, resulted in increased Crs, decreased Rrs, diminished O_2 requirement, and earlier extubation. However, treatment with glucocorticoids does not appear to have a substantial impact on long-term pulmonary outcomes, such as duration of supplemental O_2 requirement, length of hospital stay, or mortality. Subsequent trials of earlier treatment, recurrent pulses, and lower doses have yielded inconsistent results as either a prophylactic or attenuating agent. Randomized trials of inhaled glucocorticoids also did not demonstrate improved pulmonary outcome. In addition to short-term side effects, including hypertension, hyperglycemia, and spontaneous GI perforation, long-term follow-up of infants treated with postnatal corticosteroids, primarily dexamethasone, has raised concerns about impaired neurodevelopment and growth. Because of this potential harm and lack of well-established long-term benefit, routine use of corticosteroids is discouraged and reserved only for infants with progressive respiratory failure that is refractory to all other therapies. If treatment with glucocorticoids is undertaken, we discuss the potential neurodevelopmental harm with parents before use. Although this regimen has not been tested in clinical trials, we use a short course and relatively low dose of hydrocortisone to potentially reduce ventilator settings and facilitate extubation.

Hydrocortisone can be started at 5 mg/kg/day for 3 days, with weaning over 7 to 10 days. If no response is seen by 2 to 3 days, we stop treatment.

   a. Common acute complications of glucocorticoids include glucose intolerance, systemic hypertension, and transient catabolic state. Total neutrophil counts, band counts, and platelet counts increase during steroid treatment. Hypertrophic cardiomyopathy has been reported, but is transient and does not appear to affect cardiac function. Intestinal perforation and gastric ulcerations can occur. Adrenal suppression is transient.

   b. Postextubation airway edema, with stridorous obstruction (see VI.A.) leading to respiratory failure, may be attenuated with 3 doses dexamethasone, 0.25 mg/kg/dose every 12 hours starting 8 to 12 hours before the next extubation. Edema also may be acutely diminished with nebulized racemic epinephrine.

5. Cromolyn acts on both airway and pulmonary vascular tone. Prophylactic treatment of reactive airways attenuates symptoms in infants with CLD who develop asthma during the first year of life. Use in the NICU setting has not been well evaluated. Dosing can be with either MDI and spacer or nebulized (10–20 mg every 6–8 hours).

6. Pain management. Pain management and sedation are used for physical or autonomic signs of pain or discomfort. These responses may interfere with the ability to ventilate and oxygenate. Oral sucrose, morphine sulfate or fentanyl, short-acting benzodiazepines, or chloral hydrate is used (see Chap. 67).

7. Electrolyte supplements. Hyponatremia, hypokalemia, and hypochloremia with secondary hypercarbia are common side effects of chronic diuretic therapy that are corrected by lowering the diuretic dose or adding NaCl and KCl supplements. Adequate sodium intake should be provided. Serum sodium level can fall below 130 mEq/L before intervention is required. Although hypochloremia may occur with compensated respiratory acidosis, low serum chloride concentration from diuretic-induced loss and inadequate intake can cause metabolic alkalosis and $PaCO_2$ elevation. Hypochloremia may also contribute to poor growth. Chloride deficit can be corrected with KCl. Monitoring should be carried out at regular intervals until equilibrium is reached (see Chap. 23).

H. Nutrition (see Chap. 21)

1. Metabolic rate and energy expenditure are elevated in BPD although caloric intake is poor. Providing more calories by the administration of lipids instead of carbohydrates lowers the respiratory quotient, thereby diminishing CO_2 production. To optimize growth, wasteful energy expenditure should be minimized and caloric intake maximized. Prolonged parenteral nutrition is often required. As enteral feeding is started, we feed by orogastric or nasogastric tube and limit oral feeding to avoid tiring the infant. We advance to 30 cal/oz human milk or formula, if required, to maintain daily growth of at least 10 to 15 mg/kg.

2. Vitamin, trace element, and other dietary supplementation. Vitamin E and antioxidant enzymes diminish oxidant toxicity, although vitamin E supplementation does not prevent BPD. Vitamin A may promote epithelial repair and minimize fibrosis. Selenium, zinc, and copper are trace elements vital to antioxidant enzyme function, and inadequate intake may interfere with protection (see Chap. 25).

I. **Blood transfusions.** We generally maintain hematocrit approximately 30% to 35% (hemoglobin 8–10 g/dL) as long as supplemental O_2 is needed. Fluid-sensitive patients may benefit from furosemide given immediately following the transfusion. Improved O_2 delivery may allow better reserves for growth in the infant with increased metabolic demands.

J. **Behavioral factors.** As with all sick infants, care is best provided with individualized attention to behavioral and environmental factors (see Chap. 14).

VI. ASSOCIATED COMPLICATIONS

A. **Upper airway obstruction.** Trauma to the nasal septum, larynx, trachea, or bronchi is common after prolonged or repeated intubation and suctioning. Abnormalities include laryngotracheobronchomalacia, granulomas, vocal cord paresis, edema, ulceration with pseudomembranes, subglottic stenosis, and congenital structural anomalies. Stridor may develop when postextubation edema is superimposed on underlying stenosis. Abnormalities are not excluded by the absence of stridor and may be asymptomatic, becoming symptomatic at the time of a viral upper respiratory tract infection. Flexible fiberoptic bronchoscopy should be used to evaluate stridor, hoarseness, persistent wheezing, recurrent obstruction, or repeated extubation failure.

B. **Pulmonary hypertension.** Pulmonary hypertension may have reversible and fixed components. Chronic hypoxemia leads to hypoxic vasoconstriction, pulmonary hypertension, and eventual right ventricular hypertrophy and failure. Decrease in cross-sectional perfusion area and abnormal muscularization of more peripheral vessels have been documented. Left ventricular function also can be affected. Supplemental O_2 is used to maintain the PaO_2 >55 mm Hg. The ECG should be followed. Further studies may be required to define the dysfunction and evaluate therapy. Pulmonary vasodilators, including hydralazine and nifedipine, have variable efficacy and should only be tried during pulmonary artery pressure and PaO_2 monitoring. Echocardiographic studies can exclude structural heart disease, assess left ventricular function, and estimate pulmonary vascular resistance and right ventricular function. We obtain an echocardiogram at 36 to 37 weeks' PMA in infants with BPD who still require assisted ventilation or an inspired O_2 concentration of >30% to maintain adequate O_2 saturation, or have a PCO_2 of ≥60 mm Hg.

C. **Systemic hypertension,** sometimes with left ventricular hypertrophy, may develop in BPD infants receiving prolonged O_2 therapy and should be treated (see Chap. 28).

D. **Systemic-to-pulmonary shunting.** Left-to-right shunt through collateral vessels (e.g., bronchial arteries) can occur in BPD. The risk factors include chest tube placement, thoracic surgery, and pleural inflammation. When left-to-right shunt is suspected and echocardiography fails to show intracardiac or PDA shunting, collaterals may be demonstrated by angiography. Occlusion of large vessels has been associated with clinical improvement.

E. **Metabolic imbalance** secondary to diuretics (see V.G.2. and 8)

F. **Infection.** Because these chronically ill and malnourished infants are at increased risk, episodes of pulmonary and systemic decompensation should be evaluated for infection. Monitoring by Gram stain of tracheal aspirates may help distinguish endotracheal tube colonization from tracheobronchitis or pneumonia (presence of organisms and neutrophils). Viral and fungal infections should be considered when fevers or pneumonia develops. In infants with more severe clinical courses, we frequently culture tracheal aspirates for possible infection with *Ureaplasma* sp. and *Mycoplasma hominis* and may treat if these organisms are identified.

G. Central nervous system (CNS) dysfunction. A neurologic syndrome presenting with extrapyramidal signs has been described in infants with CLD.

H. Hearing loss. Ototoxic drugs (furosemide, gentamicin) and ischemic or hypoxemic CNS injury increase the risk of sensorineural hearing loss. Screening with auditory brain stem responses should be performed at discharge (see Chap. 65).

I. ROP (see Chap. 64). ELBW infants with BPD are at highest risk for developing ROP. The use of phenylephrine-containing eyedrops before eye examinations can cause an increase in airway resistance in some infants with CLD.

J. Nephrocalcinosis is frequently documented on ultrasonographic examination and has been linked to the use of furosemide and possibly steroids. Hematuria and passage of stones may occur. Most infants are asymptomatic, with eventual spontaneous resolution, but renal function should be followed (see Chap. 28).

K. Prematurity, inadequate calcium and phosphorus retention, and prolonged immobilization can lead to osteopenia. Calcium loss due to furosemide and corticosteroids may also contribute. Supplementation with vitamin D, calcium, and phosphorus should be optimized (see Chaps. 21 and 59).

L. Gastroesophageal reflux (GER). We try to document and treat GER in older infants when reflux or aspiration may contribute to pulmonary decompensation, apnea, or feeding intolerance with poor growth. Because trials have not shown acid neutralization and propulsive agents to be effective, we generally manage with optimized positioning, avoidance of excessive feeding volumes, and thickening of feeds. If decompensations associated with feeding may be related to swallow dyscoordination and microaspiration, we obtain fluoroscopic evaluations of swallowing during feeding of contrast-laced feeds to rule out aspiration. If aspiration is present, we test modification of feed viscosity. If thickening agents do not eliminate aspiration, we temporarily halt oral feeding and revert to nasogastric feeding until we confirm that aspiration with feeding has resolved. In some cases, placement of a gastrostomy tube is required until swallow coordination has adequately matured.

M. The incidence of inguinal hernia is increased by the presence of the patent processus vaginalis in VLBW infants, particularly boys, with CLD. If the hernia is reducible, surgical correction should be delayed until respiratory status is improved. Spinal, rather than general anesthesia, avoids reintubation and postoperative apnea.

N. Early growth failure may result from inadequate intake and excessive energy expenditure and may persist after clinical resolution of pulmonary disease. Premature withdrawal of supplemental O_2 should be avoided because it may contribute to slowing of growth.

VII. DISCHARGE PLANNING. The timing of discharge depends on the availability of home care support systems and parental readiness (see Chap. 18).

A. Weight gain and oxygen therapy. Supplemental O_2 should be weaned when the SaO_2 is maintained >92% to 94%; no significant periods of desaturations occur during feedings and/or sleep; good weight gain has been established; and respiratory status is stable (see V.B. and VI.N.). We prefer to delay discharge until O_2 has been discontinued. However, if long-term O_2 supplementation seems likely in an infant who is stable, growing, and has capable caretakers, we offer the option of home O_2 therapy.

B. **Teaching.** The involvement of parents in caregiving is vital to the smooth transition from hospital to home care. Parents should be taught cardiopulmonary resuscitation and early signs of decompensation. Teaching about equipment use, medication administration, and nutritional guidelines should begin when discharge planning is initiated.

C. **Baseline values.** Baseline values of vital signs, daily weight gain, discharge weight and head circumference, blood gases, SaO_2, hematocrit, electrolytes, and the baseline appearance of the chest radiograph and ECG are documented at discharge. Echocardiograms are obtained in more severely affected infants, as discussed previously (see VI.B.). This information is useful to evaluate subsequent changes in clinical status. An eye examination and hearing screening should be performed before discharge.

VIII. OUTPATIENT THERAPY

A. **Oxygen.** Supplemental O_2 can be delivered by tanks or O_2 concentrator. Portable tanks allow mobility. Weaning is based on periodic assessment of SaO_2.

B. **Medications.** Infants receiving diuretics require monitoring of electrolytes. When the infant is stable, we allow him or her to outgrow the diuretic dose by 50% before discontinuing the drug. Bronchodilators are tapered when respiratory status is stable in room air. Nebulized medications are tapered last. Discontinued medications should remain available for early use when symptoms recur.

C. **Immunizations.** In addition to standard immunizations, infants with CLD should receive pneumococcal and influenza vaccines and palivizumab (Synagis) (see Chaps. 16, 48, and 49).

D. **Nutrition.** Weight gain is a sensitive indicator of well-being and should be closely monitored. Caloric supplementation is often required to maintain good growth after discharge. At discharge, we supplement calories in a transitional formula or, optimally, breast milk.

E. **Passive smoke exposure.** Because smoking in the home increases respiratory tract illness in children, parents of CLD infants should be discouraged from smoking and should minimize the child's exposure to smoke-containing environments.

IX. OUTCOME

A. **Mortality.** Mortality is estimated at 10% to 20% during the first year of life. The risk increases with duration of O_2 exposure and level of ventilatory support. Death is frequently caused by infection. The risk of sudden, unexpected death may be increased, but the cause is unclear.

B. **Long-term morbidity**

1. **Pulmonary.** Tachypnea, retractions, dyspnea, cough, and wheezing can be seen for months to years in seriously affected children. Although complete clinical recovery can occur, underlying pulmonary function, gas exchange, and radiographic abnormalities may persist beyond adolescence. The impact of

persistent minor abnormalities of function and growth on long-term morbidity and mortality is not known. Reactive airway disease occurs more frequently, and infants with CLD are at increased risk for bronchiolitis and pneumonia. The rehospitalization rate for respiratory illness during the first 2 years of life is approximately twice that of matched-control infants. CRM measures at 6 and 12 months PMA are being evaluated as potentially more relevant outcomes to assess in the study of early therapeutic interventions aimed at preventing or attenuating BPD.

2. **Neurodevelopmental delay/neurologic deficits.** BPD is not clearly an independent predictor of adverse neurologic outcome. Early behavioral differences do exist, however, between VLBW infants with CLD and RDS controls. Later outcome varies widely; one-third to two-thirds of infants with BPD are normal by 2 years, and subsequent improvement may occur in some of the remaining infants. Cerebral palsy is markedly increased in infants born at <28 weeks' gestation and still treated with both mechanical ventilation and supplemental O_2 at 36 weeks' PMA, although not in those treated with O_2 alone. Children with BPD have higher rates of cognitive, educational, and behavioral impairments.

3. **Growth failure.** The degree of long-term growth delay is inversely proportional to birth weight and probably is influenced by the severity and duration of CLD. Weight is most affected, and head circumference is least affected. Significantly, delayed growth (<2 standard deviations below the mean) persists for weight in ~20% and length or head circumference in ~10% at 20 months corrected age.

Suggested Readings

Jobe AH. The new bronchopulmonary dysplasia. *Curr Opin Pediatr* 2011;23(2):167–172.

Kinsella JP, Greenough A, Abman SH. Bronchopulmonary dysplasia. *Lancet* 2006;367(9520):1421–1431.

Watterberg KL; American Academy of Pediatrics, Committee on Fetus and Newborn. Policy statement—postnatal corticosteroids to prevent or treat bronchopulmonary dysplasia. *Pediatrics* 2010;126(4):800–808.

35 Meconium Aspiration
Heather H. Burris

I. BACKGROUND

A. **Cause.** Acute or chronic hypoxia and/or infection can result in the passage of meconium *in utero*. In this setting, gasping by the fetus or newly born infant can cause aspiration of amniotic fluid contaminated by meconium. Meconium aspiration before or during birth can obstruct airways, interfere with gas exchange, and cause severe respiratory distress (Fig. 35.1).

B. **Incidence.** Meconium-stained amniotic fluid (MSAF) complicates delivery in approximately 8% to 25% of live births. The incidence of MSAF in preterm infants is very low. Most babies with MSAF are 37 weeks or older, and many meconium-stained infants are postmature and small for gestational age. Approximately 5% of neonates born through MSAF develop meconium aspiration syndrome (MAS) and approximately 50% of these infants require mechanical ventilation.

II. PATHOPHYSIOLOGY.
Meconium is a sterile, thick, black-green, odorless material that results from the accumulation of debris in the fetal intestine during the third month of gestation. The components of meconium include water (72%–80%), desquamated cells from the intestine and skin, gastrointestinal mucin, lanugo hair, fatty material from the vernix caseosa, amniotic fluid, intestinal secretions, blood-group–specific glycoproteins, bile, and drug metabolites.

A. **Passage of meconium *in utero*.** MSAF may result from a postterm fetus with rising motilin levels and normal gastrointestinal function, vagal stimulation produced by cord or head compression, or *in utero* fetal stress. Amniotic fluid that is thinly stained is described as *watery*. Moderately stained fluid is opaque without particles, and fluid with thick meconium with particles is sometimes called *pea soup*.

B. **Aspiration of meconium.** In the presence of fetal stress, gasping by the fetus can result in aspiration of meconium before, during, or immediately following delivery. Severe MAS appears to be caused by pathologic intrauterine processes, primarily chronic hypoxia, acidosis, and infection. Meconium has been found in the lungs of stillborn infants and infants who died soon after birth without a history of aspiration at delivery.

C. **Effects of meconium aspiration.** When aspirated into the lung, meconium may stimulate the release of cytokines and vasoactive substances that result in cardiovascular and inflammatory responses in the fetus and newborn. Meconium itself, or the resultant chemical pneumonitis, mechanically obstructs the small airways and causes atelectasis and a "ball-valve" effect with resultant air trapping and possible air leak. Aspirated meconium leads to vasospasm, hypertrophy of the pulmonary arterial musculature, and pulmonary hypertension that lead to extra-pulmonary right-to-left shunting through the ductus arteriosus or the foramen

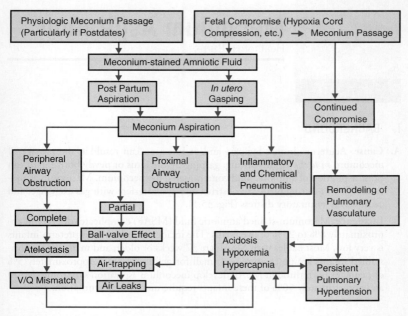

Figure 35.1. Pathophysiology of meconium aspiration. V/Q, ventilation–perfusion ratio. (From Wiswell T, Bent RC. Meconium staining and the meconium aspiration syndrome: unresolved issues. *Pediatr Clin North Am* 1993;40:955. Used with permission.)

ovale resulting in worsened ventilation–perfusion (V/Q) mismatch and severe arterial hypoxemia. Approximately one-third of infants with MAS develop persistent pulmonary hypertension of the newborn (PPHN), which contributes to the mortality associated with this syndrome (see Chap. 36). Aspirated meconium also inhibits surfactant function.

D. **Classification of respiratory disease.** Mild MAS is a disease requiring <40% oxygen for <48 hours. Moderate MAS is a disease requiring >40% oxygen for >48 hours without air leak. Severe MAS is a disease requiring assisted ventilation for >48 hours, often associated with PPHN.

E. **Sequelae.** *In utero* passage of meconium in term infants has been associated with an increased risk of perinatal and neonatal mortality, severe acidemia, need for caesarean section delivery, need for intensive care and oxygen administration, and adverse neurologic outcome. Preterm infants who pass meconium before delivery have similar adverse effects, as well as an increased incidence of severe intraventricular hemorrhage, cystic periventricular leukomalacia, and cerebral palsy.

III. PREVENTION OF MAS

A. **Prevention of passage of meconium *in utero*.** Mothers at risk for uteroplacental insufficiency and, thus, MSAF include those with preeclampsia or increased blood pressure, chronic respiratory or cardiovascular disease, poor intrauterine fetal growth, postterm pregnancy, and heavy smokers. These women should be carefully monitored during pregnancy.

B. **Amnioinfusion.** The use of amnioinfusion in women whose labor is complicated by MSAF does not reduce neonatal morbidity related to meconium aspiration, although the technique effectively treats repetitive variable fetal heart rate decelerations by relieving umbilical cord compression in labor. A large randomized trial of amnioinfusion for women with thick meconium-stained fluid with or without variable fetal heart rate decelerations showed no reduction of the risk of moderate or severe MAS, perinatal death, or caesarean delivery. However, the study did not have adequate power to determine definitively if amnioinfusion may benefit the group with variable decelerations.

C. **Timing and mode of delivery.** In pregnancies that continue past the due date, induction as early as 41 weeks may help prevent MAS by avoiding passage of meconium. Delivery mode does not appear to significantly impact the risk of aspiration.

IV. MANAGEMENT OF INFANTS DELIVERED THROUGH MECONIUM-STAINED FLUID.

Oropharyngeal and nasopharyngeal suctioning on the perineum and routine tracheal intubation and aspiration of meconium in vigorous infants are not effective in preventing MAS. Infants should be assessed and intervention reserved for infants who are depressed or have respiratory distress.

A. **Initial assessment.** At a delivery complicated by MSAF, the clinician should determine whether the infant is vigorous, demonstrated by heart rate >100 beats per minute, spontaneous respirations, and good tone (spontaneous movement or some degree of flexion). The infant will be depressed approximately 20% to 30% of the time.

1. If the infant appears vigorous, routine care should be provided, regardless of the consistency of the meconium.

2. If respiratory distress develops or the infant becomes depressed, the trachea should be intubated under direct laryngoscopy and intratracheal suctioning performed. Visualization of the cords without suctioning is not adequate because significant meconium may be present below the cords.

B. **Suctioning technique for the nonvigorous meconium-stained infant**

1. The infant should be placed on a radiant warmer and given free-flow oxygen.

2. Delay drying, stimulating, and gastric suctioning.

3. A clinician (e.g., pediatrician, anesthesiologist, advanced practice nurse) should intubate the trachea under direct laryngoscopy, preferably before inspiratory efforts have been initiated. A 3.0-mm or 3.5-mm internal diameter endotracheal tube is used in term infants.

4. After intubation, the tube is attached to wall suction at a pressure of 80 to 100 mm Hg by means of a plastic adapter (Neotech Meconium Aspirator, Neotech Products, Chatsworth, CA). Alternatively, an endotracheal tube specifically made for suctioning of meconium (Kurtis Meconium Suction Device, Vital Signs, Inc., Totowa, NJ) may be used. Continuous suction is applied as the tube is being withdrawn; the procedure is repeated until the trachea is cleared or resuscitation needs to be initiated.

5. Avoid positive pressure ventilation, if possible, until tracheal suctioning is accomplished. Postpone emptying gastric contents until the infant has stabilized.

C. **Complications of intubation** include bleeding, laryngospasm, stridor, apnea, and cyanosis. This procedure should be accomplished rapidly, and ventilation with oxygen should be initiated before significant bradycardia occurs. The infant's general condition must not be ignored in persistent attempts to clear the trachea. Because a few inspiratory efforts by the infant will move the meconium from the trachea to the smaller airways, exhaustive attempts to remove it are unwise.

V. MANAGEMENT OF MAS

A. **Observation.** Infants who are depressed at birth and have had meconium suctioned from the trachea are at risk for meconium aspiration pneumonia and should be observed closely for respiratory distress.

1. A chest radiograph may help determine those infants who are most likely to develop respiratory distress, although a significant number of asymptomatic infants will have an abnormal-appearing chest film. The classic roentgenographic findings are diffuse, asymmetric patchy infiltrates; areas of consolidation, often worse on the right; and hyperinflation.

2. Monitoring of oxygen saturation during this period aids assessment of the severity of the infant's condition and avoids hypoxemia.

B. **Care for neonate with MAS**

1. The infant should be maintained in a neutral thermal environment and tactile stimulation should be minimized.

2. Blood glucose and calcium levels should be assessed and corrected if necessary. Severely depressed infants may have severe metabolic acidosis that may need to be corrected, although we recommend only gentle, judicious use of alkali (see Chap. 36).

3. Fluids should be restricted as much as possible to prevent cerebral and pulmonary edema.

4. Infants may also require specific therapy for hypotension and poor cardiac output, including cardiotonic medications such as dopamine.

5. Circulatory support with normal saline or packed red blood cells should be provided in patients with marginal oxygenation. In infants with substantial oxygen and ventilator requirements, we usually maintain a hemoglobin concentration above 15 g (hematocrit above 40%).

6. Renal function should be continuously monitored (see Chap. 28).

7. We favor avoiding chest physiotherapy because of the potential adverse effect of exacerbating PPHN (see Chap. 36).

8. Airway and oral suctioning may be required to facilitate airway clearance, but potential benefits must be balanced against the risk of hypoxic episodes and subsequent worsening of PPHN.

C. **Oxygen therapy.** Management of hypoxemia should be accomplished by increasing the inspired oxygen concentration and by monitoring blood gases and pH. An indwelling arterial catheter is usually required for blood sampling. It is crucial to provide sufficient oxygen, because repeated hypoxic insults may result in ongoing pulmonary vasoconstriction and contribute to the development of PPHN.

D. **Assisted ventilation**

1. **Continuous positive airway pressure (CPAP).** If FiO_2 requirements exceed 0.40, a trial of CPAP may be considered. CPAP is often helpful, and the appropriate pressures must be individualized for each infant. However, CPAP may sometimes aggravate air trapping and should be instituted with caution if hyperinflation is apparent clinically or radiographically.

2. **Mechanical ventilation.** Infants with severe disease may have substantial gas exchange abnormalities. Mechanical ventilation is indicated for excessive carbon dioxide retention ($PaCO_2$ >60 mm Hg) or for persistent hypoxemia (PaO_2 <50 mm Hg).

   a. In these infants, higher inspiratory pressures (approximately 30–35 cm H_2O) are more often required than in infants with respiratory distress syndrome; the positive end-expiratory pressure (PEEP) selected (usually 3–6 cm H_2O) should depend on the individual's response. Adequate expiratory time should be permitted to prevent air trapping behind partly obstructed airways.

   b. Useful starting points are an inspiratory time of 0.4 to 0.5 seconds at a rate of 20 to 25 breaths per minute. Some infants may respond better to conventional ventilation at more rapid rates with inspiratory times as short as 0.2 seconds.

   c. High-frequency ventilation with jet or oscillatory ventilators may be effective in infants with severe MAS who fail to improve with conventional ventilation, and in those who develop air-leak syndromes. There are no prospective, randomized controlled trials comparing the efficacy of the various ventilator modes in MAS.

3. **Extracorporeal membrane oxygenation (ECMO)** may be required for infants with refractory respiratory failure.

E. **Medications**

1. **Antibiotics.** Differentiating between bacterial pneumonia and meconium aspiration by clinical course and chest x-ray findings may be difficult. Although few infants with MAS have documented infections, the use of broad-spectrum antibiotics (e.g., ampicillin and gentamicin) is usually indicated in infants when an infiltrate is seen on chest radiograph. Blood cultures should be obtained to identify bacterial disease, if present, and to determine length of antibiotic course.

2. **Surfactant.** Endogenous surfactant activity may be inhibited by meconium. Surfactant treatment of MAS may improve oxygenation and reduce pulmonary complications and the need for ECMO. We do not routinely use surfactant to treat infants with MAS. However, in infants whose clinical status continues to deteriorate and who require escalating support, surfactant administration may be helpful. We do not recommend washing meconium from the lungs with bronchoalveolar surfactant lavage.

3. **Corticosteroids.** We do not recommend the use of corticosteroids in MAS, although this approach has been proposed to reduce inflammation induced by meconium and minimize prostaglandin-mediated pulmonary vasoconstriction.

4. **Sedatives.** The use of sedation and muscle relaxation may be warranted in infants who require mechanical ventilation (see Chap. 36 and 67).

F. Complications

1. **Air leak.** Pneumothorax or pneumomediastinum occurs in approximately 15% to 33% of patients with MAS. Air leaks occur more frequently with mechanical ventilation, especially in the setting of air trapping. A high index of suspicion for air leak is necessary. Equipment should be available to evacuate a pneumothorax promptly (see Chap. 38).

2. **PPHN** is associated with MAS in approximately one-third of cases and contributes to the mortality associated with this syndrome (see Chap. 36). Depending on the extent of hypoxemia, echocardiography should be performed to ascertain the degree to which the right-to-left shunting is contributing to the infant's overall hypoxemia and to exclude congenital heart disease as the etiology. In severely ill infants with MAS and PPHN, inhaled nitric oxide (iNO) reduces the need for ECMO.

3. **Pulmonary sequelae.** Approximately 5% of survivors require supplemental oxygen at 1 month, and a substantial proportion may have abnormal pulmonary function, including increased functional residual capacity, airway reactivity, and higher incidence of pneumonia.

Suggested Readings

Fanaroff AA. Meconium aspiration syndrome: historical aspects. *J Perinatol* 2008;28:S3–S7.

Fraser WD, Hofmeyr J, Lede R, et al, for the Amnioinfusion Trial Group. Amnioinfusion for the prevention of the meconium aspiration syndrome. *N Engl J Med* 2005;353:909–917.

Vain NE, Szydl EG, Prudent LM, et al, for the Meconium Study Network. Oropharyngeal and nasopharyngeal suctioning of meconium-stained neonates before delivery of their shoulders: multicentre, randomised controlled trial. *Lancet* 2004;364:597–602.

Wiswell TE, Gannon CM, Jacob J, et al. Delivery room management of the apparently vigorous meconium-stained neonate: results of the multicenter, international collaborative trial. *Pediatrics* 2000;105:1–7.

36 Persistent Pulmonary Hypertension of the Newborn

Linda J. Van Marter

I. DEFINITION. Persistent pulmonary hypertension of the newborn (PPHN) results from disruption of the normal perinatal fetal to neonatal circulatory transition. The disorder is characterized by sustained elevation in pulmonary vascular resistance (PVR), rather than the decrease in PVR that normally occurs at birth. Survivors of PPHN are at risk for adverse sequelae including chronic pulmonary disease and neurodevelopmental disabilities. Contemporary ventilator management, treatment with inhaled nitric oxide (iNO), and extracorporeal membrane oxygenation (ECMO) have improved survival among infants with PPHN.

A. Perinatal circulatory transition. The normal perinatal circulatory transition is characterized by a rapid fall in PVR accompanying the first breath and a marked increase in systemic vascular resistance (SVR) associated with clamping of the umbilical cord. Circulating biochemical mediators released in response to increased arterial oxygen content and pH and lowered $PaCO_2$ cause constriction of the ductus arteriosus and vasorelaxation of the pulmonary circulation. These physiologic events raise SVR relative to PVR, cause functional closure of the foramen ovale, and signal the normal perinatal transition in pulmonary and systemic circulations. PPHN physiology mimics the fetal circulation in which PVR exceeds SVR and right-to-left hemodynamic shunting occurs through the foramen ovale and/or ductus arteriosus. Thus, PPHN also has been called "persistent fetal circulation." Before birth, this circulatory configuration results in systemic delivery of oxygenated blood from the placental circulation; in postnatal life, it causes diminished pulmonary perfusion and systemic hypoxemia.

II. EPIDEMIOLOGIC ASSOCIATIONS. PPHN occurs at a rate of 1 to 2 per 1,000 live births and is most common among full-term and postterm infants. Perinatal risk factors reported in association with PPHN include meconium-stained amniotic fluid and maternal conditions such as fever, anemia, and pulmonary disease. Case-control studies of risk factors for PPHN suggest associations between PPHN and a number of antenatal and perinatal factors, including maternal diabetes mellitus, urinary tract infection during pregnancy, selective serotonin reuptake inhibitors (SSRIs), aspirin, nonsteroidal anti-inflammatory drug consumption during pregnancy, and cesarean section delivery. Although mechanisms of antenatal pathogenesis remain uncertain, there are a number of perinatal and neonatal conditions that have well-established links with PPHN.

A. Severe fetal hypoxemia ("asphyxia") is the most common associated diagnosis. Some speculate that prolonged fetal stress and hypoxemia lead to remodeling and abnormal muscularization of pulmonary arterioles. Acute birth asphyxia also causes release of vasoconstricting humoral factors and suppression of pulmonary vasodilators, thus contributing to pulmonary vasospasm.

B. Pulmonary parenchymal diseases, including surfactant deficiency, pneumonia, and aspiration syndromes, such as meconium aspiration, are also associated with increased risk of PPHN. In most such cases, the pulmonary hypertension is reversible, suggesting a vasospastic contribution; however, concomitant pulmonary vascular remodeling cannot be excluded. The risk of pulmonary hypertension appears to be greater when the fetus is of more advanced gestational age, suggesting that the stage of pulmonary vascular development might play a role in susceptibility to PPHN.

C. Abnormalities of pulmonary development contribute structurally to PPHN, either by pruning of the vascular tree, as occurs in congenital diaphragmatic hernia, Potter syndrome, and other forms of pulmonary parenchymal hypoplasia, or malalignment of pulmonary veins and arteries, as is seen in alveolar capillary dysplasia.

D. Myocardial dysfunction, myocarditis, intrauterine constriction of the ductus arteriosus, and several forms of congenital heart disease, including left- and right-sided obstructive lesions, can lead to pulmonary hypertension.

E. Pneumonia and/or sepsis of bacterial or viral origin can initiate PPHN. Underlying pathophysiologic mechanisms that contribute to pulmonary hypertension in this clinical setting include suppression of endogenous nitric oxide (NO) production, endotoxin-mediated myocardial depression, and pulmonary vasoconstriction associated with release of thromboxanes.

F. Although familial recurrence of PPHN is uncommon, genetic predisposition might influence PPHN risk. Infants with PPHN have low plasma levels of arginine and NO metabolites and have a greater likelihood of specific polymorphisms at position 1,405 of the carbamoyl-phosphate synthetase gene. Further, although no specific polymorphisms of NO synthase genes have been reported in association with PPHN, diminished endothelial NO synthase (eNOS) expression has been observed among infants with PPHN. In addition, several recent case reports have linked a mutation of the ABCA3 gene with PPHN.

III. PATHOLOGY AND PATHOPHYSIOLOGY

A. **Pulmonary vascular remodeling** is pathognomonic of idiopathic PPHN and has been reported among a series of infants with fatal PPHN. Abnormal muscularization of the normally nonmuscular intra-acinar arteries, with increased medial thickness of the larger muscular arteries, results in a decreased cross-sectional area of the pulmonary vascular bed and elevated PVR. Mechanisms leading to the vascular remodeling of PPHN are under investigation. One possible stimulus to pulmonary vascular remodeling is fetal hypoxemia. Humoral growth factors released by hypoxia-damaged endothelial cells promote vasoconstriction and overgrowth of the pulmonary vascular muscular media. Laboratory and limited clinical data suggest that vascular changes might also occur following fetal exposure to nonsteroidal anti-inflammatory agents that cause constriction of the fetal ductus arteriosus and associated fetal pulmonary overcirculation.

B. **Pulmonary hypoplasia** affects both alveolar and pulmonary arteriolar development. It may be seen as an isolated anomaly or with congenital diaphragmatic hernia, oligohydramnios syndrome, renal agenesis (i.e., Potter syndrome), or remodeling or vasoconstriction of impaired fetal breathing.

C. **Reversible pulmonary vasospasm** is the likely pathophysiologic mechanism among infants with nonfatal PPHN. The underlying disease process, the associated conditions, and the developmental stage of the host each appear to modulate the pathophysiologic response. Hypoxia induces profound pulmonary vasoconstriction, and this response is exaggerated by acidemia. Neural and humoral vasoactive substances each might contribute to the pathogenesis of PPHN, the response to hypoxemia, or both. These include factors associated with platelet activation and production of arachidonic acid metabolites. Suppression of endogenous NO, prostacyclin, or bradykinin production and release of thromboxanes (A_2 and its metabolite, B_2) and leukotrienes (C_4 and D_4) appear to mediate the increased PVR seen with sepsis and hypoxemia.

D. **Myocardial dysfunction with elevated PVR**

1. **Right ventricular (RV) dysfunction** can be caused by intrauterine constriction of the ductus arteriosus, which results in altered fetal hemodynamics, postnatal pulmonary hypertension, RV failure, and an atrial right-to-left shunt. Furthermore, RV failure resulting in altered diastolic compliance causes right-to-left atrial shunting even in the absence of elevated PVR.

2. **Left ventricular (LV) dysfunction** causes pulmonary venous hypertension and secondary pulmonary arterial hypertension, often to suprasystemic levels, contributing to right-to-left hemodynamic shunting through the ductus arteriosus. Treating this form of pulmonary hypertension requires an approach that improves LV function, rather than simply lowering PVR.

E. **Mechanical factors** that influence PVR include cardiac output and blood viscosity. Low cardiac output recruits fewer pulmonary arteriolar channels and raises PVR by this mechanism as well as by its primary effect of lowering mixed venous oxygen content. Hyperviscosity, associated with polycythemia, reduces pulmonary microvasculature perfusion.

IV. DIAGNOSIS. PPHN should be routinely considered in evaluating the cyanotic newborn.

A. Among cases of suspected PPHN, the most common **alternative diagnoses** are congenital heart disease, sepsis, and severe pulmonary parenchymal disease.

B. The infant with PPHN appears distressed and has a **physical examination** that is most remarkable for evidence of cyanosis. In some infants, the extent of cyanosis might be appreciably different between regions perfused by preductal and postductal vasculature. The cardiac examination is notable for a prominent precordial impulse, a single or narrowly split and accentuated second heart sound, and sometimes a systolic murmur consistent with tricuspid regurgitation.

C. A **gradient of 10% or more in oxygenation saturation** between simultaneous preductal (right upper extremity) and postductal (lower extremity) arterial blood gas (ABG) values or transcutaneous oxygen saturation (SaO_2) measurements documents the presence of a ductus arteriosus right-to-left hemodynamic shunt and, in the absence of structural heart disease, suggests PPHN. Because a subset of infants with PPHN has hemodynamic shunting only at the foramen ovale, the absence of differential cyanosis or SaO_2 does not exclude pulmonary hypertension.

D. The **chest radiograph** usually appears normal or shows associated pulmonary parenchymal disease. The cardiothymic silhouette is normal, and pulmonary blood flow is normal or diminished.

E. The **electrocardiogram (ECG)** most commonly shows RV predominance that is within the range considered normal for age. Less commonly, the ECG might reveal signs of myocardial ischemia or infarction.

F. An **echocardiographic study** should be performed in all infants with suspected PPHN to document hemodynamic shunting, evaluate ventricular function, and exclude congenital heart disease. Color Doppler examination is useful to assess the presence of intracardiac or ductal hemodynamic shunting. Additional echocardiographic markers, such as tricuspid valve regurgitation or a ventricular septum that is flattened or bowed to the left, suggest pulmonary hypertension. Pulmonary artery pressure can be estimated using continuous-wave Doppler sampling of the velocity of the tricuspid regurgitation jet, if present.

G. Other diagnostic considerations. A number of disorders, some of which are associated with secondary pulmonary hypertension, may be misdiagnosed as PPHN. Therefore, an important aspect of the evaluation of the infant with presumed PPHN is to rule out competing conditions, including the following:

1. Structural cardiovascular abnormalities associated with right-to-left ductal or atrial shunting include the following:

a. Obstruction to pulmonary venous return: infradiaphragmatic total anomalous pulmonary venous return, hypoplastic left heart, cor triatriatum, congenital mitral stenosis

b. Myopathic LV disease: endocardial fibroelastosis, Pompe disease

c. Obstruction to LV outflow: critical aortic stenosis, supravalvar aortic stenosis, interrupted aortic arch, coarctation of the aorta

d. Obligatory left-to-right shunt: endocardial cushion defect, arteriovenous malformation, hemitruncus, coronary arteriovenous fistula

e. Miscellaneous disorders: Ebstein anomaly, transposition of the great arteries

2. Primary LV or RV dysfunction associated with right-to-left hemodynamic shunting. LV dysfunction, due to ischemia or obstruction caused by myopathic LV disease or obstruction to LV outflow, might present with a right-to-left ductus arteriosus shunt. RV dysfunction may be associated with right-to-left atrial shunting as a result of decreased diastolic compliance and elevated end-diastolic pressure. These diagnoses must be differentiated from idiopathic PPHN caused by pulmonary vascular remodeling or vasoconstriction.

H. Signs favoring cyanotic congenital cardiac disease over PPHN include cardiomegaly, grade 3+ murmur, weak pulses, active precordium, pulse differential between upper and lower extremities, pulmonary edema, and persistent preductal and postductal arterial oxygen tension (PaO_2) ≤40 mm Hg.

V. MANAGEMENT. The infant with PPHN constitutes a medical emergency in which immediate, appropriate intervention is critical to reverse hypoxemia, improve pulmonary and systemic perfusion, and preserve end-organ function. Adequate respiratory support providing normoxemia and neutral to slightly alkalotic acid–base balance facilitate the normal perinatal circulatory transition. Once stability is achieved, cardiorespiratory support should be tapered conservatively with careful attention to the infant's tolerance of each step in reducing support.

A. **Supplemental oxygen.** Hypoxia is a powerful pulmonary vasoconstrictor. Therefore, in the infant with suspected or documented PPHN, preductal and postductal SaO_2 should be continuously monitored. The use of supplemental oxygen to achieve normoxia is the most important therapy used to reduce abnormally elevated PVR. In the presence of hypoxemia, sufficient supplemental oxygen should be administered to any late preterm, near-term, or full-term newborn to maintain adequate oxygenation and minimize end-organ underperfusion and lactic acidemia. Laboratory data suggest that excessive oxygen exposure releases free radicals that worsen pulmonary hypertension; therefore, debate exists regarding the optimal set point for SaO_2. We aim to maintain postductal SaO_2 greater than 90% to ensure adequate tissue oxygenation and less than 98% to avoid hyperoxemia. Arterial access is indicated for blood gas and blood pressure monitoring.

B. **Intubation and mechanical ventilation.** Mechanical respiratory support is instituted when hypoxemia persists despite maximal administration of supplemental oxygen and/or respiratory failure is demonstrated by marked hypercapnia and acidemia. Specific approaches to respiratory support and mechanical ventilation vary among medical centers. Our approach maintains physiologic PaO_2 and $PaCO_2$ values but avoids hyperoxia and hyperventilation. Because infants with PPHN demonstrate marked lability, a conservative approach to tapering support is indicated until stability is achieved for 12 to 24 hours. Suggested target goals are as follows: SaO_2 90% to 98%, $PaCO_2$ 40 to 50 mm Hg, and pH 7.30 to 7.40.

   1. Both the nature of the underlying pulmonary parenchymal abnormality, if any, and the infant's clinical lability or stability are important factors to consider when choosing a specific respiratory management strategy.

      a. In the absence of pulmonary alveolar disease, high intrathoracic pressure impedes cardiac output and elevates PVR. The optimal strategy for this group of infants involves mechanical ventilation with rapid, low-pressure, and short inspiratory time in an effort to minimize elevated intrathoracic pressure and modulate effects of ventilation on pulmonary venous return and cardiac output.

      b. When PPHN complicates parenchymal pulmonary disease, ventilator strategies should optimize treatment of the infant's primary pulmonary disease. High-frequency oscillatory ventilation (HFOV) or high-frequency jet ventilation (HFJV) is often useful in treating infants whose PPHN is associated with severe pulmonary parenchymal disease. HFJV appears to be very useful for meconium aspiration pneumonitis and air leak. HFOV has proved to be more effective than conventional mechanical ventilation in delivering iNO to infants whose PPHN is complicated by parenchymal disease.

C. **iNO.** NO is a naturally occurring substance produced by endothelial cells. Whether produced by pulmonary endothelium or delivered through the ventilator circuit, NO diffuses into smooth muscle cells, increases intracellular cyclic guanosine monophosphate (cGMP), relaxes the vascular smooth muscle, and causes pulmonary vasodilation. In the circulation, NO is bound by hemoglobin and biologically inactivated and, therefore, when delivered by inhalation, it causes little or no systemic vasodilation or hypotension. iNO administered by conventional or high-frequency ventilation in doses of 1 to 20 parts per million (ppm) causes pulmonary but not systemic vasodilation and, thus, selectively decreases PVR. In a systematic review conducted by the Cochrane Collaboration, iNO was deemed useful in reducing the need for ECMO among term infants with severe respiratory failure. Methemoglobinemia is a serious potential toxicity of iNO treatment that is rare at doses of 20 ppm and below. We measure methemoglobin (metHb) levels 24 hours after the start of treatment. If metHb levels >7% are detected, we reduce iNO. If high levels persist despite reducing the dose or discontinuing iNO, immediate intervention should be instituted to reduce metHb levels. We continue to monitor metHb levels in infants being treated with high dose iNO for prolonged periods. Another potential complication of iNO treatment is rebound hypoxemia that occurs when iNO is discontinued abruptly. For this reason, iNO should be tapered very gradually and not discontinued entirely until adequate oxygenation can be maintained at an iNO dose of 1 ppm with an oxygen concentration of less than 50%. Because not all infants with PPHN respond to iNO and some may deteriorate rapidly, we recommend treatment of critically ill infants with PPHN at a center in which both iNO and ECMO are readily accessible.

1. The usual starting dose of iNO is 20 ppm, and it is delivered via the ventilator circuit. As the baby improves and inspired oxygen concentration is less than 50%, iNO is tapered by approximately halving the dose (e.g., 20 to 10 to 5 ppm over a 12- to 24-hour period as tolerated) and then more gradually to 2 then 1 ppm. The infant's oxygen saturation in response to each step down is observed before further weaning and/or discontinuing the medication.

2. iNO is most effective when administered after adequate alveolar recruitment. This can be accomplished among infants with PPHN and diffuse pulmonary disease by the concomitant use of HFOV and/or surfactant treatment.

3. Recent case series data suggest sildenafil, a phosphodiesterase-5 inhibitor that increases endogenous NO by inhibiting its metabolism, offers promise for the treatment of PPHN. The results of randomized clinical trials are awaited before this therapy can be recommended.

D. **ECMO.** In the absence of pulmonary hypoplasia, ECMO is lifesaving therapy for approximately 75% to 85% of infants with PPHN who fail conventional management and/or iNO treatment (see Chap. 39). Among term or near-term infants meeting ECMO criteria (alveolar-arterial oxygen difference [AaDO$_2$] >600 or oxygenation index [OI] >30 on two ABGs ≥30 minutes apart), both iNO and HFOV appear to reduce the need for ECMO treatment. Therefore, when the infant's clinical status permits, a brief trial of HFOV and/or iNO is generally instituted before commencing ECMO.

E. **Sedation and analgesia.** Because catecholamine release activates pulmonary α-adrenergic receptors, thereby potentially raising PVR, a narcotic analgesic that blocks the stress response, such as fentanyl (1–4 μg/kg/hour infusion), is a useful adjunct therapy. Morphine sulfate (0.05–0.1 mg/kg/hour infusion) is an alternative sedative that is best used when the infant is not hypotensive. Infants with PPHN rarely require neuromuscular blockade with pancuronium (0.1 mg/kg/dose; every 1–4 hours PRN) to accomplish muscle relaxation and fully synchronize the infant's breathing with mechanical ventilation (see Chap. 67).

F. **Metabolic alkalosis.** Neutral acid–base balance (pH 7.30–7.40) also mitigates hypoxic pulmonary hypertension. Neutral to alkalotic pH, rather than low PaCO$_2$, is the physiologic stimulus that reduces PVR. This can be achieved by normalizing pulmonary gas exchange and/or conservative use of metabolic therapy with sodium bicarbonate with careful attention to the associated risks of excessive sodium load and raising $PaCO_2$ levels among infants who are inadequately ventilated. Because of past reports of adverse effects of the use of tromethamine (THAM) in neonates, we do not recommend its use for treatment of infants with PPHN.

G. **Hemodynamic support** (see Chap. 40). Optimal cardiac output is necessary to maximize tissue oxygenation and mixed venous oxygen content. A limitation of current neonatal practice is the deficit of universally available technologies to assess cardiac output and end-organ perfusion. Although noninvasive means of assessing cardiac output are under development, at present, these are not widely available. In the absence of direct measures of cardiac output, hemodynamic support of infants with PPHN is generally guided by the systemic blood pressure needed to override the elevated PVR and reduce or eliminate the right-to-left hemodynamic shunt. End-organ perfusion is assessed indirectly via acid–base balance (i.e., presence or absence of lactic acidosis). Because many infants with PPHN experience PVR that is at or near normal systemic blood pressure, we usually set initial treatment goals of gradually raising systemic blood pressure to levels of 50 to 70 mm Hg (systolic) and 45 to 55 mm Hg (mean) and assessing the hemodynamic shunt at each interval increase. As the infant improves and PVR falls, he or she will tolerate lower blood pressures without exhibiting a hemodynamic shunt; thus, ongoing reassessment of hemodynamic status and related revision of the treatment plan are essential components of the management of the infant with PPHN.

1. **Volume expansion.** Intravascular volume support can be an important adjunctive therapy for infants with PPHN accompanied by pathophysiologic conditions associated with intravascular volume depletion (e.g., hemorrhage, hydrops, capillary leak) or decreased SVR (e.g., septic shock) or systemic hypotension. Normal saline (0.9% NS 10 mL/kg over 20–30 minutes) is used most often; in the case of hemorrhage or excessive capillary leak, packed red blood cells are used in addition. In treating infants with evidence of marked capillary leak, we avoid the use of 5% albumin because, under these circumstances, albumin also leaks from capillaries and worsens interstitial edema.

2. **Pharmacologic treatment.** In the clinical setting of PPHN, cardiotonic agents, such as dobutamine and vasopressors such as dopamine and/or epinephrine, often are useful. When cardiac function is very poor and the infant is unresponsive to dobutamine, milrinone—an agent that both enhances cardiac output and lowers PVR—might prove useful.

   a. **Dobutamine**, a synthetic catecholamine with a chemical structure similar to that of isoproterenol, has an inotropic more than a chronotropic effect on the heart primarily via β1-adrenergic stimulation.

   b. **Dopamine** is often used in moderate (3–5 μg/kg/minute) to high (6–20 μg/kg/minute) doses for support of systemic blood pressure and improved cardiac output by means of α- and β-adrenergic receptor stimulation. Dopamine in low doses (1–2 μg/kg/minute) also offers the benefit of enhanced mesenteric and renal blood flow. Dopamine may increase PVR, through α-adrenergic effects, especially at higher infusion rates (>10 μg/kg/minute).

   c. **Epinephrine** (0.03–0.10 μg/kg/minute) stimulates both α- and β-adrenergic receptors; therefore, it is primarily useful in raising systemic blood pressure through enhanced cardiac output and marked peripheral vasoconstriction. Caution is advised in using epinephrine infusion because pulmonary α-adrenergic receptor stimulation might result in pulmonary vasoconstriction and elevated PVR and other end-organ perfusion (e.g., renal and mesenteric) might be reduced.

H. Correction of metabolic abnormalities. Biochemical abnormalities might contribute to right-to-left shunting by impairing cardiac function. Correction of hypoglycemia and hypocalcemia is important in treating infants with PPHN in order to provide adequate substrates for myocardial function and appropriate responses to inotropic agents (see Chaps. 24 and 25).

I. Correction of polycythemia. Hyperviscosity, associated with polycythemia, increases PVR and is associated with release of vasoactive substances through platelet activation. Partial exchange transfusion to reduce the hematocrit to 50% to 55% should be considered in the infant with PPHN whose central hematocrit exceeds 65% (see Chap. 46).

J. Additional pharmacologic agents. Pharmacologic therapy is directed at the simultaneous goals of optimizing cardiac output, enhancing systemic blood pressure, and reducing PVR. Consideration of associated and differential diagnoses and the known or hypothetical pathogenesis of the right-to-left hemodynamic shunt might prove helpful in selecting the best agent or combination of agents for a particular infant. At the present time, data are insufficient to support the use of other proposed medical therapies for PPHN, including sildenafil, adenosine, magnesium sulfate, calcium channel blockers, inhaled prostacyclin, inhaled ethyl nitrite, and inhaled or intravenous tolazoline.

K. Treatment controversies. There is substantial interinstitutional variation in approaches to diagnosis and management of PPHN. A few centers have reported successful treatment of PPHN without the use of mechanical ventilation, iNO, or ECMO.

VI. POSTNEONATAL OUTCOMES AMONG INFANTS WITH PPHN.
The combined availability of iNO and ECMO led to reductions in PPHN-associated mortality from 25%–50% to 10%–15%. Survivors of PPHN remain at risk for medical and neurodevelopmental sequelae. Controlled clinical trials suggest that the risk of morbid sequelae is not affected by specific PPHN treatment(s). Infants who develop PPHN are at approximately 20% risk of rehospitalization within 1 year of discharge, and have a 20% to 46% risk of audiologic, neurodevelopmental, or cognitive impairments.

Suggested Readings

Abman SH. Recent advances in the pathogenesis and treatment of persistent pulmonary hypertension of the newborn. *Neonatology* 2007;91(4):283–290.

Konduri GG, Kim UO. Advances in the diagnosis and management of persistent pulmonary hypertension of the newborn. *Pediatr Clin North Am* 2009;56(3):579–600.

Steinhorn RH. Neonatal pulmonary hypertension. *Pediatr Crit Care Med* 2010;11 (Suppl 2):S79–S84.

37 Pulmonary Hemorrhage
Kirsten A. Kienstra

I. DEFINITION. Pulmonary hemorrhage is defined on **pathologic** examination as the presence of erythrocytes in the alveoli and/or lung interstitium, with those infants surviving longer than 24 hours showing a predominance of interstitial hemorrhage. Confluent hemorrhage involving at least two lobes of the lung is termed *massive* pulmonary hemorrhage. There is less agreement regarding the **clinical** definition. Commonly, pulmonary hemorrhage is defined as the presence of hemorrhagic fluid in the trachea accompanied by respiratory decompensation requiring increased respiratory support or intubation within 60 minutes of the appearance of fluid.

II. PATHOPHYSIOLOGY. The precise mechanisms underlying pulmonary hemorrhage remain uncertain. Pulmonary hemorrhage likely results from heterogeneous conditions converging in a common final physiologic pathway.

A. Pulmonary hemorrhage is believed to result from hemorrhagic pulmonary edema rather than direct bleeding into the lung, based on studies of lung effluent demonstrating relatively low erythrocyte concentration compared to whole blood.

B. Acute left ventricular failure, caused by hypoxia and other conditions, may lead to increased pulmonary capillary pressure and injury to the capillary endothelium. This may result in increased transudation and leak into the interstitium, and ultimately, pulmonary airspace.

C. Factors that alter the integrity of the epithelial–endothelial barrier in the alveolus or that change the filtration pressure across these membranes may predispose infants to pulmonary hemorrhage.

D. Disorders of coagulation may worsen pulmonary hemorrhage, but are not thought to initiate the condition.

III. EPIDEMIOLOGY. Clinically apparent pulmonary hemorrhage occurs at a rate of 1 to 12 per 1,000 live births. Accurate incidence rates are difficult to ascertain as the clinical definition is not uniform and definitive diagnosis requires pathologic examination (which may be unavailable because the event was not fatal or permission for pathologic examination was not obtained). In high-risk groups such as premature and growth-restricted infants, the incidence increases to as many as 50 per 1,000 live births. In autopsy studies, pulmonary hemorrhage is much more prevalent. Some studies report hemorrhage in up to 68% of autopsied neonates, with severe pulmonary hemorrhage occurring in 19% of infants dying in the first week of life. In most cases, death occurred 2 to 4 days after birth.

This is the revision of a chapter in the previous edition written by Nancy A. Louis.

IV. PREDISPOSING FACTORS. Pulmonary hemorrhage has been linked to many predisposing factors and conditions, including respiratory distress syndrome (RDS), intrauterine growth restriction, intrauterine and intrapartum asphyxia, infection, congenital heart disease, oxygen toxicity, maternal blood aspiration, severe hypothermia, diffuse pulmonary emboli, and urea cycle defects accompanied by hyperammonemia. Risk factors include conditions predisposing the infant to increased left ventricular filling pressures, increased pulmonary blood flow, compromised pulmonary venous drainage, or poor cardiac contractility. The following factors have been linked to pulmonary hemorrhage:

A. **Patent ductus arteriosus (PDA).** The presence of a PDA is a significant risk factor for pulmonary hemorrhage. Increased pulmonary blood flow and compromised ventricular function accompany decreasing pulmonary vascular resistance, leading to pulmonary microvascular injury and hemorrhagic pulmonary edema.

B. **Exogenous surfactant.** Pulmonary hemorrhage appears to be a complication of surfactant therapy; however, the overall benefits of surfactant treatment outweigh the risks. A Cochrane meta-analysis of four studies using prophylactic protein-free synthetic surfactant showed an increased incidence of PDA and pulmonary hemorrhage compared to placebo-treated controls. A Cochrane meta-analysis of 11 surfactant trials using synthetic or animal-derived surfactants also demonstrated a significant increase in pulmonary hemorrhage. However, this finding was primarily the result of an increase in pulmonary hemorrhage in infants treated with prophylactic synthetic surfactant preparations. The risk of pulmonary hemorrhage was not increased in infants treated with natural or synthetic surfactant using a rescue strategy. The reported increase in pulmonary hemorrhage likely results from surfactant-associated changes in hemodynamics and lung compliance with left-to-right shunting across a PDA and an increase in pulmonary blood flow.

C. **Sepsis.** Overwhelming sepsis appears to increase the risk of pulmonary hemorrhage, likely the result of increased pulmonary capillary permeability, and potentially exacerbated by the associated thrombocytopenia and coagulopathy.

V. CLINICAL PRESENTATION. The clinical diagnosis of pulmonary hemorrhage is made when sudden cardiorespiratory decompensation occurs in the setting of hemorrhagic fluid in the upper respiratory tract. Only a small percentage of pulmonary hemorrhages observed at autopsy are evident clinically. This is most likely due to the difficulty in diagnosing hemorrhage confined to the interstitial space without spread to the airways. In the absence of hemorrhagic secretions, respiratory deterioration is usually attributed to other causes.

VI. EVALUATION

A. **History and physical examination.** A thorough history may help identify predisposing factors such as risks of infection or the presence of a PDA. On physical examination, infants with pulmonary hemorrhage have pink or red frothy fluid in the airway and signs of respiratory decompensation. Isolated bleeding, in the absence of respiratory deterioration, may result from erosion or ulceration in the upper airway and not represent pulmonary hemorrhage.

B. **Radiographic evaluation.** The clinical diagnosis of pulmonary hemorrhage may be facilitated by the radiographic changes that accompany it. Nonspecific changes on chest radiograph include diffuse fluffy infiltrates or opacification of one or both lungs with air bronchograms.

C. **Laboratory studies.** The laboratory evaluation reflects the cardiopulmonary compromise with associated metabolic or mixed acidosis, a drop in hematocrit, and sometimes evidence of coagulopathy. In most cases, the coagulopathy is probably a result of the hemorrhage rather than a precipitating factor.

VII. TREATMENT.
Because the underlying pathogenesis remains unclear, treatment remains supportive. The general approach involves clearing the airways of hemorrhagic fluid and restoring adequate ventilation.

A. **Provide positive end-expiratory pressure (PEEP).** The use of elevated PEEP of 6 to 8 cm of H_2O helps to decrease the efflux of interstitial fluid into the alveolar space.

B. **Restore hemodynamic stability.** Correct hemodynamic instability with volume resuscitation including packed red blood cell replacement, and consider the addition of vasoactive medications, as needed.

C. **Correct acidosis.** Restore both adequate ventilation and blood pressure to improve acidosis.

D. **Consider echocardiogram.** An echocardiographic evaluation may assist in the evaluation of ventricular function, the need for vasoactive medications, and the possible contribution of a PDA. Consider pharmacologic or surgical closure of the PDA if hemodynamically significant.

E. **Identify other predisposing factors.** Additional potential contributing factors such as sepsis and coagulopathy must be addressed.

F. **Strategy for ventilation.** It is uncertain whether using high-frequency ventilation to provide high mean airway pressure while limiting tidal volume excursions is more effective than conventional ventilation to minimize further interstitial and alveolar fluid accumulation.

G. **Role of surfactant therapy.** Surfactant therapy after pulmonary hemorrhage has been considered for continued treatment of primary surfactant deficiency in RDS, or for treatment of secondary surfactant deficiency resulting from hemorrhagic airway edema. Following pulmonary hemorrhage, hemoglobin, plasma proteins, and cell membrane lipids present in the airspace may inactivate surfactant. Exogenous surfactant replacement may reverse the inhibition, as demonstrated in the setting of meconium aspiration. A small retrospective case review revealed a decrease in the oxygenation index (OI) of infants treated with surfactant following pulmonary hemorrhage, although the OI remained elevated above the level prior to hemorrhage. Decreased lung compliance following a hemorrhage may prevent or attenuate further surfactant-associated changes in pulmonary perfusion that conferred an increased risk of pulmonary edema before the hemorrhage. The potential benefits of surfactant therapy in these cases require further investigation, and treatment should be decided on a case-by-case basis.

VIII. PROGNOSIS.
The prognosis is difficult to establish in part due to the difficulty in establishing a clinical diagnosis for this condition. Pulmonary hemorrhage was thought to be uniformly fatal before mechanical ventilation, although this was based on pathologic diagnosis and, therefore, excluded infants with milder hemorrhages who survived. A small retrospective case study of very low birth weight infants with pulmonary hemorrhage suggests that although mortality remains high, the occurrence of pulmonary hemorrhage does not significantly increase the risk of later pulmonary or neurodevelopmental disabilities among survivors.

38 Pulmonary Air Leak
Mohan Pammi

I. BACKGROUND

A. **Risk factors.** The primary risk factors for air leak are mechanical ventilation and lung disorders. Risk factors common in premature infants include respiratory distress syndrome (RDS), sepsis, and pneumonia. Surfactant therapy for RDS has markedly decreased the incidence of pneumothorax. Risk factors common in term infants are aspiration of meconium, blood, or amniotic fluid; pneumonia; and congenital malformations.

B. **Pathogenesis.** Air leak syndromes arise via a common mechanism. Transpulmonary pressures that exceed the tensile strength of the noncartilaginous terminal airways and alveolar saccules can damage the respiratory epithelium. Loss of epithelial integrity permits air to enter the interstitium, causing pulmonary interstitial emphysema. Persistent elevation in transpulmonary pressure facilitates the dissection of air toward the visceral pleura and/or the hilum via the peribronchial and perivascular spaces. In rare circumstances, air can enter the pulmonary veins and result in air embolism. Rupture of the pleural surface allows the adventitial air to decompress into the pleural space, causing pneumothorax. Following a path of least resistance, air can dissect from the hilum and into the mediastinum, resulting in pneumomediastinum, or into the pericardium, resulting in pneumopericardium. Air in the mediastinum can decompress into the pleural space, the fascial planes of the neck and skin (subcutaneous emphysema), or the retroperitoneum. In turn, retroperitoneal air can rupture into the peritoneum (pneumoperitoneum) or dissect into the scrotum or labial folds.

1. **Elevations in transpulmonary pressure.** The infant's first breaths may cause a negative inspiratory pressure up to 100 cm H_2O. Uneven ventilation due to atelectasis, surfactant deficiency, pulmonary hemorrhage, or retained fetal lung fluid can increase transpulmonary pressure. In turn, this leads to alveolar overdistention and rupture. Similarly, aspiration of blood, amniotic fluid, or meconium can facilitate alveolar overdistention by a ball valve mechanism.

2. **In the presence of pulmonary disease, positive pressure ventilation increases the risk of air leak.** The high airway pressure required to achieve adequate oxygenation and ventilation in infants with poor pulmonary compliance (e.g., pulmonary hypoplasia, RDS, inflammation, pulmonary edema) further increases this risk. Excessive transpulmonary pressures can occur when ventilator pressures are not decreased as pulmonary compliance improves. This situation sometimes occurs in infants with RDS who improve rapidly after surfactant treatment. Mechanically ventilated preterm infants who make expiratory efforts against ventilator breaths are also at increased risk for pneumothorax.

3. **Direct trauma to the airways can also cause air leak.** Laryngoscopes, endotracheal tubes, suction catheters, and malpositioned feeding tubes can damage the lining of the airways and provide a portal for air entry.

II. TYPES OF AIR LEAKS

A. Pneumothorax. Spontaneous pneumothorax occurs in 0.07% of otherwise healthy appearing neonates. One in 10 of these infants is symptomatic. The high inspiratory pressures and uneven ventilation that occur in the initial stages of lung inflation may contribute to this phenomenon. Pneumothorax is more common in newborns treated with mechanical ventilation for underlying pulmonary disease.

Clinical signs of pneumothorax range from insidious changes in vital signs to the complete cardiovascular collapse that frequently accompanies a tension pneumothorax. As intrathoracic pressure rises, there is decreased lung volume, mediastinal shift, compression of the large intrathoracic veins, and increased pulmonary vascular resistance. The net effect is an increase in central venous pressure, a decrease in preload, and, ultimately, diminished cardiac output. A pneumothorax must be considered in mechanically ventilated infants who develop unexplained alterations in hemodynamics, pulmonary compliance, or oxygenation and ventilation.

1. Diagnosis

   a. Physical examination

      i. Signs of respiratory distress include tachypnea, grunting, flaring, and retractions.

      ii. Cyanosis.

      iii. Chest asymmetry with expansion of the affected side.

      iv. Episodes of apnea and bradycardia.

      v. Shift in the point of maximum cardiac impulse.

      vi. Diminished or distant breath sounds on the affected side.

      vii. Abdominal distension from displacement of the diaphragm.

      viii. Alterations in vital signs. With smaller collections of extrapulmonary air, compensatory increases may occur in heart rate and blood pressure. As the amount of air in the pleural space increases, central venous pressure rises; and severe hypotension, bradycardia, apnea, hypoxia, and hypercapnia may occur.

   b. Arterial blood gases. Changes in arterial blood gas measurements are nonspecific and demonstrate a decreased PO_2 and increased PCO_2 (and decreased pH).

   c. Chest radiograph. Anteroposterior (AP) views may show a hyperlucent hemithorax, a separation of the visceral from the parietal pleura, flattening of the diaphragm, and mediastinal shift. Smaller collections of intrapleural air can be detected beneath the anterior chest wall by obtaining a cross-table lateral view; however, an AP view is needed to identify the affected side. The lateral decubitus view, with the side of suspected pneumothorax up, may be helpful in detecting a small pneumothorax and may help differentiate skin folds, congenital lobar emphysema, cystic adenomatoid malformations, and surface blebs that occasionally give the appearance of intrapleural air.

   d. Transillumination. A high-intensity fiberoptic light source may demonstrate a pneumothorax. This technique is less sensitive in infants with chest wall edema or severe pulmonary interstitial edema (PIE), in extremely small infants with thin chest walls, or in full-term infants with thick chest walls or dark skin. We often obtain a baseline transillumination in infants at high risk for air leak.

   e. Needle aspiration. In a rapidly deteriorating clinical situation, thoracentesis may confirm the diagnosis and be therapeutic (see II.A.2.b.).

2. Treatment

   a. Conservative therapy. Close observation may be adequate for infants who have no underlying lung disease or complicating therapy (such as mechanical ventilation), have no significant respiratory distress, and have no continuous air leak. The extrapulmonary air will usually resolve in 24 to 48 hours. Although some of these infants may require an increase in their ambient O_2 concentration, we do not routinely administer 100% oxygen.

   b. Needle aspiration. Thoracentesis with a "butterfly" needle or intravenous (IV) catheter with an inner needle can be used to treat a symptomatic pneumothorax. Needle aspiration may be curative in infants not receiving mechanical ventilation and is frequently a temporizing measure in mechanically ventilated infants. In infants with severe hemodynamic compromise, thoracentesis may be a life-saving procedure.

   i. Attach a 23-G or 25-G butterfly needle or 22-G or 24-G IV catheter to a 10- to 20-mL syringe previously fitted with a 3-way stopcock.

   ii. Identify the second or third intercostal space in the midclavicular line, and prepare the overlying skin with an antibacterial solution.

   iii. Insert the needle firmly into the intercostal space and pass it just above the top of the third rib. This will minimize the chance of lacerating an intercostal artery, as these vessels are located on the inferior surface of the ribs. As the needle is inserted, have an assistant apply continuous suction with the syringe. A rapid flow of air into the syringe occurs when the needle enters the pleural space. Once the pleural space has been entered, stop advancing the needle. This will reduce the risk of puncturing the lung while the remaining air is evacuated.

   iv. A continuous air leak can be aspirated while a chest tube is being inserted (see II.A.2.c.). The "butterfly" needle can be left in place and if an IV catheter is used, the needle can be removed and the plastic catheter left in place for further aspiration. A short piece of IV extension tubing, for example, a "T" connector, attached to the IV catheter hub will allow flexibility during repeated aspirations. Otherwise, withdraw the needle after the air flow has ceased.

   c. Chest tube drainage. Chest tube drainage is generally needed to evacuate pneumothoraces that develop in infants receiving positive pressure ventilation. Frequently, these air leaks are continuous and will result in severe hemodynamic compromise if left untreated.

   i. Insertion of a chest tube

   a) Select a chest tube of the appropriate size; French size 10 (smaller) and 12 (larger) catheters are adequate for most infants.

   b) Prepare the chest area with an antiseptic solution. Infiltrate the subcutaneous tissues overlying the fourth to sixth rib at the midaxillary line with a 1% lidocaine solution. We administer an appropriate dose of narcotic for pain management.

   c) In the midaxillary line in the sixth intercostal space (ICS), parallel to the rib, make a small incision (1.0–1.5 cm) through the skin. Incisions of breast tissue should be avoided by locating the position of the nipple and surrounding tissue. An alternative site is in the anterior-superior portion of the chest wall; however, due to the possible complications of injury to the internal mammary artery and other regional vessels, we do not routinuely use this approach.

d) With a small curved hemostat, dissect the subcutaneous tissue overlying the rib. Make a subcutaneous track to the fourth ICS. Care should be taken to avoid the nipple area, the pectoralis muscle, and the axillary artery.

e) Enter the pleural space in the fourth ICS at the intersection of the nipple line just anterior to the midclavicular line with the closed hemostat. Guide the tip over the top of the rib to avoid trauma to the intercostal artery. Push the hemostat through the intercostal muscles and parietal pleura. Listen for a rush of air to indicate pleural penetration. Spread the tips to widen the opening and leave the hemostat in place. We rarely use trochars since the use of these instruments may increase the risk of lung perforation.

f) Grasp the end of the chest tube with the tips of the mosquito hemostat. The chest tube and the hemostat should be in a parallel orientation. Direct the chest tube through the skin incision, into the pleural opening, and between the opened tips. After the pleural space has been entered, direct the chest tube anteriorly and cephalad by rotating the curved points of the hemostat. Release the hemostat and advance the chest tube a few centimeters. Be certain that the side ports of the chest tube are in the pleural space.

g) The chest tube will "steam up" once it has been placed into the pleural space.

h) Direct the chest tube to the location of the pleural air. The anterior pleural space is generally most effective for infants in the supine position.

i) Palpate the chest wall around the entry site to confirm that the chest tube is not in the subcutaneous tissues.

j) Attach the chest tube to a Heimlich valve (for transport) or an underwater drainage system such as a Pleur-evac. Apply negative pressure (10–20 cm H_2O) to the underwater drainage system.

k) Using 3-0 or 4-0 silk, close the skin incision. We place a purse-string suture around the tube or a single interrupted suture on either side of the tube. Secure the chest tube by wrapping and then tying the skin suture tails around the tube. A second loop may be placed around the chest tube at a position 2 to 4 cm from the skin surface.

l) Cover the insertion site with petrolatum gauze and a small, clear, plastic, adhesive surgical dressing. We avoid extensive taping or large dressings, as they interfere with chest examination and may delay the discovery of a displaced chest tube.

m) AP and lateral chest radiographs are obtained to confirm tube position and ascertain drainage of the pleural air.

n) Radiographs may reveal chest tubes that are ineffective in evacuating extrapulmonary air. The most common cause of failure is tube placement in the posterior pleural space or the subcutaneous tissue. Other causes for ineffective drainage are tubes that perforate the lung, diaphragm, or mediastinum. Extrapulmonary air not in the pleural space, such as a pneumomediastinum or a subpleural pulmonary pseudocyst, will not be drained by a chest tube. Complications of chest tube insertion include hemorrhage, lung perforation, cardiac tamponade, and phrenic nerve injury.

ii. Insertion of a pigtail catheter

a) Pigtail catheters may be a less traumatic and faster way to relieve a pneumothorax and may be preferred to chest tube placement in premature infants.

b) Pigtail catheters 8 or 10 french gauge are inserted using a modified Seldinger technique. After locating and sterilizing the insertion site, an 18G needle or an 18G IV catheter is inserted into the pleural space. The guide wire is advanced through the catheter. The needle or the IV catheter is removed, keeping the guide wire in place and a dilator is advanced over the wire. The pigtail catheter is then inserted in the pleural space over the guide wire. The catheter is advanced until the curve of the catheter is inside the chest.

iii. Removal of a chest tube.
When the infant's lung disease has improved and the chest tube has not drained air for 24 to 48 hours, we discontinue suction and leave the tube under water seal. If radiographic examination shows no reaccumulation of extrapulmonary air in the next 12 to 24 hours, the chest tube is removed. A narcotic is given for pain control prior to the chest tube removal. To reduce the chance of introducing air into the pleural space, cover the chest wound with a small occlusive dressing while removing the tube. Remove the chest tube during expiration in spontaneously breathing infants and during inspiration in mechanically ventilated infants. A manual mechanical or bagged breath can insure removing the chest tube during the inspiratory phase.

d. Persistent pneumothorax refractory to routine measures. We often initiate high-frequency oscillatory ventilation (HFOV) to minimize mean airway pressure and resolve airleaks in mechanically ventilated infants. In patients with severe air leaks, oxygen supplementation is often increased so that mean airway pressure can be minimized. Interventional radiology may be needed to place catheters under ultrasound or fluoroscopic guidance to drain air collections that are inaccessible by standard techniques. Rare infants with refractory airleaks require extracorporeal membrane oxygenation (ECMO) (see Chap. 39).

3. Complications

a. Profound ventilatory and circulatory compromise can occur and, if untreated, result in death.

b. Intraventricular hemorrhage may result, possibly secondary to a combination of fluctuating cerebrovascular pressures, impaired venous return, hypercapnia, hypoxia, and acidosis.

c. Inappropriate antidiuretic hormone secretion may occur.

B. PIE occurs most often in mechanically ventilated, extremely preterm infants with RDS or sepsis. Interstitial air can be localized or can spread to involve significant portions of one or both lungs. Interstitial air can dissect toward the hilum and the pleural surface via the adventitial connective tissue surrounding the lymphatics and pulmonary vessels. This can compromise lymphatic drainage and pulmonary blood flow. PIE alters pulmonary mechanics by decreasing compliance, increasing residual volume and dead space, and enhancing ventilation/perfusion mismatch. Rupture of interstitial air into the pleural space and mediastinum can result in pneumothorax and pneumomediastinum, respectively.

1. **Diagnosis**
   a. PIE frequently develops in the first 48 hours after birth.
   b. PIE may be accompanied by hypotension, bradycardia, hypercarbia, hypoxia, and acidosis.
   c. PIE has two radiographic patterns: cystlike and linear. Linear lucencies radiate from the lung hilum. Occasionally, large cystlike blebs give the appearance of a pneumothorax.

2. **Treatment**
   a. If possible, attempt to decrease mean airway pressure by lowering peak inspiratory pressure, positive end-expiratory pressure (PEEP), and inspiratory time. We generally use HFOV in infants with PIE to avoid large swings in lung volume.
   b. Unilateral PIE may improve if the infant is positioned with the affected lung dependent.
   c. Endotracheal suctioning and manual positive pressure ventilation should be minimized.
   d. Severe localized PIE that has failed to improve with conservative management may require collapse of the affected lung by selective bronchial intubation or occlusion or, rarely, surgical resection.

3. **Complications.** PIE may precede more severe complications such as pneumothorax, pneumopericardium, or an air embolism.

C. **Pneumomediastinum.** Mediastinal air can develop when pulmonary interstitial air dissects into the mediastinum or when direct trauma occurs to the airways or the posterior pharynx.

1. **Diagnosis**
   a. **Physical examination.** Heart sounds may appear distant.
   b. **Chest radiograph.** Air collections are central and usually elevate or surround the thymus. This results in the characteristic "spinnaker sail" sign. A pneumomediastinum is best seen on a lateral view.

2. **Treatment**
   a. Pneumomediastinum is of little clinical importance, and specific drainage procedures are usually unnecessary.
   b. Rarely, cardiorespiratory compromise may develop if the air is under tension and does not decompress into the pleural space, the retroperitoneum, or the soft tissues of the neck. This situation may require mediastinostomy drainage. If the infant is mechanically ventilated, reduce mean airway pressure, if possible.

3. **Complications.** Pneumomediastinum may be associated with other air leaks.

D. **Pneumopericardium** is the least common form of air leak in newborns but the most common cause of cardiac tamponade. Asymptomatic pneumopericardium is occasionally detected as an incidental finding on a chest radiograph. Most cases occur in preterm infants with RDS treated with mechanical ventilation, preceded by PIE and pneumomediastinum. The mortality rate for critically ill infants who develop pneumopericardium is 70% to 80%.

1. **Diagnosis.** Pneumopericardium should be considered in mechanically ventilated newborn infants who develop acute or subacute hemodynamic compromise.
   a. **Physical examination.** Although infants may initially have tachycardia and decreased pulse pressure, hypotension, bradycardia, and cyanosis may ensue

rapidly. Auscultation reveals muffled or distant heart sounds. A pericardial knock (Hamman sign) or a characteristic mill wheel–like murmur (bruit de moulin) may be present.

b. Chest radiograph. Anteroposterior views show air surrounding the heart. Air under the inferior surface of the heart is diagnostic.

c. Transillumination. A high-intensity fiberoptic light source may illuminate the substernal region. Flickering of the light with the heart rate may help differentiate pneumopericardium from pneumomediastinum or a medial pneumothorax.

d. Electrocardiogram (ECG). Decreased voltages, manifest by a shrinking QRS complex, are consistent with pneumopericardium.

2. Treatment. We frequently consult cardiology for infants who require intervention.

a. Conservative management. Asymptomatic infants not receiving positive pressure ventilation can be managed expectantly. Vital signs are closely monitored (especially changes in pulse pressure). Frequent chest radiographs are obtained until the pneumopericardium resolves.

b. Needle aspiration. Cardiac tamponade is a life-threatening event that requires immediate pericardiocentesis.

   i. Prepare the subxiphoid area with antiseptic solution.

   ii. Attach a 20G to 22G IV catheter with an inner needle to a short piece of IV extension tubing that, in turn, is connected to a 3-way stopcock and a 20-mL syringe.

   iii. In the subxiphoid space, insert the catheter at a 30 to 45 degree angle and toward the infant's left shoulder.

   iv. Have an assistant aspirate with the syringe as the catheter is advanced.

   v. Once air is aspirated, stop advancing the catheter.

   vi. Slide the plastic catheter over the needle and into the pericardial space.

   vii. Remove the needle, reattach the IV tubing to the hub of the plastic catheter, evacuate the remaining air, and withdraw the catheter.

   viii. If air leak persists, prepare for pericardial tube placement.

   ix. If blood is aspirated, immediately withdraw the catheter to avoid lacerating the ventricular wall.

   x. The complications of pericardiocentesis include hemopericardium and laceration of the right ventricle or left anterior descending coronary artery.

c. Continuous pericardial drainage. Pneumopericardium often progresses to cardiac tamponade and may recur. A pericardial tube may be needed for continuous drainage. We manage the pericardial tube like a chest tube, although less negative pressure (5–10 cm H_2O) is used for suction.

3. Complications. Ventilated infants who have a pneumopericardium drained by needle aspiration frequently (80%) have a recurrence. Recurrent pneumopericardium can occur days after apparent resolution of the initial event.

E. Other types of air leaks

1. Pneumoperitoneum. Intraperitoneal air may result from extrapulmonary air that decompresses into the abdominal cavity. Usually, the pneumoperitoneum is of little clinical importance, but it must be differentiated from intraperitoneal air resulting from a perforated viscus. Rarely, pneumoperitoneum can impair diaphragmatic excursion and compromise ventilation. In these cases, continuous drainage may be necessary.

2. **Subcutaneous emphysema.** Subcutaneous air can be detected by palpation of crepitus in the face, neck, or supraclavicular region. Large collections of air in the neck, although usually of no clinical significance, can partially occlude or obstruct the compressible, cartilaginous trachea of the premature infant.

3. **Systemic air embolism.** An air embolism is a rare but usually fatal complication of pulmonary air leak. Air may enter the vasculature either by disruption of the pulmonary venous system or by inadvertent injection through an intravascular catheter. The presence of air bubbles in blood withdrawn from an umbilical artery catheter can be diagnostic.

Suggested Reading

Cates LA. Pigtail catheters used in the treatment of pneumothoraces in the neonate. *Adv Neonatal Care* 2009;9:7–16.

39 Extracorporeal Membrane Oxygenation

Gerhard K. Wolf and John H. Arnold

I. BACKGROUND. Extracorporeal membrane oxygenation (ECMO) is a technique of life support for neonates in cardiac or respiratory failure not responding to conventional therapy.

ECMO has been offered to >23,000 neonates worldwide to date (see Tables 39.1 and 39.2). The use of ECMO for neonatal respiratory failure has been declining since the early 1990s, whereas the use of ECMO for cardiac failure is increasing. This trend is associated with improved ventilator management and the institution of surfactant and inhaled nitric oxide for neonatal respiratory failure.

II. INDICATIONS AND CONTRAINDICATIONS

A. Respiratory failure. The indications for neonatal ECMO are (i) reversible respiratory failure and (ii) a predicted mortality with conventional therapy great enough to warrant the risks of ECMO. ECMO is also considered in patients with life-threatening air leaks not manageable with optimal ventilatory support and chest drainage. **Oxygenation index (OI)** is a measure of the severity of respiratory failure and is calculated as OI = mean airway pressure (MAP) × FiO_2/ PaO_2 × 100. It is essential to document OIs from serial blood gases over time, as the OI may vary. ECMO indications vary among different centers. Commonly used criteria include two OIs of >40 within 1 hour, one OI of 60 on high frequency ventilation, or one OI of 40 combined with cardiovascular instability. An OI of 20 should prompt an early outreach to an ECMO center for potential transfer.

B. Cardiac failure. ECMO provides biventricular support for neonates with cardiac failure. ECMO for congenital heart defects (hypoplastic left heart syndrome, coarctation of the aorta, pulmonary atresia, total anomalous pulmonary venous return [TAPVR]) is offered as a bridge to definitive treatment until the neonate's condition has stabilized. Other cardiac indications are failure to wean from cardiopulmonary bypass, cardiomyopathy, and pulmonary hypertension. In any neonate with respiratory failure, hypoxia, and bilateral opacities on chest radiograph, TAPVR should be excluded prior to initiating ECMO support. Once venoarterial (VA) ECMO support is initiated, pulmonary blood flow is reduced and the diagnosis of TAPVR may be difficult to make using echocardiography alone; those patients may require cardiac catheterization on ECMO to demonstrate presence or absence of pulmonary veins entering the left atrium.

C. Rapid-response ECMO (ECMO-cardiopulmonary resuscitation [E-CPR]). In the setting of a witnessed cardiorespiratory arrest, ECMO can be offered in centers with a rapid response team. Response times from the arrest to cannulation are ideally 15 to 30 minutes. A readily "clear-primed circuit" (an ECMO circuit

Table 39.1	Overall Outcomes for Neonatal ECMO by Indication, Extracorporeal Life Support Organization (ELSO) 2010		
Neonatal	Total patients	Survived ECLS	Survival to discharge or transfer
Respiratory	23,558	19,964 (85%)	17,720 (75%)
Cardiac	3,909	2,338 (60%)	1,515 (39%)
E-CPR	537	340 (63%)	203 (38%)

CPR = cardiopulmonary resuscitation; ECLS = extracorporeal life support; ECMO = extracorporeal membrane oxygenation.
ECLS, January 2010, Published by the Extracorporeal Life Support Organization, Ann Arbor, Michigan. "Total Patients" refers to all neonatal ECMO therapies reported in the ELSO registry. "E-CPR" refers to neonatal patients placed emergently on ECMO during cardiopulmonary resuscitation.

primed with normal saline rather than with blood products) and an ECMO team must be available 24 hours per day in order to offer E-CPR. Effective CPR before cannulation is essential for a favorable outcome during rapid-response ECMO.

D. *Ex utero* intrapartum treatment (EXIT) to ECMO procedure. The vessels are cannulated during a cesarean section while the neonate remains on placental

Table 39.2	Neonatal Respiratory Runs by Diagnosis, Extracorporeal Life Support Organization (ELSO) 2010	
Neonatal categories	Total runs	Percentage survived
MAS	7,584	94
CDH	5,929	51
PPHN/PFC	3,870	78
Sepsis	2,617	75
RDS	1,484	84
Pneumonia	327	57
Air leak syndrome	117	74
Other	1,939	63

MAS = meconium aspiration syndrome; CDH = congenital diaphragmatic hernia; PPHN = persistent pulmonary hypertension of the newborn; PFC = persistent fetal circulation; RDS = respiratory distress syndrome.

support. Indications include severe congenital diaphragmatic hernia, lung tumors, and airway-obstructing lesions, such as large neck masses and mediastinal tumors.

E. **Contraindications.** ECMO should only be offered for reversible conditions. Absolute contraindications are considered to be irreversible brain damage, significant intraventricular or intraparenchymal hemorrhage, weight <1,500 g, gestational age <34 weeks, lethal congenital abnormality, severe coagulopathy, progressive chronic lung disease, and continuous CPR for more than an hour before ECMO support.

III. PHYSIOLOGY

A. **Flow.** Venous drainage is always passive from the patient to the ECMO circuit. The cessation of venous drainage (hypovolemia, cardiac tamponade, pneumothorax) causes an automatic shutdown of the circuit, as any negative pressure could introduce air into the circuit. Flow is determined by venous return and by the ECMO pump.

B. **VA ECMO** supports the cardiac and the respiratory system, and is indicated for primary cardiac failure or respiratory failure combined with secondary cardiac failure. In VA ECMO, the blood is drained from a vein (internal jugular vein, femoral vein) and returned into the arterial system (internal carotid artery). The patient's total cardiac output (CO) is the sum of the native CO and the pump flow generated by the circuit: $CO_{total} = CO_{native} + CO_{circuit}$

C. **Venovenous (VV) ECMO.** VV ECMO supports only the respiratory system and is indicated for isolated respiratory failure. VV ECMO can also be considered in respiratory failure with hemodynamic instability, when hypotension and cardiovascular instability are thought to be caused by hypoxemia alone, as VV ECMO usually leads to rapid reversal of hypoxia and acidosis. VV ECMO spares accessing the carotid artery. In VV ECMO, the blood is drained as well as returned to the jugular vein through a double-lumen cannula. Some of the blood is immediately recirculated into the ECMO circuit. The rest of the oxygenated blood goes to the right side of the heart, into the pulmonary vascular bed, into the left side of the heart, and into the systemic circulation. As a requirement for VV ECMO, the internal jugular vein has to be large enough for a 14-French double-lumen cannula. Converting to VA ECMO is considered in the presence of additional hypotension, cardiac failure, or metabolic acidosis. Technical difficulties related to large recirculation in the venous cannula can also lead to the need to convert to VA ECMO. In our institution, the carotid artery is already identified at the time of VV cannulation. For conversion to VA ECMO, the venous cannula is left in place and an additional arterial cannula is inserted into the internal carotid artery.

D. **Oxygen delivery** is the product of CO and arterial oxygen content. During ECMO, many factors contribute to oxygen delivery. Arterial oxygen content is determined by the gas exchange in the membrane oxygenator and the gas exchange from the neonate's lung. CO is only altered during VA ECMO and is determined by the ECMO flow and the infant's native CO.

E. **Carbon dioxide removal.** Carbon dioxide (CO_2) removal is achieved by the membrane of the ECMO circuit and the patient's lung. The amount of CO_2 removed is dependent on the $PaCO_2$ of blood circulating through the membrane, the surface area of the membrane, and the gas flow through the membrane lung ("sweep gas flow"). As physiologic pulmonary function and tidal volume improve, the $PaCO_2$ decreases further and ECMO settings have to be adjusted. CO_2 removal is extremely efficient during ECMO, to the point that additional CO_2 has to be added into the circuit in order to prevent hypocarbia and respiratory alkalosis.

F. Cerebral perfusion. Cerebral perfusion during shock is rapidly restored after initiation of VA ECMO. On the other hand, cerebral venous drainage and arterial perfusion to the brain are impaired by large bore venous cannulas during ECMO. Collateral circulation to the brain during VA ECMO in neonates is maintained through the circle of Willis. The carotid artery is frequently ligated after decannulation from ECMO, although reconstruction of the carotid artery has been successfully performed. Impairments to arterial reconstructions are an intimal flap, arterial thrombosis, infections, or excessive tension on attempt of reconstruction. In our institution, the carotid artery was successfully reconstructed in 25% of patients. It is unclear whether carotid arterial reconstruction improves neurologic outcome.

G. Renal perfusion. During VA ECMO, the arterial pulse-pressure wave may become dampened as the roller pump contributes significantly to the patient's CO. Animal models suggest that renal perfusion is not different during VA compared to VV ECMO. Unclamping the bridge during VA ECMO directs the flow away from the patient and may be associated with a decrease in blood pressure and renal perfusion.

IV. MANAGEMENT

A. Pre-ECMO. In preparation for cannulation, the following should be available: central venous access to the patient, postductal arterial catheter, cross-matched blood in the blood bank, complete blood count, coagulation profile, and head ultrasonographic examination. An echocardiogram should be done before ECMO in order to rule out structural cardiac abnormalities. During VA ECMO, it may be difficult to quantify pulmonary hypertension or identify certain congenital lesions, such as total anomalous venous return, as the right atrium is decompressed and blood flow through the lung is decreased. Platelets should be transfused for a platelet count <100,000/mL.

B. Membrane. The appropriate membrane for a neonate is either a 0.8 m^2 or 1.5 m^2 silicone membrane oxygenator or a 0.8 m^2 Quadrox-i D hollow-fiber pediatric oxygenator. The resulting total volume of a neonatal ECMO circuit is 600 mL.

C. Saline priming. Patients who are placed on ECMO emergently can be started on a saline-primed circuit. Instead of blood products, the circuit is primed with normal saline. In centers with rapid-response ECMO, a saline-primed, sterile circuit is always available, minimizing the time to initiate ECMO therapy. The neonate's own blood volume is initially diluted with the normal saline from the ECMO circuit. This causes a drop in hematocrit and a transient decrease in oxygen carrying capacity. The hematocrit is later restored by using ultrafiltration and transfusing packed red blood cells (PRBCs).

D. Blood priming. Patients who are placed on ECMO non-emergently are started on a blood-primed circuit. Orders for the initial prime of a neonatal circuit are as follows: 500 mL of PRBC (cytomegalovirus [CMV] negative, <7 days old), 200 mL of fresh frozen plasma, 2 units of cryoprecipitate, and 2 units of platelets (not concentrated). Heparin and THAM (Tris-hydroxymethyl-aminomethane, also "Tris") buffer and calcium gluconate are added to the circuit. Once the circuit is fully primed with blood, the following labs (with target ranges in parentheses) are obtained prior to connecting the patient to the ECMO circuit: pH (7.35–7.45), PCO_2 (35–45 mm Hg), PO_2 (>300 mm Hg), HCO_3 (22–24 mEq/L). Na^+ (>125 mEq/L), K^+ (<8 mEq/L), ionized Ca^{++} (>0.8 mEq/L). ACT target: (>400 seconds). This lab sample should be marked clearly, indicating that the results are from the ECMO circuit prior to connection with the patient. Hyperkalemia of the circuit is treated with calcium and bicarbonate.

E. **Cannulation.** The ECMO cannulation is performed by cardiac or pediatric surgeons at the bedside, in the cardiac catheterization laboratory, or in the operating room. A surgical cutdown approach is preferred over transcutaneous cannulation. The neonate is anesthetized and paralyzed with fentanyl, midazolam, and pancuronium. Heparin 30 units/kg is administered 3 minutes before cannulation. The following cannula sizes can be used: 8 to 14 Fr for the venous side, 8 to 10 Fr for the arterial side. The vein is cannulated first. The catheter is introduced approximately 6.5 cm to the right atrium and sutured in place. In VA ECMO, the artery is cannulated in a similar manner. In full-term neonates, the arterial cannula is introduced 3.5 cm into the aortic arch. Once the patient is on ECMO, 2 units of platelets and 2 units of cryoprecipitate are administered. On initiation of ECMO, vasopressors can be rapidly weaned. The neonate may become markedly hypertensive on initiation of ECMO therapy. As hypertension in the setting of pre-ECMO acidosis and anticoagulation during ECMO is a significant risk factor for intracerebral hemorrhage, any significant hypertension has to be anticipated and treated without delay. Hydralazine 0.1 to 0.4 mg/kg/dose can be administered to treat hypertension.

F. **ECMO therapy.** ECMO pump flow rate is generally 100 to 120 mL/kg/min in neonates. Sweep gas flow rate is 1 to 2.5 L/minute for a 0.8 m^2 and 1 to 4.5 L/min for 1.5 m^2 membrane. A safety check is conducted every 4 hours. This safety check includes searching for blood clots and circuit inspection for leaks. Normothermia is maintained and temperature is regulated by adjustments in the heat exchanger water temperature. Laboratory studies are suggested to be sent at the following schedule: (i) activated clotting time hourly; (ii) lactate levels twice daily; (iii) complete blood count, platelets, whole blood electrolytes, ionized calcium, and creatinine twice daily; (iv) antithrombin III twice daily, and, prior to FFP administration and 3 hours post FFP administration; (v) liver function tests, alkaline phosphatase, LDH, bilirubin, albumin, prealbumin, and total protein every week.

G. **Blood gas monitoring.** Arterial blood gas targets are PaO_2 greater than 60 mm Hg and $PaCO_2$ 40 to 45 mm Hg. If PaO_2 is less than 60 mm Hg, the sweep gas to the ECMO membrane can be increased. If the fraction of delivered oxygen (FDO_2) is already maximized at 1.0, increasing the ECMO pump flow rate or increasing the patient's hematocrit may be helpful to increase oxygen delivery. On VV ECMO, it may be necessary to increase the ventilator settings to assist with oxygenation and ventilation.

H. **Anticoagulation.** Heparin is used in all patients to prevent clot formation. The whole blood activated clotting time (ACT) is used to monitor heparin infusion and avoid hemorrhagic complications. ACT is kept at 180 to 200 seconds. Antithrombin III (AT III) levels may decrease during ECMO, and decreased AT III levels may result in heparin resistance and clotting of the ECMO circuit. Since the interpretation of AT III levels can be difficult during ECMO, some centers administer daily infusions of fresh frozen plasma to supplement AT III. Heparin-induced thrombocytopenia (HIT) has been described in children on ECMO support. If HIT is confirmed, Argatroban, a synthetic direct thrombin inhibitor, can be used as an alternative anticoagulant.

I. Blood products. Prothrombin time is maintained at <17 seconds using fresh frozen plasma, fibrinogen is kept above 150 mg/dL using cryoprecipitate, and the platelet count is maintained above 100,000 using concentrated platelets. The hematocrit is kept above 35% to facilitate oxygen delivery.

J. Amicar®. ε-Aminocaproic acid lowers the incidence of hemorrhagic complications associated with ECMO, including intracranial and postoperative hemorrhage. Negative effects are increased clot formation in the circuit. Patients who are considered to be at high risk for bleeding complications are given Amicar®. They include infants who (i) are <37 weeks' gestational age, (ii) have sepsis, (iii) have prolonged hypoxia or acidosis (pH 7.1) before ECMO, or (iv) have grade I or II intraventricular hemorrhage. A loading dose of Amicar® (100 mg/kg) is given followed by a 30 mg/kg/hour infusion. After 72 hours of Amicar®, the patient is assessed for further risks of bleeding complications. If these risks still exist, Amicar® is continued and the circuit is changed at 120 hours. Otherwise, the Amicar® infusion is discontinued.

K. Antibiotics. Broad-spectrum antibiotics are routinely administered to lower the risk of infection while on ECMO therapy.

L. Analgesia and sedation. Patients are sedated with an opioid–benzodiazepine combination. Drugs of choice are morphine, 0.05 mg/kg/hour, and lorazepam, 0.05 to 0.1 mg/kg/dose every 4 to 6 hours. Note that fentanyl is absorbed in large quantities by the ECMO membrane, leading to suboptimal analgesia. Fentanyl can be used during ECMO cannulation, but should not be used during ECMO.

M. Fluids and nutrition. Nutrition is administered through the parenteral route. Gastric feeding during ECMO is avoided, as it may increase the risk of necrotizing enterocolitis. Lipid administration should not exceed 1 g/kg/day to prevent lipid accumulation and embolism in the circuit. Lipids should be administered directly to the patient and not to the circuit. Dextrose and amino acid solution (parenteral nutrition) can be administered through the circuit.

N. Ultrafiltration. An ultrafilter is placed in line with the ECMO circuit. The goal is to normalize fluid balance in patients who have excessive positive fluid balance. Indications are urine output of <0.5 mL/kg/hour, positive fluid balance >500 mL/24 hours and failed diuretic therapy.

O. Neurologic assessment. Head ultrasonographic examinations are performed within 24 hours of cannulation and every other day while the patient is receiving ECMO support. Electroencephalograms are performed when seizure activity is suspected.

P. Ventilator strategy. The goal of the ventilator strategy on VA ECMO is to let the lung "rest," yet not to allow total lung collapse. Typical settings are peak inspiratory pressure (PIP) = 25 cm H_2O, positive end-expiratory pressure (PEEP) = 5 cm H_2O, rate = 10, inspiratory time 1 second, and FiO_2 = 0.4. With a patient on VA ECMO for pneumothorax and air leak, apneic oxygenation with FiO_2 = 1 should be considered starting at continuous positive airway pressure (CPAP) settings of 12 cm H_2O and decreasing until no further air leaks are present. On VV ECMO, ventilator settings may have to be adjusted to achieve adequate gas exchange, since the patient's own lungs contribute to a greater degree to oxygenation and ventilation compared to VA ECMO.

Endotracheal suctioning is performed every 4 hours. During ECMO, lung function is assessed as follows: (i) As lung function improves, CO_2 removal increases and oxygenation by the lung improves, resulting in better gas exchange. Sweep gases can be adjusted accordingly; (ii) chest radiographs show gradual resolution of pulmonary edema; (iii) as pulmonary edema resolves, lung mechanics improve and expired tidal volumes increase.

Q. **Conditioning and cycling.** "Conditioning" means challenging the patient by reducing the ECMO support to evaluate the gas exchange accomplished by the lungs. Sweep gas flow is reduced; FiO_2 is increased to 1 and the respiratory rate is increased to 25 per minute; the flow of the ECMO pump is weaned to 100 mL/minute in 50 mL increments; and serial arterial blood gases are obtained. If the postductal saturation falls below 95%, the ECMO settings are resumed. "Cycling" refers to transiently removing the patient from the ECMO circuit. In VA ECMO, the venous and arterial cannulae are clamped, the bridge is opened, and the ECMO blood flow "cycles" from the arterial to the venous side through the bridge, without perfusing the patient. In VV ECMO, the sweep gas flow is interrupted ("capped"), while the circuit continues to flow.

R. **Decannulation.** The patient's lung disease has to be improved enough to tolerate moderate ventilator settings. Our criteria for decannulation are as follows: PIP = 30 cm H_2O; PEEP = 5 cm H_2O; rate = 25 breaths/minute; and FiO_2 = 0.35; PaO_2 over 60 mm Hg; $PaCO_2$ = 40 to 50 mm Hg; pH <7.5. When these criteria are used, patients rarely require recannulation. At the time of decannulation from VA ECMO, we attempt to reconstruct the common carotid artery. The jugular vein is routinely ligated. Two units of concentrated platelets are given following decannulation.

Discontinuation of ECMO support is also considered in the following situations: when the disease process becomes irreversible, failure to wean successfully, neurologic events (devastating neurologic examination, significant intracranial hemorrhage), or multiorgan system failure.

V. SPECIAL SITUATIONS DURING ECMO SUPPORT

A. **ECMO-circuit change.** A change of the entire ECMO circuit is considered (i) if premembrane pressures exceed 350 mm Hg with no change in postmembrane pressure, or if the circuit is extensively thrombosed by visual inspection of the tubing; (ii) if CO_2 removal is impaired despite maximum sweep gas flow rate and the circuit is extensively clotted; (iii) if there is a gas-to-blood leak and the circuit is extensively clotted; and (iv) if there is extensive platelet consumption. A new ECMO circuit may help to correct a persistent coagulopathy or platelet consumption. If a circuit needs to be changed, a new circuit is primed, the patient is cycled off ECMO, the old circuit is cut away, and the new circuit is connected, with care being taken to keep air out of the system and to maintain strict sterile barriers.

B. **Lung biopsy.** Irreversible causes of respiratory failure, such as alveolar capillary dysplasia (ACD) or other forms of pulmonary hypoplasia, are usually not known prior to ECMO support. If pulmonary function does not improve after a prolonged period (usually 1 to 2 weeks of ECMO support), a lung biopsy can be performed through a thoracotomy. Lung biopsy during ECMO and anticoagulation carries a significant risk of hemorrhage and should be performed by an experienced pediatric surgical team.

C. **Left-sided heart failure and left atrial decompression.** If left ventricular contractility is severely impaired, arterial blood will not be ejected through the left ventricular outflow tract, leading to an increase in both left ventricular end-diastolic pressure and left atrial pressures. This may lead to significant pulmonary edema from left atrial hypertension, and to intravascular and intracardiac thrombosis secondary to stasis. In this circumstance, the left atrium may have to be decompressed ("vented") into the venous side of the ECMO circuit. This can either be achieved by creating an atrial septostomy in the cardiac catheterization lab or, if the patient is already cannulated through the open chest, by inserting a cannula directly into the left atrium.

VI. COMPLICATIONS

A. **Neurologic.** Sequelae resulting in neurologic damage often originate from acidosis and hypoxia before commencement of ECMO. According to the extracorporeal life support (ECLS) registry, intracranial hemorrhage occurred in 6.8% and infarction of the central nervous system (CNS) occurred in 7.7% of neonates during ECMO therapy for respiratory indications. Small intracranial hemorrhages are managed by optimizing clotting factors and by using Amicar®. Larger intracranial hemorrhages may force discontinuation of ECMO.

B. **Mechanical.** Poor venous return to the circuit causes the pump to shut down in order to avoid air entrainment. Causes for poor venous return from the patient to the ECMO circuit include hypovolemia, pneumothorax, or tamponade physiology. Mechanical reasons for poor venous return related to the ECMO circuit are poor catheter position, small venous catheter diameter, excessive catheter length, kinked tubing, and insufficient hydrostatic column length (height of patient above pump head). Initially, fluids are administered while other reasons for poor return are ruled out.

C. **Cardiovascular.** Hemodynamic instability during ECMO may be a result of hypovolemia, vasodilation during septic inflammatory response, arrhythmias, and pulmonary embolism. Volume overload, especially in the setting of capillary leak, may worsen chest wall compliance and further compromise gas exchange.

VII. OUTCOME

A. **Survival.** The ECLS database has reported the outcomes of ECMO therapies worldwide since 1985. A total of 23,558 ECMO runs (85% survival) for neonatal respiratory support were reported for neonatal respiratory disorders through January 2010 (Table 39.1). Survival rate for various indications are shown in Table 39.2. For cardiac ECMO in neonates, 3,909 cases were reported, with 39% surviving to hospital discharge. For E-CPR in neonates (total 537 cases), the survival to hospital discharge was 38% (Tables 39.1 and 39.2). Mortality at 7 years of age after completion of the UK-collaborative ECMO trial was 33% in the ECMO group and 59% in the conventional group (see Table 39.3).

Table 39.3	UK Neonatal ECMO Trial; Overall Status by 7 Years of Age		
Overall status by 7 yrs of age	ECMO (n = 93) (%)	Conventional (n = 92) (%)
Deaths	31 (33)	54 (59)
Lost to follow-up	6 (6)	4 (4)
Children with:		
Severe disability	3 (3)	0
Moderate disability	9 (10)	6 (7)
Mild disability	13 (14)	11 (12)
Children with:		
Impairment only	21 (23)	15 (16)
No abnormal signs or disability	10 (11)	2 (2)
Assessed survivors with no disability	31/56 (55)	17/34 (50)

ECMO = extracorporeal membrane oxygenation.
Follow-up after completion of the McNally H, Bennett CC, Elbourne D, et al.
United Kingdom collaborative randomized trial of neonatal extracorporeal membrane oxygenation: follow-up to age 7 years. *Pediatrics* 2006;117(5):e845–e854.

B. **Neurodevelopment.** Neurologic follow-up was assessed 7 years after completion of the UK-collaborative ECMO trial (Table 39.3). Both the ECMO and conventional therapy groups had problems and impaired neurologic outcome, but the ECMO group performed better in each task. Both groups had notable difficulties with learning and processing tasks. Progressive sensorineural hearing loss was observed in both groups. There was no difference in cognitive skills, 76% of the children in each group recorded a cognitive level within the normal range. Comparing the survivors in both groups, 55% in the ECMO group versus 50% in the conventional group survived without disabilities. This study suggests that the underlying disease is the major influence on morbidity, and that the beneficial effect of ECMO is still present after 7 years.

Suggested Readings

ELSO Guidelines. Available at: http://www.elso.med.umich.edu/Guidelines.html.

McNally H, Bennett CC, Elbourne D, et al. United Kingdom collaborative randomized trial of neonatal extracorporeal membrane oxygenation: follow-up to age 7 years. *Pediatrics* 2006;117(5):e845–e854.

Short BL, Williams L, eds. *ECMO Specialist Training Manual*, 3rd ed. Ann Arbor, MI: ELSO, 2009. Available at: http://www.elso.med.umich.edu/Publications.html.

Van Meurs K, Lally KP, Peek G, et al., eds. *ECMO: extracorporeal cardiopulmonary support in critical care*, 3rd ed. Ann Arbor, MI: ELSO, 2005. Available at: http://www.elso.med.umich.edu/Publications.html.

Shock

Pankaj B. Agrawal

I. DEFINITION. Shock is an acute, complex state of circulatory dysfunction resulting in insufficient oxygen and nutrient delivery to the tissues relative to their metabolic demand leading to cellular dysfunction that may eventually cause cell death. Initially, shock may be compensated with reduction in blood supply to the skin, muscle, and splanchnic vessels and adequate blood flow to the vital organs. This may be followed by an uncompensated phase when signs of poor perfusion are accompanied by hypotension. In premature neonates, extremely low systemic perfusion can occur with normal blood pressure (BP). Lowest acceptable normal BPs are not well established, particularly for premature infants. Recent studies indicate that a mean arterial pressure (MAP) <30 mm Hg in extremely low birth weight neonates is associated with reduced cerebral blood flow and lack of cerebral autoregulation, which, in turn, may lead to white matter injury and cerebral hemorrhage.

II. ETIOLOGY. In the immediate postnatal period, abnormal regulation of peripheral vascular resistance with or without myocardial dysfunction is the most frequent cause of hypotension underlying shock, especially in preterm infants. Hypovolemia must also be considered as an underlying cause of shock in the setting of fluid loss (blood, plasma, excessive urine output, or transepidermal water losses).

A. Distributive shock secondary to:

1. Abnormal peripheral vasoregulation in neonates secondary to:
   a. Increased or dysregulated endothelial nitric oxide (NO) production in the perinatal transitional period, particularly in the preterm neonate
   b. Immature neurovascular pathways
2. Sepsis-related with release of proinflammatory cascades that lead to vasodilation
3. Rare causes include anaphylactic and neurogenic shock in neonates

B. Hypovolemic shock. Common scenarios of fluid loss in the neonatal period include the following:

1. Placental hemorrhage, as in abruptio placentae or placenta previa
2. Fetal-to-maternal hemorrhage (diagnosed by the Kleihauer-Betke test of the mother's blood for fetal erythrocytes)
3. Twin-to-twin transfusion
4. Intracranial hemorrhage
5. Massive pulmonary hemorrhage (often associated with patent ductus arteriosus [PDA])
6. Disseminated intravascular coagulation (DIC) or other severe coagulopathies

7. Plasma loss into the extravascular compartment, as seen with low oncotic pressure states or capillary leak syndrome (e.g., sepsis)

8. Excessive extracellular fluid losses, as seen with volume depletion from excess insensible water loss or inappropriate diuresis, as commonly seen in extremely low birth weight infants

C. **Cardiogenic shock due to myocardial dysfunction.** Although an infant's myocardium usually exhibits good contractility, various perinatal insults, congenital abnormalities, or arrhythmias can result in heart failure.

1. Intrapartum asphyxia can cause poor contractility and papillary muscle dysfunction with tricuspid regurgitation, resulting in low cardiac output.

2. Myocardial dysfunction can occur secondary to infectious agents (bacterial or viral) or metabolic abnormalities such as hypoglycemia. Cardiomyopathy can be seen in infants of diabetic mothers (IDMs) with or without hypoglycemia.

D. **Obstructive shock.** Obstruction to blood flow resulting in decreased cardiac output. Types of obstructions to blood flow include:

1. Inflow obstructions
   a. Cardiac anomalies including total anomalous pulmonary venous return, cor triatriatum, tricuspid atresia, and mitral atresia
   b. Acquired inflow obstructions can occur from intravascular air or thrombotic embolus, or from increased intrathoracic pressure caused by high airway pressures, pneumothorax, pneumomediastinum, or pneumopericardium.

2. Outflow obstructions
   a. Cardiac anomalies including pulmonary stenosis or atresia, aortic stenosis or atresia, and coarctation of the aorta or interrupted aortic arch
   b. Hypertrophic subaortic stenosis seen in IDMs with compromised left ventricular outflow
   c. Arrhythmias, if prolonged

III. DIAGNOSIS

A. **Clinical presentation.** Clinical presentation is based on the compensatory mechanisms that are activated to maintain oxygen delivery to tissues. The shock is initially compensated when clinical findings are consistent with inadequate tissue perfusion but systolic BP is within normal range. Clinical findings during compensated shock include tachycardia to maintain cardiac output; increased systemic vascular resistance (SVR) presenting as cold, pale skin, delayed capillary refill, and weak peripheral pulses with narrow pulse pressure (raised diastolic BP); and increased splanchnic vascular resistance manifesting as oliguria and ileus.

The physiologic response of increased SVR is altered in septic shock with release of inflammatory mediators causing vasodilation and increased capillary permeability. In such cases, hypotension and wide pulse pressure are early indicators of shock.

When inadequate tissue perfusion is associated with systolic hypotension, the infant is noted to be in hypotensive shock. This indicates that physiologic attempts to maintain systolic BP and perfusion are no longer effective, and this may signal irreversible organ injury or impending cardiac arrest. As brain perfusion declines, the infant becomes lethargic. In preterm infants, the associated decrease in brain blood flow and oxygen supply during hypotension predisposes to intraventricular/cerebral hemorrhages and periventricular leukomalacia with long-term neurodevelopmental abnormalities. In addition, in extremely low birth weight infants, the vasculature of the cerebral cortex may respond to transient myocardial dysfunction/shock with vasoconstriction rather than vasodilation, further diminishing cerebral perfusion and increasing the risk of neurologic injury.

IV. INVESTIGATIONS

Measurement of **central venous pressure** (CVP) may help management, especially in term or late preterm infants. CVP is measured using a catheter with its tip in the right atrium or in the intrathoracic superior vena cava. The catheter can be placed through the umbilical vein or percutaneously through the external or internal jugular or subclavian vein. In many infants, maintaining CVP at 5 to 8 mm Hg with volume infusions is associated with improved cardiac output. If CVP exceeds 5 to 8 mm Hg, additional volume will usually not be helpful. CVP is influenced by noncardiac factors such as ventilator pressures and by cardiac factors such as tricuspid valve function. Both factors may affect the interpretation and usefulness of CVP measurements.

Organ dysfunction occurs because of inadequate blood flow and oxygenation, and cellular metabolism becomes predominantly anaerobic, producing lactic and pyruvic acid. Hence, metabolic acidosis often indicates inadequate circulation. Serum lactate measurements can help predict the outcome, especially if done periodically.

Functional echocardiography provides objective assessment of cardiac function and helps assess response to therapeutic interventions. Flow in the superior vena cava provides an excellent assessment of the blood flow to the upper body.

Near-infrared spectroscopy (NIRS) can be used to assess the peripheral perfusion and cerebral oxygenation. A strong inverse correlation was recently reported between serum lactate values and regional oxyHb saturation values measured at various sites (cerebral, splanchnic, and renal). NIRS can help detect low cardiac output states, although it is still predominantly used in the research settings.

V. TREATMENT.
Fluids, supportive therapy, inotropes, vasopressors, and hydrocortisone replacement are used to treat shock in the neonate.

A. **Fluid therapy.** The initial approach is usually to administer crystalloids such as normal saline. Small, randomized controlled trials support the usefulness of isotonic crystalloid rather than albumin-containing solutions for acute volume expansion as they are more readily available, have lower cost, and have lesser risk of infection-related complications. Importantly, albumin has not been shown to be more efficacious than saline in treating hypotension. An infusion of 10 to 20 mL/kg isotonic saline solution is used to treat suspected hypovolemia. Blood cell transfusions or fresh frozen plasma is recommended in cases of blood loss or DIC.

B. **Supportive treatment.** Correction of negative inotropic factors such as hypoxia, acidosis, hypoglycemia, and other metabolic derangements will improve cardiac output. In addition, hypocalcemia frequently occurs in infants with circulatory failure, especially if they have received large amounts of volume resuscitation. In this setting, calcium frequently produces a positive inotropic response. Calcium gluconate 10% (100 mg/kg) can be infused slowly if ionized calcium levels are low.

C. Medications

1. Inotropes

a. Sympathomimetic amines are commonly used in infants. The advantages include rapidity of onset, ability to control dosage, and ultrashort half-life.

    i. Dopamine is a naturally occurring catecholamine. Exogenous dopamine activates receptors in a dose-dependent manner. At low doses (0.5–2 mcg/kg/minute), dopamine stimulates peripheral dopamine receptors and increases renal, mesenteric, and coronary blood flow with little effect on cardiac output. In intermediate doses (5–9 mcg/kg/minute), dopamine has positive inotropic and chronotropic effects. The increase in myocardial contractility depends in part on myocardial norepinephrine stores.

    ii. Dobutamine is a synthetic catecholamine with relatively cardioselective inotropic effects. In doses of 5 to 15 mcg/kg per minute, dobutamine increases cardiac output with little effect on heart rate. Dobutamine can decrease SVR and is often used with dopamine to improve cardiac output in cases of decreased myocardial function as its inotropic effects, unlike those of dopamine, which are independent of norepinephrine stores. However, because hypotension is a result of decreased SVR in the majority of nonasphyxiated newborns, dopamine remains the first-line pressor therapy.

    iii. Epinephrine has potent inotropic and chronotropic effects in the 0.05 to 0.3 mcg/kg/minute doses. In these doses, it has greater β-2 adrenergic effects in the peripheral vasculature with little α-adrenergic effect leading to fall in SVR. It is not a first-line drug in newborns; however, it may be effective in patients who do not respond to dopamine. Epinephrine is an effective adjunct therapy to dopamine because cardiac norepinephrine stores are readily depleted with prolonged and high rate dopamine infusions.

b. Milrinone is a phosphodiesterase-III inhibitor that enhances intracellular cyclic adenosine monophosphate (cAMP) content preferentially in the myocardium leading to increase in cardiac contractility. It improves diastolic myocardial function more readily than dobutamine. Milrinone also lowers pulmonary vascular resistance (PVR) and SVR by increasing cAMP levels in vascular smooth muscle, often necessitating the use of volume and dopamine (see Appendix A for dosage).

2. Vasopressor therapy includes high-dose dopamine, high-dose epinephrine, norepinephrine, and vasopressin.

a. Dopamine in high doses (10–20 mcg/kg/minute) causes vasoconstriction by releasing norepinephrine from sympathetic vesicles as well as acting directly on α-adrenergic receptors. Neonates have reduced releasable stores of norepinephrine. Dopamine-resistant shock commonly responds to **norepinephrine** or high-dose **epinephrine**. Norepinephrine may be the preferred agent in shock associated with low SVR. It is recommended by many as the first-line agent in adults with fluid-refractory, hypotensive, hyperdynamic shock.

b. Vasopressin has been primarily studied in adults for the treatment of shock, although recent reports suggest a therapeutic efficacy in the treatment of shock associated with vasodilation in children. Vasopressin is a hormone that is not only primarily involved in the postnatal regulation of fluid homeostasis but also plays an important role in maintaining vascular tone in the setting of hemodynamic instability. Vasopressin deficiency may occur in catecholamine-resistant hypotension in the evolution of sepsis, and hence its reported efficacy in vasodilatory shock. Vasopressin is not routinely used to treat shock in the neonate but may be a therapeutic option to consider in the setting of abnormal peripheral vasoregulation. An added beneficial effect may be its inhibitory action on NO-induced increases in the second messenger cyclic guanosine monophosphate (cGMP), a potent vasodilatory signal that predominates in the setting of sepsis from the increased endotoxin/inflammation-induced NO synthesis (usual dose of vasopressin is 0.0002–0.006 mcg/kg/minute).

3. **Hydrocortisone replacement.** Corticosteroids may be useful in extremely premature infants with hypotension refractory to volume expansion and vasopressors. In a randomized, double-blind controlled study, stress-dose hydrocortisone was effective in treating refractory hypotension in very low birth weight (VLBW) infants. Hydrocortisone stabilizes BP through multiple mechanisms. It induces the expression of the cardiovascular adrenergic receptors that are downregulated by prolonged use of sympathomimetic agents and also inhibits catecholamine metabolism. After hydrocortisone administration, there is a rapid increase in intracellular calcium availability, resulting in enhanced responsiveness to adrenergic agents. The BP response is evident as early as 2 hours after hydrocortisone treatment. For refractory hypotension, hydrocortisone can be used at a dose of 1 mg/kg. If efficacy is noted, the dose can be repeated every 8 hours for 2 to 3 days, especially if low serum cortisol levels are documented before hydrocortisone treatment.

VI. TYPICAL CLINICAL SCENARIOS OF SHOCK IN THE NEONATE AND THEIR MANAGEMENT

A. **Very low birth weight (VLBW) neonate in the immediate postnatal period**

1. Physiology includes poor vasomotor tone, immature myocardium that is more sensitive to changes in afterload, and dysregulated NO production.

2. Recommended therapy is dopamine and judicious use of volume if hypovolemia is suspected. It is important not to give large volume infusions due to their association with increased risk of bronchopulmonary dysplasia and intraventricular hemorrhage reported in the premature infants. Hydrocortisone may be considered for dopamine-resistant hypotension.

B. **Perinatal depression in preterm or full-term neonate**

1. Physiology involves release of endogenous catecholamines leading to normal or increased SVR clinically manifested by pallor, mottled appearance, and poor perfusion and myocardial dysfunction. The baby is likely to be euvolemic and may have associated pulmonary hypertension.

2. Recommended therapy is dopamine with or without dobutamine up to 10 mcg/kg/minute. Milrinone can be considered to provide afterload reduction and inotropy effects without the risk of further myocardial injury due to excess catecholamine exposure. In cases with associated pulmonary hypertension, the use of inhaled NO is warranted for infants >34 weeks' gestation. Some infants may manifest vasodilatory shock and would benefit from increased doses of dopamine. The patient's skin color and perfusion on physical examination can be used to guide therapy.

C. Preterm neonate with PDA

1. Physiology includes ductal "steal" compromising vital organ perfusion and increase in left-to-right shunt with increased risk of pulmonary hemorrhage.

2. Recommended therapy includes avoiding high-dose dopamine (>10 mcg/kg/minute) as its use will further increase left-to-right shunting and reduce vital organ perfusion. Use dobutamine to enhance cardiac inotropy. Target ventilation management to increase PVR by increasing positive end-expiratory pressure (PEEP), maintaining permissive hypercarbia, and avoiding hyperoxygenation.

D. Septic shock

1. Physiology involves relative hypovolemia, myocardial dysfunction, peripheral vasodilation, and increased pulmonary pressures secondary to acidosis and hypoxia.

2. Therapy includes volume resuscitation with crystalloid (10–30 mL/kg), which should be repeated as needed, and administration of dopamine 5 to 20 mcg/kg/minute, with or without epinephrine 0.05 to 0.3 mcg/kg/minute. A cardiac echocardiogram can be obtained to evaluate cardiac function, superior vena cava flow, cardiac output, and intracardiac shunting. Consider extracorporeal membrane oxygenation (ECMO) in infants >34 weeks' gestation if they do not respond to these interventions.

E. Preterm neonates with "pressor-resistant" hypotension

1. A proportion of VLBW infants become dependent on medium to high doses of vasopressors (usually dopamine) beyond the first postnatal days. Etiologies include relative cortisol deficiency, adrenal insufficiency, and downregulation of adrenergic receptors.

2. Consider low-dose hydrocortisone (3 mg/kg/day for 2–5 days in three divided doses) after drawing serum cortisol level. Studies support the efficacy of hydrocortisone in raising BP within 2 hours of administration, yet the long-term neurologic effects of this treatment in the VLBW infant remain to be investigated. Due to a published report of possible increased incidence of intestinal perforation in infants who have been treated with indomethacin who are also treated with hydrocortisone, the concurrent use of these drugs cannot be recommended until larger trials are conducted.

Suggested Readings

Brierley J, Carcillo JA, Choong K, et al. Clinical practice parameters for hemodynamic support of pediatric and neonatal septic shock: 2007 update from the American College of Critical Care Medicine. *Crit Care Med* 2009;37(2):666–688.

Dempsey EM, Barrington KJ. Evaluation and treatment of hypotension in the preterm infant. *Clin Perinatol* 2009;36(1):75–85.

Munro MJ, Walker AM, Barfield CP. Hypotensive extremely low birth weight infants have reduced cerebral blood flow. *Pediatrics* 2004;114(6):1591–1596.

Seri I, Noori S. Diagnosis and treatment of neonatal hypotension outside the transitional period. *Early Hum Dev* 2005;81(5):405–411.

Short BL, Van Meurs K, Evans JR, et al. Summary proceedings from the cardiology group on cardiovascular instability in preterm infants. *Pediatrics* 2006;117(3 Pt 2):S34–S39.

41 Cardiac Disorders
Stephanie Burns Wechsler and Gil Wernovsky

I. INTRODUCTION. At the beginning of the 20th century, Dr. William Osler wrote in his textbook of medicine that congenital heart disease was of "limited clinical interest as in a large proportion of cases the anomaly is not compatible with life, and in others, nothing can be done to remedy the defect or even relieve the symptoms." In the years since 1938, when Dr. Robert Gross first successfully ligated a patent ductus arteriosus (PDA) in a 7-year-old girl at Children's Hospital, Boston (with a 17-day postoperative stay, 12 of which were for "general interest in the case"), the outlook for children with congenital heart disease has improved dramatically. This remarkable progress is due to synergistic advances in pediatric and fetal cardiology, cardiac surgery, neonatology, cardiac anesthesia, intensive care, and nursing.

In critical lesions, the ultimate prognosis for the patient depends in part on (i) a timely and accurate assessment of the structural anomaly and (ii) the evaluation and resuscitation of secondary organ damage. It is therefore crucial that pediatricians and neonatologists be able to rapidly evaluate and participate in the initial medical management of neonates with congenital heart disease. A multidisciplinary approach involving several subspecialty services is frequently required, especially because one-fifth of patients with severe congenital heart disease may be premature and/or weigh <2,500 g at birth. Although neonates (as a group) may have a slightly higher surgical mortality than term infants, the secondary effects of the unoperated lesion on the heart, lung, and brain may be quite severe. These secondary changes may include chronic congestive heart failure (CHF), failure to thrive, frequent infections, irreversible pulmonary vascular changes, delayed cognitive development, or focal neurologic deficits. For these reasons, at Children's Hospital in Boston, primary surgical correction is carried out early in life, often in the neonatal period. This chapter is intended as a practical guide for the initial evaluation and management, by pediatricians and neonatologists, of neonates and infants suspected of having congenital heart disease. For a detailed discussion of the individual lesions, the clinician should consult current textbooks of pediatric cardiology and cardiac surgery.

II. INCIDENCE AND SURVIVAL. The incidence of moderate to severe structural congenital heart disease in live born infants is 6 to 8 per 1,000 live births. This incidence has been relatively constant over the years and in different areas around the world. More recent higher incidence figures appear to be due to the inclusion of more trivial forms of congenital heart disease, such as tiny ventricular septal defects that are detected more frequently by highly sensitive echocardiography. Data from the New England Regional Infant Cardiac Program suggest that approximately 3 per 1,000 live births have heart disease that results in death or requires cardiac catheterization or surgery during the first year of life. Most of these infants with congenital heart disease are identified by the end of the neonatal period. The most common congenital heart lesions presenting in the first weeks of life are summarized in Table 41.1. Recent

Table 41.1	Top Five Diagnoses Presenting at Different Ages[a]
Diagnosis	**Percentage of patients**
Age on admission: 0–6 days (n = 537)	
D-Transposition of great arteries	19
Hypoplastic left ventricle	14
Tetralogy of Fallot	8
Coarctation of aorta	7
Ventricular septal defect	3
Others	49
Age on admission: 7–13 days (n = 195)	
Coarctation of aorta	16
Ventricular septal defect	14
Hypoplastic left ventricle	8
D-Transposition of great arteries	7
Tetralogy of Fallot	7
Others	48
Age on admission: 14–28 days (n = 177)	
Ventricular septal defect	16
Coarctation of aorta	12
Tetralogy of Fallot	7
D-Transposition of great arteries	7
Patent ductus arteriosus	5
Others	53

[a]Reprinted with permission from Flanagan MF, Yeager SB, Weindling SN. Cardiac disease. In: MacDonald MG, Mullett MD, Seshia MMK, eds. *Avery's Neonatology: Pathophysiology and Management of the Newborn.* 6th ed. Philadelphia, PA: Lippincott Williams & Wilkins, 2005.

advances in diagnostic imaging, cardiac surgery, and intensive care have reduced the operative risks for many complex lesions; the hospital mortality following all forms of neonatal cardiac surgery has significantly decreased in the past decade.

III. CLINICAL PRESENTATIONS OF CONGENITAL HEART DISEASE IN THE NEONATE.

The timing of presentation and accompanying symptomatology depends on (i) the nature and severity of the anatomic defect, (ii) the *in utero* effects (if any) of the structural lesion, and (iii) the alterations in cardiovascular physiology secondary to the effects of the transitional circulation: **closure of the ductus arteriosus** and the **fall in pulmonary vascular resistance**. This chapter focuses primarily on cardiovascular abnormalities with critical effects in the neonatal period.

In the first few weeks of life, many heterogeneous forms of heart disease present in a surprisingly limited number of ways (in no particular order nor mutually exclusive): (i) cyanosis; (ii) CHF (with the most extreme presentation being cardiovascular collapse or shock); (iii) an asymptomatic heart murmur; and (iv) arrhythmia. With increasing frequency, neonates with congenital heart disease have been diagnosed before delivery by fetal echocardiography and are therefore born with a presumptive diagnosis into an expectant team of physicians and nurses. In many neonates, however, congenital heart disease is not suspected until after birth. The clinician may be diverted away from a diagnosis of heart disease because of the report of a "normal" prenatal ultrasonography performed for screening purposes. Finally, the diagnosis of "heart disease" should never divert the clinician from a complete noncardiac evaluation with a thorough search for additional or secondary medical problems—occasionally, the neonate with complex congenital heart disease and hypoxemia has inadequate attention paid to an initial and continued assessment of an adequate airway and ventilation.

A. Cyanosis

1. **Clinical findings.** Cyanosis (bluish tinge of the skin and mucous membranes) is one of the most common presenting signs of congenital heart disease in the neonate. Although cyanosis usually indicates underlying hypoxemia (diminished level of arterial oxygen saturation), there are a few instances when cyanosis is associated with a normal arterial oxygen saturation. Depending on the underlying skin complexion, clinically apparent cyanosis is usually not visible until there is >3 g/dL of **desaturated** hemoglobin in the arterial system. Therefore, the degree of visible cyanosis depends on both the severity of hypoxemia (which determines the percentage of oxygen saturation), as well as the hemoglobin concentration. For example, consider two infants with similar degrees of hypoxemia—each having an arterial oxygen saturation of 85%. The polycythemic newborn (hemoglobin of 22 g/dL) will have 3.3 g/dL (15% of 22) desaturated hemoglobin and be more easily appreciated to be cyanotic than the anemic infant (hemoglobin of 10 g/dL) who will only have 1.5 g/dL (15% of 10) desaturated hemoglobin. An additional note, true central cyanosis should be a generalized finding (i.e., not acrocyanosis, blueness of the hands and feet only, which is a normal finding in a neonate).

Because determining cyanosis by visual inspection can be challenging for the reasons mentioned, there has been recent interest in adding routine lower extremity pulse oximetry measurement as a screening test for otherwise asymptomatic congenital heart disease. There is conflicting data on the efficacy and cost-effectiveness of this screening method, but it would appear that it is most effective when the pulse oximetry reading is done in a lower extremity in infants >24 hours old with further evaluation by echocardiogram for readings <95% in room air.

2. **Differential diagnosis.** Differentiation of cardiac from respiratory causes of cyanosis in the neonatal intensive care unit (NICU) is a common problem. Pulmonary disorders are frequently the cause of cyanosis in the newborn due to intrapulmonary right-to-left shunting. Primary lung disease (pneumonia, hyaline membrane disease, pulmonary arteriovenous malformations, etc.); pneumothorax; airway obstruction; extrinsic compression of the lungs (congenital diaphragmatic hernia, pleural effusions, etc.); and central nervous system abnormalities may produce varying degrees of hypoxemia manifesting as cyanosis in the neonate. For a more complete differential diagnosis of pulmonary causes of cyanosis in the neonate, see Chapters 33 to 38. Finally, clinical cyanosis may occur in an infant without hypoxemia in the setting of methemoglobinemia or pronounced polycythemia. Table 41.2 summarizes the differential diagnosis of cyanosis in the neonate.

Cyanosis due to congenital heart disease can be broadly grouped into those lesions with (i) decreased pulmonary blood flow and intracardiac right-to-left shunting and (ii) normal to increased pulmonary blood flow with intracardiac mixing (complete or incomplete) of the systemic and pulmonary venous return. Specific lesions and lesion-specific management are covered in more detail in section V.

B. **Congestive heart failure**

1. **Clinical findings.** CHF in the neonate (or in a patient of any age) is a **clinical** diagnosis made based on the existence of certain signs and symptoms rather than on radiographic or laboratory findings (although these may be supportive evidence for the diagnosis). Signs and symptoms of CHF occur when the heart is unable to meet the metabolic demands of the tissues. Clinical findings are frequently due to homeostatic mechanisms attempting to compensate for this imbalance. In early stages, the neonate may be tachypneic and tachycardiac with an increased respiratory effort, rales, hepatomegaly, and delayed capillary refill. In contrast to adults, edema is rarely seen. Diaphoresis, feeding difficulties, and growth failure may be present. Finally, CHF may present acutely with cardiorespiratory collapse, particularly in "left-sided" lesions (see V.A.). *Hydrops fetalis* is an extreme form of intrauterine CHF (see Chap. 26).

2. **Differential diagnosis.** The age when CHF develops depends on the hemodynamics of the responsible lesion. When heart failure develops in the first weeks of life, the differential diagnosis includes (i) a structural lesion causing severe pressure and/or volume overload, (ii) a primary myocardial lesion causing myocardial dysfunction, or (iii) arrhythmia. Table 41.3 summarizes the differential diagnoses of CHF in the neonate.

C. **Heart murmur.** Heart murmurs are not uncommonly heard when examining neonates. Estimates of the prevalence of heart murmurs in neonates vary widely from <1% to >50% depending on the study. Murmurs heard in newborns in the first days of life are often associated with structural heart disease of some type, and therefore may need further evaluation, particularly if there are any other associated clinical symptoms.

Pathologic murmurs tend to appear at characteristic ages. Semilunar valve stenosis (systolic ejection murmurs) and atrioventricular valvular insufficiency (systolic regurgitant murmurs) tend to be noted very shortly after birth, on the first day of life. In contrast, murmurs due to left-to-right shunt lesions (systolic regurgitant ventricular septal defect murmur or continuous PDA murmur) may

Table 41.2	Differential Diagnosis of Cyanosis in the Neonate
Primary cardiac lesions	
Decreased pulmonary blood flow, intracardiac right-to-left shunt	
Critical pulmonary stenosis	
Tricuspid atresia	
Pulmonary atresia/intact ventricular septum	
Tetralogy of Fallot	
Ebstein anomaly	
Total anomalous pulmonary venous connection with obstruction	
Normal or increased pulmonary blood flow, intracardiac mixing	
Hypoplastic left heart syndrome	
Transposition of the great arteries	
Truncus arteriosus	
Tetralogy of Fallot/pulmonary atresia	
Complete common atrioventricular canal	
Total anomalous pulmonary venous connection without obstruction	
Other single-ventricle complexes	
Pulmonary lesions (intrapulmonary right-to-left shunt) (see Chaps. 32–38)	
Primary parenchymal lung disease	
Aspiration syndromes (e.g., meconium and blood)	
Respiratory distress syndrome	
Pneumonia	
Airway obstruction	
Choanal stenosis or atresia	
Pierre Robin syndrome	
Tracheal stenosis	
	(continued)

Table 41.2	Differential Diagnosis of Cyanosis in the Neonate *(Continued)*
Pulmonary sling	
Absent pulmonary valve syndrome	
Extrinsic compression of the lungs	
Pneumothorax	
Pulmonary interstitial or lobar emphysema	
Chylothorax or other pleural effusions	
Congenital diaphragmatic hernia	
Thoracic dystrophies or dysplasia	
Hypoventilation	
Central nervous system lesions	
Neuromuscular diseases	
Sedation	
Sepsis	
Pulmonary arteriovenous malformations	
Persistent pulmonary hypertension (see Chap. 36)	
Cyanosis with normal PO$_2$	
Methemoglobinemia	
Polycythemia[a] (see Chap. 46)	

[a]In the case of polycythemia, these infants have plethora and venous congestion in the distal extremities, which gives the appearance of distal cyanosis; these infants actually are not hypoxemic (see text).

not be heard until the second to fourth week of life, when the pulmonary vascular resistance has decreased and the left-to-right shunt increases. Therefore, the **age of the patient** when the murmur is first noted and the **character of the murmur** provide important clues to the nature of the malformation.

D. **Arrhythmias.** See section VIII (Arrhythmias) of this chapter for a detailed description of identification and management of the neonate with an arrhythmia.

E. **Fetal echocardiography.** It is increasingly common for infants to be born with a diagnosis of probable congenital heart disease due to the widespread use of

Table 41.3	Differential Diagnosis of Congestive Heart Failure in the Neonate
Pressure overload	
Aortic stenosis	
Coarctation of the aorta	
Volume overload	
Left-to-right shunt at level of great vessels	
Patent ductus arteriosus	
Aorticopulmonary window	
Truncus arteriosus	
Tetralogy of Fallot, pulmonary atresia with multiple aorticopulmonary collaterals	
Left-to-right shunt at level of ventricles	
Ventricular septal defect	
Common atrioventricular canal	
Single ventricle without pulmonary stenosis (includes hypoplastic left heart syndrome)	
Arteriovenous malformations	
Combined pressure and volume overload	
Interrupted aortic arch	
Coarctation of the aorta with ventricular septal defect	
Aortic stenosis with ventricular septal defect	
Myocardial dysfunction	
Primary	
Cardiomyopathies	
Inborn errors of metabolism	
Genetic	
Myocarditis	
	(continued)

Table 41.3	Differential Diagnosis of Congestive Heart Failure in the Neonate *(Continued)*
Secondary	
Sustained tachyarrhythmias	
Perinatal asphyxia	
Sepsis	
Severe intrauterine valvar obstruction (e.g., aortic stenosis)	
Premature closure of the ductus arteriosus	

obstetric ultrasonography and fetal echocardiography. This may be quite valuable to the team of physicians caring for mother and baby, guiding plans for prenatal care, site and timing of delivery, as well as immediate perinatal care of the infant. The recommended timing for fetal echocardiography is 18 to 20 weeks' gestation, although reasonable images can be obtained as early as 16 weeks, and transvaginal ultrasonography may be used for diagnostic purposes in fetuses in the first trimester. Indications for fetal echocardiography are summarized in Table 41.4. It is important to note, however, that most cases of prenatally diagnosed congenital heart disease occur in pregnancies without known risk factors. Most severe forms of congenital heart disease can be accurately diagnosed by fetal echocardiography. Coarctation of the aorta, small ventricular and atrial septal defects, total anomalous pulmonary venous return, and mild aortic or pulmonary stenosis are abnormalities that may be missed by fetal echocardiography. In general, in complex congenital heart disease, the main abnormality is noted; however, the full extent of cardiac malformation may be better determined on postnatal examinations.

Fetal tachyarrhythmias or bradyarrhythmias (intermittent or persistent) may be detected on routine obstetric screening and ultrasonographic examinations; this should prompt more complete fetal echocardiography to rule out associated structural heart disease, assess fetal ventricular function, and further define the arrhythmia.

Fetal echocardiography has allowed for improved understanding of the *in utero* evolution of some forms of congenital heart disease. This, in turn, has opened up the possibility of fetal cardiac intervention. Recent successes in limited, selected cases of fetal cardiac intervention suggest that this is a promising new method of treatment for congenital heart disease.

IV. EVALUATION OF THE NEONATE WITH SUSPECTED CONGENITAL HEART DISEASE. As noted, the suspicion of congenital heart disease in the neonate typically follows one of a few clinical scenarios. Circulatory collapse is, unfortunately, not an uncommon means of presentation for the neonate with congenital heart disease. It must be emphasized that **emergency treatment of shock precedes definitive anatomic diagnosis**. Although sepsis may be suspected and treated, the signs of low cardiac output should always alert the examining physician to the likely possibility of congenital heart disease.

Table 41.4	Indications for Fetal Echocardiography
Fetus-related indications	
Suspected congenital heart disease on screening ultrasonography	
Fetal chromosomal anomaly	
Fetal extracardiac anatomic anomaly	
Fetal cardiac arrhythmia	
Persistent bradycardia	
Persistent tachycardia	
Irregular rhythm	
Nonimmune hydrops fetalis	
Mother-related indications	
Congenital heart disease	
Maternal metabolic disease	
Diabetes mellitus	
Phenylketonuria	
Maternal rheumatic disease (such as systemic lupus erythematosus)	
Maternal environmental exposures	
Alcohol	
Cardiac teratogenic medications	
Amphetamines	
Anticonvulsants	
Phenytoin	
Trimethadione	
Carbamazepine	
Valproate	
	(continued)

Table 41.4	Indications for Fetal Echocardiography *(Continued)*
	Isotretinoin
	Lithium carbonate
	Maternal viral infection
	Rubella
Family-related Indications	
Previous child or parent with congenital heart disease	
Previous child or parent with genetic disease associated with congenital heart disease	

A. Initial evaluation

1. **Physical examination.** A complete physical examination provides important clues to the anatomic diagnosis. Inexperienced examiners frequently focus solely on the presence or absence of cardiac murmurs, but much more additional information should be obtained during a complete examination. A great deal may be learned from simple visual inspection of the infant. Cyanosis may first be apparent on inspection of the mucous membranes and/or nail beds (see III.A.1.). Mottling of the skin and/or an ashen, gray color are important clues to severe cardiovascular compromise and incipient shock. While observing the infant, particular attention should be paid to the pattern of respiration including the work of breathing and use of accessory muscles.

    Before auscultation, palpation of the distal extremities with attention to temperature and capillary refill is imperative. The cool neonate with delayed capillary refill should always be evaluated for the possibility of severe congenital heart disease. While palpating the distal extremities, note the presence and character of the distal pulses. Diminished or absent distal pulses are highly suggestive of obstruction of the aortic arch. Palpation of the precordium may provide an important clue to the presence of congenital heart disease. The presence of a precordial thrill usually indicates at least moderate pulmonary or aortic outflow obstruction, although a restrictive ventricular septal defect with low right ventricular (RV) pressure may present with a similar finding. A hyperdynamic precordium suggests a sizeable left-to-right shunt.

    During auscultation, the examiner should first pay particular attention to the heart rate, noting its regularity and/or variability. The heart sounds, particularly the second heart sound, can be helpful clues to the ultimate diagnosis as well. A split-second heart sound is a particularly important marker of the existence of two semilunar valves, although it is often difficult to be sure of S2 splitting with the rapid heart rate of a neonate. Differentiating an S3 from an S4 heart sound is challenging in a tachycardic newborn; however, a gallop rhythm of either type is unusual and suggests the possibility of a significant left-to-right shunt or myocardial dysfunction. Ejection clicks suggest pulmonary or aortic valvar stenosis.

The presence and intensity of systolic murmurs can be very helpful in suggesting the type and severity of the underlying anatomic diagnosis; systolic murmurs are usually due to (i) semilunar valve or outflow tract stenosis, (ii) atrioventricular valve regurgitation, or (iii) shunting through a septal defect. Diastolic murmurs are **always** indicative of cardiovascular pathology. For a more complete description of auscultation of the heart, refer to one of the cardiology texts listed at the end of the chapter.

A careful search for other anomalies is essential because congenital heart disease is accompanied by at least one extracardiac malformation 25% of the time. Table 41.5 summarizes malformation and chromosomal syndromes commonly associated with congenital heart disease.

2. **Four-extremity blood pressure.** Measurement of blood pressure should be taken in both arms and in both legs. Usually, an automated Dinamap is used, but in a small neonate with pulses that are difficult to palpate, manual blood pressure measurement with Doppler amplification may be necessary for an accurate measurement. A systolic pressure that is >10 mm Hg higher in the upper body compared to the lower body is abnormal and suggests coarctation of the aorta, aortic arch hypoplasia, or interrupted aortic arch. It should be noted that a systolic blood pressure gradient is quite specific for an arch abnormality but not sensitive; a systolic blood pressure gradient will not be present in the neonate with an arch abnormality in whom the ductus arteriosus is patent and nonrestrictive. Therefore, the lack of a systolic blood pressure gradient in newborn does **not** conclusively rule out coarctation or other arch abnormalities, but the presence of a systolic pressure gradient is diagnostic of an aortic arch abnormality.

3. **Chest x-ray.** A frontal and lateral view (if possible) of the chest should be obtained. In infants, particularly in newborns, the size of the heart may be difficult to determine due to overlying thymus. Nevertheless, useful information can be gained from the chest x-ray. In addition to heart size, notation should be made of visceral and cardiac situs (dextrocardia and *situs inversus* are frequently accompanied by congenital heart disease). The aortic arch side (right or left) can frequently be determined; a right-sided aortic arch is associated with congenital heart disease in >90% of patients. Dark or poorly perfused lung fields suggests decreased pulmonary blood flow, whereas diffusely opaque lung fields may represent increased pulmonary blood flow or significant left atrial hypertension.

4. **Electrocardiogram (ECG).** The neonatal ECG reflects the hemodynamic relations that existed *in utero*; therefore, the normal ECG is notable for RV predominance. As many forms of congenital heart disease have minimal prenatal hemodynamic effects, the ECG is frequently "normal for age" despite significant structural pathology (e.g., transposition of the great arteries, tetralogy of Fallot). Throughout the neonatal period, infancy, and childhood, the ECG will evolve due to the expected changes in physiology and the resulting changes in chamber size and thickness that occur. Because most findings on a neonate's ECG would be abnormal in an older child or adult, it is essential to refer to age-specific charts of normal values for most ECG parameters. Refer to Tables 41.6 and 41.7 for normal ECG values in term and premature neonates.

When interpreting an ECG, the following determinations should be made: (i) rate and rhythm; (ii) P, QRS, and T axes; (iii) intracardiac conduction intervals; (iv) evidence for chamber enlargement or hypertrophy; (v) evidence

Table 41.5 Chromosomal Anomalies, Syndromes, and Associations Commonly Associated with Congenital Heart Disease

	Approximate incidence or mode of inheritance	Extracardiac features	Cardiac features
Chromosomal anomalies			
Trisomy 13 (Patau syndrome)	1/5,000	SGA; facies (midfacial hypoplasia, cleft lip and palate, microophthalmia, coloboma, low-set ears); brain anomalies (microcephaly, holoprosencephaly); aplasia cutis congenita of scalp; polydactyly	≥80% have cardiac defects, VSD most common
Trisomy 18 (Edward syndrome)	1/3,000 (female–male = 3:1)	SGA; facies (dolichocephaly, prominent occiput, short palpebral fissures, low-set posteriorly rotated ears, small mandible); short sternum; rocker-bottom feet; overlapping fingers with "clenched fists"	≥95% have cardiac defects; VSD most common (sometimes multiple); redundant valvar tissue with regurgitation often affecting more than one valve (polyvalvar disease)
Trisomy 21 (Down syndrome)	1/660	Facies (brachycephaly, flattened occiput, midfacial hypoplasia, mandibular prognathism, upslanting palpebral fissures, epicanthal folds, Brushfield spots, large tongue); simian creases, clinodactyly with short fifth finger; pronounced hypotonia	40%–50% have cardiac defects, CAVC, VSD most common, also TOF, ASD, PDA; complex congenital heart disease is very rare
45,X (Turner syndrome)	1/2,500	Lymphedema of hands, feet; short stature; short webbed neck; facies (triangular with downslanting palpebral fissures, low-set ears); shield chest	25%–45% have cardiac defects, coarctation, bicuspid aortic valve most common

Single-gene defects

Noonan syndrome	AD	Facies (hypertelorism, epicanthal folds, downslanting palpebral fissures, ptosis); low-set ears; short webbed neck with low hairline; shield chest, cryptorchidism in men	50% have cardiac defect, usually valvar pulmonary stenosis, also ASD, hypertrophic CM
Holt-Oram syndrome	AD	Spectrum of upper limb and shoulder girdle anomalies	≥50% have cardiac defect, usually ASD or VSD
Alagille syndrome	AD	Cholestasis; facies (micrognathism, broad forehead, deep-set eyes); vertebral anomalies, ophthalmologic abnormalities	Cardiac findings in 90% peripheral pulmonic stenosis, most common

Gene-deletion syndromes

Williams syndrome (Deletion 7q11)	1/7,500	SGA, FIT; facies ("elfin" with short-palpebral fissures, periorbital fullness or puffiness, flat nasal bridge, stellate iris, long philtrum, prominent lips); fussy infants with poor feeding, friendly personality later in childhood; characteristic mental deficiency (motor more reduced than verbal performance)	50%–70% have cardiac defect, most commonly supravalvar aortic stenosis; other arterial stenoses also occur, including PPS, COA, renal artery and coronary artery stenoses
DiGeorge syndrome (Deletion 22q11)	1/6,000	Thymic hypoplasia/aplasia; parathyroid hypoplasia/aplasia; cleft palate or velopharyngeal incompetence	IAA and conotruncal malformations including truncus, TOF

(continued)

Table 41.5 Chromosomal Anomalies, Syndromes, and Associations Commonly Associated with Congenital Heart Disease *(Continued)*

	Approximate incidence or mode of inheritance	Extracardiac features	Cardiac features
Associations			
VACTERL		Vertebral defects; anal atresia; TE fistula; radial and renal anomalies; limb defects	Approximately 50% have cardiac defect, most commonly VSD
CHARGE		Coloboma; choanal atresia; growth and mental deficiency; genital hypoplasia (in men); ear anomalies and/or deafness	50%–70% have cardiac defect, most commonly conotruncal anomalies (TOF, DORV, truncus arteriosus)

AD = autosomal dominant; AR = autosomal recessive; CM = cardiomyopathy; CoA = coarctation of the aorta; CAVC = complete atrioventricular canal; DORV = double outlet right ventricle; FTT = failure to thrive; IAA = interrupted aortic arch; PDA = patent ductus arteriosus; PPS = peripheral pulmonary stenosis; SGA = small-for-gestational-age; TOF = tetralogy of Fallot; TEF = tracheoesophageal fistula; VSD = ventricular septal defect.

Table 41.6 ECG Standards in Newborns

Measure	Age (D)			
	0–1	1–3	3–7	7–30
Term infants				
Heart rate (beats/mm)	122 (99–147)	123 (97–148)	128 (100–160)	148 (114–177)
QRS axis (degrees)	135 (91–185)	134 (93–188)	133 (92–185)	108 (78–152)
PR interval, II (s)	0.11 (0.08–0.14)	0.11 (0.09–0.13)	0.10 (0.08–0.13)	0.10 (0.08–0.13)
QRS duration (s)	0.05 (0.03–0.07)	0.05 (0.03–0.06)	0.05 (0.03–0.06)	0.05 (0.03–0.08)
V1, R amplitude (mm)	13.5 (6.5–23.7)	14.8 (7.0–24.2)	12.8 (5.5–21.5)	10.5 (4.5–18.1)
V1, S amplitude (mm)	8.5 (1.0–18.5)	9.5 (1.5–19.0)	6.8 (1.0–15.0)	4.0 (0.5–9.7)
V6, R amplitude (mm)	4.5 (0.5–9.5)	4.8 (0.5–9.5)	5.1 (1.0–10.5)	7.6 (2.6–13.5)
V6, S amplitude (mm)	3.5 (0.2–7.9)	3.2 (0.2–7.6)	3.7 (0.2–8.0)	3.2 (0.2–3.2)

(continued)

Table 41.6 ECG Standards in Newborns *(Continued)*

Measure	Age (D)			
	0-1	1-3	3-7	7-30
Preterm infants				
Heart rate (beats/mm)	141 (109-173)	150 (127-182)	164 (134-200)	170 (133-200)
QRS axis (degrees)	127 (75-194)	121 (75-195)	117 (75-165)	80 (17-171)
PR interval (s)	0.10 (0.09-0.10)	0.10 (0.09-1.10)	0.10 (0.09-0.10)	0.10 (0.09-0.10)
QRS duration (s)	0.04	0.04	0.04	0.04
V1, R amplitude (mm)	6.5 (2.0-12.6)	7.4 (2.6-14.9)	8.7 (3.8-16.9)	13.0 (6.2-21.6)
V1, S amplitude (mm)	6.8 (0.6-17.6)	6.5 (1-0-16.0)	6.8 (0.0-15.0)	6.2 (1.2-14.0)
V6, R amplitude (mm)	11.4 (3.5-21.3)	11.9 (5.0-20.8)	12.3 (4.0-20.5)	15.0 (8.3-21.0)
V6, S amplitude (mm)	15.0 (2.5-26.5)	13.5 (2.6-26.0)	14.0 (3.0-25.0)	14.0 (3.1-26.3)

Sources: Davignon A, Rautaharja P, Boiselle E, et al. Normal ECG standards for infants and children. *Pediatr Cardiol* 1980;1(2):123–131. Sreenivasan VV, Fisher BJ, Liebman J, et al. Longitudinal study of the standard electrocardiogram in the healthy premature infant during the first year of life. *Am J Cardiol* 1973;31(1):57–63.

Table 41.7	ECG Findings in Premature Infants (Compared to Term Infants)
Rate	
Slightly higher resting rate with greater activity-related and circadian variation (sinus bradycardia to 70 with sleep, not uncommon)	
Intracardiac conduction	
PR and QRS duration slightly shorter	
Maximum QT_c <0.44 s (longer than for term infants, QT_c <0.40 s)	
QRS complex	
QRS axis in frontal plane more leftward with decreasing gestational age	
QRS amplitude lower (possibly due to less ventricular mass)	
Less right ventricular predominance in precordial chest leads	

Source: Reproduced with permission from Thomaidis C, Varlamis G, Karemperis S. Comparative study of the electrocardiograms of healthy fullterm and premature newborns. *Acta Paediatr Scand* 1988;77(5):653–657.

for pericardial disease, ischemia, infarction, or electrolyte abnormalities; and (vi) if the ECG pattern fits with the clinical picture. When the ECG is abnormal, one should also consider incorrect lead placement; a simple confirmation of lead placement may be done by comparing QRS complexes in limb lead I and precordial lead V_6—each should have a similar morphology if the limb leads have been properly placed. The ECG of the premature infant is somewhat different from that of the term infant (Table 41.7).

5. **Hyperoxia test.** In **all** neonates with suspected critical congenital heart disease (not just those who are cyanotic), a hyperoxia test should be considered. **This single test is perhaps the most sensitive and specific tool in the initial evaluation of the neonate with suspected recent disease**. In sites with timely access to echocardiography, a complete hyperoxia test may not be performed; however, it is important to realize what a valuable test this can be when echocardiography is not easily and quickly available.

To investigate the possibility of a fixed, intracardiac right-to-left shunt, the arterial oxygen tension should be measured in room air (if tolerated) followed by repeat measurements with the patient receiving 100% inspired oxygen (the "hyperoxia test"). If possible, the arterial partial pressure of oxygen (PO_2) should be measured directly through arterial puncture, although properly applied transcutaneous oxygen monitor (TCOM) values for PO_2 are also acceptable. **Pulse oximetry cannot be used** for documentation; in a neonate given 100% inspired oxygen, a value of 100% oxygen saturation may be obtained with an arterial PO_2 ranging from 80 torr (abnormal) to 680 torr (normal, see III.A.1.).

Measurements should be made (by arterial blood gas or TCOM) at both "preductal" and "postductal" sites, and the exact site of PO_2 measurement must be recorded because some congenital malformations with desaturated blood flow entering the descending aorta through the ductus arteriosus may result in "differential cyanosis" (as seen in persistent pulmonary hypertension of the newborn). A markedly higher oxygen content in the upper versus the lower part of the body can be an important diagnostic clue to such lesions, including all forms of critical aortic arch obstruction or left ventricular outflow obstruction. There are also rare cases of "reverse differential cyanosis" with elevated lower body saturation and lower upper body saturation. This occurs only in children with transposition of the great arteries with an abnormal pulmonary artery to aortic shunt due to coarctation, interruption of the aortic arch, or suprasystemic pulmonary vascular resistance ("persistent fetal circulation").

When a patient breathes 100% oxygen, an arterial PO_2 of >250 torr in both upper and lower extremities virtually eliminates the critical structural cyanotic heart disease (a "passed" hyperoxia test). An arterial PO_2 of <100 in the absence of clear-cut lung disease (a "failed" hyperoxia test) is most likely due to intracardiac right-to-left shunting and is virtually diagnostic of cyanotic congenital heart disease. Patients who have an arterial PO_2 between 100 and 250 **may** have structural heart disease with complete intracardiac mixing and greatly increased pulmonary blood flow, as is occasionally seen with single ventricle complexes, such as hypoplastic left heart syndrome. **The neonate who "fails" a hyperoxia test is very likely to have congenital heart disease involving ductal-dependent systemic or pulmonary blood flow and should receive prostaglandin E1 (PGE_1) until anatomic definition can be accomplished** (see IV.B.2.).

B. **Stabilization and transport.** On the basis of the initial evaluation, if an infant has been identified as likely to have congenital heart disease, further medical management must be planned, as well as arrangements made for a definitive anatomic diagnosis. This may involve transport of the neonate to another medical center where a pediatric cardiologist is available.

1. **Initial resuscitation.** For the neonate who presents with evidence of decreased cardiac output or shock, initial attention is devoted to the basics of advanced life support. A stable airway must be established and maintained as well as adequate ventilation. Reliable vascular access is essential, usually including an arterial line. In the neonate, this can most reliably be accomplished through the umbilical vessels. Volume resuscitation, inotropic support, and correction of metabolic acidosis are required with the goal of improving cardiac output and tissue perfusion (see Chap. 40).

2. **PGE_1.** The neonate who "fails" a hyperoxia test (or has an equivocal result in addition to other signs or symptoms of congenital heart disease) as well as the neonate who presents in shock within the first 3 weeks of life is highly likely to have congenital heart disease. These neonates are very likely to have congenital lesions that include anatomic features with ductal-dependent systemic or pulmonary blood flow, or in whom a PDA will aid in intercirculatory mixing.

PGE_1, administered as a continuous intravenous infusion, has important side effects that must be anticipated. PGE_1 causes apnea in 10% to 12% of neonates, usually within the first 6 hours of administration. Therefore, the infant who will be transferred to another institution while receiving PGE_1 should be intubated for maintenance of a stable airway before leaving the referring hospital. In infants who will not require transport, intubation may not be required but continuous cardiorespiratory monitoring is essential. In addition, PGE_1 typically causes peripheral vasodilation and subsequent hypotension in many infants. A separate intravenous line should be secured for volume administration in any infant receiving PGE_1, especially those who require transport.

Specific information regarding other adverse reactions, dose, and administration of PGE_1 is in section VII.A.

The authors cannot overemphasize the need to begin PGE_1 in **any** neonate in whom congenital heart disease is strongly suspected (i.e., a failed hyperoxia test and/or severe, acute CHF). In the neonate with ductal-dependant pulmonary blood flow, oxygen saturation will typically improve and the pulmonary blood flow remains secure until an anatomic diagnosis and plans for surgery are made. In neonates with transposition of the great arteries, maintenance of a patent ductus improves intercirculatory mixing. Most important, **neonates who present in shock in the first few weeks of life have duct-dependent systemic blood flow until proved otherwise**; resuscitation will not be successful unless the ductus is opened. In these cases, it is appropriate to begin an infusion of PGE_1 even **before** a precise anatomic diagnosis can be made by echocardiography.

It is prudent to remeasure arterial blood gases and reassess perfusion, vital signs, and acid–base status within 15 to 30 minutes of starting a PGE_1 infusion. Rarely, patients may become more unstable after beginning PGE_1. This is usually due to lesions with left atrial hypertension: hypoplastic left heart syndrome with restrictive patent foramen ovale, subdiaphragmatic total anomalous pulmonary venous return, mitral atresia with restrictive patent foramen ovale, transposition of the great arteries with intact ventricular septum with restrictive patent foramen ovale, and some cases of Ebstein anomaly (see V.B.5.). In these lesions, deterioration on PGE_1 is often a helpful diagnostic finding, and **urgent** plans for echocardiography and possible interventional catheterization or surgery should be made.

3. **Inotropic agents.** Continuous infusions of inotropic agents, usually the sympathomimetic amines, can improve myocardial performance as well as perfusion of vital organs and the periphery. Care should be taken to replete intravascular volume before institution of vasoactive agents. **Dopamine** is a precursor of norepinephrine and stimulates β-1, dopaminergic, and α-adrenergic receptors in a dose-dependent manner. Dopamine can be expected to increase mean arterial pressure, improve ventricular function, and improve urine output with a low incidence of side effects at doses <10 μg/kg/minute. **Dobutamine** is an analog of dopamine, with predominantly β-1 effects and relatively weak β-2 and α-receptor–stimulating activity. In comparison with dopamine, dobutamine lacks renal vasodilating properties, has less chronotropic effect (in adult patients), and does not depend on norepinephrine release from peripheral nerves for its effect. There are few published data available concerning the use of dobutamine in neonates, although clinical experience has been favorable. A combination of low-dose dopamine (up to 5 μg/kg/minute) and dobutamine may be used to minimize the potential peripheral vasoconstriction induced by high doses of dopamine while maximizing the dopaminergic effects on the renal circulation. See section VII.B for details of administration of inotropic agents and additional pharmacologic agents (see Chap. 40).

4. **Transport.** After initial stabilization, the neonate with suspected congenital heart disease often needs to be transferred to an institution that provides subspecialty care in pediatric cardiology and cardiac surgery. A successful transport actually involves two transitions of care for the neonate: (i) from the referring hospital staff to the transport team, and (ii) from the transport team staff to the accepting hospital staff. The need for accurate, detailed, and complete communication of information between all these teams cannot be overemphasized. If possible, the pediatric cardiologist who will be caring for the patient should be included in the discussions of care while the neonate is still at the referring hospital.

Reliable **vascular access** should be secured for the neonate receiving continuous infusions of PGE₁ or inotropic agents. Umbilical lines placed for resuscitation and stabilization should be left in place for transport; the neonate with congenital heart disease may potentially require cardiac catheterization through this route.

Particular attention should be paid to the patient's airway and respiratory effort before transport. In general, all neonates receiving a PGE₁ infusion should be **intubated for transport** (see IV.B.2.). Neonates with probable or definite congenital heart disease will most likely require surgical or interventional catheterization management during the hospitalization; therefore, it is likely that they will be intubated at some point. Because there is real risk in not intubating these infants, as a general rule, all should be intubated for transport unless there is a compelling reason not to do so. All intubated patients should have gastric decompression by nasogastric or orogastric tube.

Acid–base status and oxygen delivery should be checked with an arterial blood gas before transport. Although most noncardiac patients are transported receiving supplemental oxygen at or near 100%, this is often **not** the inspired oxygen concentration of choice for the neonate with congenital heart disease (see V for details of lesion-specific care). This management decision for transport is particularly important for those infants with duct-dependent systemic blood flow and complete intracardiac mixing with single ventricle physiology, and emphasizes the need to consult with a pediatric cardiologist before transport to achieve optimal intratransport patient care.

Finally, it is important to remember that in neonates, **hypotension** is a late finding in shock. Therefore, other signs of incipient decompensation, such as persistent tachycardia and poor tissue perfusion, are important to note and treat before transport. Before leaving the referring hospital, the patient's current hemodynamic status (distal perfusion, heart rate, systemic blood pressure, acid–base status, etc.) should be reassessed and relayed to the receiving hospital team.

C. **Confirmation of the diagnosis**

1. **Echocardiography.** Two-dimensional echocardiography, supplemented with Doppler and color Doppler has become the primary diagnostic tool for anatomic definition in pediatric cardiology. Echocardiography provides information about the structure and function of the heart and great vessels in a timely fashion. Although it is not an invasive test *per se*, a complete echocardiogram on a newborn suspected of having congenital heart disease may take an hour or more to perform, and may therefore not be well tolerated by a sick and/or premature newborn. Temperature instability due to exposure during this

extended time of examination may be a problem in the neonate. Extension of the neck for suprasternal notch views of the aortic arch may be problematic, particularly in the neonate with respiratory distress or with a tenuous airway. Therefore, in sick neonates, **close monitoring by a medical staff person other** than the one performing the echocardiogram is recommended, with attention to vital signs, respiratory status, temperature, and so on.

2. **Cardiac catheterization**

a. **Indications** (see Table 41.8). Neonatal cardiac catheterization has changed a great deal in its focus. In the current era, cardiac catheterization is rarely

Table 41.8	Indications for Neonatal Catheterization
Interventions	
Therapeutic	
Balloon atrial septostomy	
Balloon pulmonary valvuloplasty[a]	
Balloon aortic valvuloplasty[a]	
Balloon angioplasty of native coarctation of the aorta[a]	
Coil embolization of abnormal vascular communications	
Diagnostic	
Endomyocardial biopsy	
Anatomic definition (not visualized by echocardiography)	
Coronary arteries	
Pulmonary atresia/intact ventricular septum	
Transposition of the great arteries	
Tetralogy of Fallot	
Aortic to pulmonary artery collateral vessels	
Tetralogy of Fallot	
Distal pulmonary artery anatomy	
Hemodynamic measurements	

[a]These interventions have alternative surgical options and are controversial based on institutional experience (see text).

necessary for anatomic definition of intracardiac structures (although catheterization is still necessary for definition of the distal pulmonary arteries, aortic-pulmonary collaterals, and certain types of coronary artery anomalies) or for physiologic assessment as Doppler technology has assumed an increasingly important role in this regard. Increasingly, catheterization is performed for catheter-directed therapy of congenital lesions. See Figure 41.1 for normal newborn oxygen saturation and pressure measurements obtained during cardiac catheterization.

b. Interventional catheterization. Since the first balloon dilation of the pulmonary artery reported by Kan in 1982, balloon valvuloplasty has become the procedure of choice in many types of valvar lesions, even extending to critical lesions in the neonate. At Children's Hospital, balloon valvuloplasty is considered the initial treatment of choice for both pulmonary and aortic stenosis, with a >90% immediate success rate in the neonate. The application of balloon dilation of native coarctation of the aorta is controversial (see the subsequent text).

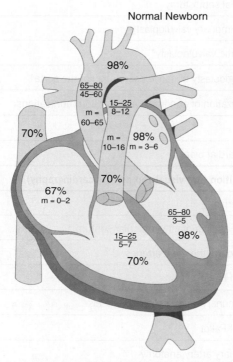

Normal Newborn

Figure 41.1. Typical hemodynamic measurements obtained at cardiac catheterization in a newborn, term infant without congenital or acquired heart disease. In this (and subsequent diagrams), oxygen saturations are shown as percentages, and typical hemodynamic pressure measurements in mm Hg are shown. In this example, the transition from fetal to infant physiology is complete; the pulmonary vascular resistance has fallen; the ductus arteriosus has closed; and there is no significant shunt at the foramen ovale. m = mean value.

c. Preparation for catheterization. Catheterization in the neonate is not without its attendant risks; young age, small size, and interventional procedures are risk factors for complications. With appropriate anticipatory care, complications can be minimized. In addition to basic medical stabilization (see IV.B.), specific attention to airway management is crucial. Sedation and analgesia are necessary, but will depress the respiratory drive in the neonate. When catheterizing a neonate, intubation and mechanical ventilation should be strongly considered, especially if an intervention is contemplated. In our institution, a **separate staff person not performing the catheterization** is present during the study, dedicated to the supervision of the infant's overall hemodynamic and respiratory status.

Supervision of the neonate undergoing catheterization should also include periodic evaluation of the patient's body temperature, acid–base status, serum glucose, and monitoring of blood loss. All infants undergoing interventional catheterization such as balloon procedures should have 10 to 25 mL/kg packed red blood cells (PRBCs) typed and crossmatched **in the catheterization laboratory** during the procedure. Intravenous lines are recommended in the upper extremities or head (because the lower body will be draped and inaccessible during the case) in order to provide unobstructed access for medications, volume infusions, and so forth. Finally, the neonate may have the catheterization performed through umbilical vessels that were previously used for the administration of fluid, glucose, PGE_1, inotropic agents, or blood administration. Therefore, a peripheral line should be started and medications changed to that site before transfer of the neonate to the cardiac catheterization laboratory.

Consultation with the pediatric cardiologist who will be performing the case beforehand will help clarify these issues and allow the infant to be well prepared and monitored during the case.

V. "LESION-SPECIFIC" CARE FOLLOWING ANATOMIC DIAGNOSIS

A. **Duct-dependent systemic blood flow.** Commonly referred to as **left-sided obstructive lesions**, this group of lesions includes a spectrum of hypoplasia of left-sided structures of the heart ranging from isolated coarctation of the aorta to hypoplastic left heart syndrome. These infants typically present in cardiovascular collapse as the ductus arteriosus closes, with resultant systemic hypoperfusion; they may also present more insidiously with symptoms of CHF (see III.B.). Although all infants with significant left-sided lesions and duct-dependent systemic blood flow require prostaglandin-induced patency of the ductus arteriosus as part of the initial management, additional care varies somewhat with each lesion.

1. **Aortic stenosis** (see Fig. 41.2). Morphologic abnormalities of the aortic valve may range from a bicuspid, nonobstructive, functionally normal valve to a unicuspid, markedly deformed, and severely obstructive valve, which greatly limits systemic cardiac output from the left ventricle. By convention, "severe" aortic stenosis is defined as a peak systolic gradient from left ventricle to ascending aorta of at least 60 mm Hg. "Critical" aortic stenosis results from severe anatomic obstruction with accompanying left ventricular failure and/or shock, regardless of the measured gradient. Patients with critical aortic stenosis have severe obstruction present *in utero* (usually due to a unicuspid, "platelike" valve), with resultant left ventricular hypertrophy and, frequently, endocardial

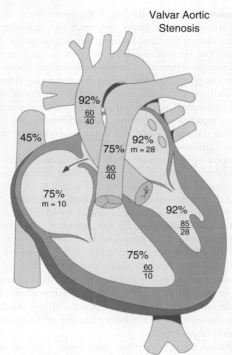

Valvar Aortic
Stenosis

Figure 41.2. Critical valvar aortic stenosis with a closed ductus arteriosus. Typical anatomic and hemodynamic findings include (i) a morphologically abnormal, stenotic valve; (ii) poststenotic dilatation of the ascending aorta; (iii) elevated left ventricular end-diastolic pressure and left atrial pressures contributing to pulmonary edema (mild pulmonary venous and arterial desaturation); (iv) a left-to-right shunt at the atrial level (note an increase in oxygen saturation from superior vena cava to right atrium); (v) pulmonary artery hypertension (also secondary to the elevated left atrial pressure); (vi) only a modest (25 mm Hg) gradient across valve. The low measured gradient (despite severe anatomic obstruction) across the aortic valve is due to a severely limited cardiac output, as evidenced by the low mixed venous oxygen saturation (45%) in the superior vena cava. m = mean value.

fibroelastosis. Associated left-sided abnormalities, such as mitral valve disease and coarctation, are not uncommon. Following closure of the ductus, the left ventricle must supply all of the systemic cardiac output. In cases of severe myocardial dysfunction, clinical CHF or shock will become apparent.

Initial management of the severely affected infant includes treatment of shock, stable vascular access, airway management and mechanical ventilation, sedation and muscle paralysis, inotropic support and institution of PGE₁. Positive end-expiratory pressure (PEEP) is helpful to overcome pulmonary venous desaturation from pulmonary edema secondary to left atrial hypertension. For a patient with critical aortic stenosis to benefit from a PGE₁ infusion, there must be a small patent foramen ovale to allow effective systemic blood flow (pulmonary venous return) to cross the atrial septum and to ultimately enter the systemic vascular bed through the ductus. Inspired oxygen should be limited to a fractional concentration of inspired oxygen (FiO_2) of 0.5 to 0.6 unless severe hypoxemia is present.

Following anatomic definition of left ventricular size, mitral valve, and aortic arch anatomy by echocardiography, cardiac catheterization or surgery should be performed as soon as possible to perform aortic valvotomy. With either type of therapy, patient outcome will depend largely on (i) the degree of relief of the obstruction, (ii) the degree of aortic regurgitation, (iii) associated cardiac lesions (especially left ventricular size), and (iv) the severity of end-organ dysfunction secondary to the initial presentation (e.g., necrotizing enterocolitis or renal failure). All patients with aortic stenosis will require lifelong follow-up, as stenosis frequently recurs. Multiple procedures in childhood are common.

2. **Coarctation of the aorta** (see Fig. 41.3) is an anatomic narrowing of the descending aorta, most commonly at the site of insertion of the ductus arteriosus (i.e., "juxtaductal"). Additional cardiac abnormalities are common, including

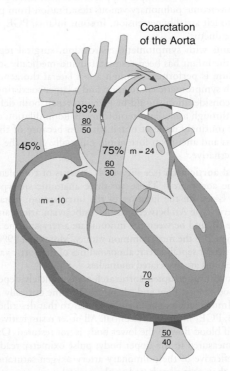

Coarctation of the Aorta

Figure 41.3. Coarctation of the aorta in a critically ill neonate with a nearly closed ductus arteriosus. Typical anatomic and hemodynamic findings include (i) "juxtaductal" site of the coarctation; (ii) a bicommissural aortic valve (seen in 80% of patients with coarctation); (iii) narrow pulse pressure in the descending aorta and lower body; (iv) a bidirectional shunt at the ductus arteriosus. As in critical aortic stenosis (see Fig. 41.2), there is an elevated left atrial pressure, pulmonary edema, a left-to-right shunt at the atrial level, pulmonary artery hypertension, and only a moderate (30 mm Hg) gradient across the arch obstruction. The low measured gradient (despite severe anatomic obstruction) across the aortic arch is due to low cardiac output. m = mean value.

bicuspid aortic valve (which occurs in 80% of patients) and ventricular septal defect (which occurs in 40% of patients). In addition, hypoplasia or obstruction of other left-sided structures including the mitral valve, the left ventricle, and the aortic valve are not uncommon and must be evaluated during the initial echocardiographic evaluation.

In utero, systemic blood flow to the lower body is through the PDA. Following ductal closure in the newborn with a critical coarctation, the left ventricle must suddenly generate adequate pressure and volume to pump the entire cardiac output past a significant point of obstruction. This sudden pressure load may be poorly tolerated by the neonatal myocardium, and the neonate may become rapidly and critically ill because of lower body hypoperfusion.

As in critical aortic stenosis, initial management of the severely affected infant includes treatment of shock, stable vascular access, airway management and mechanical ventilation, moderate supplemental oxygen, sedation and muscle paralysis, inotropic support, and institution of PGE_1. PEEP is helpful to overcome pulmonary venous desaturation from pulmonary edema secondary to left atrial hypertension. In some infants, PGE_1 is unsuccessful in opening the ductus.

In infants with symptomatic coarctation, surgical repair is performed as soon as the infant has been resuscitated and medically stabilized. Usually, the procedure is performed through a left lateral thoracotomy incision. In infants with symptomatic coarctation and a large, coexisting ventricular septal defect, consideration should be given to repair both defects in the initial procedure through a median sternotomy. Balloon dilation of native coarctation is not routinely done at our institution because of the high incidence of restenosis and aneurysm formation, especially given the safe and effective surgical alternative.

3. **Interrupted aortic arch** (see Fig. 41.4) consists of complete atresia of a segment of the aortic arch. There are three anatomic subtypes of interrupted aortic arch based on the location of the interruption: distal to the left subclavian artery (type A), between the left subclavian artery and the left carotid artery (type B), and between the innominate artery and the left carotid artery (type C). Type B is the most common variety. More than 99% of these patients have a ventricular septal defect; abnormalities of the aortic valve and narrowed subaortic regions are associated anomalies.

Infants with interrupted aortic arch are completely dependent on a PDA for lower body blood flow and, therefore, become critically ill when the ductus closes. Immediate management is similar to that described for coarctation (see V.A.2.); PGE_1 infusion is essential. All other resuscitative measures will be ineffective if blood flow to the lower body is not restored. Oxygen saturations should be measured in the upper body; pulse oximetry readings in the lower body are reflective of the pulmonary artery oxygen saturation, and are typically lower than that distributed to the central nervous system and coronary arteries. High concentrations of inspired oxygen may result in low pulmonary vascular resistance, a large left-to-right shunt, and a "runoff" during diastole from the lower body into the pulmonary circulation. Inspired oxygen levels should therefore be minimized, aiming for normal (95%) oxygen saturations in the **upper** body.

Surgical reconstruction should be performed as soon as metabolic acidosis (if present) has resolved, end-organ dysfunction has improved, and the patient

Interrupted
Aortic Arch

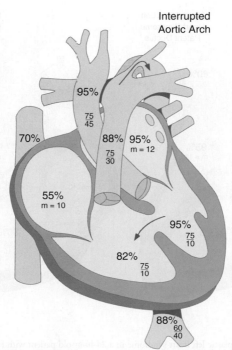

Figure 41.4. Interrupted aortic arch with restrictive patent ductus arteriosus. Typical anatomic and hemodynamic findings include (i) atresia of a segment of the aortic arch between the left subclavian artery and the left common carotid (the most common type of interrupted aortic arch—break "type B"); (ii) a posterior malalignment of the conal septum resulting in a large ventricular septal defect and a narrow subaortic area; (iii) a bicuspid aortic valve occurs in 60% of patients; (iv) systemic pressure in the right ventricle and pulmonary artery (due to the large, nonrestrictive ventricular septal defect); (v) increased oxygen saturation in the pulmonary artery due to left-to-right shunting at the ventricular level; (vi) "differential cyanosis" with a lower oxygen saturation in the descending aorta due to a right-to-left shunt at the patent ductus. Note the lower blood pressure in the descending aorta due to constriction of the ductus; opening the ductus with PGE$_1$ results in equal upper and lower extremity blood pressures but continued "differential cyanosis." PGE$_1$ indicates prostaglandin E1. m = mean value.

has been hemodynamically stabilized. The repair typically entails a corrective approach through a median sternotomy, with arch reconstruction (usually an end-to-end anastomosis) and closure of the ventricular septal defect. Arch reconstruction and a pulmonary artery band (through a lateral thoracotomy) are generally not recommended, typically reserved for patients with multiple ventricular septal defects.

4. **Hypoplastic left heart syndrome** (see Figs. 41.5A and 41.5B) represents a heterogeneous group of anatomic abnormalities in which there is a small-to-absent left ventricle with hypoplastic to atretic mitral and aortic valves. Before

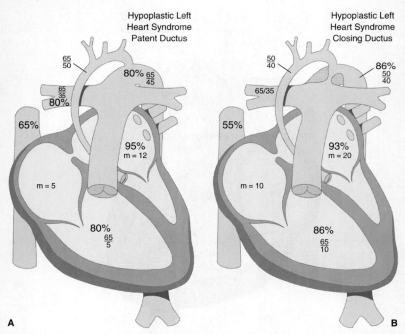

Figure 41.5. A: Hypoplastic left heart syndrome in a 24-hour-old patient with falling pulmonary vascular resistance and a nonrestrictive ductus arteriosus. Typical anatomic and hemodynamic findings include (i) atresia or hypoplasia of the left ventricle, mitral, and aortic valves; (ii) a diminutive ascending aorta and transverse aortic arch, usually with an associated coarctation; (iii) coronary blood flow is usually ***retrograde*** from the ductus arteriosus through the tiny ascending aorta; (iv) systemic arterial oxygen saturation (in FiO_2 of 0.21) of 80%, reflecting relatively balanced systemic and pulmonary blood flows—the pulmonary artery and aortic saturations are equal (see text); (v) pulmonary hypertension secondary to the nonrestrictive ductus arteriosus; (vi) minimal left atrial hypertension; (vii) normal systemic cardiac output (note the superior vena cava oxygen saturation of 65%) and blood pressure (65/45). **B:** Acute circulatory collapse following constriction of the ductus arteriosus in hypoplastic left heart syndrome. These neonates are typically in shock with poor perfusion, tachycardia, acidosis, and respiratory distress. The anatomic features are similar to those in Fig. 41.5A, with the exception of the narrowed ductus arteriosus. Note (i) the low cardiac output (as evidenced by the low mixed venous oxygen saturation in the superior vena cava of 55%); (ii) narrow pulse pressure; (iii) elevated atrial and ventricular end-diastolic pressure—elevated left atrial pressure may cause pulmonary edema (note left atrial saturation of 93%); (iv) significantly increased pulmonary blood flow, as reflected in an arterial oxygen saturation (in FiO_2 of 0.21) of 86%. m = mean value.

surgery, the right ventricle supplies both the pulmonary and systemic blood flows (through the PDA) with the proportion of cardiac output going to either circuit dependent on the relative resistances of these vascular beds.

As the pulmonary vascular resistance begins to fall (Fig. 41.5A), blood flow is preferentially directed to the pulmonary circulation at the expense of the systemic circulation. As systemic blood flow decreases, stroke volume and heart rate increase as a mechanism to preserve systemic cardiac output. The right ventricle becomes progressively volume overloaded with mildly elevated end-diastolic and left atrial pressures. The infant may be tachypneic or in respiratory distress; hepatomegaly may be present. The greater proportion of pulmonary venous return in the mixed ventricular blood results in a mildly decreased systemic arterial oxygen saturation (80%), and visible cyanosis may be mild or absent. Not infrequently, these infants are discharged from the nursery as normal newborns.

At this point, the continued fall in pulmonary vascular resistance results in a progressive increase in pulmonary blood flow and relative decrease in systemic cardiac output. As the total RV output is limited by heart rate and stroke volume, there is the onset of clinically apparent CHF, RV dilation and dysfunction, progressive tricuspid regurgitation, poor peripheral perfusion with metabolic acidosis, decreased urine output, and pulmonary edema. Arterial oxygen saturation approaches 90%.

Alternatively, a sudden deterioration takes place with rapidly progressive CHF and shock as the ductus arteriosus constricts (Fig. 41.5B). There is a decreased systemic perfusion and an increased pulmonary blood flow, which is largely independent of the pulmonary vascular resistance. The peripheral pulses are weak to absent. Renal, hepatic, coronary, and central nervous system perfusion is compromised, possibly resulting in acute tubular necrosis, necrotizing enterocolitis, or cerebral infarction or hemorrhage. A vicious cycle may also result from inadequate retrograde perfusion of the ascending aorta (coronary blood supply), with further myocardial dysfunction and continued compromise of coronary blood flow. The pulmonary to systemic flow ratio approaches infinity as systemic blood flow nears zero. Therefore, one has the paradoxical presentation of profound metabolic acidosis in the face of a relatively high PO_2 (70–100 mm Hg).

The arterial blood gas may represent the single best indicator of hemodynamic stability. Low arterial saturation (75%–80%) with normal pH indicates an acceptable balance of systemic and pulmonary blood flow with adequate peripheral perfusion, whereas elevated oxygen saturation (>90%) with acidosis represents significantly increased pulmonary and decreased systemic flow with probable myocardial dysfunction and secondary effects on other organ systems.

Resuscitation of these neonates involves pharmacologic maintenance of ductal patency with PGE_1 and ventilatory maneuvers to **increase** pulmonary resistance. In our experience, a mild respiratory acidosis (e.g., pH 7.35) is appropriate for most of these infants. It is important to note that **hyperventilation and/or supplemental oxygen is usually of no significant benefit and may be harmful** by causing excessive pulmonary vasodilation and pulmonary blood flow at the expense of the systemic blood flow.

Hypotension in these infants is more frequently caused by increased pulmonary blood flow (at the expense of systemic flow) rather than due to intrinsic myocardial dysfunction. Although small-to-moderate doses of inotropic agents are frequently beneficial, **large doses of inotropic agents may have a deleterious effect,** depending on the relative effects on the systemic and pulmonary vascular beds. Preferential selective elevations of systemic vascular tone will secondarily increase pulmonary blood flow, and careful monitoring of mean arterial blood pressure and arterial oxygen saturation is warranted.

Similar to the patient with critical aortic stenosis, in order for the neonate with hypoplastic left heart syndrome to benefit from a PGE_1 infusion, there must be at least a small patent foramen ovale to allow for effective systemic blood flow (pulmonary venous return) to cross the atrial septum and, ultimately, enter the systemic vascular bed through the ductus. An infant with hypoplastic left heart syndrome and a severely restrictive or absent patent foramen ovale will be critically ill with profound cyanosis (oxygen saturation <60%–65%) and will not improve after the institution of PGE_1. **In these neonates, emergent balloon dilation of the atrial septum may be necessary**.

Medical therapy may be briefly palliative; however, surgical therapy is necessary for survival of infants with hypoplastic left heart syndrome. After a period of medical stabilization and support to allow for recovery of ischemic organ system injury (particularly of the kidneys, liver, central nervous system, and the heart itself), surgical relief of left-sided obstruction is required. Surgical intervention involves either staged reconstruction (with a neonatal Norwood procedure followed by a Fontan operation later in childhood) or neonatal cardiac transplantation. Recent results from both reconstructive surgery and transplantation have vastly improved the outlook for infants born with this previously 100% fatal condition.

B. **Duct-dependent pulmonary blood flow.** This underlying physiology is shared by a diverse group of lesions with the common finding of restricted pulmonary blood flow due to severe pulmonary stenosis or complete pulmonary atresia. Closure of the ductus arteriosus results in marked cyanosis.

1. **Pulmonary stenosis** (see Fig. 41.6) with obstruction to pulmonary blood flow may occur at several levels: (i) within the body of the right ventricle; (ii) at the pulmonary valve (as pictured in Fig. 41.6); (iii) in the peripheral pulmonary arteries. Valvar pulmonary stenosis with an intact ventricular septum is the second most common form of congenital heart disease; "critical" obstruction occurs more rarely. Grading of the degree of pulmonary stenosis is similar to that of aortic stenosis (see V.A.1.) with severe pulmonary stenosis defined as a peak systolic gradient from right ventricle to pulmonary artery of 60 mm Hg or more. By convention, "critical" pulmonary stenosis is defined as severe valvar obstruction with associated hypoxemia due to a right-to-left shunt at the foramen ovale. Critical pulmonary stenosis may be associated with hypoplasia of the right ventricle and/or tricuspid valve and significant RV hypertrophy. The pressure in the right ventricle is often higher than the left ventricular pressure (i.e., suprasystemic) to be able to eject blood past the severe narrowing. Due to the longstanding (*in utero*) increased RV pressure, there is typically a hypertrophied, noncompliant right ventricle with a resultant increase in right atrial filling pressure. When right atrial pressure exceeds left atrial pressure, a right-to-left shunt at the foramen ovale results in cyanosis and hypoxemia. There may be an associated RV dysfunction and/or tricuspid regurgitation.

After initial stabilization of the patient and definitive diagnosis by echocardiography, transcatheter balloon valvotomy is the treatment of choice for this lesion, although surgical valvotomy may be used in specific cases. Despite successful relief of the obstruction during catheterization, cyanosis is usually not completely relieved but rather resolves gradually over the first weeks of life as the right ventricle becomes more compliant, tricuspid regurgitation lessens, and there is less right-to-left shunting at the atrial level. Successful balloon

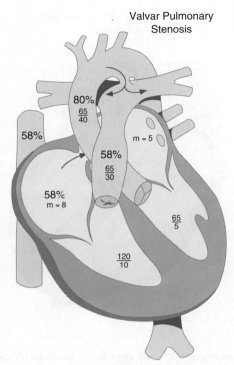

Valvar Pulmonary
Stenosis

Figure 41.6. Critical valvar pulmonary stenosis in a neonate with a nonrestrictive patent ductus arteriosus while receiving PGE₁. Typical anatomic and hemodynamic findings include (i) thickened, stenotic pulmonary valve; (ii) poststenotic dilatation of the main pulmonary artery with normal-sized branch pulmonary arteries; (iii) RV hypertrophy with suprasystemic pressure; (iv) a right-to-left shunt at the atrial level through the patent foramen ovale with systemic desaturation (80%); (v) suprasystemic RV pressure with a 55 mm Hg peak systolic ejection gradient; (vi) systemic pulmonary artery pressure (due to the nonrestrictive patent ductus); (vii) pulmonary blood flow through the patent ductus arteriosus. PGE₁ = prostaglandin E1. m = mean value.

valvuloplasty is associated with excellent clinical results among patients; the need for repeat procedures is quite low.

2. **Pulmonary atresia with intact ventricular septum ("hypoplastic right heart syndrome,"** see Fig. 41.7) is comparable to hypoplastic left heart syndrome in that there is atresia of the pulmonary valve with varying degrees of RV and tricuspid valve hypoplasia. Perhaps the most important associated anomaly is the presence of coronary artery–myocardial–RV sinusoidal connections. The coronary arteries may be quite abnormal, including areas of stenoses or complete atresia. Myocardial perfusion may therefore be dependent on a hypertensive right ventricle to supply the distal coronary arteries; surgical relief of the pulmonary atresia (with an RV-to-pulmonary artery connection) may lead to myocardial infarction and death. The presence of sinusoidal connections between the right ventricle and the coronary arteries is associated with

PA/IVS

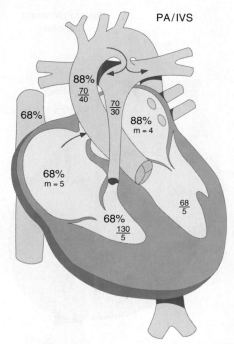

Figure 41.7. Pulmonary atresia (PA) with intact ventricular septum (IVS) in a neonate with a nonrestrictive patent ductus arteriosus while receiving PGE$_1$. Typical anatomic and hemodynamic findings include (i) hypertrophied, hypoplastic right ventricle; (ii) hypoplastic tricuspid valve and pulmonary annulus; (iii) atresia of the pulmonary valve with no antegrade flow; (iv) suprasystemic RV pressure; (v) pulmonary blood flow through the patent ductus; (vi) right-to-left shunt at the atrial level with systemic desaturation. Many patients have significant coronary abnormalities with sinusoidal or fistulous connections to the hypertensive right ventricle or significant coronary stenoses (not shown). PGE$_1$ = prostaglandin E1. m = mean value.

poorer long-term survival. Because there is no outlet of the right ventricle, there is typically suprasystemic pressure in the right ventricle and some tricuspid regurgitation. There is an obligatory right-to-left shunt at the atrial level, and pulmonary blood flow is entirely dependent on a PDA.

Although the cornerstone of initial management is PGE$_1$ infusion to maintain ductal patency, a more permanent and reliable form of pulmonary blood flow must be surgically created for the infant to survive. Surgical management is often preceded by catheterization to define the coronary artery anatomy. In patients without significant coronary abnormalities, pulmonary blood flow is established by creating an outflow for the right ventricle by pulmonary valvotomy and/or RV outflow tract augmentation. Usually, at the time of this procedure, a systemic-to-pulmonary artery shunt (most often a Blalock-Taussig shunt) is constructed to also augment pulmonary blood flow. In patients with "RV-dependent" coronary arteries, a systemic-to-pulmonary artery shunt is the typical procedure performed in the neonate.

3. Tricuspid atresia (see Fig. 41.8) involves complete absence of the tricuspid valve and, therefore, no direct communication from right atrium to right ventricle. The right ventricle may be severely hypoplastic or completely absent. More than 90% of patients have an associated ventricular septal defect, allowing blood to pass from the left ventricle to the RV outflow and pulmonary arteries. Most patients have some form of additional pulmonary stenosis. In 70% of cases, the great arteries are normally aligned with the ventricles; however, in the remaining 30%, the great arteries are transposed. An atrial level communication is necessary for blood to exit the right atrium; there is an obligatory right-to-left shunt at this level. In patients with normally related great arteries, pulmonary blood flow is derived from the right ventricle; if the right ventricle (or its connection with the left ventricle through a ventricular septal defect) is severely diminutive, the pulmonary blood flow may be duct dependent; closure of the ductus leads to profound hypoxemia and acidosis.

Immediate medical management is primarily aimed at maintenance of adequate pulmonary blood flow. In the usual case of severe pulmonary stenosis

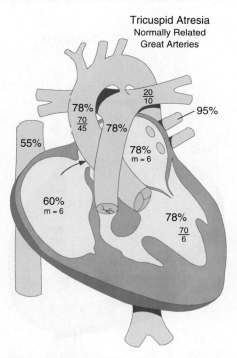

Tricuspid Atresia
Normally Related
Great Arteries

Figure 41.8. Tricuspid atresia with normally related great arteries and a small patent ductus arteriosus. Typical anatomic and hemodynamic findings include (i) atresia of the tricuspid valve; (ii) hypoplasia of the right ventricle; (iii) restriction to pulmonary blood flow at two levels: a (usually) small ventricular septal defect and a stenotic pulmonary valve; (iv) all systemic venous return must pass through the patent foramen ovale to reach the left ventricle; (v) complete mixing at the left atrial level, with systemic oxygen saturation of 78% (in FiO₂ of 0.21), suggesting balanced systemic and pulmonary blood flow ("single ventricle physiology"—see text). m = mean value.

and limited pulmonary blood flow, PGE_1 infusion maintains pulmonary blood flow through the ductus arteriosus. Surgical creation of a more permanent source of pulmonary blood flow (usually a Blalock-Taussig shunt) is undertaken as soon as possible. More complex cases (e.g., with transposition) may require more extensive palliative procedures.

4. **Tetralogy of Fallot** (see Fig. 41.9) consists of RV outflow obstruction, a ventricular septal defect (of the anterior malalignment variety), "overriding" of the aorta over the ventricular septum, and hypertrophy of the right ventricle. There is a wide spectrum of anatomic variation encompassing these findings, depending particularly on the site and severity of the RV outflow obstruction. The severely cyanotic neonate with tetralogy most likely has severe RV outflow tract obstruction and a large right-to-left shunt at the ventricular level through the large ventricular septal defect. Pulmonary blood flow may be duct dependent.

Immediate medical management involves establishing adequate pulmonary blood flow usually with PGE_1 infusion, although some have attempted balloon dilation of the RV outflow tract. Detailed anatomic definition particularly regarding

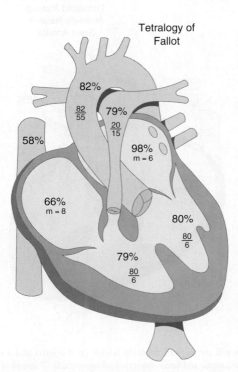

Figure 41.9. Tetralogy of Fallot. Typical anatomic and hemodynamic findings include (i) an anteriorly displaced infundibular septum, resulting in subpulmonary stenosis, a large ventricular septal defect, and overriding of the aorta over the muscular septum; (ii) hypoplasia of the pulmonary valve, main, and branch pulmonary arteries; (iii) equal right and left ventricular pressures; (iv) a right-to-left shunt at ventricular level, with a systemic oxygen saturation of 82%. m = mean value.

coronary artery anatomy, the presence of additional ventricular septal defects, and the sources of pulmonary blood flow (systemic to pulmonary collateral vessels) are necessary before surgical intervention. If echocardiography is not able to fully show these details, then diagnostic catheterization is performed. Surgical repair of the **asymptomatic** child with tetralogy of Fallot is usually recommended within the first 6 months of life. The **symptomatic** (i.e., severely cyanotic) neonate should have operative intervention. Complete repair is generally performed at our institution, although a systemic-to-pulmonary artery shunt is sometimes employed in unusual cases such as multiple ventricular septal defects or coronary anomalies.

5. **Ebstein anomaly** (see Figs. 41.10A and 41.10B) is an uncommon but grave anatomic lesion when it presents in the neonatal period. Anatomically, there is "downward displacement" of the tricuspid valve into the body of the right

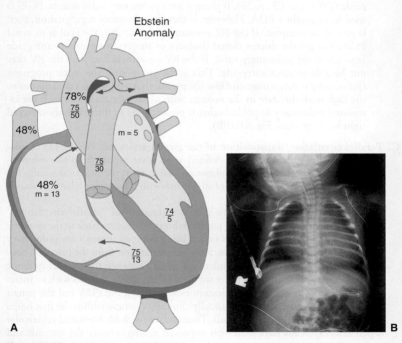

Ebstein
Anomaly

Figure 41.10. A: Ebstein anomaly (with large, nonrestrictive ductus arteriosus). Typical anatomic and hemodynamic findings include (i) inferior displacement of the tricuspid valve into the right ventricle, which may also cause subpulmonary obstruction, (ii) diminutive muscular right ventricle, (iii) marked enlargement of the right atrium due to "atrialized" portion of right ventricle as well as tricuspid regurgitation, (iv) right-to-left shunting at the atrial level (note arterial oxygen saturation of 78%), (v) a left-to-right shunt and pulmonary hypertension secondary to a large patent ductus arteriosus supplying the pulmonary blood flow, (vi) low cardiac output (note low mixed venous oxygen saturation in the superior vena cava). **B:** Chest radiograph in a neonate with severe Ebstein anomaly and no significant pulmonary blood flow from the ductus arteriosus. The cardiomegaly is due to marked dilation of the right atrium. The pulmonary vascular markings are diminished due to the decreased pulmonary blood flow. Hypoplasia of the lungs is common due to the large heart causing a "space-occupying lesion." m = mean value.

ventricle. The tricuspid valve is frequently regurgitant resulting in marked right atrial enlargement and a large right-to-left shunt at the atrial level; there is little forward flow out the RV outflow tract into the pulmonary circulation. The prognosis for neonates presenting with profound cyanosis due to Ebstein anomaly is quite grave. Surgical options are controversial and are generally reserved for the severely symptomatic child. Further complicating the medical condition, Ebstein anomaly is often associated with Wolff-Parkinson-White (WPW) syndrome and supraventricular tachycardia (SVT).

Medical management is aimed at supporting the neonate through the initial period of transitional circulation. Because of elevated pulmonary vascular resistance, pulmonary blood flow may be quite severely limited with profound hypoxemia and acidosis as a result. Medical treatment includes treatment of pulmonary hypertension with oxygen, alkalosis, and inhaled nitric oxide (iNO) (see Chap. 36). If there is total pulmonary valve atresia, PGE_1 is used to maintain a PDA. However, if there is pulmonary regurgitation, then it gets more complex. If the RV pressure is high (>20), the goal is to avoid PGE_1 and get the ductus closed (Indocin or surgery) to promote antegrade flow across the pulmonary valve. If the RV pressure is low, then the RV may not be able to eject antegrade. This is the group with the worst prognosis (pulmonary regurgitation and low RV pressure). An important contributor to the high mortality rate in the neonate with severe Ebstein anomaly is the associated pulmonary hypoplasia that is present (due to the massively enlarged right heart *in utero*, Fig. 41.10B).

C. **Parallel circulation/transposition of the great arteries** (see Fig. 41.11). **Transposition of the great arteries** is defined as an aorta arising from the morphologically right ventricle and the pulmonary artery from the morphologically left ventricle. Approximately one-half of all patients with transposition have an associated ventricular septal defect.

In the usual arrangement, this creates a situation of "parallel circulations" with systemic venous return being pumped through the aorta back to the systemic circulation and pulmonary venous return being pumped through the pulmonary artery to the pulmonary circulation. Following separation from the placenta, neonates with transposition are dependent on mixing between the parallel systemic and pulmonary circulations in order for them to survive. In patients with an intact ventricular septum, this communication exists through the PDA and the patent foramen ovale. These patients are usually clinically cyanotic within the first hours of life leading to their early diagnosis. Those infants with an associated ventricular septal defect typically have somewhat improved mixing between the systemic and pulmonary circulations and may not be as severely cyanotic.

In neonates with transposition of the great arteries and an intact ventricular septum, a very low arterial PaO_2 (15–20 torr) with high $PaCO_2$ (despite adequate chest motion and ventilation) and metabolic acidosis are markers for severely decreased effective pulmonary blood flow and need urgent attention. The initial management of the severely hypoxemic patient with transposition includes (i) **ensure adequate mixing** between the two parallel circuits and (ii) **maximize mixed venous oxygen saturation**.

In patients who do not respond with an increased arterial oxygen saturation to the opening of the ductus arteriosus with prostaglandin (usually these neonates have very restrictive atrial defects and/or pulmonary hypertension), **the foramen ovale should be emergently enlarged by balloon atrial septostomy.**

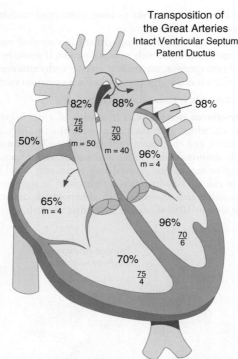

Figure 41.11. Transposition of the great arteries with an intact ventricular septum, a large patent ductus arteriosus (on PGE_1) and atrial septal defect (status post balloon atrial septostomy). Note the following: (i) the aorta arises from the anatomic right ventricle, and the pulmonary artery from the anatomic left ventricle; (ii) "transposition physiology," with a higher oxygen saturation in the pulmonary artery than in the aorta; (iii) "mixing" between the parallel circulations (see text) at the atrial (after balloon atrial septostomy) and ductal levels; (iv) shunting from the left atrium to the right atrium through the atrial septal defect (not shown) with equalization of atrial pressures; (v) shunting from the aorta to the pulmonary artery through the ductus arteriosus; (vi) pulmonary hypertension due to a large ductus arteriosus. m = mean value, PGE_1 = prostaglandin E_1.

Hyperventilation and treatment with sodium bicarbonate are important maneuvers to promote alkalosis, lower pulmonary vascular resistance, and increase pulmonary blood flow (which increases atrial mixing following septostomy).

In transposition of the great arteries, most of the systemic blood flow is recirculated systemic venous return. In the presence of poor mixing, much can be gained by increasing the mixed venous oxygen saturation, which is the **major determinant of systemic arterial oxygen saturation**. These maneuvers include (i) decreasing the whole body oxygen consumption (muscle relaxants, sedation, mechanical ventilation) and (ii) improving oxygen delivery (increase cardiac output with inotropic agents, increase oxygen-carrying capacity by treating anemia). Coexisting causes of pulmonary venous desaturation (e.g., pneumothorax) should also be sought and treated. Increasing the FiO_2 to 100% will have little effect on the arterial PO_2, unless it serves to lower pulmonary vascular resistance and increase pulmonary blood flow.

In the current era, definitive management is a surgical correction with an arterial switch operation in the early neonatal period. If severe hypoxemia persists despite medical management, mechanical support with extracorporeal membrane oxygenation (ECMO) or an urgent arterial switch operation may be indicated.

D. Lesions with complete intracardiac mixing

1. **Truncus arteriosus** (see Fig. 41.12) consists of a single great artery arising from the heart, which gives rise to (in order) the coronary arteries, the pulmonary arteries, and the brachiocephalic arteries. The truncal valve is often anatomically abnormal (only 50% are tricuspid), and is frequently thickened, stenotic, and/or regurgitant. A coexisting ventricular septal defect is present in >98% of cases. The aortic arch is right-sided in approximately one-third of the cases; other arch anomalies such as hypoplasia, coarctation, and interruption are seen in 10% of cases. Extracardiac anomalies are present in 20%

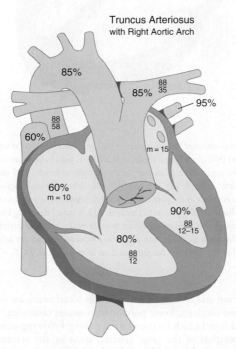

Figure 41.12. Truncus arteriosus (with right aortic arch). Typical anatomic and hemodynamic findings include (i) a single artery arises from the conotruncus giving rise to coronary arteries (not shown), pulmonary arteries, and brachiocephalic vessels; (ii) abnormal truncal valve (quadricuspid shown) with stenosis and/or regurgitation common; (iii) right-sided aortic arch (occurs in ~30% of cases); (iv) large conoventricular ventricular septal defect; (v) pulmonary artery hypertension with a large left-to-right shunt (note superior vena cava oxygen saturation of 60% and pulmonary artery oxygen saturation of 85%); (vi) complete mixing (of the systemic and pulmonary venous return) occurs at the great vessel level. m = mean value.

to 40% of cases. Thirty-five percent of the patients with truncus arteriosus have a deletion of chromosome 22 at 22q11, detectable by fluorescence *in situ* hybridization (FISH) testing.

The overwhelming majority of infants with truncus arteriosus present with symptoms of CHF in the first weeks of life. The infants may be somewhat cyanotic, but CHF symptoms and signs are usually dominant. The pulmonary blood flow is increased, with significant pulmonary hypertension common. The natural history of truncus arteriosus is quite bleak. Left unrepaired, only 15% to 30% survive the first year of life. Furthermore, in survivors of the immediate neonatal period, the occurrence of accelerated irreversible pulmonary vascular disease is common, making surgical repair in the neonatal period (or as soon as the diagnosis is made) the treatment of choice. "Medical management" of heart failure would be considered only a temporizing measure until surgical correction can be accomplished.

2. **Total anomalous pulmonary venous connection** (see Figs. 41.13A and 41.13B) occurs when all pulmonary veins drain into the systemic venous system with complete mixing of pulmonary and systemic venous return usually in the right atrium. The systemic blood flow is therefore dependent on an obligate shunt through the patent foramen ovale into the left heart. The anomalous connections of the pulmonary veins may be (i) supracardiac (usually into the right superior vena cava or to the innominate vein through a persistent vertical vein), (ii) cardiac (usually to the right atrium or coronary sinus), (iii) subdiaphragmatic (usually into the portal system), or (iv) mixed drainage.

   In patients with total connection below the diaphragm, the pathway is frequently obstructed with severely limited pulmonary blood flow, pulmonary hypertension, and profound cyanosis. This form of total anomalous pulmonary venous connection is a surgical emergency, with minimal beneficial effects from medical management. Although PGE_1 will maintain ductal patency, the limitation of pulmonary blood flow in these patients is **not** due to limited antegrade flow into the pulmonary circuit, but rather due to outflow obstruction at the pulmonary veins. In the current era of prostaglandin, ventilatory support, and advanced medical intensive care, obstructed total anomalous pulmonary venous connection represents one of the few remaining lesions that require emergent, "middle of the night" surgical intervention. Early recognition of the problem (Fig. 41.13B) and prompt surgical intervention (surgical anastomosis of the pulmonary venous confluence to the left atrium) are necessary for the infant to survive. Patients with a mild degree of obstruction typically have minimal symptoms, with many neonates escaping recognition until later in infancy when they present with signs and symptoms of CHF.

3. **Complex single ventricles.** There are multiple complex anomalies that share the common physiology of complete mixing of the systemic and pulmonary venous return, frequently with anomalous connections of the systemic and/or pulmonary veins, and with obstruction to one of the great vessels (usually the pulmonary artery). In cases with associated polysplenia or asplenia and abnormalities of visceral situs, the term *heterotaxy syndrome* is frequently applied. Physiologically, systemic blood flow and pulmonary blood flow is determined by the balance of anatomic and/or vascular resistance in the systemic and pulmonary circulations. In the well-balanced single ventricle, the oxygen saturation in the pulmonary artery and the aorta will be essentially the same (usually in the high 70% to low 80% range) with a normal pH on

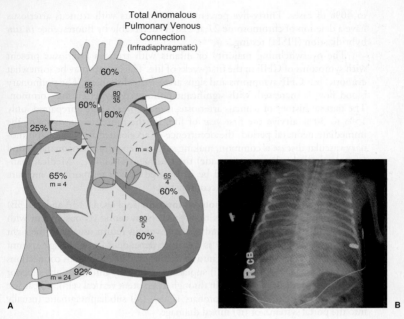

Total Anomalous
Pulmonary Venous
Connection
(Infradiaphragmatic)

A **B**

Figure 41.13. A: Infradiaphragmatic total anomalous pulmonary venous connection. Note the following: (i) pulmonary venous confluence does not connect with the left atrium but descends to connect with the portal circulation below the diaphragm. This connection is frequently severely obstructed; (ii) obstruction to pulmonary venous return results in significantly elevated pulmonary venous pressures, decreased pulmonary blood flow, pulmonary edema, and pulmonary venous desaturation (92%); (iii) systemic to suprasystemic pressure in the pulmonary artery (in the absence of a patent ductus arteriosus, pulmonary artery pressures may exceed systemic pressures when severe pulmonary venous obstruction is present); (iv) all systemic blood flow must be derived through a right-to-left shunt at the foramen ovale; (v) nearly equal oxygen saturations in all chambers of the heart (i.e., complete mixing at right atrial level), with severe hypoxemia (systemic oxygen saturation 60%) and low cardiac output (mixed venous oxygen saturation 25%). **B:** Chest radiograph in a 16-hour-old neonate with severe infradiaphragmatic obstruction to pulmonary venous return. Note the pulmonary edema, small heart, and hyperinflated lungs (on mechanical ventilation). Despite high inflating and positive end-expiratory pressures and an FiO_2 of 1, the arterial blood gas revealed a pH of 7.02, arterial carbon dioxide tension ($PaCO_2$) of 84, and an arterial oxygen tension (PaO_2) of 23 torr. Emergent surgical management is indicated. m = mean value.

arterial blood gas ("single ventricle physiology"). It is beyond the scope of this chapter to define this heterogeneous group of patients further. Although all will fail a hyperoxia test, most have significantly abnormal ECGs, and the diagnosis of complex congenital heart disease is rarely in doubt (even before anatomic confirmation with echocardiography). As there is a complete mixing of venous return and essentially a single pumping chamber, initial management is similar to that described for hypoplastic left heart syndrome (see V.A.4.).

E. **Left-to-right shunt lesions.** For the most part, infants with pure left-to-right shunt lesions are not diagnosed because of severe systemic illness but rather due to the finding of a murmur or symptoms of CHF usually occurring in the late neonatal period or beyond. The lesion of this group most likely to require attention in the neonatal nursery is that of a PDA.

1. **PDA** is not particularly common in term newborns and rarely causes CHF. However, the frequency that a premature neonate will develop a hemodynamically significant left-to-right shunt through a PDA is inversely proportional to advancing gestational age and weight.

The typical presentation of a PDA begins with a harsh systolic ejection murmur heard over the entire precordium, but loudest at the left upper sternal border and left infraclavicular areas. As the pulmonary vascular resistance decreases, the intensity of the murmur increases and later becomes continuous (i.e., extends through the second heart sound). The peripheral pulses increase in amplitude ("bounding pulses"), the pulse pressure widens to >25 mm Hg, the precordial impulse becomes hyperdynamic, and the patient's respiratory status deteriorates (manifesting as tachypnea or apnea, carbon dioxide retention, and an increasing mechanical ventilation requirement). Serial chest x-rays show an increase in heart size, and the lungs may appear more radiopaque.

It is important to remember that this typical progression of clinical signs is **not specific** only for a hemodynamically significant PDA. Other lesions may produce bounding pulses, a hyperdynamic precordium, and cardiac enlargement (e.g., an arteriovenous fistula or an aorticopulmonary window). Generally, however, the clinical assessment of a premature infant with the typical findings of a hemodynamically significant ductus is adequate to guide therapeutic decisions. If the diagnosis is in doubt, an echocardiogram will clarify the anatomic diagnosis.

Initial medical management includes increased ventilatory support, fluid restriction, and diuretic therapy. In symptomatic patients, indomethacin is initially used for nonsurgical closure of PDA in the premature neonate and is effective in approximately 80% of cases. Birth weight does not affect the efficacy of indomethacin, and there is no increase in complications associated with surgery after unsuccessful indomethacin therapy. In asymptomatic patients, the efficacy of prophylactic administration of indomethacin is controversial. Adverse reactions to indomethacin include transient oliguria, electrolyte abnormalities, decreased platelet function, and hypoglycemia. Contraindications to use of indomethacin and dosing information are noted in Appendix A.

Indications for closure of a PDA vary from institution to institution. In general, we recommend medical treatment for mechanically ventilated premature infants weighing <1,000 g when a patent ductus first becomes apparent, regardless of the presence of signs or symptoms of a significant left-to-right shunt. For infants larger than 1,000 g, we recommend treatment with indomethacin only after cardiovascular or respiratory signs of a hemodynamically significant ductus develop. Some infants who fail to respond to the first course of treatment with indomethacin may respond to a second course.

Symptomatic patients who do not respond to a second treatment with indomethacin or cannot tolerate indomethacin therapy due to side effects should undergo surgical ligation following echocardiographic documentation of the patent ductus.

Ibuprofen has been recently approved for use in the newborn in the United States. It is as effective in closing a PDA as indomethacin but appears to have a better safety profile (more normal urine output, less elevation of blood urea nitrogen [BUN] and creatinine, less decrease in mesenteric blood flow, and improved autoregulation of cerebral blood flow). Rates of necrotizing enterocolitis, gastrointestinal bleeding, and intraventricular hemorrhage were not significantly diminished in the group treated with ibuprofen compared with those treated with indomethacin. Unlike indomethacin, early prophylactic use of ibuprofen has not been found to reduce the rate of intraventricular hemorrhage. The ibuprofen lysine has not been associated with an increased incidence of pulmonary hypertension and chronic lung disease reported with the use of the ibuprofen tris-hydroxymethyl aminomethane (THAM) preparation. Pharmacokinetic studies have not shown that ibuprofen lysine displaces bilirubin from albumin. We are now using ibuprofen lysine (NeoProfen) as an option for PDA closure after the first day of life (see Appendix A).

2. **Complete atrioventricular canal** (see Fig. 41.14) consists of a combination of defects in the (i) endocardial portion of the atrial septum, (ii) the inlet portion

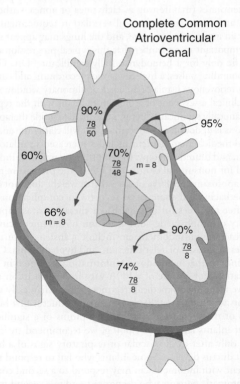

Figure 41.14. Complete common atrioventricular canal. Typical anatomic and hemodynamic findings include (i) large atrial and ventricular septal defects of the endocardial cushion type; (ii) single, atrioventricular valve; (iii) pulmonary artery hypertension (due to large ventricular septal defect); (iv) bidirectional shunting (with mild hypoxemia) at atrial and ventricular level when pulmonary vascular resistance is elevated in the initial neonatal period. With subsequent fall in pulmonary vascular resistance, the shunt becomes predominantly left-to-right with symptoms of congestive heart failure. m = mean value.

of the ventricular septum, and (iii) a common, single atrioventricular valve. Because of the large net left-to-right shunt, which increases as the pulmonary vascular resistance falls, these infants typically present early in life with CHF. There may be some degree of cyanosis as well, particularly in the immediate neonatal period before the pulmonary vascular resistance has fallen. In the absence of associated RV outflow tract obstruction, pulmonary artery pressures are at systemic levels; pulmonary vascular resistance is frequently elevated, particularly in patients with trisomy 21.

Approximately 70% of infants with complete atrioventricular canal have trisomy 21; notation of the phenotypic findings of Down syndrome often lead to evaluation of the patient for possible congenital heart disease (Table 41.5). In the immediate neonatal period, these infants may have an equivocal hyperoxia test because there may be some right-to-left shunting through the large intracardiac connections. Symptoms of congestive failure ensue during the first weeks of life as the pulmonary vascular resistance falls, and the patient develops a marked left-to-right shunt. These patients have a characteristic ECG finding of a "superior axis" (QRS axis from 0 to 180 degrees; see Fig. 41.15) which can be a useful clue for the presence of congenital heart disease in an infant with trisomy 21.

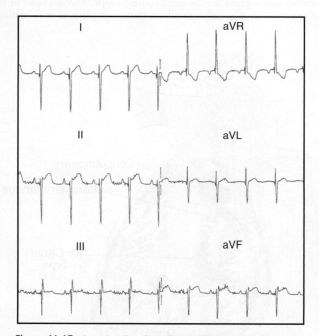

Figure 41.15. Superior ("northwest") axis as seen on the electrocardiogram (only frontal plane leads shown) in a newborn with complete atrioventricular canal. Note the initial upward deflection of the QRS complex (and subsequent predominantly negative deflection) in leads I and aVF. A superior axis (0–180 degrees) is present in 95% of patients with endocardial cushion defects.

Most patients with complete atrioventricular canal will require medical treatment for symptomatic CHF, although prolonged medical therapy in patients with failure to thrive and symptomatic heart failure is not warranted. Complete surgical repair is undertaken electively approximately from 4 to 6 months of age, with earlier repair in symptomatic patients. In our experience, corrective surgery for complete atrioventricular canal can be performed successfully in early infancy with good results.

3. **Ventricular septal defect** is the most common cause of CHF after the initial neonatal period. Moderate-to-large ventricular septal defects become hemodynamically significant as the pulmonary vascular resistance decreases and pulmonary blood flow increases due to a left-to-right shunt across the defect. As this usually takes 2 to 4 weeks to develop, term neonates with ventricular septal defect and symptoms of CHF should be investigated for coexisting anatomic abnormalities, such as left ventricular outflow tract obstruction, coarctation of the aorta, or PDA. Premature infants, who have a lower initial pulmonary vascular resistance, may develop clinical symptoms of heart failure earlier or require longer mechanical ventilation compared with term infants.

Ventricular septal defects may occur anywhere in the ventricular septum and are usually classified by their location (see Fig. 41.16). Defects in the membranous septum are the most common type. The diagnosis of ventricular septal defect is usually initially suspected on physical examination of the

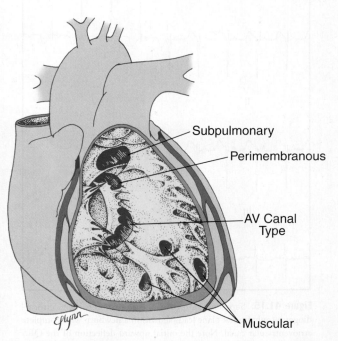

Figure 41.16. Diagram of types of ventricular septal defects as viewed from the right ventricle. AV = arteriovenous (From Fyler DC, ed. *Nadas' Pediatric Cardiology*. 1st ed. Philadelphia, PA: Hanley & Belfus, Inc., 1992.)

infant; echocardiography confirms the diagnosis and localizes the defect in the ventricular septum. Because a large number (as many as 90% depending on the anatomic type and size) of ventricular septal defects may close spontaneously in the first few months of life, surgery is usually deferred beyond the neonatal period. In large series, only 15% of all patients with ventricular septal defects ever become clinically symptomatic. Medical management of CHF includes digoxin, diuretics, and caloric supplementation. Growth failure is the most common symptom of CHF not fully compensated by medical management. When it occurs, failure to thrive is an indication for surgical repair of the defect.

F. **Cardiac surgery in the neonate.** In the past, because of the perceived high risk of open-heart surgery early in life, critically ill neonates were mostly subjected to palliative procedures or prolonged medical management. The unrepaired circulation and residual hemodynamic abnormalities frequently resulted in secondary problems of the heart, lungs, and brain, as well as in more nonspecific problems of failure to thrive, frequent hospitalizations, and infections. In addition, there are difficult-to-quantitate psychologic burdens to the family of a chronically ill infant.

   Low birth weight should not be considered as absolute contraindication for surgical repair. In one series, prolonged medical therapy in low birth weight infants to achieve further weight gain in the presence of a significant hemodynamic burden did not improve the survival rate, and prolonged intensive care management was associated with nosocomial complications. We feel that the symptomatic neonate with congenital heart disease should be repaired as early as possible, to prevent the secondary sequelae of the congenital lesion on the heart, lungs, and brain.

   Recently, improvements in surgical techniques, cardiopulmonary bypass, and intensive care of the neonate and infant have resulted in significant improvements in surgical mortality and quality of life in the survivors. It is beyond the scope of this chapter to describe the multiple surgical procedures currently employed in the management of congenital heart disease; the reader is referred to Table 41.9 and general texts of cardiac surgery.

VI. ACQUIRED HEART DISEASE

A. **Myocarditis** may occur in the neonate as an isolated illness or as a component of a generalized illness with associated hepatitis and/or encephalitis. Myocarditis is usually the result of a viral infection (coxsackie, rubella, and varicella are most common), although other infectious agents, such as bacteria and fungi, as well as noninfectious conditions, such as autoimmune diseases also may cause myocarditis. Although the clinical presentation (and in some cases endomyocardial biopsy) makes the diagnosis, specific identification of the etiologic agent is currently not made in most cases.

   The infant with acute myocarditis presents with signs and symptoms of CHF (see III.B.1.) and/or arrhythmia (see VIII.). The course of the illness is frequently fulminant and fatal; however, full recovery of ventricular function may occur if the infant can be supported and survive the acute illness. Supportive care, including supplemental oxygen, diuretics, inotropic agents, afterload reduction, and mechanical ventilation is frequently used. In severe cases, mechanical support of the myocardium with ECMO or ventricular assist devices can be considered. Care should be used when administering digoxin, due to the potential for the potentiation of arrhythmias or complete heart block (CHB).

Table 41.9	Common Neonatal Operations and Their Early Sequelae			
		Early postoperative sequelae		
Lesion	Surgical repair (eponym)	Common		Rare
Corrective procedures				
TGA	Arterial switch procedure (Jatene) 1. Division and reanastomosis of PA to RV and aorta to LV (anatomically correct ventricles) 2. Translocation of coronary arteries 3. Closure of septal defects if present	Transient decrease in cardiac output 6–12 hour after surgery		Coronary ostial stenosis or occlusion/sudden death Hemidiaphragm paresis Chylothorax
	Atrial switch procedure (Senning or Mustard) 1. Intra-atrial baffling of systemic venous return to LV (to PA) and pulmonary venous return to RV (to AO) 2. Closure of septal defects if present	Supraventricular tachycardia Sick sinus syndrome Tricuspid regurgitation		Pulmonary or systemic venous obstruction
TOF	1. Patch closure of VSD through ventriculotomy or right atrium 2. Enlargement of RVOT with infundibular patch or muscle bundle resection 3. ± Pulmonary valvotomy 4. ± Transannular RV to PA patch 5. ± RV to PA conduit	Pulmonary regurgitation (if transannular patch, valvotomy, or nonvalved conduit) Transient RV dysfunction Right-to-left shunt through PFO, usually resolves postoperatively as RV function improves		Residual left-to-right shunt at VSD patch Residual RVOT obstruction Junctional ectopic tachycardia Complete heart block

COA	Resection with end-to-end anastomosis, or Subclavian flap (Waldhaussen), or Patch augmentation	Systemic hypertension Absent left-arm pulse (if Waldhaussen)	Ileus Hemidiaphragm paresis Vocal cord paresis Chylothorax
PDA	Ligation (± division) of PDA using open thoracotomy and direct visualization or video-assisted thoracoscopic visualization	—	Hemidiaphragm paresis Vocal cord paresis Chylothorax Interruption of left PA or descending aorta
TAPVC	1. Reanastomosis of pulmonary venous confluence to posterior aspect of left atrium 2. Division of connecting vein	Pulmonary hypertension Transient low cardiac output	Residual pulmonary venous obstruction
Truncus arteriosus	1. Closure of VSD; baffling LV to truncus (neoaorta) 2. Removal of PAs from truncus 3. Conduit placement from RV to Pas	Reactive pulmonary hypertension Transient RV dysfunction with right-to-left shunt through PFO Hypocalcemia (DiGeorge syndrome)	Truncal valve stenosis or regurgitation Residual VSD Complete heart block
Palliative procedure HLHS[a]	Stage I (Norwood) 1. Connection of main PA to aorta with reconstruction of aortic arch 2. Systemic-to-pulmonary shunt 3. Atrial septectomy	Low systemic cardiac output due to excessive pulmonary blood flow	Aortic arch obstruction Restrictive atrial septal defect

(continued)

Table 41.9   Common Neonatal Operations and Their Early Sequelae *(Continued)*

Lesion	Surgical repair (eponym)	Early postoperative sequelae	
		Common	Rare
Complex lesions with decreased pulmonary blood flow[a]	Systemic-to-pulmonary shunt (using prosthetic tube = modified Blalock-Taussig shunt; using subclavian artery = classic Blalock-Taussig shunt)	Excessive pulmonary blood flow and mild congestive heart failure	Hemidiaphragm paresis Vocal cord paralysis Chylothorax Seroma
Complex lesions with excessive pulmonary blood flow[a]	Ligation of main PA, creation of systemic-to-pulmonary shunt PA band (prosthetic or Silastic constriction of main PA)		PA distortion Aneurysm of main PA

TGA = transposition of the great arteries; PA = pulmonary artery; RV = right ventricle; LV = left ventricle; AO = aorta; TOF = tetralogy of Fallot; VSD = ventricular septal defect; RVOT = right ventricular outflow tract; PFO = patent foramen ovale; PDA = patent ductus arteriosus; COA = coarctation of the aorta; TAPVC = total anomalous pulmonary venous connection; HLHS = hypoplastic left heart syndrome.
[a]In patients with a single ventricle, the goal is to separate pulmonary and systemic venous return, rerouting systemic venous blood directly to pulmonary arteries (Fontan operation) although this is done in late infancy or early childhood.
Source: Adapted from Wernovsky G, Erickson LC, Weasel DL. Cardiac emergencies. In: May HL, ed. *Emergency Medicine.* Boston, MA: Little, Brown and Company, 1992.

B. **Transient myocardial ischemia** with myocardial dysfunction may occur in any neonate with a history of perinatal asphyxia. Myocardial dysfunction may be associated with maternal autoimmune disease such as systemic lupus erythematosus. A tricuspid or mitral regurgitant murmur is often heard. An elevated serum creatine kinase MB fraction or cardiac troponin level may be helpful in determining the presence of myocardial damage. Supportive treatment is dictated by the severity of myocardial dysfunction.

C. **Hypertrophic and dilated cardiomyopathies** represent a rare and multifactorial complex of diseases, complete discussion of which is beyond the scope of this chapter. The differential diagnoses includes primary diseases (e.g., genetic causes as well as metabolic, storage, and neuromuscular disorders) or secondary diseases (e.g., end-stage infection, ischemic, endocrine, nutritional, drugs). The reader is referred to texts of pediatric cardiology for more complete discussion.

The most common hypertrophic cardiomyopathy presenting in neonates is that type seen in **infants born to diabetic mothers**. Echocardiographically and hemodynamically, these infants are indistinguishable from patients with other types of hypertrophic cardiomyopathy. They are different in one important respect: Their cardiomyopathy will completely resolve in 6 to 12 months. Noting a systolic ejection murmur, with or without CHF, in the infant of a diabetic mother should raise the question of congenital heart disease including hypertrophic cardiomyopathy. Treatment is supportive addressing the infant's particular symptoms of CHF. Propranolol has been used successfully in some patients with severe obstruction. Most patients require no specific care and no long-term cardiac follow-up (see Chap. 2).

VII. PHARMACOLOGY

A. **PGE$_1$.** PGE$_1$ has been used since the late 1970s to pharmacologically maintain patency of the ductus arteriosus in patients with duct-dependent systemic or pulmonary blood flow. PGE$_1$ must be administered as a continuous parenteral infusion. The usual starting dose is 0.05 to 0.1 μg/kg/minute. Once a therapeutic effect has been achieved, the dose may often be decreased to as low as 0.025 μg/kg/minute without loss of therapeutic effect. The response to PGE$_1$ is often immediate if patency of the ductus is important for the hemodynamic state of the infant. Failure to respond to PGE$_1$ may mean that the initial diagnosis was incorrect, the ductus is unresponsive to PGE$_1$ (usually only in an older infant), or the ductus is absent. The infusion site has no significant effect on the ductal response to PGE$_1$. Adverse reactions to PGE$_1$ include apnea (10%–12%), fever (14%), cutaneous flushing (10%), bradycardia (7%), seizures (4%), tachycardia (3%), cardiac arrest (1%), and edema (1%). See Table 41.10 for recommended mixing and dosing protocol for PGE$_1$.

B. **Sympathomimetic amine infusions** are the mainstay of pharmacologic therapies aimed at improving cardiac output and are discussed in detail elsewhere in this book (see Chap. 40). Catecholamines, endogenous (dopamine, epinephrine) or synthetic (dobutamine, isoproterenol), achieve an effect by stimulating myocardial and vascular adrenergic receptors. These agents must be given as a continuous parenteral infusion. They may be given in combination to the critically ill neonate in an effort to maximize the positive effects of each agent while minimizing the negative effects. While receiving catecholamine infusions, patients should be closely monitored, usually with an electrocardiographic monitor and an arterial catheter. Before beginning sympathomimetic amine

Table 41.10	Suggested Preparation of Prostaglandin E$_1$	
Add 1 ampule (500 μg/1 mL) to:	Concentration (μg/mL)	mL/hour × weight (kg), needed to infuse 0.1 μg/kg/min
200 mL	2.5	2.4
100 mL^a	5	1.2
50 mL	10	0.6

^{a}Usually, the most convenient dilution provides one-fourth of maintenance fluid requirement. Usually mix in dextrose-containing solution for newborns.
Source: Adapted from Wernovsky G, Erickson LC, Wessel DL. Cardiac emergencies. In: May HL, ed. Emergency Medicine, Boston: Little, Brown and Company, 1992.

infusions, intravascular volume should be repleted if necessary, although this may further compromise a congenital lesion with coexisting volume overload. Adverse reactions to catecholamine infusions include tachycardia (which increases myocardial oxygen consumption), atrial and ventricular arrhythmias, and increased afterload due to peripheral vasoconstriction (which may decrease cardiac output). See Table 41.11 for recommended mixing and dosing of the sympathomimetic amines.

Table 41.11	Sympathomimetic Amines	
Drug	Usual dose (μg/kg/min)	Effect
Dopamine	1–5	↑ urine output, ↑ HR (slightly), ↑ contractility
	6–10	↑ HR, ↑ contractility, ↑ BP
	11–20	↑ HR, ↑ contractility, ↑ SVR, ↑ BP
Dobutamine	1–20	↑ HR (slightly), ↑ contractility, ↓ SVR
Epinephrine	0.05–0.50	↑ HR, ↑ contractility, ↑ SVR, ↑ BP
Isoproterenol	0.05–1.00	↑ HR, ↑ contractility, ↓ SVR, ↓ PVR

These infusions may be mixed in intravenous solutions containing dextrose and/or saline. For neonates, dextrose-containing solutions with or without salt should usually be chosen. Calculation for convenient preparation of IV infusions:

$$6 \times \frac{\text{desired dose (μg/kg/min)}}{\text{desired rate (mL/h)}} \times \text{weight (kg)} = \frac{\text{mg drug}}{100 \text{ mL fluid}}$$

HR = heart rate; BP = blood pressure; SVR = systemic vascular resistance; PVR = pulmonary vascular resistance.

C. Afterload reducing agents

1. **Phosphodiesterase inhibitors** such as **milrinone** are **bipyridine** compounds that selectively inhibit cyclic nucleotide phosphodiesterase. These nonglycosidic and nonsympathomimetic agents exert their effect on cardiac performance by increasing cyclic adenosine monophosphate (cAMP) in the myocardial and vascular muscle, but do so independently of β-receptors. Cyclic AMP promotes improved contraction through calcium regulation by means of two mechanisms: (i) activation of protein kinase (which catalyzes the transfer of phosphate groups from adenosine triphosphate [ATP]) leading to faster calcium entry through the calcium channels, and (ii) activation of calcium pumps in the sarcoplasmic reticulum resulting in release of calcium.

   There are three major effects of phosphodiesterase inhibitors: (i) increased inotropy, with increased contractility and cardiac output as a result of cAMP-mediated increase in trans-sarcolemmal calcium flux; (ii) vasodilatation, with increase in arteriolar and venous capacitance as a result of cAMP-mediated increase in uptake of calcium and decrease in calcium available for contraction; and (iii) increased lusitropy, or improved relaxation properties during diastole.

   Indications for use include low cardiac output with myocardial dysfunction and elevated systemic vascular resistance (SVR) not accompanied by severe hypotension. Side effects have been minimal and are typically the need for volume infusions (5–10 mL/kg) following loading dose administration. See Appendix A for dosing information.

   The use of phosphodiesterase inhibitors after cardiac surgery in the pediatric patient population has been shown to increase cardiac index and decrease SVR without a significant increase in heart rate. Phosphodiesterase inhibitors are the second-line drug (after dopamine) in the treatment of low cardiac output in neonates, infants, and children following cardiopulmonary bypass in our institution.

2. **Other vasodilators** improve low cardiac output principally by decreasing impedance to ventricular ejection; these effects are especially helpful after cardiac surgery in children and in adults when SVR is particularly elevated.

   Sodium nitroprusside is the most widely used afterload reducing agent. It acts as a nitric oxide donor, increasing intracellular cyclic guanosine monophosphate (cGMP), which effects relaxation of vascular smooth muscle in both arterioles and veins. The overall effect is a decrease in atrial filling pressure and SVR with a concomitant increase in cardiac output. The vasodilatory effects of nitroprusside occur within minutes with intravenous administration. The principal metabolites of sodium nitroprusside are thiocyanate and cyanide; thiocyanate toxicity is unusual in children with normal hepatic and renal function, and monitoring of cyanide and thiocyanate concentrations in children may not be correlated with clinical signs of toxicity.

   In neonates with low cardiac output, there may be an increase in urine output and an improvement in perfusion with institution of nitroprusside, but there can also be a significant drop in blood pressure necessitating care in its use.

   Many other agents have been used as arterial and venous vasodilators to treat hypertension, reduce ventricular afterload and SVR, and improve cardiac output. A second nitrovasodilator, **nitroglycerine**, principally **a venous dilator**, also has a rapid onset of action and a short half-life (<2 minutes). Tolerance may develop after several days of continuous infusion. Nitroglycerine is used extensively in adult cardiac units for patients with ischemic heart disease; experience in pediatric patients is more limited. **Hydralazine** is more typically used for acute hypertension; its relatively long half-life limits its use in postoperative patients with labile hemodynamics. The angiotensin-converting enzyme inhibitor **enalapril** similarly has a relatively long half-life (2–4 hours), which limits its use in the acute setting. **β-blockers** (e.g., propranolol, esmolol, labetolol), although excellent in reducing blood pressure, may have deleterious effects on ventricular function. **Calcium channel blockers** (e.g., verapamil) may cause acute and severe hypotension and bradycardia in the neonate and should **rarely be used**. All intravenous vasodilators must be used cautiously in patients with moderate-to-severe lung disease; their use has been associated with increased intrapulmonary shunting and acute reductions of PaO_2.

D. Digoxin (see Appendix A) remains important for the treatment of CHF and arrhythmia. A "digitalizing dose" (with a total dose of 30 μg/kg in 24 hours for term infants and 20 μg/kg in 24 hours in premature infants) is usually used only for treatment of arrhythmias or severe heart failure. One-half of this **total digitalizing dose (TDD)** may be given IV, IM, or PO, followed by one-fourth of the TDD every 8 to 12 hours for the remaining two doses. An initial maintenance dose of one-fourth to one-third of the TDD (range 5–10 μg/kg/day) may then be adjusted according to the patient's clinical response, renal function, and tolerance for the drug (see Appendix A for further details). Infants with mild symptoms, primary myocardial disease, renal dysfunction, or the potential for atrioventricular block may be digitalized using only the maintenance dose (omitting the loading dose). The maintenance dose is divided into equal twice daily doses, 12 hours apart.

Digoxin toxicity most commonly manifest with gastrointestinal upset, somnolence, and sinus bradycardia. More severe digoxin toxicity may cause high-grade atrioventricular block and ventricular ectopy. Infants suspected of having digoxin toxicity should have a digoxin level drawn and further doses withheld. The therapeutic level is <1.5 ng/mL with probable toxicity occurring at levels >4.0 ng/mL. In infants particularly, however, digoxin levels do not always correlate well with therapeutic efficacy or with toxicity.

Digoxin toxicity in neonates is usually manageable by withholding further doses until the signs of toxicity resolve and by correcting electrolyte abnormalities (such as hypokalemia), which can potentiate toxic effects. Severe ventricular arrhythmias associated with digoxin toxicity may be managed with phenytoin, 2 to 4 mg/kg over 5 minutes, or lidocaine, 1 mg/kg loading dose, followed by an infusion at 1 to 2 mg/kg per hour. Atrioventricular block is usually unresponsive to atropine. Severe bradycardia may be refractory to these therapies and require temporary cardiac pacing.

The use of digoxin-specific antibody Fab (antigen-binding fragments) preparation (Digibind; Burroughs Wellcome) is reserved for those patients with evidence of severe digoxin intoxication and clinical symptoms of refractory arrhythmia and/or atrioventricular block; in these patients, it is quite effective. Calculation of the Digibind dose in milligrams is as follows: (serum digoxin concentration in nanograms per milliliter × 5.6 × the body weight in kilograms/1,000) × 64. The dose is given as a one-time intravenous infusion. A second dose of Digibind may be given to those patients who continue to have clinical evidence of residual toxicity. Skin testing for hypersensitivity is recommended before the first dose.

E. **Diuretics** (see Appendix A) are frequently used in patients with CHF often in combination with digoxin. **Furosemide**, 1 to 2 mg/kg per dose, usually results in a brisk diuresis within an hour of administration. If no response is noted in an hour, a second dose (double the first dose) may be given. Chronic use of furosemide may produce urinary tract stones as a result of its calciuric effects. A more potent diuretic effect may be achieved using a combination of a thiazide and a "loop" diuretic such as furosemide. Combination diuretic therapy may be complicated by hyponatremia and hypokalemia. Oral or intravenous potassium supplementation (3–4 mEq/kg/day) or an aldosterone antagonist usually should accompany the use of thiazide and/or "loop" diuretics to avoid excessive potassium wasting. It is important to carefully monitor serum potassium and sodium levels when beginning or changing the dose of diuretic medications. When changing from an effective parenteral to oral dose of furosemide, the dose should be increased by 50% to 80%. Furosemide may increase the nephro toxicity and ototoxicity of concurrently used aminoglycoside antibiotics. Detailed discussion of alternative diuretics (e.g., chlorothiazide, spironolactone) is found elsewhere in the text (see Appendix A).

VIII. ARRHYTHMIAS

A. **Initial evaluation.** When evaluating any infant with an arrhythmia, it is essential to simultaneously assess the electrophysiology and hemodynamic status. If the baby is poorly perfused and/or hypotensive, reliable intravenous access should be secured and a level of resuscitation should be employed appropriately for the degree of illness. As always, **emergency treatment of shock should precede definitive diagnosis**. It should be emphasized, however, that there is **rarely** a situation in which it is justified to omit a 12-lead ECG from the evaluation of an infant with an arrhythmia, the exceptions being ventricular fibrillation or torsade de pointes with accompanying hemodynamic instability. These arrhythmias frequently require immediate defibrillation but are extremely rare arrhythmias in neonates and young infants.

In nearly all circumstances, appropriate therapy (short term and long term) depends on an accurate electrophysiologic diagnosis. Determination of the mechanism of a rhythm disturbance is most often made from a 12-lead ECG in the abnormal rhythm compared to the patient's baseline 12-lead ECG in sinus rhythm. Although rhythm strips generated from a cardiac monitor can be helpful supportive evidence of the final diagnosis, they are typically **not** diagnostic and should **not** be the only documentation of arrhythmia if at all possible.

The three broad categories for arrhythmias in neonates are (i) tachyarrhythmias, (ii) bradyarrhythmias, and (iii) irregular rhythms. An algorithm for approaching the differential diagnosis of tachyarrhythmias can be consulted (see Fig. 41.17) in most cases. When analyzing the ECG for the mechanism of arrhythmia, a stepwise approach should be taken in three main areas: (i) rate (variable, too fast, or too slow); (ii) **rhythm** (regular or irregular, paroxysmal or gradual); and (iii) **QRS morphology**.

B. **Differential diagnosis and initial management in the hemodynamically stable patient**

1. **Narrow QRS complex tachycardias**
   a. **SVTs** are the most common symptomatic arrhythmias in all children including neonates. SVTs usually have (i) a rate >200 beats/minute, frequently

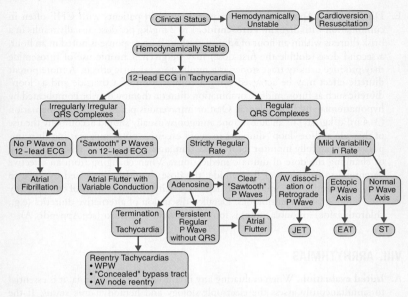

Figure 41.17. Algorithm for bedside differential diagnosis of narrow complex tachycardias, the most common type of arrhythmia in neonates. Note that, regardless of the mechanism of tachycardia, if the patient is hemodynamically unstable, immediate measures to resuscitate the infant including cardioversion are required. In addition, treatment with adenosine is helpful therapeutically as well as diagnostically. In general, tachycardias that terminate (even briefly) after adenosine are of the reentry type. ECG = electrocardiogram; JET = junctional ectopic tachycardia; EAT = ectopic atrial tachycardia; ST = sinus tachycardia; WPW = Wolff-Parkinson-White syndrome.

"fixed" with no beat-to-beat variation in rate; (ii) rapid onset and termination (in reentrant rhythms); and (iii) normal ventricular complexes on the surface ECG. The infant may initially be asymptomatic but later may become irritable, fussy, and may refuse feedings. CHF usually does not develop before 24 hours of continuous SVT; however, heart failure is seen in 20% of patients after 36 hours and in 50% after 48 hours.

SVT in the neonate is almost always "reentrant," involving either an accessory atrioventricular pathway and the atrioventricular node, or due to atrial flutter. Approximately, half the number of these patients will manifest preexcitation (delta wave) on the ECG when not in tachycardia (WPW syndrome, see Fig. 41.18). In rarer cases, the reentrant circuit may be within the atrium itself (atrial flutter) or within the atrial ventricular (AV) node (AV node reentrant tachycardia). Patients with SVT may have associated structural heart disease; evaluation for structural heart disease should be considered in all neonates with SVT. Another rare cause of SVTs in a neonate is ectopic atrial tachycardia in which the distinguishing features are an abnormal P wave axis, normal QRS axis, and significant variability in the overall rate.

Long-term medical therapy for SVT in the neonate is based on the underlying electrophysiologic diagnosis. For patients without demonstrable WPW syndrome, **digoxin** is the initial therapy in patients without CHF.

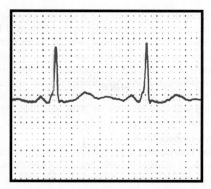

Figure 41.18. Wolff-Parkinson-White syndrome. Note the characteristic "slurred" initial QRS deflection and short PR interval that can occur in any lead; lead I only pictured here.

Digitalization is described in section VII.D and Appendix A. Vagal maneuvers (facial/malar ice wrapped in a towel to elicit the "diving reflex") may be tried in stable neonates. Direct pressure over the eyes should be avoided. Parenteral digitalization usually abolishes the arrhythmia within 10 hours. If digoxin successfully maintains the patient in sinus rhythm, it is typically continued for 6 to 12 months. Although digoxin has long been the mainstay of treatment for SVT, reliance on this drug acutely has decreased, as more efficacious and faster-acting agents have become available such as β-blockers.

Digoxin is avoided in chronic management of WPW syndrome because of its potential for enhancing antegrade conduction across the accessory pathway. **Propranolol** is used as the initial and chronic drug therapy for patients with SVT due to the WPW syndrome, to avoid the potential facilitation of antegrade (atrioventricular) conduction through the accessory pathway. Treatment with propranolol may be associated with apnea and hypoglycemia; therefore, neonates started on propranolol, especially premature infants, should be observed on a continuous cardiac monitor and have serial serum glucose checks for 1 to 2 days.

The addition or substitution of other antiarrhythmic drugs such as amiodarone, alone or in combination, may be necessary and should be done only in consultation with a pediatric cardiologist. In neonates, **verapamil should only rarely be used** because it has been associated with sudden death in babies.

In utero **SVT** may be suspected when a very rapid fetal heart rate is noted by the obstetrician during prenatal care. The diagnosis is confirmed by fetal echocardiography. At that time, an initial search for congenital heart disease and fetal hydrops may be made. *In utero* treatment of the immature fetus with SVT may be accomplished by treatment of the mother with antiarrhythmic drugs that cross the placenta. Digoxin, flecainide, and other anti-arrhythmic drugs have been successful therapies. Failure to control the fetal SVT in the presence of fetal hydrops is an indication for delivery. Cesarean delivery of an infant in persistent SVT may be necessary, as the fetal heart rate will not be a reliable indicator of fetal distress.

b. Sinus tachycardia in the neonate is defined as persistent heart rate >2 standard deviations above the mean for age with normal ECG complexes including a normal P wave morphology and axis. Sinus tachycardia is common and occurs particularly in response to systemic events such as anemia, stress, fever, high levels of circulating catecholamines, hypovolemia, and xanthine (e.g., aminophylline) toxicity. An important clue to the existence of sinus tachycardia, in addition to its normal ECG morphology, is that the rate is not fixed but rather will vary by 10% to 20% over time. Medical management consists of identifying and treating the underlying cause.

2. **Wide-complex tachycardias**

   a. Ventricular tachycardia in the neonate is relatively rare and is usually associated with severe medical illnesses, including hypoxemia, shock, electrolyte disturbances, digoxin toxicity, and catecholamine toxicity. It may rarely be due to an abnormality of the electrical conducting system of the heart such as prolonged QTc syndrome and intramyocardial tumors. Wide and frequently bizarre QRS complexes with a rapid rate are diagnostic; this ECG pattern may be simulated by SVT in patients with WPW syndrome in whom there is antegrade conduction through the anomalous pathway (SVT with "aberration"). Ventricular tachycardia is a potentially unstable rhythm commonly with hemodynamic consequences. The underlying cause should be rapidly sought and treated. The hemodynamically stable patient should be treated with a lidocaine bolus, 1 to 2 mg/kg, followed by a lidocaine infusion, 20 to 50 μg/kg/minute. Direct current cardioversion (starting dose of 1–2 J/kg) should be used if the patient is hemodynamically compromised, although it will frequently be ineffective in the presence of acidosis. If a severe acidosis (pH <7.2) is present, it should be treated with hyperventilation and/or sodium bicarbonate before cardioversion. Phenytoin, 2 to 4 mg/kg, may be effective if the arrhythmia is due to digoxin toxicity (see VII.D.).

   b. Ventricular fibrillation in the neonate is almost always an agonal (preterminal) arrhythmia. There is a coarse irregular pattern on ECG with no identifiable QRS complexes. There are no peripheral pulses or heart sounds on examination. Cardiopulmonary resuscitation should be instituted and defibrillation (starting dose of 1–2 J/kg) should be performed. A bolus of lidocaine, 1 mg/kg, followed by a lidocaine infusion should be started. Once the infant has been resuscitated, the underlying problems should be evaluated and treated.

3. **Bradycardia**

   a. Sinus bradycardia in the neonate is not uncommon especially during sleep or during vagal maneuvers, such as bowel movements. If the infant's perfusion and blood pressure are normal, transient bradycardia is not of major concern. Persistent sinus bradycardia may be secondary to hypoxemia, acidosis, and elevated intracranial pressure. Finally, a stable sinus bradycardia may occur with digoxin toxicity, hypothyroidism, or sinus node dysfunction (usually a complication of cardiac surgery).

   b. Heart block

   i. **First-degree atrioventricular block** occurs when the PR interval is >0.15 seconds. In the neonate, first-degree atrioventricular block may be due to a nonspecific conduction disturbance; medications (e.g., digoxin); myocarditis; hypothyroidism; or associated with certain types of congenital heart disease (e.g., complete atrioventricular canal or ventricular inversion). No specific treatment is generally indicated.

ii. **Second-degree atrioventricular block.** Second-degree atrioventricular block refers to **intermittent** failure of conduction of the atrial impulse to the ventricles. Two types have been described: (i) Mobitz I (Wenckebach phenomenon) and (ii) Mobitz II (intermittent failure to conduct P waves, with a constant PR interval). Second-degree atrioventricular block may occur with SVT, digitalis toxicity, or a nonspecific conduction disturbance. No specific treatment is usually necessary other than diagnosis and treatment of the underlying cause.

iii. **CHB** refers to **complete** absence of conduction of any atrial activity to the ventricles. CHB typically has a slow, constant ventricular rate that is independent of the atrial rate. CHB is frequently detected *in utero* as fetal bradycardia. Although CHB may be secondary to surgical trauma, **congenital** CHB falls into two main categories. The most common causes include (i) anatomic defects (ventricular inversion and complete atrioventricular canal) and (ii) fetal exposure to maternal antibodies related to systemic rheumatologic disease such as lupus erythematosus. The presence of CHB without structural heart disease should alert the clinician to investigate the mother for rheumatologic disease. In cases of *in utero* CHB caused by maternal antibodies related to lupus erythematosus, the prognosis may be poor. If there is a high risk of developing CHB (previous fetus with CHB, miscarriage, abnormal fetal echocardiography) treatment in pregnancy with dexamethasone, azathioprine, IV γ-globulin or plasmapheresis should be considered.

Symptoms related to CHB are related to both the severity of the associated cardiac malformation (when present) and the degree of bradycardia. Fortunately, the fetus with CHB adapts well by increasing stroke volume and will usually come to term without difficulty. Infants with isolated congenital CHB usually have a heart rate >50 beats/minute, are asymptomatic, and grow normally.

4. **Irregular rhythms**
   a. **Premature atrial contractions (PACs, see Fig. 41.19)** are common in neonates, are usually benign, and do not require specific therapy. Most PACs result in a normal QRS morphology (Fig. 41.19A), distinguishing them from premature ventricular contractions (PVCs). If the PAC occurs while the atrioventricular node is partially repolarized, an aberrantly conducted ventricular depolarization pattern may be observed on the surface ECG (Fig. 41.19B). If the premature beat occurs when the atrioventricular node is refractory (i.e., early in the cardiac cycle, occurring soon after the normal sinus beat), the impulse will not be conducted to the ventricle ("blocked") and may therefore give the appearance of a marked sinus bradycardia (Fig. 41.19C).
   b. **Premature ventricular contractions (PVCs, see Fig. 41.20)** are "wide QRS complex" beats that occur when a ventricular focus stimulates a spontaneous beat before the normally conducted sinus beat. Isolated PVCs are not uncommon in the normal neonate and do not generally require treatment. Although PVCs frequently occur sporadically, they are occasionally grouped, such as every other beat (bigeminy, Fig. 41.20A), every third beat (trigeminy), and so on. These more frequent PVCs are typically no more worrisome than isolated PVCs, although their greater frequency usually prompts a more extensive diagnostic workup. PVCs may be caused by digoxin toxicity, hypoxemia, electrolyte disturbances, catecholamine, or xanthine toxicity. PVCs occurring

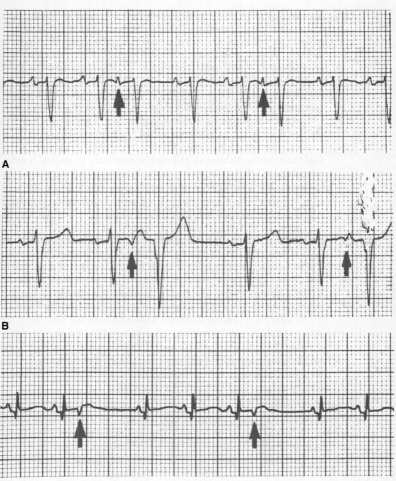

Figure 41.19. Premature atrial contractions (*arrows*) causing: **(A)** early ventricular depolarization with a normal QRS complex; **(B)** early ventricular depolarization with "aberration" of the QRS complex; **(C)** block at the atrioventricular node. (From Fyler DC, ed. *Nadas' Pediatric Cardiology*. 1st ed. Hanley & Belfus, Inc., 1992.)

in groups of two or more (i.e., couplets, triplets, etc.; Fig. 41.20B) are pathologic and are "high grade"; they may be a marker for myocarditis or myocardial dysfunction, and further evaluation should be strongly considered.

C. Emergency treatment in the hemodynamically compromised patient. With all therapies described in the following, it is important to have easily accessible resuscitation equipment available before proceeding with these antiarrhythmic interventions.

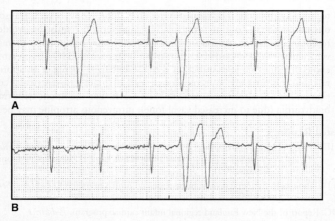

Figure 41.20. Premature ventricular contractions. **A:** PVCs alternating with normal sinus beats (ventricular bigeminy) are usually not indicative of significant pathology. **B:** Paired PVCs ("couplet") are a potentially more serious rhythm and require further investigation.

1. **Tachycardias**
   a. Adenosine. Adenosine has become the drug of choice for acute management. Adenosine transiently blocks AV node conduction, allowing termination of rapid reentrant rhythms involving the AV node. It must be given by very rapid intravenous push because its half-life is 10 seconds or less. Due to this short half-life, adenosine is a relatively safe medication; however, it has been reported to cause transient AV block severe enough to require pacing (albeit briefly) so it should be used with caution and in consultation with a pediatric cardiologist. Adenosine, by virtue of its acute action on the AV node, is frequently **diagnostic** as well. Patients who respond with abrupt termination of the SVT have reentrant tachycardias involving the AV node; those with SVT due to atrial flutter will have acute AV block and easily visible flutter waves with reappearance of SVT in 10 to 15 seconds.
   b. Cardioversion. In the hemodynamically unstable patient, the **first** line of therapy is synchronized direct current cardioversion. The energy should start at 1 J/kg and be increased by a factor of 2 if unsuccessful. Care should be taken to avoid skin burns and arcing of the current outside the body by only using electrical transmission gel with the paddles. Paddle position should be anterior–posterior if possible.
   c. Transesophageal pacing. When available, esophageal overdrive pacing is a very effective maneuver for terminating tachyarrhythmias. The proximity of the left atrium to the distal esophagus allows electrical impulses generated in the esophagus to be transmitted to atrial tissue; burst pacing may then terminate reentrant tachyarrhythmias.

2. **Bradycardias.** Therapeutic options for treating a symptomatic bradyarrhythmia are more limited. A transvenous pacemaker is a temporary measure in severely symptomatic neonates while preparing for placement of permanent epicardial pacemaker leads; however, transvenous pacing in a small neonate is

technically difficult and frequently requires fluoroscopy. Several transcutaneous pacemakers (Zoll) are available but long-term use must be avoided due to cutaneous burns. An isoproterenol infusion may temporarily increase the ventricular rate and cardiac output in an infant with CHF. The treatment of choice for sinus node dysfunction is transesophageal pacing at an appropriate rate, but this can only be accomplished with an intact atrioventricular conduction and is not effective in patients with CHB. For the infant with transient bradycardia (due to increased vagal tone), intravenous atropine may be used.

Suggested Readings

Allen HD, Gutgesell HP, Clark EB, et al. *Moss and Adams' Heart Disease in Infants, Children and Adolescents Including the Fetus and Young Adult*, 6th ed. Philadelphia: Lippincott Williams & Wilkins, 2001.

Aranda JV, Thomas R. Systemic review: intravenous ibuprofen in preterm newborns. *Semin Perinatol* 2006;30(3):114–120.

Fyler DC. Report of the New England regional infant cardiac program. *Pediatrics* 1980;65(suppl):377–461.

Hoffman JI, Kaplan S. The incidence of congenital heart disease. *J Am Coll Cardiol* 2002; 39(12):1890–1900.

Jonas RA, DiNardo J, Laussen PC, et al. *Comprehensive Surgical Management of Congenital Heart Disease*. London: Arnold Publishers, 2004.

Keane JF, Fyler DC, Lock JE. *Nadas' Pediatric Cardiology*. 2nd ed. Philadelphia: Hanley and Belfus, 2006.

Kovalchin JP, Silverman NH. The impact of fetal echocardiography. *Pediatr Cardiol* 2004;25(3):299–306.

Liske MR, Greeley CS, Law DJ, et al. Report of the Tennessee task force on screening newborn infants for critical congenital heart disease. *Pediatrics* 2006;118(4):e1250–e1256.

Mavroudis C, Backer CL. *Pediatric Cardiac Surgery*. 3rd ed. Philadelphia, PA: Mosby, 2003.

Rein AJ, Omokhodion SI, Nir A. Significance of a cardiac murmur as the sole clinical sign in the newborn. *Clin Pediatr* 2000;39(9):511–520.

Saar P, Hermann W, Müller-Ladner U. Connective tissue diseases and pregnancy. *Rheumatology* 2006;45(suppl 3):iii30–iii32.

Shah SS, Ohlsson A. Ibuprofen for the prevention of patent ductus arteriosus in preterm and/ or low birth weight infants. *Cochrane Database Syst Rev* 2006;25(1):CD004213.

Tworetzky W, Wilkins-Haug L, Jennings RW, et al. Balloon dilation of severe aortic stenosis in the fetus: potential for prevention of hypoplastic left heart syndrome: candidate selection, technique, and results of successful intervention. *Circulation* 2004;110(15):2125–2131.

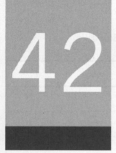

42 Blood Products Used in the Newborn

Steven R. Sloan

I. WHOLE BLOOD AND BLOOD COMPONENT TRANSFUSIONS

A. **General principles.** Routine blood components consist of packed red blood cells (RBCs), platelets, frozen plasma, fresh frozen plasma, cryoprecipitate (CRYO), and granulocytes. In some cases, whole blood, usually in the form of reconstituted whole blood, can be used. However, in most cases, blood components are preferred because each component has specific optimal storage conditions, and component therapy maximizes the use of blood donations. Other blood products include those used for transplants, such as umbilical cord blood and derivatives purified from blood, such as intravenous immunoglobulin (IVIG).

B. **Side effects**

1. **Infectious diseases.** A variety of infectious diseases can be transmitted by blood transfusion. HIV, Hepatitis B virus, Hepatitis C virus, Syphilis, human T-lymphotropic virus types I or II (HTLV I/II), and West Nile virus are screened by medical history questionnaires and laboratory tests. The risk of acquiring a transfusion-transmitted infectious disease is very low and too low to accurately measure but has been calculated in the United States and are shown in Table 42.1. The risks vary depending on the prevalence of the disease and the testing performed and thus differ in other countries.

   Cytomegalovirus (CMV) can also be transmitted by blood, but this is rare if the blood is leukoreduced and/or it tests negative for antibodies to CMV (3). Other diseases known to be capable of being transmitted by blood transfusions include malaria, babesiosis, and Chagas disease. Animal studies suggest that variant Creutzfeldt-Jakob disease (vCJD) can also be transmitted by blood transfusion, and some probable cases of transfusion-transmitted vCJD in humans have been reported.

C. **Special considerations.** Whole blood, platelets, and RBCs can be leukoreduced by filtration or irradiated to reduce the incidence of specific complications.

1. **Leukoreduction** filters remove approximately 99.9% of the white blood cells (WBCs) from RBCs and platelets. In addition, most platelets collected by apheresis are leukoreduced even without additional filtration. Benefits of leukoreduction include the following:

   a. Decreased rate of febrile transfusion reactions.

   b. Decreased rate of CMV transmission.

   c. Minimization of a possible (and controversial) immunomodulatory effects of blood transfusions.

Table 42.1	Current Infectious Disease Risks from Blood Transfusions (2)
Pathogen	**Risk per Unit**
Human immunodeficiency virus (HIV)	1 in 2,135,000
Hepatitis C virus (HCV)	1 in 1,935,000
Hepatitis A virus	1 in 1,000,000
Hepatitis B virus (HBV)	1 in 205,000–488,000
West Nile virus (WNV)	none
Parvovirus B19	1 in 10,000

 d. Decreased immunization to antigens on leukocytes such as human leukocyte antigen (HLA). This has only been shown for some oncology patients and its importance for neonates is unknown.

 Although the first three indications are not essential for neonates, neonates often receive leukoreduced blood components to decrease CMV transmission.

2. Irradiation prevents transfusion-associated graft-versus-host disease (TA-GVHD) from transfused leukocytes in cellular blood components. Among those at risk are premature infants and children with certain congenital immunodeficiencies. To ensure that nobody gets this fatal consequence of transfusion, all RBCs, platelets, and granulocytes are irradiated at Children's Hospital Boston, unless blood is emergently needed.

 Some people donate blood for specific patients, providing what is commonly known as directed or designated blood. Directed donations have a small increase in rate of infectious disease transmission. The difference is minimal and parents often want to donate for their children. Transfusion of paternal RBCs or platelets is contraindicated if the neonate's plasma contains antibodies directed against antigens expressed on paternal erythrocytes or platelets, respectively. If a first-degree relative does donate blood, the cellular blood components must be irradiated since they are at increased risk for causing TA-GVHD.

II. PACKED RED BLOOD CELLS (RBC)

A. General principles

 1. Mechanism. RBCs provide oxygen carrying capacity for patients whose blood lacks sufficient oxygen carrying capacity due to anemia, hemorrhage, or hemoglobinopathy. Transfusion for hemoglobinopathies is unusual in the neonatal period when most patients will have significant amounts of fetal hemoglobin.

 Several types of RBC units are available that vary in the preservatives added. Chemical additives delay storage damage to RBCs allowing for extended storage times. The types of units that are currently available in the United States are:

 a. Anticoagulant-preservative solution units. These units contain approximately 250 mL of a concentrated solution of RBCs. The average hematocrit of these units is 70% to 80%. In addition, these units contain 62 mg of sodium, 222 mg of citrate, and 46 mg of phosphate. Three types of units are currently approved for use in the United States. These are:

    i. CPD. This contains 773 mg of dextrose and has a 21-day shelf life.

    ii. CP2D. This contains 1,546 mg of dextrose and has a 21-day shelf life.

    iii. CPDA-1. This contains 965 mg of dextrose and 8.2 mg of adenine and has a 35-day shelf life. This is the most widely used of the anticoagulant-preservative solution units.

  b. Additive solution units. Most RBC units used in the United States are additive units. Three additive solutions are currently approved for use in the United States. Each of these units contains approximately 350 mL, has an average hematocrit of 50% to 60%, and has a 42-day shelf life. Contents of these units are shown in Table 42.2.

2. Several changes occur in PRBCs during storage:

  a. The pH decreases from 7.4–7.55 to pH 6.5–6.6 at the time of expiration.

  b. Potassium is released from the RBC. The initial plasma K+ concentration is 4.2 mM and increases to 78.5 mM in CPDA-1 units at day 35 and 45 to 50 mM in additive solution units on day 42. CPDA-1 units contain about one-third the plasma volume as additive units so the total amount of extracellular potassium is similar in all units of the same age.

  c. 2,3-diphosphoglycerol (2,3-DPG) levels drop rapidly during the first 2 weeks of storage. This increases the affinity of the hemoglobin for oxygen and decreases its efficiency in delivering oxygen to tissue. The 2,3-DPG levels replenish over several hours after being transfused.

3. Toxicity. Although there are theoretical concerns that mannitol may cause a rapid diuresis and adenine may be a nephrotoxin in the premature infant, case reports and case series have found no risk associated with additive solution units. Hence, some hospitals transfuse additive solution units to neonates. In general, we prefer to use nonadditive solution units or washed additive solution units for larger transfusions such as exchange transfusions or transfusions for surgical procedures with substantial blood loss for young infants. For transfusions of 5 to 20 mL/kg, additive units can be used.

Table 42.2	Contents of Additive Solution RBC Units		
	AS-1	**AS-3**	**AS-5**
Dextrose (mg)	2,973	2,645	1,673
Sodium (mg)	962	406	407
Citrate (mg)	222	711	222
Phosphate (mg)	46	233	46
Adenine (mg)	27	30	30
Mannitol (mg)	750	0	525

B. **Indications/contraindications.** RBC transfusions are indicated for neonates who have signs or symptoms of hypoxia or who require an exchange transfusion (see Chap. 45, Anemia). Additionally, two studies suggest that more liberal RBC transfusion protocols may decrease the incidence of short- and long-term neurologic complications in premature infants. The liberal transfusion triggers varied between studies and depended on a premature infant's oxygen support needs and in one study, an infant's age. These studies suggest that a transfusion trigger as high as 15 g/dL Hb may be beneficial for intubated premature infants, while a transfusion trigger as low as 8 to 10 g/dL Hb may be sufficient for a premature infant requiring no oxygen support (1,3).

C. **Dosing and administration.** The usual dose for a simple transfusion is 5 to 15 mL/kg transfused at a rate of 5 mL/kg/hour. This may be adjusted depending on the severity of the anemia and/or the patient's ability to tolerate increases in intravascular volume.

D. **Side effects**

1. Acute transfusion reactions

   a. **Acute hemolytic transfusion reactions.** These reactions are usually due to incompatibility of donor RBCs with antibodies in the patient's plasma. The antibodies usually responsible for acute hemolytic transfusion reactions are iso-hemagglutinins (anti-A, anti-B). These reactions are rare in neonates because they do not make isohemagglutinins until they are 4 to 6 months old. However, maternal isohemagglutinins can be present in the neonatal circulation.

      i. **Symptoms.** Possible symptoms include hypotension, fever, tachycardia, infusion site pain, and hematuria.

      ii. **Treatment.** Administer fluids and furosemide to protect kidneys. If necessary, treat hypotension with pressors and use hemostatic agents for bleeding. May need to transfuse compatible PRBCs.

   b. **Allergic transfusion reactions.** These are unusual in neonates. Allergic reactions are due to antibodies in the patient's plasma that react with proteins in donor plasma.

      i. **Symptoms.** Mild allergic reactions are characterized by hives and possibly wheezing. More severe reactions can present such as anaphylaxis.

      ii. **Treatment.** These reactions can be treated with antihistamines, bronchodilators, and corticosteroids as needed. These reactions are usually specific to individual donors. If they are serious or re-occur, RBCs and platelets can be washed.

   c. **Volume overload.** Blood components have high oncotic pressure and rapid infusion can cause excessive intravascular volume. This can cause a sudden deterioration of vital signs. Chronically anemic neonates can be especially susceptible to volume overload from transfusions.

   d. **Hypocalcemia.** Rapid infusion of components, especially FFP, can cause transient hypocalcemia, usually manifested by hypotension.

   e. **Hypothermia.** Cool blood can cause hypothermia. Transfusion through blood warmers can prevent this.

   f. **Transfusion-associated acute lung injury (TRALI).** This is often due to antibodies in donor plasma that react with the patient's histocompatibility (HLA) antigens. These reactions present as respiratory compromise and are more likely to occur with blood components containing significant amounts of plasma such as platelets or FFP.

g. Hyperkalemia. Extracellular potassium dosage is not significant for simple transfusions of 5 to 20 mL/kg. However, hyperkalemia can be important in large transfusions such as exchange transfusions or transfusions for major surgery. Ideally, fresher PRBC units can be provided for these transfusions. At Children's Hospital Boston, RBCs no more than 7 days old are transfused to children less than 1 year old undergoing surgery. If fresh RBCs are unavailable, washing blood will temporarily reduce the extracellular potassium.

h. Febrile Nonhemolytic transfusion reactions are usually due to cytokines released from leukocytes in the donor unit. These occur less frequently if the unit is leukoreduced.

i. Bacterial contamination can occur but is relatively rare with RBC transfusions.

j. Transfusion-associated graft-versus-host disease (TA-GVHD). Lymphocytes from donor blood components can mount an immune response against the patient. Patients are at risk if they are unable to mount immune responses against the transfused lymphocytes. Such patients include premature infants, infants with congenital immune deficiencies, and patients sharing HLA types with blood donors as often occurs when people donate blood for relatives. TA-GVHD can be prevented by irradiation. Leukoreduction filters do not remove enough lymphocytes to prevent TA-GVHD.

E. Special considerations. Donor exposures can be minimized by reserving a fresh unit of PRBCs for a neonate at his or her first transfusion and transfusion of *aliquots* of that unit for each subsequent transfusion. This is useful for premature infants who are expected to require multiple simple transfusions for anemia of prematurity.

III. FRESH FROZEN PLASMA, THAWED PLASMA

A. General principles. The two frozen plasma products that are most frequently available are fresh frozen plasma (FFP) and thawed plasma. Both components are used to administer all clotting factors. The contents are:

1. Each component has approximately 1 unit/mL of each coagulation factor except that thawed plasma may have approximately two-thirds the levels of the least stable factors, V and VIII.

2. 160 to 170 mEq/L sodium and 3.5 to 5.5 mEq/L potassium

3. All plasma proteins, including albumin and antibodies

4. 1,440 g sodium citrate

B. Indications. FFP and frozen plasma are indicated to correct coagulopathies due to factor deficiencies. Although plasma contains proteins and albumins, these components are not indicated for intravascular volume expansion or for antibody replacement since other components are safer and better for those indications (see Chap. 43).

C. Dosing and administration. 10 to 20 mL/kg is usually an adequate dose, and this may need to be repeated every 8 to 12 hours depending on the clinical situation.

D. Side effects. The side effects of RBC transfusion can also occur with plasma transfusions, with some different risks when compared to RBC transfusions:

1. Hyperkalemia will not occur.

2. TRALI is more likely since more plasma containing antibodies is transfused.

3. Acute hemolytic reactions involving hemolysis of transfused RBCs is extremely unlikely. However, if the plasma contains incompatible antibodies (e.g., group O plasma transfused to a group A patient), an acute hemolytic reaction can rarely occur. For this reason, transfused plasma should be compatible with the patient's blood group.

4. **Citrate-induced hypocalcemia** is a risk with plasma infusions. The amount of citrate is unlikely to cause transient hypocalcemia in most situations, but this can happen with rapid infusions of large amounts of plasma.

IV. PLATELETS

A. **General principles.** Platelets can be prepared from whole blood donations or collected by apheresis. If they are collected by apheresis, an *aliquot* is obtained for a neonatal transfusion. Often only, a portion of a whole blood-derived platelet unit is transfused to neonates, but we do not find it worthwhile to *aliquot* whole blood-derived platelets.

B. **Contents.** Each unit of whole blood-derived platelets contains at least 5×10^{10} platelets in 50 mL of anticoagulated plasma including proteins and electrolytes. Because platelets are stored at room temperature for up to 5 days, there may be relatively low levels of the least stable coagulation factors V and VIII.

C. **Indications.** No good studies exist, but NICU patients at increased risk for intracranial hemorrhage should probably be maintained at a platelet count of 50,000 to 100,000 platelets/mm^3. For additional information, see Chapter 47, Thrombocytopenia.

D. **Dosing and administration.** A dose of 5 mL/kg should raise the platelet count by 30,000/mm^3.

E. **Side effects.** The side effects of FFP transfusions can also occur with platelet transfusions. Additionally:

1. Platelets are more likely to be contaminated with bacteria causing septic reactions since platelets are stored at room temperature. For this reason, many blood banks test platelet units for bacterial contamination.

2. Inventory issues can limit the ability to match ABO types of platelets and patients. ABO-incompatible plasma in a platelet unit can rarely cause a hemolytic transfusion reaction. For this reason, Children's Hospital, Boston, concentrates group O or B platelets to be transfused to group A patients if the platelet supernatants have a high anti-A titer.

F. **Special considerations.** Platelets can be concentrated by centrifugation resulting in a volume of 15 to 20 mL. This may damage the platelets.

V. GRANULOCYTES

A. **Indications.** Granulocyte transfusions are a controversial therapy that may benefit patients with severe neutropenia or dysfunctional neutrophils and a bacterial or fungal infection not responding to antimicrobial therapy. Most granulocytes are given to patients who are neutropenic secondary to hematopoietic progenitor cell (HPC) transplants. However, septic infants with chronic granulomatous disease may also benefit from granulocyte transfusions. Granulocyte transfusions can only be used as a temporary therapy until the patient starts producing neutrophils or until another curative therapy can be instituted (see Chap. 49).

B. **Dosing and administration.** 10 to 15 mL/kg. This may need to be repeated every 12 to 24 hours.

C. **Side effects.** In addition to all the potential adverse effects associated with RBC transfusions, granulocyte transfusions can cause pulmonary symptoms and must be administered slowly to minimize the chances of severe reactions. Additionally, granulocytes can transmit CMV. Hence, donors should be serologically negative for CMV if the patient is at risk for CMV disease.

D. **Special considerations.** Granulocyte collections need to be specially scheduled, and the granulocytes should be transfused as soon as possible after collection and no later than 24 hours after the collection.

VI. WHOLE BLOOD

A. **General principles.** Whole blood contains RBCs and plasma clotting factors. Few units are stored as whole blood. Whole blood can be reconstituted from a unit of RBCs and FFP.

B. **Indications.** Whole blood is usually used for neonatal exchange transfusions. It may also be used as a substitute for blood components in priming circuits for extracorporeal membrane oxygenation (ECMO) or cardiopulmonary bypass, but this may cause increased fluid retention and longer postoperative recovery times. Whole blood may be useful for neonates immediately following disconnection from a cardiopulmonary bypass circuit for cardiac surgery.

C. **Side effects.** All of the adverse effects of individual blood components can occur with whole blood.

D. **Special considerations.** Whole blood should be transfused when it is relatively fresh since whole blood is stored at 1° to 6°C and coagulation factors decay at this temperature. When used just after cardiopulmonary bypass, the blood should be no more than 2 to 3 days old. When used in other situations, the whole blood should be no more than 5 to 7 days old.

Platelets in whole blood will be cleared rapidly following transfusion and reconstituted whole blood lacks significant quantities of platelets.

VII. IVIG

A. **General principles.** IVIG is a concentrated purified solution of immunoglobulins with stabilizers such as sucrose. Most products contain over 90% immunoglobulin G (IgG), with small amounts of immunoglobulin M (IgM) and immunoglobulin A (IgA). Several brands of IVIG are available.

B. **Indications.** IVIG can have an immunosuppressive effect that is useful for alloimmune disorders such as neonatal alloimmune thrombocytopenia and, possibly, alloimmune hemolytic anemia. Both of these disorders are due to maternal antibodies to antigens on the neonate's cells (see Chaps. 26 and 47).

IVIG can also be used to replace immunoglobulins for patients who are deficient in immunoglobulins as occurs with some congenital immunodeficiency syndromes.

Some studies have attempted to determine whether IVIG is useful as a prophylaxis or treatment for neonatal sepsis. Results from these studies are mixed and not enough evidence exists for routine use of IVIG for general sepsis (see Chap. 49).

1. **Hyperimmune Immunoglobulins.** High titer disease-specific immunoglobulins are available for several infectious agents, including varicella zoster virus and respiratory syncytial virus. These immunoglobulins may be useful for infants at high risk for these infections (see Chap. 48).

C. **Dosing and administration.** IVIG (non-disease-specific) is usually given at a dose of 500 to 900 mg/kg. Doses for the disease-specific immunoglobulins should follow manufacturer's recommendations.

D. **Side effects.** Rare complications include transient tachycardia or hypertension. Because of the purification processes, current IVIG has a very low risk of transmitting infectious diseases.

VIII. UMBILICAL CORD BLOOD (UCB)

A. **General principles.** Umbilical cord blood (UCB) is the only blood that is derived from neonatal blood. UCB contains HPCs and is used for HPC transplants. UCB can be used for autologous transplants in which the patient receives the same blood that he or she donated or can be used for allogeneic transplants in which the UCB is transplanted into an individual who did not donate the UCB.

B. **UCB donations.** UCB is collected from the placenta and umbilical cord immediately following delivery and clamping of the umbilical cord. If the mother and baby are healthy, the cord blood can be collected without any impact on the neonate.

UCB can be collected for processing, freezing, and storage by private UCB banks which charge families for this service. A UCB unit stored in a private bank may be used by the neonate that donated the UCB or by other people designated by the family. The UCB has a very low chance of being needed by the neonate since he would only be able to use the UCB if he were to develop a malignancy for which an autologous transplant is indicated when he or she is a child. A single UCB unit has an insufficient dose for transplants for adolescents or adults.

UCB can be collected, processed, frozen, and stored by a public UCB bank. Such banks do not charge for this service. A UCB unit in a public bank is available for any patient who could use it and can be a valuable source of stem cells for a child with a malignancy or with some types of inherited diseases.

C. **Dosing and administration.** An entire cord blood is used for younger children and two cord bloods may be used for adult transplants. Cord bloods are usually infused into central veins as part of a hematopoietic cell transplant protocol.

D. **Side effects.** All of the side effects for other blood components can occur for UCB transplants. However, the plasma content is low and TRALI is unlikely. Because UCB cannot be leukoreduced, febrile reactions are more common than with other blood components. Because UCB cannot be irradiated and patients are immunosuppressed, graft-versus-host disease (GVHD) risk is significant. Since the transplanted HPCs are not attacked by the UCB lymphocytes GVHD from UCB is usually not fatal.

REFERENCES

1. Bell EF, Strauss RG, Widness JA, et al. Randomized trial of liberal versus restrictive guidelines for red blood cell transfusion in preterm infants. *Pediatrics* 2005;115(6):1685–1691.
2. Stramer SL. Current risks of transfusion-transmitted agents: a review. *Arch Pathol Lab Med* 2007;131(5):702–707.
3. Vamvakas EC. Is white blood cell reduction equivalent to antibody screening in preventing transmission of cytomegalovirus by transfusion? A review of the literature and meta-analysis. *Transfus Med Rev* 2005;19(3):181–199.
4. Whyte RK, Kirpalani H, Asztalos EV, et al. Neurodevelopmental outcome of extremely low birth weight infants randomly assigned to restrictive or liberal hemoglobin thresholds for blood transfusion. *Pediatrics* 2009;123(1):207–213.

43 Bleeding

Ellis J. Neufeld

The hemostatic mechanism in the neonate differs from that in the older child. In neonates, there is decreased activity of several clotting factors, diminished platelet function, and suboptimal defense against clot formation. A detailed review of the subject is provided in reference (1).

I. ETIOLOGY

A. Deficient clotting factors

1. **Transitory deficiencies** of the procoagulant vitamin K–dependent factors II, VII, IX, and X and anticoagulant proteins C and S are characteristic of the newborn period and may be accentuated by the following:

   a. The administration of total parenteral alimentation or antibiotics or the lack of administration of vitamin K to premature infants.

   b. Term infants may develop vitamin K deficiency by day 2 or 3 if they are not supplemented with vitamin K parenterally because of negligible stores and inadequate intake.

   c. The mother might have received certain drugs during pregnancy that can cause bleeding in the first 24 hours of the infant's life.

   i. Phenytoin (Dilantin), phenobarbital, and salicylates interfere with the vitamin K effect on synthesis of clotting factors.

   ii. **Warfarin** and related compounds given to the mother interfere with the synthesis of vitamin K–dependent clotting factors by the livers of both the mother and the fetus, and the bleeding may not be immediately reversed by administration of vitamin K.

2. **Disturbances of clotting** may be related to associated diseases, such as disseminated intravascular coagulation (DIC), due to infection, shock, anoxia, necrotizing enterocolitis (NEC), renal vein thrombosis (RVT), or the use of vascular catheters. Any significant liver disease may interfere with the production of clotting factors by the liver.

   a. Extracorporeal membrane oxygenation (ECMO) in neonates with critical cardiopulmonary disease is a special case of coagulopathy related to consumption of clotting factors in the bypass circuit plus therapeutic anticoagulation (2,3) (see Chap. 39).

3. **Inherited abnormalities of clotting factors**

   a. X-linked recessive (expressed predominantly in males; affected females should raise concern for Turner syndrome, partial X deletions, or nonrandom X-chromosome inactivation):

   i. Factor VIII levels are decreased in the newborn with hemophilia A (1 in 5,000 boys) (4).

   ii. Hemophilia B or Christmas disease is due to an inherited deficiency of factor IX (1 in 25,000 boys) (4).

One-third of patients with severe hemophilia express "new mutations," so family history alone cannot rule out the problem.

b. **Autosomal dominant** (expressed in boys and girls with one parent affected):

   i. Von Willebrand disease (VWD) is due to decreased levels or functional activity of von Willebrand factor (VWF), which acts as a carrier for factor VIII and as a platelet-aggregation agent. VWD is the most common inherited coagulation defect (up to 1% of the population as assayed by factor levels) (4). Neonatal levels of VWF are elevated in normal babies compared with older children and nonpregnant adults because of maternal estrogen.

   ii. Dysfibrinogenemia (very rare) is due to fibrinogen structural mutations.

c. **Autosomal recessive** (occurs in both boys and girls born to carrier parents). In order of frequency, deficiencies of factors XI, VII, V, X, II, fibrinogen, and XIII are all encoded by autosomal genes. Factor XII is a special case because deficiency causes long partial thromboplastin time (PTT) but never causes bleeding. Combined factors V and VIII deficiency is caused by defect in the common processing protein ERGIC-53 (5).

   i. Severe factor VII or factor XIII deficiency can present as intracranial hemorrhage in neonates.

   ii. Factor XI deficiency is incompletely recessive because heterozygotes may have unpredictable bleeding problems with surgery or trauma.

   iii. VWD type III (rare, complete absence of VWF) (4).

B. **Platelet problems** (see Chap. 47)

1. **Qualitative disorders** include hereditary conditions (e.g., storage pool defects, Glanzmann thrombasthenia, Bernard-Soulier syndrome, platelet-type VWD (6) and transient disorders that result from the mother's use of antiplatelet agents.

2. **Quantitative disorders** include the following:

   a. Immune thrombocytopenia (maternal idiopathic thrombocytopenic purpura [ITP] or neonatal alloimmune thrombocytopenia [NAIT]) (7).

   b. Maternal preeclampsia or HELLP syndrome (see Chap. 4), or severe uteroplacental insufficiency.

   c. DIC due to infection or asphyxia.

   d. **Inherited marrow failure syndromes, including Fanconi anemia** and congenital amegakaryocytic thrombocytopenia.

   e. **Congenital** leukemia.

   f. Inherited thrombocytopenia syndromes, including gray platelet syndrome and the macrothrombocytopenias, such as May-Hegglin syndrome (6).

   g. Consumption of platelets in clots or vascular lesions without DIC. Examples include vascular malformations, notably Kasabach-Merritt phenomenon from kaposiform hemangioendotheliomas; thrombosis from catheters; RVT; and NEC.

   h. Heparin-induced thrombocytopenia (HIT) deserves special consideration for several reasons. First, this condition leads to platelet activation and risk of thrombosis more than bleeding. Second, it is probably rare in neonates, although the antibody can be detected by ELISA assays after cardiac surgery. Finally, in neonates, the antibody may be maternal, as with other antibodies passed across the placenta.

C. **Other potential causes of bleeding** are vascular in etiology and may include central nervous system hemorrhage, pulmonary hemorrhage, arterio-venous malformations, and hemangiomas.

D. **Miscellaneous problems**

1. **Trauma** (see Chap. 6)
   a. Rupture of spleen or liver associated with breech delivery.
   b. Retroperitoneal or intraperitoneal bleeding may present as scrotal ecchymosis.
   c. Subdural hematoma, cephalhematoma, or subgaleal hemorrhage (the latter may be associated with vacuum extraction).

2. **Liver dysfunction.**

II. DIAGNOSTIC WORKUP OF THE BLEEDING INFANT

A. The **history** includes (i) family history of excessive bleeding or clotting, (ii) maternal medications (e.g., aspirin, phenytoin), (iii) pregnancy and birth history, (iv) maternal history of a birth of an infant with a bleeding disorder, and (v) any illness, medication, anomalies, or procedures done to the infant.

B. **Examination.** The crucial decision in diagnosing and managing the bleeding infant is determining whether the infant is sick or well (see Table 43.1).

1. **Sick infant.** Consider DIC, viral or bacterial infection, or liver disease (hypoxic/ischemic injury may lead to DIC).

2. **Well infant.** Consider vitamin K deficiency, isolated clotting factor deficiencies, or immune thrombocytopenia. Maternal blood in the infant's gastrointestinal (GI) tract will not cause symptoms in the infant.

3. **Petechiae, small superficial ecchymosis, or mucosal bleeding** suggests a platelet problem.

4. **Large bruises** suggest deficiency of clotting factors, DIC, liver disease, or vitamin K deficiency.

5. **Enlarged spleen** suggests possible congenital infection or erythroblastosis.

6. **Jaundice** suggests infection, liver disease, or resorption of a large hematoma.

7. **Abnormal retinal findings** suggest infection (see Chap. 48).

C. **Laboratory tests** (see Table 43.2)

1. **The Apt test** is used to rule out maternal blood. If the child is well and only GI bleeding is noted, an Apt test is performed on gastric aspirate or stool to rule out the presence of maternal blood swallowed during labor or delivery or from a bleeding breast. A breast pump can be used to collect milk to confirm the presence of blood in the milk, or the infant's stomach can be aspirated before and after breastfeeding.
   a. **Procedure.** Mix one part bloody stool or vomitus with five parts water; centrifuge it and separate the clear pink supernatant (hemolysate); add 1 mL of sodium hydroxide 1% (0.25 M) to 4 mL of hemolysate.
   b. **Result.** Hemoglobin A (HbA) changes from pink to yellow brown (maternal blood); hemoglobin F (HbF) stays pink (fetal blood).

2. **Peripheral blood smear** is used to assess the number, size, and granulation of platelets and the presence of fragmented red blood cells (RBCs) as seen in

Table 43.1	Differential Diagnosis of Bleeding in the Neonate			
Clinical evaluation	Laboratory studies			Likely diagnosis
	Platelets	PT	PTT	
"Sick"	D−	I+	I+	DIC
	D−	N	N	Platelet consumption (infection, necrotizing enterocolitis, renal vein thrombosis)
	N	I+	I+	Liver disease
	N	N	N	Compromised vascular integrity (associated with hypoxia, prematurity, acidosis, hyperosmolality)
"Healthy"	D−	N	N	Immune thrombocytopenia, occult infection, thrombosis, bone marrow hypoplasia (rare), or bone marrow infiltrative disease
	N	I+	I+	Hemorrhagic disease of newborn (vitamin K deficiency)
	N	N	I+	Hereditary clotting factor deficiencies
	N	N	N	Bleeding due to local factors (trauma, anatomic abnormalities); qualitative platelet abnormalities (rare); factor XIII deficiency (rare)

PT = prothrombin time; PTT = partial thromboplastin time; D− = decreased; I+ = increased; DIC = disseminated intravascular coagulation; N = normal.
(Modified from Glader BE, Amylon MD. Bleeding disorders in the newborn infant. In: Taeusch HW, Ballard RA, Avery ME, eds. *Diseases of the Newborn*. Philadelphia: WB Saunders; 1991.)

DIC. Large platelets reflect either young platelets (implying an immune cause of destructive thrombocytopenia) or congenital macrothrombocytopenias.

3. **Significant bleeding** from thrombocytopenia **is usually associated with platelet counts under 20,000 to 30,000/mm³ or less**, except in alloimmune thrombocytopenia due to antibodies against the platelet alloantigen, HPA1 (also known as PLA1), which may cause bleeding in platelet counts up to 50,000 platelets/mm³ because the antibody interferes with platelet surface fibrinogen receptor, glycoprotein IIb to IIIa (see Chap. 47).

4. **Prothrombin time (PT)** is a test of the poorly named "extrinsic" clotting system. Factor VII and tissue factor activate factor X; Factor Xa activates prothrombin (II) to form thrombin, with factor Va as a cofactor. Thrombin cleaves fibrinogen to fibrin.

Table 43.2	Normal Values for Laboratory Screening Tests in the Neonate		
Laboratory test	Premature infant having received vitamin K	Term infant having received vitamin K	Child 1–2 mo of age
Platelet count/μL	150,000–400,000	150,000–400,000	150,000–400,000
PT (s)*	14–22	13–20	12–14
PTT (s)*	35–55	30–45	25–35
Fibrinogen (mg/dL)	150–300	150–300	150–300

PT = prothrombin time; PTT = partial thromboplastin time.
*Normal values may vary from laboratory to laboratory, depending on the particular reagent employed. In full-term infants who have received vitamin K, the PT and PTT values generally fall within the normal "adult" range by several days (PT) to several weeks (PTT) of age. Small premature infants (under 1,500 g) tend to have longer PT and PTT than larger babies. In infants with hematocrit levels >60%, the ratio of blood to anticoagulant (sodium citrate 3.8%) in tubes should be 19:1 rather than the usual ratio of 9:1; otherwise, spurious results will be obtained, because the amount of anticoagulant solution is calculated for a specific volume of plasma. Blood drawn from heparinized catheters should not be used. The best results are obtained when blood from a clean venipuncture is allowed to drip directly into the tube from the needle or scalp vein set. Factor levels II, VII, IX, and X are decreased. Three-day-old full-term baby not receiving vitamin K has levels similar to a premature baby. Factor XI and XII levels are lower in preterm infants than in term infants and account for prolonged PTT. Fibrinogen, factor V, and factor VII are normal in premature and term infants. Factor XIII is variable.
(Data from normal laboratory values at the Hematology Laboratory, The Children's Hospital Boston; Alpers JB, Lafonet MT, eds. *Laboratory Handbook*. Boston: The Children's Hospital, 1984.)

5. **PTT** is a test of the so-called "intrinsic" clotting system and of the activation of factor X by factors XII, XI, IX, and VIII, as well as the factors of the common coagulation pathway (factors V and II and fibrinogen).

6. **Fibrinogen** can be measured on the same sample as that used for PT and PTT. It may be decreased in liver disease and consumptive states, and the usual functional assay is low in dysfibrinogenemia.

7. **D-Dimer assays** measure degradation products of fibrin found in the plasma of patients with DIC and in patients with liver disease who have problems clearing fibrin split products. D-Dimers are formed from the action of plasmin on the fibrin clot, generating derivatives of cross-linked fibrin containing pairs of D-domains from adjacent fibrinogen molecules. Normal levels depend on the type of assay used, which vary from hospital to hospital. Levels are high in DIC and any significant venous thromboembolism. False-positive D-dimers are common in the intensive care unit setting, because trivial clotting from catheter tips and other causes give positive results in this sensitive assay.

8. **Specific factor assays and von Willebrand panels** for patients with positive family history **can be measured in cord blood, or by venipuncture after birth.** Age-specific norms must be consulted.

9. **Bleeding times are to be discouraged in all patients, but especially in neonates.** This test measures response to a standardized razor blade cut and does not predict surgical bleeding. The apparatus is not well suited to infants and should never be used.

10. Platelet function analysis using instruments such as the PFA100 may be useful as a screening test for VWD or platelet dysfunction in some settings, but confirmatory specific assays are required for positive tests. Because functional platelet assays are best drawn through large bore needles, assessment later than the newborn period, or in affected family members, is preferable to testing neonates if possible.

III. TREATMENT OF NEONATES WITH ABNORMAL BLEEDING PARAMETERS WHO HAVE NOT HAD CLINICAL BLEEDING.
In one study, preterm infants with respiratory distress syndrome or term infants with asphyxia were treated for abnormal bleeding parameters (without DIC) to correct the hemostatic defect. Although the treatment was successful in correcting the defect, no change in mortality was seen in comparison with controls (8).

In general, we treat clinically ill infants or infants weighing <1,500 g with fresh frozen plasma (FFP; 10 mL/kg) if the PT or PTT or both are more than two times normal for age, or with platelets (1 unit) (see IV.C.) if the platelet count is under 20,000/mm^3 (see Chaps. 42 and 47). This will vary with the clinical situations, trend of the laboratory values, impending surgery, and so forth. Some babies will receive platelets if their platelet count is <50,000/mm^3, particularly in known NAIT with HPA1 (PLA1) sensitization.

IV. TREATMENT OF BLEEDING

A. **Vitamin K$_1$ (Aquamephyton).** An intravenous or intramuscular dose of 1 mg is administered in case the infant was not given vitamin K at birth. Infants receiving total parenteral nutrition and infants receiving antibiotics for more than 2 weeks should be given at least 0.5 mg of vitamin K$_1$ (IM or IV) weekly to prevent vitamin K depletion. Ideally, vitamin K (rather than FFP) should be given for long PT and PTT due to vitamin K deficiency with minimal bleeding, while plasma should be reserved for significant bleeding or emergencies because correction with vitamin K can take 12 to 48 hours.

B. **FFP** (see Chap. 42) (10 mL/kg) is given intravenously for active bleeding and is repeated every 8 to 12 hours as needed or as a drip of 1 cc/kg/hour. FFP replaces the clotting factors immediately.

C. **Platelets** (see Chap. 47). If there is no increased platelet destruction (as a result of DIC, immune platelet problem, or sepsis), 1 unit of platelets given to a 3-kg infant will raise the platelet count by 50,000 to 100,000/mm^3. If no new platelets are made or transfused, the platelet count will drop slowly over 3 to 5 days. If available, platelets from the mother or from a known platelet-compatible donor should be used if the infant has an alloimmune platelet disorder. The blood of the donor should be matched for Rh factor and type and washed, because RBCs will be mixed in the platelet concentrates. Platelets are irradiated before transfusion.

D. **Fresh whole blood** (see Chaps. 42 and 45). The baby is given 10 mL/kg; more is given as needed. Reconstituted components (FFP, PRBC, cryoprecipitate, and platelets) are more flexible and readily dosed than fresh whole blood.

E. **Clotting factor concentrates** (see Chap. 42). When there is a known deficiency of factor VIII or IX, the plasma concentration should be raised to normal adult levels (50% to 100% of pooled normal control plasma, or 0.5 to 1 unit/mL) to stop serious bleeding. Recombinant DNA-derived factors VIII and IX should be used if the diagnosis is clear. If severe VWD is considered, a VWF-containing plasma-derived factor VIII concentrate should be used. For other factor deficiencies, 10 mL/kg of FFP will transiently raise the factor level approximately to 20% of adult control. Cryoprecipitate is the most practical source of fibrinogen or factor XIII for neonates until a specific diagnosis is made.

F. **Disorders due to problems other than hemostatic proteins.** Diagnosis and treatment should be aimed at the underlying cause (e.g., infection, liver rupture, catheter, or NEC).

G. **Treatment of specific disorders**

1. **DIC.** The baby usually appears sick and may have petechiae, GI hemorrhage, oozing from venipunctures, infection, asphyxia, or hypoxia. The platelet count is decreased, and PT and PTT are increased. Fragmented RBCs are seen on the blood smear. Fibrinogen is decreased, and D-dimers are increased. Treatment involves the following steps:

   a. **The underlying cause should be treated** (e.g., sepsis, NEC, herpes). This is **always** the most important factor in treatment of DIC and determines success of overall treatment.

   b. **Confirm that vitamin K_1 has been given.**

   c. **Platelets and FFP are given** as needed to keep the platelet count over 50,000/mL and to stop the bleeding. FFP contains anticoagulant proteins, which may slow down or stop ongoing consumption.

   d. **If the bleeding persists**, one of the following steps should be taken, depending on the availability of blood, platelets, or FFP:

      i. Exchange transfusion with fresh citrated whole blood or reconstituted whole blood (packed RBCs, platelets, FFP).

      ii. Continued transfusion with platelets, packed RBCs, and FFP as needed.

      iii. Administration of cryoprecipitate (10 mL/kg) for hypofibrinogenemia.

   e. If consumption coagulopathy is associated with thrombosis of large vessels and not with concurrent bleeding, **heparinization without a bolus may be considered** (e.g., 10 to 15 units/kg/hour as a continuous infusion). Platelets and plasma are continued to be given after the heparin has been started. Platelet counts should be kept at or above 50,000/mL. Heparin is best monitored by functional heparin levels, with a goal of 0.3 to 0.7 units/mL, aiming on the lower side in patients with mild concurrent bleeding. The plasma is essential to provide antithrombin III (AT III) and other anticoagulant proteins. Heparinization is generally contraindicated in the presence of intracranial hemorrhage, and if bleeding accompanies DIC and thrombosis concurrently, heparinization is complicated. Consult an expert immediately (see Chap. 44).

2. **Hemorrhagic disease of the newborn** (HDN) occurs in 1 out of every 200 to 400 neonates not given vitamin K prophylaxis.

   a. In the healthy infant, **HDN may occur when the infant is not given vitamin K.** The infant may have been born in a busy delivery room, at home, or transferred from elsewhere. Bleeding and bruising may occur after the infant is 48 hours old. The platelet level is normal, and PT and PTT are prolonged. If there is active bleeding, 10 mL/kg of FFP and an IV dose of 1 mg of vitamin K are given.

b. If the mother has been treated with phenytoin (Dilantin), primidone (Mysoline), methsuximide (Celontin), or phenobarbital, the infant may be vitamin K deficient and bleed during the first 24 hours. The mother should be given vitamin K 24 hours before delivery (10 mg of vitamin K_1 IM). The newborn should have PT, PTT, and platelet counts monitored if any signs of bleeding occur. The usual dose of vitamin K_1 (1 mg) should be given to the baby postpartum and repeated in 24 hours. Repeated infusions of FFP are given if any bleeding occurs.

c. Delayed HDN from vitamin K deficiency can occur at 4 to 12 weeks of age. This may happen in breastfed infants who are not receiving supplementation. Infants who are undergoing treatment with broad-spectrum antibiotics or infants with malabsorption (liver disease, cystic fibrosis) are at greater risk for hemorrhagic disease. Vitamin K_1, 1 mg/week orally for the first 3 months of life, may prevent late hemologic disease of the newborn. Although blood tests show that breastfed infants are at potential risk for HDN, HDN has not been reported in infants who received intramuscular vitamin K at birth (1,9).

REFERENCES

1. Monagle P, Andrew M. Developmental hemostasis: relevance to newborns and infants. In: Nathan DG, Orkin SH, Ginsburg D, eds. *Hematology of infancy and childhood*. Philadelphia: WB Saunders; 2003:121–168.
2. Plötz FB, van Oeveren W, Bartlett RH, et al. Blood activation during neonatal extracorporeal life support. *J Thorac Cardiovasc Surg* 1993;105(5):823–832.
3. Robinson TM, Kickler TS, Walker LK, et al. Effect of extracorporeal membrane oxygenation on platelets in newborns. *Crit Care Med* 1993;21(7):1029–1034.
4. Montgomery RR, Gill JC, Scott JP. Hemophilia and von Willebrand disease. In: Nathan DG, Orkin SH, Ginsburg D, eds. *Hematology of infancy and childhood*. Philadelphia: WB Saunders; 2003:1547–1576.
5. Bauer K. Rare hereditary coagulation factor abnormalities. In: Nathan DG, Orkin SH, Ginsburg D, eds. *Hematology of infancy and childhood*. Philadelphia: WB Saunders; 2003:1577–1596.
6. Poncz M. Inherited platelet disorders. In: Nathan DG, Orkin SH, Ginsburg D, eds. *Hematology of infancy and childhood*. Philadelphia: WB Saunders; 2003:1527–1546.
7. Wilson DB. Acquired platelet defects. In: Nathan DG, Orkin SH, Ginsburg D, eds. *Hematology of infancy and childhood*. Philadelphia: WB Saunders; 2003:1597–1630.
8. Turner T. Treatment of premature infants with abnormal clotting parameters. *Br J Hematol* 1981;47:65.
9. American Academy of Pediatrics Committee on Fetus and Newborn. Controversies concerning vitamin K and the newborn. American Academy of Pediatrics Committee on Fetus and Newborn. *Pediatrics* 2003;112(1 pt 1):191–192.

Suggested Readings

Andrew M, Paes B, Milner R, et al. Development of the human coagulation system in the full-term infant. *Blood* 1987;70(1):165–172.

Cantor AB. Developmental hemostasis: relevance to newborns and infants. In: Orkin SH, Nathan DG, Ginsburg D, et al., eds. *Hematology of infancy and childhood*. 7th ed. Philadelphia: Saunders Elsevier; 2009:147–191.

Monagle P, Barnes C, Ignjatovic V, et al. Developmental haemostasis. Impact for clinical haemostasis laboratories. *Thromb Haemost* 2006;95(2):362–372.

Rajpurkar M, Lusher JM. Clinical and laboratory approach to the patient with bleeding. In: Orkin SH, Nathan DG, Ginsburg D, et al. *Hematology of infancy and childhood*. 7th ed. Philadelphia: Saunders Elsevier; 2009:1449–1461.

Trenor CC, Neufeld EJ. In: Hoffman R, Benz EJ, Shattil SJ, et al., eds. *Hematology: Basic Principles and Practice*. 5th ed. Linn, MO: Churchill Livingstone; 2009:2010–2019.

Neonatal Thrombosis

Munish Gupta

I. PHYSIOLOGY

A. Physiology of thrombosis

1. **Thrombin is the primary procoagulant protein,** converting fibrinogen into a fibrin clot. The intrinsic and extrinsic pathways of the coagulation cascade result in formation of active thrombin from prothrombin.

2. **Inhibitors of coagulation** include antithrombin, heparin cofactor I, protein C, protein S, and tissue factor pathway inhibitor (TFPI). Antithrombin activity is potentiated by heparin.

3. **Plasmin is the primary fibrinolytic enzyme,** degrading fibrin in a reaction that produces fibrin degradation products and D-dimers. Plasmin is formed from plasminogen by numerous enzymes, most important of which is tissue plasminogen activator (tPA).

4. In neonates, factors affecting blood flow, blood composition (leading to hypercoagulability), and vascular endothelial integrity can all contribute to thrombus formation.

B. Unique physiologic characteristics of hemostasis in neonates

1. *In utero*, coagulation proteins are synthesized by the fetus and do not cross the placenta.

2. Both thrombogenic and fibrinolytic pathways are altered in the neonate compared with the older child and adult, resulting in increased vulnerability to both hemorrhage and pathologic thrombosis. However, under normal physiologic conditions, the hemostatic system in premature and term newborns is in balance, and healthy neonates do not clinically demonstrate hypercoagulable or bleeding tendencies.

3. Concentrations of most procoagulant proteins are reduced in neonates compared with adult values, although fibrinogen levels are normal or even increased. Compared with adults, neonates have a decreased ability to generate thrombin, and values for the prothrombin time (PT) and the activated partial thromboplastin time (PTT) are prolonged.

4. Concentrations of most antithrombotic and fibrinolytic proteins are also reduced, including protein C, protein S, plasminogen, and antithrombin. Thrombin inhibition by plasmin is diminished compared with adult plasma.

5. Platelet number and life span appear to be similar to that of adults. The bleeding time, an overall assessment of platelet function and interaction with vascular endothelium, is shorter in neonates than in adults, suggesting more rapid platelet adhesion and aggregation.

II. EPIDEMIOLOGY AND RISK FACTORS

A. Epidemiology

1. Thrombosis occurs more frequently in the neonatal period than at any other age in childhood.

2. The presence of an indwelling vascular catheter is the single greatest risk factor for arterial or venous thrombosis. Indwelling catheters are responsible for more than 80% of venous and 90% of arterial thrombotic complications.

3. Autopsy studies show 20% to 65% of infants who expire with an umbilical venous catheter (UVC) in place are found to have a thrombus associated with the catheter. Venography suggests asymptomatic thrombi are present in 30% of newborns with a UVC.

4. Umbilical arterial catheterization (UAC) appears to result in clinically severe symptomatic vessel obstruction requiring intervention in approximately 1% of patients. Asymptomatic catheter-associated thrombi have been found in 3% to 59% of cases by autopsy and 10% to 90% of cases by angiography or ultrasound.

5. Other risk factors for thrombosis include infection, increased blood viscosity, polycythemia, dehydration, hypoxia, hypotension, maternal preeclampsia, maternal diabetes, chorioamnionitis, and intrauterine growth restriction (IUGR).

6. Infants undergoing surgery involving the vascular system, including repair of congenital heart disease, are at increased risk for thrombotic complications. Diagnostic or interventional catheterizations also increase the risk of thrombosis.

7. **Renal vein thrombosis (RVT)** is the most common type of noncatheter-related pathologic thrombosis in newborns.

8. Registries from Canada, Germany, and the Netherlands have described series of cases of neonatal thrombosis.

   a. Incidence of clinically significant thrombosis were estimated as 2.4 per 1,000 admissions to the neonatal intensive care unit in Canada, 5.1 per 100,000 births in Germany, and 14.5 per 10,000 neonates aged 0 to 28 days in the Netherlands.

   b. Two series examined both venous and arterial thromboses. Among all thrombotic events, percentage of RVT, other venous thrombosis, and arterial thrombosis were 44%, 32%, and 24%, respectively, in one series; and 22%, 40%, and 34% in the other series.

   c. Excluding cases of RVT, 89% and 94% of venous thromboses were found to be associated with indwelling central lines in two of the studies.

   d. Other commonly identified risk factors included sepsis, perinatal asphyxia, congenital heart disease, and dehydration.

   e. Mortality was uncommon, but present, and was generally restricted to very premature infants or infants with large arterial or intracardiac thromboses.

B. Inherited thrombophilias

1. **Inherited thrombophilias** are characterized by positive family history, early age of onset, recurrent disease, and unusual or multiple locations of thromboembolic events. It is estimated that a genetic risk factor can be identified in approximately 70% of patients with thrombophilia.

2. Important inherited thrombophilias include:

    a. Deficiencies of protein C, protein S, and antithrombin, which appear to have the largest increase in relative risk for thromboembolic disease, but are relatively rare.

    b. Activated protein C resistance, including the factor V Leiden mutation, and the prothrombin G20210A mutation, which have high incidence, particularly in certain populations, but appear to have a low risk of thrombosis in neonates.

    c. Hyperhomocysteinemia, increased lipoprotein(a) levels, and polymorphism in the methylene tetrahydrofolate reductase (MTHFR) gene, which are relatively common but whose significance in neonatal thrombosis is still poorly understood.

3. Multiple other defects in the anticoagulation, fibrinolytic, and antifibrinolytic pathways have been identified, including abnormalities in thrombomodulin, TFPI, fibrinogen, plasminogen, tPA, and plasminogen-activator inhibitors. The frequency and importance of these defects in neonatal thrombosis is poorly understood.

4. The incidence of thrombosis in patients heterozygous for most inherited thrombophilias is small; however, increasing evidence suggests that the presence of a second risk factor substantially increases the risk of thrombosis. This second risk factor can be an acquired clinical condition or illness, or another inherited defect. Patients with single defects for inherited prothrombotic disorders rarely present in neonatal period, unless another pathologic process or event occurs.

5. Patients who are homozygous for a single defect or double heterozygotes for different defects can present in the neonatal period, often with significant illness due to thrombosis. The classic presentation of homozygous prothrombotic disorders is **purpura fulminans** with homozygous protein C or S deficiency, which presents within hours or days of birth, often with evidence of *in utero* cerebral damage.

6. Overall, the importance of inherited thrombophilias as independent risk factors for neonatal thrombosis is still undetermined. It appears that the absolute risk of thrombosis in the neonatal period in all patients with inherited thrombophilia (nonhomozygous) is actually quite small; however, among neonates with thrombotic disease, the incidence of an inherited thrombophilia appears to be substantially increased compared with incidence in the general population, and evaluation for thrombophilia should be considered (see V.A.).

C. Acquired thrombophilias

1. Newborns can acquire significant coagulation factor deficiencies due to placental transfer of maternal antiphospholipid antibodies, including the lupus anticoagulant and anticardiolipin antibody.

2. These neonates can present with significant thrombosis, including purpura fulminans.

III. SPECIFIC CLINICAL CONDITIONS

A. Venous thromboembolic disorders

1. General considerations

    a. Most venous thrombosis occur secondary to **central venous catheters.** Spontaneous (i.e., noncatheter-related) venous thrombosis can occur in renal veins, adrenal veins, inferior vena cava, portal vein, hepatic veins, and the venous system of the brain.

b. Spontaneous venous thrombi usually occur in the presence of another risk factor. Less than 1% of significant venous thromboembolic events in neonates are idiopathic.

c. Thrombosis of the **sinovenous system of the brain** is an important cause of neonatal cerebral infarction.

d. Short-term complications of venous catheter-associated thrombosis include loss of access, pulmonary embolism, superior vena cava syndrome, and specific organ impairment.

e. It is likely that the frequency of pulmonary embolism in sick neonates is underestimated, as signs and symptoms would be similar to multiple other common pulmonary diseases.

f. Long-term complications of venous thrombosis are poorly understood. Inferior vena cava thrombosis, if extensive, can be associated with a high rate of persistent partial obstruction and symptoms such as leg edema, abdominal pain, lower extremity thrombophlebitis, varicose veins, and leg ulcers. Other complications can include chylothorax, portal hypertension, and embolism.

2. Major venous thrombosis—signs and symptoms

a. Initial sign of catheter-related thrombosis is usually difficulty infusing through or withdrawing from the line.

b. Signs of venous obstruction include swelling of the extremities, possibly including the head and neck, and distended superficial veins.

c. The onset of thrombocytopenia in the presence of a central venous line (CVL) also raises the suspicion of thrombosis.

3. Major venous thrombosis—diagnosis

a. Ultrasound is diagnostic in most cases of significant venous thrombosis. In smaller infants or low-flow states, however, the ultrasound may not provide sufficient information about the size of the thrombus, and a significant false-negative rate for ultrasound diagnosis has been documented.

b. Contrast studies. A radiographic line study can be helpful for diagnosis of catheter-associated thrombosis. Venography through peripheral vessels may be needed for diagnosis of thrombosis proximal to the catheter tip, for spontaneous thrombosis in the upper body, and for thrombosis not seen by other methods (see IV.).

4. Prevention of catheter-associated venous thrombosis

a. Heparin 0.5 units/mL is added to all infusions (compatability permitting) through CVLs.

b. UVCs should be removed as soon as clinically feasible and should not remain in place for longer than 10 to 14 days. Our usual practice is to place a peripherally inserted central catheter (PICC) line if anticipated need for central access is more than 7 days.

5. Management of major venous thrombosis

a. Nonfunctioning CVL

    i. If fluid can no longer be easily infused through the catheter, remove the catheter unless the CVL is absolutely necessary.

    ii. If continued central access through the catheter is judged to be clinically necessary, clearance of the blockage with thrombolytic agents or HCl can be considered (see V.F.).

b. Local obstruction. If a small occlusive catheter-related thrombosis is documented, a low-dose infusion of thrombolytic agents through the catheter can be considered for localized site-directed thrombolytic therapy (see V.E.). If infusion through the catheter is not possible, the CVL should be removed and heparin therapy should be considered.

c. Extensive venous thrombosis. Consider leaving the catheter in place and attempting local site-directed thrombolytic therapy. Otherwise, remove the catheter and begin heparin therapy. Systemic thrombolytic therapy should be reserved for extensive non–catheter-related venous thrombosis and for venous thrombosis with significant clinical compromise.

d. In cases of catheter-related venous thrombosis, some clinicians suggest delaying catheter removal until after 3 to 5 days of anticoagulation in order to reduce risk of paradoxical emboli at time of catheter removal. Data is limited to evaluate this practice.

B. Aortic or major arterial thrombosis

1. General considerations

a. Spontaneous arterial thrombi in absence of a catheter are unusual but may occur in ill neonates.

b. Acute complications of catheter-related and spontaneous arterial thrombi depend on location, and can include renal hypertension, intestinal necrosis, peripheral gangrene, and other organ failure.

c. Thrombosis of cerebral arteries is an important cause of neonatal cerebral infarction.

d. Long-term effects of symptomatic and asymptomatic arterial thrombi are not well studied, but may include increased risk for atherosclerosis at the affected area and chronic renal hypertension.

2. Aortic thrombosis—signs and symptoms

a. Initial sign is often isolated dysfunction of umbilical arterial catheter (UAC).

b. Mild clinical signs include hematuria in absence of transfusions or hemolysis, hematuria with red blood cells (RBCs) on microscopic analysis, hypertension, and intermittent lower extremity decreased perfusion or color change.

c. Strong clinical signs include persistent lower extremity color change or decreased perfusion, blood pressure differential between upper and lower extremities, decrease or loss of lower extremity pulses, signs of peripheral thrombosis, oliguria despite adequate intravascular volume, signs of necrotizing enterocolitis (NEC), and signs of congestive heart failure.

3. Aortic thrombosis—diagnosis

a. Ultrasound with Doppler flow imaging should generally be performed in all cases of suspected aortic thrombosis; if signs of thrombosis are mild and resolve promptly after removal of the arterial catheter, an ultrasound may not be necessary. Ultrasound is diagnostic in most cases, although a significant false-negative rate has been documented.

b. Contrast study. If an ultrasound is negative or inconclusive, and major arterial thrombosis is suspected, a radiographic contrast study can be performed via the arterial catheter.

4. Prevention of catheter-associated arterial thrombosis

a. Heparin 0.5 to 1 unit/mL is added to all infusions (compatibility permitting) through arterial catheters; heparin infusion through arterial catheters has been shown to prolong patency and to likely reduce incidence of local thrombus, without the risk of significant complications.

b. Review of the literature suggests **"high" umbilical arterial lines** (tip in descending aorta below left subclavian artery and above diaphragm) are preferable to "low" lines (tip below renal arteries and above aortic bifurcation), with fewer clinically evident ischemic complications, an apparent trend to reduced incidence of thrombi, and no difference in serious complications such as NEC and renal dysfunction (see Chap. 66).

c. Consider placing a **peripheral arterial line** rather than an umbilical arterial line in infants weighing >1,500 g.

d. Monitor carefully for clinical evidence of thrombus formation when an UAC is present.

  i. Monitor for evidence of UAC dysfunction, including waveform dampening and difficulty flushing or withdrawing blood.

  ii. Monitor lower extremity color and perfusion.

  iii. Check all urine for heme.

  iv. Check upper and lower extremity blood pressure three times daily.

  v. Monitor for hypertension and decreased urine output.

e. UACs should be removed as soon as clinically feasible. Our general practice is to leave UACs in place for no longer than 5 to 7 days, and to place a peripheral arterial line should continued arterial access be needed.

5. **Management of aortic and major arterial thrombosis**

  a. Minor aortic thrombi. Small aortic thrombi with limited mild symptoms can often be managed with prompt removal of the UAC, with rapid resolution of symptoms.

  b. Large but nonocclusive thrombus. For large thrombi that are nonocclusive to blood flow (as demonstrated by ultrasound or contrast study) and that are not accompanied by signs of significant clinical compromise, the arterial catheter should be removed and anticoagulation with heparin considered. Close follow-up with serial imaging studies is indicated.

  c. Occlusive thrombus or significant clinical compromise. Large occlusive aortic thrombi or thrombi accompanied by signs of significant clinical compromise, including renal failure, congestive heart failure, NEC, and signs of peripheral ischemia, should be managed aggressively:

    i. If catheter is still present and patent, consider local thrombolytic therapy through the catheter (see V.E.).

    ii. If catheter has already been removed or is obstructed, consider systemic thrombolytic therapy. The catheter should be removed if still in place and obstructed.

  d. Surgical thrombectomy is generally not indicated, since the mortality and morbidity are considered to exceed that of current medical management. Some recent experience suggests thrombectomy and subsequent vascular reconstruction may have utility in significant peripheral arterial thrombosis, although this experience is limited.

6. **Peripheral arterial thrombosis**

  a. Congenital occlusions of large peripheral arteries are seen, although rare, and can present with symptoms ranging from a poorly perfused, pulseless extremity to a black, necrotic limb, depending on duration and timing of occlusion.

    i. Common symptoms include decreased perfusion, decreased pulses, pallor, and embolic phenomena that may manifest as skin lesions or petechiae.

    ii. Diagnosis can often be made by Doppler flow ultrasound.

b. Peripheral arterial catheters, including radial, posterior tibial, and dorsalis pedis catheters, are rarely associated with significant thrombosis.

    i. Poor perfusion to the distal extremity is frequently seen, and usually resolves with prompt removal of the arterial line.

    ii. We infuse heparin 0.5 to 1 unit/mL at 1 to 2 mL/hour through all peripheral arterial lines.

    iii. Treatment of significant thrombosis or persistently compromised extremity perfusion associated with a peripheral catheter should consist of heparin anticoagulation and consideration of systemic thrombolysis for extensive lesions. Removal of the catheter should be considered but sometimes it is left in for thrombolysis. Close follow-up with serial imaging is indicated.

C. Renal vein thrombosis (see Chap. 28)

  1. RVT occurs primarily in newborns and young infants, and most often presents in the first week of life. A significant proportion of cases appear to result from *in utero* thrombus formation.

  2. Affected neonates are usually term and are often large for gestational age (LGA). There is an increased incidence among infants of diabetic mothers, and males are more often affected than females. Other associated conditions and risk factors include perinatal asphyxia, hypotension, polycythemia, increased blood viscosity, and cyanotic congenital heart disease.

  3. Presenting symptoms in the neonatal period include flank mass, hematuria, proteinuria, thrombocytopenia, and renal dysfunction. Coagulation studies may be prolonged, and fibrin degradation products are usually increased. Complications can include adrenal hemorrhage and extension of the thrombus into the inferior vena cava.

  4. A recent review demonstrated that bilateral disease occurs in 30% of cases.

  5. Retrospective studies have demonstrated that 43% to 67% of neonates with RVT had at least one or more prothrombotic risk factors. An evaluation of infants presenting with RVT for thrombophilia is warranted.

  6. Diagnosis is usually by ultrasound.

  7. Management is generally based on extent of thrombosis.

    a. Unilateral RVT without significant renal dysfunction and without extension into the inferior vena cava is often managed with supportive care alone.

    b. Unilateral RVT with renal dysfunction or extension into the inferior vena cava and bilateral RVT should be considered for anticoagulation with heparin.

    c. Bilateral RVT with significant renal dysfunction should be considered for thrombolysis followed by anticoagulation.

    d. There may be hypertension requiring treatment (see Chap. 28).

D. Portal vein thrombosis (PVT)

  1. PVT is primarily associated with sepsis/omphalitis and UVC use.

  2. Diagnosis is made by ultrasound; reversal of portal flow is an indication of severity.

  3. Spontaneous resolution is common. However, PVT can be associated with later development of portal hypertension.

E. Cerebral sinovenous thrombosis

  1. Thrombosis of the sinovenous system of the brain is an important cause of neonatal cerebral infarction.

2. Major presenting clinical features of cerebral sinovenous thrombosis (CSVT) in neonates include seizures, lethargy, irritability, and poor feeding. The majority present within the first week of life.

3. The superior sagittal sinus, transverse sinuses, and the straight sinus are most commonly affected.

4. Hemorrhagic infarctions are frequent complications of sinovenous thrombosis.

5. The majority of cases of neonatal sinovenous thrombosis are associated with maternal conditions (including preeclampsia, diabetes, and chorioamnionitis) and/or acute systemic illness in the neonate.

6. Inherited thrombophilias have been reported in 15% to 20% of neonates with sinovenous thrombosis.

7. Ultrasound and CT scan can detect sinovenous thrombosis and associated complications, but MRI with venography is the imaging modality of choice for the best detection of sinovenous thrombosis and cerebral injury.

8. Data on management is limited. In general, neonates with CSVT without associated hemorrhage can be considered for anticoagulation therapy. If significant hemorrhage is present, anticoagulation should be reserved for cases in which thrombus is noted to propagate.

IV. DIAGNOSTIC CONSIDERATIONS

A. **Ultrasound with Doppler flow analysis is the most commonly used diagnostic modality.**

1. Advantages include relative ease of performance, noninvasiveness, and ability to perform sequential scans to assess progression of thrombosis or response to treatment.

2. Sensitivity of ultrasound may be somewhat limited: several recent studies suggest that significant venous and arterial thrombi may be missed by ultrasonography. Ultrasound remains our test of first choice, but if it is inconclusive or negative in the context of significant clinical suspicion of thrombosis, a contrast study should be considered.

B. **Radiographic line study.** Imaging after injection of contrast material through a central catheter often is diagnostic for catheter-associated thrombi and has the advantage of relative ease of performance.

C. **Venography.** Venography with injection of contrast through peripheral vessels may be necessary when other diagnostic methods fail to demonstrate the extent and severity of thrombosis.

1. A contrast line study will not provide information on venous thrombosis proximal to catheter tip (i.e., along the length of the catheter).

2. Upper extremity and upper chest venous thromboses, either catheter-related or spontaneous, are particularly difficult to visualize with ultrasound.

V. MANAGEMENT

A. **Evaluation for thrombophilia**

1. Consider evaluating for congenital or acquired thrombophilias in those neonates with severe or unusual manifestations of thrombosis or with positive

family histories of thrombosis. The benefit of evaluation in infants with known risk factors such as indwelling central catheters is uncertain.

2. Initial evaluation should include consideration of deficiencies of protein C, protein S, or antithrombin; presence of activated protein C resistance and the factor V Leiden mutation; presence of the prothrombin G20210A mutation; and passage of maternal antiphospholipid antibodies.

   a. Protein C, protein S, and antithrombin deficiencies can be evaluated by measurement of antigen or activity levels. Results of testing of neonates should be compared with standard gestational age-based reference ranges, as normal physiologic values can be as low as 15% to 20% of adult values. In addition, levels will be physiologically depressed in the presence of active thrombosis and may be difficult to interpret; we therefore generally wait until 2 to 3 months after the thrombotic episode before performing these measurements in the infant. As an alternative to or in conjunction with testing of the neonate, parents can be tested for carrier status by measurement of protein C, protein S, and antithrombin levels.

   b. Factor V Leiden and prothrombin G20210A mutations can be assayed by specific genetic tests in the neonate. Parents can be tested for carrier status.

   c. The mother can be tested for antinuclear antibodies, lupus anticoagulant, and anticardiolipin antibodies.

3. If all of the above are negative, subsequent specialized laboratory evaluation includes consideration of abnormalities or deficiencies of homocysteine, lipoprotein(a), MTHFR, plasminogen, and fibrinogen. Very rarely seen are abnormalities or deficiencies of heparin cofactor II, thrombomodulin, plasminogen activator inhibitor-1, platelet aggregation, and tPA.

B. General considerations

1. Precautions

   a. Avoid intramuscular (IM) injections and arterial punctures during anticoagulation or thrombolytic therapy.

   b. Avoid indocin or other antiplatelet drugs during therapy.

   c. Use minimal physical manipulation of patient (i.e., no physical therapy) during thrombolytic therapy.

   d. Thrombolytic therapy should not be initiated in the presence of active bleeding or significant risk for local bleeding and should be carefully considered if there is a history of recent surgery of any type (particularly neurosurgery).

   e. Monitor clinical status carefully for signs of hemorrhage, including internal hemorrhage and intracranial hemorrhage.

   f. Consider giving fresh frozen plasma (FFP) 10 mL/kg to any patient who needs anticoagulation.

2. **Guidelines for choice of therapy**

   a. Small asymptomatic nonocclusive arterial or venous thrombi related to catheters can often be treated with catheter removal and supportive care alone.

   b. Large or occlusive venous thrombi can be treated with anticoagulation with heparin or low-molecular-weight (LMW) heparin. Usually, relatively short courses (7–14 days) of anticoagulation are sufficient, but occasionally, long-term treatment may be necessary.

   c. Most arterial thrombi should be treated with anticoagulation with heparin or LMW heparin.

   d. In cases of massive venous thrombi or arterial thrombi with significant clinical compromise, treatment with local or systemic thrombolysis should be considered.

C. Heparin

1. General considerations

a. Term newborns generally have increased clearance of heparin compared with adults, and thus require relatively increased heparin dosage. This increased clearance is significantly diminished, however, in premature neonates.

b. Heparin should be infused through a dedicated IV line that is not used for any other medications or fluids, if possible.

c. Prior to starting heparin therapy, obtain a complete blood count (CBC), PT, and PTT.

d. Adjustment of heparin infusion rate is based on clinical response, serial evaluation of thrombus (usually by ultrasound), and monitoring of laboratory parameters.

e. Significant patient-to-patient variability in heparin dosage requirements is seen.

f. Use of PTT to monitor heparin effect is problematic in neonates due to significant variability of coagulation factor concentrations and baseline prolongation of the PTT. **Heparin activity level** is generally considered to be a more reliable marker.

g. Therapeutic heparin activity for treatment of most thromboembolic events is considered to be an antifactor Xa level of 0.35 to 0.7 unit/mL or a heparin level by protamine titration of 0.2 to 0.4 unit/mL. Most laboratories report heparin activity levels as an antifactor Xa level.

h. Follow CBC frequently while on heparin treatment to monitor for heparin-associated thrombocytopenia, which can be diagnosed by an assay of heparin-associated antiplatelet antibodies.

i. Heparin activity is dependent on presence of antithrombin. Consider administration of FFP (10 mL/kg) when effective anticoagulation with heparin is difficult to achieve. Administration of antithrombin concentrate should also be considered, although evidence for its benefits in neonates is limited; doses of 40 to 50 units/kg have been used in neonates.

    i. Antithrombin levels can be measured directly to aid in therapy, although administration of exogenous antithrombin can increase sensitivity to heparin even in patients with near-normal antithrombin levels.

    ii. Note that measurement of heparin activity levels, unlike measurement of PTT, is independent of presence of antithrombin. Therefore, measured heparin activity levels may be therapeutic even though effective anticoagulation is not seen due to antithrombin deficiency.

2. Dosing guidelines

a. Standard unfractionated heparin is given as an initial bolus of 75 units/kg, followed by a continuous infusion that is begun at 28 units/kg/hour. In premature infants under 37 weeks' gestation, lower dosing of 25 to 50 units/kg bolus followed by 15 to 20 units/kg/hour can be considered.

b. Heparin activity levels and/or PTT should be measured 4 hours after initial bolus and 4 hours after each change in infusion dose, and every 24 hours once a therapeutic infusion dose has been achieved (see Table 44.1).

3. Duration of therapy.
Anticoagulation with heparin may continue up to 10 to 14 days. Oral anticoagulants are generally not recommended in neonates. If long-term anticoagulation is needed, consult hematology.

4. Reversal of anticoagulation

a. Termination of heparin infusion will quickly reverse anticoagulation effects of heparin therapy, and is usually sufficient.

Table 44.1	Heparin Dosing Monitoring and Adjustment				
PTT (s)*	Heparin activity (U/mL)	Bolus (U/kg)	Hold	Rate	Recheck
<50	0–0.2	50	—	+10%	4 h
50–59	0.21–0.34	0	—	+10%	4 h
60–85	0.35–0.7	0	—	—	24 h
86–95	0.71–0.8	0	—	−10%	4 h
96–120	0.81–1.0	0	30 min	−10%	4 h
>120	>1	0	60 min	−15%	4 h

*PTT values may vary by laboratory depending on reagents used. Generally, PTT values of 1.5 to 2.5 × the baseline normal for a given laboratory correspond to heparin activity levels of 0.35 to 0.7 U/mL.
Source: Adapted from Monagle P, Chalmers E, Chan A, et al. Antithrombotic therapy in neonates and children. *Chest* 2008;133:887S–968S.

    b. If rapid reversal is necessary, protamine sulfate may be given IV. Protamine can be given in a concentration of 10 mg/mL at a rate not to exceed 5 mg/minute. Hypersensitivity can occur in patients who have received protamine-containing insulin or previous protamine therapy.
    c. Dosing of protamine (see Table 44.2).

D. Low-molecular-weight heparin
    1. General considerations
        a. Although data on LMW heparin usage in neonatal patients is limited, growing evidence of safety and efficacy in adult and pediatric patients has led to increased use in neonatal populations.
        b. Several **advantages of LMW heparins** over standard unfractionated heparin exist: more predictable pharmacokinetics, decreased need for laboratory monitoring, subcutaneous BID dosing, probable reduced risk of heparin-induced thrombocytopenia, and possible reduced risk of bleeding at recommended dosages.
        c. Therapeutic dosage of LMW heparins are titrated to antifactor Xa levels. **Target antifactor Xa levels** for treatment of most thromboembolic events are 0.50 to 1.0 unit/mL, measured 4 to 6 hours after a subcutaneous injection. In patients at particularly high risk for bleeding, target levels of 0.4 to 0.6 unit/mL can be considered. When used for prophylaxis, target levels are 0.1 to 0.3 unit/mL. After therapeutic levels have been achieved for 24 to 48 hours, levels should be followed at least weekly.
        d. Infants under 2 months of age have a higher dose requirement than older children. In addition, some studies suggest higher initial doses for preterm infants. Dosage requirements to maintain target levels in preterm infants may be quite variable.

Table 44.2	Protamine Dosage to Reverse Heparin Therapy* (Based on Total Amount Heparin Received in Prior 2 hours)
Time since last heparin dose (min)	Protamine dose (mg/100 U heparin received)
<30	1.0
30–60	0.5–0.75
60–120	0.375–0.5
>120	0.25–0.375

*Maximum dosage is 50 mg. Maximum infusion rate is 5 mg/min of 10 mg/mL solution.
Source: Adapted from Monagle P, Chalmers E, Chan A, et al. Antithrombotic therapy in neonates and children. *Chest* 2008;133:887S–968S.

    e. Several different LMW heparins are available, and the dosages are not interchangeable. Enoxaparin (Lovenox) has the most widespread pediatric usage.
    f. Follow CBCs, as thrombocytopenia can occur.
  2. Dosing guidelines (see Tables 44.3 and 44.4)
  3. Reversal of anticoagulation
    a. Termination of subcutaneous injections usually is sufficient to reverse anticoagulation when clinically necessary.
    b. If rapid reversal is needed, protamine sulfate can be given within 3 to 4 hours of last injection, although protamine may not completely reverse anticoagulant effects. Administer 1 mg protamine sulfate per 1 mg LMW heparin given in last injection. See V.C.4. for administration guidelines.

E. Thrombolysis
  1. General considerations
    a. Thrombolytic agents act by converting endogenous plasminogen to plasmin. Plasminogen levels in neonates are reduced compared with adult values, and thus effectiveness of thrombolytic agents may be diminished. Cotreatment with plasminogen can increase thrombolytic effect of these agents.

Table 44.3	Initial Dosing of Enoxaparin, Age-dependent (in mg/kg/dose SQ)	
Age	Initial treatment dose	Initial prophylactic dose
<2 mo	1.5 q12h	0.75 q12h
>2 mo	1.0 q12h	0.5 q12h

Initial dose of 2 mg/kg q12h can be considered in preterm infants.
Source: Adapted from Young TE, Mangum B. *Neofax 2008.* Montvale, NJ: Thompson-Reuters; 2008 and Monagle P, Chalmers E, Chan A, et al. Antithrombotic therapy in neonates and children. *Chest* 2008;133:887S–968S.

Table 44.4	Monitoring and Dosage Adjustment of Enoxaparin Based on Antifactor Xa Level Measured 4 h After Dose of Enoxaparin		
Antifactor Xa level (U/mL)	Hold dose	Dose change	Repeat AntiXa level
<0.35	—	+25%	4 h after next dose
0.35–0.49	—	+10%	4 h after next dose
0.5–1.0	—	—	24 h
1.1–1.5	—	−20%	Before next dose
1.6–2.0	3 h	−30%	Before next dose, then 4 h after next dose
>2	Until level is 0.5 U/mL	−40%	Before next dose; if level not <0.5 U/mL, repeat q12h

Adapted from Monagle P. et al. Antithrombotic therapy in children. *Chest* 2001;110: 344S–370S.

b. Indications include recent arterial thrombosis, massive thrombosis with evidence of organ dysfunction or compromised limb viability, and life-threatening thrombosis. Thrombolytic agents can also be used to restore patency to thrombosed central catheters (see V.F.), and local infusions of low-dose thrombolytic agents can be used for small to moderate occlusive thrombosis near a central catheter.

c. Minimal data exist in newborn populations regarding all aspects of thrombolytic therapy, including appropriate indications, safety, efficacy, choice of agent, duration of therapy, use of heparin, and monitoring guidelines. Recommendations for use are generally based on small series and case reports, which overall suggest that thrombolytic therapy in neonates can be effective with limited significant complications.

d. Consider evaluating all patients for intraventricular hemorrhage prior to initiating thrombolytic therapy.

e. Contraindications to thrombolytic therapy include active bleeding, major surgery or hemorrhage within past 7 to 10 days, neurosurgery within the last 3 weeks, severe thrombocytopenia, and, generally, prematurity under 32 weeks.

2. Treatment guidelines
  a. Preparation for thrombolytic therapy
   i. Place sign at head of bed indicating thrombolytic therapy.
   ii. Have topical thrombin available in unit refrigerator.
   iii. Notify blood bank to insure availability of cryoprecipitate.
   iv. Notify pharmacy to ensure availability of aminocaproic acid (Amicar).
   v. Obtain good venous access; consider access to allow frequent blood draws to minimize need for phlebotomy.
   vi. Consider hematology consult.

b. Thrombolysis can be achieved by local, site-directed administration of thrombolytic agents in low doses directly onto or near a thrombosis via a central catheter or by **systemic** administration of thrombolytic agents in higher doses. Local therapy is generally limited to small or moderate-sized thromboses. Minimal data exist supporting one method over the other.

c. tPA versus streptokinase versus urokinase. Minimal data exist comparing safety, efficacy, and cost of different thrombolytic agents in children. **tPA has become the agent of choice,** although significantly more expensive, for several reasons:

    i. Streptokinase has the greatest potential for allergic reactions, whereas tPA has the lowest.

    ii. tPA has the shortest half-life.

    iii. tPA theoretically has less stimulation of a systemic proteolytic state due to its poor binding of circulating plasminogen and its maximal impact on fibrin-bound plasminogen.

    iv. The production of urokinase has faced difficulties in the past due to manufacturing concerns.

d. Obtain CBC, platelets, PT, PTT, and fibrinogen prior to initiating therapy.

e. Monitor PT, PTT, and fibrinogen every 4 hours initially and then at least every 12 to 24 hours. Monitor hematocrit and platelets every 12 to 24 hours. Monitor thrombosis by imaging every 6 to 24 hours.

f. Expect fibrinogen to decrease by 20% to 50%. If no decrease in fibrinogen is seen, obtain D-dimers or fibrinogen split products to show evidence that a thrombolytic state has been initiated.

g. Maintain fibrinogen level above 100 mg/dL and platelets above 50,000 to 100,000/mm^3 to minimize the risks of clinical bleeding. Administer cryoprecipitate 10 mL/kg (or 1 unit/5 kg) or platelets 10 mL/kg as needed. If fibrinogen level drops below 100, decrease the dose of thrombolytic agent by 25%.

h. If no improvement in clinical condition or thrombosis size is seen after initiating therapy, and if fibrinogen levels remain high, **consider giving FFP 10 mL/kg,** which may correct deficiencies of plasminogen and other thrombolytic factors.

i. Duration of therapy. Thrombolytic therapy is usually provided for a brief period (i.e., 6–12 hours), but longer durations can be used for refractory thromboses with appropriate monitoring. Overall, therapy should balance resolution of the thrombus and improvement in clinical status against signs of clinical bleeding.

j. Concomitant heparin therapy. Heparin therapy, usually without the loading bolus dose, should be initiated during or immediately after completion of thrombolytic therapy.

3. Dosing (see Tables 44.5 and 44.6)

4. Treatment of bleeding during thrombolytic therapy

    a. Localized bleeding: apply pressure, administer topical thrombin, and provide supportive care; thrombolytic therapy does not necessarily need to be stopped if bleeding is controlled.

    b. Severe bleeding: stop infusion and administer cryoprecipitate (1 unit/5 kg).

    c. Life-threatening bleeding: stop infusion, give cryoprecipitate, and infuse aminocaproic acid (Amicar) (at usual dose of 100 mg/kg IV every 6 hours); consult hematology prior to giving Amicar.

Table 44.5	Systemic Thrombolytic Therapy		
Agent	**Load**	**Infusion**	**Notes**
tPA	none	0.1–0.6 mg/kg/h for 6 h	Duration usually 6 h; can continue for 12 h or repeat after 24 h, although lysis of clot will continue for hours after infusion stops. Lower dose appears to be as effective as higher dose.
Streptokinase	2,000 U/kg over 10 min	1,000–2,000 U/kg/hr for 6–12 h	Only one course should be given for 6 h. Consider premedication with tylenol and benadryl.
Urokinase	4,400 U/kg over 10 min	4,400 U/kg/h for 6–12 h	Longer duration may be necessary based on clinical response.
Consider concomitant heparin therapy at 5–20 U/kg/h without bolus dose for all three agents. Optimal duration of therapy is uncertain and can be individualized based on clinical response.			

5. **Post-thrombolytic therapy.** Consider initiating heparin therapy, but without the initial loading dose. Consider discontinuing heparin if no reaccumulation of the thrombus occurs after 24 to 48 hours.

F. **Treatment of central catheter thrombosis**

1. **Treatment guidelines**

a. Central catheters may become occluded because of thrombus or a chemical precipitate, which is usually secondary to parenteral nutrition.

Table 44.6	Local Site-directed Thrombolytic Therapy	
Agent	**Infusion**	**Notes***
tPA	0.01–0.05 mg/kg/h	Duration of therapy is based on clinical response. Systemic thrombolysis has been reported at doses of 0.05 mg/kg/h.
Urokinase	150 U/kg/h	Increase infusion by 200 U/kg/h if no clinical effect.
*Monitor laboratory studies as for systemic treatment.		

Table 44.7	Local Installation of Agents for Catheter Blockage
Agent	**Dosing**
tPA	0.5 mg/lumen diluted in NS to volume needed to fill line, to max 3 mL.
Urokinase	5,000 U/mL, 1–2 mL/lumen. Comes in unit doses prepared expressly for catheter clearance.
HCl	0.1 M, 0.1–1 mL/lumen.

    b. Nonfunctioning central catheters should be removed whenever possible, unless continued access through that catheter is absolutely necessary.

    c. Thrombolytic agents may be used for thrombosis and hydrochloric acid (HCl) may be attempted for chemical blockage.

    d. General procedure

        i. Instill chosen agent at volume needed to fill catheter (up to 1–2 mL) with gentle pressure; agent should not be forced in if resistance is too high. If instillation is difficult, a three-way stopcock can be used to create a vacuum in the catheter: attach catheter, 10-mL empty syringe, and 1-mL syringe containing agent to the stopcock, and create vacuum by gently drawing back several milliliter in the 10-mL syringe while the stopcock is off to the 1-mL syringe. While holding pressure, turn stopcock off to the 10-mL syringe and allow vacuum in catheter to draw in infusate from the 1-mL syringe.

        ii. Use of HCl for catheter clearance in neonates is based on limited clinical data and experience and should be performed with caution. Suggested volumes to use range from 0.1 mL to 1 mL of 0.1 molar solution. As severe tissue damage may result from peripheral administration or extravasation of HCl, consultation with a surgeon prior to HCl use should be considered.

        iii. Wait 1 to 2 hours for thrombolytic agents and 30 to 60 minutes for HCl and attempt to withdraw fluid through the catheter.

        iv. If unsuccessful, above steps can be repeated once. Urokinase can also be left in place for 8 to 12 hours if shorter intervals are unsuccessful.

        v. If clearance of catheter is not successful after two attempts or longer urokinase infusion, the catheter should be removed or contrast study performed to delineate extent of blockage.

    e. Low-dose continuous infusion of thrombolytic agents can be considered for local thrombosis occluding catheter tip (see above).

  2. **Dosing guidelines (see Table 44.7).**

Suggested Readings

Barrington KJ. Umbilical artery catheters in the newborn: effects of position of the catheter tip. *Cochrane Database of Syst Rev* 1999;(1).

Cantor AB. Developmental hemostasis: relevance to newborns and infants. In: Orkin SH, Nathan DG, Ginsburg D, Look AT, Fisher DE, Lux SE, eds. *Nathan and Oski's Hematology of Infancy and Childhood*. 7th ed. Philadelphia: Saunders Elsevier; 2009:147–191.

Chalmers EA. Epidemiology of venous thromboembolism in neonates and children. *Thromb Res* 2006;118:3–12.

Duffy LF, Kerzner B, Gebus V, et al. Treatment of central venous catheter occlusions with hydrochloric acid. *J Pediatr* 1989;114:1002–1004.

Hartmann J, Hussein A, Trowitzsch E, et al. Treatment of neonatal thrombus formation with recombinant tissue plasminogen activator: six years experience and review of the literature. *Arch Dis Child Fetal Neonatal Ed* 2001;85(1):F18–F22.

Häusler M, Hübner D, Delhaas T, et al. Long-term complications of inferior vena cava thrombosis. *Arch Dis Child* 2001;85(3):228–233.

Heleen van Ommen C, Heijboer H, Büller HR, et al. Venous thromboembolism in childhood: a prospective two-year registry in the Netherlands. *J Pediatr* 2001;139:676–681.

Lau KK, Stoffman JM, Williams S, et al. Neonatal renal vein thrombosis: review of the English-language literature between 1992 and 2006. *Pediatrics* 2007;120: e1278–e1284.

Manco-Johnson MJ, Grabowski EF, Hellgreen M, et al. Recommendations for tPA thrombolysis in children. *Thromb Haemost* 2002;88(1):157–158.

Michaels LA, Gurian M, Hegyi T, et al. Low molecular weight heparin in the treatment of venous and arterial thromboses in the premature infant. *Pediatrics Sept* 2004;114(3):703–707.

Monagle P, Chalmers E, Chan A, et al. Antithrombotic therapy in neonates and children. *Chest* 2008;133:887S–968S.

Nowak-Göttl U, von Kries R, Göbel U. Neonatal symptomatic thromboembolism in Germany: two-year survey. *Arch Dis Child Fetal Neonatal Ed* 1997;76(3):F163–F167.

Roy M, Turner-Gomes S, Gill G, et al. Incidence and diagnosis of neonatal thrombosis associated with umbilical venous catheters. *Thromb Haemost* 1997;78(suppl):724.

Saxonhouse MA, Burchfield DJ. The evaluation and management of postnatal thromboses. *J Perinat* 2009;29(7):467–478.

Schmidt B, Andrew M. Neonatal thrombosis: report of a prospective Canadian and international registry. *Pediatrics* 1995(5);96:939–943.

Werlin SL, Lausten T, Jessen S, et al. Treatment of central venous catheter occlusions with ethanol and hydrochloric acid. *J Parent Ent Nutr* 1995;19:416–418.

Yang JY, Chan AK, Callen DJ, et al. Neonatal cerebral sinovenous thrombosis: sifting the evidence for a diagnostic plan and treatment strategy. *Pediatrics* 2010;126(3): e693–e700.

Young TE, Mangum B. *Neofax 2008*. Montvale, NJ: Thompson-Reuters; 2008.

Anemia

Helen A. Christou

I. HEMATOLOGIC PHYSIOLOGY OF THE NEWBORN (1–5). Significant changes occur in the red blood cell (RBC) mass of an infant during the neonatal period and ensuing months. The evaluation of anemia must take into account this developmental process, as well as the infant's physiologic needs.

A. **Normal development: The physiologic anemia of infancy** (1)

1. *In utero*, the fetal aortic oxygen saturation is 45%, the erythropoietin levels are high, and the RBC production is rapid. The fetal liver is the major site of erythropoietin production.

2. After birth, the oxygen saturation is 95%, and the erythropoietin is undetectable. RBC production by day 7 is <1/10th the level *in utero*. Reticulocyte counts are low, and the hemoglobin level falls (see Table 45.1).

3. Despite dropping hemoglobin levels, the ratio of hemoglobin A to hemoglobin F increases and the levels of 2,3-diphosphoglycerate (2,3-DPG) (which interacts with hemoglobin A to decrease its affinity for oxygen, thereby enhancing oxygen release to the tissues) are high. As a result, oxygen delivery to the tissues actually increases. This physiologic "anemia" is not a functional anemia in that oxygen delivery to the tissues is adequate. Iron from degraded RBCs is stored.

4. At 8 to 12 weeks, hemoglobin levels reach their nadir (see Table 45.2), oxygen delivery to the tissues is impaired, renal erythropoietin production is stimulated, and RBC production increases.

5. Infants who have received transfusions in the neonatal period have lower nadirs than normal because of their higher percentage of hemoglobin A (1).

6. During this period of active erythropoiesis, iron stores are rapidly utilized. The reticuloendothelial system has adequate iron for 15 to 20 weeks in term infants. After this time, the hemoglobin level decreases if iron is not supplied.

B. **Anemia of prematurity** is an exaggeration of the normal physiologic anemia (Tables 45.1 and 45.2).

1. RBC mass and iron stores are decreased because of low birth weight; however, hemoglobin concentrations are similar in preterm and term infants.

2. The hemoglobin nadir is reached earlier than in the term infant because of the following:
   a. RBC survival is decreased in comparison with the term infant.
   b. There is a relatively more rapid rate of growth in premature babies than in term infants. For example, a premature infant gaining 150 g/week requires approximately a 12 mL/week increase in total blood volume.

Table 45.1	Hemoglobin Changes in Babies in the First Year of Life		
	Hemoglobin level		
Week	Term babies	Premature babies (1,200–2,500 g)	Small premature babies (<1,200 g)
0	17.0	16.4	16.0
1	18.8	16.0	14.8
3	15.9	13.5	13.4
6	12.7	10.7	9.7
10	11.4	9.8	8.5
20	12.0	10.4	9.0
50	12.0	11.5	11.0

Source: Glader B, Naiman JL. Erythrocyte disorders in infancy. In: Taeusch HW, Ballard RA, Avery ME, eds. *Diseases of the Newborn*. Philadelphia: WB Saunders; 1991.

  c. Many preterm infants have reduced red cell mass and iron stores because of iatrogenic phlebotomy for laboratory tests. This has been somewhat ameliorated with the use of microtechniques.

  d. Vitamin E deficiency is common in small premature infants, unless the vitamin is supplied exogenously.

 3. The hemoglobin nadir in premature babies is lower than in term infants, because erythropoietin is produced by the term infant at a hemoglobin level of 10 to 11 g/dL and is produced by the premature infant at a hemoglobin level of 7 to 9 g/dL.

 4. Iron administration before the age of 10 to 14 weeks does not increase the nadir of the hemoglobin level or diminish its rate of reduction. However, this iron is stored for later use.

 5. Once the nadir is reached, RBC production is stimulated, and iron stores are rapidly depleted because less iron is stored in the premature infant than in the term infant.

Table 45.2	Hemoglobin Nadir in Babies in the First Year of Life	
Maturity of baby at birth	Hemoglobin level at nadir	Time of nadir (wk)
Term babies	9.5–11.0	6–12
Premature babies (1,200–2,500 g)	8.0–10.0	5–10
Small premature babies (<1,200 g)	6.5–9.0	4–8

Source: Glader B, Naiman JL. Erythrocyte disorders in infancy. In: Taeusch HW, Ballard RA, Avery ME, eds. *Diseases of the Newborn*. Philadelphia: WB Saunders; 1991.

II. ETIOLOGY OF ANEMIA IN THE NEONATE (6)

A. **Blood loss** is manifested by a decreased or normal hematocrit (Hct), increased or normal reticulocyte count, and a normal bilirubin level (unless the hemorrhage is retained) (4,5). If blood loss is recent (e.g., at delivery), the Hct and reticulocyte count may be normal, and the infant may be in shock. The Hct will fall later because of hemodilution. If the bleeding is chronic, the Hct will be low, the reticulocyte count will go up, and the baby will be normovolemic.

1. **Obstetric causes of blood loss,** including the following malformations of placenta and cord:
   a. Abruptio placentae
   b. Placenta previa
   c. Incision of placenta at cesarean section
   d. Rupture of anomalous vessels (e.g., vasa previa, velamentous insertion of cord, or rupture of communicating vessels in a multilobed placenta)
   e. Hematoma of cord caused by varices or aneurysm
   f. Rupture of cord (more common in short cords and in dysmature cords)

2. **Occult blood loss**
   a. **Fetomaternal bleeding** may be chronic or acute. It occurs in 8% of all pregnancies; and in 1% of pregnancies, the volume may be as large as 40 mL. The diagnosis of this problem is by Kleihauer-Betke stain of maternal smear for fetal cells (2). Chronic fetal-to-maternal transfusion is suggested by a reticulocyte count >10%. Many conditions may predispose to this type of bleeding:
      i. Placental malformations—chorioangioma or choriocarcinoma
      ii. Obstetric procedures—traumatic amniocentesis, external cephalic version, internal cephalic version, breech delivery
      iii. Spontaneous fetomaternal bleeding
   b. **Fetoplacental bleeding**
      i. Chorioangioma or choriocarcinoma with placental hematoma
      ii. Cesarean section, with infant held above the placenta
      iii. Tight nuchal cord or occult cord prolapse
   c. **Twin-to-twin transfusion**

3. Bleeding in the neonatal period may be due to the following causes:
   a. **Intracranial bleeding** associated with:
      i. Prematurity
      ii. Second twin
      iii. Breech delivery
      iv. Rapid delivery
      v. Hypoxia
   b. **Massive cephalhematoma,** subgaleal hemorrhage, or hemorrhagic caput succedaneum
   c. **Retroperitoneal bleeding**
   d. **Ruptured liver or spleen**
   e. **Adrenal or renal hemorrhage**
   f. **Gastrointestinal bleeding** (maternal blood swallowed from delivery or breast should be ruled out by the Apt test) (see Chap. 43):
      i. Peptic ulcer
      ii. Necrotizing enterocolitis
      iii. Nasogastric catheter
      [b]leeding from umbilicus

4. **Iatrogenic causes.** Excessive blood loss may result from blood sampling with inadequate replacement.

B. **Hemolysis** is manifested by a decreased Hct, increased reticulocyte count, and an increased bilirubin level (1,2).

1. **Immune hemolysis** (see Chap. 26)
   a. **Rh incompatibility**
   b. **ABO incompatibility**
   c. **Minor blood group incompatibility** (e.g., c, E, Kell, Duffy)
   d. **Maternal disease** (e.g., lupus), autoimmune hemolytic disease, rheumatoid arthritis (positive direct Coombs test in mother and newborn, no antibody to common red cell antigen Rh, AB, etc.), or drugs

2. **Hereditary RBC disorders**
   a. **RBC membrane defects** such as spherocytosis, elliptocytosis, or stomatocytosis.
   b. **Metabolic defects.** Glucose-6-phosphate dehydrogenase (G6PD) deficiency (significant neonatal hemolysis due to G6PD deficiency is seen only in Mediterranean or Asian G6PD-deficient men; blacks in the United States have a 10% incidence of G6PD deficiency but rarely have significant neonatal problems, unless an infection or drug is operative), pyruvate kinase deficiency, 5'-nucleotidase deficiency, and glucose-phosphate isomerase deficiency.
   c. **Hemoglobinopathies**
      i. α- and γ-Thalassemia syndromes
      ii. α- and γ-Chain structural abnormalities

3. **Acquired hemolysis**
   a. **Infection:** bacterial or viral
   b. **Disseminated intravascular coagulation**
   c. **Vitamin E deficiency** and other nutritional anemias[1]
   d. **Microangiopathic hemolytic anemia,** cavernous hemangioma, renal artery stenosis, and severe coarctation of the aorta

C. **Diminished RBC production** is manifested by a decreased Hct, decreased reticulocyte count, and normal bilirubin level.

1. **Diamond-Blackfan syndrome**
2. **Congenital leukemia** or other tumor
3. **Infections,** especially rubella and parvovirus (see Chap. 48)
4. **Osteopetrosis,** leading to inadequate erythropoiesis
5. **Drug-induced suppression of RBC production**
6. **Physiologic anemia or anemia of prematurity** (see I.A. and I.B.)

III. DIAGNOSTIC APPROACH TO ANEMIA IN THE NEWBORN (SEE TABLE 45.3)

A. The **family history** should include questions about anemia, jaundice, g
and splenectomy.

B. The **obstetric history** should be evaluated.

Table 45.3	Classification of Anemia in the Newborn			
Reticulocytes	Bilirubin	Coombs test	RBC morphology	Diagnostic possibilities
Normal or ↓	Normal	Negative	Normal	Physiologic anemia of infancy or prematurity; congenital hypoplastic anemia; other causes of decreased production
Normal or ↑	Normal	Negative	Normal	Acute hemorrhage (fetomaternal, placental, umbilical cord, or internal hemorrhage)
↑	Normal	Negative	Hypochromic microcytes	Chronic fetomaternal hemorrhage
↑	↑	Positive	Spherocytes Nucleated RBC	Immune hemolysis (blood group incompatibility or maternal autoantibody)
Normal or ↑	↑	Negative	Spherocytes	Hereditary spherocytosis
Normal or ↑	↑	Negative	Elliptocytes	Hereditary elliptocytosis
Normal or ↑	↑	Negative	Hypochromic microcytes	α- or γ-Thalassemia syndrome
↑	↑	Negative	Spiculated RBCs	Pyruvate kinase deficiency
Normal or ↑	Normal or ↑	Negative	Schistocytes and RBC fragments	Disseminated intravascular coagulation; other microangiopathic processes
↑	↑	Negative	Bite cells (Heinz bodies with supravital stain)	Glucose-6-phosphate dehydrogenase deficiency
Normal, ↑ or ↓	↑	Negative	Normal	Infections; enclosed hemorrhage (cephalhematoma)

↓ = decreased; ↑ = increased; RBC = red blood cell.
Source: Adapted from the work of Dr. Glader B. Director of Division of hematology-oncology. California: Children's Hospital at Stanford, 1991.[3]

C. The **physical examination** may reveal an associated abnormality and provide clues to the origin of the anemia.

   1. **Acute blood loss** leads to shock, with cyanosis, poor perfusion, and acidosis.

   2. **Chronic blood loss** produces pallor, but the infant may exhibit only mild symptoms of respiratory distress or irritability.

   3. **Chronic hemolysis** is associated with pallor, jaundice, and hepatosplenomegaly.

D. **Complete blood cell count.** Capillary blood Hct is 2.7% to 3.9% higher than venous Hct. Warming the foot reduced the difference from 3.9% to 1.9% (1,2).

E. **Reticulocyte count** (elevated with chronic blood loss and hemolysis, depressed with infection and production defect).

F. **Blood smear** (Table 45.3).

G. **Coombs test and bilirubin level** (see Chap. 26).

H. **Apt test** (see Chap. 43) on gastrointestinal blood of uncertain origin.

I. **Kleihauer-Betke preparation** of the mother's blood. A 50-mL loss of fetal blood into the maternal circulation will show up as 1% fetal cells in the maternal circulation.[2]

J. **Ultrasound of abdomen and head.**

K. **Parental testing.** Complete blood cell count, smear, and RBC indices are useful screening studies. Osmotic fragility testing and RBC enzyme levels (e.g., G6PD, pyruvate kinase) may be helpful in selected cases.

L. **Studies for infection.** Toxoplasmosis, rubella, cytomegalovirus (CMV), and herpes simplex (see Chap. 48).

M. **Bone marrow** (rarely used, except in cases of bone marrow failure from hypoplasia or tumor).

IV. THERAPY

A. **Transfusion** (see Chap. 42)

   1. **Indications for transfusion.** The decision to transfuse must be made in consideration of the infant's condition and physiologic needs (8).

      a. Infants with significant respiratory disease or congenital heart disease (e.g., large left-to-right shunt) may need their Hct maintained above 40%. Transfusion with adult RBCs provides the added benefit of lowered hemoglobin oxygen affinity, which augments oxygen delivery to tissues. Blood should be fresh (3–7 days old) to ensure adequate 2,3-DPG levels.

      b. Healthy, asymptomatic newborns will self-correct a mild anemia, provided that iron intake is adequate.

      c. Infants with ABO incompatibility who do not have an exchange transfusion may have protracted hemolysis and may require a transfusion several weeks after birth. This may be ameliorated with the use of intravenous immune globulin (IVIG). If they do not have enough hemolysis to require treatment with phototherapy, they will usually not become anemic enough to need a transfusion (see Chap. 26).

      d. Premature babies may be quite comfortable with hemoglobin levels of 6.5 to 7 mg/dL. The level itself is not an indication for transfusion. Although one study suggested a possible increased risk for NEC in anemic infants, several studies also suggested an unanticipated relationship between late onset necrotizing enterocolitis and elective transfusion in stable growing premature infants (7). Sick infants (e.g., with sepsis, pneumonia, or bronchopulmonary dysplasia) may require increased oxygen-carrying capacities and therefore need transfusion. Growing premature infants may also manifest a need for transfusion by exhibiting poor weight gain, apnea, tachypnea, or poor feeding (8). Transfusion guidelines are shown in Table 45.4. Despite efforts to adopt uniform transfusion criteria, significant variation in transfusion practices among neonatal intensive care units (NICUs) has been reported (9).

2. **Blood products and methods of transfusion**[2] (see Chap. 42)

    a. **Packed RBCs.** The volume of transfusion may be calculated as follows:

$$\frac{\text{Weight in kilogram} \times \text{blood volume per kilogram} \times (\text{Hct desired} - \text{Hct observed})}{\text{Hct of blood to be given}} = \text{volume of transfusion}$$

    The average newborn blood volume is 80 mL/kg; the Hct of packed RBCs is 60% to 80% and should be checked before transfusion. We generally transfuse 15 to 20 mL/kg; larger volumes may need to be divided.

    b. **Whole blood** is indicated when there is acute blood loss.

    c. **Isovolemic transfusion** with high Hct-packed RBCs may be required for severely anemic infants, when routine transfusion of the volume of packed RBCs necessary to correct the anemia would result in circulatory overload (see Chap. 26).

    d. **Irradiated RBCs** are recommended in premature infants weighing <1,200 g. Premature infants may be unable to reject foreign lymphocytes in transfused blood. **We use irradiated blood for all neonatal transfusions. Leukocyte depletion** with third-generation transfusion filters has substantially reduced the risk of exposure to foreign lymphocytes and CMV. (4,10). However, blood from CMV-negative donors for neonatal transfusion is preferable (see Chap. 42).

Table 45.4	Transfusion Guidelines for Premature Infants

1. Asymptomatic infants with Hct <21% and reticulocytes <100,000/UL (2%)

2. Infants with Hct <31% and hood O_2 <36% or mean airway pressure <6 cm H_2O by CPAP or IMV or >9 apneic and bradycardic episodes per 12 h or 2/24 h requiring bag-and-mask ventilation while on adequate methylxanthine therapy or HR >180/min or RR >80/min sustained for 24 h or weight gain of <10 g/d for 4 d on 100 Kcal/kg/d or having surgery

3. Infants with Hct <36% and requiring >35% O_2 or mean airway pressure of 6–8 cm H_2O by CPAP or IMV

CPAP = continuous positive airway pressure by nasal or endotracheal route; HR = heart rate; Hct = hematocrit; IMV = intermittent mandatory ventilation; RR = respiratory rate. From the multicenter trial of recombinant human erythropoietin for preterm infants. *Source*: Data from Strauss RG. Erythropoietin and neonatal anemia. *N Engl J Med* 1994;330(17):1227–1228.

    e. Directed-donor transfusion is requested by many families. Irradiation of directed-donor cells is especially important, given the human leukocyte antigen (HLA) compatibility among first-degree relatives and the enhanced potential for foreign lymphocyte engraftment.

    f. Because of concern for multiple exposure risk associated with repeated transfusions in extremely low birth weight (ELBW) infants, **we recommend transfusing stored RBCs from a single unit reserved for an infant** (1).

B. Prophylaxis

    1. Term infants should be sent home from the hospital on iron-fortified formula (2 mg/kg/day) if they are not breastfeeding (12).

    2. Premature infants (preventing or ameliorating the anemia of prematurity). The following is a description of our usual nutritional management of premature infants from the point of view of providing RBC substrates and preventing additional destruction:

        a. Iron supplementation in the preterm infant prevents late iron deficiency (13). We routinely supplement iron in premature infants at a dose of 2 to 4 mg of elemental iron/kg/day once full enteral feeding is achieved (see Chap. 21).

        b. Mother's milk or formulas similar to mother's milk, in that they are low in linoleic acid, are used to maintain a low content of polyunsaturated fatty acids in the RBCs (3).

        c. Vitamin E (15 to 25 IU of water-soluble form) is given daily until the baby is 38 to 40 weeks' postconceptional age (this is usually stopped at discharge from the hospital) (see Chap. 21).

        d. These infants should be followed up carefully, and additional iron supplementation may be required.

        e. Methods and hazards of transfusion are described in Chap. 42.

        f. Recombinant human erythropoietin (rh-EPO) has been evaluated as a promising measure in ameliorating anemia of prematurity (14–19). Studies in which we participated showed that rh-EPO stimulates RBC production and decreases the frequency and volume of RBC transfusions administered to premature infants. However, many studies have shown that erythropoietin treatment is of limited benefit in reducing the number of transfusions once strict transfusion criteria are instituted. In addition, a Cochrane Review meta-analysis showed that early EPO use increased the risk of retinopathy of prematurity, therefore we do not recommend it as a routine procedure (16,17,20). Complementary strategies to reduce phlebotomy losses and the use of conservative standardized transfusion criteria have contributed to significant reductions in transfusions.

REFERENCES

1. Bifano EM, Ehrenkranz Z, eds. Perinatal hematology. *Clin Perinatol* 1995:23(3).
2. Blanchette V, Doyle J, Schmidt B, et al. Hematology. In: Avery GB, Fletcher MA, MacDonald MG, eds. *Neonatology*. 4th ed. Philadelphia: Lippincott–Raven Publishers; 1994:952–999.
3. Glader B, Naiman JL. Erythrocyte disorders in infancy. In: Taeusch HW, Ballard RA, Avery ME, eds. *Diseases of the Newborn*. Philadelphia: WB Saunders; 1991.
4. Nathan DG, Oski FA. *Hematology of Infancy and Childhood*. 4th ed. Philadelphia: WB Saunders; 1993.

5. Oski FA, Naiman JL. *Hematologic Problems in the Newborn*. 3rd ed. Philadelphia: WB Saunders; 1982.

6. Molteni RA. Perinatal blood loss. *Pediatr Rev* 1990;12(2):47–54.

7. Singh R, Visitainer PF, Frantz ID, et al. Association of Necrotizing Enterocolitis with anemia and packed red blood transfusions in preterm infants. *J Perinatol* 2011;31:176–182.

8. Ross MP, Christensen RD, Rothstein G, et al. A randomized trial to develop criteria for administering erythrocyte transfusions to anemic preterm infants 1 to 3 months of age. *J Perinatol* 1989;9:246.

9. Ringer SA, Richardson DK, Sacher RA, et al. Variations in transfusion practice in neonatal intensive care. *Pediatrics* 1998;101(2):194–200.

10. Andreu G. Role of leukocyte depletion in the prevention of transfusion-induced cytomegalovirus infection. *Semin Hematol* 1991;28(3 suppl 5):26–31.

11. Strauss RG. Blood banking issues pertaining to neonatal red blood cell transfusions. *Transfus Sci* 1999;21(1):7–19.

12. American Academy of Pediatrics Committee on Nutrition: Iron-fortified infant formulas. *Pediatrics* 1989;84(6):1114–1115.

13. Hall RT, Wheeler RE, Benson J, et al. Feeding iron-fortified premature formula during initial hospitalization to infants less than 1800 grams birth weight. *Pediatrics* 1993;92(3):409–414.

14. Shannon KM, Keith JF III, Mentzer WC, et al. Recombinant human erythropoietin stimulates erythropoiesis and reduces erythrocyte transfusions in very low birth weight preterm infants. *Pediatrics* 1995;95(1):1–8.

15. Maier RF, Obladen M, Scigalla P, et al. The effect of epoetin beta (recombinant human erythropoietin) on the need for transfusion in very low birth weight infants. European Multicentre Erythropoietin Study Group. *N Engl J Med* 1994;330(17):1173–1178.

16. Strauss RG. Erythropoietin and neonatal anemia. *N Engl J Med* 1994;330(17):1227–1228.

17. Wilimas JA, Crist WM. Erythropoietin—not yet a standard treatment for anemia of prematurity. *Pediatrics* 1995;95(1):9–10.

18. Soubasi V, Kremenopoulos G, Diamandi E, et al. In which neonates does early recombinant human erythropoietin treatment prevent anemia of prematurity? Results of a randomized, controlled study. *Pediatr Res* 1993;34(5):675–679.

19. http://www2.cochrane.org/reviews/en/ab004863.html. Accessed 2011.

20. Ohlsson A, Aher SM. Early erythropoietin for preventing red blood cell transfusion in preterm and/or low birth weight infants. *Cochrane Database of Syst Rev* 2006;19(3):CD004863. DOI:10.1002/14651858.CD004863.PUB2

Polycythemia

Deirdre O'Reilly

As the central venous hematocrit rises, there is increased viscosity and decreased blood flow. When the hematocrit increases to >60%, there is decreased oxygen delivery (1) (see Figure 46.1). Newborns have larger, irregularly shaped red blood cells (RBC) with different membrane characteristics than the RBCs of adults (1–3). As viscosity increases, there is impairment of tissue oxygenation and decreased glucose in plasma, leading to increased risk of microthrombus formation. If these events occur in the cerebral cortex, kidneys, or adrenal glands, significant damage may result. Hypoxia and acidosis increase viscosity and deformity further. Poor perfusion increases the possibility of thrombosis.

I. DEFINITIONS

A. **Polycythemia** is defined as venous hematocrit of at least 65% (2,3). Hematocrit measurements vary greatly with site of sample, and capillary hematocrit may be up to 20% higher than venous (2). Hematocrit initially rises after birth from placental transfer of RBCs, then decreases to baseline by approximately 24 hours (4). The mean venous hematocrit of term infants is 53% in cord blood, 60% at 2 hours of age, 57% at 6 hours of age, and 52% at 12 to 18 hours of age (2).

B. **Hyperviscosity** is defined as viscosity >2 standard deviations greater than the mean (3). Blood viscosity, as described by Poiseuille, is the ratio of shear stress to shear rate and is dependent on such factors as the pressure gradient along the vessel, radius, length, and flow (4). The relationship between hematocrit and viscosity is nearly linear below a hematocrit of 60%, but viscosity increases exponentially at a hematocrit of 70% or greater (Figure 46.1) (4,5).

Other factors affect blood viscosity, including plasma proteins such as fibrinogen, local blood flow, and pH (3,4). The hyperviscosity syndrome is usually seen only in infants with venous hematocrits above 60%.

II. INCIDENCE.
The incidence of polycythemia is 1% to 5% in term newborns (1,3,6,7). Polycythemia is increased in babies that have intrauterine growth restriction (IUGR), are small for gestational age (SGA), and are born postterm.

III. CAUSES OF POLYCYTHEMIA

A. **Placental red cell transfusion**
1. **Delayed cord clamping** may occur either intentionally or in unattended deliveries.
   a. When the cord is clamped within 1 minute after birth, the blood volume of the infant is approximately 80 mL/kg.

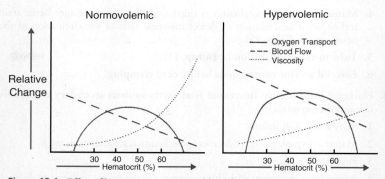

Figure 46.1. Effect of hematocrit on viscosity, blood flow, and oxygen transport. (Adapted from Glader B, Naiman JL. Erythrocyte disorders in infancy. In: Taeusch HW, Ballard RA, Avery ME, eds. *Diseases of the Newborn*. Philadelphia: WB Saunders; 1991.)

    b. When the cord is clamped 2 minutes after delivery, the blood volume of the infant is 90 mL/kg.

    c. In newborns with polycythemia, blood volume per kilogram of body weight varies inversely in relation to birth weight (see Figure 46.2).

2. Cord stripping (thereby pushing more blood into the infant).

3. Holding the baby below the mother at delivery.

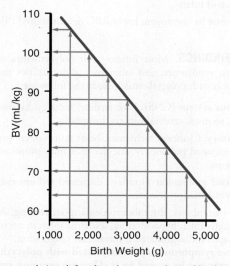

Figure 46.2. Nomogram designed for clinical use, correlating blood volume per kilogram with birth weight in polycythemic neonates; BV = blood volume. (From Rawlings JS, Pettett G, Wiswell T, et al. Estimated blood volumes in polycythemic neonates as a function of birth weight. *J Pediatr* 1982;101[4]:594–599.)

4. **Maternal-to-fetal transfusion** is diagnosed with the Kleihauer-Betke stain technique of acid elution to detect maternal cells in the circulation of the newborn (see Chap. 45).

5. **Twin-to-twin transfusion** (see Chap. 11).

6. **Forceful uterine contractions before cord clamping.**

B. **Placental insufficiency (increased fetal erythropoiesis secondary to chronic intrauterine hypoxia)**

1. SGA and IUGR infants.

2. Maternal hypertension syndromes (preeclampsia, renal disease, etc.).

3. Postterm infants.

4. Infants born to mothers with chronic hypoxia (heart disease, pulmonary disease).

5. Pregnancy at high altitude.

6. Maternal smoking.

C. **Other conditions**

1. Infants of diabetic mothers (increased erythropoiesis).

2. Some large-for-gestational-age (LGA) babies.

3. Infants with congenital adrenal hyperplasia, Beckwith-Wiedemann syndrome, neonatal thyrotoxicosis, congenital hypothyroidism, trisomy 21, trisomy 13, trisomy 18.

4. Drugs (maternal use of propranolol).

5. Dehydration of infant.

6. Sepsis (increase in fibrinogen, lower RBC deformability) (4).

IV. CLINICAL FINDINGS. Most infants with polycythemia are asymptomatic. Clinical symptoms, syndromes, and laboratory abnormalities that have been described in association with polycythemia include the following:

A. **Central nervous system (CNS).** Poor feeding, lethargy, hypotonia, apnea, tremors, jitteriness, seizures, cerebral venous thrombosis.

B. **Cardiorespiratory.** Cyanosis, tachypnea, heart murmur, congestive heart failure, cardiomegaly, elevated pulmonary vascular resistance, prominent vascular markings on chest x-ray.

C. **Renal.** Decreased glomerular filtration, decreased sodium excretion, renal vein thrombosis, hematuria, proteinuria.

D. **Other.** Other thrombosis, thrombocytopenia, poor feeding, increased jaundice, persistent hypoglycemia, hypocalcemia, testicular infarcts, necrotizing enterocolitis (NEC), priapism, disseminated intravascular coagulation.

All of these symptoms may be associated with polycythemia and hyperviscosity but may not be caused by it. They are common symptoms in many neonatal disorders.

V. SCREENING. The routine screening of all newborns for polycythemia and/or hyperviscosity has been advocated by some authors (8,9). The timing and site of blood sampling alter the hematocrit value (3,10,11). We do not routinely screen well term newborns for this syndrome, because there are few data showing that treatment of asymptomatic patients with partial exchange transfusion is beneficial in the long term (3,11,12).

VI. DIAGNOSIS. The capillary blood or peripheral venous hematocrit level should be determined in any baby who appears plethoric, who has any predisposing cause of polycythemia, who has any of the symptoms mentioned in IV, or who is not well for any reason.

A. Warming the heel before drawing blood for a capillary hematocrit determination will give a better correlation with the peripheral venous or central hematocrit. If the capillary blood hematocrit is above 65%, the peripheral venous hematocrit should be determined.

B. Few hospitals are equipped to measure blood viscosity. If the equipment is available, the test should be done, because some infants with venous hematocrits under 65% will have hyperviscous blood (7).

VII. MANAGEMENT

A. Once other causes of illness have been considered and excluded (e.g., sepsis, pneumonia, hypoglycemia), any child with symptoms that could be due to hyperviscosity should be considered for **partial exchange transfusion if the peripheral venous hematocrit is >65%.**

B. **Asymptomatic infants** with a peripheral venous hematocrit between 60% and 70% **can usually be managed by increasing fluid intake and repeating the hematocrit in 4 to 6 hours.**

C. Many neonatologists perform an **exchange transfusion when the peripheral venous hematocrit is >70% in the absence of symptoms, but this is a controversial** issue (10–13).

D. The following formula can be used to calculate the exchange with normal saline that will bring the hematocrit to 50% to 60%. In infants with polycythemia, the blood volume varies inversely with the birth weight (see Fig. 46.2). **Usually we take the blood from the umbilical vein and replace it with normal saline in a peripheral vein.** Because randomized trials show no advantage with albumin and there is less chance of infection, nonhuman products, such as saline, are preferred (14). There are many methods of exchange (see Chap. 26).

Volume of exchange in mL

$$= \frac{(\text{blood volume/kg} \times \text{weight in kg}) \times (\text{observed hematocrit} - \text{desired hematocrit})}{\text{observed hematocrit}}$$

Example: A 3-kg infant, hematocrit 75%, blood volume 80 mL/kg—to bring hematocrit to 50%:

$$\text{Volume of exchange (in mL)} = \frac{(80 \text{ mL} \times 3 \text{ kg}) \times (75 - 50)}{75}$$

$$= \frac{240 \text{ mL} \times 25}{75}$$

$$= 80\text{-mL exchange}$$

The total volume exchanged is usually 15 to 20 mL/kg of body weight. This will depend on the observed hematocrit. (Blood volume may be up to 100 mL/kg in polycythemic infants.)

VIII. OUTCOME

A. **Infants with polycythemia and hyperviscosity who have decreased cerebral blood flow velocity and increased vascular resistance develop normal cerebral blood flow following partial exchange transfusion** (12). They also have improvement in systemic blood flow and oxygen transport (2,5,11,13).

B. **The long-term neurologic outcome** in infants with asymptomatic polycythemia and/or hyperviscosity, whether treated or untreated, **remains controversial.**

1. One trial with small numbers of randomized patients showed decreased IQ scores in school-age children who had neonatal hyperviscosity syndrome, in both treated and untreated newborns (10,15).

2. Another retrospective study, with small numbers of patients, showed no difference in the neurologic outcome of patients with asymptomatic neonatal polycythemia, including both treated and untreated newborns (16).

3. A small prospective study showed no difference at follow-up between control infants and those with hyperviscosity, between those with symptomatic and asymptomatic hyperviscosity, and between asymptomatic infants treated with partial exchange transfusion and those who were observed. Analysis revealed that other perinatal risk factors and race, rather than polycythemia or partial exchange transfusion, significantly influenced the long-term outcome (2,11).

4. An increased incidence of NEC following partial exchange transfusions by umbilical vein has been reported (15,17). NEC was not seen in one retrospective analysis of 185 term polycythemic babies given partial exchange transfusions with removal of blood from the umbilical vein and reinfusion of a commercial plasma substitute through peripheral veins (18).

5. A larger prospective, randomized clinical trial comparing partial exchange transfusion with symptomatic care (increased fluid intake, etc.) equally balanced for risk factors and the etiologies of the polycythemia will be necessary to give guidelines for treatment of the asymptomatic newborn with polycythemia and/or hyperviscosity.

6. Partial exchange transfusion will lower hematocrit, decrease viscosity, and reverse many of the physiologic abnormalities associated with polycythemia and/or hyperviscosity but has not been shown to significantly change the long-term outcome of these infants (2).

REFERENCES

1. Glader B. Erythrocyte disorders in infancy. In: Taeusch HW, Ballard RA, Avery ME, eds. *Diseases of the newborn*. 6th ed. Philadelphia: WB Saunders; 1991.
2. Werner EJ. Neonatal polycythemia and hyperviscosity. *Clin Perinatol* 1995;22(3):693–710.
3. Linderkamp O. Blood Viscosity of the Neonate. *NeoReviews* 2004;5:406–415.
4. Rosenkrantz TS. Polycythemia and hyperviscosity in the newborn. *Semin Thromb Hemost* 2003;29(5):515–527.
5. Swetnam SM, Yabek SM, Alverson DC. Hemodynamic consequences of neonatal polycythemia. *J Pediatr* 1987;110:443–447.

6. Lindermann R, Haines L. Evaluation and treatment of polycythemia in the neonate. In: Christensen RD, ed. *Hematologic problems of the neonate*. Philadelphia: WB Saunders; 2000.

7. Wirth FH, Goldberg KE, Lubchenco LO. Neonatal hyperviscosity: I. Incidence. *Pediatrics* 1979;63(6):833–886.

7.5. Ramamurthy RS, Berlanga M. Postnatal alteration in hematocrit and viscosity in normal and polycythemic infants. *J Pediatr* 1987;110(6):929–934.

8. Drew JH, Guaran RL, Cichello M, et al. Neonatal whole blood hyperviscosity: the important factor influencing later neurologic function is the viscosity and not the polycythemia. *Clin Hemorheol Microcirc* 1997;17(1):67–72.

9. Wiswell TE, Cornish JD, Northam RS. Neonatal polycythemia: frequency of clinical manifestations and other associated findings. *Pediatrics* 1986;78(1):26–30.

10. Delaney-Black VD, Camp BW, Lubchenco LO, et al. Neonatal hyperviscosity association with lower achievement and IQ scores at school age. *Pediatrics* 1989;83(5):662–667.

11. Bada H, Korones SB, Pourcyrous M, et al. Asymptomatic syndrome of polycythemic hyperviscosity: effect of partial plasma exhange transfusion. *J Pediatr* 1992;120(4 pt 1): 579–585.

12. Oski FA, Naiman JL. *Hematologic problems in the newborn*. 3rd ed. Philadelphia: WB Saunders; 1982:87–96.

13. Phibbs RH, Clapp DW, Shannon KM. Hematologic problems. In: Klaus MH, Fanaroff AA, Eds. *Care of the high risk neonate*. Philadelphia: WB Saunders; 1993:421.

14. de Waal KA, Baerts W, Offringa M. Systematic review of the optimal fluid for dilutional exchange transfusion in neonatal polycythaemia. *Arch Dis Child Fetal Neonatal Ed* 2006;91(1):F7–F10.

15. Black VD, Lubchenco LO. Neonatal polycythemia and hyperviscosity. *Pediatr Clin North Am* 1982;5:1137–1148.

16. Høst A, Ulrich M. Late prognosis in untreated neonatal polycythemia with minor or no symptoms. *Acta Paediatr Scand* 1982;71(4):629–633.

17. Black VD, Rumack CM, Lubchenco LO, et al. Gastrointestinal injury in polycythemic term infants. *Pediatrics* 1985;76(2):225–231.

18. Hein HA, Lathrop SS. Partial exchange transfusion in term, polycythemic neonates: absence of association with severe gastrointestinal injury. *Pediatrics* 1987;80(1):75–78.

47 Neonatal Thrombocytopenia

Chaitanya Chavda, Matthew Saxonhouse, and
Martha Sola-Visner

I. INTRODUCTION. Thrombocytopenia in neonates is traditionally defined as a platelet count of less than $150 \times 10^3/\text{mcL}$ and is classified as mild ($100-150 \times 10^3/\text{mcL}$), moderate ($50-99 \times 10^3/\text{mcL}$), or severe ($<50 \times 10^3/\text{mcL}$). However, platelet counts in the $100-150 \times 10^3/\text{mcL}$ range are somewhat more common among healthy neonates than among healthy adults. For that reason, careful follow-up and expectant management in an otherwise healthy-appearing neonate with mild, transient thrombocytopenia is an acceptable approach, although lack of quick resolution, worsening of thrombocytopenia, or changes in clinical condition should prompt further evaluation. The incidence of thrombocytopenia in neonates varies significantly, depending on the population studied. Specifically, while the *overall* incidence of neonatal thrombocytopenia is relatively low (0.7%–0.9%) (1), the incidence among neonates admitted to the Neonatal Intensive Care Unit (NICU) is very high (22%–35%) (2–4). Within the NICU, mean platelet counts are lower among preterm neonates than among neonates born at or near term (5), and the incidence of thrombocytopenia is inversely correlated to the gestational age, reaching approximately 70% among neonates born with a weight $<1,000$ g (6).

II. APPROACH TO THE THROMBOCYTOPENIC NEONATE. When evaluating a thrombocytopenic neonate, the first step to narrow the differential diagnosis is to classify the thrombocytopenia as either **early onset (within the first 72 h of life)** or **late onset (after the initial 72 h of life)**, and to determine whether the infant is clinically ill or well. Importantly, infection and sepsis should always be considered near the top of the differential diagnosis (regardless of the time of presentation and the infant's appearance), as any delay in diagnosis and treatment can have life-threatening consequences.

A. **Early-onset thrombocytopenia (Figure 47.1).** The most frequent cause of early-onset thrombocytopenia in a well-appearing neonate is placental insufficiency, as occurs in infants born to mothers with pregnancy-induced hypertension/pre-eclampsia or diabetes and in those with intrauterine growth restriction (IUGR) (7,8). This thrombocytopenia is always mild to moderate, presents immediately or shortly after birth, and resolves within 7 to 10 days. If an infant with a prenatal history consistent with placental insufficiency and mild-to-moderate thrombocytopenia remains clinically stable and the platelet count normalizes within 10 days, no further evaluation is necessary. However, if the thrombocytopenia becomes severe and/or persists >10 days, further investigation is necessary.

Severe early-onset thrombocytopenia in an otherwise healthy infant should trigger suspicion for an immune-mediated thrombocytopenia, either autoimmune

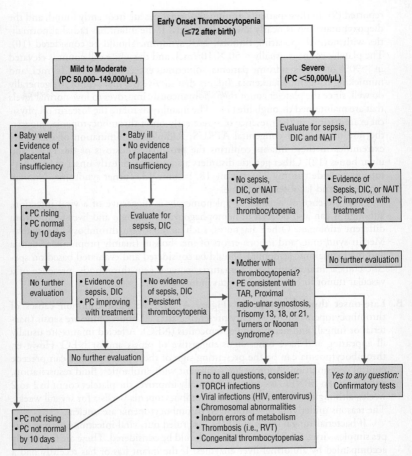

Figure 47.1. Guidelines for the evaluation of neonates with early-onset thrombocytopenia (≤72 hours of life). PC = platelet count; DIC = disseminated intravascular coagulation; NAIT = neonatal alloimmune thrombocytopenia; RVT = renal vein thrombosis.

(i.e., the mother is also thrombocytopenic) or alloimmune (i.e., the mother has a normal platelet count). These varieties of thrombocytopenia are discussed in detail below.

Early-onset thrombocytopenia of any severity in an *ill-appearing* term or preterm neonate should prompt evaluation for sepsis, congenital viral or parasitic infections, or disseminated intravascular coagulation (DIC). DIC is most frequently associated with sepsis but can also be secondary to birth asphyxia.

In addition to these considerations, the affected neonate should be carefully examined for any radial abnormalities (suggestive of thrombocytopenia-absent radius (TAR) syndrome, amegakaryocytic thrombocytopenia with radioulnar synostosis (ATRUS), or Fanconi anemia). Although thrombocytopenia associated with Fanconi almost always presents later (during childhood), neonatal cases have been reported (9). In these patients, thumb abnormalities are frequently found, and the diepoxybutane test is nearly always diagnostic. If the infant has radial abnormalities with normal appearing thumbs, TAR syndrome should be considered (10). The platelet count is usually $<50 \times 10^3$/mcL and the white cell count is elevated in $>90\%$ of TAR syndrome patients, sometimes exceeding 100×10^3/mcL and mimicking congenital leukemia. Infants that survive the first year of life generally do well, since the platelet count then spontaneously improves to low-normal levels that are maintained through life (11). The inability to rotate the forearm on physical examination, in the presence of severe early-onset thrombocytopenia, suggests the rare diagnosis of congenital ATRUS. Radiologic examination of the upper extremities in these infants confirms the proximal synostosis of the radial and ulnar bones (12). Other genetic disorders associated with early-onset thrombocytopenia include trisomy 21, trisomy 18, trisomy 13, Turner syndrome, Noonan syndrome, and Jacobsen syndrome.

The presence of hepato- or splenomegaly is suggestive of a viral infection, although it can also be seen in hemophagocytic syndrome and liver failure from different etiologies. Other diagnoses, such as renal vein thrombosis, Kasabach–Merritt syndrome, and inborn errors of metabolism (mainly propionic acidemia and methylmalonic acidemia), should be considered and evaluated based on specific clinical indications (i.e., hematuria in renal vein thrombosis, presence of a vascular tumor in Kasabach-Merritt syndrome).

B. **Late-onset thrombocytopenia (Figure 47.2).** The most common causes of thrombocytopenia of any severity presenting after 72 hours of life are sepsis (bacterial or fungal) and necrotizing enterocolitis (NEC). Affected infants are usually ill appearing and have other signs suggestive of sepsis and/or NEC. However, thrombocytopenia can be the presenting sign of these processes and can precede clinical deterioration. Appropriate treatment with antibiotics, fluid resuscitation, and bowel rest (if NEC is considered) usually improves the platelet count in 1 to 2 weeks, although in some infants, the thrombocytopenia persists for several weeks. The reasons underlying this prolonged thrombocytopenia are unclear.

If bacterial/fungal sepsis and NEC are ruled out, viral infections such as herpes simplex virus, CMV, or enterovirus should be considered. These are frequently accompanied by abnormal liver enzymes. If the infant has or has recently had a central venous or arterial catheter, thromboses should be part of the differential diagnosis. Finally, drug-induced thrombocytopenia should be considered if the infant is clinically well and is receiving heparin, antibiotics (penicillins, ciprofloxacin, cephalosporins, metronidazole, vancomycin, and rifampin), indomethacin, famotidine, cimetidine, phenobarbital, or phenytoin, among others (13,14). Other less common causes of late-onset thrombocytopenia include inborn errors of metabolism and Fanconi anemia (rare).

Novel tools to evaluate platelet production and aid in the evaluation of thrombocytopenia have been recently developed and are likely to become widely available to clinicians in the near future. Among those, the immature platelet fraction (IPF) measures the percentage of newly released platelets (<24 hrs). The IPF can be measured in a standard hematologic cell counter (Sysmex XE-2100 hematology analyzer) as part of the complete cell count and can help differentiate thrombocytopenias associated with decreased platelet production from those with increased platelet destruction in a manner similar to the use of reticulocyte counts to evaluate anemia (15). Recent studies have shown the usefulness of the IPF to evaluate mechanisms of thrombocytopenia and to predict platelet recovery in

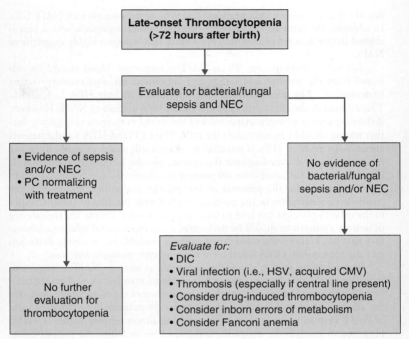

Figure 47.2. Guidelines for the evaluation of neonates with late-onset thrombocytopenia (>72 hours of life). PC = platelet count; NEC = necrotizing enterocolitis; HSV = herpes simplex virus; CMV = cytomegalovirus.

neonates (16,17). The IPF should be particularly helpful to guide the diagnostic evaluation of infants with thrombocytopenia of unclear etiology.

III. IMMUNE THROMBOCYTOPENIA. Immune thrombocytopenia occurs due to the passive transfer of antibodies from the maternal to the fetal circulation. There are two distinctive types of immune mediated thrombocytopenia: (i) neonatal alloimmune thrombocytopenia (NAIT) and (ii) autoimmune thrombocytopenia. In NAIT, the antibody is produced in the mother against a specific human platelet antigen (HPA) present in the fetus but absent in the mother. The antigen is inherited from the father of the fetus. The anti-HPA antibody produced in the maternal serum crosses the placenta and reaches the fetal circulation, leading to platelet destruction and thrombocytopenia. In autoimmune thrombocytopenia, the antibody is directed against an antigen on the mother's own platelets (autoantibody) as well as on the baby's platelets. The maternal autoantibody also crosses the placenta, resulting in destruction of fetal platelets and thrombocytopenia.

A. Neonatal alloimmune thrombocytopenia. NAIT should be considered in any neonate who presents with severe thrombocytopenia at birth or shortly thereafter, particularly in the absence of other risk factors, clinical signs, or abnormalities in the physical exam or in the other blood cell counts. In a study of more than 200 neonates with thrombocytopenia, using a platelet count $<50 \times 10^3$/mcL in the first day of life as a screening indicator identified 90% of the patients with NAIT (18). In addition, the combination of severe neonatal thrombocytopenia with a parenchymal (rather than intraventricular) intracranial hemorrhage is highly suggestive of NAIT.

Laboratory Investigation: When NAIT is suspected, blood should be collected from the mother and father and submitted for confirmatory testing (if accessible). The initial antigen screening should include HPA 1, 3, and 5. This evaluation should identify approximately 90% of cases of NAIT. However, if the diagnosis is strongly suspected and the initial evaluation is negative, further testing should be undertaken for HPA 9 and 15 (and HPA 4 if the parents are of Asian descent) (19). If positive, these tests will reveal an antibody in the mother's plasma directed against the specific platelet antigen in the father. If blood cannot be collected from the parents in a timely fashion, neonatal serum may be screened for the presence of anti-platelet antibodies. However, a low antibody concentration in the neonate coupled with binding of the antibodies to the infant's platelets can lead to false-negative results. Due to the complexity of testing, evaluations should be performed in an experienced reference laboratory that has a large number of typed controls available for antibody detection and the appropriate DNA-based technology to type multiple antigens.

Brain imaging studies should be performed as soon as NAIT is suspected, regardless of the presence or absence of neurologic manifestations, because findings from these studies will dictate the aggressiveness of the treatment regimen for the affected infant and for the mother's future pregnancies. The clinical course of NAIT is short in most cases, often resolving almost entirely within 2 weeks. However, to confirm the diagnosis, it is important to follow the platelet count frequently until a normal count is achieved.

Management: The management of NAIT differs depending on the specific clinical scenario:

1. Suspected NAIT in an unknown pregnancy
2. Known case of NAIT
3. Antenatal management of pregnant woman with previous history of NAIT

   a. Management of the neonate with suspected NAIT in an unknown pregnancy. Based on recent data demonstrating that a large proportion of infants with NAIT respond to **random-donor platelet transfusions, this is now considered the first line of therapy for infants in whom NAIT is suspected** (20).

   i. If the patient is clinically stable and does not have evidence of an intracranial hemorrhage, platelets are usually given when the platelet count is less than $30 \times 10^3/\text{mcL}$, although this is arbitrary.

   ii. If the patient has evidence of an intracranial hemorrhage, the goal is to maintain a platelet count greater than $100 \times 10^3/\text{mcL}$. This can be challenging in neonates with NAIT.

   iii. In addition to platelets, if the diagnosis of NAIT is confirmed or strongly suspected, intravenous immune globulin (IVIG) (1 g/kg/day for up to 2 consecutive days) may be infused to increase the patient's own platelets and potentially to protect the transfused platelets (21). Because in NAIT the platelet count usually falls after birth, IVIG can be infused when the platelet count is between 30 and $50 \times 10^3/\text{mcL}$, to try to prevent a further drop.

iv. It is important to keep in mind that some infants with NAIT fail to respond to random-donor platelets and IVIG. For that reason, the blood bank should be immediately alerted about any infant with suspected NAIT, and arrangements should be made to secure a source of antigen-negative platelets (either from HPA-1b1b and 5a5a donors, which should be compatible in >90% of cases, or from the mother) as soon as possible if there is no response to the initial therapies. If maternal platelets are used, they need to be concentrated to decrease the amount of anti-platelet antibodies (present in the mother's plasma) infused into the infant. Platelets can also be washed to eliminate the plasma, but this induces more damage to the platelets than concentrating them (19). Of note, in some European countries, HPA-1b1b and 5a5a platelets are maintained in the blood bank inventory and are immediately available for use. In those cases, these are preferable to random-donor platelets and/or IVIG and should be the first line of therapy.

v. Methylprednisolone (1 mg/kg bid for 3–5 days) has also been used in individual case reports and small series, but should only be considered if the infant does not respond to random platelets and IVIG, there is no suspicion of bacterial or viral infection, and antigen-matched platelets are not readily available. Some experts recommend IV methylprednisolone at a low dose (1 mg q8h) on the days that IVIG is given (19).

b. **Management of the neonate with known NAIT.** When a neonate is born to a mother who had a previous pregnancy affected by confirmed NAIT, genotypically matched platelets (e.g., HPA-1b1b platelets) should be available in the blood bank at the time of delivery and should be the first line of therapy if the infant is thrombocytopenic.

c. **Antenatal management of pregnant women with previous history of NAIT.** Mothers who delivered an infant with NAIT should be followed in high-risk obstetric clinics during all future pregnancies. The intensity of prenatal treatment will be based on the severity of the thrombocytopenia and the presence or absence of intracranial hemorrhage (ICH) in the previously affected fetus. This is particularly important to assess the risk of developing an ICH in the current pregnancy and to minimize this risk. Current recommendations involve maternal treatment with IVIG (1–2 g/kg/wk) ± steroids, starting at 12 or at 20 to 26 weeks' gestation, depending on whether the previously affected fetus suffered an ICH, and if so, at what time during pregnancy (19).

B. **Autoimmune thrombocytopenia.** The diagnosis of neonatal autoimmune thrombocytopenia should be considered in any neonate who has early-onset thrombocytopenia and a maternal history of either idiopathic thrombocytopenic purpura (ITP) or an autoimmune disease (with or without thrombocytopenia). A retrospective study of obstetric patients who had ITP (including a high number of mothers who had thrombocytopenia during their pregnancies) demonstrated a relatively high incidence of affected babies: 25% of neonates exhibited thrombocytopenia at birth; the thrombocytopenia was severe in 9%, and 15% received treatment for it (22). Other large studies confirmed an incidence of severe neonatal thrombocytopenia in this population ranging from 8.9% to 14.7%, with ICH occurring in 0% to 1.5% of affected neonates (23–25). Based on these data, it is recommended that all neonates born to mothers who have autoimmune diseases undergo a screening platelet count at or shortly after birth. If the platelet count is normal, no further evaluation is necessary. If the infant has mild thrombocytopenia, however, the platelet count should be repeated in 2 to 3 days, since it usually reaches the nadir between days 2 and 5 after birth. If the platelet count is less than 30×10^3/mcL, IVIG (1 g/kg, repeated if necessary) is the first line of therapy. Random-donor platelets, in addition to IVIG, should be provided only if the infant has evidence of active bleeding. Cranial imaging should be obtained in all infants with platelet counts $<50 \times 10^3$/mcL to evaluate for intracranial hemorrhage. Importantly, neonatal thrombocytopenia secondary to maternal ITP may last for months and requires long-term monitoring and sometimes a second dose of IVIG at 4 to 6 weeks of life.

Maternal management. Even if the mother has true ITP, it appears that fetal hemorrhage *in utero* is very rare compared with the small but definite risk of such hemorrhage in alloimmune thrombocytopenia. Because of that, treatment of ITP during pregnancy is mostly based on the risk of maternal hemorrhage (26). A small prospective randomized trial of low-dose betamethasone (1.5 mg/day orally) failed to prevent thrombocytopenia in newborns (27). IVIG given prenatally to the mother with ITP has also not been clearly shown to affect the fetal platelet count.

There is in general little correlation between fetal platelet counts and either maternal platelet counts, platelet antibody levels, or history of maternal splenectomy. However, attempts to measure the fetal platelet count before delivery are not recommended due to the risk associated with such attempts. In regard to the mode of delivery, there is no evidence that cesarean section is safer for the fetus with thrombocytopenia than uncomplicated vaginal delivery. Given this fact, combined with the difficulty predicting severe thrombocytopenia in neonates and the very low risk of serious hemorrhage, the 2010 International Consensus Report on the Investigation and Management of Primary Immune Thrombocytopenia concluded that the mode of delivery in ITP patients should be determined by purely obstetric indications (26).

IV. PLATELET TRANSFUSIONS IN THE NICU (see Chapter 42). Recent

studies have shown that there is great variability in neonatal transfusion practices in the United States and worldwide (28,29). To a large extent, this is attributable to the paucity of scientific evidence in the field. Only one randomized trial has compared different platelet transfusion thresholds in neonates, and it was limited to very low birth weight (VLBW) infants in the first week of life (30). This study found no differences in the incidence or severity of intraventricular hemorrhages (IVHs) between a group of neonates transfused for any platelet count less than 150×10^3/mcL and a group transfused only for counts below 50×10^3/mcL. Based on these findings, the investigators concluded that transfusing VLBW infants with platelet counts $>50 \times 10^3$/mcL did not reduce the risk of IVH. A more recent retrospective study evaluated whether platelet counts $<50 \times 10^3$/mcL could be safely tolerated in neonates. This study concluded that using a platelet count of 30×10^3/mcL as a transfusion threshold was a safe practice for stable neonates with no prior hemorrhages (31). Based on this limited evidence, we currently propose administering platelet transfusions to neonates according to the criteria shown in Table 47.1.

There is more consensus in regard to the platelet product that should be transfused. Most experts agree that neonates should receive 10 to 15 mL/kg of a standard platelet suspension, either a platelet concentrate ("random-donor platelets") or apheresis platelets. Each random-donor platelet unit has approximately 50 mL of volume and contains approximately 10×10^9 platelets per 10 ml (32). There is no need to pool

Table 47.1	Guidelines for Platelet Transfusion
Platelet Count (× 10³/mcL)	
<30	*Transfuse all*
30–49	*Transfuse if:* • BW <1,500g and ≤7 days old • Clinically unstable • Concurrent coagulopathy • Previous significant hemorrhage (i.e., grade 3 or 4 IVH) • Prior to surgical procedure • Postoperative period (72 hours)
50–100	*Transfuse if:* • Active bleeding • NAIT with intracranial bleed • Before or after neurosurgical procedures
BW = birth weight; NAIT = neonatal alloimmune thrombocytopenia.	

more than one random-donor unit for a neonatal transfusion, a practice that (while still somewhat prevalent) only increases donor exposures and induces platelet activation without any benefit. Two additional important considerations in neonatology are the prevention of transfusion-transmitted CMV infections and graft-versus-host disease (GVHD). Most blood banks provide either CMV-negative or leukoreduced products to neonates, both of which significantly reduce (but do not eliminate) the risk of transfusion transmitted CMV. GVHD is effectively prevented by irradiating cellular blood products prior to transfusion. Of note, most neonatal cases of GVHD have been reported in neonates with underlying immunodeficiencies, receiving intrauterine or large volume transfusions (i.e., double exchange transfusions) or receiving blood products from a first-degree relative. These are all absolute indications for irradiating blood products (32).

When making platelet transfusion decisions, it is important for neonatologists to be aware of the risks associated with these transfusions. In the case of platelet suspensions, the risk of bacterial contamination is higher than the combined risk of all viral infections for which platelets are routinely tested. In addition, platelet transfusions can induce transfusion-associated lung injury (TRALI), a process characterized by the onset of hypoxemia and bilateral pulmonary infiltrates within 6 hours of a transfusion (33). Given that neonates have frequent episodes of respiratory decompensation due to different causes, TRALI is likely to be underrecognized in the NICU. Several recent publications have also shown a strong association between the number of platelet transfusions and the mortality rate among NICU patients (34–37). It is unclear from these studies whether this association simply reflects sicker patients receiving more platelets or whether platelet transfusions adversely affect outcomes. Nevertheless, while we await for data from well-designed randomized controlled studies, platelet transfusion decisions in neonates should be made thoughtfully, carefully balancing the risks and benefits in each individual patient.

REFERENCES

1. Burrows RF, Kelton JG. Fetal thrombocytopenia and its relation to maternal thrombocytopenia. *N Engl J Med* 1993;329(20):1463–1466.
2. Andrew M, Castle V, Saigal S, et al. Clinical impact of neonatal thrombocytopenia. *J Pediatr* 1987;110(3):457–464.
3. Castle V, Andrew M, Kelton J, et al. Frequency and mechanism of neonatal thrombocytopenia. *J Pediatr* 1986;108(5 pt 1):749–755.
4. Mehta P, Vasa R, Neumann L, et al. Thrombocytopenia in the high-risk infant. *J Pediatr* 1980;97(5):791–794.
5. Wiedmeier SE, et al. Platelet reference ranges for neonates, defined using data from over 47,000 patients in a multihospital healthcare system. *J Perinatol* 2009;29(2):130–136.
6. Christensen RD, et al. Thrombocytopenia among extremely low birth weight neonates: data from a multihospital healthcare system. *J Perinatol* 2006;26(6):348–353.
7. Murray NA, Roberts IA. Circulating megakaryocytes and their progenitors in early thrombocytopenia in preterm neonates. *Pediatr Res* 1996;40(1):112–119.
8. Murray NA, Watts TL, Roberts IA. Endogenous thrombopoietin levels and effect of recombinant human thrombopoietin on megakaryocyte precursors in term and preterm babies. *Pediatr Res* 1998;43(1):148–151.
9. Gershanik JJ, Morgan SK, Akers R. Fanconi's anemia in a neonate. *Acta Paediatr Scand* 1972;61(5):623–625.
10. Hedberg VA, Lipton JM. Thrombocytopenia with absent radii. A review of 100 cases. *Am J Pediatr Hematol Oncol* 1998;10(1):51–64.
11. Geddis AE. Inherited thrombocytopenia: congenital amegakaryocytic thrombocytopenia and thrombocytopenia with absent radii. *Semin Hematol* 2006;43(3):196–203.
12. Sola MC, Slayton WB, Rimsza LM, et al. A neonate with severe thrombocytopenia and radio-ulnar synostosis. *J Perinatol* 2004;24(8):528–530.
13. Aster RH, Bougie DW. Drug-induced immune thrombocytopenia. *N Engl J Med* 2007;357(6):580–587.
14. Aster RH, Curtis BR, McFarland, et al. Drug-induced immune thrombocytopenia: pathogenesis, diagnosis, and management. *J Thromb Haemost* 2009;7(6):911–918.
15. Abe Y, Wada H, Tomatsu H, et al. A simple technique to determine thrombopoiesis level using immature platelet fraction (IPF). *Thromb Res* 2006;118(4):463–469.
16. Cremer M, Paetzold J, Schmalisch G, et al. Immature platelet fraction as novel laboratory parameter predicting the course of neonatal thrombocytopenia. *Br J Haematol* 2008;144(4):619–621.
17. Cremer M, Weimann A, Schmalisch G, et al. Immature platelet values indicate impaired megakaryopoietic activity in neonatal early-onset thrombocytopenia. *Thromb Haemost* 2010;103(5):1016–1021.
18. Bussel JB, Zacharoulis S, Kramer K, et al. Clinical and diagnostic comparison of neonatal alloimmune thrombocytopenia to non-immune cases of thrombocytopenia. *Pediatr Blood Cancer* 2005;45(2):176–183.
19. Bussel JB, Sola-Visner M. Current approaches to the evaluation and management of the fetus and neonate with immune thrombocytopenia. *Semin Perinatol* 2009;33(1):35–42.
20. Kiefel V, Bassler D, Kroll H, et al. Antigen-positive platelet transfusion in neonatal alloimmune thrombocytopenia (NAIT). *Blood* 2006;107(9):3761–3763.
21. Mueller-Eckhardt C, Kiefel V, Grubert A. High-dose IgG treatment for neonatal alloimmune thrombocytopenia. *Blut* 1989;59(1):145–146.
22. Webert KE, Mittal R, Sigoun C, et al. A retrospective 11-year analysis of obstetric patients with idiopathic thrombocytopenic purpura. *Blood* 2003;102(13):4306–4311.
23. Kaplan C, Daffos F, Forestier F, et al. Fetal platelet counts in thrombocytopenic pregnancy. *Lancet* 1990;336(8721):979–982.
24. Samuels P, Bussel JB, Braitman LE, et al. Estimation of the risk of thrombocytopenia in the offspring of pregnant women with presumed immune thrombocytopenic purpura. *N Engl J Med* 1990;323(4):229–235.

25. Burrows RF, Kelton JG. Pregnancy in patients with idiopathic thrombocytopenic purpura: assessing the risks for the infant at delivery. *Obstet Gynecol Surv* 1993;48(12):781–788.

26. Provan D, Stasi R, Newland AC, et al. International consensus report on the investigation and management of primary immune thrombocytopenia. *Blood* 2010;115(2):168–186.

27. Christiaens GC, Nieuwenhuis HK, von dem Borne AE, et al. Idiopathic thrombocytopenic purpura in pregnancy: a randomized trial on the effect of antenatal low dose corticosteroids on neonatal platelet count. *Br J Obstet Gynaecol* 1990;97(10):893–898.

28. Josephson CD, Su LL, Christensen RD, et al. Platelet transfusion practices among neonatologists in the United States and Canada: results of a survey. *Pediatrics* 2009;123(1):278–285.

29. Kahn DJ, Richardson DK, Billett HH. Inter-NICU variation in rates and management of thrombocytopenia among very low birth weight infants. *J Perinatol* 2003;23(4):312–316.

30. Andrew M, Vegh P, Caco C, et al. A randomized, controlled trial of platelet transfusions in thrombocytopenic premature infants. *J Pediatr* 1993;123(2):285–291.

31. Murray NA, Howarth LJ, McCoy MP, et al. Platelet transfusion in the management of severe thrombocytopenia in neonatal intensive care unit patients. *Transfus Med* 2002;12(1):35–41.

32. Strauss RG. Blood banking and transfusion issues in perinatal medicine. In: Christensen R, ed. *Hematologic Problems of the neonate.* Philadelphia: WB Saunders; 2000:405–425.

33. Goldman M, Webert KE, Arnold DM, et al. Proceedings of a consensus conference: towards an understanding of TRALI. *Transfus Med Rev* 2005;19(1):2–31.

34. Baer VL, Lambert DK, Henry E, et al. Do platelet transfusions in the NICU adversely affect survival? Analysis of 1600 thrombocytopenic neonates in a multihospital healthcare system. *J Perinatol* 2007;27(12):790–796.

35. Del Vecchio A, Sola MC, Theriaque DW, et al. Platelet transfusions in the neonatal intensive care unit: factors predicting which patients will require multiple transfusions. *Transfusion* 2001;41(6):803–808.

36. Garcia MG, Duenas E, Sola MC, et al. Epidemiologic and outcome studies of patients who received platelet transfusions in the neonatal intensive care unit. *J Perinatol* 2001;21(7):415–420.

37. Stanworth SJ, Clarke P, Watts T, et al. Prospective, observational study of outcomes in neonates with severe thrombocytopenia. *Pediatrics* 2009;124(5):826–834.

48 Viral Infections
Sandra K. Burchett

I. INTRODUCTION. Vertically transmitted (mother-to-child) viral infections of the fetus and newborn can generally be divided into two major categories. The first are **congenital infections**, which are transmitted to the fetus *in utero*. The second are **perinatal infections**, which are acquired intrapartum or in the postpartum period. Infections acquired through breastfeeding are in the latter category. Classifying these infections into congenital and perinatal categories highlights aspects of their pathogenesis in the fetus and newborn infant. Generally, when these infections occur in older children or adults, they are benign. However, if the host is immunocompromised or if the immune system is not yet developed, such as in the neonate, clinical symptoms may be quite severe or even fatal. Congenital infections can have manifestations that are clinically apparent antenatally by ultrasonography or when the infant is born, whereas perinatal infections may not become clinically obvious until after the first few days or weeks of life. Although, classically, the congenital infections have gone by the acronym TORCH (T = toxoplasmosis, O = other, R = rubella, C = cytomegalovirus, H = herpes simplex virus), this term is now archaic and should be avoided. When congenital or perinatal infections are suspected, the diagnosis of each of the possible infectious agents should be considered separately and the appropriate most rapid diagnostic test requested in order to implement therapy as quickly as possible. Useless information is often obtained when the diagnosis is attempted by drawing a single serum sample to be sent for measurement of TORCH titers. These immunoglobulin G (IgG) antibodies are acquired by passive transmission to the fetus and merely reflect the maternal serostatus. Pathogen-specific IgM antibodies do reflect fetal/infant infection status but with variable sensitivity and specificity. The following discussion is divided by pathogen as to the usual timing of acquisition of infection (congenital or perinatal) and in approximate order of prevalence. A summary of the diagnostic evaluation for separate viral infections is shown in Table 48.1.

II. CYTOMEGALOVIRUS (CMV: CONGENITAL AND PERINATAL). CMV is a double-stranded enveloped DNA virus with lifelong infection. It is a member of the herpesvirus family, is found only in humans, and derives its name from the histopathologic appearance of infected cells, which have abundant cytoplasm and both intranuclear and cytoplasmic inclusions.

A. **Epidemiology.** CMV is present in saliva, urine, genital secretions, breast milk, and blood or blood products of infected persons and can be transmitted by exposure to any of these sources. Primary infection (acute infection) is usually asymptomatic in older infants, children, and adults, but may manifest with mononucleosis-like symptoms, including a prolonged fever and a mild hepatitis. Latent infection is asymptomatic unless the host becomes immunocompromised. CMV infection is very common, with seroprevalence in the United States between 50% and 85% by age 40. Forty percent or more of pregnant women in the United States are

Table 48.1	Diagnostic Techniques for Diagnosis of Perinatal Infections			
Pathogen	**Test of Choice**	**Sensitivity**	**Expense**	**Turnaround**
HSV	DFA skin lesion	High	Moderate	Hours
Parvovirus	PCR blood	High	Moderate	Hours*
Parvovirus	IgM	Moderate	Low	Days
CMV	PCR urine/saliva	High	Moderate	Hours*
CMV	Spin-enhanced urine culture (shell vial)	High	Moderate	Days
HIV	DNA PCR if mother known HIV-infected	High	High	Hours*
HIV	RNA PCR if mother not treated	High	Moderate	Hours*
HBV	HBVSAg	High	Low	Hours
HBV	DNA PCR	High	Moderate	Hours*
HCV	RNA PCR <12 mo	High	Moderate	Hours*
HCV	RIBA >15 mo	High	Low	Hours*
V-ZV	DFA skin lesion	Moderate	Moderate	Hours
EV	RNA PCR blood	High	Moderate	Hours*
EV	Culture urine, oropharynx, stool	Moderate	High	Days
Rubella	Culture urine	Moderate	High	Many days
RSV	DFA	Moderate	Moderate	Hours

HSV = herpes simplex virus; DFA = direct fluorescent antibody; PCR = polymerase chain reaction; IgM = immunoglobulin M; CMV = cytomegalovirus; HBV = hepatitis B virus; HCV = hepatitis C virus; V-ZV = varicella-zoster virus; EV = enterovirus; RSV = respiratory syncytial virus.
*PCRs in general are done within a half day but often are a send-out test to a central lab requiring days to ship and retrieve data.

infected, with the lowest infection prevalence in young primigravidas. Primary CMV infection occurs in 1% to 3% of pregnant women, with a fetal attack rate of 30% to 40%. About 30,000 infants are born annually in the United States with congenital CMV infection (1 in 150 births) with more than 5,000 infants with permanent problems (1 in 750 births). Eighty percent of infants with congenital

CMV infection will remain asymptomatic. The risk of transmission to the fetus as a function of gestational age is uncertain, but infection during early gestation likely carries a higher risk of severe fetal disease. Vertical transmission can occur at any time in gestation or in the perinatal period, and infants are usually asymptomatic, especially if born to women seropositive before pregnancy. However, as many as 17% of infants with symptomatic CMV are born to women with prior seropositivity. Congenital CMV occurs in at least 1% of all live births in the United States and is the leading infectious cause of sensorineural hearing loss (SNHL) and developmental delay. Annually, of these 40,000 CMV-infected infants, 10% will have symptomatic disease at birth. Additionally, 10% of the asymptomatic neonates will develop significant sequelae in the first year of life. Therefore, at least 8,000 infants are severely affected or die from CMV infection in the United States each year. CMV infection is more common among HIV-1 infected infants, and coinfected infants may have more rapid progression of HIV-1 disease. Therefore, screening for CMV in HIV-exposed infants is advised.

B. **Clinical disease** in congenital infection may present at birth, while both congenital and perinatal infection can manifest with symptoms later in infancy.

1. **Congenital early** symptomatic disease can present as an acute **fulminant** infection involving multiple organ systems with as high as 30% mortality. **Signs** include petechiae or purpura (79%), hepatosplenomegaly (HSM) (74%), jaundice (63%), prematurity and/or "blueberry muffin spots" reflecting extramedullary hematopoiesis. **Laboratory abnormalities** include elevated hepatic transaminases and bilirubin levels (as much as half conjugated), anemia, and thrombocytopenia. Hyperbilirubinemia may be present at birth or develop over time and usually persists beyond the period of physiologic jaundice. Approximately one-third of these infants are preterm, and one-third have intrauterine growth restriction (IUGR).

   A second early presentation includes infants who are symptomatic but without life-threatening complications. These babies may have IUGR or disproportionate microcephaly (48%) with or without intracranial calcifications. These calcifications may occur anywhere in the brain, but are classically found in the periventricular area. Other findings of central nervous system (CNS) disease can include ventricular dilatation, cortical atrophy, migrational disorders such as lissencephaly, pachygyria, and demyelination as well as chorioretinitis in approximately 10% to 15% of infants. Babies with CNS manifestations almost always have developmental abnormalities and neurologic dysfunction. These range from mild learning and language disability or mild hearing loss to intelligence quotient (IQ) scores below 50, motor abnormalities, deafness, and visual problems. Because SNHL is the most common sequela of CMV infection (60% in symptomatic and 5% in asymptomatic infants at birth), any infant failing the newborn hearing screen also should be screened for CMV infection. Conversely, infants with documented congenital CMV infection should be assessed for hearing loss as neonates and throughout the first year of life.

2. **Asymptomatic congenital** infection at birth in 5% to 15% of neonates can manifest as **later disease** in infancy. Abnormalities include developmental abnormalities, hearing loss, mental retardation, motor spasticity, and acquired microcephaly. Other problems that can be detected later in life include inguinal hernia and dental defects due to abnormal enamel production.

3. **Perinatally acquired** CMV infection may occur (i) from intrapartum exposure to the virus within the maternal genital tract, (ii) from postnatal exposure to infected breast milk, (iii) from exposure to infected blood or blood products, or (iv) nosocomially through urine or saliva. The time from infection to disease presentation varies from 4 to 12 weeks. Almost all term infants who are infected perinatally remain asymptomatic, especially if the infection arose from a mother with reactivated viral excretion. While long-term developmental and neurologic abnormalities are rarely seen, an acute infection syndrome, including neutropenia, anemia, HSM, lymphadenopathy, and hearing loss can be found, especially in preterm infants. Data suggest that all infants, regardless of gestational age, should have hearing testing over the first year of life if documented to have acquired CMV.

4. **CMV pneumonitis.** CMV has been associated with pneumonitis occurring especially in preterm infants <4 months old. Symptoms and radiographic findings in CMV pneumonitis are similar to those seen in afebrile pneumonia of other causes in neonates and young infants, including *Chlamydia trachomatis*, *Ureaplasma urealyticum*, and respiratory syncytial virus (RSV). Symptoms include tachypnea, cough, coryza, and nasal congestion. Intercostal retractions and hypoxemia may be present, and apnea may occur. Radiographically, there is hyperinflation, diffusely increased pulmonary markings, thickened bronchial walls, and focal atelectasis. A small number of infants may have symptoms that are severe enough to require mechanical ventilation, and historically, approximately 3% of infants die if untreated. Laboratory findings in CMV pneumonitis are nonspecific. Long-term sequela includes recurrent pulmonary problems, including wheezing and, in some cases, repeated hospitalizations for respiratory distress. Whether this presentation reflects congenital or perinatal CMV infection is unclear. Conversely, merely finding CMV in respiratory secretions of a preterm infant does not prove causality of symptomatology because CMV is present in saliva of infected infants.

5. **Transfusion-acquired CMV infection.** In the past, significant morbidity and mortality could occur in newborn infants receiving CMV-infected blood or blood products. Since both the cellular and humoral maternal immune systems are helpful in preventing infection or in ameliorating clinical disease, those most severely affected were preterm, low birth weight infants born to CMV-seronegative women. Mortality was estimated to be 20% in very low birth weight infants. Symptoms typically developed 4 to 12 weeks after transfusion, lasted for 2 to 3 weeks, and consisted of respiratory distress, pallor, and HSM. Hematologic abnormalities were also seen, including hemolysis, thrombocytopenia, and atypical lymphocytosis. Transfusion-acquired CMV is now rare, prevented by using blood or blood products from CMV-seronegative donors or filtered, leukoreduced products (see Chap. 42).

C. **Diagnosis.** CMV infection should be suspected in any infant having typical symptoms of infection or if there is a maternal history of seroconversion or a mononucleosis-like illness in pregnancy. The diagnosis is made if CMV is identified in urine, saliva, blood, or respiratory secretions and defined as *congenital* infection if found within the first 2 weeks of life and as *perinatal* infection if negative in the first 2 weeks and positive after 4 weeks of life. Depending upon when the fetus or infant infection occurred, blood is the earliest specimen to become positive, but urine is likely to give the highest sensitivity for diagnosis as CMV is concentrated in high titers in the urine. CMV is also shed in saliva. A negative viral test from blood cannot rule out CMV infection, but a negative urine test in an untreated infant symptomatic for 4 weeks or more does rule out infection. There are three rapid diagnostic techniques:

1. **CMV polymerase chain reaction (PCR).** CMV may be detected by PCR in urine or blood. The sensitivity of using this test for diagnosis is quite high for urine, but a negative PCR in blood does not rule out infection.

2. **Spin-enhanced culture or "shell vial."** Virus can be isolated from saliva and in high titer from urine. Depending upon local laboratory specifications, the specimen is collected with a Dacron swab, inoculated into viral transport medium, and then inoculated into viral tissue culture medium containing a coverslip on which tissue culture cells have been grown and incubated. Viable CMV infects the cells, which are then lysed and stained with antibody to CMV antigens. Virus can be detected with high sensitivity and specificity within 24 to 72 hours of inoculation. It is much more rapid than standard tissue culture, which may take from 2 to 6 weeks for replication and identification. A negative result generally rules out CMV infection except in infants who may have acquired infection within the prior 2 to 3 weeks.

3. **CMV antigen.** Peripheral blood can be centrifuged and the buffy coat spread on a slide. The neutrophils are then lysed and stained with an antibody to CMV pp65 antigen. Positive results confirm CMV infection and viremia; however, negative results do not rule out CMV infection. This test is usually used to follow efficacy of therapy.

4. **CMV IgG and IgM.** The determination of serum antibody titers to CMV has limited usefulness for the neonate, although negative IgG titers in both maternal and infant sera are sufficient to exclude congenital CMV infection. The interpretation of a positive IgG titer in the newborn is complicated by the presence of transplacentally derived maternal IgG. Uninfected infants usually show a decline in IgG within 1 month and have no detectable titer by 4 to 12 months. Infected infants continue to produce IgG throughout the same time period. Tests for CMV-specific IgM have limited specificity but can help in the diagnosis of an infant infection.

   If the diagnosis of congenital CMV infection is made, the infant should have a thorough physical and neurologic examination, magnetic resonance imaging (MRI) or computed tomography (CT) scan of the brain, an ophthalmologic examination, and a hearing test. Laboratory evaluation should include a complete blood count, liver function tests, and cerebrospinal fluid (CSF) examination. In CMV-infected infants with symptomatic disease, approximately 90% with abnormal brain imaging will have CNS sequelae. However, about 30% of infants with normal brain imaging will also have sequelae.

D. Treatment. Ganciclovir (9-[(1,3-dihydroxy-2-propoxy)methyl]guanine) and the oral prodrug, valganciclovir, have been effective in the treatment of and prophylaxis against dissemination of CMV in immunocompromised patients. The earliest studies of infants with symptomatic CMV disease showed a strong trend toward efficacy in the ganciclovir-treated infants as assessed by stabilization or improvement of SNHL. Randomized studies are ongoing using oral valganciclovir treatment for symptomatic, congenitally infected infants. Most treated infants will have thrombocytopenia and neutropenia during the course of therapy. Families should be advised that while evidence is increasing as to antiviral efficacy, questions remain about the potential for future reproductive system effects as testicular atrophy and gonadal tumors were found in some animals treated with pharmacologic doses of ganciclovir. Additionally, although there have been no controlled trials, hyperimmune CMV immunoglobulin (CMVIG) might conceivably benefit infants with congenital CMV, especially those with a fulminant presentation. Treatment should be supervised by a pediatric infectious disease specialist.

E. Prevention

1. **Screening.** Because only 1% to 3% of women acquire primary CMV infection during pregnancy, with the overall risk of symptomatic fetal infection, only 0.2%, screening for women at risk for seroconversion is generally not recommended. Isolation of virus from the cervix or urine of pregnant women cannot be used to predict fetal infection. In cases of documented primary maternal infection or seroconversion, quantitative PCR testing of amniotic fluid can determine whether the fetus acquired infection. However, counseling about a positive finding of fetal infection is difficult because 85% of infected fetuses will only have mild or asymptomatic disease. Some investigators have found that higher CMV viral loads from the amniotic fluid tended to correlate with abnormal neurodevelopmental outcome. One study suggested a protective benefit against severe neonatal disease by administering hyperimmune CMVIG antenatally to women with low-affinity antibody to CMV. Presently, there is not enough information about fetal transmission and outcome to provide guidelines for obstetric management, such as recommendations for therapeutic abortion, even if primary maternal CMV infection is documented. The Centers for Disease Control and Prevention (CDC) recommends that (i) pregnant women practice hand washing with soap and water after contact with diapers or oral secretions; and not share food, utensils, toothbrushes, pacifiers with children; and avoid saliva when kissing a child; (ii) pregnant women who develop a mononucleosis-like illness during pregnancy should be evaluated for CMV infection and counseled about risks to the unborn child; (iii) antibody testing can confirm prior CMV infection; (iv) recovery of CMV from the cervix or urine of women near delivery does not warrant a cesarean section; (v) the benefits of breastfeeding outweigh the minimal risk of acquiring CMV; and (vi) there is no need to screen for CMV or exclude CMV-excreting children from schools or institutions.

2. **Immunization.** Passive immunization with hyperimmune anti-CMVIG and active immunization with a live-attenuated CMV vaccine represent attractive therapies for prophylaxis against congenital CMV infections. However, data from clinical trials are lacking. Immune globulin might be considered as prophylaxis of susceptible women against primary CMV infection in pregnancy. Two live-attenuated CMV vaccines have been developed, but their efficacy has not been clearly established. The possibility of reactivation of vaccine-strain CMV in pregnancy with subsequent infection of the fetus must be considered carefully before adequate field trials can be completed in women of childbearing age.

3. **Breast milk restriction.** Although breast milk is a common source for perinatal CMV infection in the newborn, symptomatic infection is rare, especially in term infants. In this setting, protection against disseminated disease may be provided by transplacentally derived maternal IgG or antibody in breast milk.

However, there may be insufficient transplacental IgG to provide adequate protection in preterm infants. It remains unclear whether mothers of preterm infants should be recommended to offer breast milk without prior screening for CMV seropositivity. In mothers of extremely premature infants known to be CMV positive, pasteurizing breast milk at 220°C, or freezing breast milk, will reduce the titer of CMV but will not eliminate active virus. At present, there is no recommended method of minimizing the risk of exposure to CMV in infected breast milk.

4. **Environmental restrictions.** Day care centers and hospitals are potential high-risk environments for acquiring CMV infection. Not surprisingly, a number of studies confirmed an increased risk for infection in day care workers. However, there does not appear to be an increased risk of infection in hospital personnel. Good hand-washing and infection-control measures practiced in hospital settings generally are sufficient to control the spread of CMV to workers. Unfortunately, such control may be difficult to achieve in day care centers. Good hand-washing technique should be suggested to pregnant women with children in day care, especially if the women are known to be seronegative. The determination of CMV susceptibility of these women by serology may be useful for counseling.

5. **Transfusion product restrictions.** The risk of transfusion-acquired CMV infection in the neonate has been almost eliminated by the use of CMV anti-body-negative donors, by freezing packed red blood cells (PRBCs) in glycerol or by removing the white blood cells. It is particularly important to use blood from one of these sources in preterm, low birth weight infants (see Chap. 42).

III. HERPES SIMPLEX VIRUS (HSV: PERINATAL).
HSV, a life-long infection, is a double-stranded, enveloped DNA virus with two virologically distinct types: types 1 and 2. HSV-2 is the predominant cause of neonatal disease (75%–80%), but both types produce clinically indistinguishable neonatal syndromes. The virus can cause localized disease of the skin, eye; or mouth, or may disseminate by cell-to-cell contiguous spread or viremia. After adsorption and penetration into host cells, viral replication proceeds, resulting in cellular swelling, hemorrhagic necrosis, formation of intranuclear inclusions, cytolysis, and cell death.

A. **Epidemiology.** At least 80% of the U.S. population is infected with HSV type 1, the cause of recurrent orolabial disease and an increasing cause of genital disease. According to the 2005–2008 National Health and Nutrition Examination Survey, the overall seroprevalence of HSV-2, the predominant cause of recurrent genital disease, is 16.2%, increasing with age and number of sexual partners to as high as 48% in African American women and about 21% in Caucasian and Hispanic women. The majority of seropositive persons are unaware of their HSV-2 infection status. Infection in the newborn occurs as a result of direct exposure, most commonly in the perinatal period from maternal genital disease. HSV-2 is more likely to recur in the genital tract and, therefore, accounts for most neonatal HSV infections. In one study, the characteristic ulcerations of the genitalia were present only in two-thirds of the genital tracts from which HSV could be isolated. Others had asymptomatic shedding or atypical lesions. It is estimated that up to 0.4% of all women presenting for delivery are shedding virus, and approximately 1% of all women with a history of recurrent HSV infection asymptomatically shed HSV at delivery. However, when the birth canal is carefully visualized and those with asymptomatic lesions excluded, this rate of shedding is nearer to 0.5%. **It is critical to recognize that most mothers of infants with neonatal HSV do not have a history of HSV.** Approximately 30% to 50% of infants will acquire HSV infection if maternal primary infection occurs near delivery; whereas <1% of infants are infected if born to a woman seropositive (recurrent) prior to pregnancy or who acquired infection in the first half of pregnancy. Additionally, one-third of infants born to mothers with newly acquired HSV-2, although already infected with HSV-1 (nonprimary, first episode), may acquire HSV infection. This may well be due to protective maternal type-specific antibodies in the infant's serum or the birth canal. The overall incidence of newborn infection with HSV is estimated to be from 1 in 3,000 to 1 in 20,000, or from 200 to 1,333 infants per year in the United States.

B. **Transmission**

1. **Intrapartum transmission** is the most common cause of neonatal HSV infection. It is primarily associated with active shedding of virus from the cervix or vulva at the time of delivery. As many as 95% of newborn infections occur as a result of intrapartum transmission. The amount and duration of maternal virus shedding is likely to be a major determinate of fetal transmission. These are greatest with primary maternal infections. Maternal antibody to HSV is also important and is associated with a decreased risk of fetal or neonatal transmission. In fact, when maternal antibody is present, the risk of acquisition of HSV, even for the newborn exposed to HSV in the birth canal, is very low. The exact mechanism of action of maternal antibody in preventing perinatal infection is not known, but transplacentally acquired antibody has been shown to reduce the risk of severe newborn disease following perinatal HSV exposure. The risk of intrapartum infection increases with ruptured membranes, especially when ruptured longer than 4 hours. Finally, direct methods for fetal monitoring, such as with scalp electrodes, increase the risk of fetal transmission in the setting of active shedding. It is best to avoid these techniques in women with a history of recurrent infection or suspected primary HSV disease.

2. **Antenatal transmission.** *In utero* infection has been documented but is uncommon. Spontaneous abortion has occurred with primary maternal infection before 20 weeks' gestation, but the true risk to the fetus of early-trimester primary infection is not known. Fetal infections may occur by either transplacental or ascending routes and have been documented in the setting of both primary and rarely recurrent maternal disease. There may be a wide range of clinical manifestations, from localized skin or eye involvement to multiorgan disease and congenital malformations. Chorioretinitis, microcephaly, and hydranencephaly may be found in a small number of patients.

3. **Postnatal transmission.** A small percentage of neonatal HSV infections result from postnatal exposure. Potential sources include symptomatic and asymptomatic oropharyngeal shedding by either parent, hospital personnel, or other contacts, and maternal breast lesions. Measures to minimize exposure from these sources are discussed in the subsequent text.

C. **Clinical manifestations.** Data from the National Institute of Allergy and Infectious Diseases (NIAID) Collaborative Antiviral Study Group (CASG) indicate that morbidity and mortality of neonatal HSV best correlates with three categories of disease. These are infections localized to the skin, eye, and/or mouth; encephalitis with or without localized mucocutaneous disease; and disseminated infection with multiple organ involvement. The NIAID CASG reported on the outcome of

210 infants with HSV infection who were randomized to receive either acyclovir or vidarabine antiviral therapy. Eight babies had congenital infection with signs (chorioretinitis, skin lesions, hydrocephalus) at birth with very high mortality. More than 50% mortality was seen in infants having disseminated disease, with hemorrhagic shock and pneumonitis as the principal causes of death. Of the survivors for whom follow-up was available, significant neurologic sequelae were seen in a high percentage of the infants with encephalitis and disseminated disease.

1. **Skin, eye, and mouth infection.** Approximately 50% of infants with HSV have disease localized to the skin, eye, or mucocutaneous membranes. Vesicles typically appear on the sixth to ninth day of neonatal life. A cluster of vesicles often develops on the presenting part of the body, where extended direct contact with virus may occur. Vesicles occur in 90% of infants with localized mucocutaneous infection, and recurrent disease is common. Significant morbidity can occur in these infants despite the absence of signs of disseminated disease at the time of diagnosis. Up to 10% of infants later show neurologic impairment, and infants with keratoconjunctivitis can develop chorioretinitis, cataracts, and retinopathy. Thus, ophthalmologic and neurologic follow-up is important in all infants with mucocutaneous HSV. Infants with three or more recurrences of vesicles, likely reflecting poor cellular or humoral viral control, have an increased risk of neurologic complications.

2. **CNS infection.** Approximately one-third of neonates with HSV present with encephalitis in the absence of disseminated disease, and as many as 60% of these infants do not have mucocutaneous vesicles. These infants usually become symptomatic at 10 to 14 days of life with lethargy, seizures, temperature instability, and hypotonia. In the setting of disseminated disease, HSV is thought to invade the CNS from hematogenous spread. However, CNS infection in the absence of disseminated disease can occur, most often in infants having transplacentally derived viral-neutralizing antibodies, which may protect against widespread dissemination but not influence intraneuronal viral replication. Mortality is high without treatment and is approximately 15% with treatment. Late treatment is associated with increased mortality. Approximately two-thirds of surviving infants have impaired neurodevelopment. Long-term sequelae from acute HSV encephalitis include microcephaly, hydranencephaly, porencephalic cysts, spasticity, blindness, deafness, chorioretinitis, and learning disabilities.

3. **Disseminated infection.** This is the most severe form of neonatal HSV infection. It accounts for approximately 22% of all infants with neonatal HSV infection and ends in mortality for over half. Pneumonitis and fulminant hepatitis are associated with greater mortality. Symptoms usually begin within the first week of neonatal life. The liver, adrenals, and other visceral organs are usually involved. Approximately two-thirds of infants also have encephalitis. Clinical findings include seizures, shock, respiratory distress, disseminated intravascular coagulation (DIC), and respiratory failure. A typical vesicular rash may be absent in as many as 20% of infants. Forty percent of the infants who survive have long-term morbidity.

D. **Diagnosis.** HSV infection should be considered in the differential diagnosis of ill neonates with a variety of clinical presentations. These include CNS abnormalities, fever, shock, DIC, and/or hepatitis. HSV should also be considered in infants with respiratory distress without an obvious bacterial cause or a clinical course and findings consistent with prematurity. The possibility of concomitant HSV infection with other commonly encountered problems of the preterm infant should be considered. **Viral isolation** or fluorescent antibody **detection of viral proteins** in the appropriate clinical setting remains critical to the diagnosis. For the infant with mucocutaneous lesions, tissue should be scraped from vesicles, placed in the appropriate viral transport medium, and promptly processed for culture by a diagnostic virology laboratory. Alternatively, virus can be detected directly when tissue samples are swabbed onto a glass slide and evaluated by direct fluorescent antibody (DFA) technique. Virus can also be isolated from the oropharynx and nasopharynx, conjunctivae, stool, urine, and CSF. In the absence of a vesicular rash, viral isolation from these sites may aid in the diagnosis of disseminated HSV or HSV encephalitis. With encephalitis, an elevated CSF protein level and pleocytosis are often seen, but initial values may be within normal limits. Therefore, serial CSF examinations may be very important. Electroencephalography and CT/MRI are also useful in the diagnosis of HSV encephalitis. Viral isolation from CSF is reported to be successful in as many as 40% of cases, and rates of detection in CSF by PCR may reach close to 100%. Combined HSV-1 and -2 serology is of little value, because many women are infected with HSV-1 and because these tests usually have a relatively slow turnaround time; however, obtaining type-specific antibody (glycoprotein specific) has an 80% to 98% sensitivity and >96% specificity for identifying maternal infection and infant prognosis. Specific IgM is not useful. The number of different viral antigen-specific antibodies produced seems to correlate with the extent of disseminated disease, and the presence of certain antigen-specific antibodies may have long-term prognostic value. Laboratory abnormalities seen with disseminated disease include elevated hepatic transaminase levels, direct hyperbilirubinemia, neutropenia, thrombocytopenia, and coagulopathy. A diffuse interstitial pattern is usually observed on radiographs of infants with HSV pneumonitis.

E. **Treatment.** Effective antiviral therapy (acyclovir, a nucleoside analog that selectively inhibits HSV replication) exists, but the timing of therapy is critical. Treatment is indicated for all forms of neonatal HSV disease. Initially, NIAID CASG studies were carried out with vidarabine, which reduced morbidity and mortality. Mortality with encephalitis was reduced from 50% to 15% and in disseminated disease from 90% to 70%. Later, studies from the CASG found that acyclovir is as efficacious as vidarabine for the treatment of neonatal HSV. Furthermore, acyclovir is a selective inhibitor of viral replication with minimal side effects on the host and can be administered in relatively small volumes over short infusion times. Recommendations include treating infants with disease limited to the skin, eye, and mouth disease with 20-mg acyclovir/kg every 8 hours for 14 days, and those with CNS or disseminated disease for at least 21 days, or longer if the CSF PCR remains positive. Infants with ocular involvement should have an ophthalmologic evaluation and treatment with topical ophthalmic agents (1% trifluridine, 0.1% iododeoxyuridine, or 3% vidarabine) in addition to parenteral therapy. Oral therapy such as with valacyclovir is not recommended at this time for initial treatment. Some experts recommend acyclovir suppressive therapy at 300 mg/m^2/dose three times a day after the initial treatment period until 6 months of life with careful monitoring for neutropenia and anemia.

F. **Prevention**

1. **Pregnancy strategies.** Pregnant women known to be HSV-2 seronegative should avoid genital sexual intercourse with a known HSV-2 seropositive

partner in the third trimester. Some experts also suggest avoiding oral–genital contact with partners known to have HSV-2 or -1 if the woman is known to be seronegative since HSV-1 can also result in maternal recurrent genital disease. For women who do acquire primary HSV during pregnancy, several trials have shown efficacy and safety of treating pregnant women with clinically symptomatic primary HSV infection with a 10-day course of acyclovir (oral therapy or IV if more severe disease). It is also recommended that women with HSV-2 be tested for HIV since HSV-2 seropositive persons have a twofold greater risk for acquisition of HIV than those who are seronegative for HSV-2.

2. **Delivery strategies.** Women with known clinical or serologic evidence of HSV-2 are often offered acyclovir near term until delivery, enabling a vaginal delivery if there are no visible lesions.

3. **Management of the newborn at risk for HSV (see Table 48.**2). The principal problem in developing strategies for the prevention of HSV transmission is the inability to identify maternal shedding of virus at the time of delivery. Viral identification requires isolation in tissue culture, so any attempt to identify

Table 48.2	Management of the Child Born to a Woman with Active Genital Herpes Simplex Virus Infection
Maternal primary or first-episode infection:	
■ Consider offering an elective cesarean section, regardless of lesion status at delivery, or if membranes ruptured less than 4 h	
■ Swab infant's conjunctive and nasopharynx, and possibly collect urine for DFA and culture to determine exposure to HSV	
■ Treat with acyclovir if DFA or culture positive or signs of neonatal HSV	
If cesarean section performed after 24 h of ruptured membranes or if vaginal delivery unavoidable:	
■ Swab infant's conjunctivae and nasopharynx, and collect urine for DFA and culture to determine exposure to HSV	
■ Consider initiation of acyclovir while pending culture and DFA results or if signs of neonatal HSV	
Recurrent infection, active at delivery: **If cesarean section after 4 h of ruptured membranes or unavoidable vaginal delivery:**	
■ Swab infant's conjunctivae and nasopharynx, and possibly collect urine for DFA and culture to determine exposure to HSV	
■ Treat with acyclovir if culture positive or if with signs of HSV infection	
DFA = direct fluorescent antibody; HSV = herpes simplex virus.	

women who may be shedding HSV at delivery would require antenatal cervical cultures. Unfortunately, such screening cultures taken before labor fail to predict active excretion at delivery. Until more rapid techniques such as a screening PCR are made available for the identification of HSV, the only clear recommendation that can be made is to deliver infants by cesarean section if genital lesions are present at the start of labor. The efficacy of this approach may diminish when membranes are ruptured beyond 4 hours. Nevertheless, it is generally recommended that cesarean section be considered even with membrane rupture of longer durations, although data showing efficacy beyond 4 hours are lacking. For women with a history of genital herpes, careful examination should be performed to determine whether lesions are present when labor commences. If lesions are observed, cesarean section should be offered. If no lesions are identified, vaginal delivery is appropriate, but a cervical swab should be obtained for culture. At this time, there are no data to support the prophylactic use of antiviral agents or immunoglobulin to prevent transmission to the newborn infant. Infants inadvertently delivered vaginally in the setting of cervical lesions should be isolated from other infants in the nursery, and cultures should be obtained from the oropharynx/nasopharynx and conjunctivae. If the mother can be identified as having recurrent infection, the resultant neonatal infection rate is low, and parents should be instructed to consult their pediatrician if a rash or other clinical changes (lethargy, tachypnea, poor feeding) develop. Weekly pediatric follow-up during the first month is recommended. Infants with a positive culture from any site or the evolution of clinical symptomatology should immediately have cultures repeated and antiviral therapy started. Before starting acyclovir therapy, the infant should have conjunctival, nasopharyngeal swabs for DFA and culture, urine for culture, and a CSF evaluation for pleocytosis and HSV DNA PCR. Evidence of dissemination should be evaluated with hepatic transaminases and a chest radiograph if respiratory symptoms develop.

4. **Postnatal strategies.** Infants and mothers with HSV lesions should be in contact isolation. Careful hand washing and preventing the infant from having direct contact with lesions should be emphasized. Breastfeeding should be avoided if there are breast lesions, and women with oral HSV should wear a mask while breastfeeding. Hospital personnel with orolabial HSV infection represent a low risk to the newborn, although the use of face masks should be recommended if active lesions are present. Of course, hand washing or use of gloves should again be emphasized. The exception to these guidelines is nursery personnel with herpetic whitlows. Because they have a high risk of viral shedding, and as transmission can occur despite the use of gloves, these individuals should not care for newborns.

IV. PARVOVIRUS (CONGENITAL). Parvoviruses are small, unenveloped single-stranded DNA viruses. Humans are the only known host. The cellular receptor for parvovirus B19 is the P blood group antigen, which is found on erythrocytes, erythroblasts, megakaryocytes, endothelial cells, placenta, and fetal liver and heart cells. This tissue specificity correlates with sites of clinical abnormalities (which are usually anemia with or without thrombocytopenia and sometimes fetal myocarditis). Lack of the P antigen is extremely rare, but these persons are resistant to infection with parvovirus.

A. **Epidemiology.** Parvovirus transmission results after contact with respiratory secretions, blood or blood products, or by vertical transmission. Cases can occur sporadically or in outbreak settings (especially in schools in late winter and early spring). Secondary spread occurs in at least half of susceptible household contacts. Infection is very common, such that 90% of elderly persons are seropositive. The prevalence of infection increases throughout childhood, such that approximately one-half of women of childbearing age are immune and the other half are susceptible to primary infection. The annual seroconversion rate in these women is 1.5%; however, because assessment of parvovirus infection status is not part of routine prenatal testing and because clinical infection is often asymptomatic, the rate of fetal infection in women who seroconvert during pregnancy is unknown. Women who are parents of young children, elementary school teachers, or childcare workers may be at greatest risk for exposure. Unfortunately, the time of greatest transmissibility of parvovirus is before the onset of symptoms or rash. Additionally, 50% of contagious contacts may not have a rash, and 20% may be asymptomatic. The incubation period is usually 4 to 14 days but can be as long as 21 days. Rash and joint symptoms occur 2 to 3 weeks after infection. The virus is probably spread by means of respiratory secretions, which clear in patients with typical erythema infectiosum at or shortly after the onset of rash. The epidemiology of community outbreaks of erythema infectiosum suggests that the risk of infection to susceptible schoolteachers is approximately 19% (compared with 50% for household contacts). This would lower the risk of B19 fetal disease in pregnant schoolteachers to <1%. Therefore, special precautions are not necessary in this setting. In fact, there is likely to be widespread inapparent infection in both adults and children, providing a constant background exposure rate that cannot be altered. The overall rate of vertical transmission of parvovirus from the mother with primary infection to her fetus is approximately one-third. The risk of fetal loss (3%–6%) is greatest when maternal infection occurs in the first half of pregnancy. Fetal death usually occurs within 6 weeks of maternal infection. The risk of fetal hydrops is approximately 1%. Therefore, parvovirus B19 could be the cause of as many as 1,400 cases of fetal death or hydrops fetalis each year in the United States.

B. **Transmission** is from mothers to fetuses antenatally.

C. **Clinical manifestations**

1. **Disease in children.** Parvovirus B19 has been associated with a variety of rashes, including the typical "slapped-cheek" rash of erythema infectiosum (fifth disease). In approximately 60% of school-age children with erythema infectiosum, fever occurs 1 to 4 days before the facial rash appears. Associated symptoms include myalgias, upper respiratory or gastrointestinal symptoms, and malaise, but these symptoms generally resolve with the appearance of the rash. The rash is usually macular, progresses to the extremities and trunk, and may involve the palms and soles. The rash may be pruritic and may recur. These children are likely most infectious before the onset of fever or rash. In group settings such as classrooms, the appearance of one clinically symptomatic child could reinforce the need for good hand-washing practices among potentially seronegative pregnant women.

2. **Disease in adults.** The typical school-age presentation of erythema infectiosum can occur in adults, but arthralgias and arthritis are more common. As many as 60% of adults with parvovirus B19 infection may have acute joint

swelling, most commonly involving peripheral joints (symmetrically). Rash and joint symptoms occur 2 to 3 weeks after infection. Arthritis may persist for years and may be associated with the development of rheumatoid arthritis.

3. **Less common manifestations of parvovirus B19 infection**
   a. **Infection in patients with severe anemia or immunosuppression.** Parvovirus B19 has been identified as a cause of persistent and profound anemia in patients with rapid red blood cell turnover, including those with sickle cell (SC) disease, hemoglobin SC disease, thalassemia, hereditary spherocytosis, and cellular enzyme deficits, such as pyruvate kinase deficiency. Parvovirus B19 has also been associated with acute and chronic red blood cell aplasia in immunosuppressed patients.

   b. **Fetal infection.** Although parvovirus B19 has genotypic variation, no antigenic variation between isolates has been demonstrated. Parvoviruses tend to infect rapidly dividing cells and can be transmitted across the placenta, posing a potential threat to the fetus. Based primarily on the demonstration of viral DNA in fetal tissue samples, parvovirus B19 has been implicated in approximately 10% of cases of fetal nonimmune hydrops. The presumed pathogenic sequence is as follows: Maternal primary infection → Transplacental transfer of B19 virus → Infection of red blood cell precursors → Arrested red blood cell production → Severe anemia (Hb <8 g/dL) → Congestive heart failure → Edema. Furthermore, B19 DNA has been detected in cardiac tissues from aborted fetuses. B19 may cause fetal myocarditis, which can contribute to the development of hydrops. Finally, fetal hepatitis with severe liver disease has been documented. Although there have been rare case reports of infants with fetal anomalies and parvovirus infection, it is unlikely that parvovirus causes fetal anomalies. Hence, therapeutic abortion should not be recommended in women infected with parvovirus during pregnancy. Rather, the pregnancy should be followed carefully by frequent examination and ultrasonography for signs of fetal involvement.

D. **Diagnosis.** Parvovirus B19 will not grow in standard tissue cultures because humans are the only host. Determination of serum IgG and IgM levels is the most practical test. Serum B19 IgG is absent in susceptible hosts, and IgM appears by day 3 of an acute infection. Serum IgM may be detected in as many as 90% of patients with acute B19 infection, and serum levels begin to fall by the second to third month after infection. Serum IgG appears a few days after IgM and may persist for years. Serum or plasma can also be assessed for viral DNA by PCR and defines recent infection. Viral antigens may be directly detected in tissues by radioimmunoassay, enzyme-linked immunosorbent assay (ELISA), immunofluorescence, *in situ* nucleic acid hybridization, or PCR. These techniques may be valuable for certain clinical settings, such as the examination of tissues from fetuses with nonimmune hydrops or determination of infection (PCR).

E. **Treatment.** Treatment is generally supportive. Intravenous immunoglobulin (IVIG) has been used with reported success in a limited number of patients with severe hematologic disorders related to persistent parvovirus infection. The rationale for this therapy stems from the observations that (i) the primary immune response to B19 infection is the production of specific IgM and IgG, (ii) the appearance of systemic antibody coincides with the resolution of clinical symptoms, and (iii) specific antibody prevents infection. However, no controlled studies have been performed to establish the efficacy of IVIG prophylaxis or therapy for B19 infections. There are no recommendations for use of IVIG in pregnancy. In the carefully followed pregnancy in which hydrops fetalis is worsening, intrauterine blood transfusions may be considered, especially if the fetal hemoglobin is <8 g/dL. The risk/benefit of this procedure to the mother and fetus should be assessed since some hydropic fetuses will improve without intervention. In some cases, if there is also fetal myocardiopathy secondary to parvovirus infection, the cardiac function may be inadequate to handle transfusion. Attempts to identify other causes of fetal hydrops are obviously important (see Chap. 26).

F. **Prevention.** Three groups of pregnant women of interest when considering the potential risk of fetal parvovirus disease are those exposed to an infected household contact, schoolteachers, and health care providers. In each, the measurement of serum IgG and IgM levels may be useful to determine who is at risk or acutely infected after B19 exposure. The risk of fetal B19 disease is apparently very small for asymptomatic pregnant women in communities where outbreaks of erythema infectiosum occur. In this setting, no special diagnostic tests or precautions may be indicated. However, household contacts with erythema infectiosum place pregnant women at increased risk for acute B19 infection. The estimated risk of B19 infection in a susceptible adult with a household contact is approximately 50%. Considering an estimated risk of 5% for severe fetal disease with acute maternal B19 infection, the risk of hydrops fetalis is approximately 2.5% for susceptible pregnant women exposed to an infected household contact during the first 18 weeks of gestation. Management of these women may include the following:

1. **Determination of susceptibility of acute infection** by serum IgG and IgM and PCR.

2. For susceptible or acutely infected women, **serial fetal ultrasonography** to monitor fetal growth and the possible evolution of hydrops.

3. Serial determinations of **maternal serum α-fetoprotein (AFP)** (AFP may rise up to 4 weeks before ultrasonography evidence of fetal hydrops), although this use is of uncertain value.

4. Determination of **fetal IgM or DNA PCR** by percutaneous umbilical blood sampling (PUBS). The utility of this is questionable given the relatively high risk–benefit ratio at present, especially because it is unclear that obstetric management will be altered by results. It may be useful to confirm B19 etiology when hydrops fetalis is present.

    Considering the high prevalence of B19, the low risk of severe fetal disease, and the fact that attempts to avoid potential high-risk settings only reduce but do not eliminate exposure, exclusion of pregnant schoolteachers from the workplace is not recommended. A similar approach may be taken for pregnant health care providers where the principal exposure will be from infected children presenting to the emergency room or physician's office. However, in many cases, the typical rash of erythema infectiosum may already be present, at which time infectivity is low. Furthermore, precautions directed at minimizing exposure to respiratory secretions may be taken to decrease the risk of transmission. Particular care should be exercised on pediatric wards where there are immunocompromised patients or patients with hemolytic anemias in whom B19 disease is suspected. These patients may shed virus well beyond the period of initial clinical symptoms, particularly when presenting with aplastic crisis. In this setting, there may be a significant risk for the spread of B19 to susceptible health care workers or other patients at risk for B19-induced aplastic crisis. To minimize this risk, patients with aplastic crises from B19 infections should be maintained on contact precautions, masks should be worn for close contact, and pregnant health care providers should not care for these patients.

V. HUMAN IMMUNODEFICIENCY VIRUS (HIV: CONGENITAL AND PERI-NATAL).

HIV is a cytopathic RNA retrovirus for which there is no cure presently. The virus binds to the host $CD4^+$ cell. This virus/receptor complex then binds to a coreceptor, and the viral core enters the host cell cytoplasm. The virus uses reverse transcriptase to synthesize DNA from its viral RNA, and this viral DNA integrates into the host genome. On cell activation, the viral DNA is transcribed to RNA, and viral proteins are synthesized. The virion acquires its outer envelope coat on budding from the host cell surface and is then infectious for other $CD4^+$ cells. HIV contains genomic RNA within a core that is surrounded by an inner protein shell and an outer lipid envelope. The genome consists of the three genes found in all retroviruses (*gag, pol, env*), along with at least six additional genes, including gp120, which is necessary for the binding of virus to target cells, and p24, which is the major core protein. When HIV-infected lymphocytes are activated, such as in intercurrent illnesses, many virions may be transcribed, and the cell can be lysed or apoptosis enhanced, each resulting in host cell death. Because $CD4^+$ lymphocytes are central to developing an appropriate immune response to almost all pathogens, the host with $CD4^+$ counts below $200/mm^3$ is susceptible to opportunistic infections and malignancies. In initial HIV infection, virus may first infect dendritic cells, viremia is present, and the lymphoid tissue is seeded. The host immune response is triggered, viremia is cleared, and 80% of patients become asymptomatic; for 20%, a rapidly progressive course ensues.

A. **Epidemiology.** HIV-1 is the principal cause of HIV infection in the United States and throughout the world.

1. **Domestically**, in the United States and its five dependencies, AIDS diagnoses and deaths are confidentially reported to the CDC. Approximately 1,150,000 AIDS cases had been reported by 2009: 78% in men and adolescent boys and 19% in women and adolescent girls. These data include more than 50,000 cases reported in youth between 13 and 24 years old. It was estimated that 80,000 people died yearly from AIDS from 1993 to 1997, and 15,000 to 20,000 have died yearly since 1997, with cumulative deaths of more than 600,000 infected people by the end of 2008. The decreased death rate in recent years is in large part attributed to access to more potent antiretroviral therapies since 1996. In the year 2009, there were about 35,000 AIDS cases reported, but only 13 in children younger than 13 in the United States. Estimates included 1,100,000 people living with HIV in the United States in 2006, with an additional 56,300 acquiring new infection yearly. Of these, about one-third acquired HIV through heterosexual transmission. These estimates are difficult because only AIDS is mandatorily reported in all states, with HIV infection (not progressed to AIDS) not reported in 10 states or the District of Columbia when these data were collected. Additionally, many persons who are HIV infected have not been tested and therefore do not know their infection status; they are at high risk for horizontal or vertical transmission. Approximately 20% of persons living with AIDS and 27% of those with HIV infection are **women**, most are of childbearing age. For 85% of these women, the leading risk behavior is heterosexual contact with a known HIV-infected person or unknown risk behavior (presumably

heterosexual contact with a person of unknown positive status). Whereas enormous successes in reduction of mother-to-child transmission have been realized with introduction of exposure prophylaxis (zidovudine in 1994 and potent antiretrovirals in 1996), it is estimated that 100 to 200 infants still acquire perinatal HIV infection yearly. The vast majority of these infected infants are born to women who were unaware of their diagnosis, either because counseling and testing was not offered or because women did not consent to testing. One study found that the majority of **pregnant women** were unaware that antenatal antiretroviral agents could prevent more than 99% of neonatal HIV infections. Consequently, the CDC recommends routine antenatal "opt-out" HIV testing, which has been shown to be far more effective in identifying HIV-infected persons than systems in which written informed consent is required. At present, 80% to 90% of HIV-infected pregnant women receive antiretroviral therapy at or before delivery. Those who do not receive therapy are thought not to know their diagnosis.

2. **Globally**, the World Health Organization (WHO) estimated that by the end of 2008, there were 33.4 million persons living with AIDS (15.7 million women and 2.1 million children younger than 15 years). New HIV infections were estimated in 2008 to be 2.7 million, including 430,000 children. Deaths in 2008 were 2 million (280,000 in children). All of these numbers are far less than the 2006 statistics and is reflective of the global response to HIV prevention and treatment access. Breastfeeding has been found to increase the rate of perinatal transmission by approximately 14%; therefore, it is highly discouraged where safe formula-feeding alternatives exist. Trials of continued maternal and/or infant prophylaxis with antiretroviral therapy as well as with early weaning and alternatives to breastfeeding are continuing. Increasingly, countries are able to offer antiretroviral therapy to HIV-infected women postpartum and the fathers of these babies, recognizing that even if the infant escapes HIV infection, he or she may become orphaned and therefore have a lower life expectancy unless the parents are treated. Contributions from wealthy foundations and governments in developed countries have helped to put these treatment programs in place. Unquestionably, HIV has posed one of the most serious and challenging health problems of the late 20th and early 21st centuries. Although there are still many remaining challenges, significant progress is being made.

B. **Transmission.** There are three principal routes for HIV transmission: sexual contact, parenteral inoculation, and maternal–fetal or maternal–newborn transfer.

1. **Sexual contact.** This remains the principal mode of transmission of HIV in the United States and worldwide. Both semen and vaginal secretions have been found to contain HIV. The principal risk behavior for 85% of mothers of children reported with AIDS is heterosexual contact.

2. **Parenteral inoculation.** Parenteral transmission of HIV results from the direct inoculation of infected blood or blood products. The groups affected have been intravenous drug users and patients receiving transfusions or factor concentrates. Screening of blood donors for risk factors for infection, universal HIV antibody and viral testing of donated blood, and the special preparation of clotting factor to eliminate the risk of viral contamination have greatly reduced the incidence of transfusion-acquired HIV. The most likely reason for false-negative HIV serology is the seronegative window that occurs between

the time of initial infection and the production of antiviral antibody. The odds of transfusion-acquired HIV infection from the transfusion of a single unit of tested blood have been estimated to be from 1:250,000 to 1:150,000.

3. **Congenital and perinatal transmission.** More than 92% of pediatric AIDS cases have resulted from maternal blood exposure antenatally, at birth, or post-natally through breast milk. The rate of transmission of HIV from untreated infected mothers to their fetuses and newborn infants has been estimated to be between 15% and 40%. HIV has been isolated from cord blood specimens, and products of conception have demonstrated HIV infection as early as 14 to 20 weeks' gestation; however, it is believed that most of the infection is transmitted in late third trimester or at delivery. The mechanism of transplacental transfer of HIV is not known, but HIV can infect trophoblast and placental macrophage cell lines. Neither infection nor quantity of virus present in the placenta correlates with congenital infection. This may suggest that the placenta in general acts as a protective barrier to transmission or conversely as a focus of potential transmission. In a study of 100 sets of twins delivered to HIV-infected mothers, twin A was infected in 50% delivered vaginally and 38% delivered by cesarean. Twin B was infected in 19% of both vaginal and cesarean deliveries. This study, as well as the Women and Infants Transmission Study and a meta-analysis of transmission studies, suggests that intrapartum infection occurs as a correlate of duration of ruptured membranes and that elective (without onset of labor) cesarean section deliveries may be preventive, especially if the maternal HIV viral load is not controlled at delivery.

C. **Clinical disease.** In untreated patients, $CD4^+$ cell loss progresses, with the median duration of the asymptomatic phase being approximately 10 years in adults. After this phase, the patient becomes symptomatic, generally with opportunistic infections, especially tuberculosis, and death occurs within 5 years.

1. **HIV in infants** manifests with an initially high viral load, which declines over the first 5 years of life as the immune system develops. Current U.S. and WHO guidelines suggest treating all infants diagnosed with HIV infection in the first year of life so that the immune system can develop normally, and many experts continue treatment to ensure suppression of HIV. After 1 year of age, suggestions for initiation of therapy based on $CD4^+$ cell count and HIV viral load are less specific, but include treating children with symptomatic infection and for those with the lowest $CD4^+$ cell percentages, regardless of age. Issues of when to initiate antiretroviral therapy must be individualized, and willingness of the care provider to ensure that the infant or child receives every dose every day is a critical component of success.

2. **HIV in pregnancy.** The HIV-infected pregnant woman should be counseled that completion of pregnancy probably does not worsen her prognosis. HIV-infected women should be screened for other sexually transmitted diseases (gonorrhea, herpes, chlamydia, hepatitis B and C, and syphilis), as well as being tested for infection with CMV and toxoplasmosis. The mother should also have a tuberculin skin test and, when appropriate, be offered hepatitis B, pneumococcal, and influenza vaccines. If the $CD4^+$ count is below 350 per μL, she should be offered antiretroviral therapy, including zidovudine, for her own health care. Additionally, guidelines suggest that pregnant women should be treated with the same antiretroviral combinations and with the same goal of suppression of HIV viral load and maintenance or increase of $CD4^+$

lymphocytes as nonpregnant women. Exceptions to these recommendations include efavirenz, which has shown teratogenic effects in animal studies; the combination of didanosine and stavudine, which has been associated with rare cases of maternal hepatic steatosis and death; and nevirapine, which has resulted in fulminant hepatitis in women with higher CD4$^+$ lymphocyte counts. Therefore, these agents should be used cautiously in pregnancy. All HIV-infected pregnant women should be offered at least zidovudine throughout pregnancy, even if the HIV viral load and CD4$^+$ cell count would not warrant initiation of therapy for their own health care. Currently in the United States, the rate of vertical transmission is <2% in women who are diagnosed and who take antiretroviral therapy before delivery. This rate is <1% when the HIV viral load is suppressed at delivery. This essentially makes perinatal transmission of HIV a preventable disease when women have antenatal counseling and testing and receive antiretroviral therapy for themselves and their infants. HIV testing is not a mandatory component of antenatal care; hence, every obstetric provider and pediatrician should offer testing and counseling to all pregnant women so they may consider therapeutic options for themselves and prophylactic options for their fetuses. Data have shown that instituting zidovudine as a component of antiretroviral therapy antenatally, intrapartum, or even neonatally reduces transmission compared with that seen (~25%) when no antiretroviral therapy is received by the mother or the infant. *Pneumocystis jirovecii* and possibly *Mycobacterium avium* intracellulare prophylaxis also should be considered. Currently, prospective studies on HIV in pregnancy, such as through the International Maternal Pediatric Adolescent AIDS Clinical Trials (IMPAACT) Group, a National Institutes of Health-sponsored multicenter trial, are under way.

3. **HIV infection in children.** Most pediatric AIDS cases occur in infants and young children, reflecting the preponderance of congenital and perinatally acquired infections. Where HIV infection is undiagnosed, 50% of pediatric AIDS cases are reported in the first year of life, and approximately 80% are reported by the age of 3. Of these patients, HIV-related symptoms occur in >80% in the first year of life (median age at onset of symptoms is 9 months). It is estimated that 20% of untreated infants with congenital/perinatal HIV infection will die within the first year of life, and 60% will have severe symptomatic disease by the age of 18 months. These patients are defined as "rapid progressors." These statistics reflect only pediatric AIDS cases reported to the CDC and may reflect only the part of the spectrum of disease that is identified. Statistics are also heavily influenced by the natural disease progression in untreated children. It is possible that many infected children are undiagnosed and remain asymptomatic for years. Children should be prescribed antiretroviral regimens based on the goal of maintaining a CD4$^+$ lymphocyte percentage >15%, and many experts would suggest 25%, along with a moderately low or suppressed HIV viral load. As of this writing, in developed countries, pediatric HIV infection should be considered a treatable chronic infection, not a disease with a limited life span or poor quality of life. The clinical presentation differs in children compared with adults. The HIV-infected newborn is usually asymptomatic but may present with lymphadenopathy and/or HSM. Generally, the infant-infected peripartum does not develop signs or symptoms until after the first 2 weeks of life. These include lymphadenopathy and HSM (as in adults); poor weight gain, as might be found in chronic viral infection; and occasionally neuromotor abnormalities or encephalopathy. Before

antiretroviral therapy was available to children, 50% to 90% of HIV-infected children had CNS involvement characterized by an encephalopathy that was often clinically devastating. Although the clinical presentation may vary, developmental delay or loss of developmental milestones and diminished cognitive function are common features. All too often, an infant is diagnosed with AIDS between the ages of 2 and 6 months when he or she presents with *P. jirovecii* pneumonia. This is an interstitial pneumonia often without auscultatory findings. Patients present with low-grade fever, tachypnea, and often, tachycardia. Progressive hypoxia ensues and may result in mortality as high as 90%. This is the AIDS-defining illness at presentation in 37% of pediatric patients, with a peak incidence at the age of 4 months. Treatment is intravenous trimethoprim-sulfamethoxazole and steroids. Prophylaxis to prevent such life-threatening possibilities is of course preferable to acquisition of disease. It is now recommended by the Public Health Service that all HIV-infected infants be started on *P. jirovecii* pneumonia prophylaxis at the age of 1 month. A second condition, possibly unique to pediatric AIDS, is the development of chronic interstitial lung disease, referred to as *lymphoid interstitial pneumonitis* (LIP). LIP is characterized by a diffuse lymphocytic and plasma cell infiltrate. The clinical course of LIP is quite variable but may be progressive, resulting in marked respiratory distress (tachypnea, retractions, wheezing, and hypoxemia). There is an association with Epstein-Barr virus infection, but the significance of this is uncertain. After the initial presentation, the prognosis appears to be more favorable for children with symptomatic HIV infection when the AIDS-defining illness is LIP. In addition to LIP, recurrent bacterial infections are a frequent feature of pediatric AIDS, owing in part to the early occurrence of B-cell dysfunction with dysfunctional hypergammaglobulinemia. Both focal and disseminated infections are encountered, with sepsis being most common. The organism, usually isolated from the bloodstream, is *Streptococcus pneumoniae*, but a variety of other bacteria have been recovered, especially from hospitalized patients. Pneumococcal disease is less common now that conjugated pneumococcal vaccines are standard of care for infants in the first 6 months of life. Other manifestations of HIV infection that may be more common in children are parotitis and cardiac dysfunction. Older children present with the more typical AIDS-defining opportunistic infections when the $CD4^+$ count wanes.

D. Diagnosis. The diagnosis of HIV infection in adults is made by the detection of specific antibody by an ELISA with confirmation by Western blot analysis. Infants who are culture or DNA PCR or high-level RNA PCR positive in the first 3 days of life are considered to have been infected *in utero*; infants who test negative in the first 3 days and positive for HIV thereafter are considered to have peripartum-acquired HIV. This differentiation is relevant because offering potent antiretroviral therapy at the time of delivery, even in undiagnosed and/or untreated mothers, may be highly effective in reducing vertical transmission. Rapid diagnostic testing for HIV in previously untested women at presentation for delivery with institution of prophylactic therapy has been shown to reduce transmission. On the basis of this kind of information, investigators are targeting the intrapartum interval to offer potent, rapidly active preventive treatments such as antiretroviral therapy (especially using nevirapine). Intrapartum transmission is likely to account for at least 50% of HIV infections in infants. Testing should be offered to anyone engaging in risk behaviors for HIV transmission and for all pregnant women. Serology is of limited value in diagnosing vertically transmitted HIV infection in infants <15 months old, because maternal IgG crosses the placenta and can persist in infants throughout the first year or more of life. In the presence of an AIDS-defining illness and a positive antibody test, the diagnosis is made even if the infant is <15 months of age. However, the picture is less clear in infants with minimal or no symptomatology. Therefore, viral detection tests must be used to identify infected infants born to HIV-seropositive mothers. These include the following:

1. PCR to detect viral DNA in peripheral blood cells.

2. PCR for viral RNA in plasma, or viral load: must be >10,000 copies/mL to be diagnostic.

3. *In vitro* cell culture of mononuclear cells.

    The blood samples for these tests should be collected in anticoagulant but not heparin. Sometimes, the diagnosis is made with a positive p24 antigen detection in peripheral blood or *in situ* hybridization to detect HIV-specific DNA in infected cells. Culture is sensitive and specific but is expensive, is technically difficult, and may require weeks before results are obtained, hence is infrequently done. In contrast, PCR is sensitive and quickly obtained. The mainstay of early viral diagnostic testing of the infant born to an HIV-infected mother remains HIV PCR to detect both viral RNA and DNA. The p24 antigen assay suffers from a lack of sensitivity, particularly in infants, and can be replaced by acid-dissociated p24 antigen detection, which has a much greater sensitivity. The importance of obtaining an early diagnosis is clear: to provide even very young infants the benefit of antiretroviral therapy, which is hoped to reduce viral load and possibly prevent or reduce the viral burden at sites such as the CNS, as well as to maintain normal numbers of $CD4^+$ cells.

E. **Treatment.** The major part of the management of HIV infection is antiretroviral therapy. This should be offered to all symptomatic patients regardless of $CD4^+$ cell count. At present, there is no cure for HIV infection, but the goal of antiretroviral therapy is to suppress the HIV viral load and to maintain or reconstitute $CD4^+$ cell numbers to >25%. Generally, these agents are of four classes:

1. Nucleoside or nucleotide analog reverse transcriptase inhibitors (NRTIs) (e.g., zidovudine/AZT). These agents prevent viral RNA from being reverse-transcribed to DNA; therefore, infection of cells can be aborted.

2. Non-nucleoside analog reverse transcriptase inhibitors (NNRTIs) (e.g., nevirapine). These agents also act to prevent reverse transcription, but at a slightly different site on the enzyme. They are generally more potent than the NRTIs, but resistance can develop rapidly if the viral load is not controlled.

3. Protease inhibitors (PIs) act to prevent processing of viral proteins. These agents are quite potent but are highly protein bound and, therefore, little crosses the placenta, making these excellent agents to treat maternal viral load but limit exposure of the fetus.

4. Integrase inhibitors act to prevent virion production and are increasingly a component of antiretroviral therapy.

    Generally, initial therapy is with two NRTIs and either a PI or an NNRTI. Other possible therapies being investigated include other sites of action in the retroviral life cycle such as fusion inhibitors, viral entry inhibitors, and immune-based therapies.

Optimization of nutrition, routine immunizations, prophylaxis against opportunistic infections (most notably *P. jirovecii*), and the prompt recognition and treatment of HIV-related complications (e.g., opportunistic infections, cardiac dysfunction) are paramount to the improvement in the longevity and the quality of life for HIV-infected patients. In the newborn, special attention should be given to the possibility of congenitally and perinatally transmitted pathogens, such as tuberculosis, toxoplasmosis, and sexually transmitted diseases, which may have a relatively high prevalence in HIV-infected adults.

F. **Prevention.** In this chapter, we will only focus on prevention strategies to reduce **maternal-to-child transmission** both in the United States and globally.

1. **Domestically,** efforts to prevent mother-to-child transmission of HIV have been highly successful in the United States. Combined information from the randomized Pediatric AIDS Clinical Trials Group (PACTG) studies PACTG 076 and PACTG 185 found that HIV-infected pregnant women who received zidovudine antenatally, intrapartum intravenously at 2 mg/kg for the first hour of labor followed by 1 mg/kg/hour until delivery, and to their infants orally at 2 mg/kg every 6 hours for the first 6 weeks of life had a markedly lower transmission compared to placebo recipients (8.3% of the infants in the zidovudine-receiving group were infected vs. 25.5% in the placebo group for 076). Therefore, since February 1994, it has been the standard of care to offer the 076 algorithm as a backbone of antiretroviral regimens for pregnant women. Elective cesarean section (before onset of labor) can further reduce transmission if the HIV viral load remains >1,000 copies/mL. There is no added benefit to elective cesarean if the HIV viral load is suppressed below this value. Several studies have shown that higher maternal viral load, along with lower $CD4^+$ T-cell counts, is a strong correlate of vertical transmission; therefore, it is imperative to treat pregnant women with an optimized antiretroviral regimen to suppress viral load. Resistance testing should also be performed even for women who have never been treated, as it is estimated that as many as 15% of previously untreated persons will have an HIV isolate that has resistance to one or more antiretrovirals. It is advised that care of HIV-infected pregnant women be offered in concert with obstetricians, internists, and pediatricians with experience in taking care of HIV-infected patients for optimal outcome. Current standard of care in the United States is to suppress maternal viral load to nondetectable levels during pregnancy (and after pregnancy to optimize maternal health) using combinations of the approved agents to treat HIV infection. The rate of vertical transmission is <1% for women with a nondetectable viral load.

Frequently, mothers may learn for the first time that they are HIV infected during their pregnancy. The appropriate social, nonjudgmental support network must be effectively in place to achieve the best pregnancy outcome possible. The mother's health, both medical and emotional, should not be subjugated to that of the fetus; rather, optimization of the mother–baby pair is key in effecting the best possible outcome. Any instrumentation, including fetal scalp electrodes and pH sampling, during the intrapartum period that would expose the fetus to maternal blood and secretions should be avoided in HIV-positive women. Postpartum, the mother should be advised to avoid allowing her infant to contact her blood or secretions. At present, prevention of horizontal transmission relies on barrier protection for known HIV-infected persons and on reduction of viral load in genital fluids with antiretroviral therapy.

2. **Globally**, there has also been progress in limiting perinatal HIV infection. A trial in Uganda (HIVNET 012) offered a single dose of nevirapine to HIV-infected women in labor and followed this with a single dose of nevirapine at 3 days of life to the infants. The rate of perinatal transmission was markedly reduced in the nevirapine arm. Nevirapine was found to readily cross the placenta, and with the two-dose regimen for the mother–infant pair, the nevirapine level in the infant's blood is above the level needed to reduce HIV viral load for at least a week. However, by 18 months of age, the infant mortality in the nevirapine-treated group equaled that in the other group, most likely because of HIV transmission from breast milk feeding. Data from Thailand have shown a transmission rate of 2%, using a combination of zidovudine as per 076 and nevirapine as per HIVNET 012, along with exclusive bottle feeding. Birth canal washes with a virostatic agent have been disappointing to date. WHO 2010 guidelines recommend that HIV-seropositive women be offered antenatal and intrapartum maternal antiretroviral treatment or infant prophylaxis. Additional recommendations include that each country should decide whether HIV-seropositive women should exclusively formula feed their infants or breastfeed with concomitant antiretroviral therapy. If the latter, the recommendations are for exclusive breastfeeding for the first 6 months with complementary foods added and rapid weaning at 12 months, if adequate nutrition is available for the baby. Studies have also suggested that in countries where breastfeeding is near universal, the transmission rate may be as much as 14% over the presumed rate seen that is due to *in utero* or intrapartum transmission. In studies of women in endemic areas who were not HIV infected at the time of delivery but who seroconverted postpartum, some infants seroconverted almost simultaneously with their mothers. It may be that infants who do not have maternally derived, passively transferred antibody to HIV or those infants whose mothers acquire primary HIV infection during lactation are at a higher risk of acquisition of HIV exposure through breast milk than are those who are probably exposed to virions and antibody together. Therefore, breastfeeding is contraindicated in countries in which formula preparations are safe and nutritionally replete.

VI. HEPATITIS. Acute viral hepatitis is defined by the following clinical criteria: (i) symptoms consistent with viral hepatitis, (ii) elevation of serum aminotransaminase levels to >2.5 times the upper limit of normal, and (iii) the absence of other causes of liver disease. At least five agents have been identified as causes of viral hepatitis: hepatitis A virus (HAV) has no vertical transmission and will not be discussed; hepatitis B virus (HBV); hepatitis C virus (HCV) (post-transfusion non-A, non-B [NANB] hepatitis virus); hepatitis D virus (HDV); and hepatitis E virus (HEV) (enteric, epidemic NANB hepatitis virus). HDV, also referred to as the *delta agent*, is a defective virus that requires coinfection or superinfection with HBV. HDV is coated with hepatitis B surface antigen (HBsAg). Specific antibodies to HDV can be detected in infected individuals, but there is no known therapy to prevent infection in exposed HBsAg-positive patients. For the newborn, therapy directed at the prevention of HBV infection should also prevent HDV infection because coinfection is required.

A. **HBV (perinatal and congenital).** This DNA virus is one of the most common causes of acute and chronic hepatitis worldwide.

1. **Epidemiology.** In endemic populations, the carrier state is high, and perinatal transmission is a common event. The risk of chronic infection is inversely

proportional to age, with a 90% carriage rate following infection in neonates. The overall incidence of HBV infections in the United States is relatively low. Approximately 300,000 infections occur yearly, with 250 deaths from fulminate disease. The incubation period for HBV infection is approximately 120 days (range 45–160 days). **High-risk groups for HBV infection** in the United States include the following:

a. Persons born in endemic areas. Alaskan natives and Pacific Islanders and natives of China, Southeast Asia, most of Africa, parts of the Middle East, and the Amazon basin; descendants of individuals from endemic areas.

b. Persons with high-risk behavior. Men who have sex with men, intravenous drug use, and multiple sex partners.

c. Close contacts with HBV-infected persons (sex partners, family members).

d. Selected patient populations, particularly those receiving multiple blood or blood product transfusions.

e. Selected occupational groups, including health care providers.

2. **Transmission** occurs by percutaneous or permucosal routes from infected blood or body fluids. The transmission of HBV from infected mothers to their newborns is thought to result primarily from exposure to maternal blood at the time of delivery. Transplacental transfer appears to occur in Taiwan, but this has not been found in other parts of the world, including the United States. In Taiwan, there is a high chronic carrier rate that may be related to the transplacental transfer observed in that country. When acute maternal HBV infection occurs during the first and second trimesters of pregnancy, there is generally little risk to the newborns because antigenemia is usually cleared by term and anti-HBs is present. Acute maternal HBV infection during late pregnancy or near the time of delivery, however, may result in a 50% to 75% transmission rate.

3. **Clinical disease with chronic active hepatitis** is seen in approximately 25% of the 1 million individuals who are chronic carriers. Symptoms include anorexia, malaise, nausea, vomiting, abdominal pain, and jaundice. Patients with chronic active hepatitis are at increased risk for developing cirrhosis and hepatocellular carcinoma, and approximately 5,000 of these patients die each year from HBV-related hepatic complications (primarily cirrhosis).

4. Diagnosis. The diagnosis is made by specific serology and by the detection of viral antigens. The specific tests are as follows:

a. HBsAg determination. Usually found 1 to 2 months after exposure and lasts a variable period of time.

b. Anti-HB surface (anti-HBs) antigen. Appears after resolution of infection or immunization and provides long-term immunity.

c. Anti-HB core (anti-HBc) antigen. Present with all HBV infections and lasts for an indefinite period of time.

d. Anti-HBc IgM. Appears early in infection, is detectable from 4 to 6 months after infection and is a good marker for acute or recent infection.

e. HB early antigen (HBeAg). Present in both acute and chronic infections and correlates with viral replication and high infectivity.

f. Anti-HBe antigen (anti-HBe). Develops with resolution of viral replication and correlates with reduction in infectivity. Infectivity correlates best with HBeAg positivity, but any patient positive for HBsAg is potentially infectious. Acute infection can be diagnosed by the presence of clinical symptoms and a positive HBsAg or anti-HBc IgM. The chronic carrier state is defined as the presence of HBsAg on two occasions, 6 months apart, or the presence of HBsAg without anti-HBc IgM.

5. **Treatment.** Treatments such as lamivudine, tenofovir, or etanercept may be suggested by infectious disease specialists to further reduce the possibility of transmission, especially in women with higher HBV viral loads.

6. **Prevention.** The principal strategy for the prevention of neonatal HBV disease has been to use immunoprophylaxis for **newborns** at high risk for infection. Vaccination of these infants is also an important part of perinatal prevention and safeguards against postnatal exposure as well (Table 48.3). Immunization of infants effectively reduced the risk of chronic HBV infection in Taiwan. Universal immunization of infants promises to be one of the best options for disease control in the United States and is now recommended for all infants born to HBsAg-negative mothers. Three doses before the age of 18 months should be given. High-risk populations, such as Alaskan natives, Pacific Islanders, and infants of immigrant mothers from areas where HBV is endemic, should receive the three-dose series by the age of 6 to 9 months. The recommended schedule is begun during the newborn period; the second dose is given 1 to 2 months later; and the third dose is given at the age of 6 months for infants of mothers with HBsAg positive or unknown status and between 6 and 18 months for infants of mothers with negative HBsAg status. The preterm infant born to an HBsAg-positive mother should be started on the immunization series and given treatment with hepatitis B immune globulin (HBIG) immediately (see Table 48.3). The *Red Book, Report of the Committee on Infectious Diseases, American Academy of Pediatrics* is the best source for dosing based on gestational age and birth weight. Other methods of disease control have been considered; these include delivery by cesarean section. In one study in Taiwan, cesarean delivery in conjunction with maternal immunization dramatically reduced the incidence of perinatally acquired HBV from highly infective mothers. These results are promising and may offer a potential adjunctive therapy for very high-risk situations (e.g., HBsAg/HBe-positive women).

It is recommended that all pregnant women be screened for HBsAg. Screening should be done early in gestation. If the test result is negative, no

Table 48.3	Doses of Hepatitis B Vaccines in Neonates*		
	Active Immunization: Either		
	Recombivax HB (Merck)	Engerix-B (SmithKline Beecham)	Passive Immunization HBIG
Infants of HBsAg-negative mothers	5 μg (0.5 mL)	10 μg (0.5 mL)	—
Infants of HBsAg-positive mothers	5 μg (0.5 mL)	10 μg (0.5 mL)	0.5 mL

HBIG = hepatitis B immunoglobulin; HBsAg = hepatitis B surface antigen.
*Both vaccine regimens use a three-dose schedule.

further evaluation is recommended unless there is a potential exposure history. When there is any concern about a possible infectious contact, development of acute hepatitis, or high-risk behavior in a nonimmunized woman, testing should be repeated. All infants born to mothers confirmed to be positive for HBsAg should receive HBIG in addition to recombinant hepatitis B vaccine. The first immunization and HBIG are given within the first 12 hours of life, and the vaccine is repeated at the ages of 1 and 6 months. If the mother has emigrated from an endemic area, HBIG also should be given unless the mother is found to be HBsAg-negative. Postnatal transmission of HBV by the fecal–oral route probably occurs, but the risk appears to be small. Nevertheless, this possibility adds further support to the need for the immunization of infants born to HBsAg-positive women. Another potential route of infection is by means of breast milk. This mode of transmission appears to be very uncommon in developed countries; there has been no documented increase in the risk of HBV transmission by breastfeeding mothers who are HBsAg positive. This is true, although HBsAg can be detected in breast milk. Recommendations regarding breastfeeding in developed countries should be individualized, depending on how strongly breastfeeding is desired by the mother. The risk is certain to be negligible in infants who have received HBIG and hepatitis vaccine. **Prevention of nosocomial spread** from HBsAg-positive infants in the nursery is minimized if nursery personnel wear gloves and gowns when caring for infected infants. Of course, with current precautions, the risk of exposure to blood and body secretions already should be minimized. Immunization of health care workers is also strongly recommended, but if exposure should occur in a nonimmunized person, blood samples should be sent for hepatitis serology and HBIG administered as soon as possible unless the individual is known to be anti-HBs positive. This should apply to personnel having close contact without appropriate precautions, as well as those exposed parenterally (e.g., from a contaminated needle).

B. **HCV (perinatal and congenital).** Hepatitis C is the agent responsible for most NANB hepatitis in transfusion or organ transplant recipients and is a single-strand RNA virus related to the flavivirus family.

   1. **Epidemiology.** At least five HCV subtypes have been characterized based on sequence heterogeneity of the viral genome. HCV is found worldwide, and different subtypes have been identified from the same area. Subtype 1 is the most common in the United States and has a poorer prognosis than other subtypes.

      a. **Horizontal transmission.** Injection drug use is now the most common risk behavior for infection. In addition to injection drug users and transfusion recipients, dialysis patients and sexual partners of HCV-infected persons may also be infected, but 50% of identified persons are unable to define a risk factor.

      b. **Vertical transmission.** Overall rate of transmission is approximately 5% from known hepatitis C–infected women to their infants. The transmission rate may well be much higher and may approach 70% when the pregnant mother has a high viral load as assessed by semiquantitative PCR. HCV is transmitted at a higher frequency if the mother is also HIV infected, but this has not been assessed in women with a controlled HIV viral load and lower semiquantitative HCV viral load. The mode of transmission is also unknown. Detection of HCV by RNA PCR in cord blood would suggest that at least in some cases *in utero* transmission occurs. There is also a case report of one infant having been infected with an HCV strain different from all maternal strains at the time of delivery, suggesting *in utero* transmission. Conversely, PCR-negative infants at birth may develop PCR positivity later in infancy, suggesting perinatal infection. One study found 50% of vaginal samples collected at 30 weeks' gestation from HCV-positive mothers to contain HCV, suggesting the possibility of infection by passage through the birth canal. The potential risk of breastfeeding is not well defined. HCV has been detected in breast milk by PCR, but vertical transmission rates in breastfed and bottle-fed infants are similar. The CDC currently states that maternal HCV infection is not a contraindication to breastfeeding. The decision to breastfeed should be discussed with the mother on an individual basis.

2. **Clinical manifestations.** HCV accounts for 20% to 40% of viral hepatitis in the United States. The incubation period is 40 to 90 days after exposure, and manifestations often present insidiously. Serum transaminase levels may fluctuate or remain chronically elevated for as long as 1 year. Chronic disease may result in as many as 60% of community-acquired HCV infections. Cirrhosis may result in as many as 20% of chronic disease cases, but may be less likely in pediatric patients.

3. **Diagnosis.** ELISA detects antibodies to three proteins (c100–3, c22–3, and c33c) that are components of HCV. This test may be able to detect infection as early as 2 weeks after exposure. Another serologic assay with even greater sensitivity is the radioimmunoblot assay, which detects antibodies to the three antigens detected by the ELISA and a fourth antigen, 5–5–1. Infants born to HCV-infected mothers will show evidence of passively acquired maternal antibody; therefore, to determine infection in the infant, RNA PCR, which detects the viral genome itself, must be performed. This assay can detect viremia within 1 week of infection in adults. In adults, approximately 70% of samples with detectable antibody will also be positive by PCR. This is a curious finding in that a serologic response does not provide adequate protection. Persons who have had an acute infection that resolves will become antibody negative. Infants born to known seropositive women should be tested for HCV antibody and HCV RNA by PCR at the age of 1, and possibly by RNA PCR earlier, to determine which infants to follow more closely. If both are negative, the infant is likely uninfected; if the PCR is negative, but the antibody is positive, the infant should be retested at 18 months.

4. **Treatment.** Clinical trials suggest that symptomatic persons with chronic HCV infection may benefit from treatment with α-interferon and ribavirin, as well as newer agents, given for as long as a year. Side effects of this therapy include fever and myalgias, and the risk–benefit ratio must be carefully weighed; and none of these agents have been approved in pregnancy.

5. **Prevention.** Blood products are screened for antibody to HCV. Presence of the antibody likely also indicates presence of virus, and the unit is discarded if antibody positive. **There is *no* benefit to immune globulin given to the exposed infant or to the needlestick recipient, as products containing antibody are excluded from the lot.**

C. **HEV.** Enterically transmitted NANB viral hepatitis (HEV) is a single-stranded RNA virus that is similar to a calcivirus. It is primarily spread by fecal-contaminated water supplies. Epidemics have been documented in parts of Asia, Africa, and Mexico, and shellfish have been implicated as sources of infection. Incubation is 15 to 60 days.

The clinical picture in infected individuals is similar to that of HAV infection, with fever, malaise, jaundice, abdominal pain, and arthralgia. HEV infection has an unusually high incidence of mortality in pregnant women. Treatment is supportive. The efficacy of immunoglobulin prophylaxis against this form of hepatitis is unknown, but because the infection is not endemic in the United States, commercial preparations in the United States would not be expected to be helpful.

D. **Hepatitis G virus (HGV).** HGV is a single-stranded RNA virus in the Flaviviridae family that shares 27% homology with HCV. HGV can be found worldwide and is found in approximately 1.5% of blood donors in the United States. Coinfection with HBV or HCV may be as much as 20%, suggesting common routes of transmission, such as transfusion or organ transplantation. Transplacental transmission is probably rare and may be associated with higher maternal viral loads. HGV is diagnosed by RNA PCR in research settings, and there is no current treatment or prophylactic therapy.

VII. VARICELLA-ZOSTER VIRUS (V-ZV: CONGENITAL OR PERINATAL). The
causative agent of varicella (chickenpox) is a DNA virus member of the herpesvirus family. The same agent is responsible for herpes zoster (shingles); hence, this virus is referred to as V-ZV. Chickenpox results from primary V-ZV infection, following which the virus may remain latent in sensory nerve ganglia. Zoster results from reactivation of latent virus later in life or if the host becomes immunosuppressed.

A. **Epidemiology.** Before the use of varicella vaccine, there were approximately 3 million cases of varicella yearly in the United States, most occurring in school-age children. Most adults have antibodies to V-ZV, indicating prior infection, even when there is thought to be no history of chickenpox. It follows that varicella is an uncommon occurrence in pregnancy. The precise incidence of gestational varicella is uncertain, but is certainly less than it was before the widespread use of varicella vaccine. There are recommendations to immunize nonimmune adults unless they are pregnant. Alternatively, zoster is primarily a disease of adults. The incidence of zoster in pregnancy is also unknown, but the disease is likely to be uncommon as well. The overall risk of the congenital varicella syndrome following maternal infection is 0.4% in the first 12 weeks of pregnancy, and 2% from 13 to 20 weeks' gestation. It is primarily seen with gestational varicella but may rarely occur with maternal zoster. The primary mode of transmission of V-ZV is through respiratory droplets from patients with chickenpox. Spread through contact with vesicular lesions also can occur. Typically, individuals with chickenpox are contagious from 1 to 2 days before and 5 days after the onset of rash. Conventionally, a patient is no longer considered contagious when all vesicular lesions have dried and crusted over. The incubation period for primary disease extends from 10 to 21 days, with most infections occurring between 13 and 17 days. Transplacental transfer of V-ZV may take place, presumably secondary to maternal viremia, but its frequency is unknown. Varicella occurs in approximately 25% of newborns whose mothers developed varicella within the peripartum period. The onset of disease usually occurs 13 to 15 days after the onset of maternal rash. When the rash develops in the newborn within 10 days, it is presumed to result from *in utero* transmission. The greatest risk for severe disease is seen when maternal varicella occurs 5 days before or 2 days after delivery. In these cases, there is insufficient time for the fetus to acquire transplacentally derived V-ZV–specific antibodies. Symptoms generally begin 5 to 10 days after delivery, and the expected mortality is approximately 30%. When *in utero* transmission of V-ZV occurs before the peripartum period, there is no obvious clinical impact in most fetuses; however, congenital varicella syndrome can occur.

B. Clinical manifestations

1. **Congenital varicella syndrome.** There is a strong association between gestational varicella and a spectrum of congenital defects comprising a unique syndrome. Characteristic findings include cicatricial skin lesions, ocular defects, CNS abnormalities, IUGR, and early death. The syndrome most commonly occurs with maternal V-ZV infection in weeks 7 to 20 of gestation.

2. **Zoster.** Zoster is uncommon in young infants but may occur as a consequence of *in utero* fetal infection with V-ZV. Similarly, children who develop zoster but have no history of varicella most likely acquired V-ZV *in utero*. Zoster in childhood is usually self-limiting, with only symptomatic therapy indicated in otherwise healthy children.

3. **Postnatal varicella.** Varicella acquired in the newborn period as a result of postnatal exposure is generally a mild disease. Rarely, severe disseminated disease occurs in newborns exposed shortly after birth. In these instances, treatment with acyclovir may be beneficial. Varicella has been detected in breast milk by PCR; therefore, it may be prudent to defer breastfeeding at least during the period of time in which the mother is likely to be viremic and/or infectious.

C. Diagnosis. Infants with congenital varicella resulting from *in utero* infection occurring before the peripartum period do not shed virus, and the determination of V-ZV–specific antibodies is often confusing. Therefore, the diagnosis is made on the basis of clinical findings and maternal history. With neonatal disease, the presence of a typical vesicular rash and a maternal history of peripartum varicella or postpartum exposure are all that is required to make the diagnosis. Laboratory confirmation can be made by (i) culture of vesicular fluid, although the sensitivity of this method is not optimal because the virus is quite labile; (ii) demonstration of a fourfold rise in V-ZV antibody titer by the fluorescent antibody to membrane antigen (FAMA) assay or by ELISA. Antigen can also be detected from cells at the base of a vesicle by immunofluorescent antibody detection. The latter is sensitive, specific, and rapid and should be the preferred method of diagnosis when vesicles are present.

D. Treatment. Infants with congenital infection, resulting from *in utero* transmission before the peripartum period, are unlikely to have active viral disease, so antiviral therapy is not indicated. However, infants with perinatal varicella acquired from maternal infection near the time of delivery are at risk for severe disease. In this setting, therapy with acyclovir is generally recommended. Data are not available on the most efficacious and safe dose of acyclovir for the treatment of neonatal varicella, but minimal toxicity has been shown with the administration of 60 mg/kg/day divided every 8 hours for 14 to 21 days for the treatment of neonatal HSV infection. At present, there is no U.S. Food and Drug Administration (FDA)-approved immunotherapy for the treatment of V-ZV infections or postexposure prophylaxis. However, VariZIG, a hyperimmune gammaglobulin product, currently is available under an expanded use Investigational New Drug (IND) protocol for postexposure prophylaxis. It can be obtained by calling the 24-hour telephone number at FFF Enterprises (800-843-7477). It must be administered within 96 hours of exposure. The dose is 125 units intramuscularly. Alternatively, if VariZIG is unavailable, IVIG at a dose of 400 mg/kg may be given as postexposure prophylaxis.

E. **Prevention**

1. **Vaccination** of women who are not immune to varicella should decrease the incidence of congenital and perinatal varicella. Women should not receive the vaccine if they are pregnant or in the 3 months before pregnancy. If this inadvertently occurs, the women should be enrolled in the National Registry. Additionally, acyclovir should also be considered for seronegative women exposed to varicella during pregnancy beginning 7 to 9 days postexposure and continuing 7 days. Women who acquire primary varicella during pregnancy should be treated with acyclovir for their own health, as well as to prevent fetal infection.

2. **Management of varicella in the nursery.** The risk of horizontal spread of varicella following exposure in the nursery appears to be low, possibly because of a combination of factors, including (i) passive protection resulting from transplacentally derived antibody in infants born to varicella-immune mothers and (ii) brief exposure with a lack of intimate contact. Nevertheless, nursery outbreaks do occur, so steps should be taken to minimize the risk of nosocomial spread. The infected infant should be isolated in a separate room, and visitors and caregivers should be limited to individuals with a history of varicella. A new gown should be worn on entering the room, and good hand-washing technique should be used. Bedding and other materials should be bagged and sterilized. VariZIG can be given to all other exposed neonates, but this can be withheld from full-term infants whose mothers have a history of varicella. Neonates at <28 weeks' gestation should be given VariZIG or IVIG postexposure regardless of maternal status. Exposed personnel without a history of varicella should be tested for V-ZV antibodies, and patient care by these individuals should be restricted as outlined subsequently. In the regular nursery, all exposed infants will ordinarily be discharged home before they could become infectious. Occasionally, an exposed infant needs to remain in the nursery for >8 days, and in this circumstance, isolation may be required. In the neonatal intensive care unit, exposed neonates are generally cohorted and isolated from new admissions within 8 days of exposure. If there is antepartum exposure within 21 days of hospital admission for a mother without a history of varicella, the mother and infant should be discharged as soon as possible from the hospital. If the exposure occurred 6 days or less before admission and the mother is discharged within 48 hours, no further action is required. Otherwise, mothers hospitalized between 8 and 21 days after exposure should be kept isolated from the nursery and other patients. Personnel without a history of varicella should be kept from contact with a potentially infectious mother. If such an individual is inadvertently exposed, serologic testing (FAMA or ELISA) should be performed to determine susceptibility, and further contact should be avoided until immunity is proved. If the mother who is at risk for infection has not developed varicella 48 hours after the staff member was exposed, no further action is required. Alternatively, if a susceptible staff member is exposed to any individual with active varicella lesions or in whom a varicella rash erupts within 48 hours of the exposure, contact with any patients should be restricted for that staff member from day 8 through day 21 after exposure. Personnel without a history of varicella should have serologic testing, and if not immune, they should be vaccinated. For mothers in whom varicella has occurred in the 21 days before

delivery, if there were resolution of the infectious stage before hospitalization, maternal isolation is not required. The newborn should be isolated from other infants (room in with mother). If the mother has active varicella lesions on admission to the hospital, isolate the mother and administer VariZIG to the newborn if maternal disease began <5 days before delivery or within 2 days postpartum (not 100% effective, and may consider acyclovir in addition). The infant should be isolated from the mother until she is no longer infectious. If other neonates were exposed, VariZIG may be administered; these infants may require isolation if they are still hospitalized by day 8 after exposure.

VIII. ENTEROVIRUSES (CONGENITAL). The enteroviruses are RNA viruses belonging to the Picornaviridae family. They are classified into four major groups: coxsackieviruses group A, coxsackieviruses group B, echoviruses, and polioviruses. All four groups cause disease in the neonate. Infections occur throughout the year, with a peak incidence between July and November. The viruses are shed from the upper respiratory and gastrointestinal tracts. In most children and adults, infections are asymptomatic or produce a nonspecific febrile illness.

A. **Epidemiology.** Most infections in newborns are caused by coxsackieviruses B and echoviruses. The mode of transmission appears to be primarily transplacental, although this is less well understood for echoviruses. Clinical manifestations are most commonly seen with transmission in the perinatal period.

B. **Clinical manifestations.** Symptoms in the newborn often appear within the first week postpartum. Clinical presentations vary from a mild nonspecific febrile illness to severe life-threatening disease. There are three major clinical presentations in neonates with enterovirus infections. Approximately 50% have meningoencephalitis, 25% have myocarditis, and 25% have a sepsis-like illness. The mortality (approximately 10%) is lowest for the group with meningoencephalitis. With myocarditis, there is a mortality of approximately 50%. The mortality from the sepsis-like illness is essentially 100%. Most (70%) of severe enteroviral infections in neonates are caused by echovirus 11.

C. **Diagnosis.** The primary task in symptomatic enterovirus infections is differentiating between viral and bacterial sepsis and meningitis. In almost all cases, presumptive therapy for possible bacterial disease must be initiated. Obtaining a careful history of a recent maternal viral illness, as well as that of other family members, particularly young siblings, and especially during the summer and fall months, may be helpful. The principal diagnostic laboratory aid generally available at this time is viral culture or PCR. Material for cultures should be obtained from the nose, throat, stool, blood, urine, and CSF and from blood, urine, stool, or CSF for PCR. Usually, evidence of viral growth can be detected within 1 week, although a longer time is required in some cases.

D. **Treatment.** In general, treatment of symptomatic enteroviral disease in the newborn is supportive only. There are no approved specific antiviral agents known to be effective against enteroviruses. However, protection against severe neonatal disease appears to correlate with the presence of specific transplacentally derived antibody. Furthermore, the administration of immune serum globulin appears to be beneficial in patients with agammaglobulinemia who have chronic enteroviral infection. Given these observations, it has been recommended that high-dose immune serum globulin be given to infants with severe, life-threatening enterovirus infections. It may also be beneficial to delay the time of delivery if acute maternal enteroviral infection is suspected, provided there are no maternal or fetal contraindications. This is done to allow transplacental passage of maternal antibody. The clinical presentation in infants with a sepsis-like syndrome frequently evolves into shock, fulminant hepatitis with hepatocellular necrosis, and DIC. In the initial stages of treatment, broad-spectrum antibiotic therapy is indicated for possible bacterial sepsis. Later, with the recognition of progressive viral disease, some form of antibiotic prophylaxis to suppress intestinal flora may be helpful. Neomycin (25 mg/kg every 6 hours) has been recommended. Drugs designed to prevent attachment of enterovirus to the host cell (e.g., pleconaril) are under study for neonatal enteroviral sepsis, but not clinically available.

IX. RUBELLA (CONGENITAL). This human-specific RNA virus is a member of the togavirus family. It causes a mild self-limiting infection in susceptible children and adults, but its effects on the fetus can be devastating.

A. **Epidemiology.** Before widespread immunization beginning in 1969, rubella was a common childhood illness: 85% of the population was immune by late adolescence and approximately 100% by ages 35 to 40 years. Epidemics occurred every 6 to 9 years, with pandemics arising with a greater and more variable cycle. During pandemics, susceptible women were at significant risk for exposure to rubella, resulting in a high number of fetal infections. A worldwide epidemic from 1963 to 1965 accounted for an estimated 11,000 fetal deaths and 20,000 cases of congenital rubella syndrome (CRS). Childhood immunization has dramatically reduced the number of cases of rubella in the United States. In fact, some states have omitted rubella serologic screening from standard antenatal diagnostic recommendations because the very few cases of CRS in recent years have been reported from unimmunized immigrants. The relative risk of fetal transmission and the development of CRS as a function of gestational age have been studied. With maternal infection in the first 12 weeks of gestation, the rate of fetal infection was 81%. The rate dropped to 54% for weeks 13 to 16, 36% for weeks 17 to 22, and 30% for weeks 23 to 30. During the last 10 weeks of gestation, the rate of fetal infection again rose 60% for weeks 31 to 36 and 100% for weeks 36 and beyond. Fetal infection can occur at any time during pregnancy, but early-gestation infection may result in multiple organ anomalies. When maternofetal transmission occurred during the first 10 weeks of gestation, 100% of the infected fetuses had cardiac defects and deafness. Deafness was found in one-third of fetuses infected at 13 to 16 weeks, but no abnormalities were found when fetal infection occurred beyond the 20th week of gestation. There are also case reports of vertical transmission with maternal reinfection.

B. **Clinical manifestations.** Classically, CRS is characterized by the constellation of cataracts, SNHL, and congenital heart disease. The most common cardiac defects are patent ductus arteriosus and pulmonary artery stenosis. Common early features of CRS are IUGR, retinopathy, microphthalmia, meningoencephalitis, electroencephalographic abnormalities, hypotonia, dermatoglyphic abnormalities, HSM, thrombocytopenic purpura, radiographic bone lucencies, and diabetes mellitus. The onset of some of the abnormalities of CRS may be delayed months to years. Many additional rare complications have been described, including myocarditis, glaucoma, microcephaly, chronic progressive panencephalitis, hepatitis, anemia, hypogammaglobulinemia, thymic hypoplasia, thyroid abnormalities, cryptorchidism, and polycystic kidney disease. A 20-year follow-up study of 125 patients with congenital rubella from the 1960s epidemic found ocular disease to be the most common disorder (78%), followed by sensorineural hearing deficits (66%), psychomotor retardation (62%), cardiac abnormalities (58%), and mental retardation (42%).

C. **Diagnosis**

1. **Maternal infection.** The diagnosis of acute rubella in pregnancy requires serologic testing. This is necessary because the clinical symptoms of rubella are nonspecific and can be seen with infection by other viral agents (e.g., enteroviruses, measles, and human parvovirus). Furthermore, a large number of individuals may have subclinical infection. Several sensitive and specific assays exist for the detection of rubella-specific antibody. Viral isolation from the nose, throat, and/or urine is possible, but this is costly and not practical in most instances. **Symptoms** typically begin 2 to 3 weeks after exposure and include malaise, low-grade fever, headache, mild coryza, and conjunctivitis occurring 1 to 5 days before the onset of rash. The rash is a salmon-pink macular or maculopapular exanthem that begins on the face and behind the ears and spreads downward over 1 to 2 days. The rash disappears in 5 to 7 days from onset, and posterior cervical lymphadenopathy is common. Approximately one-third of women may have arthralgias without arthritis. In women suspected of having acute rubella infection, confirmation can be made by demonstrating a fourfold or higher rise in serum IgG titers when measured at the time of symptoms and approximately 2 weeks later. The results of some assays may not directly correlate with a fourfold rise in titer, so other criteria for a significant increase in antibody may be required. When there is uncertainty about the interpretation of assay results, advice should be obtained from the laboratory running the test and an infectious diseases consultation.

2. **Recognized or suspected maternal exposure.** Any individual known to have been immunized with rubella vaccine after his or her first birthday is generally considered immune. However, it is best to determine immunity by measuring rubella-specific IgG, which has become a standard of practice in obstetric care. If a woman exposed to rubella is known to be seropositive, she is immune, and the fetus is considered not to be at risk for infection. Reinfections in previously immune women have been rarely documented, but the risk of fetal damage appears to be very small. If the exposed woman is known to be seronegative, a serum sample should be obtained 3 to 4 weeks after exposure for determination of titer. A negative titer indicates that no infection has occurred, whereas a positive titer indicates infection. Women with an uncertain immune status and a known exposure to rubella should have serum samples obtained as soon as possible after exposure. If this is done within 7 to 10 days of exposure, and the titer is positive, the patient is rubella immune and no further testing is required. If the first titer is negative or was determined on serum taken more than 7 to 10 days after exposure, repeat testing (~3 weeks later) and careful clinical follow-up are necessary. When both the immune status and the time of exposure are uncertain, serum samples for titer determination should be obtained 3 weeks apart. If both titers are negative, no infection has occurred. Alternatively, infection is confirmed if seroconversion or a fourfold increase in titer is observed. Further testing and close clinical follow-up are required if titer results are inconclusive. In this situation, specific IgM determination may be helpful. It should be emphasized that all serum samples should be tested simultaneously by the same laboratory when one is determining changes in titers with time. This can be accomplished by saving a portion of each serum

sample before sending it for titer determination. The saved portion can be frozen until convalescent serum samples have been obtained.

3. **Congenital rubella infection**

   a. Antenatal diagnosis. The risk of severe fetal anomalies is highest with acute maternal rubella infection during the first 16 weeks of gestation. However, not all early-gestation infections result in adverse pregnancy outcomes. Approximately 20% of fetuses may not be infected when maternal rubella occurs in the first 12 weeks of gestation, and as many as 45% of fetuses may not be infected when maternal rubella occurs closer to 16 weeks of gestation. Unfortunately, there is no foolproof method of determining infected from uninfected fetuses early in pregnancy, but *in utero* diagnosis is being investigated. One method that has been used with some success is the determination of specific IgM in fetal blood obtained by PUBS. Direct detection of rubella antigen and RNA in a chorionic villus biopsy specimen also has been used successfully. Although these techniques offer promise, their use may be limited by sensitivity and specificity or the lack of widespread availability.

   b. Postnatal diagnosis. Guidelines for the establishment of congenital rubella infection or CRS in neonates have been summarized by the CDC. The diagnosis of congenital infection is made by one of the following:

   i. Isolation of rubella virus (oropharynx, urine). Notify the laboratory in advance as special culture medium needs to be prepared.

   ii. Detection of rubella-specific IgM in cord or neonatal blood.

   iii. Persistent rubella-specific titers over time (i.e., no decline in titer as expected for transplacentally derived maternal IgG). If, in addition, there are congenital defects, the diagnosis of CRS is made.

D. **Treatment.** There is no specific therapy for either maternal or congenital rubella infection. Maternal disease is almost always mild and self-limiting. If primary maternal infection occurs during the first 5 months of pregnancy, termination options should be discussed with the mother. More than one-half of newborns with congenital rubella may be asymptomatic at birth. If infection is known to have occurred beyond the 20th week of gestation, it is unlikely that any abnormalities will develop, and parents should be reassured. Nevertheless, hearing evaluations should be repeated during childhood. Closer follow-up is required if early-gestation infection is suspected or the timing of infection is unknown. This is true for asymptomatic infants as well as those with obvious CRS. The principal reason for close follow-up is to identify delayed-onset abnormalities or progressive disorders. In some cases, early interventions, such as therapy for glaucoma, may be critical. Unfortunately, there is no specific therapy to halt the progression of most of the complications of CRS.

E. **Prevention.** The primary means of prevention of CRS is by immunization of all susceptible persons. Immunization is recommended for all nonimmune individuals 12 months or older. Documentation of maternal immunity is an important aspect of good obstetric management. When a susceptible woman is identified, she should be reassured of the low risk of contracting rubella, but she should also be counseled to avoid contact with anyone known to have acute or recent rubella infection. Individuals with postnatal infection typically shed virus for 1 week before and 1 week after the onset of rash. On the other hand, infants with congenital infection may shed virus for many months, and contact should be avoided during the first year. Unfortunately, once exposure has occurred, little can be done to alter the chances of maternal and subsequently fetal disease. Although hyperimmune globulin has not been shown to diminish the risk of maternal rubella following exposure or the rate of fetal transmission, it should be given in large doses to any woman who is exposed to rubella and who does not wish to terminate her pregnancy. The lack of proven efficacy must be emphasized in these cases. Susceptible women who do not become infected should be immunized soon after pregnancy. There have been reports of acute arthritis occurring in women immunized in the immediate postpartum period, and a small percentage of these women developed chronic joint or neurologic abnormalities or viremia. Vaccine-strain virus may also be shed in breast milk and transmitted to breastfed infants, some of whom may develop chronic viremia. Therefore, it is best to avoid breastfeeding in women receiving rubella vaccine. Conception also should be avoided for 3 months following immunization. Immunization during pregnancy is not recommended because of the theoretical risk to the fetus. Inadvertent immunizations during pregnancy have occurred, and fetal infection has been documented in a small percentage of these pregnancies. However, no cases of CRS have been identified. In fact, the rubella registry at the CDC has been closed, with the following conclusions: The number of inadvertent immunizations during pregnancy is too small to be able to state with certainty that no adverse pregnancy outcomes will occur, but these would appear to be very uncommon. Therefore, it is still recommended that immunization not be carried out during pregnancy, but when this has occurred, reassurance of little risk to the fetus can be given.

X. RSV (NEONATAL). RSV is an enveloped RNA paramyxovirus that is the leading cause of bronchiolitis and can cause severe or even fatal lower respiratory tract disease, especially in preterm infants. Conditions that increase the risk of severe disease include cyanotic or complicated congenital heart disease, pulmonary hypertension, chronic lung disease, and immune-compromised states.

A. **Epidemiology.** Humans are the only source of infection, spread by respiratory secretions as droplets or fomites, which can survive on environmental surfaces for hours. Spread by hospital workers to infants occurs, especially in the winter and early spring months in temperate climates. Viral shedding is from 3 to 8 days, but in very young infants, it may last for weeks. The incubation period is from 2 to 8 days.

B. **Diagnosis.** Rapid diagnosis is made by immunofluorescent antigen testing of respiratory secretions. This test can have up to 95% sensitivity and is quite specific. Viral culture usually requires 3 to 5 days.

C. **Treatment.** Treatment is largely supportive, with hydration, supplemental oxygen, and mechanical ventilation as needed. Controversy exists as to whether nebulized bronchodilator therapy is beneficial. Ribavirin has been marketed for treatment of infants with RSV infection because it does have *in vitro* activity; however, efficacy has never been repeatedly proven in randomized trials. This makes the risk of ribavirin (aerosol route, potentially toxic side effects to health care personnel, and high cost) important to consider on a case-by-case basis. The use of palivizumab may be considered along with your infectious disease consultant for the most severely affected infants.

D. **Prevention.** Palivizumab (Synagis), a humanized mouse monoclonal antibody given intramuscularly, has been approved by the FDA for prevention of RSV disease in children younger than 2 years of age with chronic lung disease or who were <35 weeks' gestation. Palivizumab is easy to administer, has a low volume, and is given (15 mg/kg intramuscularly) just before and monthly throughout the RSV season (typically mid-November to March or April). Because the drug supply is limited, its protection incomplete, and is costly, the American Academy of Pediatrics has made the following recommendations regarding which high-risk infants should receive palivizumab:

1. **Infants who have required therapy for chronic lung disease** within 6 months of the RSV season.

2. **Infants who are born at <32 weeks' gestation** without chronic lung disease up to 12 months of age if born at 28 weeks' gestation or less; up to 6 months of age if born at 29 to 32 weeks' gestation.

3. **Children** who are 24 months of age or younger with hemodynamically significant cyanotic or acyanotic congenital heart disease.

4. **Preterm infants 32 to 35 weeks** <6 months of age who have two or more of the following risk factors: attending day care, with school-aged siblings in household, exposure to environmental pollutants, congenital abnormalities of the airways, or severe neuromuscular disease.

   If an RSV outbreak is documented in a high-risk unit (e.g., pediatric intensive care unit), primary emphasis should be placed on proper infection-control practices. The need for and efficacy of antibody prophylaxis in these situations has not been documented. Each unit should evaluate the risk to its exposed infants and decide on the need for treatment. If the patient stays hospitalized, this may only require one dose. Palivizumab does not interfere with the routine immunization schedule.

E. **Antibody preparations are not recommended for the following:**

1. Healthy preterm babies greater than 32 weeks' gestation without other risk factors.

2. Patients with hemodynamically insignificant heart disease.

3. Infants with lesions adequately corrected by surgery, unless they continue to require medication for congestive heart failure.

Suggested Readings

American Academy of Pediatrics, Committee on Infectious Diseases. *2009 Red Book: Report of the Committee on Infectious Diseases.* 28th ed. Elk Grove Village, IL: American Academy of Pediatrics; 2009.

James SH, Kimberlin DW, Whitley R. Antiviral therapy for herpesvirus central nervous system infections: neonatal herpes simplex infection, herpes simplex encephalitis, and congenital cytomegalovirus infection. *Antiviral Res* 2009;83:207–213.

Kimberlin DW, Lin CY, Jacobs RF, et al. Natural history of neonatal herpes simplex virus infections in the acyclovir era. *Pediatrics* 2001;108:223–229.

Mofenson LM. Antiretroviral drugs to prevent breastfeeding HIV transmission. *Antiviral Ther.* 2010;15:537–553.

Panel on Antiretroviral Therapy and Medical Management of HIV-Infected Children. Guidelines for the use of antiretroviral agents in pediatric HIV infection. August 16, 2010; pp. 1–219. Available at: http://aidsinfo.nih.gov/ContentFiles/PediatricGuidelines.pdf.

Panel on Treatment of HIV-Infected Pregnant Women and Prevention of Perinatal Transmission. Recommendations for use of antiretroviral drugs in pregnant HIV-1 infected women for maternal health and interventions to reduce perinatal HIV transmission in the United States. May 24, 2010, pp. 1–117. Available at: http://aidsinfo.nih.gov/ContentFiles/Perinatal LG.pdf.

UNAIDS Global Report on the AIDS Epidemic, 2010. Available at unaids.org/globalreport/global.

49 Bacterial and Fungal Infections

Karen M. Puopolo

I. BACTERIAL SEPSIS AND MENINGITIS

A. **Introduction.** Bacterial sepsis and meningitis continue to be major causes of morbidity and mortality in newborns, particularly in premature infants. Although improvements in neonatal intensive care have decreased the impact of early-onset sepsis (EOS) in term infants, preterm infants remain at high risk for both EOS and its sequelae. Very low birth weight (VLBW) infants are also at risk for late-onset (hospital-acquired) sepsis. Neonatal survivors of sepsis can have severe neurologic sequelae due to central nervous system (CNS) infection, as well as from secondary hypoxemia resulting from septic shock, persistent pulmonary hypertension, and severe parenchymal lung disease.

B. **Epidemiology of EOS.** The overall incidence of EOS has decreased significantly since the Centers for Disease Control and Prevention (CDC) first published recommendations for intrapartum antibiotic prophylaxis (IAP) against group B *Streptococcus* (GBS) in 1996. Studies conducted afterwards showed the overall incidence of EOS to be approximately 1 to 2 cases per 1,000 live births. The incidence is twice as high among moderately premature infants, and highest among VLBW (<1,500 g) infants with recent reports ranging from 15 to 23 cases per 1,000 VLBW births.

C. **Risk factors for EOS.** Maternal and infant characteristics associated with the development of EOS have been most rigorously studied with respect to GBS EOS. Maternal factors predictive of GBS disease include documented maternal GBS colonization, intrapartum fever (>38°C) and other signs of chorioamnionitis, and prolonged rupture of membranes (ROM) (>18 hours). Neonatal risk factors include prematurity (<37 weeks' gestation) and low birth weight (LBW) (<2,500 g).

D. **Clinical presentation of EOS.** Early-onset disease can manifest as asymptomatic bacteremia, generalized sepsis, pneumonia, and/or meningitis. The clinical signs of EOS are usually apparent in the first hours of life; 90% of infants are symptomatic by 24 hours of age. Respiratory distress is the most common presenting symptom. Respiratory symptoms can range in severity from mild tachypnea and grunting, with or without a supplemental oxygen requirement, to respiratory failure. Persistent pulmonary hypertension of the newborn (PPHN) can also accompany sepsis. Other less specific signs of sepsis include irritability, lethargy, temperature instability, poor perfusion, and hypotension. Disseminated intravascular coagulation (DIC) with purpura and petechiae can occur in more severe septic shock. Gastrointestinal (GI) symptoms can include poor feeding, vomiting, and ileus. Meningitis may present with seizure activity, apnea, and depressed sensorium, but may complicate sepsis without specific neurologic symptoms, underscoring the importance of the lumbar puncture (LP) in the evaluation of sepsis.

Other diagnoses to be considered in the immediate newborn period in the infant with signs of sepsis include transient tachypnea of the newborn, meconium aspiration syndrome, intracranial hemorrhage, congenital viral disease, and congenital cyanotic heart disease. In infants presenting at more than 24 hours of age, closure of the ductus arteriosus in the setting of a ductal-dependent cardiac anomaly (such as critical coarctation of the aorta or hypoplastic left heart syndrome) can mimic sepsis. Other diagnoses that should be considered in the infant presenting beyond the first few hours of life with a sepsis-like picture include bowel obstruction, necrotizing enterocolitis (NEC), and inborn errors of metabolism.

E. **Evaluation of the symptomatic infant for EOS. Laboratory evaluation** of the symptomatic infant suspected of EOS includes at minimum a complete blood count (**CBC**) with differential and blood culture. Other laboratory abnormalities can include hyperglycemia and metabolic acidosis. Thrombocytopenia as well as evidence of DIC (elevated prothrombin time [PT], partial thromboplastin time [PTT], and international normalized ratio [INR]; decreased fibrinogen) can be found in more severely ill infants. For infants with a strong clinical suspicion of sepsis, **a LP for cerebrospinal fluid (CSF) cell count, protein and glucose concentration, Gram stain, and culture** should be performed before the administration of antibiotics if the infant is clinically stable. The LP may be deferred until after the institution of antibiotic therapy if the infant is clinically unstable, or if later culture results or clinical course demonstrate that sepsis was present.

Infants with respiratory symptoms should have a **chest radiograph** as well as other indicated evaluation such as arterial blood gas measurement. Radiographic abnormalities caused by retained fetal lung fluid or atelectasis usually resolve within 48 hours. **Neonatal pneumonia** will present with persistent focal or diffuse radiographic abnormalities and variable degrees of respiratory distress. Neonatal pneumonia (particularly that caused by GBS) can be accompanied by primary or secondary surfactant deficiency.

F. **Treatment of EOS.** Empiric **antibiotic therapy** includes a broad coverage for organisms known to cause EOS, usually a β-lactam antibiotic and an aminoglycoside. In our institutions, we use ampicillin and gentamicin as initial therapy. We add a third-generation cephalosporin (cefotaxime or ceftazidime) to the empiric treatment of critically ill infants for whom there is a strong clinical suspicion for sepsis to optimize therapy for ampicillin-resistant, enteric gram-negative organisms, primarily ampicillin-resistant *Escherichia coli*. (See Table 49.1 for treatment recommendations.) **Supportive treatments for sepsis** include the use of mechanical ventilation, exogenous surfactant therapy for pneumonia and respiratory distress syndrome (RDS), volume and pressor support for hypotension and poor perfusion, sodium bicarbonate for metabolic acidosis, and anticonvulsants for seizures. **Echocardiography** may be of benefit in the severely ill, cyanotic infant to determine if significant pulmonary hypertension or cardiac failure is present. Infants born at ≥34 weeks with symptomatic pulmonary hypertension may benefit from treatment with inhaled nitric oxide (**iNO**). Extracorporeal membrane oxygenation (**ECMO**) can be offered to infants ≥34 weeks if respiratory and circulatory failure occurs despite all conventional measures of intensive care. ECMO is not generally available to infants less than 34 weeks' gestation.

Table 49.1	Suggested Antibiotic Regimens for Sepsis and Meningitis*		
Organism	**Antibiotic**	**Bacteremia**	**Meningitis**
GBS	Ampicillin or penicillin G	10 d	14–21 d
E. coli	Cefotaxime or ampicillin and gentamicin	10–14 d	21 d
CONS	Vancomycin	7 d	14 d
Klebsiella, Serratia[†]	Cefotaxime or meropenem and gentamicin	10–14 d	21 d
Enterobacter, Citrobacter[‡]	Cefepime or meropenem and gentamicin	10–14 d	21 d
Enterococcus[§]	Ampicillin or vancomycin and gentamicin	10 d	21 d
Listeria	Ampicillin and gentamicin	10–14 d	14–21 d
Pseudomonas	Ceftazidime or piperacillin/ tazobactam and gentamicin or tobramycin	14 d	21 d
S. aureus[¶]	Nafcillin	10–14 d	21 d
MRSA	Vancomycin	10–14 d	21 d

GBS = group B *Streptococcus*; CONS = coagulase-negative staphylococci; MRSA = Methicillin-resistant *Staphylococcus aureus*.

*All treatment courses are counted from the first documented negative blood culture and assume that that antibiotic sensitivity data are available for the organisms. In late-onset infections, all treatment courses assume central catheters have been removed. With CONS infections, the clinician may choose to retain the catheter during antibiotic treatment, but if repeated cultures remain positive, the catheters must be removed. Many infectious disease specialists recommend repeat lumbar punctures at the completion of therapy for meningitis to ensure eradication of the infection.

†The spread of plasmid-borne extended-spectrum beta-lactamases (ESBL) among enteric pathogens such as *E. coli, Klebsiella*, and *Serratia* is an increasing clinical problem. Recent literature suggests that ESBL-containing organisms can be effectively treated with cefepime or meropenem. Reports of carbapenemase-producing organisms are of concern and infection with these requires consultation with an infectious disease specialist.

‡*Enterobacter* and *Citrobacter* species have inducible, chromosomally-encoded cephalosporinases. Cephalosporins other than the fourth generation cefepime should not be used to treat infections with these organisms **even if** initial *in vitro* antibiotic sensitivity data suggest sensitivity to third-generation cephalosporins such as cefotaxime. There are some reports in the literature of cefepime-resistant *Enterobacter*.

§Enterococci are resistant to all cephalosporins. Ampicillin-resistant strains of enterococci are common in hospitals, and require treatment with vancomycin. Treatment of vancomycin resistant strains (VRE) requires consultation with an infectious disease specialist.

¶Uncomplicated methicillin-sensitive *S. aureus* and MRSA bacteremias may be treated for only 10 days if central catheters have been removed. Persistent bacteremias can require treatment for 3 to 4 weeks. Bacteremias complicated by deep infections such as osteomyelitis or infectious arthritis often require surgical drainage and treatment for up to 6 weeks. The use of additional agents such as linezolid, daptomycin and rifampin to eradicate persistent *S. aureus* infection; or to treat vancomycin-intermediately susceptible (VISA) and resistant (VRSA) strains requires consultation with an infectious disease specialist.

A variety of **adjunctive immunotherapies** for sepsis have been trialed since the 1980s to address deficits in immunoglobulin and neutrophil number and function. Double-volume exchange transfusions, granulocyte infusions, the administration of intravenous immunoglobulin (IVIG), and treatment with granulocyte-colony stimulating factor (G-CSF) and granulocyte macrophage-colony stimulating factor (GM-CSF) have all been investigated with variable results.

1. **Double-volume exchange transfusion and granulocyte infusion.** Several experimental approaches have been taken to replete neutrophils in neutropenic septic infants: (i) double-volume exchange transfusion with fresh whole blood, (ii) infusion of fresh buffy-coat preparations, or (iii) infusion of granulocytes collected by leukopheresis. Two small, randomized controlled trials of exchange transfusion with whole blood in infants with (largely gram-negative) sepsis were published in the 1990s. Both reported a 50% reduction in mortality of the infants undergoing exchange, and demonstrated increases in neutrophil number, improvement in neutrophil function, and increases in immunoglobulin concentration in the exchanged infants. A Cochrane review of four small trials of granulocyte transfusion in neutropenic neonates with sepsis concluded that there is insufficient evidence of survival benefit with this therapy. Both whole blood exchange transfusion and granulocyte infusion present significant risks, including graft-versus-host disease, blood-group sensitization, and transmission of infections such as cytomegalovirus (CMV), HIV, and viral hepatitis. In addition, the emergent availability of these blood products (especially leukopheresed granulocytes) is limited in most centers. We do not currently use either of these treatments in the treatment of early- or late-onset sepsis.

2. **IVIG.** The use of IVIG in the acute treatment of neonatal sepsis is controversial. It is likely that any efficacy of IVIG would be highest in EOS, which in the United States is largely due to the encapsulated organisms such as GBS and *E. coli* K1, and in premature infants, who are most likely to have inadequate immunoglobulin reserves. IVIG trials reported to date have been conducted in several different countries, using different dosing regimens and/or immunoglobulin preparations. Meta-analysis of randomized trials of the use of IVIG in the acute treatment of suspected or proven neonatal sepsis shows a decrease in mortality of borderline significance. IVIG is expensive and has potential infectious risks, and based on the current marginal evidence of benefit, most authorities have not endorsed the routine use of IVIG in the treatment of neonatal sepsis.

3. **Cytokines.** Recombinant G-CSF and GM-CSF have been shown to restore neutrophil levels in small studies of neutropenic growth-restricted infants, ventilator-dependent neutropenic infants born to mothers with preeclampsia, and in neutropenic infants with sepsis. A rise in the absolute neutrophil count (ANC) above 1,500/mm^3 occurred in 24 to 48 hours. To date, seven randomized controlled trials of recombinant colony-stimulating factors have been reported, all enrolling small numbers of infants. Assessment of these trials is complicated by the use of different preparations, dosages, and durations of therapy, as well as variable enrollment criteria (differing gestational age ranges, presumed and culture-proven sepsis, neutropenic and non-neutropenic infants, early- and late-onset of infection). None of the trials included neurodevelopmental follow-up. These studies suggest that G-CSF may result in lower mortality among neutropenic, septic VLBW infants; but, overall, there

is currently insufficient evidence to support the routine use of these preparations in the acute treatment of neonatal sepsis.

   4. **Activated protein C (APC) and pentoxifylline.** Both of these immunomodulatory preparations have been studied in adults with severe sepsis. Both are active in preventing the microvascular complications of sepsis, by promoting fibrinolyis (APC) and improving endothelial cell function (pentoxifylline), and both decrease the production of tumor necrosis factor (TNF). APC has not been studied in neonates in randomized trials. Pentoxifylline has been studied in a small number of preterm infants with late-onset sepsis with improvement in mortality. Neither medication can be recommended for use in neonates without further study.

G. **Evaluation of the asymptomatic infant at risk for EOS.** There are a number of clinical factors that place infants at risk for EOS. These factors also identify a group of asymptomatic infants who may have colonization or bacteremia that places them at risk for the development of symptomatic EOS. These infants include those born to mothers who have received inadequate intrapartum antibiotic prophylaxis (IAP) for GBS (see subsequent text) and those born to mothers with suspected chorioamnionitis. Blood cultures are the definitive determination of bacteremia. A number of laboratory tests have been evaluated for their ability to predict which of the at-risk infants will go on to develop symptomatic or culture-proven sepsis, but no single test has adequate sensitivity and specificity.

   1. **Blood culture.** With advances in the development of computer-assisted, continuous-read culture systems, most blood cultures will be positive within 24 to 36 hours of incubation if organisms are present. Most institutions, including ours, empirically treat infants for sepsis for a minimum of 48 hours with the assumption that true positive cultures will turn positive within that period. At least 0.5 mL (and preferably 1 mL) of blood should be placed in most pediatric blood culture bottles. We use two culture bottles, one aerobic and one anaerobic. Certain organisms causing EOS (such as *Bacteroides fragilis* [*B. fragilis*]) will only grow under anaerobic conditions; 5% of culture-proven EOS in our institution is due to strictly anaerobic species. Additionally, GBS, *Staphylococcus* species, and many gram-negative organisms grow in a facultative fashion, and the use of two culture bottles increases the likelihood of detecting low-level bacteremia with these organisms.

   2. **White blood count (WBC).** The WBC and differential is readily available and commonly used to evaluate both symptomatic and asymptomatic infants at risk for sepsis. Interpretation of neonatal WBC has been compromised by the relatively small size of studies used to determine normal values and by a lack of data quantifying the impact of differences mediated by gestational age, postnatal age, mode of delivery, and maternal conditions. Maternal fever, neonatal asphyxia, meconium aspiration syndrome, pneumothorax, and hemolytic disease have all been associated with neutrophilia; maternal pregnancy-induced hypertension and preeclampsia are associated with neonatal neutropenia as well as thrombocytopenia.
   One finding common to all published neonatal WBC data is the "roller coaster" shape of the WBC, ANC, and immature to total neutrophil ratio (I:T) curves in the first 72 hours of life. This suggests that optimal interpretation of WBC data to predict EOS should account for the natural rise and fall in WBC during this period. A recent study supports the use of CBC

only after the first few hours of life, when placed in the proper clinical context and used as part of an algorithm to evaluate infants for sepsis risk. In this study, both the WBC and ANC were most predictive of infection when these values were low (WBC <5,000 and ANC <2,000) and when obtained at more than 4 hours of age. An elevated WBC (>20,000) was neither worrisome nor reassuring in neonates. The I:T ratio was most informative if measured beyond 1 to 4 hours after birth, with low values (<0.15) reassuring, whereas elevated values (>0.3) were weakly associated with EOS.

Although studies demonstrate that no component of the WBC is very sensitive among term and late preterm infants for the prediction of sepsis, there are little data to guide interpretation of the WBC among VLBW infants at risk for EOS. It is possible that the WBC and its components may be of more value in the VLBW infant and/or in the evaluation of late-onset infection. Finally, some centers combine WBC values in a "sepsis screen" (e.g., the use of an algorithm incorporating total WBC, I:T ratio, total band count, with or without C-reactive protein [CRP] values) to guide treatment decisions.

3. **CRP** is a nonspecific marker of inflammation or tissue necrosis. Elevations in CRP are found in bacterial sepsis and meningitis. A single determination of CRP at birth lacks both sensitivity and specificity for infection, but serial CRP determinations at birth and at 12 hours and beyond have been used to manage infants at risk for sepsis. Some centers use serial CRP measurements to determine length of antibiotic treatment for infants with culture-negative clinical sepsis. We do not use CRP measurements in the evaluation of infants at risk for sepsis.

4. **Cytokine measurements.** Advances in the understanding of the immune responses to infection and in the measurement of small peptide molecules have allowed investigation into the utility of these inflammatory molecules in predicting infection in neonates at risk. Serum levels of interleukin-6, interleukin-8, interleukin-10, interleukin-1 β, G-CSF, TNF-α, and procalcitonin, as well as measurements of inflammatory cell-surface markers such as CD64, have been variably correlated with culture-proven, clinical, and viral sepsis. The need for serial measurements and the availability of the specific assays so far limit the use of cytokine markers in diagnosing neonatal infection. In addition, most studies have been performed on infants who are symptomatic and being evaluated for sepsis. None of these have yet proven useful in predicting infection in initially well-appearing infants.

5. **Other strategies. Urine latex particle agglutination testing for GBS** remains available at some institutions, but we have given up the use of this test due to very poor predictive value. Latex particle testing of CSF for both GBS and *E. coli* K1 can be of use in evaluating CSF after the institution of antibiotic treatment.

6. **LP.** The use of routine LP in the evaluation of **asymptomatic neonates** at risk for EOS remains controversial. A retrospective review of 9,111 infants born at ≥34 weeks' gestation from 150 neonatal intensive care unit (NICU) on whom a LP was performed found 95 cases of culture-proven meningitis. In 38% of these cases, the accompanying blood culture was sterile. Another retrospective study of CSFs taken from a population of 169,849 infants identified eight infants with culture-positive CSF, but with negative blood cultures and no CNS symptoms. In both studies, the authors concluded that the selective use of LP in the evaluation of EOS may lead to missed diagnoses of meningitis. However, in both studies, infants were not all evaluated for sepsis in the absence

of symptoms, and the subjects were drawn from large numbers of hospitals with likely disparate culture systems. Another study reviewed the results of sepsis evaluations in a population of 24,452 infants from a single institution. This study found 11 cases of meningitis, all in symptomatic infants; 10 of 11 corresponding blood cultures were positive for the same organism. No cases of meningitis were found in 3,423 asymptomatic infants evaluated with LP.

We do not perform LP's for the evaluation of **asymptomatic term infants** at risk for EOS. A review of our own data from 1996 to 2009, a period during which IAP for GBS was implemented using a screening-based approach, revealed 20 cases of culture-positive meningitis from a population of over 70,000 deliveries. Only two cases occurred in term infants; both infants grew GBS from both blood and CSF cultures and both infants were symptomatic. **It is our current policy to perform LPs only** on (i) infants with positive blood cultures and (ii) symptomatic infants with negative blood cultures who are treated empirically for the clinical diagnosis of sepsis. Whenever clinically feasible, LPs are performed on symptomatic infants with a high suspicion for sepsis before administering antibiotics.

When LPs are performed after the administration of antibiotics, a clinical evaluation of the presence of meningitis is made, taking into account the blood culture results, the CSF cell count, protein, and glucose levels, as well as the clinical scenario. We recommend sending two separate CSF samples for cell count from the same LP in these circumstances to account for the role of possible fluctuation in CSF cell count measurements. Interpretation of CSF WBC values can be challenging. **Normal CSF WBC counts** in term, noninfected infants are variable, with most studies reporting a mean of <20 cells per mm^3, with ranges of up to 90 cells, and widely varying levels of polymorphonuclear cells on the differential. One recent study defined "noninfected" infants by negative bacterial blood, CSF and urine cultures, and negative viral CSF culture, as well as negative enteroviral CSF polymerase chain reaction (PCR). This study reported a mean CSF WBC 7.3 (±14) per mm^3 with a range of 0 to 130 cells. Another study of culture-proven, early-onset meningitis demonstrated only 80% sensitivity and specificity for CSF WBC values >20. The presence of blood in the CSF, due to subarachnoid or intraventricular hemorrhage, or to blood contamination of CSF samples by "traumatic" LPs, can yield abnormal cell counts that may be due to the presence of blood in the CSF rather than true infection. Adjustment of the WBC in traumatic LP results (those with >500 RBC per mm^3) using different algorithms has not been shown to substantially improve the sensitivity and specificity of the WBC in predicting culture-confirmed meningitis.

H. **Algorithm for the evaluation of the infant born at ≥35 weeks' gestation at risk for EOS.** At the Brigham and Women's Hospital (BWH), to ensure consistency amongst caregivers, an algorithm is used for the evaluation of asymptomatic, ≥35-week gestation infants who are at risk for developing EOS (Figure 49.1). This algorithm incorporates both the evaluation of infants based on maternal GBS colonization, and an evaluation of infants at risk for EOS due to maternal intrapartum risk factors. A total WBC of $<5,000$ or an I:T ratio of >0.3 is used to guide treatment decisions in the evaluation of the well-appearing infant at risk for sepsis. A single CBC determination is used in most cases to avoid multiple blood draws from otherwise asymptomatic infants; as noted previously, WBC values may have better predictive value when performed after 1 to 4 hours of age.

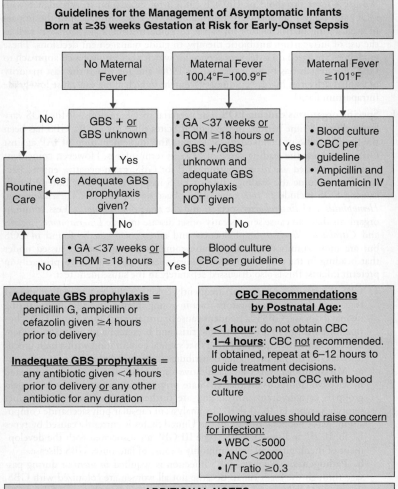

Guidelines for the Management of Asymptomatic Infants Born at ≥35 weeks Gestation at Risk for Early-Onset Sepsis

No Maternal Fever

Maternal Fever 100.4°F–100.9°F

Maternal Fever ≥101°F

GBS + or GBS unknown

- GA <37 weeks or
- ROM ≥18 hours or
- GBS +/GBS unknown and adequate GBS prophylaxis NOT given

- Blood culture
- CBC per guideline
- Ampicillin and Gentamicin IV

Routine Care

Adequate GBS prophylaxis given?

- GA <37 weeks or
- ROM ≥18 hours

Blood culture CBC per guideline

Adequate GBS prophylaxis = penicillin G, ampicillin or cefazolin given ≥4 hours prior to delivery

Inadequate GBS prophylaxis = any antibiotic given <4 hours prior to delivery or any other antibiotic for any duration

CBC Recommendations by Postnatal Age:

- **<1 hour**: do not obtain CBC
- **1–4 hours**: CBC not recommended. If obtained, repeat at 6–12 hours to guide treatment decisions.
- **≥4 hours**: obtain CBC with blood culture

Following values should raise concern for infection:
- WBC <5000
- ANC <2000
- I/T ratio ≥0.3

ADDITIONAL NOTES

1. Chorioamnionitis is an obstetrical clinical diagnosis made on the basis of clinical findings, laboratory data and fever. If obstetrical staff diagnose chorioamnionitis, the infant should be evaluated for sepsis and receive empiric antibiotic treatment.
2. Maternal fever that occurs within one hour of delivery should be treated like intrapartum fever.
3. Women with a previous infant with GBS disease should receive intrapartum GBS prophylaxis.
4. Blood cultures should consist of aerobic and anaerobic bottles with minimum 1 cc blood in each bottle.

Figure 49.1 Algorithm for Sepsis Evaluations in at risk Asymptomatic Infants ≥35 weeks gestation.

We use a fever threshold of 100.4°F (38°C) for evaluation in accordance with CDC and other published recommendations. We take into account the impact of a clustering of risk factors for sepsis to guide treatment decisions, as well as the use of intrapartum antibiotic therapy, to guide management decisions. These guidelines are based on a delivery service for which a screening-based approach to GBS prophylaxis has been in place since 1996, and for which the vast majority of vaginal deliveries involve epidural placement (which alone can cause low-grade intrapartum fever).

I. **Specific organisms causing EOS.** The bacterial species responsible for EOS vary by locality and time period. In the United States since the 1980s, GBS has been the leading cause of neonatal EOS. Despite the implementation of IAP against GBS, it remains the leading cause of EOS in term infants. However, coincident with the increased use of intrapartum IAP for GBS, gram-negative enteric bacteria have become the leading cause of EOS in preterm infants. Enteric bacilli causing EOS include *E. coli*, other Enterobacteriaceae (*Klebsiella*, *Pseudomonas*, *Hemophilus*, and *Enterobacter* species) and the anaerobe *B. fragilis*. Less common organisms that can cause serious early-onset disease include *Listeria monocytogenes* and *Citrobacter diversus*. Staphylococci and enterococci can be found in EOS but are more commonly causes of nosocomial sepsis and are discussed under that heading in the subsequent text. Fungal species can cause EOS primarily in preterm infants; this is also discussed separately in the subsequent text.

1. **GBS** (*Streptococcus agalactiae*) frequently colonizes the human genital and GI tracts and the upper respiratory tract in young infants. In addition to causing neonatal disease, GBS is a frequent cause of urinary tract infection (UTI), chorioamnionitis, postpartum endometritis, and bacteremia in pregnant women. There is some evidence suggesting that vaginal colonization with a high inoculum of GBS during pregnancy contributes to premature birth.

   a. **Microbiology.** GBS are facultative diplococci that are easily cultivated in selective laboratory media. GBS are primarily identified by the Lancefield group B carbohydrate antigen and are further subtyped into nine distinct serotypes (types Ia, Ib, II–VIII) by analysis of capsular polysaccharide composition. Most neonatal disease in the United States is currently caused by types Ia, Ib, II, III and type V GBS. Type III GBS are associated with the development of meningitis and are commonly a cause of late-onset GBS disease.

   b. **Pathogenesis.** Neonatal GBS infection is acquired *in utero* or during passage through the birth canal. Because not all women are colonized with GBS, documented colonization with GBS is the strongest predictor of GBS EOS. Approximately 20% to 30% of American women are colonized with GBS at any given time. A longitudinal study of GBS colonization in a cohort of primarily young, sexually active women demonstrated that 45% of initially GBS-negative women acquired colonization at some time over a 12-month period. In the absence of IAP, approximately 50% of infants born to mothers colonized with GBS are found to be colonized with this organism at birth. Approximately 1% to 2% of all colonized infants develop invasive GBS disease, with clinical factors such as gestational age and duration of ROM contributing to risk for any individual infant (see subsequent text). Lack of maternally derived protective capsular polysaccharide-specific antibody is associated with the development of invasive GBS disease. Other factors predisposing the newborn to GBS disease are less well understood, but relative deficiencies in complement, neutrophil function and innate immunity may be important.

Table 49.2	Risk Factors for Early-onset Group B *Streptococcus* (GBS) Sepsis in the Absence of Intrapartum Antibiotic Prophylaxis
Risk factor	**Odds ratio (95% CI)**
Maternal GBS colonization	204 (100–419)
BW <1,000 g	24.8 (12.2–50.2)
BW <2,500 g	7.37 (4.48–12.1)
Prolonged ROM >18 h	7.28 (4.42–12.0)
Chorioamnionitis	6.42 (2.32–17.8)
Intrapartum fever >37.5°C	4.05 (2.17–7.56)

CI = confidence interval; BW = birth weight; ROM = rupture of membranes.
Data from Benitz WE, Gould JB, Druzin ML. Risk factors for early-onset group B streptococcal sepsis: estimation of odds ratios by critical literature review. *Pediatrics* 1999;103(6):e77.

c. **Clinical risk factors for GBS EOS (see Table 49.2).** GBS bacteriuria during pregnancy is associated with heavy colonization of the rectovaginal tract and is considered a significant risk factor for EOS. Black race and maternal age <20 years are associated with higher rates of GBS EOS, although it is not entirely clear whether this reflects only higher rates of GBS colonization in these populations. Multiple gestation is **not** an independent risk factor for GBS EOS.
d. **Prevention of GBS infection.** Multiple trials have demonstrated that the use of intrapartum penicillin or ampicillin significantly reduces the rate of neonatal colonization with GBS and the incidence of early-onset GBS disease. IAP for the prevention of GBS EOS can be administered to pregnant women during labor based on (i) specific risk factors for early-onset GBS infection or on (ii) the results of antepartum screening of pregnant women for GBS colonization. In 2002, the CDC issued guidelines recommending universal screening of pregnant women for GBS by rectovaginal culture at 35 to 37 weeks' gestation and management of IAP based on screening results. Pregnant women with documented GBS bacteriuria during pregnancy or who previously delivered an infant who developed invasive GBS disease need not be screened as these women should be given IAP **regardless of current GBS colonization status.** The CDC guidelines for the prevention of early-onset GBS disease were revised in 2010 to address recent data on neonatal and obstetrical infection management and outcomes (http://www.cdc.gov/groupbstrep/guidelines/guidelines.html).

Highlights of the new guidelines included revised recommendations for the management of neonates at risk for EOS, changes in recommended antibiotic choices for GBS IAP, specific recommendations for mothers who experience preterm labor and premature ROM, expanded laboratory methods for the detection of GBS, including use of alternate culture-based detection methods, and intrapartum nucleic acid amplification testing as an alternative to culture-based detection.

In the 2010 revised guidelines, penicillin and ampicillin remain the recommended antibiotics for GBS IAP. The document addresses the challenges of providing adequate IAP to the roughly 10% of women who reported having penicillin allergy. There is no data directly supporting the efficacy of any antibiotic other than pencillin, ampicillin, or cefazolin for GBS IAP. Erythromycin and clindamycin are frequently given to penicillin-allergic women, but an increasing proportion of GBS isolates (15%–40%) are resistant to these antibiotics. In the penicillin-allergic woman, it is recommended that any GBS isolates identified on screening be tested for antibiotic susceptibility, including specific testing for inducible clindamycin resistance. For the woman with a non–life-threatening penicillin allergy, cefazolin is the recommended antibiotic for IAP. If a woman has a documented history of anaphylactic penicillin or cephalosporin allergy (including urticaria, angioedema, and/or respiratory distress), clindamycin is recommended if the colonizing isolate is fully susceptible to this antibiotic; otherwise vancomycin is the recommended agent. For the purpose of infant management, however, the 2010 guideline does not consider the administration of clindamycin or vancomycin to constitute fully adequate IAP.

e. Current status of GBS EOS. The CDC active surveillance data for the United States in 2007 to 2008 demonstrates that the overall incidence of GBS EOS has fallen to 0.28 cases per 1,000 live births (compared with 1.7 cases per 1,000 live births in 1993). There is ongoing racial disparity with the incidence among black infants roughly four times that of white infants. Approximately one-quarter of all GBS EOS now occurs among infants born at <37 weeks' gestation. We evaluated the reasons for persistent GBS EOS despite the use of a screening-based approach to IAP at the Brigham and Women's Hospital (BWH). We found that most GBS EOS in term infants now occurs in infants born to women with **negative** antepartum screens for GBS colonization. Subsequent CDC multistate surveillance studies from 2003 to 2004 found that 61% of GBS disease among term infants occurred in infants born to mothers who screened GBS negative. These "false-negative" screens may be due to improper culture technique or acquisition of GBS between the time of culture and start of labor.

Bacterial culture remains the CDC-recommended standard for detection of maternal GBS colonization. The 2010 revision includes new recommendations for the use of chromogenic GBS detection media and for the use of direct broth detection methods by latex agglutination, probe detection, or nucleic acid amplification testing (NAAT) methods. These approaches may shorten the time to GBS identification. In 2002, the U.S. Food and Drug Administration (FDA) approved the first **PCR-based** rapid NAAT diagnostic for detection of maternal GBS colonization directly from vaginal/rectal swab specimens. Different kits are now commercially available, and the 2010 guideline endorses the optional use of these NAATs for the management of women whose GBS status is unknown at the time of delivery. Recent data demonstrates that NAATs are more sensitive than antenatal culture in predicting intrapartum GBS status but real-time use is compromised by a 10% incidence of nonresults due to technical issues. Due to the costs and technicalities of providing continuous support for a real-time, PCR-based diagnostic, as well as the inherent time delay in an intrapartum diagnostic, most obstetric services continue to rely on antenatal culture-based screening programs.

f. Evaluation of infants after maternal GBS IAP. The 2010 revised CDC guidelines include a recommended algorithm for the evaluation of infants born to mothers exposed to IAP. As in prior versions, the algorithm recommends a full diagnostic evaluation (CBC with white cell differential, LP, CSF and blood cultures, and chest radiograph) and empiric antibiotic therapy for any infant with clinical signs of infection. For asymptomatic infants, a limited evaluation, including CBC/differential and blood culture, and empiric antibiotic therapy are recommended if there were intrapartum signs of maternal chorioamnionitis. **Different from previous guidelines, the 2010 version considers only the administration of penicillin, ampicillin, or cefazolin ≥4 hours prior to delivery to constitute adequate IAP. If GBS IAP was indicated but not adequately administered, the revised guideline recommends limited diagnostic evaluation only if other risk factors for EOS are present (gestational age <37 weeks and or ROM ≥18 hours).**

g. Treatment of infants with invasive GBS disease. When GBS is identified as the sole causative organism in EOS, empiric antibiotic treatment should be narrowed to ampicillin (200 to 300 mg/kg/day) or penicillin G (250,000 to 450,000 U/kg/day) alone, with the higher dosing reserved for cases complicated by meningitis. The total duration of therapy should be at least 10 days for sepsis without a focus, 14 to 21 days for meningitis, and 28 days for osteomyelitis. Bone and joint infections that involve the hip or shoulder require surgical drainage in addition to antibiotic therapy.

h. Recurrent GBS infection. Recurrent GBS infections are infrequent, with reported incidences ranging from 1% to 6%. Infants usually fail to have a specific antibody response after infection with GBS, and GBS can be isolated from mucosal surfaces of infants even after appropriate antibiotic treatment for invasive disease. Occasionally, reinfection with a new strain of GBS occurs. Treatment of recurrent GBS infections is the same as for primary infection except that susceptibility testing of the GBS strain to penicillin is recommended if not routinely performed. Rifampin, which eliminates colonization in other infections such as meningococcal disease, does not reliably eradicate mucous membrane colonization with GBS.

2. *E. coli* **and other enteric gram-negative bacilli.** With the implementation of IAP against GBS, an **increasing proportion** of EOS cases are caused by gram-negative organisms. Whether GBS IAP policies are contributing to an absolute increase in the **incidence** of EOS caused by gram-negative organisms and, in particular, of ampicillin-resistant gram-negative organisms, is a matter of ongoing controversy. In 2003, CDC researchers published a review of 23 reports of EOS in the era of GBS prophylaxis. This review concluded that there is no evidence of an increase in non-GBS EOS among term infants. **However, increases in non-GBS EOS and ampicillin-resistant EOS are reported in among VLBW infants.** We have analyzed EOS at the BWH from 1990 to 2007, comparing the period from 1990 to 1992 (no GBS IAP policy) with 1997 to 2007 (screening-based GBS IAP policy). We found an **absolute decrease in the incidence** of all-cause EOS in both term and VLBW infants, and no increases in non-GBS EOS, *E. coli* EOS, or ampicillin-resistant EOS in term or VLBW infants. Because GBS IAP prevents gram-positive, ampicillin-sensitive infections, the proportion of remaining EOS cases caused by ampicillin-resistant, gram-negative organisms is increased. Trends in the microbiology of EOS likely vary to some extent by institution and may be influenced by local obstetrical practices as well as by local variation in indigenous bacterial flora. The outcomes at our institution may be, in part, due to the exclusive use of penicillin G (and not ampicillin) for GBS IAP by our obstetricians.

a. Microbiology and pathogenesis. *E. coli* are aerobic gram-negative rods found universally in the human intestinal tract and commonly in the human vagina and urinary tract. There are hundreds of different lipopolysaccharide (LPS), flagellar, and capsular antigenic types of *E. coli*, but EOS *E. coli* infections, particularly those complicated by meningitis, are primarily due to strains with the K1-type polysaccharide capsule. *E. coli* with the K1 antigen are resistant to the bactericidal effect of normal human serum; strains that possess both a complete LPS and K1 capsule have been shown to specifically evade both complement-mediated bacteriolysis and neutrophil-mediated killing. The K1 antigen has been shown to be a primary factor in the development of meningitis in a rat model of *E. coli* infection. The K1 capsule is a poor immunogen, however, and despite widespread carriage of this strain in the population, there is usually little protective maternal antibody available to the infant. In addition to the K1 antigen, surface fimbriae, or pili are have been associated with adherence to vaginal and uroepithelial surfaces and may also function as a virulence mechanism in EOS.

b. Treatment. When there is a strong clinical suspicion for sepsis in a critically ill infant, the possibility of ampicillin-resistant *E. coli* must be considered. The addition of a third-generation cephalosporin such as cefotaxime or ceftazidime is recommended in this setting. *E. coli* bacteremia should be treated with a total of 14 days of antibiotic according to the identified sensitivities. *E. coli* meningitis is treated with a 21-day course of cefotaxime (see Appendix A).

3. *Listeria monocytogenes.* Although uncommon, *L. monocytogenes* deserves a special note due to its unique role in pregnancy. *L. monocytogenes* are gram-positive, β-hemolytic, motile bacteria that frequently cause disease in animals, and most commonly infect humans through the ingestion of contaminated food. These bacteria do not cause significant disease in immunocompetent adults, but can cause severe illness in the elderly, in immunocompromised patients, in pregnant women and their fetuses, and in newborns. There is human epidemiologic evidence and evidence in animal models of listeriosis that indicate that *L. monocytogenes* is particularly virulent in pregnancy. The bacteria readily invades the placenta and can infect the developing fetus by either ascending infection, direct tissue invasion, or hematogenous spread, causing spontaneous abortion or preterm labor and delivery, and often fulminant early-onset disease. Like GBS, *L. monocytogenes* can also cause late-onset neonatal infection, the pathogenesis of which is not fully understood. Over 90% of late-onset infections are complicated by meningitis.

Listeriosis is a reportable disease, and the CDC data for the United States in 2009 revealed an overall incidence of 0.34 cases per 100,000 population, with most cases occurring among persons ≥65 years old. The true incidence of listeriosis in pregnancy is difficult to determine because many cases are undiagnosed when they result in spontaneous abortion of the previable fetus. The incidence of EOS due to *L. monocytogenes* in the CDC active surveillance effort in Atlanta and San Francisco was 2.4 cases per 100,000 live births; at our institution over the past 20 years, the incidence was 1.7 cases per 100,000 live births. Listeriosis can result from ingestion of contaminated food such as soft cheeses, deli meat, and hot dogs. Infection in pregnant woman may not be recognized or may cause a mild febrile illness with or without GI symptoms before resulting in pregnancy loss or preterm labor. Epidemic outbreaks of listeriosis affecting both pregnant and nonpregnant adults are reported. An epidemic outbreak in Massachusetts in 2008 resulted in three elderly deaths, a premature delivery, and a term stillbirth. This outbreak was notable in that the source of infection was pasteurized milk produced a single dairy, highlighting the potential for postpasteurization contamination of processed foods with *Listeria*.

a. **Microbiology and pathogenesis.** *L. monocytogenes* are distinguished from other gram-positive rods by tumbling motility that is most prominent at room temperature. The organisms can be gram-variable and depending on growth stage, can also appear cocci-like, and can therefore be initially misdiagnosed on a Gram stain. *L. monocytogenes* is an intracellular pathogen that can invade cells as well as persist in phagocytic cells (monocytes, macrophages). *Listeria* possess a variety of virulence factors, including surface proteins that promote cellular invasion, and enzymes (listeriolysin O, phospholipase) that enhance the ability of the organism to persist intracellularly. On pathologic examination of tissues infected with *Listeria*, miliary granulomas and areas of necrosis and suppuration are seen. The liver is prominently involved. Both T cell-mediated killing as well as immunoglobulin M (IgM) complement-mediated killing are involved in host response to listeriosis. Deficiencies in both of these arms of the newborn immune system may contribute to the virulence of *L. monocytogenes* in the neonate; similarly, it is hypothesized that local downregulation of the immune response in the pregnant uterus may account for proliferation of the bacteria in the placenta.

b. **Treatment.** EOS due to *L. monocytogenes* is treated with ampicillin and gentamicin for 14 days; meningitis is treated for 21 days. *L. monocytogenes* is resistant to cephalosporins. In the case of meningitis, it is recommended that LPs be repeated daily until sterilization of the CSF is achieved. Additional therapy with rifampin or trimethoprim-sulfamethoxazole, as well as cerebral imaging is recommended if the organism persists in the CSF for longer than 2 days. *L. monocytogenes* can persist in the stool of preterm infants even after adequate systemic treatment of the infection, thus proper infection control measures must be observed to prevent nosocomial spread of the organism.

4. **Other organisms responsible for EOS.** Bacteria causing EOS vary with time and locality. Beyond GBS and *E. coli*, there are a number of pathogens that cause EOS in the United States in the era of IAP for GBS. Viridans streptococci (species such as *Streptococcus mitis*, *Streptococcus oralis*, and *Streptococcus sanguis*, which are part of the oral flora), enterococci, and *Staphylococcus aureus* are next in frequency. *Listeria*, a variety of gram-negative organisms (*Klebsiella*, *Hemophilus*, *Enterobacter*, and *Pseudomonas* species) and the anaerobe *B. fragilis* cause most of the remaining infections. Gram-negative organisms, especially *Hemophilus influenzae* and *Klebsiella*, predominate in some Asian and South American countries.

J. **Late-onset sepsis (LOS).** Late-onset neonatal sepsis is defined as occurring from 8 to 90 days of life. LOS can be divided into two distinct entities: disease occurring in otherwise healthy term infants in the community, and disease affecting premature infants in the NICU. The latter is often referred to as hospital-acquired sepsis, as the risk factors for LOS in premature infants are related to the necessities of their care (i.e., the presence of central lines), and the bacteria that cause LOS are often acquired in the NICU. For epidemiologic purposes, LOS infections occurring in VLBW infants in the NICU are defined as those occurring at >72 hours of life.

This section is primarily devoted to LOS in the NICU population, but disease in otherwise **healthy term and near-term infants** deserves mention. In these infants, LOS is largely caused by GBS and gram-negative species such as *E. coli* and *Klebsiella* species. Causes of bacteremia in older infants (such as *Streptococcus pneumoniae*, and *Neisseria meningitidis*) occur less frequently. The **risk factors for late-onset GBS disease** are not as well defined as for early-onset disease, but like early-onset disease are related to prematurity, colonization of the infant from maternal and community (or less commonly, hospital) sources, gestational age and lack of maternally derived protective antibody. The use of IAP for GBS has had no significant impact on the rate of GBS LOS, remaining at 0.33 cases per 1,000 live births from 1999 to 2005. Preterm infants account for a disproportionate number of GBS late-onset infections; from 1999 to 2005 CDC surveillance revealed that 52% of late-onset GBS cases occurred in infants born at <37 weeks' gestation with a median gestational age of 30 weeks among the preterm cases. GBS LOS is more often complicated by meningitis than early-onset disease and is predominantly caused by polysaccharide serotype III strains. Although mortality from GBS LOS is low (1%–5% in term and preterm infants, respectively), sequelae in survivors of GBS meningitis can be severe. A recent study of GBS meningitis occurring in infants born at ≥36 weeks' gestation from 1998 to 2006 revealed that a quarter of all infants died or survived with significant neurologic impairment.

Gram-negative bacteremia is often associated with UTI. Different series report 20% to 30% of UTIs in infants under 1 month of age are complicated by bacteremia. Mortality is low if promptly treated, and sequelae are few unless meningitis occurs. *L. monocytogenes* can also cause late-onset disease, with onset commonly by 30 days of life, and can account for up to 20% of LOS in some centers. Late-onset listeriosis is frequently complicated by meningitis, but unlike late-onset GBS meningitis, the morbidity and long-term sequelae are infrequent if the disease is diagnosed and treated in a timely fashion.

Term infants with LOS generally present with fever and/or poor feeding and lethargy to the private pediatrician or emergency department. Evaluation in the infant younger than 3 months old in most centers includes at minimum a CBC, urinalysis, CSF cell count, glucose and protein, and cultures of blood, urine, and CSF. Infants under 1 month are generally hospitalized for empiric IV therapy that includes coverage for GBS, *Listeria*, and gram-negative organisms (commonly ampicillin and cefotaxime); for infants over 1 month, management varies in different centers.

K. **Epidemiology of LOS in premature infants.** Most LOS occurs in the NICU among LBW infants. The National Institute of Child Health and Human Development (NICHD) Neonatal Research Network (NRN) data from 2003 to 2007 revealed that 36% of their VLBW cohort (birth weight of <1,500 g and gestational age of 22–28 weeks) had at least one episode of blood culture-proven sepsis beyond 3 days of life. There was considerable variability in the incidence of LOS, ranging from 18% to 51% among the 20 NICHD network centers. NICHD network LOS data from 1998 to 2000 demonstrated overall mortality from LOS was 18% of infected infants versus 7% of uninfected infants. The mortality among infants with gram-negative infections was about 40%, and 30% with fungal infections.

L. **Risk factors for LOS.** A number of clinical factors are associated with an increased risk of LOS (Table 49.3). The incidence of LOS is inversely related to birth weight. The risk of developing LOS associated with central catheters, parenteral nutrition, and mechanical ventilation are all increased with longer duration of these therapies.

M. **Microbiology of LOS.** Nearly half of cases of LOS are caused by coagulase-negative staphylococci (CONS). In the NICHD study, 22% of cases of LOS were

Table 49.3	Risk Factors for Late-onset Sepsis in Infants with Birth Weight Less Than 1,500 g
Birth weight <750 g	
Presence of central venous catheters (umbilical, percutaneous, and tunneled)	
Delayed enteral feeding	
Prolonged hyperalimentation	
Mechanical ventilation	
Complications of prematurity	
Patent ductus arteriosus	
Bronchopulmonary dysplasia	
Necrotizing enterocolitis	

Data from Stoll BJ, Hansen N, Fanaroff AA, et al. Late onset sepsis in very low birth weight neonates: the experience of the NICHD Neonatal Research Network. *Pediatrics* 2002;110(2 pt 1):285–291 and Makhoul IR, Sujov P, Smolkin T, et al. Epidemiologic, clinical, and microbiologic characteristics of late-onset sepsis among very low birth weight infants in Israel: a national survey. *Pediatrics* 2002;109(1):34–39.

caused by other gram-positive organisms (*S. aureus*, *Enterococcus*, GBS), 18% by gram-negative organisms (*E. coli*, *Klebsiella*, *Pseudomonas*, *Enterobacter*, *Serratia*), and 12% by fungal species (*Candida albicans* and *Candida parapsilosis*). The distribution of organisms causing LOS may vary significantly at individual centers. We reviewed cases of LOS occurring in the BWH's NICU from 1995 to 2009. Although the overall incidence of LOS among VLBW infants did not differ between the BWH and the NICHD network centers, the **distribution of pathogens** causing LOS in our population differs from that reported by the NICHD Network. These differences are primarily due to a higher incidence of *S. aureus* infections, and a lower incidence of fungal infections. Awareness of local variation in the microbiology of LOS is important in choosing empiric antibiotic therapy for the acutely ill infant in whom LOS is suspected.

1. **Coagulase negative *Staphylococcus* (CONS).** CONS are a heterogeneous group of gram-positive organisms with a structure similar to *S. aureus*, but these organisms lack protein A and have different cell wall components. *Staphylococcus epidermidis* is the primary cause of NICU disease. CONS universally colonize the skin of NICU patients. They are believed to cause bacteremia by first colonizing the surfaces of central catheters. A polysaccharide surface adhesin (PSA), as well as several other surface components, has been implicated in adherence to and colonization of the catheter surface; subsequent biofilm and slime production inhibit the ability of the host to eliminate the organism. Most CONS are resistant to penicillin, semisynthetic penicillins, and gentamicin, and empiric treatment for LOS in the NICU usually includes vancomycin. CONS disease is rarely fatal even

to the VLBW infant, and rarely if ever causes meningitis or site-specific disease. However, CONS disease can cause systemic instability resulting in temporary cessation of enteral feeding and/or escalation of ventilatory support, and is associated with prolonged hospitalization and poorer neurodevelopmental outcome.

2. *S. aureus* is an encapsulated gram-positive organism that elaborates multiple adhesins, virulence-associated enzymes, and toxins to cause a wide range of serious disease, including bacteremia, meningitis, cellulitis, omphalitis, osteomyelitis, and arthritis. *S. aureus* is distinguished from CONS by the production of coagulase, and by the presence of protein A, a component of the cell wall that contributes to virulence by binding to the Fc portion of immunoglobulin G (IgG) antibody and blocking opsonization. LOS caused by *S. aureus* can result in significant morbidity. Disease is frequently complicated by focal site infections (soft tissue, bone, and joint infections are commonly observed in neonates) and marked by persistent bacteremia despite antibiotic administration. Joint infections often require open surgical drainage and can lead to joint destruction and permanent disability. The treatment of methicillin-sensitive *S. aureus* (MSSA) requires the use of semisynthetic penicillins such as nafcillin or oxacillin.

   Methicillin-resistant *Staphylococcus aureus* (MRSA) is an increasingly recognized pathogen in NICUs. National Nosocomial Infection Surveillance (NNIS) System data from 1995 to 2004 demonstrates >300% increase in the incidence of MRSA infections among NICU infants with the greatest incidence among infants with a birth weight of <1,000 g. Resistance to semisynthetic penicillins is mediated by chromosomal acquisition of the *mecA* gene, found on different types of staphylococcal chromosomal cassette *mec* (SCC*mecA*) elements. The *mecA* gene encodes a modified penicillin-binding protein (PBP) with a low affinity for methicillin. Once acquired, the modified PBP replaces similar proteins on the bacterial cell membrane and results in resistance to all β-lactam antibiotics. The emergence of MRSA infections in NICUs appears to track the increase in these infections in both general hospital settings and in the community. MRSA isolates can be grouped as hospital-associated (HA-MRSA) or community-associated (CA-MRSA) in origin. Uniform resistance to all common antibiotics except for vancomycin characterizes HA-MRSA. Community-acquired isolates are usually resistant only to β-lactam antibiotics and erythromycin. CA-MRSA has emerged as the dominant form of MRSA causing infection among NICU infants, but distinguishing between the two types of organisms can be important for determining the source of epidemic outbreaks of MRSA disease within individual units as well as for developing effective infection control measures. Whatever the source of the organism, however, it can be rapidly spread within the NICU by nosocomial transmission on the hands of caregivers. Infection control measures, including identification of colonized infants by routine surveillance and cohorting and isolation of colonized infants, may be required to prevent spread and persistence of the organism. MRSA infections usually require treatment with **vancomycin.** As with methicillin-sensitive *S. aureus*, MRSA infections can be complicated by deep tissue involvement and persistent bacteremia that may require surgical debridement for resolution. Although it cannot be used as a single agent, rifampin can be a helpful adjunctive therapy for persistent MRSA infection. Consultation with an infectious diseases specialist is recommended regarding the utility of adding newer gram-positive antibiotics (the oxazolidinone antibiotic linezolid or the lipopeptide antibiotic daptomycin) to eradicate persistent MRSA bacteremia.

3. **Enterococci.** Formerly categorized as members of Group D streptococci, both *Enterococcus faecalis* and *Enterococcus faecium* cause LOS in premature infants. These organisms are associated with indwelling catheters; they are encapsulated organisms that produce both biofilm and slime and can adhere to and persist on catheter surfaces as described in the preceding text for CONS. Although disease can be complicated by meningitis and is sometimes associated with NEC, enterococcal LOS is associated with low overall mortality. Enterococci are resistant to cephalosporins and often resistant to penicillin G and ampicillin; treatment requires the synergistic effect of an aminoglycoside with ampicillin or vancomycin. Vancomycin-resistant enterococci (VRE) present a significant problem in adult intensive care settings, and outbreaks have occurred in NICUs as well. Linezolid, daptomycin and quinupristin/dalfopristin (Synercid) have variable activity against VRE. Linezolid is approved for use in neonates and is effective against vancomycin-resistant *E. faecalis* and *E. faecium*. VRE of *faecium* origin can be treated with quinupristin/dalfopristin but this combination is not effective against *E. faecalis*. Treatment decisions should be made in consultation with infectious diseases experts. VRE outbreaks may also require the institution of infection control measures (surveillance to identify colonized infants, isolation and cohorting of those colonized) to control spread and persistence of the organism.

4. **Gram-negative organisms.** LOS caused by gram-negative organisms is complicated by a 40% mortality rate in the NICHD cohort. *E. coli* were discussed under EOS (see I.I.2.).

   a. *Pseudomonas aeruginosa.* Mortality associated with *P. aeruginosa* sepsis in LBW infants is high (76% in the NICHD cohort). A number of bacterial factors, including LPS, mucoid capsule, adhesins, invasins, and toxins (notably exotoxin A), contribute to its extreme virulence in premature infants as well as in debilitated adults and burn victims. Both LPS and the mucoid capsule help the organism avoid opsonization and secreted proteases inactivate complement, cytokines, and immunoglobulin. The lipid A moiety of LPS (endotoxin) causes the typical aspects of gram-negative septicemia (i.e., hypotension, DIC). Exotoxin A is antigenically distinct from diphtheria toxin, but acts by the same mechanism: adenovirus death protein (ADP)-ribosylation of eukaryotic elongation factor 2 results in inhibition of protein synthesis and cell death. *P. aeruginosa* is present in the intestinal tract of approximately 5% of healthy adults, but colonizes premature infants at much higher rates due to nosocomial acquisition of the bacteria. Selection of the bacteria, likely due to the resistance of *Pseudomonas* to most common antibiotics, also plays a role in colonization; prolonged exposure to IV antibiotics is an identified risk factor for LOS with *Pseudomonas*. *Pseudomonas* can be found in environmental reservoirs in ICUs (i.e., sinks, respiratory equipment), and outbreaks of nosocomial disease have been linked to both environmental sources and spread by the hands of health care workers.

   Treatment requires a combination of two agents active against *Pseudomonas*, such as ceftazidime, piperacillin/tazobactam, gentamicin, or tobramycin. Generally a β-lactam–based antibiotic combined with an aminoglycoside is preferred; however, both extended-spectrum beta-lactamases (ESBL) and constitutive AmpC-type β-lactamases are emerging in pseudomonal species (see subsequent text) and treatment must be guided by isolate antibiotic sensitivity testing. A survey of neonatologists' practices in the treatment of LOS reveals that the most common antibiotics empirically used are vancomycin and gentamicin. When an infant presents as severely ill, or when the infant becomes acutely sicker during or after standard antibiotic treatment, consideration should be given to empiric coverage for *Pseudomonas* until blood culture results are available.

b. *Enterobacter* species. Like *Escherichia coli*, *Enterobacter* species are LPS-containing, gram-negative rods that are normal constituents of colonic flora that can cause overwhelming sepsis in LBW infants. The most common isolates are *Enterobacter cloacae* and *Enterobacter aerogenes*. *Enterobacter sakazakii* has received publicity due to outbreaks of disease caused by contamination of powdered infant formulas with this organism. Although *Enterobacter* species account for <5% of total infections in NICHD and our local data, there are multiple reports of epidemic outbreaks of cephalosporin-resistant *Enterobacter* in NICUs. *Enterobacter* species contain chromosomally encoded, inducible β-lactamases (AmpC-encoded cephalosporinases), and treatment with third-generation cephalosporins, even if the initial isolate appears to be sensitive, can result in the emergence of cephalosporin-resistant organisms. In addition, stably derepressed, high-level, constitutive, AmpC-producing strains of *Enterobacter*, *Citrobacter* and *Serratia* have been reported. The fourth-generation cephalosporin cefepime is relatively stable against AmpC-type β-lactamases. ESBLs (discussed in the subsequent text) have also been reported in the *Enterobacter* species. Given the increasing concern about cephalosporin resistance among infectious disease experts, cefepime or meropenem and gentamicin is usually recommended for treatment of infections caused by *Enterobacter* species. Infection control measures and restriction of cephalosporin use can be effective in controlling outbreaks of resistant organisms.

N. Symptoms and evaluation of LOS. Lethargy, an increase in the number or severity of apneic spells, feeding intolerance, temperature instability, and/or an increase in ventilatory support all may be early signs of LOS—or may be part of the variability in the course of the VLBW infant. The difficulty in distinguishing between these two in part explains the frequency of evaluation for LOS; in the NICHD study, 62% of VLBW infants had at least one blood culture drawn after the third day of life. With mild symptoms and a low suspicion for the presence of sepsis, it is reasonable to draw a CBC with differential and a blood culture and wait for the results of the CBC (while monitoring the infant's symptoms closely) before beginning empiric antibiotic therapy. If the CBC is abnormal or the infant's status worsens, empiric antibiotic therapy should be started. If the suspicion for sepsis is still low, and/or the clinical impression is that a CONS infection is likely, it is not unreasonable to obtain a blood culture only. Ideally cultures of urine and CSF should also be obtained before antibiotic therapy, both to guide empiric therapy and to ensure proper follow-up (such as renal imaging if a UTI is present). A study of late-onset infection in VLBW infants underscores the importance of **performing a LP in the evaluation of LOS** in this population. Two-thirds of a cohort of over 9,000 infants had one or more blood cultures drawn after 72 hours of life; one-third had a LP. Culture-proven meningitis was diagnosed in 134 infants (5% of those on whom a LP was performed) and in 45 out of 134 cases, the coincident blood culture was negative.

If a previously well, convalescing premature infant presents primarily with increased apnea with or without URI symptoms, consideration should be given to a viral source of infection as well. Tracheal or nasal aspirate should be sent for rapid analysis and culture to rule out respiratory syncytial virus (RSV), parainfluenzae, and influenzae A and B if seasonally appropriate.

O. Treatment of LOS. Table 49.1 lists suggested antibiotic regimens for selected organisms. Note that for many antibiotics, dosing is dependent on gestational and postnatal age (see Appendix A). A study of **central line removal** in culture-proven LOS demonstrated that bacteremic infants experience fewer complications of infection if central lines are removed promptly upon identification of a positive culture. This was particularly true for infections caused by *S. aureus* and gram-negative organisms.

ESBLs are plasmid-encoded bacterial enzymes that confer resistance to a variety of penicillins and cephalosporins. ESBLs are distinguished from the generally chromosomally encoded AmpC-type enzymes by sensitivity to clavulanate. Nosocomial gram-negative pathogens that commonly colonize and cause disease in VLBW infants (such as *E. coli*, *Enterobacter*, *Klebsiella*, *Pseudomonas*, and *Serratia*) are increasingly found to harbor these resistance enzymes. ESBL organisms have become a significant problem in adult ICUs. Multiple international reports document an increasing impact of ESBL-producing organisms in NICUs. The magnitude of the problem in American NICUs is limited to case reports of outbreaks, primarily with ESBL-containing *Klebsiella* species. Risk factors for acquiring ESBL organisms include low gestational age and use of third-generation cephalosporins. Current recommendations to control outbreaks of these organisms include restriction of third-generation cephalosporin use and the same infection control measures (routine surveillance for colonization, cohorting and isolation of colonized infants) that are needed for control of MRSA. Treatment of ESBL infections should ideally include consultation with infectious diseases specialists; carbapenems, cefepime, and piperacillin/tazobactam are currently most effective, with increasing rates of coresistance reported for aminoglycosides and fluoroquinolones.

Carbapenemase-producing organisms and other multidrug-resistant organisms (MDROs) have been recently recognized in hospital settings. Carbapenem resistance can occur in gram-negative organisms by either the acquisition of specific enzymes such as the transposon-mediated *Klebsiella pneumoniae* carbapenemase (KPC), or by reduced carbapenem influx caused by the loss of outer membrane protein porins in ESBL organisms. Early recognition of these organisms is critical both for proper individual treatment and to prevent nosocomial spread. This is complicated by the fact that carbapenemase-producing isolates can demonstrate elevated but susceptible carbapenem minimal inhibitory concentrations (MICs) using traditional laboratory methods. The modified Hodge test is recommended for carbapenemase surveillance. Current treatment of infections with most carbapenemase-producing organisms requires the use of the polymyxin B, an antibiotic with significantly toxicity. Recent reports of hospital-acquired infections by extensively drug-resistant *Acinetobacter baumannii* raise the specter of infection with organisms for which no effective treatment exists, underscoring the importance of good infection control practices and responsible use of antibiotics in all intensive care settings.

P. Prevention of LOS. In addition to significant mortality, LOS is associated with prolonged hospitalization and overall poorer outcome in VLBW infants compared to those that remain uninfected. A number of strategies to lower rates of LOS have been studied. These include administration of specific medications and biologics for infection prophylaxis, antibiotic restriction and surveillance policies to prevent antibiotic-resistant infections, and "bundled" implementation of multiple care practices to prevent central-line associated bloodstream infections (CLABSI).

1. **IVIG.** Multiple studies have been conducted using prophylactic administration of IVIG to address the relative deficiency of immunoglobulin in LBW infants and prevent LOS. A meta-analysis of these 19 trials revealed that

although the use of IVIG to prevent LOS resulted in a 3% to 4% decrease in LOS, IVIG was not associated with a decrease in mortality or other serious outcomes and is generally not recommended.

2. **G-CSF.** G-CSF has been shown to resolve preeclampsia-associated neutropenia and may thereby decrease the rate of LOS in this population of infants. One trial of GM-CSF in premature neonates with the clinical diagnosis of early-onset disease did not improve mortality but was associated with acquiring fewer nosocomial infections over the subsequent 2 weeks.

3. **Prophylactic vancomycin.** A meta-analysis of several trials of low-dose vancomycin administration to VLBW infants demonstrated that the administration of prophylactic vancomycin reduced the incidence of both total LOS and CONS-associated infections, but did not improve mortality or length of hospitalization. Prophylactic vancomycin IV lock solution has been studied with some success in decreasing CONS infection. Antibiotic-impregnated catheters are not currently available for VLBW infants. There is concern that widespread use of vancomycin in these ways will lead to the increased emergence of vancomycin-resistant organisms.

4. **Probiotics.** Several clinical trials have evaluated the administration of probiotic formulations in the prevention of both LOS and necrotizing enterocolitis (NEC). A recent meta-analysis of 11 randomized, placebo-controlled trials (most were published since 2005) concluded that probiotic administration significantly reduced the risk of death or NEC among VLBW infants, but found no significant effect on the incidence of LOS. The bacterial formulations and doses used varied among the studies; all included some form of *Lactobacillus* or *Bifidobacterium* species. Some experts feel this evidence is strong enough to offer probiotic formulations to all VLBW infants without further placebo-controlled trials. Others argue that the lack of standardized, regulated probiotic products and the relative lack of data among infants with birth weights of <1,000 g suggest that further study is required.

5. **Lactoferrin.** Lactoferrin is the major whey protein in both human and cow's milk. Present in high concentration in human colostrum, lactoferrin is important to innate immune defense against microbial pathogens, acting by sequestering iron and by impacting microbial membrane integrity. A recent randomized, placebo-controlled trial of oral administration of bovine lactoferrin with or without a *Lactobacillus* probiotic preparation demonstrated a 70% reduction in the incidence of LOS among VLBW infants. Larger trials are needed to determine optimal dose, as well as to define interactions with breast milk feeding and probiotic administration, to determine the full value of this protein in LOS prevention.

6. **Establishment of early enteral feedings** in VLBW infants may have the greatest effect on reducing LOS by reducing exposure to parenteral nutrition and allowing for decreased use of central catheters. **Breast milk** feeding may also help decrease nosocomial infection rates among VLBW infants, both by its numerous infection-protective properties (i.e., secretory immunoglobulin A [IgA], lactoferrin, lysozyme) and by aiding in the establishment of enteral feeds. A retrospective cohort study of 212 VLBW infants from a single center revealed lower rates of LOS in infants receiving breast milk (29%) versus infants receiving formula (47%). Later systematic review of nine studies of the human milk feeding and risk of LOS could not establish that human milk prevents LOS

among VLBW infants. Human milk feeding may impact the risk of LOS by decreasing the time to full enteral feeding and, thus, decreasing the duration of central venous access and use of total parenteral nutrition (TPN).

7. **Antibiotic restriction.** Limitation of the use of broad-spectrum antibiotics in neonatal, pediatric, and adult ICUs has been inconsistently associated with decreased rates of patient colonization with antibiotic-resistant organisms. Cycling of antibiotics used for empiric treatment has not been successful in preventing neonatal LOS or impacting colonization patterns. **However, the widespread emergence of MRSA, VRE and multi drug resistant gram-negative organisms (MDROs) has led to an increased awareness of the risk of empiric use of vancomycin and third-generation cephalosporins among infectious diseases experts.** Some studies suggest that substitution of oxacillin for vancomycin in the empiric treatment of LOS is not likely to cause significant morbidity in VLBW infants because of the low virulence of the organism, and may decrease the acquisition and spread of VRE and other antibiotic-resistant organisms.

8. **Surveillance practices.** Concerns over emergence of MRSA, VRE, and gram-negative MDROs has led to increased interest in the effect of ongoing surveillance to detect neonatal colonization. Multiple reports document the combined use of bacterial surveillance cultures, cohorting, isolation, and in some cases, attempts at decolonization, to control outbreaks of infection with specific pathogens within NICUs. The impact of ongoing, longitudinal surveillance practices is less certain. We have shown that ongoing use of a weekly MRSA surveillance program in our NICU may help prevent patient-to-patient spread of MRSA but did not completely eliminate the introduction of MRSA into the NICU, likely due to the prevalence of this pathogen in the general population. Surveillance programs must be accompanied by strict hand hygiene practices for optimal impact, including reinforcement of hand-washing policies, routine use of waterless hand disinfectants, and restriction of artificial fingernails, natural nails over 1/4-inch length, nail polish, and wearing of rings, watches and bracelets in the NICU setting.

9. **Implementation of recommended best practices to prevent CLABSI.** Most bloodstream infections that occur in VLBW infants are associated with the presence of central venous catheters. CLABSI are defined as culture-proven bloodstream infections occurring in the presence of a central catheter for which there is no other obvious source of infection (i.e., perinatal exposures in EOS, or perforated bowel in NEC). The recognition of significant inter-NICU variation in the incidence of these infections has led to efforts to define optimal care practices associated with lower rates of infection.

Multiple resources are now available to guide optimal care practices for the prevention of CLABSI. The basic components of CLABSI prevention bundles are shown in Table 49.4. The **California Perinatal Quality Care Collaborative (CPQCC)** summarizes and provides critical review of evidence-based practices for neonatal infection prevention in their toolkit, **"Neonatal Hospital-Acquired Infection Prevention,"** last revised in 2008 and available at www.cpqcc.org.

II. ANAEROBIC BACTERIAL INFECTIONS. Anaerobic bacteria comprise a significant portion of the oral, vaginal, and GI flora. Although many anaerobes are of low virulence, a few anaerobic organisms can cause both EOS and LOS. These organisms include the *Bacteroides species* (primarily *B. fragilis*), *Peptostreptococcus*, and

Table 49.4	Components of Neonatal CLABSI Prevention

Hand Hygiene

- Before and after any patient contact
- Before and after donning gloves
- Before central line placement or adjustment

Central Line Care Practices

- Maximal barrier precautions/sterile procedure for insertion
- Formalized daily use and dressing maintenance procedures
- Preparation of parenteral fluids in pharmacy under laminar flow hood
- Standards for timing of administration set changes
- Daily review of central line necessity

Diagnostic Criteria and Reporting Practices

- Optimize practices for obtaining and interpreting blood culture results
- Collect accurate data to determine CLABSI per 1,000 line days
- Communicate CLABSI data and trends to local caregivers
- Benchmark local data against appropriate national standards

Data from: Bowles, Pettitt J, Mickas N, Nisbet C, Proctor T, Wirtschafter D, for the Perinatal Quality Improvement Panel, California Perinatal Quality Care Collaborative. *Neonatal hospital-acquired infection prevention.* Updated March 2008. Available at www.cpqcc.org and O'Grady NP, Alexander M, Dellinger EP, et al. Guidelines for the prevention of intravascular catheter-related infections. *Pediatrics* 2002;110(5):e51.

Clostridia perfringens. NEC and/or bowel perforation can be complicated by anaerobic sepsis alone or by a polymicrobial infection. In addition to bacteremia, *B. fragilis* can cause abdominal abscesses, meningitis, omphalitis, cellulitis at the site of fetal scalp monitors, endocarditis, osteomyelitis, and arthritis in the neonate.

A. **Treatment of anaerobic infections.** Bacteremia and/or meningitis are treated with IV antibiotics; abscesses and other focal infections often require surgical drainage. *B. fragilis* is a gram-negative rod, and although oral *Bacteroides* species are sensitive to penicillin, *B. fragilis* usually requires treatment with drugs such as metronidazole, clindamycin, cefoxitin, or imipenem. Occasional strains of *B. fragilis* are also resistant to clindamycin, cefoxitin, and/or imipenem. Most other cephalosporins and vancomycin are ineffective against *B. fragilis*. *Peptostreptococcus* and *Clostridia* are gram-positive organisms that are sensitive to penicillin G. NEC and intestinal perforations are treated with ampicillin, gentamicin, and clindamycin (or metronidazole) to provide coverage for the spectrum of organisms that can complicate these illnesses.

B. **Neonatal tetanus.** This syndrome is caused by the effect of a neurotoxin produced by the anaerobic bacterium *Clostridium tetani*. Infection can occur by invasion of the umbilical cord due to unsanitary childbirth or cord care practices. It has historically been a significant cause of neonatal mortality in developing countries. An estimated 787,000 deaths due to neonatal tetanus occurred worldwide in 1988. The World Health Organization (WHO) has set multiple target dates for the worldwide elimination of neonatal tetanus since 1989. Elimination has been achieved in many developing countries, but neonatal tetanus persists in remote and poverty-ridden regions, associated with lack of adequate maternal tetanus toxoid immunization and unsanitary delivery settings. WHO estimates 59,000 deaths still occurred worldwide from neonatal tetanus in 2008. This disease is virtually nonexistent in the United States; only three cases were reported to the CDC from 1990 to 2004, associated with inadequately vaccinated mothers; none have been recorded since. Infected infants develop hypertonia and muscle spasms including trismus and consequent inability to feed. Treatment consists of the administration of tetanus toxoid (500 U IM) and penicillin G (100 to 300,000 U/kg/day for 10 to 14 days) as well as supportive care with mechanical ventilation, sedatives, and muscle relaxants. Neonatal tetanus does not result in immunity to tetanus and infants require standard tetanus immunizations after recovery.

III. FUNGAL INFECTIONS

A. **Mucocutaneous candidiasis.** Fungal infections in the well term infant are generally limited to mucocutaneous disease involving *C. albicans*. *Candida* species are normal commensal flora beyond the neonatal period and rarely cause serious disease in the immunocompetent host. Immaturity of host defenses and colonization with *Candida* before complete establishment of normal intestinal flora probably contribute to the pathogenicity of *Candida* in the neonate. Oral and GI colonization with *Candida* occurs before the development of oral candidiasis (thrush) or diaper dermatitis. *Candida* can be acquired through the birth canal, or through the hands or breast of the mother. Nosocomial transmission in the nursery setting has been documented, as has transmission from feeding bottles and pacifiers.

Oral candidiasis in the young infant is treated with a nonabsorbable oral antifungal medication, which has the advantages of little systemic toxicity and concomitant treatment of the intestinal tract. **Nystatin** oral suspension (100,000 U/mL) is standard treatment (1 mL is applied to each side of the mouth every 6 hours, for a minimum of 10 to 14 days). Ideally, treatment is continued for several days after lesions resolve. **Gentian violet** (1%, applied once or twice) is an effective treatment for thrush, but it does not eliminate intestinal fungal colonization. This topical dye has fallen out of favor in the United States: it stains skin and clothing, can irritate the mucosa with prolonged use, and has been shown to be mutagenic *in vitro*. **Miconazole** oral gel (20 mg/g) is also effective, but is only approved for use in the United States in patients 16 years of age and older. Systemic **fluconazole** is highly effective in treating chronic mucocutaneous candidiasis in the immunocompromised host. A 2002 pilot study demonstrated the superiority of oral fluconazole over nystatin suspension in curing thrush in otherwise healthy infants, but fluconazole is not currently approved for this use.

Infants with chronic, severe thrush refractory to treatment should be evaluated for an underlying congenital or acquired immunodeficiency.

Oral candidiasis in the **breastfed infant** is often associated with superficial or ductal candidiasis in the mother's breast. Concurrent treatment of both the mother and infant is necessary to eliminate continual cross-infection. Breastfeeding of term infants can continue during treatment. Mothers with breast ductal candidiasis who are providing expressed breast milk for VLBW infants should be advised to withhold expressed milk until treatment has been instituted. *Candida* can be difficult to detect in breast milk as lactoferrin inhibits the growth of *Candida* in culture. Freezing does not eliminate *Candida* from expressed breast milk.

Candidal diaper dermatitis is effectively treated with topical agents such as 2% nystatin ointment, 2% miconazole ointment, or 1% clotrimazole cream. Concomitant treatment with oral nystatin to eliminate intestinal colonization is often recommended, but not well studied. It is reasonable to use simultaneous oral and topical therapy for refractory candidal diaper dermatitis.

B. **Systemic candidiasis.** Systemic candidiasis is a serious form of nosocomial infection in VLBW infants. Recent data on late-onset candidal sepsis from the NICHD NRN showed that 9% of a cohort of 1,515 infants with birth weights of <1,000 g developed candidal sepsis or meningitis, primarily caused by *C. albicans* and *C. parapsilosis*. One-third of these infants died. Invasive candidiasis is associated with overall poorer neurodevelopmental outcomes and higher rates of threshold retinopathy of prematurity, compared to matched VLBW control infants. GI tract colonization of the LBW infants often precedes invasive infection, and **risk factors for colonization and invasive disease** are similar. The most significant epidemiologic factors specific to candidal LOS in the NICHD cohort studies were birth weights of <1,000 g, presence of a central catheter, delay in enteral feeding, and days of broad-spectrum antibiotic exposure. Other clinical factors included in a recent clinical predictive model for invasive candidiasis in the population with birth weights of <1,000 g include the presence of candidal diaper dermatitis, vaginal delivery, lower gestational age, and significant hypoglycemia and thrombocytopenia. The use of H_2 blockers or systemic steroids has also been identified as independent risk factors for the development of invasive fungal infection.

1. **Microbiology.** Disseminated candidiasis is primarily caused by *C. albicans* and *C. parapsilosis* in preterm infants, but infection with *Candida tropicalis*, *Candida lusitaniae*, *Candida guilliermondii*, *Candida glabrata* and *Candida krusei* are reported less frequently in neonates. The pathogenicity of *C. albicans* is associated with the variable production of a number of toxins, including an endotoxin. *C. albicans* can be acquired perinatally as well as postnatally. *C. parapsilosis* has emerged as the second most common cause of disseminated neonatal candidiasis in recent years. Studies suggest that *C. parapsilosis* is primarily a nosocomial pathogen, in that it is acquired at a later age than *C. albicans* and is associated with colonization of health care workers' hands. In NICHD studies, fungal species (primarily *C. albicans* vs. *C. parapsilosis*) did not independently predict death or later neurodevelopmental impairment, and a delay in removal of central catheters was associated with higher mortality rates from *Candida* LOS regardless of species.

2. **Clinical manifestations.** Candidiasis due to *in utero* infection can occur. Congenital cutaneous candidiasis can present with severe, widespread, and desquamating skin involvement. Pulmonary candidiasis can occur in isolation or with disseminated infection and presents as a severe pneumonia. Most cases of systemic candidiasis, however, present as LOS in VLBW infants, most often after

the second or third week of life. The initial clinical features of **late-onset invasive candidiasis** are often nonspecific, and can include lethargy, increased apnea or need for increased ventilatory support, poor perfusion, feeding intolerance, and hyperglycemia. Both the total WBC and the differential can be normal early in the course of infection, and although thrombocytopenia is a consistent feature, it is not universally found at presentation. The clinical picture is initially difficult to distinguish from sepsis caused by CONS infection, and contrasts with the abrupt onset of septic shock that often accompanies LOS caused by gram-negative organisms. Candidemia can be complicated by meningitis and brain abscess, as well as end-organ involvement of the kidneys, heart, joints, and eyes (endophthalmitis). The fatality rate of disseminated candidiasis is high relative to that found in CONS infections, and increases in the presence of CNS involvement.

3. **Diagnosis.** *Candida* can be cultured from standard pediatric blood culture systems; the time to identification of a positive culture is usually by 48 hours, although late identification (beyond 72 hours) does occur more frequently than with bacterial species. Specialized fungal isolator tubes can aid in the identification of fungal infection if it is suspected by allowing for direct culture on selective media. Both fungal culture and fungal staining (KOH preparation) of urine obtained by suprapubic aspiration can be helpful in making the diagnosis of systemic candidiasis. Specimens obtained by bag urine collection or bladder catheterization are difficult to interpret as they can be readily contaminated with colonizing species. We have obtained urine by SPA from VLBW infants under bedside ultrasound guidance for maximal safety. Before the initiation of antifungal therapy, CSF should be obtained for cell count and fungal culture.

4. **Treatment.** Systemic candidiasis is treated with **amphotericin B**, 0.5 to 1 mg/kg/day for durations of 7 to 14 days after a documented negative blood culture if the infection is considered to be catheter associated and the catheter has been promptly removed. Otherwise, recommended length of treatment for neonatal candidemia is 3 weeks, and for longer periods if specific end-organ infection is present. All common strains of *Candida* other than some strains of *C. lusitaniae*, *C. glabrata*, and *C. krusei* are sensitive to amphotericin. This medication is associated with a variety of dose-dependent immediate and delayed toxicities in older children and adults and can cause phlebitis at the site of infusion. Febrile reactions to the infusion do not usually occur in the LBW infant (although renal and electrolyte disturbances can occur), and we start infants at the higher 1 mg/kg dose from the beginning of treatment. The medication is given slowly (over 4–6 hours) to minimize the risk of seizures and arrhythmias during the infusion. There is increased experience in VLBW babies with **liposomal preparations of amphotericin B**, and we now use this formulation routinely for invasive candidiasis if urinary tract and CNS involvement are excluded. Doses of 5 mg/kg/day can be used without toxicity, and the medication can be given over 2 hours with less irritation at the site of infusion. It is recommended that CNS disease be treated with an additional second agent, commonly **5-fluorocytosine (flucytosine 5-FC) (50–150 mg/kg/day) or fluconazole (6 mg/kg/day).** Flucytosine achieves good CNS penetration and appears to be safe in infants, but is only available for enteral administration, limiting its utility in sick VLBW infants. Bone marrow and liver toxicity has occurred in adults and correlates with elevated serum levels of the medication. Serum levels can be monitored (40–60 μg/mL is desirable). Fluconazole is safe for use in infants and can be

successfully used for primary treatment of candidemia. It should not be used until candidal speciation is completed, because *C. krusei* and *C. glabrata* are frequently resistant to fluconazole.

Removal of central catheters in place, when candidemia is identified, is essential to the eradication of the infection. Delayed catheter removal is associated with persistent candidemia and increased mortality.

Further evaluation of the infant with invasive candidiasis should include renal and brain ultrasonography to rule out fungal abscess formation and opthalmologic examination to rule out endophthalmitis. In infants who are persistently fungemic despite catheter removal and appropriate therapy, an echocardiogram to rule out endocarditis or vegetation formation is warranted.

5. **Prevention.** Minimizing use of broad-spectrum antibiotics (particularly cephalosporins and carbapenems) and H_2 blockers may be helpful in preventing disseminated candidiasis. The CDC recommends changing infusions of lipid suspensions every 12 hours to minimize microbial contamination; solutions of parenteral nutrition and lipid mixtures should be changed every 24 hours. Several randomized, placebo-controlled trials of **prophylactic fluconazole administration** to prevent invasive fungal infection in VLBW infants have been published since 2001. All the trials demonstrated decreased rates of colonization with fungal species and most also demonstrated decreased rates of invasive fungal infection. The largest randomized trial of infants with birth weights of <1,000 g demonstrated a 63% decrease in colonization and statistically significant decrease in invasive fungal disease (from 20% in placebo group to 0% in treatment group), with no adverse effects. Different meta-analyses of fluconazole prophylaxis studies differ in the assessment of the impact on mortality, but most evidence supports a decrease in the overall risk of death, in death from *Candida* infection, and in the combined outcome of death or invasive candidiasis. The widespread implementation of any fluconazole prophylaxis regimen has been limited by the concern that when infants receiving prophylaxis do become colonized or develop invasive fungal disease, the isolates are more likely to be less fluconazole-sensitive *Candida* species. However, a 2002 to 2006 study of fluconazole prophylaxis in 362 infants with birth weights of <1,000 g found no evidence for the emergence of fluconazole resistance. The impact of fluconazole itself on long-term neurodevelopmental outcome is uncertain and also of concern. These risks must be balanced with the potentially severe consequences of invasive fungal infection (in the NICHD cohort, 73% of infants with LOS fungal sepsis died or survived with significant neurodevelopmental impairment), as well as the frequency of LOS fungal infection in an individual NICU in making a decision to implement a fluconazole prophylaxis policy.

C. **Malassezia furfur.** This organism is a lipophilic dermatophyte that readily colonizes infants in neonatal units and is found in 30% to 60% of neonates over time. *M. furfur* requires exogenous long-chain fatty acids for growth and readily contaminates and proliferates in IV lipid preparations, as well as on the catheters used for administration of lipids. It causes a nonspecific sepsis syndrome. *M. furfur* grows poorly in standard pediatric blood culture bottles, but isolation is optimized by the addition of a lipid source to the bottles or by the use of fungal isolator systems and the addition of sterile olive oil to the selective media. In most reported cases, removal of the contaminated central catheter results in a cure; amphotericin B is effective when catheter removal alone does not resolve the fungemia.

IV. FOCAL BACTERIAL INFECTIONS (see Chap. 63)

A. **Skin Infections.** The newborn may develop a variety of rashes associated with both systemic and focal bacterial disease. Responsible organisms include all of the usual causes of EOS (GBS, enteric gram-negative rods, and anaerobes) as well as gram-positive organisms that specifically colonize the skin—staphylococci and other streptococci. Colonization of the newborn skin occurs with organisms acquired from vaginal flora as well as from the environment. **Sepsis** can be accompanied by skin manifestations such as maculopapular rashes, erythema multiforme, and petechiae or purpura. **Localized infections** can arise in any site of traumatized skin: in the scalp at lesions caused by intrapartum fetal monitors or blood gas samples, in the penis and surrounding tissues due to circumcision, in the extremities at sites of venipuncture or IV placement, or in the umbilical stump (omphalitis.) Generalized pustular skin infections can occur due to *S. aureus*, occasionally in epidemic fashion.

1. **Cellulitis** usually occurs at traumatized skin sites as noted in the preceding text. Localized erythema and/or drainage in a term infant (e.g., at a scalp electrode site) can be treated with careful washing and local antisepsis with antibiotic ointment (bacitracin or mupirocin ointment) and close monitoring. Cellulitis at sites of IV access or venipuncture in premature infants must be addressed in a more aggressive fashion due to the risk of local and systemic spread, particularly in the VLBW infant. If the premature infant with a localized cellulitis is well appearing, a CBC and blood culture should be obtained and IV antibiotics administered to provide coverage primarily for skin flora (i.e., oxacillin or nafcillin and gentamicin). If MRSA is a concern in a particular setting, vancomycin should be substituted for nafcillin. If blood cultures are negative, the infant can be treated for a total of 5 to 7 days with resolution of the cellulitis. If an organism grows from the blood culture, a LP should be performed to rule out meningitis, and careful physical examination should be performed to rule out accompanying osteomyelitis or septic arthritis. Therapy is guided by the organism identified (see Table 49.1).

2. **Pustulosis.** Infectious pustulosis is usually caused by *S. aureus* and must be distinguished from the benign neonatal rash erythema toxicum and transient pustular melanosis. The pustules are most commonly found in the axillae, groin, and periumbilical area; both erythema toxicum and transient pustular melanosis have a more generalized distribution. Lesions can be unroofed after cleansing in sterile fashion with betadine or 4% chlorhexidine, and contents aspirated and analyzed by a Gram stain and culture. Gram stain of infectious pustules will reveal neutrophils and gram-positive cocci, whereas Wright stain of erythema toxicum lesions will reveal predominantly eosinophils and no (or a few contaminating) organisms. Gram stain of transient pustular melanosis lesions will reveal neutrophils but no organisms. Cultures of the benign rashes will be sterile or grow contaminating organisms such as *S. epidermidis*. Treatment of pustulosis caused by *S. aureus* is tailored to the degree of involvement and condition of the infant. A few lesions in a healthy term infant may be treated with topical mupirocin and oral therapy with medications such as amoxicillin/clavulanate, dicloxacillin, or cephalexin. More extensive lesions, systemic illness, or pustulosis occurring in the premature infant requires IV therapy with nafcillin or oxacillin.

Some strains of *S. aureus* produce toxins that can cause **bullous lesions or scalded skin syndrome.** The cutaneous changes are due to local and systemic spread of toxin. Although blood cultures may be negative, IV antibiotics should be given (nafcillin or oxacillin) until the progression of disease stops and skin lesions are healing.

Pediatricians who diagnose infectious pustulosis in an infant under 2 weeks of age should report the case to the birth hospital; **epidemic outbreaks due to nosocomial acquisition in newborn nurseries** are often recognized in this way because the rash may not occur until after hospital discharge. This has become particularly important with the emergence of MRSA infections among infants <1 month in the community. When such outbreaks are recognized in the nursery or NICU, hospital infection control experts should be consulted. Appropriate steps may include surveillance cultures of staff members and newborns and cohorting of colonized infants.

3. **Omphalitis.** Omphalitis is characterized by erythema and/or induration of the periumbilical area with purulent discharge from the umbilical stump. The infection can progress to widespread abdominal wall cellulitis or necrotizing fasciitis; complications such as peritonitis, umbilical arteritis or phlebitis, hepatic vein thrombosis, and hepatic abscess have all been described. Responsible organisms include both gram-positive and gram-negative species. Treatment consists of a full sepsis evaluation (CBC, blood culture, LP) and empiric IV therapy with oxacillin or nafcillin and gentamicin. With serious disease progression, broader spectrum gram-negative coverage with a cephalosporin or piperacillin/tazobactam should be considered. As noted in II.A, Treatment of Anaerobic Infections, invasion of the umbilical stump by *C. tetani* under conditions of poor sanitation can result in neonatal tetanus in the infant of an unimmunized mother.

B. **Conjunctivitis (ophthalmia neonatorum).** This condition refers to the inflammation of the conjunctiva within the first month of life. Causative agents include topical medications (chemical conjunctivitis), bacteria, and herpes simplex viruses. Chemical conjunctivitis is most commonly seen with silver nitrate eye prophylaxis, requires no specific treatment, and usually resolves within 48 hours. Bacterial causes include *Neisseria gonorrhoeae* and *Chlamydia trachomatis*, as well as staphylococci, streptococci, and gram-negative organisms. In the United States, where routine birth prophylaxis against opthalmia neonatorum is practiced, the incidence of this disease is very low. In developing countries in the absence of prophylaxis, the incidence is 20% to 25% and remains a major cause of blindness.

1. **Prophylaxis against infectious conjunctivitis.** One percent silver nitrate solution (1–2 drops to each eye), 0.5% erythromycin opthalmic ointment or 1% tetracycline ointment (1-cm strip to each eye), and 2.5% povidone-iodine solution (1 drop to each eye) administered within 1 hour of birth are all effective in the prevention of opthalmia neonatorum. In a trial comparing the use of these three agents conducted in Kenya, povidone-iodine was shown to be slightly more effective against both *C. trachomatis* and other causes of infectious conjunctivitis, and equally effective against *N. gonorrhoeae* and *S. aureus*. Povidone-iodine was associated with less noninfectious conjunctivitis and is less costly than the other two agents; in addition, this agent is not associated with the development of bacterial resistance. However, an ophthalmic preparation of povidone-iodine solution is not currently available in the United States. In our institution, where most mothers receive prenatal care and the incidences of chlamydia and gonorrhea are low, we use erythromycin ointment. Silver nitrate or povidone-iodine are the preferred agents in areas where the incidence of penicillinase-producing *N. gonorrhoeae* is high.

2. **N. gonorrhoeae.** Pregnant women should be screened for *N. gonorrhoeae* as part of routine prenatal care. High-risk women or women without prenatal care should be screened at delivery. If a mother is known to have untreated *N. gonorrhoeae* infection, the infant should receive **ceftriaxone 25 to 50 mg/kg IV or IM (not to exceed 125 mg) or one dose of cefotaxime (100 mg/kg IV or IM) at birth.**

   Gonococcal conjunctivitis presents with chemosis, lid edema, and purulent exudate beginning 1 to 4 days after birth. Clouding of the cornea or panophthalmitis can occur. Gram stain and culture of conjunctival scrapings will confirm the diagnosis. The treatment of infants with uncomplicated gonococcal conjunctivitis requires only a single dose of ceftriaxone (25–50 mg/kg IV or IM, not to exceed 125 mg). Additional topical treatment is unnecessary. However, infants with gonococcal conjunctivitis should be hospitalized and screened for invasive disease (i.e., sepsis, meningitis, arthritis). Scalp abscesses can result from internal fetal monitoring. Treatment of these complications is ceftriaxone (25–50 mg/kg/day IV or IM q24h) or cefotaxime (25 mg/kg IV or IM q12h) for 7 to 14 days (10–14 days for meningitis). The infant and mother should be screened for coincident chlamydial infection.

3. **C. trachomatis.** Pregnant women should be screened for **C. trachomatis** as part of routine prenatal care. Prophylaxis for infants born to mothers with untreated chlamydial infection is not indicated. Chlamydial conjunctivitis is the most common identified cause of infectious conjunctivitis in the United States. It presents with variable degrees of inflammation, yellow discharge, and eyelid swelling 5 to 14 days after birth. Conjunctival scarring can occur, although the cornea is usually not involved. DNA hybridization tests or shell vial culture are used to detect *Chlamydia* in conjunctival specimens. NAATs are commercially available and more sensitive than direct hybridization or culture methods, but NAATs are not currently FDA-approved for detecting *Chlamydia* in conjunctival specimens. Chlamydial conjunctivitis is treated with oral **erythromycin base or ethylsuccinate 40 mg/kg/day divided into 4 doses for 14 days.** Topical treatment alone is not adequate and is unnecessary when systemic therapy is given. An association of oral erythromycin therapy and infantile hypertrophic pyloric stenosis has been reported in infants younger than 6 weeks. Infants should be monitored for this condition. The efficacy of treatment is approximately 80%, and infants must be evaluated for treatment failure and the need for a second course of treatment. Infants should also be evaluated for the concomitant presence of chlamydial pneumonia. The treatment for pneumonia is the same as for conjunctivitis, in addition to necessary supportive respiratory care.

4. **Other bacterial conjunctivitis.** Other causes are generally diagnosed by culture of eye exudate. *S. aureus*, *E. coli*, and *H. influenzae* can cause conjunctivitis that is usually easily treated with local ophthalmic ointments (erythromycin or gentamicin) without complication. Very severe cases caused by *H. influenzae* may require parenteral treatment and evaluation for sepsis and meningitis. *P. aeruginosa* can cause a rare and devastating form of conjunctivitis that requires parenteral treatment.

C. **Pneumonia.** The diagnosis of **neonatal pneumonia** is challenging. It is difficult to distinguish primary (occurring from birth) neonatal bacterial pneumonia clinically from sepsis with respiratory compromise, or radiographically from other causes of respiratory distress (hyaline membrane disease, retained fetal lung fluid, meconium aspiration, amniotic fluid aspiration). Persistent focal opacifications on chest radiograph due to neonatal pneumonia are uncommon, and their presence should prompt some consideration of noninfectious causes of focal lung opacification (such as congenital cystic lesions or pulmonary sequestration). The causes of neonatal bacterial pneumonia are the same as for EOS, and antibiotic treatment is generally the same as for sepsis. The infant's baseline risk for infection, radiographic and laboratory studies, and, most important, the clinical progression must all be taken into account when making the diagnosis of neonatal pneumonia.

The diagnosis of **nosocomial, or ventilator-associated pneumonia** in neonates who are ventilator dependent due to chronic lung disease or other illness, is equally challenging. Culture of tracheal secretions in infants who are chronically ventilated can yield a variety of organisms, including all the causes of EOS and LOS as well as (often antibiotic-resistant) gram-negative organisms that are endemic within a particular NICU. A distinction must be made between colonization of the airway and true tracheitis or pneumonia. Culture results must be taken together with the infant's respiratory and systemic condition, as well as radiographic and laboratory studies when making the diagnosis of nosocomial pneumonia.

Ureaplasma urealyticum deserves mention with respect to chronically ventilated infants. This mycoplasmal organism frequently colonizes the vagina of pregnant women and has been associated with chorioamnionitis, spontaneous abortion, and premature delivery, and infection of the premature infant. Infection with *Ureaplasma* has been studied as a contributing factor to the development of chronic lung disease, but the role of the organism and the value of diagnosis and treatment is unclear and controversial. *Ureaplasma* requires special culture conditions and will grow within 2 to 5 days. PCR-based diagnostics have been developed but are not widely available. It will not be identified on routine bacterial culture. It is sensitive to erythromycin, but is difficult to eradicate, and few data are available on the dosing, treatment duration, and efficacy of treatment when this organism is found in tracheal secretions. Only two small randomized trials of erythromycin treatment to prevent chronic lung disease have been published and neither demonstrated a change in the incidence or severity of bronchopulmonary dysplasia (BPD).

D. **Urinary Tract Infection (UTI)** may occur secondary to bacteremia, or bacteremia may occur secondary to primary UTI. UTI is a common cause of infection among febrile infants less than 3 months of age. The incidence is slightly higher in females, but highest among uncircumcised males. Among community infants who present with febrile UTI, the prevalence of vesicoureteral reflux (VUR) diagnosed on subsequent vesico urethrocystogram (VCUG) is approximately 20%. The incidence of UTI among VLBW infants in the NICU is much less well documented. Evaluation for infection in this population often excludes urine culture, focusing on central line, pulmonary, and GI sources of infection. A recent single-center study found culture-proven UTI occurred in 1.6% of all NICU admissions during a 10-year period. The infants with UTI had a mean gestational age of 28 weeks, were predominantly male and only 8% had a concurrent bacteremia. Less than 5% had identified anomalies on subsequent renal imaging.

The most common causative organisms are gram-negative, such as *E. coli*, but enterococci and staphylococci can also cause UTI, especially among VLBW NICU infants. Culture of urine is not routinely recommended as part of the evaluation for EOS but is an essential part of the evaluation for LOS (see section I.N.). The most common presenting symptoms in term and older preterm infants are fever, lethargy, and poor feeding; younger preterm infants will present as for LOS. Diagnosis is made by urinalysis and urine culture. Culture of urine obtained from a bag collection or diaper is of little value as it will commonly be contaminated with skin and fecal flora. Specimens should be obtained by bladder catheterization or suprapubic bladder aspiration with sterile technique. Ultrasound guidance can be useful in performing suprapubic aspirate in the VLBW infant. Empiric treatment in term and preterm infants is as for LOS (see I. J.); antibiotic choice and treatment duration is guided by blood, urine, and CSF culture results. If the urine culture **alone** is positive in a term infant, treatment is completed with oral therapy once the infant is afebrile. Treatment duration in the absence of a positive blood or CSF culture is 10 to 14 days. It is recommended that infants with UTI undergo renal ultrasound and vesico urethrocystogram (VCUG) imaging to identify any underlying anatomic or functional abnormalities (i.e., VUR) that may have contributed to the development of the UTI. Traditionally infants have received UTI prophylaxis with amoxicillin (10 to 20 mg/kg once per day) after completing UTI treatment until imaging studies are performed and have continued with prophylaxis if VUR is documented. Several recent meta-analyses have found little to no value in antibiotic prophylaxis for VUR, although it remains widely used.

E. **Osteomyelitis and septic arthritis.** These focal infections are rare in newborns and may result from hematogenous seeding in the setting of bacteremia, or direct extension from a skin source of infection. The most common organisms are *S. aureus*, GBS, and gram-negative organisms including *N. gonorrhoeae*. Symptoms include localized erythema, swelling, and apparent pain or lack of spontaneous movement of the involved extremity. The hip, knee, and wrist are commonly involved in septic arthritis, and the femur, humerus, tibia, radius, and maxilla are the most common bone sites of infection. The evaluation should be as for sepsis, including blood, urine, and CSF culture, and culture of any purulent skin lesions. Needle aspiration of an infected joint is sometimes possible, and plain film and ultrasound can aid in diagnosis. Empiric treatment is with nafcillin or oxacillin and gentamicin, and/or vancomycin if MRSA is a concern and is later tailored to any identified organisms. Joint infections commonly require surgical drainage; material can be sent for Gram stain and culture at surgery. Duration of therapy is 3 to 4 weeks. Significant disability can result from joint or growth plate damage.

Suggested Readings

Benjamin DK, Stoll BJ, Gantz MG, et al. Neonatal candidiasis: epidemiology, risk factors and clinical judgment. *Pediatrics* 2010;126(4):e865–e873.

Isenberg SJ, Apt L, Wood M. A controlled trial of povidone-iodine as prophylaxis against ophthalmia neonatorum. *N Engl J Med* 1995;332(9):562–566.

Kaufman D, Boyle R, Hazen KC, et al. Fluconazole prophylaxis against fungal colonization and infection in preterm infants. *N Engl J Med* 2001;345(23):1660–1666.

Moore MR, Schrag SJ, Schuchat A. Effects of intrapartum antimicrobial prophylaxis for prevention of group-B-streptococcal disease on the incidence and ecology of early-onset neonatal sepsis. *Lancet Infect Dis* 2003;3:201–213.

Newman TB, Puopolo KM, Wi S, et al. Interpreting complete blood counts soon after birth in newborns at risk for sepsis. *Pediatrics* 2010;126(5):903–909.

O'Grady NP, Alexander M, Dellinger EP, et al. Guidelines for the prevention of intravascular catheter-related infections. *Pediatrics* 2002;110(5):e51.

Puopolo KM, Eichenwald EC. No change in the incidence of ampicillin-resistant, neonatal, early-onset sepsis over 18 years. *Pediatrics* 2010;125(5):e1031–e1038.

Stoll BJ, Hansen N, Fanaroff AA, et al. Late-onset sepsis in very low birth weight neonates: the experience of the NICHD Neonatal Research Network. *Pediatrics* 2002;110(2 pt 1): 285–291.

50 Congenital Toxoplasmosis

Lucila Marquez and Debra Palazzi

I. EPIDEMIOLOGY. *Toxoplasma gondii*—an obligate, intracellular protozoan parasite—is an important human pathogen, especially for the fetus, newborn, and immunocompromised patient.

A. Transmission

1. The cat, the only definitive host, is usually asymptomatic. During acute infection, millions of oocysts are shed daily in the stool for 2 weeks or longer. Oocysts may remain viable in the soil for over 1 year in some climates. Other animals become infected by ingesting the oocysts resulting in tissue cysts containing viable organisms, predominately in muscle and brain.

2. *Toxoplasma* can be acquired through food, water, or soil contaminated with oocysts or through ingestion of cysts in undercooked meat. The meat products most often implicated include pork and lamb. Food products that have been implicated include mussels, produce such as raspberries, and unpasteurized milk.

3. Congenital infection can occur through transplacental transmission.

B. The **prevalence** of *Toxoplasma* antibody increases with age and varies by geographic location and population. Data from one area or population may not accurately be generalized to other areas or populations. Based on data from the National Health and Nutrition Examination Survey (NHANES), the seroprevalence in persons ages 12 to 49 in the United States is 15.8%. The reported prevalence of *T. gondii* antibodies in women of childbearing age ranges from 4% to 80% worldwide. Women without antibodies are at risk for acute toxoplasmosis during pregnancy.

C. Seroconversion during pregnancy also varies by geographic location. Rates range from 1.5% in France, a high prevalence country, to 0.17% in Norway, a low prevalence country. The National Collaborative Perinatal Project (National Institutes of Health) estimated the rate at 1.1 in 1,000 in the United States.

D. The reported **incidence** of congenital toxoplasmosis in the United States has decreased during the last 20 years, from a high of 20 in 10,000 to 1 in 10,000. In the United States, an estimated 500 to 5,000 infants are born each year with congenital toxoplasmosis.

II. PATHOPHYSIOLOGY

A. Normal children and adults are susceptible to acute infection if they lack specific antibody to the organism. Both humoral and cell-mediated immunity are important in the control of infection. Transmission usually occurs by direct ingestion of oocysts or ingestion of the cysts in undercooked meat. After acute parasitemia, the organism forms tissue cysts, which probably persist for life in multiple organs including muscle and brain. Usually, these are of little consequence to the normal host, but progressive, localized, or reactivated disease may occur.

B. Human congenital infection

1. Placental pathology suggests that parasites from the maternal circulation invade and multiply within placental cells before reaching the fetal circulation. This delay in transmission from the placenta to the fetus, called the *prenatal incubation period*, ranges from under 4 weeks to over 16 weeks.

2. The risk of congenital infection increases with gestational age, occurring in 6% of infants whose mothers seroconvert at 13 weeks' gestation and 72% at 36 weeks. The fetal disease severity, however, is inversely proportional to gestational age; 61% of infants will have clinical manifestations when seroconversion occurs at 13 weeks' gestation in contrast to 9% at 36 weeks. Without prenatal therapy, most fetuses infected in the first trimester die *in utero* or in the neonatal period or have severe central nervous system (CNS) and ophthalmologic disease. Conversely, most fetuses infected in the second trimester, and almost all infants infected in the third trimester have mild or subclinical disease in the newborn period. Therefore, the period of highest risk for severe congenital disease is thought to be between 10 and 24 weeks.

3. Congenital infection due to serologic relapse in chronic maternal infection is extremely rare. Maternal immune dysfunction, including human immunodeficiency virus (HIV) infection, should be suspected if this occurs.

III. MATERNAL/FETAL INFECTION

A. Clinical manifestations

1. Maternal infection is asymptomatic in more than 90% of women. However, symptoms can include fatigue, painless lymphadenopathy, and chorioretinitis.

2. Fetal findings on ultrasound include hydrocephalus, brain and hepatic calcifications, hepatosplenomegaly, and ascites.

B. Diagnosis

1. **Recommended maternal tests**
   a. Screening: Serum immunoglobulin G (IgG) and immunoglobulin M (IgM)
   i. After infection, IgG is detectable in 1 to 2 weeks, peaks in 3 to 6 months, and persists at low titers for life. The Sabin-Feldman dye test is the most reliable IgG assay but available in only a few reference labs. Direct agglutination tests are accurate. Immunofluorescent assay (IFA) test and enzyme-linked immunosorbent assay (ELISA) are not consistently reliable. Indirect hemagglutination should not be used for screening pregnant women.
   ii. IgM appears within 2 weeks after infection, peaks at 1 month, and usually declines to undetectable levels within 6 to 9 months. However, IgM may persist for more than 1 year after initial infection and, thus, does not necessarily indicate an acute infection.

    iii. It is recommended that a *Toxoplasma* reference laboratory confirm all positive or equivocal IgM test results. The serologic tests discussed here are available as panels and are performed by the Toxoplasma Serology Laboratory at Palo Alto, California (available at: http://www.pamf.org/serology).

  b. Confirmatory: IgG; IgM; immunoglobulin A (IgA); immunoglobulin E (IgE). A series of IgG tests can help differentiate acute vs. remote infection.

    i. Avidity testing (IgG) may differentiate acute vs. remote infection. IgG antibodies produced early in infection have low avidity, but avidity increases over time. The presence of high-avidity antibodies indicates that infection occurred 12 to 16 weeks prior; thus, testing is useful in early pregnancy. The test has limitations, however, as slow maturation of this high-avidity response has been reported in pregnant women. This test is not commercially available in the United States.

    ii. Differential agglutination detects rising IgG titers. Rising titers indicate acute infection.

    iii. Differential agglutination test AC/HS compares IgG titers for sera against formalin (HS) vs. acetone (AC)-fixed tachyzoites. The AC preparation is recognized by antibodies early in infection.

  2. Fetal testing

    a. Ultrasound is recommended monthly in women suspected of having acute infection.

    b. Amniotic fluid polymerase chain reaction (PCR) is recommended to diagnose fetal infection in cases where there is serologic evidence of acute infection, ultrasound evidence of fetal damage, or severe maternal immunocompromise. High parasite DNA levels can be found in cases in which infection occurred earlier in gestation or sequelae are more severe. A negative amniotic fluid PCR does not rule out fetal infection as the accuracy range is wide and parasite transmission from the mother to the fetus may be delayed. PCR sensitivity for the B1 gene is high (>90%) when maternal infection occurs between 17 to 21 weeks' gestation, and is lower (29%–68%) before 17 weeks and after 21 weeks. In suspected or probable cases, antenatal maternal therapy to prevent or treat fetal infection should extend until delivery, even with a negative PCR result.

C. Treatment

  1. Medications. Treatment should be instituted for mothers with acute infections and immunocompromised mothers with evidence of distant infection. In some studies, treatment has reduced fetal infection by 50%. Prompt treatment may prevent irreversible *in utero* retinal and brain damage.

    a. Spiramycin (prophylaxis) can prevent placental transmission of *Toxoplasma* but does not treat the fetus. It is recommended for women suspected of having acquired infection before 18 weeks' gestation. This macrolide antibiotic reduces or delays vertical transmission to the fetus through high placental drug levels (3–5 times maternal serum levels). However, if transmission occurs, disease severity may be unaltered. Spiramycin should be continued until delivery if the fetus is uninfected by amniotic fluid PCR (usually performed at 15–17 weeks). Spiramycin is available in the United States as an *investigational new drug* through the Food and Drug Administration.

b. Pyrimethamine, sulfadiazine, and folinic acid treatment cannot be used prior to 18 weeks' gestation. Therefore, these drugs are recommended for infections acquired after 18 weeks' gestation or when fetal infection is confirmed by amniotic fluid PCR starting at 18 weeks' gestation (or if amniocentesis cannot be performed). Pyrimethamine can cause bone marrow suppression.

2. Therapeutic abortion is considered by some families. When infection occurs before 16 weeks' gestation, prognosis can be severe with brain necrosis despite lack of ventricular dilation by ultrasonography.

IV. NEONATAL INFECTION

A. Clinical manifestations

1. **There are four recognized patterns of presentation for congenital toxoplasmosis**
   a. Subclinical infection. At present, the outcome of a newborn that is asymptomatic cannot be predicted. Most infants with congenital toxoplasmosis (80%–90%) do not have overt signs of infection at birth but may have retinal and CNS abnormalities when further testing is performed. The New England Regional Newborn Screening Program (1986–1992) identified 52 cases of congenital toxoplasmosis in 635,000 infants screened for IgM antibody to *T. gondii*. Fifty infants were full term, asymptomatic, and had normal physical examinations. After confirming congenital infection, CNS or retina abnormalities were identified in 19 of 48 infants.
   b. Neonatal symptomatic disease is usually severe, can be generalized, and neurologic signs are invariably present. Common generalized symptoms include fever, hepatosplenomegaly, and jaundice. CNS abnormalities include hydrocephalus, microcephaly, seizures, cerebral calcifications, cerebrospinal fluid (CSF) abnormalities, and chorioretinitis.
   c. Delayed onset is most often seen with premature infants and occurs within the first 3 months of age. It can behave like neonatal symptomatic disease.
   d. Sequelae or relapse in infancy through adolescence of a previously undiagnosed infection occurs in 24% to 85% of infected patients. Most commonly, eye (chorioretinitis) or neurologic (seizures, late CSF obstruction) findings develop. Close to 30% of congenitally infected adults will have retinal damage. The peak presentation of chorioretinitis from congenital infection occurs between the ages of 15 to 20 years.

2. **Specific symptoms.** Hydrocephalus, chorioretinitis, and intracranial calcifications are the classic triad, but disease is usually a clinical spectrum.
   a. Neurologic. These can include signs of CSF obstruction (bulging fontanelle, increased head circumference), seizures, motor deficits, and deafness. Encephalitis may be present with CSF abnormalities or cerebral calcifications. The neonate may have evidence of endocrine dysfunction or difficulties with temperature regulation depending on the areas of the brain that are affected. Active encephalitis and obstructive hydrocephalus from edema and inflammation may respond well to treatment.
   b. Ophthalmologic. Toxoplasmosis is one of the most common causes of chorioretinitis and can lead to visual impairment. In congenital toxoplasmosis, lesions are usually bilateral. External findings can include strabismus, nystagmus, cataracts, and microcornea. Fundoscopic findings include focal

necrotizing retinitis; yellow–white, cotton-like patches; and edema. Macular lesions are more common than peripheral lesions. Vitreous exudates may prevent visualization of the fundus. In the National Collaborative Congenital Toxoplasmosis (NCCT) study of patients with eye disease, 22% of patients had active lesions if not treated in the first year compared with 8% of treated patients. Chorioretinal scars were seen in 100% of untreated patients vs. 74% of treated patients. Other manifestations include phthisis (destruction of the globe), retinal detachment, optic atrophy, iritis, scleritis, uveitis, and vitreitis.

   c. Other common symptoms include hepatosplenomegaly, persistent conjugated hyperbilirubinemia (from liver damage or hemolysis), and thrombocytopenia. Dermatologic findings include a maculopapular rash. Some patients have lymphadenopathy, anemia, and hypogammaglobulinemia.

   d. Rare presentations include erythroblastosis and hydrops fetalis, myocarditis, pneumonitis, and nephritic syndrome.

   e. Special cases. Infected infants are commonly born premature (25%–50%). Monozygotic twins often have similar patterns of infection in contrast to dizygotic twins. Neonates born to HIV-infected mothers are often asymptomatic, only to develop severe disseminated infection during the first weeks or months of age.

3. Differential diagnosis

   a. The clinical and laboratory findings are common to congenital infections caused by rubella, cytomegalovirus (CMV), syphilis, neonatal herpes simplex virus, HIV, and lymphocytic choriomeningitis virus (LCMV).

   b. Other disorders to be considered include hepatitis B, varicella, bacterial sepsis, hemolytic diseases, metabolic disorders, immune thrombocytopenia, histiocytosis, and congenital leukemia.

B. Diagnosis. All neonates suspected of having congenital toxoplasmosis based on symptoms, maternal acute *Toxoplasma* infection during pregnancy, or maternal HIV with a history of chronic *Toxoplasma* infection should be evaluated. Diagnosis may be made by serology, PCR, histology, or isolation of the parasite. Currently, only Massachusetts, New Hampshire, and Vermont screen all neonates.

1. Recommended neonatal tests: IgG, IgM, IgA, and IgE. Sabin-Feldman dye test (IgG), IgM immunosorbent agglutination assay (ISAGA), IgA ELISA, IgE ISAGA or ELISA.

   a. IgG appears within 1 to 2 weeks, peaks at 1 to 2 months, and persists throughout life. Transplacental IgG antibody disappears by 6 to 12 months of age. For patients with seroconversion or a fourfold rise in IgG antibody titer, perform IgM testing.

   b. Because **IgM** and **IgA** do not cross the placenta, they are useful in determining congenital infection. If maternal blood contamination is possible, repeat the IgM, IgA, and IgE testing in a few days. In infants who are IgM and IgA negative, the traditional means of diagnosis is to wait for clearance of transplacental IgG at about 12 months of age.

   c. The sensitivity of some IgM assays is poor and dependent on the gestational age at infection; a sensitivity of 50% is reached at 30 weeks' gestation. ELISA and ISAGA are more sensitive than IFA, which has a sensitivity of 25%. IFA is also fraught with false-positives from antinuclear antibodies.

d. IgA rises rapidly, and it usually disappears by 7 months (uncommonly, more than 1 year). IgA may have greater sensitivity for neonates compared with IgM assays. IgE rises rapidly and does not persist as long as IgM and IgA (under 4 months).

e. In congenital toxoplasmosis, antibody production varies significantly and is affected by treatment.

2. **Description of serologic assays**

   a. The Sabin-Feldman dye test (IgG) uses the uptake of methylene blue by *Toxoplasma* tachyzoites (organisms appear swollen and blue). The tachyzoite membranes lyse in the presence of complement and IgG-specific antibody (organisms appear thin and unstained). There is extensive experience with this test, particularly as an antenatal screen for maternal seroconversion in pregnancy.

   b. IFA (IgG, IgM) uses fluorescein-tagged antiserum against Ig to detect antibody binding to *Toxoplasma* slide preparations. In general, IgG IFA and the dye test qualitatively agree.

   c. Double-sandwich ELISA (IgM, IgA, IgE) uses wells coated with specific antibody to IgM to detect IgM in serum. A second antibody to IgM linked to an enzyme is added. The enzyme converts substrate into a fluorescent signal.

   d. The ISAGA (IgM, IgA, IgE) measures *Toxoplasma*-specific antibody captured from sera by the agglutination of a particulate antigen preparation. Sensitivity is 75% to 80%.

3. Other diagnostic testing

   a. **Labs**: Complete blood count (CBC), creatinine (Cr), uric acid (UA), liver function tests (LFTs), glucose-6-phosphate dehydrogenase (G6PD)

      i. A peripheral blood count often demonstrates leukocytosis or leukopenia. Early manifestations include lymphocytopenia or monocytosis. Eosinophilia may be seen (may be >30%), as well as thrombocytopenia.

      ii. Serum G6PD screen should be performed prior to starting sulfadiazine.

      iii. Quantitative IgG levels are recommended to determine a baseline.

   b. **CSF** findings include xanthochromia, mononuclear pleocytosis, and elevated protein content (may be very high). Persistence of *Toxoplasma*-specific immunoglobulin (IgM) may indicate active infection. *Toxoplasma*-specific IgG has been seen, and quantitative IgG levels should be determined as a baseline. Treatment may decrease these findings. PCR is the preferred method to detect parasite from CSF.

   c. Auditory brain stem response to 20 dB is recommended.

4. Head **computed tomography** (CT) scan without contrast is the preferred study. One study reported a clear relationship between the lesions on CT scan, neurologic signs, and the date of maternal infection.

   a. CT scan may detect calcifications not seen by ultrasonography. They may be single or multiple and are usually limited to intracranial structures. Common locations include periventricular, scattered in the white matter, and the basal ganglia (often caudate). The pattern may be indistinguishable from that seen with CMV infection. Lesions can decrease or resolve with treatment.

   b. Hydrocephalus is usually due to periaqueductal obstruction. Massive hydrocephalus may develop in as quickly as 1 week.

   c. Cortical atrophy, as well as porencephalic cysts, can be seen.

5. Pathologic findings

   a. Histology may demonstrate tachyzoites (acute toxoplasmosis) or cysts (acute or chronic toxoplasmosis) in the placenta, tissue, or body fluids.

b. Tissue or mouse culture can be performed to isolate the parasite from peripheral blood buffy coat or the placenta, but may require 1 or 6 weeks, respectively, for results.

6. Multidisciplinary **consultation** is usually helpful for patient management. Specialty consultation is typically required for the following:

a. Infectious diseases. Congenital infection is frequently subclinical, has symptoms similar to other infections and diseases, and serologic diagnosis may be difficult.

b. Ophthalmology. Retinal evaluation is recommended.

c. Neurosurgery. Recommended for ventricular dilation.

d. Neurodevelopmental pediatrics. Follow-up is suggested every 3 to 6 months for 1 year, then as needed.

C. Treatment

1. Medications. Therapy is recommended, regardless of symptoms, to prevent the high incidence of sequelae, resolve acute symptoms, and improve outcomes. Improved outcomes occur if infants are treated in the first year of life. As current medications do not eradicate *T. gondii* and primarily act against the tachyzoite form not tissue cysts (especially from neural tissue and the eye), extended therapy until 1 year of age is recommended.

a. **Pyrimethamine** (1 mg/kg every 12 hours for 2 days, then daily until 2 to 6 months of age, then 3 times weekly until 1 year of age), and **sulfadiazine** (50 mg/kg every 12 hours until 1 year of age) act synergistically and can result in symptom resolution within the first few weeks of therapy.

b. Pyrimethamine (a dihydrofolate reductase inhibitor) can induce bone marrow suppression; patients should be monitored by a CBC, differential, and platelet count twice weekly. Neutropenia is more frequent than megaloblastic anemia or thrombocytopenia. Other less frequent side effects include gastrointestinal distress, convulsions, and tremor. Folinic acid (10 mg 3 times weekly until 1 week after pyrimethamine is stopped) helps prevent bone marrow suppression, but temporary cessation of therapy with pyrimethamine or dose modification may be required. Side effects of sulfadiazine include bone marrow suppression, crystalluria, hematuria, and hypersensitivity. Alternative medications for atopy or severe intolerance of sulfadiazine include clindamycin, azithromycin, and atovaquone.

c. Treatment for congenital infection is usually continued through 1 year of age.

d. **Prednisone** (0.5 mg/kg every 12 hours) is recommended for active CNS disease (CSF protein exceeding 1 g/dL) or active chorioretinitis, which threatens vision. The dose can be tapered and discontinued when symptoms improve.

e. The same treatment regimen is recommended for infants born to mothers infected with both HIV and *T. gondii*. However, combining these agents with antiretrovirals, such as zidovudine, may increase bone marrow toxicity. Treatment may be discontinued after 1 year if the infant's CD_4+ count is >200 cells/mm^3.

2. Ventricular shunting for ventricular dilation is recommended, although systematic outcome data is unavailable. A perioperative head CT scan to assess adequacy of drainage and subdural bleeding (after pressure reduction) may help with prognosis. After treatment with ventricular shunt and medications, some patients experience significant improvement in hydrocephalus with brain cortical expansion and growth. Intelligence quotient (IQ) may be within the normal range.

V. OUTCOMES. The NCCT study has reported outcomes in a series of children with congenital infection. Treatment improved early outcomes for many congenitally infected children. All children who died had severe infection at birth.

A. With treatment, chorioretinitis usually resolved within 1 to 2 weeks and did not relapse during therapy. Relapse after treatment may occur, often during adolescence. Risk factors for relapse are unknown. Visual impairment at 5 years of age is a prominent sequela, even with treatment in 85% of patients who had severe disease at birth and 15% of neonates with mild or asymptomatic disease. Most retinal disease causing impairment was present at birth. Acuity may be adequate for reading and daily activities even with large macular scars. Poor acuity has affected school performance and cognitive development for some patients. Retinal scarring can cause retinal detachment. Ophthalmologic examinations are recommended every 3 months until 18 months of age, and then yearly.

B. With treatment, 80% of patients with **severe** disease at birth had normal motor function, and 73% had an IQ over 70 at follow-up compared with >80% of untreated children who had IQ scores under 70 at 4 years. All treated patients with **asymptomatic to moderate disease** at birth had normal motor and cognitive function. Despite the good cognitive outcomes, patients' IQ scores often are 15 points lower than their closest sibling ($p < .05$). Children asymptomatic at birth may have varying degrees of impairment. No hearing impairment was observed compared with previous reports. With treatment, the head CT scan findings improved. After the resolution of encephalitis with treatment, antiepileptic medications could be discontinued in some patients.

C. With treatment, other signs of infection, including thrombocytopenia, hepatitis, and rashes, resolved within 1 month.

RESOURCES

Congenital toxoplasmosis study group (US) 773-834-4152

Toxoplasma Serology Laboratory at the Palo Alto Medical Foundation Research Institute, Ames Bldg, 795 El Camino Real, Palo Alto, CA 94301-2302 (Tel: [650] 853-4828; Fax [650] 614-3292); E-mail: toxolab@pamf.org; Website: http://www.pamf.org/serology)

Suggested Readings

McLeod R, Boyer K, Karrison T, et al. Outcome of treatment for congenital toxoplasmosis, 1981–2004: the National Collaborative Chicago-based, Congenital Toxoplasmosis Study. *Clin Infect Dis* 2006;42(10):1383–1394.

Montoya JG, Remington JS. Management of Toxoplasma gondii infection during pregnancy. *Clin Infect Dis* 2008;47(4):554–566.

Montoya JG, Rosso F. Diagnosis and management of toxoplasmosis. *Clin Perinatol* 2005;32(3):705–726.

Remington JS, Mcleod R, Thulliez P, et al. Toxoplasmosis. In: Remington JS, Klein JO, Wilson CB, et al. eds. *Infectious Diseases of the Fetus and the Newborn Infant*. 6th ed, pp. 947–1091. Philadelphia: Elsevier Saunders; 2006.

Tamma P. Toxoplasmosis. *Pediatr Rev* 2007;28(12):470–471.

Syphilis
Louis Vernacchio

I. PATHOPHYSIOLOGY

A. **Acquired syphilis** is a sexually transmitted infection caused by the spirochete *Treponema pallidum*. The incubation period is typically about 3 weeks but can range from 9 to 90 days. The disease has three clinically recognizable stages.

1. **Primary syphilis** is manifested by one or more chancres (painless indurated ulcers) at the site of inoculation, typically the genitalia, anus, or mouth. It is often accompanied by regional lymphadenopathy.

2. **Secondary syphilis** occurs 3 to 6 weeks after the appearance of the chancre, often after the chancre has resolved. The secondary stage is characterized by a polymorphic rash, most commonly maculopapular, generalized, and involving the palms and soles. Sore throat, fever, headache, diffuse lymphadenopathy, myalgias, arthralgias, alopecia, condylomata lata, and mucous membrane plaques may also be present. The symptoms resolve without treatment. Some patients develop recurrences of the manifestations of secondary syphilis.

3. **Latent syphilis** is defined as those periods of time with no clinical symptoms but with positive serologic evidence of infection. A variable latent period usually follows the manifestations of secondary syphilis, sometimes interrupted by recurrences of the secondary symptoms.

4. **Tertiary syphilis** usually occurs 4 to 12 years after the secondary stage and is characterized by gummata—nonprogressive, localized lesions that may occur in the skin, bones, or viscera. These lesions are thought to be due to a pronounced immunologic reaction. The tertiary stage can also be marked by cardiovascular syphilis, especially inflammation of the great vessels.

5. **Neurosyphilis** may occur at any stage of the disease. Early manifestations include meningitis and neurovascular disease. Late manifestations include dementia, posterior column disease (tabes dorsalis), and seizures, among others.

B. **Congenital syphilis** results from transplacental passage of *T. pallidum* or contact with infectious lesions during birth. The risk of transmission to the fetus correlates largely with the duration of maternal infection—the more recent the maternal infection, the more likely transmission to the fetus will occur. During the primary and secondary stages of syphilis, the likelihood of transmission from an untreated woman to her fetus is extremely high, approaching 100%. After the secondary stage, the likelihood of transmission to the fetus declines steadily until it reaches approximately 10% to 30% in late latency. Transplacental transmission of *T. pallidum* can occur throughout pregnancy.

Congenital infection may result in stillbirth, hydrops fetalis, or premature delivery. Most affected infants will be asymptomatic at birth, but clinical signs usually develop within the first 3 months of life. The most common signs of early congenital syphilis include hepatomegaly, skeletal abnormalities (osteochondritis, periostitis, and pseudoparalysis), skin and mucocutaneous lesions, jaundice, pneumonia, splenomegaly, anemia, and watery nasal discharge (snuffles). If untreated, late manifestations appear after 2 years of age and may include neurosyphilis, bony changes (frontal bossing, short maxilla, high palatal arch, Hutchinson teeth, saddle nose), interstitial keratitis, and sensorineural deafness, among others.

II. EPIDEMIOLOGY. The incidence of primary and secondary syphilis in the United States, which had increased significantly throughout the 1980s and early 1990s, underwent a dramatic decline to a historic low of 2.1 cases per 100,000 population in 2000. Since then, the infection rate has risen somewhat to 2.7 cases per 100,000 population, although this rise has been largely due to an increase among men who have sex with men. The incidence of syphilis is significantly higher in African Americans, in urban areas, and in the Southern United States.

Along with the generally decreasing incidence of primary and secondary syphilis among women, the number of cases of congenital syphilis in the United States declined from a recent high of nearly 50 cases per 100,000 live births in 1995 to a low of 8.2 cases per 100,000 live births in 2005; however, since 2005, the Centers for Disease Control and Prevention (CDC) has reported an increase to 10.1 cases per 100,000 live births in 2008. Paralleling the patterns of syphilis among women, congenital syphilis is substantially more common among infants of African American women (34.6 cases per 100,000 live births in 2008) and in the Southern United States (15.7 cases per 100,000 live births in 2008).

The most important risk factors for congenital syphilis are lack of prenatal health care and maternal illicit drug use, particularly cocaine. Clinical scenarios that contribute to the occurrence of congenital syphilis include lack of prenatal care; no serologic test for syphilis (STS) performed during pregnancy; a negative STS in the first trimester, without repeat test later in pregnancy; a negative maternal STS around the time of delivery in a woman who was recently infected with syphilis but had not converted her STS yet; laboratory error in reporting STS results; delay in treatment of a pregnant woman identified as having syphilis; and failure of treatment in an infected pregnant woman.

III. DIAGNOSIS OF SYPHILIS

A. Serologic tests for syphilis

1. **Nontreponemal tests** include the rapid plasma reagin (RPR) test, the Venereal Disease Research Laboratory (VDRL) test, and the automated reagin test (ART). These tests measure antibodies directed against a cardiolipin-lecithin-cholesterol antigen from *T. pallidum* and/or its interaction with host tissues. These antibodies give quantitative results, are helpful indicators of disease activity, and are useful for follow-up after treatment. Titers usually rise with each new infection and fall after effective treatment. A sustained fourfold decrease in titer of the nontreponemal test with treatment demonstrates adequate therapy; a similar increase after treatment suggests reinfection.

   Nontreponemal tests will be positive in approximately 75% of cases of primary syphilis, nearly 100% of cases of secondary syphilis, and 75% of cases of latent and tertiary syphilis. In secondary syphilis, the RPR or VDRL test result is usually positive in a titer >1:16. In the first attack of primary syphilis, the RPR or VDRL test will usually become nonreactive 1 year after treatment, whereas in secondary syphilis, the test will usually become nonreactive approximately 2 years after treatment. In latent or tertiary syphilis, the RPR or VDRL test may become nonreactive 4 or 5 years after treatment or may never turn completely nonreactive. A notable cause of false-negative nontreponemal tests is the prozone phenomenon, a negative or weakly positive reaction that occurs with very high antibody concentrations. In this case, dilution of the serum will result in a positive test.

In 1% of cases, a positive RPR or VDRL result is not caused by syphilis. This has been called a *biologic false-positive* (*BFP*) *reaction* and is probably related to tissue damage from various causes. Acute BFPs, which usually resolve in approximately 6 months, may be caused by certain viral infections (particularly infectious mononucleosis, hepatitis, measles, and varicella), endocarditis, intravenous drug abuse, and mycoplasma or protozoa infections. Rarely, BFPs are seen as a result of pregnancy alone. Patients with BFPs usually have low titers (1:8 or less) and nonreactive treponemal tests. Chronic BFPs may be seen in chronic hepatitis, cirrhosis, tuberculosis, extreme old age, malignancy (if associated with excess gamma globulin), connective tissue disease, or autoimmune disease. Patients with systemic lupus erythematosus may have a positive RPR or VDRL test result. The titer is usually 1:8 or less.

2. **Treponemal tests** include the fluorescent treponemal antibody absorption test (FTA-ABS) and the *T. pallidum* particle agglutination (TP-PA) test. Although these tests are more specific than nontreponemal tests, they are also more expensive and labor-intensive and are therefore not used for screening. Rather, they are used to confirm positive nontreponemal tests. The treponemal tests correlate poorly with disease activity and usually remain positive for life, even after successful therapy, and therefore should not be used to assess treatment response.

False-positive treponemal tests occur occasionally, particularly in other spirochetal diseases such as Lyme disease, yaws, pinta, leptospirosis, and ratbite fever; nontreponemal tests should be negative in these situations. In addition, in some cases where antibodies to DNA are present, such as in systemic lupus erythematosus, rheumatoid arthritis, polyarteritis, and other autoimmune diseases, a false-positive FTA-ABS test result may occur. Rarely, pregnancy itself will cause a false-positive treponemal test.

B. **Cerebrospinal fluid** (CSF) testing for neurosyphilis should be done using VDRL test. A cell count and protein concentration should also be performed. A positive CSF VDRL test result is diagnostic of neurosyphilis, but a negative CSF VDRL test result does not exclude neurosyphilis. The FTA-ABS test is recommended by some experts for CSF testing because it is more sensitive than the VDRL test; however, contamination with blood during the lumbar puncture may result in a false-positive CSF FTA-ABS test result. A negative CSF FTA-ABS test result is good evidence against neurosyphilis. The RPR test should not be used for CSF testing.

C. **New tests** under investigation for the diagnosis of syphilis include the following:

1. **Immunoglobulin M (IgM) tests.** Because IgM does not cross the placenta, a positive syphilis IgM test in newborn serum should indicate congenital syphilis. A variety of IgM tests (19S FTA-ABS, immunoblot, enzyme-linked immunosorbent assay [ELISA]) have been developed, but none are routinely clinically available or recommended at the current time by the CDC.

2. **Polymerase chain reaction (PCR)** can detect the presence of the *T. pallidum* genome in a clinical specimen and, therefore, should be helpful in diagnosing congenital syphilis and neurosyphilis. PCR is not yet widely available for clinical use but may become more so in the future.

IV. SCREENING AND TREATMENT OF PREGNANT WOMEN FOR SYPHILIS

A. **All pregnant women should be screened for syphilis with a nontreponemal STS.** Testing should be performed at the first prenatal visit and, in high-risk populations, should be repeated at 28 to 32 weeks' gestation and at delivery. When a woman presents in labor with no history of prenatal care or if results of previous testing are unknown, an STS should be performed at delivery and the infant should not be discharged from the hospital until the test results are known. In women at very high risk, consideration should be given to a repeat STS 1 month postpartum to capture the rare patient who was infected just before delivery but had not yet seroconverted. All positive nontreponemal STS in pregnant women should be confirmed with a treponemal test.

B. **Pregnant women with a reactive nontreponemal STS confirmed by a reactive treponemal STS should be treated unless previous adequate treatment is clearly documented and follow-up nontreponemal titers have declined at least fourfold.** Treatment depends on the stage of infection:

1. **Primary and secondary syphilis.** Benzathine penicillin G 2.4 million units IM in a single dose. Some experts recommend a second dose of 2.4 million units IM 1 week after the first dose.

2. **Early latent syphilis (without neurosyphilis).** Treatment is the same as in primary and secondary syphilis.

3. **Late latent syphilis over 1-year duration or syphilis of unknown duration (without neurosyphilis).** Benzathine penicillin G in a total dose of 7.2 million units given as 2.4 million units IM weekly for 3 weeks.

4. **Tertiary syphilis (without neurosyphilis).** Benzathine penicillin G in a total dose of 7.2 million units given as 2.4 million units IM weekly for 3 weeks.

5. **Neurosyphilis.** Aqueous crystalline penicillin G 18 to 24 million units daily administered as 3 to 4 million units IV every 4 hours for 10 to 14 days. If compliance can be assured, an alternative regimen of procaine penicillin 2.4 million units IM daily plus probenecid 500 mg orally 4 times a day for 10 to 14 days may be used. At the end of these therapies, some experts recommend benzathine penicillin G 2.4 million units IM weekly for up to 3 weeks.

6. **Penicillin-allergic patients.** There are no proven alternatives to penicillin for the prevention of congenital syphilis. If an infected pregnant woman has a history of penicillin allergy, she may be skin-tested against the major and minor penicillin determinants. If these test results are negative, penicillin may be given under medical supervision. If the test results are positive or unavailable, the patient should be desensitized and then given penicillin. Desensitization should be done in consultation with an expert and in a facility where emergency treatment is available.

7. **Human immunodeficiency virus (HIV)-infected pregnant women** receive the same treatment as HIV-negative pregnant women, except that treatment

for primary and secondary syphilis and early latent syphilis may be extended to 3-weekly doses of benzathine penicillin G 2.4 million units IM per week.

8. **The Jarisch-Herxheimer reaction**—the occurrence of fever, chills, headache, myalgias, and exacerbation of cutaneous lesions—may occur after treatment of pregnant women for syphilis. Fetal distress, premature labor, and stillbirth are rare but possible. Patients should be made aware of the possibility of such reactions, but concern about such complications should not delay treatment.

9. If a mother is treated for syphilis in pregnancy, **monthly follow-up should be provided.** A sustained fourfold decrease in nontreponemal titer should be seen with successful treatment. All patients with syphilis should be evaluated for other sexually transmitted diseases such as chlamydia, gonorrhea, hepatitis B, and HIV.

V. EVALUATION AND TREATMENT OF INFANTS FOR CONGENITAL SYPHILIS.

No newborn should be discharged from the hospital until the mother's serologic syphilis status is known. Screening of newborn serum or cord blood in place of screening maternal blood is not recommended because of potential false-negative results.

A. Any infant born to a mother with a reactive nontreponemal test confirmed by a treponemal test should be evaluated with the following:

1. **Complete physical examination** looking for evidence of congenital syphilis (see I.B.).

2. **Quantitative nontreponemal test (RPR or VDRL).** This test should be performed on infant serum, not on cord blood, because of potential false-negative and false-positive results. Because immunoglobulin G (IgG) is readily transported across the placenta, the infant's serum RPR or VDRL test result will be positive even if the infection was not transmitted. The infant's titer should begin to fall by 3 months and become nonreactive by 6 months if the antibody is passively acquired. If the baby was infected, the titer will not fall and may rise. The tests may be negative at birth if the infection was acquired late in pregnancy. In this case, repeating the test later will confirm the diagnosis.

3. **Pathologic examination** of the placenta or umbilical cord using specific fluorescent antitreponemal antibody staining, if available.

4. **Darkfield microscopic examination** or direct fluorescent antibody staining of any suspicious lesions or body fluids (e.g., nasal discharge).

B. The CDC recommends classifying infants evaluated for congenital syphilis into one of the following four scenarios:

1. **Scenario one**
   a. **Any** of the following is evidence of **proven or highly probable disease:**
      i. **Abnormal physical examination** consistent with congenital syphilis.
      ii. **Nontreponemal titer** that is **fourfold higher** than the mother's titer (**note** that the absence of a fourfold or greater titer does not exclude congenital syphilis).
      iii. **Positive darkfield** or **fluorescent antibody test** of body fluid(s).
   b. Further evaluation of infants with proven or highly probable disease should include the following:
      i. **CSF analysis for VDRL, cell count, and protein concentration.** Note that in the neonatal period, interpretation of CSF values may be difficult. Normal values of protein and white blood cells (WBC) are

higher in preterm infants. Values up to 25 WBC/mm^3 and 150 mg protein/dL may be normal.

    ii. Complete blood count (CBC) with differential and platelet count.

    iii. Other tests as clinically indicated, including long-bone radiographs, chest radiograph, liver function tests, cranial ultrasonography, ophthalmologic examination, and auditory brainstem responses.

  c. Treatment for infants with proven or highly probable disease should consist of either of the following:

    i. Aqueous crystalline penicillin G 100,000 to 150,000 units/kg/day IV, administered as 50,000 units/kg/dose IV every 12 hours during the first 7 days of life and every 8 hours thereafter for a total of 10 days, or

    ii. Procaine penicillin G 50,000 units/kg/dose IM daily in a single dose for 10 days.

2. Scenario two

  a. Infants who have a normal physical examination and a serum quantitative nontreponemal titer the same or less than fourfold the maternal titer and **any of** the following:

    i. Maternal treatment not given, inadequate, or not documented.

    ii. Maternal treatment with erythromycin or any other **nonpenicillin** regimen.

    iii. Maternal treatment administered **<4 weeks before delivery.**

  b. Such infants should be evaluated with the following:

    i. CSF analysis for VDRL, cell count, and protein concentration.

    ii. CBC with differential and platelet count.

    iii. Long-bone radiographs.

  c. Treatment of such infants should consist of one of the following:

    i. Aqueous crystalline penicillin G 100,000 to 150,000 units/kg/day IV, administered as 50,000 units/kg/dose IV every 12 hours during the first 7 days of life and every 8 hours thereafter for a total of 10 days, or

    ii. Procaine penicillin G 50,000 units/kg/dose IM daily in a single dose for 10 days.

    iii. If the complete evaluation is normal (CBC with differential and platelets, CSF analysis with VDRL, cell count, and protein concentration, and long-bone radiographs) and follow-up is certain, **a single dose of benzathine penicillin G** 50,000 units/kg IM **may be substituted for the full 10-day course.** If any part of the evaluation is abnormal or not interpretable (e.g., CSF sample contaminated with blood), or if follow-up is not certain, then the full 10-day course of parenteral therapy should be given.

3. Scenario three

  a. Infants who have a normal physical examination and a serum quantitative nontreponemal titer the same as or less than fourfold the maternal titer and **all of** the following:

    i. Maternal treatment during pregnancy with a penicillin regimen appropriate for the stage of infection and >4 weeks before delivery.

    ii. No evidence of maternal reinfection or relapse.

  b. Such infants require no further evaluation.

  c. Such infants should be treated with a **single dose of benzathine penicillin G** 50,000 units/kg IM.

4. **Scenario four**

   a. Infants who have a normal physical examination and a serum quantitative nontreponemal titer the same as or less than fourfold the maternal titer and **both of** the following:

   i. **Adequate maternal treatment before pregnancy.**

   ii. **Maternal nontreponemal titer remained low** and stable before and during pregnancy and at delivery (VDRL <1:2 or RPR <1:4).

   b. Such infants require no further evaluation.

   c. No treatment is required; however, some experts recommend a single dose of benzathine penicillin G 50,000 units/kg IM, particularly if follow-up is uncertain.

C. Evaluation and treatment of infants and children **older than 1 month.**

   Children identified as having a reactive STS after the neonatal period should have maternal serology and treatment records reviewed to determine if the child has congenital or acquired syphilis.

   1. If the child is at risk for congenital syphilis, **evaluation should include the following:**

      a. CSF analysis for VDRL, cell count, and protein concentration.

      b. CBC with differential and platelet count.

      c. Other tests as clinically indicated, including long-bone radiographs, chest radiograph, liver function tests, cranial ultrasonography, ophthalmologic examination, and auditory brainstem responses.

   2. **Treatment should consist of aqueous crystalline penicillin G** 200,000 to 300,000 units/kg/day IV, administered as 50,000 units/kg every 4 to 6 hours for 10 days. Some experts also suggest administering a single dose of benzathine penicillin G 50,000 units/kg IM following the 10-day course of IV therapy.

D. Some experts would treat all newborns with a positive STS because it may be difficult to document that the mother had adequate treatment and falling serologic titers, a low titer may be present in latent maternal syphilis, infected newborns may have no clinical signs at birth, and follow-up/compliance may be difficult in populations at risk for congenital syphilis. If the mother has received an appropriate penicillin regimen >1 month before delivery, the infant's clinical and laboratory examination are normal, and follow-up is assured, some would follow-up the infant without treatment.

VI. FOLLOW-UP OF INFANTS TREATED FOR CONGENITAL SYPHILIS.

All seroreactive infants should have a physical examination and nontreponemal titer every 2 to 3 months until the test becomes nonreactive or the titer decreases fourfold. If the titer is found to increase or remain reactive at 6 to 12 months, the infant should undergo reevaluation for signs of active syphilis and re-treatment should be seriously considered. Infants with possible neurosyphilis (abnormal or uninterpretable CSF results at the time of initial diagnosis) should undergo repeat CSF examination at 6-month intervals until the CSF is normal. If the CSF VDRL test result remains positive at any 6-month interval, re-treatment is recommended. If the CSF VDRL test result is negative, but the CSF cell count and/or protein concentration are not declining or remain abnormal at 2 years, re-treatment is recommended.

VII. INFECTION CONTROL. Nasal secretions and open syphilitic lesions are highly infectious. Strict bodily fluid precautions should be taken. Health care personnel as well as family members and other visitors should wear gloves when handling infants with congenital syphilis until therapy has been administered for at least 24 hours. Those who have had close contact with an infected infant or mother before precautions were taken should be examined and tested for infection, and treatment should be considered.

A. Infants and their mothers at risk for syphilis or infected with syphilis should be evaluated for other sexually transmitted diseases such as hepatitis B, gonorrhea, chlamydia, and HIV.

B. Assistance and guidance in syphilis testing and treatment are available from the CDC, Atlanta, Georgia, and state health departments.

Suggested Readings

American Academy of Pediatrics. Syphilis. In: Pickering LK, Baker CJ, Kimberlin DW, et al., eds. *Red Book: 2009 Report of the Committee on Infectious Diseases.* 28th ed. Elk Grove Village, IL: American Academy of Pediatrics; 2009:638–651.

Centers for Disease Control and Prevention. Congenital syphilis—United States, 2003–2008. *MMWR Morb Mortal Wkly Rep* 2010;59(14):413–417.

Wolff T, Shelton E, Sessions C, et al. Screening for syphilis infection in pregnant women: evidence for the U.S. Preventive Services Task Force reaffirmation recommendation statement. *Ann Intern Med* 2009;150(10):710–716.

Workowski KA, Berman S. Centers for Disease Control and Prevention (CDC). Sexually transmitted diseases treatment guidelines, 2010. *MMWR Recomm Rep.* 2010; 59(RR-12):1–110.

52 Tuberculosis

Dmitry Dukhovny and John P. Cloherty

I. INCIDENCE. The World Health Organization (WHO) estimates that one-third of the world's population is infected by the acid-fast bacillus (AFB) *Mycobacterium tuberculosis*, with 9.2 million (139 per 100,000 population) new cases and 1.7 million deaths reported in 2006 (1). Between 1985 and 1992, there was a 20% increase in the reported cases of **tuberculosis (TB)** in the United States (2,3). This increase was greatest in young adults and children and has been attributed to four factors: (i) the human immunodeficiency virus (HIV) co-epidemic; (ii) recent immigration to the United States from areas with a high prevalence of TB; (iii) increased transmission in high-risk facilities (prisons, hospitals, nursing homes, and homeless shelters); and (iv) the decrease in public health TB services and lack of access to care in persons of low socioeconomic status (4).

Intensified strategic measures initiated in 1989 have steadily reduced the incidence of TB in the United States. Indeed, there were only 11,540 cases reported in the United States in 2009, the lowest recorded since reporting was initiated in 1953 (3). However, the Centers for Disease Control and Prevention's (CDC) goal of eliminating TB from the United States by 2010 failed, in part, to deceleration in the decline of TB from 7.3% per year from 1993 to 2000 to 3.8% per year from 2000 to 2008 (of note, from 2008 to 2009, a record high decrease of 11.4% was observed). Although the rate of TB has declined among all racial and ethnic groups in the United States, the foreign-born persons remain most affected with a rate of almost 11 times higher compared to those born in the United States; among those born in the United States, blacks have the highest number of cases (3). The number of multidrug-resistant TB cases in the United States has remained low, at just over 1%, with a disproportionate burden among foreign-born persons who accounted for 81.6% of the cases in 2007 (3,5). The increasing proportion of TB among foreign-born persons is due to emigration from countries with higher rates of TB, coupled with falling rates of TB in U.S.-born persons (5). Indeed, foreign-born children younger than 5 years had the highest rate of TB between 1993 and 1998 among different age groups (5). Because the highest risk group for mortality from TB are patients <5 years of age, and untreated TB in the newborn is fatal in approximately 30% to 40% of cases (6), pediatricians and neonatologists should maintain a high index of suspicion for this disease.

II. TRANSMISSION AND PATHOGENESIS. TB is transmitted most commonly by respiratory droplet nuclei, which can remain suspended in the air for several hours. Under normal conditions, *M. tuberculosis* organisms are only transmissible from disease sites in the respiratory system: larynx, bronchi, and pulmonary parenchyma. The risk of infectivity from pulmonary TB increases if the sputum is smear positive for AFB in addition to being culture positive. In primary TB, the chest radiograph may show hilar lymphadenopathy, often with focal infiltrates, but may be normal if the focus of infection is small. In contrast, the chest radiograph in adult type reactivation disease often shows pulmonary cavities in the upper lung zones. Primary TB may have mild or nonspecific symptoms, so in some cases, there may be a prolonged period of symptoms before a diagnosis of TB is made (4,6,7). In other cases, there may be significant fever or cough, the latter often related to impingement of bronchi by enlarged lymph nodes. Extrapulmonary TB can act as a source of transmission only rarely, which is related to medical/surgical procedures that create aerosols from infected tissue. One rare but critical exception is congenital transmission, which can arise from maternal blood-borne or occult genitourinary TB (8).

The **incubation stage** occurs after a person has become infected after exposure to a person with contagious pulmonary TB (9). Usually, exposure has to be close (e.g., in an enclosed room) for an extended period. After being inspired by a new host, the respiratory droplets may travel to the alveoli, where they are ingested by alveolar macrophages. For the first several days, there is relatively unrestricted bacterial replication, and the organisms can spread to the regional lymph nodes and the bloodstream (6). During this incubation stage, the tuberculin skin test with purified protein derivative (PPD) remains negative (if the person had not been previously sensitized), and the chest x-ray (CXR) is normal. Acquired immunity typically develops within 2 to 8 weeks, at which point the individual will react to the tuberculin skin test. Sensitivity to tuberculin may take longer to evolve in neonates and young children (9). In all age groups, after the infection is established, the CXR may be normal or minimally abnormal because of enlarged lymph nodes or focal infiltrates (9).

The initial infection can then progress directly to **TB disease**. The likelihood of direct progression to disease is increased by weakened cellular immunity (HIV infection, prolonged courses of corticosteroids or other immunosuppressive therapies, substance abuse, neonatal period, chronic malabsorption syndromes, and low body weight defined as less than 10% or more below ideal weight). In the majority of infected individuals, the infection is controlled and remains asymptomatic (latent). When infection progresses to TB disease, it may occur within weeks from 1 to 2 years following infection. The reactivation of latent infection is more likely in individuals with specific underlying illnesses such as pneumosilicosis, diabetes, end-stage renal disease, and cancer of the head and neck or any form of immune suppression. In any individual who has been infected, TB disease can emerge after a quiescent (latent) period. Ten percent of those with normal immune systems and **latent tuberculosis infection (LTBI)** will convert to TB disease at some point during their lifetime. Approximately half of those cases occur within 2 years. Therefore, the treatment of latent infection is appropriate for individuals with LTBI, as demonstrated by diagnosis of infection after recent known exposure or by a skin test conversion. The disease can take decades to emerge, presumably after intercurrent declines in immunity (6). Although TB disease involves only the lungs in two-thirds of cases, it can also affect any organ system. Extrapulmonary manifestations of TB are more common in immunosuppressed patients and occur in 25% to 35% of infants and young children with disease (4).

III. MATERNAL TUBERCULOSIS.

Clear distinctions must be made between LTBI and TB disease because the diagnosis, treatment, and health implications are different. LTBI is common in populations that are at risk for exposure, and it is not an immediate threat to the mother, the fetus or newborn, or the wider community. Diagnosing LTBI creates opportunities for preventing future TB disease. Public health departments often take an active role in the diagnosis and treatment of LTBI, for example, in the setting of contact investigations, or they can provide consultation. In contrast with LTBI, TB disease is uncommon, but it is an immediate threat to the mother and the fetus or newborn, and it creates an infection-control hazard in the health care setting and the wider community.

A. Latent tuberculosis infection

1. **Diagnosis.** There should be a low threshold for obtaining a PPD in pregnant women. Skin testing should be done on all pregnant women who are exposed to a person with TB; are immigrants from areas with a high incidence of TB; have increased susceptibility to TB because of HIV infection; live in a high-prevalence area; or work in a profession with a high probability of exposure (8). Pregnancy does not alter the response to a tuberculin skin test, and there have been no adverse effects on women or their infants from tuberculin testing (10).

    · A positive PPD reaction in an asymptomatic woman is the most common method of diagnosing TB infection during pregnancy in the United States. Forty-eight to 72 hours after placement of a PPD (5 tuberculin units, 0.1 mL), a positive result is defined as follows (8,11,12):

    a. Induration ≥5 mm if the person is immunosuppressed (e.g., HIV seropositive, glucocorticoid treatment of greater than 15 mg/day, organ transplant, chemotherapy), has close contact with person(s) who have infectious TB disease, or has an abnormal CXR consistent with old TB.

    b. Induration ≥10 mm if the person is an intravenous drug user; has an underlying medical disorder (including chronic renal failure, diabetes mellitus, malnutrition, leukemia, gastrectomy); is foreign-born from high TB prevalence area; resident of long-term facility, jail, or shelter; lives in a medically underserved region; a health care worker in high-risk areas; and is less than 4 years of age.

    c. Induration ≥15 mm if the person is without risk factors and with low likelihood of true TB infection.

    Whenever there is a positive reaction to PPD, it is essential to determine if it is due to a LTBI or TB disease. A complete history and physical examination should be performed to assess for presence of clinical manifestations of TB disease. In addition, a CXR should be obtained (see III.B.1.a.).

    An alternative to a PPD is the use of an interferon-gamma release assay (IGRA), a test that measures interferon-gamma production from T-lymphocytes after specific antigen stimulation (12,13). Two IGRAs are currently approved for clinical use in the United States: the QuantiFERON Gold-TB test and the T-SPOT.TB test. These tests have a similar sensitivity, but IGRA has an increased specificity compared with the PPD due to lack of cross-reactivity in patients who may have received the Bacillus Calmette-Guérin (BCG) vaccine (13).

2. **Treatment** (6,8,10,12). The current recommendations for treating women with LTBI are (i) to wait until the postpartum period, with exceptions in the following high-risk populations: women with HIV, close contacts with a patient with active TB, and women who had a skin test conversion within the last 2 years; and (ii) to receive isoniazid (INH) with pyridoxine supplementation for 9 months. Although there is no evidence for teratogenic concerns, some experts recommend waiting until the second trimester to initiate treatment. TB disease must be excluded before undertaking treatment.

B. Tuberculosis disease

1. **Diagnosis**

    a. Chest radiography. If the tuberculin skin test is positive or there is clinical evidence of TB, a CXR should be obtained to determine if there is active disease. An abdominal shield is required to protect the fetus from the x-ray. Radiographic findings consistent with active disease include adenopathy, focal or multinodular infiltrates, cavitation, and decreased expansion of the upper lobes of the lung. Because radiographic findings may be normal despite TB disease, further evaluation (e.g., sputum cultures) is necessary if symptoms are present (8).

b. Maternal signs and symptoms (14). The clinical manifestations of TB during pregnancy are similar to those in nonpregnant women. Although many women may be asymptomatic, possible symptoms include fever, cough, weight loss, malaise and fatigue, or hemoptysis (8,15). Malaise, fatigue, and vomiting can often be mistaken for other pregnancy-associated conditions. Extrapulmonary involvement can lead to mastitis, miliary TB, TB meningitis, involvement of the lymph nodes, bones, kidneys, or the genitourinary tract. There is an increased incidence of extrapulmonary TB in patients who also have HIV (8).

c. Culture. Any pregnant woman suspected of having TB (positive PPD reaction, suspicious or positive CXR, and/or clinical manifestations) should have three early morning sputum samples obtained for acid-fast staining, culture (isolation can take up to 6 weeks), and susceptibility testing (4,8,16). Because 5% to 10% of pregnant women with TB exhibit extrapulmonary disease, a complete evaluation is essential; and, if indicated, biopsies of lymph nodes or other affected sites should be obtained for staining and culture. A peritoneal fibrinous exudate at cesarean section or an infected placenta may assist in the diagnosis of TB in the mother and/or neonate. If there is evidence of active TB, close contacts should be tested for the disease.

2. **Treatment** (8,10,12) (see Fig. 52.1). If active TB is diagnosed during pregnancy (positive culture, clinical, or radiographic evidence), prompt initial therapy with INH, rifampin (RIF), and ethambutol (EMB) is recommended. Pyridoxine (25–50 mg daily) is added to this regimen because of the increased requirement of this vitamin (B_6) during pregnancy and because it might help prevent INH-related neuropathy. The length of therapy of each drug is dependent upon the sensitivity results of the organism. If the bacilli are sensitive to INH and RIF, EMB should be discontinued after 2 months and INH and RIF continued for 9 months total. If the bacilli are resistant to INH or RIF, consultation with an expert in TB treatment should be obtained to provide effective therapy (depending on the situation, pyrazinamide [PZA] and possibly other drugs would likely be added, especially if there is RIF resistance). Additional considerations must be taken in women who are also coinfected with HIV (17). If extrapulmonary manifestations are present, as in cases of meningeal TB, or if there is slow response to treatment, prolonged therapy may be indicated. All patients with active TB should be isolated in a room with an independent air-handling system and negative air pressure, and the staff should use N95 respirator masks (7,18). According to the WHO, a woman with drug-sensitive pulmonary TB is no longer considered infectious after appropriate treatment for 2 to 3 weeks (1). However, most hospital infection control policies require a patient with active TB to remain in isolation until three consecutive negative sputum AFB smears on different days. Furthermore, for multidrug-resistant TB, isolation should be considered for the entire duration of the inpatient hospitalization (6). Notify the local health department so that a contact investigation can be done.

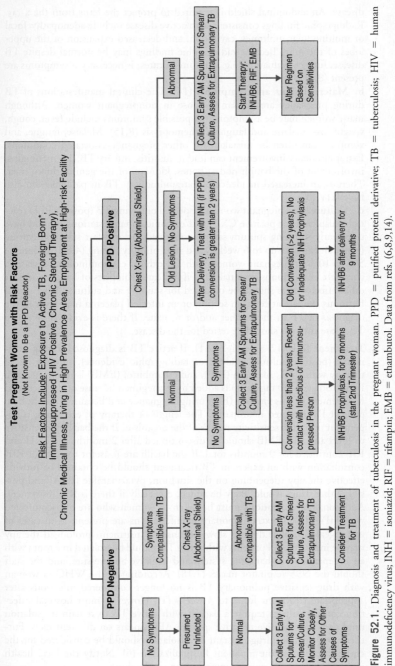

Figure 52.1. Diagnosis and treatment of tuberculosis in the pregnant woman. PPD = purified protein derivative; TB = tuberculosis; HIV = human immunodeficiency virus; INH = isoniazid; RIF = rifampin; EMB = ethambutol. Data from refs. (6,8,9,14).

*Born in countries with high prevalence of TB

For HIV positive women, the type of medications used for prophylaxis and treatment against TB may vary (please see reference 17).

INH, RIF, and EMB appear to be relatively safe for the fetus, and the benefit of treatment outweighs the potential risk to the fetus. Although streptomycin (STREP) is often used to treat TB, it is contraindicated in pregnant women because it can cause ototoxicity in the fetus. There are no data on the effects of PZA in pregnancy and, thus, it is not routinely used in the United States. However, it is part of the recommended regimen for management of TB in pregnancy by the WHO. Additional drugs contraindicated in pregnant women include kanamycin, amikacin, capreomycin, and fluoroquinolones. Consult an expert if a pregnant woman has multidrug-resistant TB and therefore requires treatment with medications that are usually contraindicated in pregnancy or have unknown fetal effects. For all patients with TB disease, supervision of treatment and the use of direct direct observation of treatment (DOT) are indicated.

Although anti-TB medications pass through breast milk, the amount transmitted is low and there is little effect on the neonate; therefore, breastfeeding is not contraindicated.

IV. TUBERCULOSIS OF THE FETUS OR NEWBORN

A. **Pathogenesis** (4,6,8,14,19,20). Although **congenital TB** is rare (~350 reported cases), it can be acquired in the following ways:

1. Hematogenous spread through the umbilical vein from an infected placenta to the fetal liver and lungs (can also involve the gastrointestinal tract, bone marrow, skin, or mesenteric nodes).

2. Inhalation or ingestion of infected amniotic fluid, *in utero* or at the time of birth, leading to primary infection in the lungs or gastrointestinal tract. Congenital TB is found at a higher incidence in neonates born to a mother with tuberculous endometritis or miliary TB (8) and in infants born to mothers with untreated TB during pregnancy (21). The risk of vertical transmission is likely independent of maternal HIV status (21).

   The diagnosis of congenital TB requires the presence of tuberculous lesion and at least one of the following: lesions in the first week of life; primary hepatic lesions; maternal, placental, or genital TB; or exclusion of postnatal transmission after an extensive investigation. If these criteria are not met, the infection was probably acquired **postnatally** in the following ways:

   a. Inhalation (most common) or ingestion of infected respiratory droplets.
   b. Contamination of traumatized skin or mucous membranes.
   c. Ingestion of infected breast milk (theoretical).

   Ultimately, it is not necessary to distinguish between the onset of TB infection in the newborn since the management and prognosis are similar, thus a title of perinatal TB may be more appropriate. However, it is important to identify the source of infection such that proper precautions are taken and the source can be appropriately treated (6,20).

B. **Neonatal signs and symptoms** (4,8,14,19,20). The clinical manifestations of TB in the neonate vary in relation to the duration, mechanism, and location of the infection in the infant. Although symptoms may be present at birth, they are more commonly observed between 2 and 4 weeks of life. The diagnosis of perinatal TB is extremely difficult to make and thus requires a high index of suspicion (20). Clinical manifestations are often nonspecific and include hepatic and splenic enlargement (76%), respiratory distress (72%), fever (48%), lymphadenopathy (38%), abdominal distension (24%), lethargy and irritability (21%), ear discharge (17%), and skin papules (14%) (19). In addition, apnea, failure to thrive, jaundice, and central nervous system (CNS) signs can occur. Infection is more likely to disseminate in neonates compared with children older than 2 years of age and adults due to a more vulnerable immune system (20).

Most infected infants will have an abnormal CXR (infiltrates or miliary pattern in 50%), and almost all infected infants will have an initial negative PPD. The PPD is more likely to be positive (defined in children <4 years of age as ≥10 mm) if infection has been present for 1 to 4 months (4,6). Due to limited evidence, the IGRA is not routinely recommended in children below 5 years of age (12).

Stains for AFB and cultures should be performed on blood, urine, three early morning gastric aspirates, tracheal aspirates, and cerebrospinal fluid (CSF). While CNS involvement is rare, 50% of the patients with CNS infection are younger than 2 years of age (7). Abnormal liver function tests suggest disseminated disease. Tissue from lymph nodes, liver, lung, bone marrow, skin lesions, and the placenta may reveal organisms on pathologic examination and culture. Drug sensitivities should be performed on any organism grown from these cultures as well as organisms grown from maternal isolates. If all direct smears are negative and the infant is ill, anti-TB therapy should be started until the diagnosis of TB is excluded. HIV testing should be done on all neonates with TB because the treatment regimen is longer for coinfection.

C. Management

1. **Congenital TB** (4,12,20) (see Table 52.1). Perinatal TB can be fatal if untreated. Neonates with suspected TB should have a tuberculin skin test, CXR, lumbar puncture, and cultures obtained as part of the initial management. In addition, the placenta should be cultured and examined histologically. Initial treatment of the neonate should include INH, RIF, PZA, and an aminoglycoside such as amikacin. This initial regimen provides broad coverage because neonates are at greater risk for developing extrapulmonary TB (e.g., meningitis, miliary TB, bone and joint disease). If the organism is drug-susceptible, the infant should receive 2 months of this broad therapy followed by 4 months of INH and RIF for *M. tuberculosis* or 9 to 12 months for *Mycobacterium bovis*. If TB meningitis is diagnosed, the infant should be treated for 2 months with the four-drug regimen followed by 7 to 10 months of INH and RIF. Corticosteroids (2 mg/kg/day of prednisone or equivalent for 4–6 weeks followed by a taper) should be added if TB meningitis is confirmed. For those infants coinfected with HIV, at least a 9-month course, should be considered. Due to the increase risk of drug–drug interactions between anti-TB and anti-retrovirals, a specialist should be consulted. If the infant has multidrug-resistant TB, a prolonged (12–18 months) four-drug regimen is often recommended in consultation with a TB specialist (7). Because the yield of culturing bacilli in the neonate is low, the clinician may need to rely on the mother's susceptibilities to determine treatment. In contrast with older children who have adequate pyridoxine levels, infants who are breastfeeding and receiving INH should be supplemented with pyridoxine owing to relatively low levels of this vitamin in breast milk. Consider isolating infants with congenital TB because they typically have a high inoculum of organisms in their tracheal aspirates (18). Consult a TB specialist during neonatal therapy.

Table 52.1   Commonly Used Medications for Treatment of TB Infection in Neonates and Children (Refs. 6,12)

Drug	Dosage (mg/kg/day)	Activity	Side effects
Isoniazid (INH) Tablets (100 or 300 mg) Syrup (10 mg/mL) (unstable at room temperature; should be kept cold) Injection (100 mg/mL), IM	10–15[1] (or 20–30 mg/kg/dose twice weekly) Max dose: 300 mg daily (900 mg twice a week)	Bactericidal	Peripheral neuropathy, hepatotoxic, allergic reactivity Need pyridoxine supplementation in exclusively breastfed infant
Rifampin (RIF) Capsules (150 or 300 mg) (syrup unstable), also IV	10–20 (or 10–20 mg/kg/ dose twice weekly) Max dose: 600 mg	Bactericidal	Orange discoloration of body fluids; hepatotoxic, vomiting, thrombocytopenia, flu-like reaction, pruritis; can alter metabolism of many other drugs due to effect on the liver
Pyrazinamide (PZA) Tablets (500 mg)	30–40 (or 50 mg/kg/dose twice weekly) Max dose: 2 g	Bactericidal	Hepatotoxic, hyperuricemia, gastrointestinal tract upset
Streptomycin (STREP) 1 g and 4 g vials IM Administration (can give IV if not tolerating)	20–40 IM (12 wk maximal use) Max Dose: 1 g	Bactericidal	Ototoxic, nephrotoxic (dose adjust with renal insuf- ficiency), rash, vestibulotoxic; monitor renal function and hearing screens
Amikacin 500 mg or 1 g vials IV or IM	15–30 IM or IV Max dose: 1 g	Bactericidal	Ototoxic, nephrotoxic (dose adjust with renal insuf- ficiency), vestibulotoxic; monitor renal function and hearing screens
Ethambutol (EMB) Tablets (100 or 400 mg)	20–25 (or 50 mg/kg/dose twice weekly) Max dose: 2.5 g	Bacteriostatic, (bactericidal at higher doses)	Optic neuritis (consider risk and benefits in infants since visual fields cannot be monitored), allergic re- activity, gastrointestinal symptoms; monthly monitor visual fields, acuity, and color discrimination

[1]When isoniazid in a dosage exceeding 10 mg/kg/day is used in combination with rifampin, the incidence of hepatoxic effects may be increased.
IM = intramuscular; IV = intravascular

2. **Asymptomatic neonate, active infection in the mother (or household contact)** (4,7,12). Assess the infant for clinical evidence of TB, place a PPD, obtain a CXR, send three gastric aspirates for smear and culture, perform a lumbar puncture, examine the placenta for organisms, and obtain an HIV test. If there is evidence of neonatal disease, treat as in congenital TB (see IV.C.1.); if there is no evidence of neonatal disease, the infant is at high risk and should receive INH daily. If the bacillus is INH resistant, use RIF in place of INH. If the bacilli are INH and RIF resistant, consult a specialist.

   Continue INH therapy in the infant until the mother is culture negative for 3 to 4 months. At that time, if the neonate has a positive PPD without evidence of clinical or radiographic TB, continue INH for a total of 9 months. In contrast, if the neonate has a negative PPD, INH can be discontinued if the mother is adherent and there is adequate clinical response to therapy. In all scenarios, close clinical monitoring of the neonate is necessary (4).

   As soon as a mother is diagnosed with active TB, notify the local health department, so that a contact investigation can be performed, and separate the infant from the mother. Once the infant is receiving chemotherapy, further isolation is not required unless the mother is severely ill, noncompliant, or has multidrug-resistant TB. When the infant and mother are reunited, breastfed infants should receive pyridoxine.

3. **Asymptomatic neonate, mother (or household contact) with positive PPD and abnormal CXR** (4,7,12). Separate the infant and mother until the mother has been evaluated. If the mother has active TB, follow protocol as in section IV.C.2. If the mother does not have active pulmonary disease, the infant is at low risk for infection and does not require therapy. If the mother has not been treated in the past, however, she requires therapy to prevent reactivation. Evaluate household members for TB.

4. **Asymptomatic neonate, mother (or household contact) with positive PPD, negative sputum, and normal CXR** (4,7,12). In this situation, if the mother is asymptomatic, the infant is not separated from the mother. Although the mother requires INH postpartum, the infant does not need therapy. Evaluate household members for TB. If disease cannot be excluded in household members, or if disease is found in the family, further skin testing is required in the neonate.

5. **Neonate with TB exposure in the nursery** (4,12). Although neonates exposed to TB in the nursery have a low risk for acquiring disease, infection can occur. If the exposure is considered to be significant, the infant should be skin tested and, even if negative, treated with INH for 3 months. The skin test should then be repeated; if it is still negative, therapy can be stopped. If the skin test is positive, the infant should be treated with INH for 9 months with close clinical monitoring. To prevent transmission of TB in the nursery, personnel should be skin tested yearly.

V. BACILLUS CALMETTE-GUÉRIN (BCG) VACCINATION (4,6,7,12,22). BCG
is a live, attenuated vaccine prepared from *M. bovis*. Although BCG vaccination has been shown to prevent disseminated TB in children, its efficacy in the prevention of pulmonary disease in adolescents and adults remains uncertain. While the vaccination is currently used in more than 100 countries and is recommended by the Expanded Programme on Immunizations of the WHO, the current indications in the United States are limited to select groups that meet defined criteria: (i) infants and

children (PPD-negative and HIV seronegative) with prolonged exposure to untreated, ineffectively treated contagious persons or exposure to multidrug-resistant contagious persons if removal from the source is not possible; or (ii) nontuberculin reactors working in homeless shelters or health care facilities in high-risk multidrug-resistant TB areas (provided infection-control precautions have not been successful). BCG vaccination is contraindicated in patients with HIV, congenital immunodeficiencies, malignancies, and burns and those receiving radiation therapy and chemotherapy (including corticosteroids). Furthermore, the WHO no longer recommends BCG vaccination in healthy, HIV-infected children. Owing to the unknown effects of BCG on the fetus, the vaccine is not recommended during pregnancy.

Before administering the BCG vaccine, consult a local TB specialist. When BCG is given, closely follow the instructions on the insert. Infants of age <2 months do not need tuberculin testing (unless congenital infection is suspected), whereas older children require a negative PPD before receiving BCG. Infants <30 days of age should receive one-half the recommended dose due to increased risk of lymphadenitis. If the indications for vaccination persist after 1 year of age, they should receive a full vaccine dose if their PPD is <5 mm. Although limited, there is some efficacy data on the use of BCG vaccine in premature infants, which could be administered 2 to 3 months postnatal age or before discharge home (23,24).

Following BCG vaccination, pustule formation often occurs at the injection site within 3 weeks and often leads to a permanent scar. Other complications are infrequent but may include ulceration at the injection site, local lymphadenitis, and, less commonly, osteitis. Disseminated BCG may occur in severely immunodeficient patients. Adverse reactions can be treated with anti-TB medications in consultation with a TB expert. Report all adverse reactions to the manufacturer.

Although BCG administration may affect the future diagnostic utility of the PPD, studies have shown that most children who receive BCG in infancy have a negative PPD at 5 to 10 years of age, and the recommendations for interpretation of the PPD are not altered in persons who have been immunized with BCG. The use of an IGRA in BCG-vaccinated persons may provide greater specificity.

ACKNOWLEDGMENTS

The authors would like to thank Robert N. Husson, MD (Division of Infectious Diseases, Children's Hospital, Boston), for his critical review of this manuscript.

REFERENCES

1. World Health Organization. WHO Report 2008. Global Tuberculosis Control: surveillance, planning, financing. Available at: http://www.who.int/tb/publications/global_report/2008/pdf/fullreport.pdf. Accessed July 7, 2010.
2. Small PM, Fujiwara PI. Management of tuberculosis in the United States. *N Engl J Med* 2001;345(3):189–200.
3. Centers for Disease Control and Prevention. Decrease in reported tuberculosis cases - United States, 2009. *MMWR Morb Mortal Wkly Rep* 2010;59(10):289–294.
4. Starke JR. Tuberculosis. In: Remington JS, Klein JO, eds. *Infectious diseases of the fetus and newborn infant.* 6th ed. Philadelphia: WB Saunders; 2006.
5. Talbot EA, Moore M, McCray E, et al. Tuberculosis among foreign-born persons in the United States, 1993–1998. *JAMA* 2000;284(22):2894–2900.
6. Centers for Disease Control and Prevention. Interactive Core Curriculum on Tuberculosis: What the Clinician Should Know. 2004. Available at: http://www.cdc.gov/tb/webcourses/CoreCurr/index.htm. Accessed July 9, 2010.

7. Cruz AT, Starke JR. Pediatric tuberculosis. *Pediatr Rev* 2010;31(1):13–25.

8. Nhan-Chang CL, Jones TB. Tuberculosis in pregnancy. *Clin Obstet Gynecol* 2010;53(2):311–321.

9. Starke JR. Tuberculosis. An old disease but a new threat to the mother, fetus, and neonate. *Clin Perinatol* 1997;24(1):107–127.

10. Centers for Disease Control and Prevention. Tuberculosis and Pregnancy. Published 2008. Available at: **http://www.cdc.gov/tb/publications/factsheets/specpop/pregnancy.htm**. Accessed July 6, 2010.

11. Centers for Disease Control and Prevention. Tuberculin skin testing. Published 2010. Available at: **http://www.cdc.gov/tb/publications/factsheets/testing/skintesting.htm**. Accessed July 7, 2010.

12. American Academy of Pediatrics. Tuberculosis. In: Pickering LK, Baker CJ, Kimberlin DW, et al., eds. *Red book: 2009 Report of the Committee on Infectious Diseases*. 28th ed. Elk Grove Village, IL: American Academy of Pediatrics; 2009:680–701.

13. Mazurek M, Jereb J, Vernon A, et al. Updated guidelines for using Interferon Gamma Release Assays to detect Mycobacterium tuberculosis infection—United States, 2010. *MMWR Recomm Rep* 59(RR-5):1–25.

14. Laibl VR, Sheffield JS. Tuberculosis in pregnancy. *Clin Perinatol* 2005;32(3):739–747.

15. Good JT Jr, Iseman MD, Davidson PT, et al. Tuberculosis in association with pregnancy. *Am J Obstet Gynecol* 1981;140(5):492–498.

16. Jacobs RF, Abernathy RS. Management of tuberculosis in pregnancy and the newborn. *Clin Perinatol* 1988;15(2):305–319.

17. Kaplan JE, Benson C, Holmes KH, et al. Guidelines for prevention and treatment of opportunistic infections in HIV-infected adults and adolescents: recommendations from CDC, the National Institutes of Health, and the HIV Medicine Association of the Infectious Diseases Society of America. *MMWR Recomm Rep* 2009;58(RR-4):1–207.

18. Jensen PA, Lambert LA, Iademarco MF, et al. Guidelines for preventing the transmission of Mycobacterium tuberculosis in health-care settings, 2005. *MMWR Recomm Rep* 2005;54(RR-17):1–141.

19. Cantwell MF, Shehab ZM, Costello AM, et al. Brief report: congenital tuberculosis. *N Engl J Med* 1994;330(15):1051–1054.

20. Whittaker E, Kampmann B. Perinatal tuberculosis: new challenges in the diagnosis and treatment of tuberculosis in infants and the newborn. *Early Hum Dev* 2008;84(12): 795–799.

21. Pillay T, Sturm AW, Khan M, et al. Vertical transmission of Mycobacterium tuberculosis in KwaZulu Natal: impact of HIV-1 co-infection. *Int J Tuberc Lung Dis* 2004;8(1):59–69.

22. Centers for Disease Control and Prevention. The role of BCG vaccine in the prevention and control of tuberculosis in the United States. A joint statement by the Advisory Council for the Elimination of Tuberculosis and the Advisory Committee on Immunization Practices. *MMWR Recomm Rep* 1996;45(RR-4):1–18.

23. Negrete-Esqueda L, Vargas-Origel A. Response to Bacillus Calmette-Guérin vaccine in full-term and preterm infants. *Am J Perinatol* 2007;24(3):183–189.

24. Okan F, Karagoz S, Nuhoglu A. Bacillus Calmette-Guérin vaccination in preterm infants. *Int J Tuberc Lung Dis* 2006;10(12):1337–1341.

Additional Web References with Most Current TB Screening and Treatment Guidelines

American Academy of Pediatrics Red Book: **http://aapredbook.aappublications.org/**

Centers for Disease Control and Prevention: **http://www.cdc.gov/tb/**

World Health Organization: **http://www.who.int/tb/en/** (also available in other languages)

53 Lyme Disease
Muhammad Aslam

I.   LYME DISEASE (Lyme borreliosis) is the most common vector-borne disease in the United States. The causative organism is the spirochete *Borrelia burgdorferi*, which is transmitted to humans through the bite of tick species including the deer tick (Ixodes scapularis). White-footed mice and deer are important in the life cycle of the tick. Distribution of Lyme disease correlates with the distribution of these hosts. Most cases in the United States are clustered in the northeast from Massachusetts to Maryland, in the midwest in Wisconsin and Minnesota, or in California. There have been cases reported from all states and also in Canada, Europe, China, Japan, and Russia. Humans are most likely to be infected in June, July, and August. The incubation period from tick bite to the appearance of skin lesion(s) ranges from 1–32 days with a median of 11 days.

The clinical manifestations of Lyme disease may be divided into three stages: In the **early localized** stage, an annular, erythematous, nonpruritic rash known as *erythema chronicum migrans* presents at site of a tick bite, usually within 1 to 2 weeks. The early localized stage may also present with multiple erythema migrans lesions, fever, myalgia, and arthralgia. Patients with **early disseminated** disease may present with multiple erythema migrans lesions, neurologic involvement (meningitis, cranial nerve palsy, and peripheral radiculopathy), and carditis (atrioventricular block and myocardial dysfunction). **Late** disease manifests as recurrent pauciarticular arthritis, peripheral neuropathy, and cognitive impairment.

Early case reports and case series confirmed that transplacental transmission of *B. burgdorferi* was possible and raised concerns about a congenital Lyme disease syndrome analogous to that seen with other spirochetal infections such as syphilis. A wide variety of clinical manifestations were noted, with most initial concerns being focused on congenital cardiac malformations and fetal death. However, epidemiologic studies have not supported an association between congenital infection and adverse fetal or neonatal outcomes. A prospective study of 2,014 pregnant women showed no association between seropositivity or history of tick bite and congenital malformations, low birth weight, and fetal death. A report by the same authors compared 2,504 infants born in an endemic region to 2,507 delivered in a nonendemic region. This study showed a significant increase in the rate of congenital cardiac malformations in the endemic compared with the nonendemic region, but notably no association within the endemic region between seropositivity and cardiac malformation. Similarly, in a retrospective case-control study of 796 patients with congenital heart disease and 704 control infants, there was no association between cardiac anomalies and clinical evidence of Lyme disease during pregnancy. Although these studies were limited by the low prevalence of Lyme disease, it appears from available evidence that any increased risk for adverse neonatal effects of prenatal Lyme borreliosis are likely to be small.

There is no evidence that *B. burgdorferi* is transmitted in human milk.

II. DIAGNOSIS. Lyme disease may be diagnosed by the appearance of a typical rash (erythema migrans) in women living in or visiting an area where cases of Lyme disease have been previously reported. However, the spectrum of clinical symptoms may be quite variable. As discussed, there is no accepted syndrome of congenital Lyme borreliosis. Serologic testing begins with acute and convalescent enzyme immunoassay (EIA) or immunofluorescence assay (IFA) to detect immunoglobulin M (IgM) antibodies against *B. burgdorferi*. The IgM titer peaks at 3 to 6 weeks after infection and may be negative for patients with isolated erythema migrans, those who are pregnant, or those who have been treated early. In addition, false-positive EIA and IFA results occur secondary to cross-reaction with other spirochetal and viral infections and autoimmune diseases. Therefore, positive or equivocal EIA or IFA test results should be confirmed with Western immunoblot. If central nervous system involvement is suspected, spinal fluid serology should also be obtained. Polymerase chain reaction for detection of *B. burgdorferi* is currently investigational.

III. TREATMENT OF MOTHERS AND THE NEWBORN. Patients known to have Lyme disease or who are suspected of having Lyme disease during pregnancy should be treated. The treatment is the same as for nonpregnant persons except that doxycycline is contraindicated.

A. **Isolation.** Standard isolation precautions are recommended.

B. **Tick bite.** Prophylactic treatment of tick bites in endemic areas is not generally recommended, although this is sometimes prescribed in nonpregnant individuals, particularly those with prolonged duration of attachment (>72 hours).

C. **Localized early Lyme disease.** Amoxicillin 500 mg PO tid for 14 to 21 days or cefuroxime axetil 500 mg PO bid for 14 to 21 days. For penicillin-allergic patients, erythromycin 500 mg PO qid for 14 to 21 days is an alternative; however, macrolides appear to be less effective, and these patients should therefore be closely followed up.

D. **Disseminated early Lyme disease or any manifestations of late disease.** Ceftriaxone 2 g IV once daily for 14 to 28 days or penicillin G 18 to 24 million units IV every day divided q4h. Patients with isolated cranial nerve palsy, first- or second-degree heart block, or arthritis without neurologic manifestations may be treated with oral therapy as for localized early Lyme disease. Jarisch-Herxheimer reaction (an acute febrile reaction accompanied by headache, myalgia, and an aggravated clinical picture lasting less than 24 hours) can occur when therapy is initiated. Symptomatic treatment, use of nonsteroidal anti-inflammatory agents (NSAIDs), and continuation of the antimicrobial agent are recommended.

E. **Newborn of mother with confirmed Lyme disease in pregnancy.** The relative risk of fetal transmission as a function of severity of maternal disease, chronicity of maternal disease, or choice of antibiotic and route of administration is not known. Similarly, data are lacking on the optimal therapy for the newborn infant with symptoms of acute Lyme disease. In one report, a 38-week fetus born to a mother who developed acute Lyme disease 1 week before delivery developed petechiae and a vesicular rash that resolved with the intravenous administration of penicillin G for 10 days. If an infant is thought to have Lyme disease, treatment with penicillin or ceftriaxone intravenously should be given for 14 to 21 days after studies are taken from blood and spinal fluid. If a mother was treated for Lyme disease with erythromycin during pregnancy, consideration should be given to treatment of the infant with penicillin or ceftriaxone.

F. Prevention of Lyme disease. A recombinant vaccine against the outer surface protein of *B. burgdorferi* was licensed by the U.S. Food and Drug Administration (FDA) in 1998 for individuals between 15 and 70 years of age. It was not recommended for use in pregnant women. The vaccine was withdrawn from the market in 2002 by the manufacturer, owing to lack of demand. In the absence of a vaccine, prevention rests on avoidance of heavily tick-infested areas, use of appropriate tick and insect repellents, and careful examination for and removal of ticks as soon as possible after attachment. Persons with acute infection should not donate blood, but persons who have been treated for Lyme disease can be considered for blood donation. Routine screening of pregnant women, whether living in endemic or non-endemic areas, is not recommended.

Suggested Readings

American Academy of Pediatrics. Committee on infectious diseases. Prevention of Lyme disease. *Pediatrics* 2000;105:142.

American Academy of Pediatrics. Lyme disease. In: Pickering LK, Baker CJ, Kimberlin DW, et al., eds. *Red book: 2009 Report of the Committee of Infectious Disease.* 28th ed. Elk Grove Village: American Academy of Pediatrics; 2009:430–435.

Silver HM. Lyme disease during pregnancy. *Infect Dis Clin North Am* 1997;11:93–97.

Strobino BA, Abid S, Gewitz M. Maternal Lyme disease and congenital heart disease: a case-control study in an endemic area. *Am J Obstet Gynecol* 1999;180:711–716.

Strobino BA, Williams CL, Abid S, et al. Lyme disease and pregnancy outcome: a prospective study of two thousand prenatal patients. *Am J Obstet Gynecol* 1993;169:367–374.

Wormser GP, Nadelman RB, Dattwyler RJ, et al. Practice guidelines for the treatment of Lyme disease. *Clin Infect Dis* 2000;31(suppl 1):1–14.

54 Intracranial Hemorrhage
Janet S. Soul

OVERVIEW

The incidence of intracranial hemorrhage (ICH) varies from 2% to >30% in newborns, depending on gestational age (GA) at birth and the type of ICH. Bleeding within the skull can occur: (i) external to the brain into the epidural, subdural, or subarachnoid spaces; (ii) into the parenchyma of the cerebrum or cerebellum; or (iii) into the ventricles from the subependymal germinal matrix or choroid plexus (Table 54.1). The incidence, pathogenesis, clinical presentation, diagnosis, management, and prognosis of ICH varies according to the ICH location and size, and the infant's GA (1,2). There is often a combination of two or more types of ICH, as an ICH in one location often extends into an adjacent compartment; for example, extension of a parenchymal hemorrhage into the subarachnoid space or ventricles. Although intraventricular hemorrhage (IVH) may be associated with parenchymal hemorrhage, this parenchymal hemorrhage is not an extension of the IVH, but a hemorrhagic venous infarction caused by obstruction of the terminal vein.

Diagnosis usually depends on clinical suspicion when an infant presents with typical neurologic signs, such as seizures, irritability, depressed level of consciousness, and/or focal neurologic deficits referable either to the cerebrum or brain stem. Diagnosis is confirmed with an appropriate neuroimaging study. MRI is the optimal imaging modality for almost all types of ICH, but ultrasound (US) is typically preferred for premature infants and critically ill infants who are not stable for transport to MRI. To avoid exposure of newborns to the ionizing radiation associated with CT, CT scan should be used only for emergent imaging studies when neither MRI or US is available/possible. The American Academy of Neurology (AAN) practice parameter states that all infants with a birth GA of <30 weeks should undergo routine cranial ultrasound (CUS) between 7–14 days and optimally repeated between 36 to 40 weeks postmenstrual age, but MRI is not recommended for routine surveillance (3). Our local practice is to obtain a CUS on every newborn with a birth GA of <32 weeks and birth weight <1,500 grams.

Management varies according to the size and location of the ICH and the presenting neurologic signs. In general, only very large hemorrhages with clinical signs require surgical intervention for removal of the ICH itself. With a large ICH, pressor support or volume replacement (with normal saline, albumin, or packed red blood cells) may be required because of significant blood loss. More commonly, management is focused on treating complications such as seizures or the development of posthemorrhagic hydrocephalus. In general, although a large ICH is more likely to result in greater morbidity or mortality than a small one, the presence and severity of parenchymal injury—whether due to hemorrhage, infarction, or other neuropathology—is usually the best predictor of outcome.

I. SUBDURAL HEMORRHAGE (SDH) AND EPIDURAL HEMORRHAGE (EH)

A. **Etiology and pathogenesis.** The pathogenesis of SDH relates to rupture of the draining veins and sinuses of the brain that occupy the subdural space.

Table 54.1	Illustrating Neonatal ICH by Location, and Whether Each ICH Type Is Predominantly Primary (1°) or Secondary (2°) Source of Bleeding, and the Relative Incidence in Preterm (PT) or Term (T) Newborns		
Type (location) of hemorrhage		Principal source of ICH	Relative Incidence in PT vs. T
1. Subdural and epidural hemorrhage		1° > 2°	T > PT
2. Subarachnoid hemorrhage (SAH)		2° > 1°*	Unknown*
3. Intraparenchymal hemorrhage			
	Cerebral	2° > 1°	PT > T
	Cerebellar	2° > 1°	PT > T
4. Germinal matrix/intraventricular hemorrhage		1° > 2°	PT > T

*True incidence unknown, small 1° SAH may be more common than is recognized in both PT and T newborns.

Vertical molding, fronto-occipital elongation, and torsional forces acting on the head during delivery may provoke laceration of dural leaflets of either the tentorium cerebelli or the falx cerebri. These lacerations can result in rupture of the vein of Galen, inferior sagittal sinus, straight sinus and/or transverse sinus, and usually a posterior fossa SDH. Breech presentation also predisposes to occipital osteodiastasis, a depressed fracture of the occipital bone or bones, which may lead to direct laceration of the cerebellum or rupture of the occipital sinus. Clinically significant SDH in the posterior fossa often results from trauma in the full-term infant, although small, inconsequential SDH is fairly common in uncomplicated deliveries (the true incidence in apparently well newborns is unknown). SDH in the supratentorial space usually results from rupture of the bridging, superficial veins over the cerebral convexity. Other risk factors for SDH include factors that increase the likelihood of significant forces on the infant's head, such as large head size; rigid pelvis (e.g., in a primiparous or older multiparous mother); nonvertex presentation (breech, face, etc.); very rapid or prolonged labor or delivery; difficult instrumented delivery; or, rarely, a bleeding diathesis. MRI is the best modality to determine age of ICH. Postnatally, SDH and EH are almost always due to direct head trauma or shaking; hence, nonaccidental injury needs to be suspected in cases of acute presentation of SDH or EH beyond the perinatal period. However, care should be taken not to confuse an old chronic effusion from a birth-related ICH with an acute postnatally acquired ICH. Careful interpretation of neuroimaging studies, particularly MRI, should distinguish acute SDH or EH from chronic effusion.

B. **Clinical presentation.** When the accumulation of blood is rapid and large, as occurs with rupture of large veins or sinuses, the presentation follows shortly after birth and evolves rapidly. This is particularly true in infratentorial SDH, where compression of the brain stem may result in nuchal rigidity or opisthotonus, obtundation or coma, apnea, other abnormal respiratory patterns, and unreactive pupils and/or abnormal extraocular movements. With increased intracranial pressure (ICP), there may be a bulging fontanelle and/or widely split sutures. With large hemorrhages, there may be systemic signs of hypovolemia and anemia. When the sources of hemorrhage are small veins, there may be few clinical signs for up to a week, at which time either the hematoma attains a critical size, imposes on the brain parenchyma and produces neurologic signs, or hydrocephalus develops. Seizures may occur in up to half of neonates with SDH, particularly with SDH over the cerebral convexity. With cerebral convexity SDH, there may also be subtle focal cerebral signs and mild disturbances of consciousness, such as irritability. Subarachnoid hemorrhage probably coexists in the majority of cases of neonatal SDH, as demonstrated by a cerebrospinal fluid (CSF) exam (4). Finally, a chronic subdural effusion may gradually develop over months, presenting as abnormally rapid head growth, with the occipitofrontal circumference (OFC) crossing percentiles in the first weeks to months after birth.

C. **Diagnosis.** The diagnosis should be suspected on the basis of history and clinical signs and confirmed with a neuroimaging study. CT scan is the study of choice for diagnosing SDH or EH for acute emergencies, if MRI cannot be obtained quickly (3). Although CUS may be valuable in evaluating the sick newborn at the bedside, **US imaging of structures adjacent to bone (i.e., the subdural space) is often inadequate.** MRI has proven to be quite sensitive to small hemorrhage and can help establish timing of ICH. MRI is also superior for detecting other lesions, such as contusion, thromboembolic infarction, or hypoxic-ischemic injury that occurs in some infants with severe hypovolemia/anemia or other risk factors for parenchymal lesions. However, a CT scan is much quicker to obtain and usually adequate in an unstable infant with elevated ICP who may require neurosurgical intervention. **When there is clinical suspicion of a large SDH, a lumbar puncture (LP) should not be performed until after the CT is obtained.** The LP may be contraindicated if there is a large hemorrhage within the posterior fossa or supratentorial compartment. If a small SDH is found, an LP should be performed to rule out infection in the newborn with seizures, depressed mental status, or other systemic signs of illness, since small SDH are often clinically silent.

D. **Management and prognosis.** Most infants with SDH do not require surgical intervention and can be managed with supportive care and treatment of any accompanying seizures. Infants with rapid evolution of a large infratentorial SDH require prompt stabilization with volume replacement (fluid and/or blood products), pressors, and respiratory support, as needed. An urgent head CT and neurosurgical consultation should be obtained in any infant with signs of progressive brain stem dysfunction (i.e., coma, apnea, cranial nerve dysfunction); opisthotonus; or tense, bulging fontanelle. Open surgical evacuation of the clot is the usual management for the minority of infants with large SDH in any location accompanied by such severe neurologic abnormalities or obstructive hydrocephalus. When the clinical picture is stable and no deterioration in neurologic function or unmanageable increase in ICP exists, supportive care and serial CT examinations instead of surgical intervention should be utilized in the management of posterior fossa SDH (5). Laboratory testing to rule out sepsis or a bleeding diathesis should be considered with large SDH. The infant should be monitored for the development of hydrocephalus, which can occur in a delayed fashion following SDH. Finally, chronic subdural effusions may occur rarely and can present weeks to months later with abnormally increased head growth. The outcome for infants with nonsurgical SDH is usually good, provided there is no other significant neurologic injury or disease. The prognosis for normal development is also good for cases in which prompt surgical evacuation of the hematoma is successful and there is no other parenchymal injury.

E. **Epidural hemorrhage (EH).** There are approximately 20 case reports of neonatal EH in the literature. EH appears to be correlated with trauma (e.g., difficult instrumented delivery), and a large cephalohematoma or skull fracture was found in about half the reported cases of EH. Removal or aspiration of the hemorrhage was performed in the majority of cases, and the prognosis was quite good except when other ICH or parenchymal pathology was present.

II. SUBARACHNOID HEMORRHAGE

A. **Etiology and pathogenesis.** Subarachnoid hemorrhage (SAH) is a common form of ICH among newborns, although the true incidence of small SAH remains unknown. Primary SAH (i.e., SAH not due to extension from ICH in an adjacent compartment) is probably frequent but clinically insignificant. In these cases, SAH may go unrecognized because of a lack of clinical signs. For example, hemorrhagic or xanthochromic CSF may be the only indication of such a hemorrhage in infants who undergo a CSF exam to rule out sepsis. Small SAH probably results from the normal "trauma" associated with the birth process. The source of bleeding is usually ruptured bridging veins of the subarachnoid space or ruptured small leptomeningeal vessels. This is quite different from SAH in adults, where the source of bleeding is usually arterial and, therefore, produces a much more emergent clinical syndrome. SAH should be distinguished from subarachnoid extension of blood from a germinal matrix hemorrhage (GMH)/IVH, which occurs most commonly in the preterm infant. SAH may also result from extension of SDH (e.g., particularly in the posterior fossa) or a cerebral contusion (parenchymal hemorrhage). Finally, subpial hemorrhage may occur, mostly in the otherwise healthy term newborn, and is usually a focal hemorrhage likely caused by local trauma resulting in venous compression or occlusion in the setting of a vaginal delivery (often instrumented) (6).

B. **Clinical presentation.** As with other forms of ICH, clinical suspicion of SAH may result because of blood loss or neurologic dysfunction. Only rarely is the blood volume loss large enough to provoke catastrophic results. More often, neurologic signs manifest as seizures, irritability, or other mild alteration of mental status, particularly with SAH or subpial hemorrhage occurring over the cerebral convexities.

Small SAH may not result in any overt clinical signs except seizures in an otherwise well-appearing baby. In these circumstance, the seizures may be misdiagnosed as abnormal movements or other clinical events.

C. **Diagnosis.** Seizures, irritability, lethargy, or focal neurologic signs should prompt investigation to determine whether there is a SAH (or other ICH). The diagnosis is best established with a MRI (or CT) scan, or by LP to confirm or diagnose small SAH. CT scans are usually adequate to diagnose SAH, but as in the case of SDH/ EH, an MRI is preferred because of the lack of radiation and is superior for the determination of whether there is evidence of any other parenchymal pathology. For example, SAH may occur in the setting of hypoxic-ischemic brain injury or meningoencephalitis, pathologies that are better detected by MRI than CT or US. CUS is not sensitive for the detection of small SAH, so should be used only if the patient is too unstable for transport to MRI/CT.

D. **Management and prognosis.** Management of SAH usually requires only symptomatic therapy, such as anticonvulsant therapy for seizures (see Chap. 56, Neonatal Seizures) and nasogastric feeds or intravenous fluids if the infant is too lethargic to feed orally. The majority of infants with small SAH do well with no recognized sequelae. In rare cases, a very large SAH will cause a catastrophic presentation with profound depression of mental status, seizures, and/or brain stem signs. In such cases, blood transfusions and cardiovascular support should be provided as needed, and neurosurgical intervention may be required. It is important to establish by MRI whether there is coexisting hypoxia-ischemia or other significant neuropathology that will be the crucial determinant of a poor neurologic prognosis, since a surgical procedure may not improve outcome if there is extensive brain injury in addition to the SAH. Occasionally, hydrocephalus will develop after a moderate-large SAH, and thus follow-up CUS scans should be performed in such infants, particularly if there are signs of increased ICP or abnormally rapid head growth.

III. INTRAPARENCHYMAL HEMORRHAGE

A. **Etiology and pathogenesis**

1. **Primary cerebral hemorrhage** is uncommon in all newborns, while cerebellar hemorrhage is found in 5% to 10% of autopsy specimens in the premature infant. An intracerebral hemorrhage may occur rarely as a primary event related to rupture of an arteriovenous malformation or aneurysm, from a coagulation disturbance (e.g., hemophilia, thrombocytopenia), or from an unknown cause. More commonly, cerebral intraparenchymal hemorrhage (IPH) occurs as a secondary event, such as hemorrhage into a region of hypoxic-ischemic brain injury. For example, IPH may occur as a result of venous infarction (since venous infarctions are typically hemorrhagic) either in relation to a large GMH/ IVH (PT > T, see IV.) or as a result of sinus venous thrombosis (T > PT). Bleeding may occur secondarily into an arterial distribution infarction (term [T] > preterm [PT]) or, rarely, into an area of necrotic periventricular leukomalacia (PT > T). IPH is found not infrequently in infants undergoing extracorporeal membrane oxygenation (ECMO) therapy. Finally, cerebral IPH may occur as an extension of a large ICH in another compartment, such as large SAH or SDH, as rarely occurs with significant trauma or coagulation disturbance, and it may sometimes be difficult to identify the original source of hemorrhage.

2. **Intracerebellar hemorrhage** occurs more commonly in preterm than term newborns and may be missed by routine CUS, since the reported incidence is significantly higher in neuropathologic than clinical studies. The use of mastoid and posterior fontanelle views during CUS examination increases the

likelihood of detection of cerebellar hemorrhage (and posterior fossa SAH). Intracerebral IPH may be a primary hemorrhage or may result from venous hemorrhagic infarction or from extension of GMH/IVH or SAH (PT > T). It is often difficult to distinguish the primary source or etiology of such hemorrhages by CUS. Cerebellar IPH rarely occurs as an extension of large SAH/SDH in the posterior fossa related to a trauma (T > PT).

B. **Clinical presentation.** The presentation of IPH is similar to that of SDH, where the clinical syndrome differs depending on the size and location of the IPH. In the preterm infant, IPH is often clinically silent in either intracranial fossa, unless the hemorrhage is quite large. In the term infant, intracerebral hemorrhage typically presents with focal neurologic signs such as seizures, asymmetry of tone/movements, or gaze preference, along with irritability or depressed level of consciousness. A large cerebellar hemorrhage (±SDH/SAH) presents as described above (see I.) and should be managed as for a large posterior fossa SDH.

C. **Diagnosis.** MRI is the best imaging modality for IPH, but CUS may be used in the preterm infant or when a rapid bedside imaging study is necessary. CT can be used for urgent evaluation when MRI is not available quickly, but the radiation exposure of CT should be avoided when possible. MRI is superior for demonstrating the extent and age of the hemorrhage and the presence of any other parenchymal abnormality. In addition, MR angiography/venography can be useful to demonstrate a vascular anomaly, lack of flow distal to an arterial embolus, or sinus venous thrombosis. Thus, MRI is more likely than CT or CUS to establish the etiology of the IPH and to determine accurately the long-term prognosis for the term infant. For the preterm infant, CUS views through the mastoid and posterior fontanelle improve the detection of hemorrhage in the posterior fossa. In cases where the etiology of IPH is unknown, an LP should be considered to rule out infection, unless there is significant mass effect or herniation.

D. **Management and prognosis**

1. Acute management of IPH is similar to that for SDH and SAH, where most small hemorrhages require only symptomatic treatment and support, while a large IPH with severe neurologic compromise should prompt neurosurgical intervention. It is important to diagnose and treat any coexisting pathology, such as infection or sinus venous thrombosis, as these underlying conditions may cause further injury that can have a greater impact on long-term outcome than the IPH itself. A large IPH, especially in association with IVH or SAH/SDH, may cause hydrocephalus, and thus head growth and neurologic status should be monitored for days to weeks following IPH. Follow-up imaging by MRI and/or CUS should be obtained in the case of large IPH, both to establish the severity and extent of injury and to rule out hydrocephalus or remaining vascular malformation.

2. The long-term prognosis largely relates to location and size of the IPH and GA of the infant. A small IPH may have relatively few or no long-term neurologic consequences. A large cerebral IPH may result in a life-long seizure disorder, hemiparesis or other type of cerebral palsy (CP), feeding difficulties, and cognitive impairments ranging from learning disabilities to significant intellectual disability, depending on the location. Cerebellar hemorrhage in the term newborn often has a relatively good prognosis, although it may result in cerebellar signs of ataxia, hypotonia, tremor, nystagmus, and mild cognitive deficits. There may be only minor deficits from small, unilateral cerebellar

IPH in either preterm or term newborns. In contrast, a large cerebellar IPH that destroys a significant portion of the cerebellum (i.e., significant bilateral cerebellar injury) in a preterm newborn may result in severe cognitive and motor impairments for those infants who survive the newborn period (such infants often die of systemic illness rather than IPH) (7).

IV. GERMINAL MATRIX HEMORRHAGE/INTRAVENTRICULAR HEMORRHAGE

A. Etiology and pathogenesis

GMH/IVH is found principally in the preterm infant, where the incidence is currently 15% to 20% in infants born at <32 weeks' GA, but is uncommon in the term newborn. The etiology and pathogenesis are different for term and preterm infants.

1. **In the term newborn,** primary IVH typically originates in the choroid plexus or in association with venous (±sinus) thrombosis and thalamic infarction, although IVH may also occur in the small remnant of the subependymal germinal matrix. The pathogenesis of IVH in the term infant is more likely to be related to trauma (i.e., from a difficult delivery) or perinatal asphyxia. However, at least 25% of infants have no identifiable risk factors. One study of CT imaging suggested that IVH might occur secondary to venous hemorrhagic infarction in the thalamus in 63% of term infants with clinically significant IVH (8). In such cases, there may be thrombosis of the internal cerebral veins, but occasionally there may be more extensive sinovenous thrombosis.

2. **In the preterm infant, GMH/IVH originates from the fragile involuting vessels of the subependymal germinal matrix, located in the caudothalamic groove.** There are numerous risk factors that have been identified in the etiology of IVH, including maternal factors such as infection/inflammation and hemorrhage, lack of antenatal steroids, external factors such as mode of delivery or neonatal transport to another hospital, and increasingly recognized genetic factors that predispose some newborns to IVH. However, these risk factors all contribute to the basic pathogenesis of GMH/IVH, which relates to alterations in blood flow and coagulation. Thus, the pathogenesis of GMH/IVH in preterm newborns has been shown to be largely related to intravascular, vascular, and extravascular factors (Table 54.2). The intravascular risk factors are probably the most important and are also the factors most amenable to preventive efforts.

   a. The intravascular risk factors predisposing to GMH/IVH include ischemia/reperfusion, increases in cerebral blood flow (CBF), fluctuating CBF, and increases in cerebral venous pressure. Ischemia/reperfusion occurs commonly when hypotension is corrected quickly, whether due to disease or to iatrogenic intervention. This scenario often occurs shortly after birth, when a premature infant may have hypovolemia or hypotension that is treated with infusion of colloid, normal saline, or hyperosmolar solutions such as sodium bicarbonate. Rapid infusions of such solutions are thought to be particularly likely to contribute to GMH/IVH. Indeed, studies of the beagle puppy model showed that ischemia/reperfusion (hypotension precipitated by blood removal followed by volume infusion) reliably produces GMH/IVH (9). Sustained increases in CBF may contribute to GMH/IVH and can be caused by seizures, hypercarbia, anemia, and hypoglycemia, which result in

Table 54.2	Factors in the pathogenesis of GMH/IVH
Intravascular factors	Ischemia/reperfusion (e.g., volume infusion after hypotension)
	Fluctuating CBF (e.g., with mechanical ventilation)
	Increase in CBF (e.g., with hypertension, anemia, hypercarbia)
	Increase in cerebral venous pressure (e.g., with high intrathoracic pressure, usually from ventilator)
	Platelet dysfunction and coagulation disturbances
Vascular factors	Tenuous, involuting capillaries with large luminal diameter
Extravascular factors	Deficient vascular support
	Excessive fibrinolytic activity

a compensatory increase in CBF. Fluctuating CBF has also been demonstrated to be associated with GMH/IVH in preterm infants. In one study, infants with large fluctuations in CBF velocity by Doppler US were much more likely to develop GMH/IVH than infants with a stable pattern of CBF velocity (10). The large fluctuations typically occurred in infants breathing out of synchrony with the ventilator, but such fluctuations have also been observed in infants with large patent ductus arteriosus or hypotension, for example. Increases in cerebral venous pressure are also thought to contribute to GMH/IVH. Sources of such increases include ventilatory strategies where intrathoracic pressure is high (e.g., high continuous positive airway pressure), pneumothorax, tracheal suctioning, and both labor and delivery, where fetal head compression likely results in significantly increased venous pressure (11). Indeed, a higher incidence of GMH/IVH is found in preterm infants with a longer duration of labor and in those delivered vaginally compared with those delivered via caesarean section. With all of these intravascular factors related to changes in cerebral arterial and venous blood flow, the role of a pressure-passive cerebral circulation is likely to be important. Several studies have shown that preterm infants, particularly asphyxiated newborns, have an impaired ability to regulate CBF in response to blood pressure changes (hence, "pressure-passive") (12,13). Such impaired autoregulation puts the infant at increased risk for rupture of the fragile germinal matrix vessels in the face of significant increases in cerebral arterial or venous pressure, and particularly when ischemia precedes such increased pressure. Finally, impaired coagulation and platelet dysfunction are also intravascular factors that can contribute to the pathogenesis of GMH/IVH.

b. Vascular factors that contribute to GMH/IVH include the fragile nature of the involuting vessels of the germinal matrix. There is no muscularis mucosa and little adventitia in this area of relatively large diameter, thin-walled vessels; all of these factors make the vessels particularly susceptible to rupture.

c. Extravascular risk factors for GMH/IVH include deficient extravascular support and likely excessive fibrinolytic activity in preterm infants.

B. Pathogenesis of complications of GMH/IVH. The two major complications of GMH/IVH are **periventricular hemorrhagic infarction (PVHI)** and **posthemorrhagic ventricular dilation (PVD). The risk of both complications increases with increased size of IVH.** The pathogeneses of these two complications are discussed here.

1. **PVHI** has previously been considered an extension of a large IVH, hence referred to as a grade IV IVH. Although this designation is still used in much of the literature, careful neuropathologic studies have shown that the finding of a large, often unilateral or asymmetric hemorrhagic lesion dorsolateral to the lateral ventricle **is not an extension of the original IVH**, but is a separate lesion consisting of a venous hemorrhagic infarction. Neuropathologic studies demonstrate the fan-shaped appearance of a typical hemorrhagic venous infarction in the distribution of the medullary veins that drain into the terminal vein, resulting from obstruction of flow in the terminal vein by the large ipsilateral IVH. Evidence supporting the notion of venous obstruction underlying the pathogenesis of PVHI includes the observation that PVHI occurs on the side of the larger IVH, and Doppler US studies show markedly decreased or absent flow in the terminal vein on the side of the large IVH (14). Further neuropathologic evidence that **PVHI is a separate lesion from the original IVH** is that the ependymal lining of the lateral ventricle separating IVH and PVHI has been observed to remain intact in some cases, demonstrating that the IVH did not "extend" into the adjacent cerebral parenchyma. Hence, PVHI is a complication of large IVH, which is why some authors refer to it as a separate lesion rather than denoting PVHI to be a "higher" grade of IVH (i.e., a grade IV IVH). Risk factors for the development of PVHI include low birth GA, low Apgar scores, early life acidosis, patent ductus arteriosus, pneumothorax, pulmonary hemorrhage, and need for significant respiratory or blood pressure support (15).

2. **Progressive posthemorrhagic ventricular dilation (PVD) or posthemorrhagic hydrocephalus (PHH—terminology varies),** may occur days to weeks following the onset of GMH/IVH. Not all ventricular dilation progresses to established hydrocephalus that requires treatment, hence the terms are used with slightly different meanings (see IV.C.3. for clinical course of PVD). The pathogenesis of *progressive posthemorrhagic ventricular dilation* likely relates at least in part to impaired CSF resorption and/or obstruction of the aqueduct or the foramina of Luschka or Magendie by particulate clot (16). Recent work suggests that other mechanisms may play a role in the pathogenesis of PVD. High levels of TGF-β1 are found in the CSF following IVH, particularly in infants with PVD; TGF-β1 upregulates genes for extracellular matrix proteins that elaborate a "scar," which may obstruct CSF flow and/or CSF reabsorption (16–18). In addition, restricted arterial pulsations (e.g., due to decreased intracranial compliance) have been proposed to underlie chronic hydrocephalus in hydrodynamic models of hydrocephalus (19). The **pathogenesis of the brain injury resulting from PVD** is probably related in large part to regional hypoxia-ischemia and mechanical distension of the

periventricular white matter, based on animal and human studies (20–23). In addition, the presence of non–protein-bound iron in the CSF of infants with PVD may lead to the generation of reactive oxygen species that in turn contribute to the injury of immature oligodendrocytes in the white matter (24). The brain injury associated with PVD is principally a bilateral cerebral white matter injury (WMI) similar to periventricular leukomalacia (PVL) with regard to both its neuropathology and long-term outcome (23,25–27).

C. **Clinical presentation**

1. **GMH/IVH in the preterm newborn is usually a clinically silent syndrome** and thus is recognized only when a routine CUS is performed. The vast majority of these hemorrhages occur within 72 hours after birth, hence the use of routine CUS within 3–4 days after birth in many nurseries for infants with a GA <32 weeks. Infants with large IVH may present with decreased levels of consciousness and spontaneous movements, hypotonia, abnormal eye movements, or skew deviation. Rarely, an infant will present with a rapid and severe neurologic deterioration with obtundation or coma, severe hypotonia and lack of spontaneous movements, and generalized tonic posturing that is often thought to be seizure, but does not have an electrographic correlate by electroencephalogram.

2. **The term newborn with IVH typically presents with signs such as seizures, apnea, irritability or lethargy, vomiting with dehydration, or a full fontanelle.** Ventriculomegaly is often present at the time of IVH diagnosis in a term newborn. It is rare to find a catastrophic presentation unless there is another ICH, such as a large SDH or parenchymal hemorrhage.

3. **Posthemorrhagic ventricular dilation (PVD) may develop over days to weeks following IVH,** particularly in premature infants, and may present with increasing head growth (crossing percentiles on the growth chart), bulging fontanelle, splitting of sutures, decreased level of consciousness, impaired upgaze or sunsetting sign, apnea, worsening respiratory status, or feeding difficulties. However, PVD may be relatively asymptomatic in preterm newborns, as ICP is often normal in this population, particularly with slowly progressive dilation. Thus, serial CUS scans are critical for diagnosis of PVD in preterm infants with known IVH. A retrospective study of infants with birth weight <1,500 g who developed IVH and survived at least 14 days showed that 50% of such infants will not show ventricular dilation, 25% will develop nonprogressive ventricular dilation (or stable ventriculomegaly), and the remaining 25% will develop PVD (28). The incidence of PVD increases with increasing severity of GMH/IVH; it is uncommon with grades I and II IVH (see Table 54.3) (up to 5% to 12%), but occurs in up to 75% of infants with grade III IVH ± PVHI. The incidence of PVD is also higher with younger GA at birth. Ventricular dilation may proceed rapidly (over a few days) or slowly (over weeks). About 40% of infants with PVD will have spontaneous resolution of PVD without any treatment. The remaining 60% generally require medical and/or surgical therapy (~15% of this latter group do not survive).

D. **Diagnosis**

1. **The diagnosis of GMH/IVH is almost invariably made by real-time portable CUS in the premature infant.** We obtain routine CUS studies in all infants born at <32 weeks' GA. In addition, CUS may be considered in

Table 54.3	Grading of GMH/IVH	
Grading system	Severity of GMH/IVH	Description of findings
Papile (29)	I	Isolated GMH (no IVH)
	II	IVH without ventricular dilatation
	III	IVH with ventricular dilatation
	IV	IVH with parenchymal hemorrhage
Volpe (2)	I	GMH with no or minimal IVH (<10% ventricular volume)
	II	IVH occupying 10%–50% of ventricular area on parasagittal view
	III	IVH occupying >50% of ventricular area on parasagittal view, usually distends lateral ventricle (*at time of IVH diagnosis*)
	Separate notation	Periventricular echodensity (location and extent)

older infants born at >32 weeks' GA who have risk factors, such as perinatal asphyxia or tension pneumothorax, or who present with abnormal neurologic signs as described above. We perform routine CUS studies on or around days 7, 30, and 60 (or just prior to discharge) for infants born at <32 weeks' GA (or birth weight <1,500 g). For unstable infants in whom the CUS may change management, we also obtain a CUS on day 3. In a very sick, very low birth weight infant, consideration should be given to performing a first CUS within 24 hours of birth, as a large IVH with/without other intracranial pathology (e.g., PVHI) may be an important factor in considering redirection of goals of care. Also, a large IVH in very sick, very preterm infants may require earlier follow-up CUS studies to determine whether there is rapidly progressive ventricular dilation. Infants found to have GMH/IVH require more frequent CUS to monitor for complications of GMH/IVH, such as PVD and PVHI, and for other lesions such as PVL (see V.). In addition, any preterm infant who develops abnormal neurologic signs or a significant risk factor for IVH at any point (such as pneumothorax, sepsis, sudden hypotension or volume loss of any etiology) should undergo CUS.

For term newborns, a CUS is sufficient to detect IVH, but MRI is superior for the demonstration of associated abnormalities frequently associated with IVH, such as thalamic infarction or sinus venous thrombosis.

2. **Grading of GMH/IVH is important for determining management and prognosis.** Two systems are accepted for grading GMH/IVH, as outlined in Table 54.3 (2,29). Grading of GMH/IVH should be assigned based on the

earliest CUS obtained when the IVH itself is of maximal size. Specifically, ventricular dilation that occurs days to weeks following GMH/IVH is **not** a grade III IVH; it represents either PVD or ventriculomegaly secondary to parenchymal volume loss. Given the variability in grading systems and in CUS interpretation, a detailed description of the CUS findings should be reported. Specifically, the description should include the following:

a. Presence or absence of blood in the germinal matrix.

b. Laterality (or bilaterality) of the hemorrhage.

c. Presence or absence of blood in each ventricle, including volume of blood in relation to ventricle size.

d. Presence or absence of blood in cerebral parenchyma, with specification of location and size of hemorrhage.

e. Presence or absence of ventricular dilation, with measurements of ventricles when dilated.

f. Presence or absence of any other hemorrhage (e.g., SAH) or parenchymal abnormalities.

3. **In the term newborn, IVH is usually diagnosed when a CUS or MRI is performed because of seizures, apnea, or abnormal mental status.** A brain MRI is superior for the demonstration of other lesions that may be associated with IVH in full-term newborns, such as thalamic hemorrhagic infarction, hypoxic-ischemic brain injury, or sinus venous thrombosis (8).

E. **Management and prognosis**

1. **Prevention of GMH/IVH should be the primary goal;** the decreased incidence of GMH/IVH since the 1980s is likely related to numerous improvements in maternal and neonatal care. Although antenatal administration of **glucocorticoids** has clearly been shown to decrease the incidence of GMH/IVH, antenatal phenobarbital, vitamin K, and magnesium sulfate have not been conclusively demonstrated to prevent GMH/IVH. Postnatal prevention of GMH/IVH should be directed toward minimizing risk factors outlined above in IV.A. In particular, infusions of colloid or hyperosmolar solutions should be given slowly, and all efforts should be directed to avoiding hypotension and large fluctuations or sustained increases in arterial blood pressure or cerebral venous pressure. Elimination of CBF fluctuation related to mechanical ventilation may be achieved by administration of sedative (or muscle relaxant) medication. This recommendation is based on the randomized trial that showed a marked reduction in the incidence of GMH/IVH in premature infants with fluctuating CBF who were muscle relaxed for the first 72 hours after birth, compared with infants who were not muscle relaxed (30). We do not routinely muscle relax our preterm infants because of the many risks associated with this intervention but do provide sedation as needed.

2. **Management of GMH/IVH in the premature newborn largely consists of supportive care** and monitoring for and treatment of complications of GMH/IVH. An increase in the size of GMH/IVH may occur, thus appropriate early care may prevent enlargement of the IVH. Supportive care should be directed toward maintaining stable cerebral perfusion by maintaining normal blood pressure, circulating volume, electrolytes, and blood gases. Transfusions of packed red blood cells may be required in cases of large IVH to restore normal blood volume and hematocrit. Thrombocytopenia or coagulation disturbances should be corrected.

3. **Management of IVH in the term newborn is directed at supportive care of the infant and treatment of seizures during the acute phase.** However, as symptomatic IVH in this group of newborns is frequently large, PVD develops in many infants and **may require serial LPs and/or eventual ventriculoperitoneal shunt placement in up to 50% of such infants.**

4. **Management of PVD consists of careful monitoring of ventricle size by serial CUS and appropriate intervention when needed to reduce CSF accumulation, such as serial LPs to remove CSF, surgical interventions to divert CSF flow, and rarely, medications to reduce CSF production (Figure 54.**1). The goals of therapy are to reduce ventriculomegaly and remove blood products, both of which may contribute to the pathogenesis of brain injury (see IV.B.2.), and potentially to prevent need for a permanent shunt. CSF removal has been shown to improve cerebral perfusion, metabolism, and neurophysiologic function in infants with PVD (20,31–33). Evidence from numerous animal studies and some human data suggest that earlier treatment of PVD can improve neurologic outcome (26,34–36), although no clinical trial has shown improved outcome from any therapy.

   a. In cases of **slowly progressive PVD** (over weeks), close monitoring of clinical status (particularly OFC, fontanelle, and sutures) and ventricle size (by CUS) may be sufficient. Many such cases will have spontaneous resolution of PVD without intervention or will prove to have stable ventriculomegaly. **It is critical to determine by serial CUS which infants have progressive dilation requiring therapy, versus which infants have stable ventriculomegaly due to other causes (such as atrophy due to PVL).**

   b. When serial CUS show persistent PVD, intervention is usually required, particularly if the infant shows clinical signs related to the PVD (e.g., worsening clinical status, bulging fontanelle, widening sutures, rapid increase in OFC). We typically begin therapy when progressive dilation persists for about 1 to 2 weeks in infants with clinical signs, although the rate of ventricular dilation and size of ventricles is assessed in each case to decide whether therapy should be initiated sooner or later. One retrospective study suggested that treatment initiated before ventricle size reached the 97th percentile + 4 mm resulted in improved long-term neurologic outcome (36). We usually rely on a combination of measures of ventricle size, rate of PVD, resistive index (see below), and the infant's clinical course to decide when to initiate treatment, rather than using a single measure of ventricle size as an upper limit (e.g., 97th percentile + 4 mm) (37). Therapy should begin with LPs performed every 1 to 3 days (removing 10–15 mL of CSF per kg body weight), depending on the rate of ventricular dilation and the effectiveness of CSF removal. The opening pressure should be measured whenever possible to help guide therapy. A CUS performed before and after CSF removal is often helpful in establishing the diagnosis of PVD and determining the effect of CSF removal in decreasing ventricle size (33). If PVD is rapidly progressive, daily taps or early surgical intervention may be needed (see IV.E.4.f.).

   c. Measurement of the resistive index (RI) can be helpful in guiding management of PVD. The RI is a measure of resistance to blood flow and may indicate when intracranial compliance is low and cerebral perfusion may be decreased. Since persistent or intermittent decreases in cerebral perfusion may result in ischemic brain injury, we have used the measurement of RI to help guide treatment of PVD. **RI is obtained by measuring systolic and**

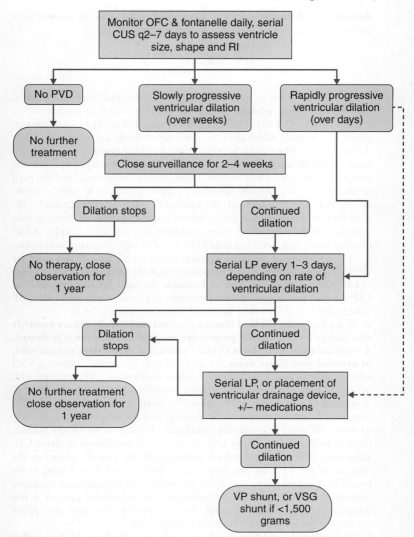

Figure 54.1. Suggested algorithm for management of posthemorrhagic ventricular dilatation (PVD) following intraventricular hemorrhage (IVH). OFC = occipital-frontal circumference; CUS = cranial ultrasound; RI = resistive index; LP = lumbar puncture; VP = ventriculo-peritoneal; VSG = ventriculosubgaleal.

diastolic blood flow velocities by Doppler US (usually in the anterior cerebral artery) and calculating the RI as given by the formula:

$$RI = \frac{(systolic - diastolic)}{systolic}$$

where "systolic" refers to systolic blood flow velocity and "diastolic" refers to diastolic blood flow velocity. Normal RI values are <0.7 in newborns, and baseline values >0.9 to 1.0 indicate that diastolic flow to the brain is compromised. Occasionally values of RI >1.0 will be recorded, due to reversal of flow during diastole, which likely puts the infant at risk for ongoing ischemic brain injury. A significant rise in RI from baseline RI values when gentle fontanelle compression is applied may indicate hemodynamic compromise and the need to remove CSF. We typically consider a >30% increase in RI with compression compared with baseline RI, or a baseline RI >0.9, as an indication for the need for CSF removal (38). Note that the interpretation of RI needs to take into account the presence of other conditions that can affect systolic and/or diastolic blood flow, such as a large PDA or use of high-frequency ventilation.
d. A combination of the infant's clinical status, ventricular size and shape by serial CUS, measurement of ICP by manometry, RI by Doppler US, and response to CSF removal should be used to determine **the need for and frequency of CSF removal procedures** or other interventions to reduce intraventricular CSF volume and reduce the risk of ischemic brain injury (see Fig. 54.1).
e. If the foregoing medical therapy does not successfully reduce ventricle size, and/or PVD is rapidly progressive, surgical intervention is indicated. A ventriculosubgaleal shunt (VSG), ventricular access device (reservoir), or external ventricular drain should be placed. We prefer to insert a VSG because (like a ventricular drain) it offers continuous CSF drainage and, hence, the potential to maintain normal ventricle size and cerebral perfusion, as opposed to intermittent CSF removal by spinal or ventricular taps. A VSG may be sufficient for adequate CSF drainage into the subgaleal space for days to weeks, although may provide insufficient drainage or eventually become blocked by particulate matter (39). If the VSG is insufficient to drain CSF adequately, CSF may be removed intermittently by a needle placed in the reservoir of the VSG (or ventricular access device) every 1 to 3 days, as for serial LPs. External ventricular drains are less favored by many neurosurgeons because of the high incidence of infection, especially if the catheter is not tunneled subcutaneously, although they do provide the ideal therapy of continuous (rather than intermittent) CSF drainage.
f. Acetazolamide and furosemide are carbonic anhydrase inhibitors that can be used to decrease CSF production. However, their combined use often produces electrolyte disturbances and nephrocalcinosis and may be associated with a worse long-term neurologic outcome (40,41). For these reasons, the use of acetazolamide and furosemide together has fallen out of favor and we rarely use these agents in our local practice. The single large multicenter trial of these two agents used together showed no improvement in neurologic outcome compared with "standard therapy," although the standard therapy group was not managed according to a standardized protocol, and treatment was initiated only once the PVD was well established (40,41). Acetazolamide could be considered for cases where intermittent CSF removal is not possible by

LP, ventricular tap or surgical drainaged procedure, or to reduce the frequency of intermittent CSF removal procedures; for example, in very small or critically ill infants in whom a tap or surgical procedure has an unacceptably high risk. However, it should be noted that the safety and efficacy of acetazolamide mono-therapy for PVD has not been demonstrated in large studies and pharmaco-therapy alone is usually ineffective in most severe cases of PVD.

   i. **Logistics.** If absolutely necessary, acetazolamide can be administered 25 to 150 mg/kg/day, given every 6 hours intravenously or orally, starting at a dose of 25 mg/kg/day increased by 25 mg/kg/day to a maximum of 150 mg/kg/day), with or without furosemide 1 to 3 mg/kg IV or PO per day, given every 6 to 12 hours, starting at a dose of 1 mg/kg/day. The lowest effective dose of acetazolamide and furosemide should be used because of potentially toxic effects of high doses of these medications.

   ii. **Side effects and risks.** Careful monitoring and specific treatment is needed for the common and significant side effects and risks associated with these agents, including metabolic acidosis, electrolyte abnormalities, dehydration, gastrointestinal upset, and hypercalciuria with a risk of neph-rocalcinosis. Infants who receive prolonged acetazolamide therapy usually require electrolyte solutions to replace sodium, potassium, and bicarbonate with a goal of maintaining serum HCO3 >10 mEq/mL. Infants receiving prolonged furosemide therapy should be monitored for nephrocalcinosis with serial renal US scans. The urine Ca^{++}:Cr ratios should be intermit-tently measured, with a ratio of greater than 0.21 suggesting a degree of hy-percalciuria that might promote nephrocalcinosis. The diagnosis of hyper-calciuria and nephrocalcinosis, made by either renal US scan or Ca^{++}:Cr ratio requires discontinuation of diuretic therapy. Nephrocalcinosis is a reversible condition; therefore, diuretic therapy may be reinstituted at a decreased dose if there are no other options for treating the PVD.

g. Fibrinolytic therapy alone has not been demonstrated to prevent PVD in five separate studies of different fibrinolytic agents (42). A preliminary trial of continuous drainage, irrigation, and fibrinolytic therapy (called "DRIFT") in 24 infants with PVD showed an apparent reduction in the incidence of shunt sur-gery, mortality, and disability compared with historical controls (43). However, when this very intensive high-risk therapy was tested in a larger multicenter trial, the side effects appeared to outweigh the benefit (44). Of 34 infants treated with DRIFT in this second trial, 2 died and 13 received a VP shunt (44%), whereas of the 36 infants treated with standard therapy (lumbar or ventricular taps), 5 died and 14 underwent a shunt placement (50%) (44). Notably, 12 of 34 patients treated with DRIFT had a secondary IVH, whereas only 3 of 36 in the standard therapy group had further IVH. This second trial showed that DRIFT may have been helpful to a subset of infants, but the overall risks of the therapy were greater than in the pilot trial, thus this therapy has not been widely adopted.

h. If PVD has persisted for >4 weeks despite medical therapy as described above, a permanent shunt will usually be needed. However, a permanent ventriculo-peritoneal (VP) shunt can usually only be placed once infants weigh >1,500 to 2,000 g and are stable enough to undergo this surgery. If the infant weighs <1,500 g, a VSG (39), external drain or ventricular access device will be needed (if not already placed) until the infant is large enough to undergo VP shunt placement. An **endoscopic third ventriculostomy combined with cho-roid plexus cauterization (ETV/CPC)** procedure may be attempted instead of VP shunt in centers that have the expertise for this procedure (45). Success of an ETV is more likely if there is no scarring in the prepontine cistern, if the aqueduct is obstructed, and if choroid plexus cauterization is performed (46). Depending on these factors, failure may occur in up to 60% of cases, usually within 6 months of the procedure, and a VP shunt will need to be placed.

i. Rarely, PVD will recur weeks to months later despite apparent resolution in the neonatal period (47). Monitoring of head growth and fontanelle should continue after discharge home for the first year of life.

5. **The long-term prognosis for infants with GMH/IVH varies considerably depending on the severity of IVH, complications of IVH or other brain lesions, the birth weight/GA, and other significant illnesses that affect neurologic outcome.** Several recent studies suggest that preterm infants with grades I and II IVH have an increased risk of CP and/or cognitive impairment compared with those without IVH (48–50). However, as many as 50% of children born at <32 weeks' GA have school difficulties whether or not they had IVH, even though the risk is clearly higher among children and adolescents with a history of IVH and lower birth GA/weight (51,52). These cognitive impairments likely relate in part to coexisting cerebral WMI (i.e., PVL; see next section), which has many of the same risk factors as GMH/IVH. Infants with ventriculomegaly by CUS with or without GMH/IVH have been shown to be at increased risk for long-term neurologic impairments, likely because mild ventriculomegaly is a consequence of WMI that results in decreased cerebral volume (53,54). Studies thus far have been unable to determine definitively the separate contributions of small GMH/IVH and cerebral WMI, especially as these lesions frequently coexist and the latter is often missed by CUS. Infants with grade III IVH are at a higher risk of cognitive and motor impairments, however, these infants frequently have complications of IVH or other neuropathologic lesions such as PVL that likely contribute significantly to their neurologic outcome. Notably, infants with grade III IVH and those with PVHI ("grade IV IVH") are often grouped together in outcome studies. Recent work shows that MRI is superior to CUS in improving detection, classification and hence, prognosis of GMH/IVH and its associated complications and other neuropathologic lesions such as periventricular WMI (55–57).

Infants with the two major complications of IVH, namely PVHI and PVD, are at much higher risk of neurologic impairments than those with IVH alone. Infants with PVD/PHH requiring significant intervention often manifest spastic diparesis and cognitive impairments due to bilateral periventricular WMI. Infants with a localized, unilateral PVHI usually develop a spastic hemiparesis affecting the arm and leg with minimal or mild cognitive impairments (55). Quadriparesis and significant cognitive deficits (including mental retardation) are more likely if the PVHI is extensive or bilateral, or if there is also coexisting PVL, which is common (58). In addition to cognitive and motor impairments, infants with severe PHH and/or PVHI are at risk for developing cerebral visual impairment and epilepsy (58).

Outcome in term newborns with IVH relates to factors other than IVH alone, as uncomplicated small IVH in this population has a favorable prognosis. Infants with a history of trauma or perinatal asphyxia, or with neuroimaging evidence of thalamic hemorrhagic infarction, hypoxic-ischemic brain injury, or other parenchymal lesions, are at high risk for significant cognitive and/or motor deficits and epilepsy.

V. PERIVENTRICULAR LEUKOMALACIA

A. **Etiology and pathogenesis.** PVL is a lesion found predominantly in the preterm infant and is the neuropathologic lesion underlying much of the cognitive, motor and sensory impairments and disabilities in children born prematurely. The true incidence of this lesion is not known, largely because detection of the mild form of this lesion is difficult using conventional neuroimaging and because the threshold for determining signal abnormality in the cerebral white matter has not been rigorously defined. *White matter injury* is a term used increasingly in place of the traditional term *periventricular leukomalacia* or periventricular leukoencephalopathy, although the term PVL is still commonly used. WMI is a somewhat broader term than PVL in that it denotes the diffuse lesion of the cerebral white matter that extends beyond the periventricular regions defined in initial neuropathologic and ultrasonographic studies and is often a noncystic lesion. An even more encompassing term, "encephalopathy of prematurity," was proposed by Volpe to include the findings of neuronal abnormalities in gray matter structures demonstrated by neuropathology and neuroimaging studies in addition to the WMI (59). This term is not yet in widespread use in the literature but is a term that reflects increasing evidence that premature newborns suffer a brain injury that affects many gray matter structures in addition to the cerebral white matter. Note that WMI with a similar imaging pattern to PVL in the preterm infant has also been reported in infants born at term (60), particularly in those who underwent surgical repair of congenital heart disease (61).

The **characteristic neuropathology** of PVL was first described in detail by Banker and Larroche in their classic 1962 report of the histologic findings in 51 autopsy specimens (62). They described the classic features of PVL to include bilateral areas of focal necrosis, gliosis, and disruption of axons, with the so-called "retraction clubs and balls." The topographical distribution of the lesions was noted to be in the periventricular white matter dorsolateral to the lateral ventricles, primarily anterior to the frontal horn (at the level of the foramen of Monro) and lateral to the occipital horns. They noted that a severe "anoxic" episode occurred in 50 of 51 infants, that the lesions were consistently observed in the location of the border zone of the vascular supply, and that 75% of the group had been born prematurely. They thus suggested two key features of the pathogenesis of PVL, namely, (i) hypoxia-ischemia affecting the watershed regions of the white matter, and (ii) a particular vulnerability of the periventricular white matter of the premature brain. Further neuropathologic studies have extended these initial observations, demonstrating that in many cases PVL consists of areas of both focal necrosis (which become cystic) and a diffuse white matter lesion. The diffuse white matter lesion consists of hypertrophic astrocytes and loss of oligodendrocytes and is followed by an overall decrease in the volume of cerebral white matter myelin. Interestingly, volumetric MRI analysis demonstrates a significant reduction in cortical and subcortical gray matter volumes (rather than white matter volume) in newborns and children born prematurely (63–65). These MRI studies have been confirmed by recent neuropathologic studies showing that there is significant neuronal loss and gliosis in the thalamus, basal ganglia, and cerebral cortex associated with WMI in infants born prematurely (66–69). Thus, these quantitative MRI and neuropathologic data confirm the notion that PVL or WMI involves a much more diffuse destructive and developmental injury to the developing brain that involves neuronal as well as white matter injury (70).

This distinctive lesion of PVL found in the immature white matter of premature newborns likely results from the interaction of multiple pathogenetic factors.

Several major factors have been identified to date: (i) hypoxia-ischemia, (ii) intrinsic vulnerability of cerebral white matter of the premature newborn, and (iii) infection/inflammation (71). These three major factors will be discussed briefly, as follows. First, Banker and Larroche originally suggested that PVL occurred in the regions of vascular border zones in the cerebral white matter and that ischemia would thus be expected to preferentially affect these zones (62). Subsequent authors have further defined these zones using postmortem injection of the blood vessels to demonstrate the presence of vascular border and end zones in the periventricular white matter, where PVL is found (72,73). It is hypothesized that these are watershed zones, which are vulnerable to ischemic injury during times of vascular compromise. In addition, there is evidence to suggest the presence of a pressure-passive circulation in a subset of premature infants, further predisposing these infants to hypoxic-ischemic brain injury (12,74). Indeed, one study of 32 infants showed a higher incidence of PVL (as well as IVH) in infants who demonstrated evidence of a pressure-passive circulation (75).

Second, Banker and Larroche first proposed the hypothesis that the periventricular white matter of the premature newborn may be more vulnerable to anoxia than the mature brain (62). A maturational vulnerability of the periventricular white matter is suggested by the finding that PVL occurs much more commonly in the premature than in the term newborn. Specifically, the observation that the diffuse lesion of PVL affects the oligodendrocyte (with resulting myelin loss) with relative preservation of other cellular elements suggests that the immature oligodendrocyte is the cell most vulnerable to injury. Immature oligodendrocytes are susceptible to injury and apoptotic cell death by free radical attack (76,77) and by glutamate receptor-mediated excitotoxic mechanisms (78). Notably, apoptosis is postulated to be the mechanism of cell death by a moderate ischemic insult, as would be expected for most cases of PVL; necrosis results from severe ischemic insults (79). Thus, there is cellular and biochemical evidence to support the original postulate that the preterm infant's white matter displays a maturational vulnerability to hypoxic-ischemic injury that results in PVL.

Finally, epidemiologic and experimental studies suggest a role for infection and inflammation in the pathogenesis of PVL. Epidemiologic studies have shown an association between maternal infection, prolonged rupture of membranes, cord blood interleukin-6 levels, and an increased incidence of PVL (80), leading to the hypothesis that maternal infection may be an etiologic factor in the development of PVL (81). Experimental work has shown that certain cytokines, such as interferon-γ, have a cytotoxic effect on immature oligodendrocytes (82). However, cytokines may also be secreted in the setting of hypoxia-ischemia (in the absence of infection). Moreover, infection and/or cytokines may lead to ischemia-reperfusion, which may cause further injury to oligodendrocytes (83). Thus, there are multiple pathways by which infection/inflammation might cause or contribute to the pathogenesis of PVL. In most cases, the pathogenesis of PVL probably involves a complex interaction of more than one of the pathogenetic mechanisms described above.

B. **Clinical presentation and diagnosis.** PVL is typically a clinically silent lesion, evolving over days to weeks with few or no outward neurologic signs until weeks to months later when spasticity is first detected, or at an even later age when children present with cognitive difficulties in school. With moderate to severe PVL, some evidence of spasticity in the lower extremities may be detected by the careful observer by term age or earlier. However, **PVL is usually diagnosed in**

the neonatal period by CUS, or less commonly by MRI (84). The evolution of echogenicity in the periventricular white matter over the first few weeks after birth, with or without echolucent cysts, is the classical description of PVL by US imaging. Ventriculomegaly due to volume loss from atrophy of the periventricular white matter is often present within weeks. Isolated ventriculomegaly is associated with an increased risk of CP (53), suggesting that ventriculomegaly without radiologically evident white matter abnormalities may also indicate the presence of PVL.

Studies correlating US and autopsy data have demonstrated that the incidence of PVL is underestimated by CUS, the technique most widely used to diagnose brain abnormalities in the preterm infant (85,86). Several studies have shown that MRI is more sensitive than CUS for the detection of PVL, especially for the noncystic form of PVL (84,87,88). Noncystic WMI detected by MRI in the newborn period is evident as high-signal intensity in the cerebral white matter by T2w MRI and low-signal intensity by T1w sequences. As for CUS studies, there is no universally accepted measure of the severity or extent of signal abnormality by MRI that defines WMI. While it is clear that greater severity of WMI is correlated with a higher incidence of later neurodevelopmental deficits, there is a broad range of outcomes for mild, moderate, and severe WMI (57), and the threshold for defining clinically significant WMI has not been determined. For example, one study reported abnormal signal intensity within the white matter by MRI exam at term age in 80% of infants born at 23 to 30 weeks' GA (89). It has not been shown that this diffuse excessive high-signal intensity on T2-weighted MRI correlates with neuropathologically proven PVL, although there was some correlation between this MRI finding and mild developmental delay at 18 months of age (89). The routine use of MRI scans to detect WMI or other lesions has not been recommended (3), although it may be useful in some high-risk premature infants. It is probably most useful to perform an MRI scan close to term age, if an MRI scan is to be obtained during the newborn period. A brain MRI is the most useful imaging modality to confirm clinically suspected WMI in an older infant or child born prematurely who presents with cognitive, motor and/or sensory impairments. In older infants and children, the brain MRI may show one or more of the following findings: abnormal signal and/or decreased volume of the periventricular white matter, a thin corpus callosum, enlarged ventricles with a square appearance to the frontal horns, and/or enlarged extra-axial CSF spaces (90).

C. **Management.** There are currently no medications or treatments available for the specific treatment of PVL during the newborn period. Current efforts are directed at prevention, based on knowledge of the various risk factors and pathogenetic mechanisms described above. Maintenance of normal cerebral perfusion should be attempted by careful management of systemic hemodynamics (e.g., blood pressure), intravascular volume, oxygenation and ventilation, and avoidance of sudden changes in systemic hemodynamics. It should be noted that there is controversy about the management of blood pressure in the premature infant, and that a normal blood pressure does not necessarily imply normal cerebral perfusion, given the known impairments of cerebral pressure autoregulation in some premature infants (74). Avoidance and prompt treatment of infection (including prompt delivery in setting of chorioamnionitis) may also minimize PVL, although no studies have shown conclusively any effect of such interventions. Management of PVL after discharge from the NICU is directed at identification of any cognitive, sensory or motor impairments, and appropriate therapies for any such impairments, as described below. Promising studies of neuroprotective strategies to prevent or minimize PVL are being conducted in animal models (76,78), but human trials of such agents are likely years away.

D. **Prognosis. PVL is the principal cause of the cognitive, behavioral, motor and sensory impairments found in children born at <32 weeks' GA** (91). There is an approximately 10% incidence of CP and up to 50% incidence of school difficulties in children born prematurely that is largely due to PVL, with PVHI being the other cerebral lesion that contributes significantly to neurologic disabilities. The incidence of neurologic impairments increases with lower GA at birth. For example, one study of extremely low birth weight infants (<1,000 g) showed that only 30% of such children were performing at grade level without extra support at 8 years of age (51). Similarly, the incidence of CP is much higher in children born extremely prematurely, occurring in ~20% of children born at <26 weeks' GA but in only 4% of children born at 32 weeks' GA (49,92). Spastic diparesis is the most common form of CP in children born prematurely (49), because PVL typically affects the periventricular white matter closest to the ventricles. The axons subserving the lower extremities are located closest to the ventricle, the axons of the upper extremities are situated lateral to them, and the axons of the facial musculature are located farthest from the ventricle. Thus, PVL produces abnormal tone (usually spasticity) and weakness predominantly in the lower extremities, with the upper extremities and face demonstrating milder abnormalities. When PVL is more severe and/or widespread, quadriplegia may result. While premature infants can have retinopathy of prematurity affecting their vision, PVL and other cerebral lesions alone can result in strabismus, nystagmus, visual field deficits, and perceptual difficulties, which may not be recognized until school age or later (93). In particular, the lower visual fields may be affected by PVL since the optic radiations subserving the lower visual field pass through the white matter dorsolateral to the occipital horns frequently affected by PVL (94). Children with WMI may manifest visual perceptual defects or other higher order visual impairments that worsen their cognitive and school function, so these are particularly important to detect (95). As visual field deficits and other types of cerebral visual impairment can be difficult to detect, routine monitoring of visual function for early detection of these problems is important. Finally, children with severe PVL may develop epilepsy, although epilepsy is more commonly related to lesions with significant direct neuronal injury such as PVHI.

REFERENCES

1. Volpe JJ. *Intracranial Hemorrhage: Subdural, Primary Subarachnoid, Cerebellar, Intraventricular (term infant), and Miscellaneous.* In: Neurology of the Newborn (pp. 483–516). Philadelphia: WB Saunders; 2008.
2. Volpe JJ. *Intracranial Hemorrhage: Serminal Matrix-Intraventricular Hemorrhage of the Premature Infant.* In: Neurology of the Newborn (pp. 517–588). Philadelphia: WB Saunders; 2008.
3. Ment LR, Bada HS, Barnes P, et al. Practice parameter: neuroimaging of the neonate: report of the Quality Standards Subcommittee of the American Academy of Neurology and the Practice Committee of the Child Neurology Society. *Neurology* 2002;58(12):1726–1738.
4. Chamnanvanakij S, Rollins N, Perlman JM. Subdural hematoma in term infants. *Pediatr Neurol* 2002;26(4):301–304.
5. Perrin RG, Rutka JT, Drake JM, et al. Management and outcomes of posterior fossa subdural hematomas in neonates. *Neurosurgery* 1997;40:1190–1199; discussion 1199–1200.
6. Huang AH, Robertson RL. Spontaneous superficial parenchymal and leptomeningeal hemorrhage in term neonates. *AJNR Am J Neuroradiol* 2004;25(3):469–475.

7. Bodensteiner JB, Johnsen SD. Cerebellar injury in the extremely premature infant: newly recognized but relatively common outcome. *J Child Neurol* 2005;20(2):139–142.

8. Roland EH, Flodmark O, Hill A. Thalamic hemorrhage with intraventricular hemorrhage in the full-term newborn. *Pediatrics* 1990;85(5):737–742.

9. Goddard-Finegold J, Armstrong D, Zeller RS. Intraventricular hemorrhage, following volume expansion after hypovolemic hypotension in the newborn beagle. *J Pediatr* 1982;100(5):796–799.

10. Perlman JM, McMenamin JB, Volpe JJ. Fluctuating cerebral blood-flow velocity in respiratory-distress syndrome: relation to the development of intraventricular hemorrhage. *N Engl J Med* 1983;309(4):204–209.

11. Hill A, Perlman JM, Volpe JJ. Relationship of pneumothorax to occurrence of intraventricular hemorrhage in the premature newborn. *Pediatrics* 1982;69(2):144–149.

12. Lou HC, Lassen NA, Friis-Hansen B. Impaired autoregulation of cerebral blood flow in the distressed newborn infant. *J Pediatr* 1979;94(1):118–121.

13. Pryds O, Greisen G, Lou H et al. Heterogeneity of cerebral vasoreactivity in preterm infants supported by mechanical ventilation. *J Pediatr* 1989;115(4):638–645.

14. Taylor GA. Effect of germinal matrix hemorrhage on terminal vein position and patency. *Pediatr Radiol* 1995;25(suppl 1):S37–S40.

15. Bassan H, Feldman HA, Limperopoulos C, et al. Periventricular hemorrhagic infarction: risk factors and neonatal outcome. *Pediatr Neurol* 2006;35(2):85–92.

16. Larroche JC. Post-haemorrhagic hydrocephalus in infancy: anatomical study. *Biol Neonate* 1972;20(3):287–299.

17. Whitelaw A, Christie S, Pople I. Transforming growth factor-beta 1: a possible signal molecule for posthemorrhagic hydrocephalus? *Pediatr Res* 1999;46(5):576–580.

18. Whitelaw A, Thoresen M, Pople I. Posthaemorrhagic ventricular dilatation. *Arch Dis Child Fetal Neonatal Ed* 2002;86(2):F72–F74.

19. Greitz D. Radiological assessment of hydrocephalus: new theories and implications for therapy. *Neurosurg Rev* 2004;27(3):145–165; discussion 166–147.

20. Bejar R, Saugstad OD, James H et al. Increased hypoxanthine concentrations in cerebrospinal fluid of infants with hydrocephalus. *J Pediatr* 1983;103(1):44–48.

21. da Silva MC, Drake JM, Lemaire C, et al. High-energy phosphate metabolism in a neonatal model of hydrocephalus before and after shunting. *J Neurosurg* 1994;81(4):544–553.

22. da Silva MC, Michowicz S, Drake JM, et al. Reduced local cerebral blood flow in periventricular white matter in experimental neonatal hydrocephalus-restoration with CSF shunting. *J Cereb Blood Flow Metab* 1995;15(6):1057–1065.

23. Del Bigio MR, Zhang YW. Cell death, axonal damage, and cell birth in the immature rat brain following induction of hydrocephalus. *Exp Neurol* 1998;154(1):157–169.

24. Savman K, Nilsson UA, Blennow M, et al. Non-protein-bound iron is elevated in cerebrospinal fluid from preterm infants with posthemorrhagic ventricular dilatation. *Pediatr Res* 2001;49(2):208–212.

25. Fukumizu M, Takashima S, Becker LE. Neonatal posthemorrhagic hydrocephalus: neuropathologic and immunohistochemical studies. *Pediatr Neurol* 1995;13(3):230–234.

26. du Plessis AJ. Posthemorrhagic hydrocephalus and brain injury in the preterm infant: dilemmas in diagnosis and management. *Semin Pediatr Neurol* 1998;5(3):161–179.

27. Whitelaw A, Rosengren L, Blennow M. Brain specific proteins in posthaemorrhagic ventricular dilatation. *Arch Dis Child Fetal Neonatal Ed* 2001;84(2):F90–F91.

28. Murphy BP, Inder TE, Rooks V, et al. Posthaemorrhagic ventricular dilatation in the premature infant: natural history and predictors of outcome. *Arch Dis Child Fetal Neonatal Ed* 2002;87(1):F37–F41.

29. Papile LA, Burstein J, Burstein R, et al. Incidence and evolution of subependymal and intraventricular hemorrhage: a study of infants with birth weights less than 1,500 gm. *J Pediatr* 1978;92(4):529–534.

30. Perlman JM, Goodman S, Kreusser KL, et al. Reduction in intraventricular hemorrhage by elimination of fluctuating cerebral blood-flow velocity in preterm infants with respiratory distress syndrome. *N Engl J Med* 1985;312(21):1353–1357.

31. Ehle A, Sklar F. Visual evoked potentials in infants with hydrocephalus. *Neurology* 1979;29(11):1541–1544.

32. De Vries LS, Pierrat V, Minami T, et al. The role of short latency somatosensory evoked responses in infants with rapidly progressive ventricular dilatation. *Neuropediatrics* 1990;21(3):136–139.

33. Soul JS, Eichenwald E, Walter G, et al. CSF removal in infantile posthemorrhagic hydrocephalus results in significant improvement in cerebral hemodynamics. *Pediatr Res* 2004;55(5):872–876.

34. Del Bigio MR, Kanfer JN, Zhang YW. Myelination delay in the cerebral white matter of immature rats with kaolin-induced hydrocephalus is reversible. *J Neuropathol Exp Neurol* 1997;56(9):1053–1066.

35. Del Bigio MR, Crook CR, Buist R. Magnetic resonance imaging and behavioral analysis of immature rats with kaolin-induced hydrocephalus: pre- and postshunting observations. *Exp Neurol* 1997;148(1):256–264.

36. de Vries LS, Liem KD, van Dijk K, et al. Early versus late treatment of posthaemorrhagic ventricular dilatation: results of a retrospective study from five neonatal intensive care units in The Netherlands. *Acta Paediatr* 2002;91(2):212–217.

37. Levene MI. Measurement of the growth of the lateral ventricles in preterm infants with real-time ultrasound. *Arch Dis Child* 1981;56(12):900–904.

38. Taylor GA, Madsen JR. Neonatal hydrocephalus: hemodynamic response to fontanelle compression—correlation with intracranial pressure and need for shunt placement. *Radiology* 1996;201(3):685–689.

39. Rahman S, Teo C, Morris W, et al. Ventriculosubgaleal shunt: a treatment option for progressive posthemorrhagic hydrocephalus. *Childs Nerv Syst* 1995;11(11):650–654.

40. International PHVD Drug Trial Group. International randomised controlled trial of acetazolamide and furosemide in posthaemorrhagic ventricular dilatation in infancy. *Lancet* 1998;352(9126):433–440.

41. Kennedy CR, Ayers S, Campbell MJ, et al. Randomized, controlled trial of acetazolamide and furosemide in posthemorrhagic ventricular dilation in infancy: follow-up at 1 year. *Pediatrics* 2001;108(3):597–607.

42. Haines SJ, Lapointe M. Fibrinolytic agents in the management of posthemorrhagic hydrocephalus in preterm infants: the evidence. *Childs Nerv Syst* 1999;15(5):226–234.

43. Whitelaw A, Pople I, Cherian S, et al. Phase 1 trial of prevention of hydrocephalus after intraventricular hemorrhage in newborn infants by drainage, irrigation, and fibrinolytic therapy. *Pediatrics* 2003;111(4 pt 1):759–765.

44. Whitelaw A, Evans D, Carter M, et al. Randomized clinical trial of prevention of hydrocephalus after intraventricular hemorrhage in preterm infants: brain-washing versus tapping fluid. *Pediatrics* 2007;119(5):e1071–e1078.

45. Warf BC. Endoscopic third ventriculostomy and choroid plexus cauterization for pediatric hydrocephalus. *Clin Neurosurg* 2007;54:78–82.

46. Warf BC, Kulkarni AV. Intraoperative assessment of cerebral aqueduct patency and cisternal scarring: impact on success of endoscopic third ventriculostomy in 403 African children. *J Neurosurg Pediatr* 2010;5(2):204–209.

47. Perlman JM, Lynch B, Volpe JJ. Late hydrocephalus after arrest and resolution of neonatal post-hemorrhagic hydrocephalus. *Dev Med Child Neurol* 1990;32(8):725–729.

48. Sherlock RL, Anderson PJ, Doyle LW. Neurodevelopmental sequelae of intraventricular haemorrhage at 8 years of age in a regional cohort of ELBW/very preterm infants. *Early Hum Dev* 2005;81(11):909–916.

49. Ancel PY, Livinec F, Larroque B, et al. Cerebral palsy among very preterm children in relation to gestational age and neonatal ultrasound abnormalities: the EPIPAGE cohort study. *Pediatrics* 2006;117(3):828–835.

50. Patra K, Wilson-Costello D, Taylor HG, et al. Grades I–II intraventricular hemorrhage in extremely low birth weight infants: effects on neurodevelopment. *J Pediatr* 2006;149(2):169–173.

51. Bowen JR, Gibson FL, Hand PJ. Educational outcome at 8 years for children who were born extremely prematurely: a controlled study. *J Paediatr Child Health* 2002;38(5):438–444.

52. van de Bor M, den Ouden L. School performance in adolescents with and without periventricular-intraventricular hemorrhage in the neonatal period. *Semin Perinatol* 2004;28(4):295–303.

53. Allan WC, Vohr B, Makuch RW, et al. Antecedents of cerebral palsy in a multicenter trial of indomethacin for intraventricular hemorrhage [see comments]. *Arch Pediatr Adolesc Med* 1997;151(6):580–585.

54. Vollmer B, Roth S, Riley K, et al. Neurodevelopmental outcome of preterm infants with ventricular dilatation with and without associated haemorrhage. *Dev Med Child Neurol* 2006;48(5):348–352.

55. De Vries LS, Groenendaal F, van Haastert IC, et al. Asymmetrical myelination of the posterior limb of the internal capsule in infants with periventricular haemorrhagic infarction: an early predictor of hemiplegia. *Neuropediatrics* 1999;30(6):314–319.

56. Valkama AM, Pääkkö EL, Vainionpää LK, et al. Magnetic resonance imaging at term and neuromotor outcome in preterm infants. *Acta Paediatr* 2000;89(3):348–355.

57. Woodward LJ, Anderson PJ, Austin NC, et al. Neonatal MRI to predict neurodevelopmental outcomes in preterm infants. *N Engl J Med* 2006;355(7):685–694.

58. Bassan H, Benson CB, Limperopoulos C, et al. Ultrasonographic features and severity scoring of periventricular hemorrhagic infarction in relation to risk factors and outcome. *Pediatrics* 2006;117(6):2111–2118.

59. Volpe JJ. Brain injury in premature infants: a complex amalgam of destructive and developmental disturbances. *Lancet Neurol* 2009;8(1):110–124.

60. Kwong KL, Wong YC, Fong CM, et al. Magnetic resonance imaging in 122 children with spastic cerebral palsy. *Pediatr Neurol* 2004;31(3):172–176.

61. Galli KK, Zimmerman RA, Jarvik GP, et al. Periventricular leukomalacia is common after neonatal cardiac surgery. *J Thorac Cardiovasc Surg* 2004;127(3):692–704.

62. Banker BQ, Larroche JG. Periventricular leukomalacia of infancy. *Arch Neurol* 1962;7:386–410.

63. Peterson BS, Vohr B, Staib LH, et al. Regional brain volume abnormalities and long-term cognitive outcome in preterm infants. *JAMA* 2000;284(15):1939–1947.

64. Abernethy LJ, Cooke RW, Foulder-Hughes L. Caudate and hippocampal volumes, intelligence, and motor impairment in 7-year-old children who were born preterm. *Pediatr Res* 2004;55(5):884–893.

65. Inder TE, Warfield SK, Wang H, et al. Abnormal cerebral structure is present at term in premature infants. *Pediatrics* 2005;115(2):286–294.

66. Pierson CR, Folkerth RD, Billiards SS, et al. Gray matter injury associated with periventricular leukomalacia in the premature infant. *Acta Neuropathol* 2007;114(6):619–631.

67. Ligam P, Haynes RL, Folkerth RD, et al. Thalamic damage in periventricular leukomalacia: novel pathologic observations relevant to cognitive deficits in survivors of prematurity. *Pediatr Res* 2008;65(5):524–529.

68. Kinney HC. The encephalopathy of prematurity: one pediatric neuropathologist's perspective. *Semin Pediatr Neurol* 2009;16(4):179–190.

69. Andiman SE, Haynes RL, Trachtenberg FL, et al. The cerebral cortex overlying periventricular leukomalacia: analysis of pyramidal neurons. *Brain Pathol* 2010;20(4):803–814.

70. Volpe JJ. The encephalopathy of prematurity—brain injury and impaired brain development inextricably intertwined. *Semin Pediatr Neurol* 2009;16(4):167–178.

71. Volpe JJ. Neurobiology of periventricular leukomalacia in the premature infant. *Pediatr Res* 2001;50(5):553–562.

72. Takashima S, Tanaka K. Development of cerebrovascular architecture and its relationship to periventricular leukomalacia. *Arch Neurol* 1978;35(1):11–16.

73. De Reuck JL. Cerebral angioarchitecture and perinatal brain lesions in premature and full-term infants. *Acta Neurol Scand* 1984;70(6):391–395.

74. Soul JS, Hammer PE, Tsuji M, et al. Fluctuating pressure-passivity is common in the cerebral circulation of sick premature infants. *Pediatr Res* 2007;61(4):467–473.

75. Tsuji M, Saul JP, du Plessis A, et al. Cerebral intravascular oxygenation correlates with mean arterial pressure in critically ill premature infants. *Pediatrics* 2000;106(4):625–632.

76. Oka A, Belliveau MJ, Rosenberg PA, et al. Vulnerability of oligodendroglia to glutamate: pharmacology, mechanisms, and prevention. *J Neurosci* 1993;13(4):1441–1453.

77. Back SA, Gan X, Li Y, et al. Maturation-dependent vulnerability of oligodendrocytes to oxidative stress-induced death caused by glutathione depletion. *J Neurosci* 1998;18(16):6241–6253.

78. Follett PL, Deng W, Dai W, et al. Glutamate receptor-mediated oligodendrocyte toxicity in periventricular leukomalacia: a protective role for topiramate. *J Neurosci* 2004;24(18):4412–4420.

79. Ankarcrona M, Dypbukt JM, Bonfoco E, et al. Glutamate-induced neuronal death: a succession of necrosis or apoptosis depending on mitochondrial function. *Neuron* 1995;15(4):961–973.

80. Yoon BH, Romero R, Yang SH, et al. Interleukin-6 concentrations in umbilical cord plasma are elevated in neonates with white matter lesions associated with periventricular leukomalacia. *Am J Obstet Gynecol* 1996;174(5):1433–1440.

81. Dammann O, Leviton A. Maternal intrauterine infection, cytokines, and brain damage in the preterm newborn. *Pediatr Res* 1997;42(1):1–8.

82. Baerwald KD, Popko B. Developing and mature oligodendrocytes respond differently to the immune cytokine interferon-gamma. *J Neurosci Res* 1998;52(2):230–239.

83. Gilles FH, Averill DR Jr, Kerr CS. Neonatal endotoxin encephalopathy. *Ann Neurol* 1977;2(1):49–56.

84. Maalouf EF, Duggan PJ, Counsell SJ, et al. Comparison of findings on cranial ultrasound and magnetic resonance imaging in preterm infants. *Pediatrics* 2001;107(4):719–727.

85. Hope PL, Gould SJ, Howard S, et al. Precision of ultrasound diagnosis of pathologically verified lesions in the brains of very preterm infants. *Dev Med Child Neurol* 1988;30(4):457–471.

86. Carson SC, Hertzberg BS, Bowie JD, et al. Value of sonography in the diagnosis of intracranial hemorrhage and periventricular leukomalacia: a postmortem study of 35 cases. *AJNR Am J Neuroradiol* 1990;11(4):677–683.

87. Roelants-van Rijn AM, Groenendaal F, Beek FJ, et al. Parenchymal brain injury in the preterm infant: comparison of cranial ultrasound, MRI and neurodevelopmental outcome. *Neuropediatrics* 2001;32(2):80–89.

88. Inder TE, Anderson NJ, Spencer C, et al. White matter injury in the premature infant: a comparison between serial cranial sonographic and MR findings at term. *AJNR Am J Neuroradiol* 2003;24(5):805–809.

89. Dyet LE, Kennea N, Counsell SJ, et al. Natural history of brain lesions in extremely preterm infants studied with serial magnetic resonance imaging from birth and neurodevelopmental assessment. *Pediatrics* 2006;118(2):536–548.

90. Okumura A, Hayakawa F, Kato T, et al. MRI findings in patients with spastic cerebral palsy, I: correlation with gestational age at birth. *Dev Med Child Neurol* 1997;39(6):363–368.

91. Volpe JJ. Cerebral white matter injury of the premature infant—more common than you think. *Pediatrics* 2003;112(1 pt 1):176–180.

92. Wood NS, Marlow N, Costeloe K, et al. Neurologic and developmental disability after extremely preterm birth. EPICure Study Group. *N Engl J Med* 2000;343(6):378–384.

93. Jacobson L, Ygge J, Flodmark O, et al. Visual and perceptual characteristics, ocular motility and strabismus in children with periventricular leukomalacia. *Strabismus* 2002;10(2):179–183.

94. Jacobson L, Lundin S, Flodmark O, et al. Periventricular leukomalacia causes visual impairment in preterm children: a study on the aetiologies of visual impairment in a population-based group of preterm children born 1989–1995 in the county of Värmland, Sweden. *Acta Ophthalmol Scand* 1998;76:593–598.

95. Jacobson L, Ek U, Fernell E, et al. Visual impairment in preterm children with periventricular leukomalacia—visual, cognitive and neuropaediatric characteristics related to cerebral imaging. *Dev Med Child Neurol* 1996;38(8):724–735.

55 Perinatal Asphyxia and Hypoxic-Ischemic Encephalopathy

Anne R. Hansen and Janet S. Soul

I. PERINATAL ASPHYXIA refers to a condition during the first and second stage of labor in which impaired gas exchange leads to fetal hypoxemia and hypercarbia. It is identified by fetal acidosis as measured in umbilical arterial blood. The umbilical artery pH that defines asphyxia is not the major determinant of brain injury. Although the most widely accepted definition of fetal acidosis is a pH <7.0, even with this degree of acidosis, the likelihood of brain injury is low. The following terms may be used in evaluating a term newborn at risk for brain injury in the perinatal period:

A. **Perinatal hypoxia, ischemia, and asphyxia.** These pathophysiologic terms describe respectively, lack of oxygen, blood flow, and gas exchange to the fetus or newborn. These terms should be reserved for circumstances when there are rigorous prenatal, perinatal, and postnatal data to support their use.

B. **Perinatal/neonatal depression** is a clinical, descriptive term that pertains to the condition of the infant on physical examination in the immediate postnatal period (i.e., in the first hour after birth). The clinical features of infants with this condition include depressed mental status, muscle hypotonia, and possibly disturbances in spontaneous respiration and cardiovascular function. This term makes no association with the prenatal or later postnatal (i.e., beyond the first hour) condition, physical exam, laboratory tests, imaging studies, or electroencephalograms (EEGs). After the first hour or so of life, neonatal encephalopathy is the preferred descriptive term for infants with abnormal mental status and associated findings.

C. **Neonatal encephalopathy** is a clinical and not an etiologic term that describes an abnormal neurobehavioral state consisting of decreased level of consciousness and usually other signs of brain stem and/or motor dysfunction. It does **not** imply a specific etiology, nor does it imply irreversible neurologic injury as it may be caused by such reversible conditions as maternal medications or hypoglycemia.

D. **Hypoxic-ischemic encephalopathy (HIE)** is a term that describes encephalopathy as defined above, with objective data to support a hypoxic-ischemic mechanism as the underlying cause for the encephalopathy.

E. **Hypoxic-ischemic (HI) brain injury** refers to neuropathology attributable to hypoxia and/or ischemia as evidenced by biochemical (such as serum creatine kinase brain bound [CK-BB]), electrophysiologic (EEG), neuroimaging (head ultrasonography [HUS], magnetic resonance imaging [MRI], computed tomography [CT]), or pathologic (postmortem) abnormalities.

The diagnosis of HIE and hypoxic ischemic brain injury is not a diagnosis of exclusion, but ruling out other etiologies of neurologic dysfunction is a critical part of the diagnostic evaluation. When making a diagnosis of HIE, the following information should be documented in the medical record:

1. **Prenatal history:** complications of pregnancy with emphasis on risk factors associated with neonatal depression, any pertinent family history

2. **Perinatal history:** concerns of labor and delivery, including FHR tracing and sepsis risk factors, scalp and/or cord pH (specify if arterial or venous), Apgar scores, resuscitative effort, immediate postnatal blood gases

3. Postnatal data
   a. Admission physical exam with emphasis on neurologic exam and presence of any dysmorphic features
   b. Clinical course including presence or absence of seizures (and time of onset), oliguria, cardiorespiratory dysfunction, and treatment (e.g., need for ventilator support, pressor medications)
   c. Laboratory testing, including blood gases, evidence of injury to end organs other than the brain (kidney, liver, heart, lung, blood, bowel), possible evaluation for inborn errors of metabolism, or transient metabolic abnormalities
   d. Imaging studies
   e. EEG and any other neurophysiologic data (e.g., evoked potentials)
   f. Placental pathology

II. INCIDENCE.
The frequency of perinatal asphyxia is approximately 1% to 1.5% of live births in developed countries with advanced obstetric/neonatal care and is inversely related to gestational age and birth weight. It occurs in 0.5% of live born newborns >36 weeks' gestation and accounts for 20% of perinatal deaths (50% if stillbirths are included). A higher incidence is noted in newborns of diabetic or toxemic mothers, those with intrauterine growth restriction, breech presentation, and newborns who are postdates.

III. ETIOLOGY.
In term newborns, asphyxia can occur in the antepartum or intrapartum period as a result of impaired gas exchange across the placenta that leads to the inadequate provision of oxygen (O_2) and removal of carbon dioxide (CO_2) and hydrogen (H^+) from the fetus. There is debate and a lack of certainty regarding the timing of asphyxia in many cases. Asphyxia can also occur in the postpartum period, usually secondary to pulmonary, cardiovascular, or neurologic abnormalities.

A. **Factors that increase the risk of perinatal asphyxia include the following:**

1. Impairment of maternal oxygenation
2. Decreased blood flow from mother to placenta
3. Decreased blood flow from placenta to fetus
4. Impaired gas exchange across the placenta or at the fetal tissue level
5. Increased fetal O_2 requirement

B. **Etiologies of hypoxia-ischemia may be multiple and include the following:**

1. Maternal factors: hypertension (acute or chronic), hypotension, infection (including chorioamnionitis), hypoxia from pulmonary or cardiac disorders, diabetes, maternal vascular disease, and *in utero* exposure to cocaine.

2. Placental factors: abnormal placentation, abruption, infarction, fibrosis

3. Uterine rupture

4. Umbilical cord accidents: prolapse, entanglement, true knot, compression

5. Abnormalities of umbilical vessels

6. Fetal factors: anemia, infection, cardiomyopathy, hydrops, severe cardiac/circulatory insufficiency

7. Neonatal factors: cyanotic congenital heart disease, persistent pulmonary hypertension of the newborn (PPHN), cardiomyopathy, other forms of neonatal cardiogenic and/or septic shock

IV. PATHOPHYSIOLOGY

A. Events that occur during the normal course of labor cause most babies to be born with little O_2 reserve. These include the following:

1. Decreased blood flow to placenta due to uterine contractions, some degree of cord compression, maternal dehydration, and maternal alkalosis due to hyperventilation

2. Decreased O_2 delivery to the fetus as a result of the reduction of placental blood flow

3. Increased O_2 consumption in both mother and fetus

B. Hypoxia-ischemia causes a number of physiologic and biochemical alterations:

1. With **brief asphyxia,** there is a transient increase, followed by a decrease in heart rate (HR), mild elevation in blood pressure (BP), an increase in central venous pressure (CVP), and essentially no change in cardiac output (CO). This is accompanied by a redistribution of CO with an increased proportion going to the brain, heart, and adrenal glands (diving reflex). When there is severe but brief asphyxia (e.g., placental abruption then stat caesarean section), it is thought that this diversion of blood flow to vital deep nuclear structures of the brain does not occur, hence results in the typical pattern of injury to the subcortical and brain stem nuclei.

2. With **prolonged asphyxia,** there can be a loss of pressure autoregulation and/or CO_2 vasoreactivity. This, in turn, may lead to further disturbances in cerebral perfusion, particularly when there is cardiovascular involvement with hypotension and/or decreased cardiac output. A decrease in cerebral blood flow results in anaerobic metabolism and eventual cellular energy failure due to increased glucose utilization in the brain and a fall in the concentration of glycogen, phosphocreatine, and adenosine triphosphate (ATP). Prolonged asphyxia typically results in diffuse injury to both cortical and subcortical structures, with greater injury to neuronal populations particularly susceptible to HI insults.

C. Cellular dysfunction occurs as a result of diminished oxidative phosphorylation and ATP production. This energy failure impairs ion pump function, causing accumulation of intracellular Na^+, Cl^-, H_2O, and Ca^{2+}; extracellular K^+; and excitatory neurotransmitters (e.g., glutamate). Impaired oxidative phosphorylation can occur during the primary HI insult(s) as well as during a secondary energy failure that usually occurs approximately 6 to 24 hours after the initiating insult. Cell death can be either immediate or delayed, and either necrotic or apoptotic.

1. **Immediate neuronal death (necrosis)** can occur due to intracellular osmotic overload of Na^+ and Ca^{2+}, from ion pump failure as above or excitatory neurotransmitters acting on inotropic receptors (such as the N-methyl-D-aspartate (NMDA) receptor.

2. **Delayed neuronal death (apoptosis)** occurs secondary to uncontrolled activation of enzymes and second messenger systems within the cell (e.g., Ca^{2+}-dependent lipases, proteases, and caspases); perturbation of mitochondrial respiratory electron chain transport; generation of free radicals and leukotrienes; generation of nitric oxide (NO) through NO synthase; and depletion of energy stores.

3. **Reperfusion** of previously ischemic tissue may cause further injury as it can promote the formation of excess reactive oxygen species (e.g., superoxide, hydrogen peroxide, hydroxyl, singlet oxygen), which can overwhelm the endogenous scavenger mechanisms, thereby causing damage to cellular lipids, proteins, and nucleic acids, as well as to the blood–brain barrier. This may result in an influx of neutrophils that, along with activated microglia, release injurious cytokines (e.g., interleukin 1-β and tumor necrosis factor α).

V. DIAGNOSIS

A. **Perinatal assessment of risk** includes awareness of preexisting maternal or fetal problems that may predispose to perinatal asphyxia (see III.) and of changing placental and fetal conditions (see Chap. 1) ascertained by ultrasonographic examination, biophysical profile, and nonstress tests.

B. **Low Apgar scores** and need for resuscitation in the delivery room are common but nonspecific findings. Many features of the Apgar score relate to cardiovascular integrity and **not** neurologic dysfunction resulting from asphyxia.

1. In addition to perinatal asphyxia, the differential diagnosis for a term newborn with an Apgar score ≤3 for ≥10 minutes includes depression from maternal anesthesia or analgesia, trauma, infection, cardiac or pulmonary disorders, neuromuscular, and other central nervous system disorders or malformations.

2. If the Apgar score is >6 by 5 minutes, perinatal asphyxia is not likely.

C. **Umbilical cord or first blood gas** determination. The specific blood gas criteria that define asphyxia causing brain damage are uncertain, however, the pH and base deficit on the cord or first blood gas is helpful for determining which infants have asphyxia that indicates need for further evaluation for the development of HIE. In the randomized clinical trials of hypothermia for neonatal HIE, severe acidosis was defined as pH ≤7.0 or base deficit ≥16 mmol/L.

D. **Clinical presentation and differential diagnosis.** HIE should be suspected in encephalopathic newborns with a history of fetal and neonatal distress and laboratory evidence of asphyxia. The diagnosis of HIE should not be overlooked in scenarios such as meconium aspiration, pulmonary hypertension, birth trauma, or fetal–maternal hemorrhage, where HIE may be missed because of the severity of pulmonary dysfunction, anemia, or other clinical manifestations. The diagnosis of neonatal encephalopathy includes a number of etiologies in addition to perinatal hypoxia-ischemia. Asphyxia may be suspected and HIE reasonably included in the differential diagnosis when there is:

1. Prolonged (>1 hour) antenatal acidosis

2. Fetal HR <60 beats/minute

3. Apgar score ≤3 at ≥10 minutes

4. Need for positive pressure ventilation for >1 minute or first cry delayed >5 minutes

5. Seizures within 12 to 24 hours of birth

6. Burst suppression or suppressed background pattern on EEG or amplitude-integrated EEG (aEEG)

VI. NEUROLOGIC SIGNS.
The clinical spectrum of HIE is described as mild, moderate, or severe (see Table 55.1, Sarnat stages of HIE). EEG is useful to provide objective data to grade the severity of encephalopathy.

A. **Encephalopathy.** Newborns with HIE must have depressed consciousness by definition, whether mild, moderate, or severe. Mild encephalopathy can consist of an apparent hyperalert or jittery state, but the newborn does not respond appropriately to stimuli, and thus consciousness is abnormal. Moderate and severe encephalopathies are characterized by more impaired responses to stimuli such as light, touch, or even noxious stimuli. The background pattern detected by EEG or aEEG is useful for determining the severity of encephalopathy.

B. **Brain stem and cranial nerve abnormalities.** Newborns with HIE may have brain stem dysfunction, which may manifest as abnormal or absent brain stem reflexes, including pupillary, corneal, oculocephalic, cough, and gag reflexes. There can be abnormal eye movements such as dysconjugate gaze, gaze preference, ocular bobbing or other abnormal patterns of bilateral eye movements, and an absence of visual fixation or blink to light. Newborns may show facial weakness (usually symmetric) and have a weak or absent suck and swallow with poor feeding. They can have apnea or abnormal respiratory patterns.

C. **Motor abnormalities.** With greater severity of encephalopathy, there is generally greater hypotonia, weakness, and abnormal posture with lack of flexor tone, which is usually symmetric. With severe HIE, primitive reflexes such as the Moro or grasp reflex may be diminished. Over days to weeks, the initial hypotonia may evolve into spasticity and hyperreflexia if there is significant HI brain injury. Note that if a newborn shows significant hypertonia within the first day or so after birth, the HI insult may have occurred earlier in the antepartum and have already resulted in established HI brain injury.

D. **Seizures** occur in up to 50% of newborns with HIE, and usually start within 24 hours after the HI insult. Seizures indicate that the severity of encephalopathy is moderate or severe, not mild.

1. Seizures may be subtle, tonic, or clonic. It can sometimes be difficult to differentiate seizures from jitteriness or clonus, although the latter two are usually suppressible with firm hold of the affected limb(s).

2. Since seizures are often subclinical (electrographic only) and abnormal movements or posture may not be seizure, EEG remains the gold standard for diagnosing neonatal seizures, particularly in HIE.

Table 55.1	Sarnat and Sarnat Stages of Hypoxic-Ischemic Encephalopathy*		
Stage	**Stage 1 (Mild)**	**Stage 2 (Moderate)**	**Stage 3 (Severe)**
Level of consciousness	Hyperalert; irritable	Lethargic or obtunded	Stuporous, comatose
Neuromuscular control:	Uninhibited, overreactive	Diminished spontaneous movement	Diminished or absent spontaneous movement
Muscle tone	Normal	Mild hypotonia	Flaccid
Posture	Mild distal flexion	Strong distal flexion	Intermittent decerebration
Stretch reflexes	Overactive	Overactive, disinhibited	Decreased or absent
Segmental myoclonus	Present or absent	Present	Absent
Complex reflexes:	Normal	Suppressed	Absent
Suck	Weak	Weak or absent	Absent
Moro	Strong, low threshold	Weak, incomplete, high threshold	Absent
Oculovestibular	Normal	Overactive	Weak or absent
Tonic neck	Slight	Strong	Absent
Autonomic function:	Generalized sympathetic	Generalized parasympathetic	Both systems depressed
Pupils	Mydriasis	Miosis	Midposition, often unequal; poor light reflex
Respirations	Spontaneous	Spontaneous; occasional apnea	Periodic; apnea
Heart rate	Tachycardia	Bradycardia	Variable
Bronchial and salivary secretions	Sparse	Profuse	Variable

(continued)

Table 55.1	(Continued)		
Stage	**Stage 1 (Mild)**	**Stage 2 (Moderate)**	**Stage 3 (Severe)**
Gastrointestinal motility	Normal or decreased	Increased, diarrhea	Variable
Seizures	None	Common focal or multifocal (6–24 hours of age)	Uncommon (excluding decerebration)
Electroen-cephalographic findings	Normal (awake)	Early: generalized low-voltage, slowing (continuous delta and theta)	Early: periodic pattern with isopotential phases
		Later: periodic pattern (awake); seizures focal or multifocal; 1.0–1.5 Hz spike and wave	Later: totally isopotential
Duration of symptoms	<24 hours	2–14 days	Hours to weeks
Outcome	About 100% normal	80% normal; abnormal if symptoms more than 5–7 days	About 50% die; remainder with severe sequelae

*The stages in this table are a continuum reflecting the spectrum of clinical states of newborns over 36 weeks' gestational age.
Source: From Sarnat HB, Sarnat MS. Neonatal encephalopathy following fetal distress: a clinical and electroencephalographics study. *Arch Neurol* 1976;33(10):696–705.

3. Seizures may compromise ventilation and oxygenation, especially in newborns who are not receiving mechanical ventilation.

E. **Increased intracranial pressure (ICP)** resulting from diffuse cerebral edema in HIE often reflects extensive cerebral necrosis rather than swelling of intact cells and indicates a poor prognosis. Treatment to reduce ICP does not affect outcome.

VII. **MULTIORGAN DYSFUNCTION.** Other organ systems in addition to the brain usually exhibit evidence of asphyxial damage. In a minority of cases (<15%), the brain may be the only organ exhibiting dysfunction following asphyxia. In most cases, multiorgan dysfunction occurs as a result of systemic hypoxia-ischemia. The frequency of organ involvement in perinatal asphyxia varies among published series, depending in part on the definitions used for asphyxia and organ dysfunction.

A. The **kidney** is the most common organ to be affected in the setting of perinatal asphyxia. The proximal tubule of the kidney is especially affected by decreased perfusion, leading to acute tubular necrosis with oliguria (see Chap. 28).

B. **Cardiac** dysfunction is caused by transient myocardial ischemia. The ECG may show ST depression in the midprecordium and T-wave inversion in the left precordium. Echocardiographic findings include decreased left ventricular contractility, especially of posterior wall; elevated ventricular end-diastolic pressures; tricuspid insufficiency and pulmonary hypertension. In severely asphyxiated newborns, dysfunction more commonly affects the right ventricle. A fixed HR may raise suspicion of severe brain stem injury.

C. **Gastrointestinal effects** include an increased risk of bowel ischemia and necrotizing enterocolitis (see Chap. 27).

D. **Hematologic effects** include disseminated intravascular coagulation due to damage to blood vessels, poor production of clotting factors due to liver dysfunction, and poor production of platelets by the bone marrow.

E. **Liver dysfunction** may be manifested by isolated elevation of hepatocellular enzymes. More extensive damage may occur, leading to DIC, inadequate glycogen stores with resultant hypoglycemia, altered metabolism, or elimination of drugs.

F. **Pulmonary effects** include increased pulmonary vascular resistance leading to PPHN, pulmonary hemorrhage, pulmonary edema due to cardiac dysfunction, and meconium aspiration.

VIII. LABORATORY EVALUATION OF ASPHYXIA

A. **Cardiac evaluation**

1. **Cardiac troponin I (cTNI) and cardiac troponin T (cTnT),** cardiac regulatory proteins that control the calcium-mediated interaction of actin and myosin, are markers of myocardial damage. Normal values in the neonate are troponin I = 0 to 0.28 ± 0.42 μg/L and troponin T = 0 to 0.097 μg/L. Elevated levels of these proteins have been described in newborns with clinical and laboratory evidence of asphyxia.

2. An elevation of **serum creatine kinase myocardial bound** (CK-MB) fraction of >5% to 10% may indicate myocardial injury.

B. **Neurologic markers of brain injury**

1. Serum CK-BB may be increased in asphyxiated newborns within 12 hours of the insult, but has not been correlated with long-term neurodevelopmental outcome. CK-BB is also expressed in placenta, lungs, gastrointestinal tract, and kidneys. Other serum markers such as protein S-100, neuron specific enolase, and urine markers have been measured in newborns with asphyxia and HIE.

2. In practice, serum and urine markers of brain injury are not routinely used to evaluate for the presence of brain injury or to predict outcome.

C. **Renal evaluation**

1. Blood urea nitrogen (BUN) and serum creatinine (Cr) may be elevated in perinatal asphyxia. Typically, elevation is noted 2 to 4 days after the insult.

2. Fractional excretion (FE) of Na$^+$ or renal failure index may help confirm renal insult (see Chap. 28).

3. Urine levels of β-2-microglobulin have been used as an indicator of proximal tubular dysfunction, although not routinely. This low molecular weight protein is freely filtered through the glomerulus and reabsorbed almost completely in the proximal tubule.

4. Renal sonographic abnormalities correlate with the occurrence of oliguria.

IX. BRAIN IMAGING

A. **Cranial sonographic** examination can demonstrate edema as loss of gray-white differentiation when severe, but is generally insensitive for the detection of HI brain injury, particularly in the first days after birth. It may be useful to rule out large intracranial hemorrhage, particularly since this may be a contraindication to therapeutic hypothermia.

B. **Computed tomography (CT)** may be used to detect cerebral edema, hemorrhage, and eventually HI brain injury. Because of the degree of radiation exposure, CT is only indicated if imaging is urgently needed to determine clinical treatment and neither ultrasound nor MRI is available on an emergency basis.

C. **Magnetic resonance imaging (MRI).** Conventional T1- and T2-weighted MRI sequences are the best modality for determining the severity and extent of HI brain injury, but the injury is often not apparent on these sequences in the first days after the HI insult (unless the injury is older than suspected or very severe). These conventional sequences are best for the detection of brain injury after 7 to 10 days, and a scan as late as 14 days or older may be needed if there are clinical signs of HI brain injury without imaging correlates at an earlier time.

1. **Diffusion-weighted imaging (DWI)** can show abnormalities within hours of an HI insult that may be useful in the diagnosis of neonatal HIE and an early indicator of possible brain injury. However, DWI can both underestimate and overestimate the location and severity of HI brain injury, depending on the timing of the study. Early DWI scans will usually show restricted diffusion in brain regions affected by hypoxia-ischemia, although this does not inevitably mean that these regions are irreversibly injured. At 7 to 10 days of age, there is pseudonormalization of diffusion, so DWI can appear normal despite the presence of HI injury. After 7 to 10 days, diffusion is usually increased in regions of HI brain injury. Thus, DWI data need to be interpreted carefully within the context of the history and clinical course of the newborn with HIE.

2. **Proton magnetic resonance spectroscopy (MRS),** also called *proton-MRS or ¹H-MRS*, measures the relative concentrations of various metabolites in tissue. Elevated lactate, decreased N-acetylaspartate (NAA), and alterations of the ratios of these two metabolites in relation to choline or creatine can indicate HIE and help prognosticate neurologic outcome.

3. **Susceptibility-weighted imaging** may be useful for the detection of hemorrhage or hemorrhagic injury.

4. **MR angiography or venography** may occasionally be useful if there is suspicion of vascular anomalies, thromboembolic disease, or sinus venous thrombosis resulting in HI injury.

X. EEG is used both to detect and monitor seizure activity and also to define abnormal background patterns such as discontinuous burst suppression, low voltage, or isoelectric patterns. When conventional 8- or 16-channel neonatal EEG is not readily available, amplitude-integrated EEG (aEEG) has been used to evaluate the background pattern, particularly when rapid assessment is needed for determination of treatment with therapeutic hypothermia. This method consists of a reduced montage with 1- or 2-channel EEG with parietal electrodes. Although aEEG may detect some seizures, there are data showing that aEEG is insufficient to detect all seizures compared with conventional EEG, and that the quality of aEEG interpretation depends very much on the experience and expertise of the reader.

XI. PATHOLOGIC FINDINGS OF BRAIN INJURY

A. Specific neuropathology may be seen after moderate or severe asphyxia.

   1. Focal or multifocal cortical necrosis affecting all cellular elements can result in cystic encephalomalacia and/or ulegyria (attenuation of depths of sulci) due to loss of perfusion in one or several vascular beds.

   2. Watershed injury occurs in boundary zones between cerebral arteries, particularly following severe hypotension. This results from poor perfusion of the vulnerable periventricular border zones in the centrum semiovale and produces predominantly white matter injury. In the term newborn, this typically results in bilateral parasagittal cortical and subcortical white matter injury or injury to the parieto-occipital cortex.

   3. Selective neuronal necrosis is the most common type of injury seen following perinatal asphyxia. It is due to differential vulnerability of specific cell types to hypoxia-ischemia; for example, neurons are more easily injured than glia. Specific regions at increased risk are CA1 region of hippocampus, Purkinje cells of cerebellum in term newborns, and brain stem nuclei. Necrosis of thalamic nuclei and basal ganglia (status marmoratus) can be considered a subtype of selective neuronal necrosis.

B. Neuropathology may reflect the type of asphyxial episode although the precise pattern is not predictable.

   1. Prolonged partial episodes of asphyxia tend to cause diffuse cerebral (especially cortical) necrosis, although there is often involvement of subcortical ± brain stem structures as well.

   2. Acute total asphyxia tends to spare the cortex in large part (except the perirolandic cortex) and instead affects primarily the brain stem, thalamus, and basal ganglia.

   3. Partial prolonged asphyxia followed by a terminal acute asphyxial event (combination) is probably present in most cases.

XII. TREATMENT

A. Perinatal management of high-risk pregnancies

   1. Fetal HR and rhythm abnormalities may provide supporting evidence of asphyxia, especially if accompanied by presence of thick meconium. However, they provide no information concerning duration or severity of an asphyxial event.

   2. Measurement of fetal scalp pH is a better determinant of fetal oxygenation than PO_2. With intermittent hypoxia-ischemia, PO_2 may improve transiently whereas the pH progressively falls. Fetal scalp blood lactate has been suggested as easier and more reliable than pH, but has not gained wide acceptance.

3. Close monitoring of progress of labor with awareness of other signs of *in utero* stress is important.

4. The presence of a constellation of abnormal findings may indicate the need to mobilize the perinatal team for a newborn that could require immediate intervention. Alteration of delivery plans may be indicated and guidelines for intervention in cases of suspected fetal distress should be designed and in place in each medical center (see Chap. 1).

B. Delivery room management (see Chap. 9)

The initial management of the HI newborn in the delivery room is described in Chapter 5.

C. Postnatal management of neurologic effects of asphyxia

1. Ventilation. CO_2 should be maintained in the normal range. Hypercapnia can cause cerebral acidosis and cerebral vasodilation. This may result in more flow to uninjured areas and relative ischemia to damaged areas ("steal phenomenon"). Excessive hypocapnia (CO_2 <25 mm Hg) may decrease CBF.

2. Oxygenation. Oxygen levels should be maintained in the normal range, although poor peripheral perfusion may limit the accuracy of continuous non-invasive monitoring. Hypoxemia should be treated with supplemental O_2 and/or ventilation. Hyperoxia may cause decreased CBF or exacerbate free radical damage.

3. Temperature. Passive cooling by turning off warming lights is an effective way to initiate therapeutic hypothermia as soon as possible after the HI insult. Hyperthermia should always be avoided.

4. Perfusion. Cardiovascular stability and adequate mean systemic arterial BP are important in order to maintain adequate cerebral perfusion pressure.

5. Maintain physiologic metabolic state

a. Hypocalcemia is a common metabolic alteration after neonatal asphyxia. It is important to maintain calcium in the normal range because hypocalcemia can compromise cardiac contractility and may cause seizures (see Chaps. 25 and 56).

b. Hypoglycemia is often seen in asphyxiated newborns. Blood glucose level should be maintained in the normal range for term newborns. Hypoglycemia may increase cerebral blood flow and exacerbate the energy deficit. Hyperglycemia may lead to increased brain lactate, damage to cellular integrity, cerebral edema, or further disturbance in vascular autoregulation.

6. Judicious fluid management is needed and both fluid overload and inadequate circulating volume should be avoided. Two processes predispose to fluid overload in asphyxiated newborns:

a. Syndrome of inappropriate antidiuretic hormone (SIADH) secretion (see Chap. 23) is often seen 3 to 4 days after the HI event. It is manifested by hyponatremia and hypo-osmolarity in combination with low urine output and inappropriately concentrated urine (elevated urine specific gravity, osmolarity, and Na^+).

b. ATN (see Chap. 28) can result from the "diving reflex" (see IV.B.1., above).

c. Fluid restriction may aid in minimizing cerebral edema although the effect of fluid restriction on long-term outcome in newborns who are not in renal failure is not known.

7. **Control of seizures.** Seizures generally start within 12 hours of birth, increase in frequency, and then usually resolve within days, although seizures may persist in severe cases. Seizures caused by HIE can be extremely difficult to control and may not be possible to eliminate completely with currently available anticonvulsants. It is important to remember that seizures in HIE are often subclinical (electrographic only), and that seizures in newborns on musculoskeletal blockade may be manifested only by abrupt changes in BP, HR, and oxygenation. In these cases, EEG is absolutely required to detect seizures and monitor the response to anticonvulsant therapy, and is superior to aEEG for this purpose (1). There is increasing evidence that seizures exacerbate brain injury (2,3), but anticonvulsants are often incompletely effective and it has not yet been proven that improved seizure control results in improved neurologic outcome (4). Metabolic perturbations such as hypoglycemia, hypocalcemia, and hyponatremia that may cause or exacerbate seizure activity and should be corrected.

   a. **Acute anticonvulsant management**

      i. **Phenobarbital** is the initial drug of choice. It is given as a loading dose of 20 mg/kg IV. If seizures continue, additional loading doses of 5 to 10 mg/kg IV may be given as needed to control seizures. A maintenance dose of 3 to 5 mg/kg/day PO or IV divided bid should be started 12 to 24 hours after the loading dose. During loading doses of phenobarbital, the newborn needs to be monitored closely for respiratory depression. Therapeutic serum levels are 15 to 40 mg/dL. Because of a prolonged serum half-life, which may be increased by hepatic and renal dysfunction, serum levels need to be monitored and maintenance dosing adjusted accordingly.

      ii. **Phenytoin** may be added when seizures are not controlled by phenobarbital. The loading dose is 15 to 20 mg/kg IV followed by a maintenance dose of 4 to 8 mg/kg/day divided q8h. In many centers, **fosphenytoin** is used in place of parent drug (phenytoin), because the risk of hypotension is less and extravasation has no adverse effects. Dosage is calculated and written in terms of phenytoin equivalents to avoid medication errors. Therapeutic serum level is typically 15 to 20 mg/dL although levels in the 20 to 25 range may be effective, and consideration should be given to measurement of the free phenytoin level.

      iii. Benzodiazepines are considered third-line drugs and include lorazepam, which can be given in doses of 0.05 to 0.1 mg/kg/dose IV. Some clinicians use midazolam boluses and IV infusions to control seizures, but there are few data regarding the safety and efficacy of this treatment.

      iv. Levetiracetam has been used recently because of its availability in IV form and relative safety and efficacy for various types of childhood epilepsy. There are a few series published reporting benefit, but no randomized controlled trials and few data regarding safety and few data regarding the appropriate dose for neonatal seizures.

   b. **Long-term anticonvulsant management.** Anticonvulsants can be weaned when the clinical exam and EEG indicate that the newborn is no longer having seizures. If a newborn is receiving more than one anticonvulsant, weaning should be in the reverse order of initiation, with phenobarbital being weaned last. There is controversy regarding when phenobarbital should be discontinued, with some favoring discontinuation shortly before discharge and some favoring continued treatment for 1 to 6 months or more. Newborns who have a high risk of recurring seizures in infancy or childhood are those with persistent neurologic deficit and those with an abnormal EEG.

8. Management of other target organ injury

a. Cardiac dysfunction should be managed with correction of hypoxemia, acidosis, and hypoglycemia and avoidance of volume overload. Diuretics may not be helpful if concomitant renal impairment is present. Newborns will require continuous monitoring of systemic mean arterial BP, CVP (if available), and urine output. Newborns with cardiovascular compromise may require inotropic drugs such as dopamine (see Chap. 40) and may need afterload reduction (e.g., with a phosphodiesterase inhibitor such as milrinone) to maintain BP and perfusion.

   i. Arterial BP should be maintained in the normal range to support adequate cerebral perfusion.

   ii. Monitoring of CVP may be helpful to assess adequacy of preload (i.e., that the newborn is not hypovolemic due to vasodilatation or third spacing); a reasonable goal is 5 to 8 mm Hg in term newborns.

b. Renal dysfunction should be monitored by measuring urine output, and with serum electrolytes, paired urine/serum osmolarity, urinalysis, urine specific gravity.

   i. In the presence of oliguria or anuria, avoid fluid overload by limiting free water administration to replacement of insensible losses and urine output (~60 mL/kg/day) and consider using low-dose dopamine infusion (≤2.5 μg/kg/minute) (see Chaps. 23 and 28).

   ii. Volume status should be evaluated before instituting strict fluid restriction. If there is no or low urine output, a 10 to 20 mL/kg fluid challenge followed by a loop diuretic such as furosemide may be helpful.

   iii. To avoid fluid overload, as well as hypoglycemia, concentrated glucose infusions delivered through a central line may be needed. Glucose levels should be monitored closely and rapid glucose boluses avoided. Infusions should be weaned slowly to avoid rebound hypoglycemia.

c. Gastrointestinal effects. Feeding should be withheld until blood pressure is stable, active bowel sounds are audible, and stools are negative for blood (see Chap. 27).

d. Hematologic abnormalities (see Chaps. 42–47). Coagulation profile should be monitored with partial thromboplastin time (PTT) and prothrombin time (PT), fibrinogen, and platelets. Abnormalities may need to be corrected with fresh frozen plasma, cryoprecipitate, and/or platelet infusions.

e. Liver function should be monitored with measurement of transaminases (ALT, AST), clotting (PT, PTT, and fibrinogen), albumin, bilirubin, and ammonia. Levels of drugs that are metabolized or eliminated through the liver must be monitored.

f. Lung (see Chaps. 29, 30, and 36). Management of the pulmonary effects of asphyxia depends on the specific etiology.

XIII. NEUROPROTECTIVE STRATEGIES. A number of neuroprotective strategies have been proposed.

A. Agents tested in animals with few or no data in human newborns include antagonists of excitotoxic neurotransmitter receptors such as NMDA receptor blockade with ketamine or MK-801; free radical scavengers such as allopurinol, superoxide dismutase, and vitamin E; Ca^{2+}-channel blockers such as magnesium sulfate, nimodipine, nicardipine; cyclooxygenase inhibitors such as indomethacin; benzodiazepine receptor stimulation such as midazolam; and enhancers of protein synthesis such as dexamethasone. There are new agents such as xenon and erythropoietin that are undergoing preliminary evaluation in Phase I trials, but there are no data supporting the use of any agent besides therapeutic hypothermia for neuroprotection.

B. **Therapeutic hypothermia** has been shown to decrease the risk of brain injury in newborns exposed to perinatal hypoxic ischemic conditions (5–7). Both total body and head cooling have been shown to be safe and effective (8–10). We offer total body cooling to newborns at risk for HIE based on the following criteria:

1. **Inclusion**
   a. Gestational age ≥36 weeks and birth weight ≥2,000 g
   b. Evidence of **fetal** distress as evidenced by at least one of the following:
      i. History of acute perinatal event (e.g., abruption placenta, cord prolapse, severe fetal heart rate abnormality, and variable or late decelerations)
      ii. Biophysical Profile <6/10 (or 4/8) within 6 hours of birth
      iii. Cord pH ≤ 7.0 **or** base deficit ≥16 mEq/L
   c. Evidence of **neonatal** distress as evidenced be at least one of the following:
      i. Apgar score ≤5 at 10 minutes
      ii. Postnatal blood gas pH at <1 hour ≤7.0 **or** base deficit ≥16 mEq/L
      iii. Continued need for ventilation initiated at birth and continued for at least 10 minutes
   d. Evidence of neonatal encephalopathy by physical exam (ideally confirmed by a neurologist)
   e. Abnormal aEEG with minimum of 20 minutes recording, one of the following:
      i. Severely abnormal: Upper margin <10 μV
      ii. Moderately abnormal: Upper margin >10 μV **and** lower margin <5 μV
      iii. Seizures identified by an aEEG
   Missing data should be considered carefully and not necessarily be presumed to be normal.

2. **Exclusion.** Patients may be excluded from this protocol according to the judgment of the attending neonatologist. If an exclusion criterion is identified during therapy, the patient should be warmed according to re-warming procedure described below.
   a. Normal initial aEEG tracing: lower margin >5 μV, no seizures
   b. Inability to initiate cooling by 6 hours of age
   c. Presence of lethal chromosomal anomaly (e.g., trisomy 13 or 18)
   d. Presence of severe congenital anomalies (e.g., complex cyanotic congenital heart disease, major central nervous system anomaly)
   e. Symptomatic systemic congenital viral infection (e.g., hepatosplenomegaly, microcephaly)
   f. Symptomatic systemic bacterial infection (e.g., meningo-encaphalitis, disseminated intravascular coagulopathy)
   g. Bleeding diathesis (platelet count <50 K, spontaneous clinical bleeding)
   h. Major intracranial hemorrhage
   Cooling should be started before 6 hours of age; therefore, early recognition is essential.

The target esophageal temperature goal during cooling is 33.5°C (33°–34°C) with acceptable range: 32.5° to 34.5°C.

Arterial access and central venous access should be obtained prior to initiation of therapeutic hypothermia protocol if able. Obtaining central access in the hypothermic state can be extremely challenging due to vasoconstrictive effects.

C. **Safety monitoring of newborns during 72 hours of therapeutic hypothermia and re-warming: Temperature**

1. Temp: Monitor skin and esophageal temperature continuously. Check for areas of skin breakdown and reposition newborn frequently given the risk of subcutaneous fat necrosis. The hypothermia blanket should be kept dry.

2. CVR/Resp: Use pulse oximetry cautiously, if at all since the reading may be inaccurate. Follow arterial blood gases (with patient temp recorded on blood gas requisition) and lactate levels.

3. FEN/Renal/GI: Monitor serum electrolytes, BUN/Cr, AST/ALT. Because of potential neuroprotective effect of magnesium, we aim for serum level at upper limits of normal range. To avoid cerebral edema, our goal Na is 140 to 148. Because many of these patients have decrease urine output, we anticipate need for relative fluid restriction.

4. Heme: Monitor PT/PTT/INR fibrinogen, platelets and treat as clinically indicated. We transfuse platelets if <100 K due to decreased platelet function.

5. ID: Monitor CBC differential and blood culture results. We treat with antibiotics for duration of cooling as prophylaxis in setting of relative immune dysfunction induced by hypothermia. We have a low threshold for changing gentamicin to cefotaxime if evidence of renal impairment.

6. aEEG to meet inclusion criteria: We continue aEEG and/or full 20-lead EEG when needed to monitor seizure activity. If unable to obtain MRI within first 24 hours of cooling, we obtain a head ultrasound to assess for any intracranial hemorrhage that would contraindicate further hypothermia therapy. We ensure adequate sedation both to optimizing comfort and avoid an increase in metabolism as the newborn attempts to increase temperature, thus decreasing the efficacy of the hypothermia therapy.

At the end of 72 hours of induced hypothermia, the newborn is re-warmed at a rate of 0.5°C every 2 hours following above procedure until reach 36.5°C. This should take approximately 10 hours.

If a patient is discovered to meet an exclusion criterion or undergoes a major adverse event while undergoing hypothermia treatment, we re-warm according to the same procedure. We obtain a brain MRI after completion of therapeutic hypothermia; ideally, this should be obtained at 7 to 10 days of age or later if possible to detect the full extent of any HI brain injury.

XIV. OUTCOME IN PERINATAL ASPHYXIA

A. The overall mortality rate is approximately 20%. The frequency of neurodevelopmental sequelae in surviving newborns is approximately 30%.

B. The risk of CP in survivors of perinatal asphyxia is 5% to 10% compared to 0.2% in the general population. **Most CP is not related to perinatal asphyxia, and most perinatal asphyxia does not cause CP.**

C. Specific outcomes depend on the severity of the encephalopathy, the presence or absence of seizures, EEG results, and neuroimaging findings.

    1. Severity of encephalopathy can be ascertained using the **Sarnat clinical stages of HIE** (Table 55.1).

        a. Stage 1 or mild HIE: 98% to 100% of newborns will have a normal neurologic outcome and <1% mortality.

        b. Stage 2 or moderate HIE: 20% to 37% die or have abnormal neurodevelopmental outcomes. Prognosis can be refined by the use of EEG and MRI studies to detect the severity of encephalopathy, seizures, and the severity and location of HI brain injury. This group may benefit the most from therapeutic hypothermia.

        c. Stage 3 or severe HIE: Death is more likely, including as a result of withdrawal of medical technology when there is evidence of severe brain injury and devastating neurologic prognosis. Survivors are likely to have one or more major neurodevelopmental disability such as CP, intellectual disability, visual impairment, or epilepsy.

    2. The presence of seizures increases a newborn's risk of CP 50 to 70 fold. Mortality and long-term morbidity are highest for seizures that begin within 12 hours of birth, are electrographic, and/or are frequent (3).

    3. The detection of low voltage activity or isoelectric background by EEG is a prognostic indicator of poor outcome. While a transient burst-suppression pattern may be associated with a good outcome, a persistent burst-suppression pattern (e.g., ≥7 days) is associated with a high risk of death or neurodevelopmental disability.

    4. MRI has added a great deal of information to the clinical and EEG data as the pattern of HI brain injury by MRI generally correlates well with neurologic outcome, when performed at the right age and interpreted by a physician with expertise in interpreting neonatal brain MRI scans. Significant injury to the cortex or subcortical nuclei is almost invariably associated with both intellectual and motor disability. However, discrete lesions in the subcortical nuclei or less severe watershed pattern injuries can be associated with a normal cognitive outcome and only mild motor impairments. Thus, these studies should be interpreted with care by physicians with experience in caring for children who had neonatal HIE.

REFERENCES

1. Shellhaas RA, Soaita AI, Clancy RR. Sensitivity of amplitude-integrated electroencephalography for neonatal seizure detection. *Pediatrics* 2007;120(4):770–777.
2. Wirrell EC, Armstrong EA, Osman LD, et al. Prolonged seizures exacerbate perinatal hypoxic-ischemic brain damage. *Pediatr Res* 2001;50(4):445–454.
3. McBride MC, Laroia N, Guillet R. Electrographic seizures in neonates correlate with poor neurodevelopmental outcome. *Neurology* 2000;55(4):506–513.
4. Rennie J, Boylan G. Treatment of neonatal seizures. *Arch Dis Child Fetal Neonatal Ed* 2007;92(2):F148–F150.
5. Gluckman PD, Wyatt JS, Azzopardi D, et al. Selective head cooling with mild systemic hypothermia after neonatal encephalopathy: multicentre randomised trial. *Lancet* 2005;365(9460):663–670.
6. Shankaran S, Laptook AR, Ehrenkranz RA, et al. Whole-body hypothermia for neonates with hypoxic-ischemic encephalopathy. *N Engl J Med* 2005;353(15):1574–1584.

7. Azzopardi DV, Strohm B, Edwards AD, et al. Moderate hypothermia to treat perinatal asphyxial encephalopathy. *N Engl J Med* 2009;361(14):1349–1358.
8. Gunn AJ, Gluckman PD, Gunn TR. Selective head cooling in newborn infants after perinatal asphyxia: a safety study. *Pediatrics* 1998;102(4 pt 1):885–892.
9. Eicher DJ, Wagner CL, Katikaneni LP, et al. Moderate hypothermia in neonatal encephalopathy: safety outcomes. *Pediatr Neurol* 2005;32(1):18–24.
10. Shankaran S, Pappas A, Laptook AR, et al. Outcomes of safety and effectiveness in a multicenter randomized, controlled trial of whole-body hypothermia for neonatal hypoxic-ischemic encephalopathy. *Pediatrics* 2008;122(4):e791–e798.

Suggested Readings

ACOG Task Force on Neonatal Encephalopathy and Cerebral Palsy. *Neonatal encephalopathy and cerebral palsy: Defining the pathogenesis and pathophysiology.* Washington, DC: American College of Obstetricians and Gynecologists, 2003.

Barkovich AJ, Westmark K, Partridge C, et al. Perinatal asphyxia: MR findings in the first 10 days. *AJNR Am J Neuroradiol* 1995;16(3):427–438.

Battin MR, Thoresen M, Robinson E, et al. Does head cooling with mild systemic hypothermia affect requirement for blood pressure support? *Pediatrics* 2009;123(3):1031–1036.

Blackmon LR, Stark AR. Hypothermia: a neuroprotective therapy for neonatal hypoxic-ischemic encephalopathy. *Pediatrics* 2006;117(3):942–948.

Edwards AD, Azzopardi DV. Therapeutic hypothermia following perinatal asphyxia. *Arch Dis Child Fetal Neonatal Ed* 2006;91(2):F127–F131.

Edwards AD, Brocklehurst P, Gunn AJ, et al. Neurological outcomes at 18 months of age after moderate hypothermia for perinatal hypoxic ischaemic encephalopathy: synthesis and meta-analysis of trial data. *BMJ* 2010;340:c363.

Groenendaal F, De Vooght KM, van Bel F. Blood gas values during hypothermia in asphyxiated term neonates. *Pediatrics* 2009;123(1):170–172.

Higgins RD, Raju TN, Perlman J, et al. Hypothermia and perinatal asphyxia: executive summary of the National Institute of Child Health and Human Development workshop. *J Pediatr* 2006;148(2):170–175.

Holmes G, Rowe J, Hafford J, et al. Prognostic value of the electroencephalogram in neonatal asphyxia. *Electroencephalogr Clin Neurophysiol* 1982;53(1):60–72.

Johnston MV, Trescher WH, Ishida A, et al. Neurobiology of hypoxic-ischemic injury in the developing brain. *Pediatr Res* 2001;49(6):735–741.

Leviton A, Nelson KB. Problems with definitions and classifications of newborn encephalopathy. *Pediatr Neurol* 1992;8(2):85–90.

Mallard EC, Williams CE, Gunn AJ, et al. Frequent episodes of brief ischemia sensitize the fetal sheep brain to neuronal loss and induce striatal injury. *Pediatr Res* 1993;33(1):61–65.

McKinstry RC, Miller JH, Snyder AZ, et al. A prospective, longitudinal diffusion tensor imaging study of brain injury in newborns. *Neurology* 2002;59(6):824–833.

Meberg A, Broch H. Etiology of cerebral palsy. *J Perinat Med* 2004;32(5):434–439.

Ment LR, Bada HS, Barnes P, et al. Practice parameter: neuroimaging of the neonate: report of the Quality Standards Subcommittee of the American Academy of Neurology and the Practice Committee of the Child Neurology Society. *Neurology* 2002;58(12):1726–1738.

Murray DM, Boylan GB, Ryan CA, et al. Early EEG findings in hypoxic-ischemic encephalopathy predict outcomes at 2 years. *Pediatrics* 2009;124(3):e459–e467.

Myers RE. Four patterns of perinatal brain damage and their conditions of occurrence in primates. *Adv Neurol* 1975;10:223–234.

Nelson KB, Leviton A. How much of neonatal encephalopathy is due to birth asphyxia? *Am J Dis Child* 1991;145(11):1325–1331.

Pryds O, Greisen G, Lou H, et al. Vasoparalysis associated with brain damage in asphyxiated term infants. *J Pediatr* 1990;117(1 pt 1):119–125.

Rutherford M, Ramenghi LA, Edwards AD, et al. Assessment of brain tissue injury after moderate hypothermia in neonates with hypoxic-ischaemic encephalopathy: a nested substudy of a randomised controlled trial. *Lancet Neurol* 2010;9(1):39–45.

Sarkar S, Bhagat I, Dechert RE, et al. Predicting death despite therapeutic hypothermia in infants with hypoxic-ischaemic encephalopathy. *Arch Dis Child Fetal Neonatal Ed* 2010;95(6):F423–F428.

Sarnat HB, Sarnat MS. Neonatal encephalopathy following fetal distress. A clinical and electroencephalographic study. *Arch Neurol* 1976;33(10):696–705.

Soul JS, Robertson RL, Tzika AA, et al. Time course of changes in diffusion-weighted magnetic resonance imaging in a case of neonatal encephalopathy with defined onset and duration of hypoxic-ischemic insult. *Pediatrics* 2001;108(5):1211–1214.

Volpe JJ. *Neurology of the Newborn*. 5th ed. Philadelphia, PA: Saunders Elsevier; 2008.

Wilkinson DJ, Thayyil S, Robertson NJ. Ethical and practical issues relating to the global use of therapeutic hypothermia for perinatal asphyxial encephalopathy. *Arch Dis Child Fetal Neonatal Ed* 2011;96(1):F75–F78.

Wu YW, Escobar GJ, Grether JK, et al. Chorioamnionitis and cerebral palsy in term and near-term infants. *JAMA* 2003;290(20):2677–2684.

Yap V, Engel M, Takenouchi T, et al. Seizures are common in term infants undergoing head cooling. *Pediatr Neurol* 2009;41(5):327–331.

Neonatal Seizures

Ann M. Bergin

I. INTRODUCTION. Seizures occur more frequently in the neonatal period than at any other time of life. Estimates of the incidence of neonatal seizures vary according to case definition, method of ascertainment and definition of the neonatal period, and range from 0.95 to 3.5 per 1,000 live births. Seizures may be symptomatic of an underlying disorder or due to a primary epileptic condition. In neonates, the vast majority of seizures are symptomatic of underlying disorders although primary epileptic disorders may also present in this age group. The occurrence of seizure may be the first clinical indication of neurologic disorder.

Developmental immaturity influences many aspects of diagnosis, management, and prognosis of seizures in the newborn:

A. Clinical seizure patterns in the neonate reflect the "reduced connectivity" in the neonatal brain, with prominence of focal ictal characteristics, and rarity of generalized patterns of clinical seizures.

B. The balance of excitatory and inhibitory processes in the immature brain is weighted toward excitation with an excess of glutamatergic synapses over inhibitory (usually GABA-ergic) synapses. In fact, in some regions of the neonatal brain, GABA may temporarily act as an excitatory neurotransmitter. These developmental features may underlie the neonate's tendency to frequently recurrent seizures.

C. Systemic processes are immature, leading to altered drug handling compared to older children.

D. The immature brain may be more susceptible to developmental effects of anticonvulsant medications.

II. DIAGNOSIS. An epileptic seizure is a change in neurologic function (motor, sensory, experiential, or autonomic) that is associated with an abnormal synchronous discharge of cortical neurons. This abnormal electrical discharge may be recorded by electroencephalography (EEG). At all ages, including in the newborn, paroxysmal behaviors may occur, which raise suspicion of electrical seizure but lack correlating patterns on scalp EEG. Management of these events is difficult at any age and controversial in the newborn. For this review, only those paroxysmal events typically associated with an electrographic seizure pattern are considered.

Early diagnosis of neonatal seizures is important to allow:
- Identification and treatment of underlying disorders
- Treatment to prevent additional seizures and seizure-related systemic effects, such as hypoxemia and hypertension
- Treatment of seizures to possibly prevent seizure-related excitotoxic neuronal injury

Diagnosis of seizures in the neonate requires knowledge of the clinical patterns associated with electrographic seizures at this age and confirmation with EEG, ideally accompanied by video telemetry. Nonepileptic paroxysmal events are common in the encephalopathic infant, and unlike seizures, lack an EEG seizure pattern and may be altered or stopped by gentle restraint and/or change in position. Nonepileptic events are often stimulus-evoked. In addition, video-EEG recordings have revealed that a large proportion of electrographic neonatal seizures (ENS) occurring in encephalopathic infants lack a clinical correlate. This also occurs following treatment with phenobarbital when the clinical events appear to cease, but EEG recordings continue to show ENS (estimates vary between 30% and 80% of cases). Whether these subclinical electrographic seizures cause additional brain injury in the newborn is unproven to date. However, a study in human neonates has correlated an increased amount of ENS with increased morbidity and mortality, especially in asphyxiated infants. In a magnetic spectroscopy study of human neonates, an increasing seizure severity score correlated with greater abnormality of the lactate:choline and N-acetylaspartate:choline ratios, reflecting impaired cerebral metabolism and possibly compromised neuronal integrity, respectively.

A. Common clinical seizure patterns

1. **Focal clonic seizures.** This pattern may occur unilaterally, sequentially in different limbs, or simultaneously but asynchronously. The movement is rhythmic, biphasic with a fast-contraction phase and a slower relaxation. A clinical correlate may be present for only a small portion of the total duration of the electrographic seizure. Face, upper or lower limbs, eyes, or trunk may be involved.

2. **Focal tonic seizures.** Patterns include a sustained posture of a single limb, tonic horizontal eye deviation or asymmetric tonic truncal postures. In contrast to focal tonic events, generalized tonic movements are generally not accompanied by seizure patterns on EEG.

3. **Myoclonic seizures.** These are characterized by a rapid movement usually of flexion. Of the varieties of myoclonus occurring in the newborn, generalized myoclonus, usually involving both upper limbs and less commonly the lower limbs, is most often associated with an EEG seizure pattern. Focal or multifocal myoclonic events are usually not associated with such patterns.

4. **Autonomic seizures.** Autonomic events such as apnea, often with associated tachycardia rather than bradycardia (particularly in term newborns), and/or pupillary dilatation. These are often also associated with hypertension.
   Many newborns may have more than one seizure type. In premature infants, a wider range of clinical behaviors can be associated with electrographic seizure patterns; for instance, self-limited short periods of otherwise unexplained tachypnea, tachycardia, and other autonomic changes may represent seizures in the preterm infant, as may chewing, sucking, and cycling movements, which usually are not associated with EEG seizures in the term infant.

B. EEG diagnosis

1. **Routine neonatal EEG recording**, typically of 1 hour duration, allows assessment of background activity, developmental maturity, and sometimes, epileptic potential. Such recordings, especially if performed serially, are useful for prognostication. However, a typical clinical event may not be captured in such a short time. If available, prolonged EEG recording (hours–days) is helpful to capture a clinical event, especially if the diagnosis of seizure is not clear. The EEG usually demonstrates a rhythmic focal correlate associated with, but typically of longer duration than the clinical event. A focus of origin and spread to adjacent areas can be seen (Figure 56.1). The more severely encephalopathic

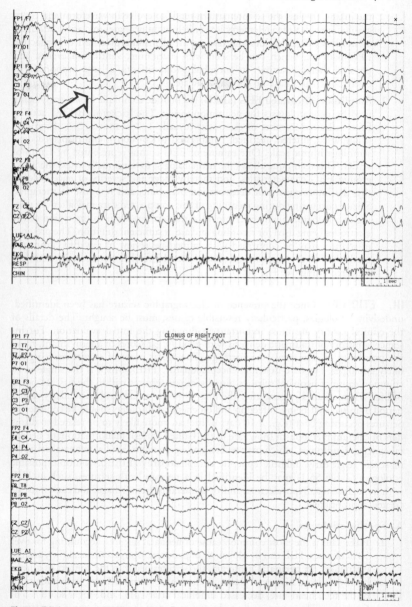

Figure 56.1 Left parasagittal neonatal seizure with focal clonic seizure. Electrographic seizure begins in the left parasagittal area (open arrow), and 12 seconds later, focal clonus of the right foot is noted.

the infant, the less the seizure pattern tends to evolve in waveform and topographic spread. Video telemetry is very helpful in neonates to clarify the nature of nonepileptic behaviors and also to avoid misinterpretation of artifactual EEG patterns, which can be seen with suctioning, ventilation events, and physical therapy/patting. In encephalopathic infants, a large proportion of electrical seizures have no clinical correlate.

2. **Amplitude-integrated EEG (aEEG)** is a bedside technique increasingly being used by neonatologists for neuromonitoring. The background EEG activity from a limited number of electrodes (usually 1–2 channels, 2–4 electrodes) is amplified, filtered, rectified, compressed (6 cm/hour), and displayed on a semi-logarithmic scale. One minute of EEG is thus represented by 1 mm of aEEG. This technique allows the neonatologist to continually assess the background EEG characteristics, and thereby judge the severity of encephalopathy, the improvement or deterioration over time, and response to therapies. Seizures occurring during recording of this compressed data may alter the tracing in a recognizable manner provided the seizures occur in the region of the electrodes being used for recording and are of sufficient duration. The presence of seizures may be confirmed with immediate review of raw EEG from the available 1 to 2 channels, and should then be further assessed with standard EEG recording (see Fig. 56.2).

III. ETIOLOGY.

Once the presence of electrographic seizure has been identified, underlying etiologies, particularly reversible causes, must be sought. The details of the clinical history are most important in directing the initial evaluation. For instance, a history of traumatic delivery, with good Apgar scores in a term infant, raises the possibility of intracranial hemorrhage. The age at onset of seizure may suggest likely etiologies. Hypoxic-ischemic encephalopathy (HIE), which is the single most common cause of neonatal seizures, usually causes seizures within the first 24 hours of life. When seizures present after the first 48 hours of life, and particularly after a period of initial well-being, infection and biochemical disorders should be considered. Seizures occurring later (e.g., >10 days of life) are more likely to be related to disorders of calcium metabolism (now rare in the United States), malformation, or neonatal epilepsy syndromes, which may be benign (e.g., benign familial neonatal seizures) or severe (e.g., early infantile epileptic encephalopathy [EIEE]). Multiple possible etiologies (Table 56.1) may be identified in a neonate with seizures, such as HIE with hypoglycemia, hypocalcemia, and/or intracranial hemorrhage, and each must be treated appropriately.

A. **Specific etiologies**

1. **HIE.** This is the most common cause of neonatal seizures, accounting for over 50% of cases. HIE can be global, as in perinatal asphyxia or focal (i.e., arterial infarction). In **perinatal asphyxia**, the seizures occur in the context of a newborn who has a history of difficulty during labor and delivery with alterations of the fetal heart rate, decreased umbilical artery pH, and Apgar score <5 at 5 minutes. There is typically early suppression of the mental status, sometimes with coma and low tone, in addition to the seizures, which are often seen within the first 12 to 24 hours. Although the insult is global, the seizures are usually focal and may be multifocal. They are typically of short duration (<1 minute) but may be very frequent and refractory, especially in the first 24 hours. Treatment is urgent and complicated in many infants by the effects of hypoxic injury

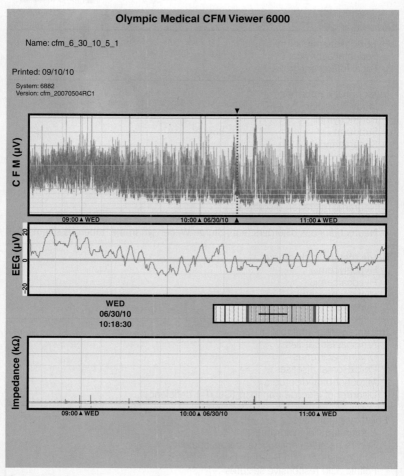

Figure 56.2 Amplitude integrated EEG

Upper panel: Compressed EEG data with wide band of activity, occasionally with sudden elevation of lower margin—a marker for possible seizure.
Middle panel: Raw EEG at the timepoint indicated by the cursor in the upper panel. Single channel EEG with rhythmicity concerning for possible seizure. Full EEG required for confirmation.
Lower panel: Indication of electrode impedance, which is appropriately low. Patterns seen in the compressed EEG data are uninterpretable in the presence of high electrode impedance.

to other organ systems (hepatic, pulmonary, renal, cardiovascular). Additionally, the anticonvulsant drugs may contribute to hypotension and hypoventilation. Another concern is the possibility of unidentified electrographic seizures in infants with HIE. This is particularly important following treatment with anticonvulsant drugs, which may eliminate clinical events but allow continuing electrographic seizures (electroclinical dissociation). Where possible, prolonged

Table 56.1	Etiologies of Neonatal Seizures

Hypoxic-ischemic injury
    Perinatal asphyxia
    Focal infarction/stroke

Intracranial hemorrhage
    Intraventricular
    Parenchymal
    Subdural
    Subarachnoid

CNS infection

Malformations and other structural lesions
    Neuronal migration disorders
    Cerebral dysgenesis
    Neurocutaneous disorders (e.g., Sturge-Weber syndrome, tuberous sclerosis)

Acute metabolic disorders
    Hypoglycemia
    Hypocalcemia
    Hypomagnesemia
    Hyponatremia

Inborn errors of metabolism
    Aminoacidopathies
    Organic acidurias
    Peroxisomal diseases
    Mitochondrial disorders
    Disorder of glucose transport (GLUT-1 deficiency)

Epilepsy syndromes
    Benign familial syndromes
    Severe neonatal epileptic encephalopathies
    Pyridoxine (Vitamin B_6)-dependent seizures
    Folinic acid responsive seizures

EEG is invaluable in identifying ongoing subclinical seizures. In **focal ischemic lesions**, such as middle cerebral artery stroke, in contrast, the infant usually appears well and presents with focal clonic seizures. Such arterial strokes may have occurred prior to, or in early labor. Asymmetries of the motor examination are often lacking in these infants, and diagnosis may be delayed until later in their first year if they do not present with neonatal seizures.

2. **Intracranial hemorrhages (ICHs)** are responsible for 10% to 15% of neonatal seizures. In the term infant, primary **subarachnoid hemorrhage** (not due to extension of a deeper cerebral or intraventricular hemorrhage) is probably more common than is realized. Most are not of clinical significance and produce no symptoms. Normal delivery or deliveries with instrumentation and/or trauma may be associated with more substantial subarachnoid hemorrhages, which

may present with seizures, usually on the second day of life. These infants appear clinically well between seizures and have a very good outcome. **Subdural hemorrhages** are related to large infant size, breech delivery, and instrumentation. They are due to tears in the falx, the tentorium, or the superficial cerebral veins. They are often associated with underlying cerebral contusions, which may be responsible for the seizures in some cases. Presenting seizures are usually focal and occur in the first few days of life. If large, subdural hematomas may be treated by surgical means making diagnosis important. In the **preterm infant, germinal matrix, intraventricular and parenchymal hemorrhages** are the prototypic manifestations of premature hypoxic injury. Seizures can occur with extension of the germinal matrix hemorrhage into the adjacent hypoxic parenchyma typically after the first 3 days of life. Generalized tonic events are usually not associated with electrographic seizure patterns, reflecting instead alterations in intracranial pressure. EEG recording may confirm seizure patterns with autonomic phenomena or cycling motor movements in these premature infants and also has identified subclinical electrographic seizures in association with these hemorrhages. Seizures occurring in the setting of premature hemorrhagic lesions are not usually associated with a good outcome.

3. **CNS infections** account for about 5% of neonatal seizures. **Congenital intrauterine infections**, such as with cytomegalovirus (CMV), toxoplasma, rubella, and herpes viruses may present early (first 2 days) with seizures in severe cases. The clinical scenario may include microcephaly, poor intrauterine growth, prematurity, and other skin, ophthalmic, and systemic findings. Meningoencephalitis, cerebral calcification, and dysgenesis (in cases of early intrauterine infection) contribute to the pathogenesis of seizures in these cases. **Postnatal sepsis**, for example, with group B *Streptococcus* or *Escherichia coli*, is often complicated by meningitis and may be associated with seizures. In this setting, the newborn has often been well for a couple of days, only to deteriorate later with seizures occurring after the first 48 to 72 hours.

4. **Acute Metabolic Disorders.** These rapidly remediable conditions are the focus of the initial investigations in neonatal seizures and include hypoglycemia, hypocalcemia, hypomagnesemia, and hyponatremia. They account for ~5% of neonatal seizures.

   a. **Hypoglycemia.** Even when it occurs in association with other potential causes of seizure, such as HIE, hypoglycemia should be treated (Table 56.2). The

Table 56.2	Initial Management of Acute Metabolic Disorders
Hypoglycemia	Dextrose 10%, 2–3 mL/kg IV
Hypocalcemia	Calcium gluconate, 5% (50 mg/mL), 100–200 mg/kg IV 10% (100 mg/mL) 50–100 mg/kg IV if inadequate time for dilation
Hypomagnesemia	Magnesium sulphate, 12.5% (125 mg/mL) 50–100 mg/kg IV
Hyponatremia	Furosemide 1 mg/kg IV 3% NaCl 1–3 mL/kg over 15 to 30 minutes

definition of hypoglycemia is controversial, but reasonable thresholds for treatment are <40 mg/dL (<2.2 mmol/L) in the first 24 hours, and <50 mg/dL (<2.8 mmol/L) after 24 hours. Most hypoglycemic infants are asymptomatic, but at any point, symptoms of neuroglycopenia should prompt immediate treatment. These are jitteriness/tremor, hypotonia, alteration of consciousness, poor feeding, apnea, and seizures. Causes of neonatal hypoglycemia include decreased glucose supply, as in the premature and small-for-gestational-age infant, as well as disorders in which pathways of gluconeogenesis are deficient or suppressed (e.g., glycogen storage disorders, aminoacidopathies such as maple syrup urine disease, fatty acid oxidation defects), and increased utilization, such as in hyperinsulinemic states, most commonly seen in the infant of the diabetic mother. Other hyperinsulinemic states include the overgrowth syndrome Beckwith-Wiedemann syndrome, erythroblastosis, and the rare hyperinsulinemic hypoglycemia.

b. Hypocalcemia. Whole blood ionized calcium (iCa) is the best measure of calcium status in ill infants. Hypocalcemia is considered present when iCa in term infants or prematures >1,500 g birth weight is <4.4 mg/dL (<1.1 mmol/L) and in premature infants <1,500 g at birth, <4.0 mg/dL (<1 mmol/L). **Early-onset** hypocalcemia occurs in the first 3 days of life and is associated with prematurity, infants of diabetic mothers, intrauterine growth retardation, and perinatal asphyxia. Most is asymptomatic. Symptoms of hypocalcemia include jitteriness, stimulus-induced muscle jerks, seizures, and rarely laryngospasm. **Late-onset** (>10 days of life) hypocalcemia can occur because of hypoparathyroidism, the feeding of high-phosphate formula, DiGeorge syndrome (chromosome 22q11-pter deletion), some mitochondrial cytopathies, and hypomagnesemia. Symptomatic or persistent cases should be treated (Table 56.2).

c. Hypomagnesemia. The most common cause is transient neonatal hypomagnesemia. It causes parathyroid hormone resistence and, so, causes hypocalcemia. Hypomagnesemia must be corrected before the hypocalcemia can be corrected (Table 2). Levels <1.4 mg/dL (<0.6 mmol/L) are considered low.

d. Hyponatremia (see Chap. 23, section IV)

5. **Malformations/structural lesions.** Five percent of neonatal seizures are caused by cerebral dysgenesis. **Cerebral dysgenesis** can cause seizures from the first day of life. This is most likely with the more severe disorders, such as hemimegalencephaly, lissencephaly, and polymicrogyrias. Seizures are often very refractory to medications. Some disorders may be amenable to surgical treatments, such as hemimegalencephaly and focal polymicrogyrias. In general, these infants are not encephalopathic interictally. On occasion, clues to neurocutaneous diseases are apparent on the newborn examination—for instance, the hemangioma in the distribution of cranial nerve V1 in Sturge-Weber syndrome, which can occasionally cause seizures in the newborn period. Depigmented "ash-leaf" macules of tuberous sclerosis may be seen, although neonatal seizures are rare in this disorder. Neuroimaging is primary in making these diagnoses.

6. **Inborn errors of metabolism.** Although individually very rare, inborn errors of metabolism as a group cause at least 1% of cases of seizures in the newborn. Typically caused by an enzyme defect in the metabolic pathways of carbohydrates, proteins, or fat, many cause disease due to accumulation of toxic products that are unable to proceed along the appropriate metabolic pathways. In these disorders, infants initially appear well due to the benefits of placental clearance of toxins until birth and only become encephalopathic and have

seizures after 2 to 3 days. Biochemical markers for these disorders include hypo-glycemia, metabolic acidosis, hyperammonemia, as well as specific patterns of alteration in amino acid or organic acid profiles. Other disorders cause disease due to a mutation-related defect in a vital function, for example in GLUT-1 deficiency, which impairs glucose transport across the blood–brain barrier, with resulting developmental delay and seizures. This disorder illustrates the importance of identifying these disorders, as it and some others are treatable, providing an opportunity to prevent brain injury. Diagnosis also allows repro-ductive counseling for later pregnancies. Among metabolic disorders, **glycine encephalopathy (nonketotic hyperglycinemia)** commonly causes myoclonic events, with or without EEG correlate, encephalopathy with depressed senso-rium, respiratory compromise, and hypotonia. The EEG background often reveals a very abnormal "burst-suppression" pattern. Glycine is elevated in the CSF, and usually, but not always, in plasma. The defect is in the glycine cleav-age system and as glycine is a co-agonist with the excitatory glutamate, results in enhanced cortical excitability. In spite of efforts to block glutamate neuro-transmission pharmacologically with dextromethorphan, most of these infants do very poorly. **Pyridoxine dependency**, although rare, is an important cause of neonatal seizures as treatment is available. The most common form is due to a defect in the ALDH7A1/antiquitin gene, which results in deficiency of alpha-aminoadipic semialdehyde (α-AASA) dehydrogenase and accumulation of α-AASA in blood, urine, and CSF, thus providing a biologic marker for the disorder. This enzyme is involved in lysine breakdown in the brain and is believed to have an impact on the metabolism of the neurotransmitters glu-tamate and γ-amino butyric acid. Seizures present early, sometimes *in utero*, and infants are irritable. A test dose of pyridoxine 100 mg IV, with EEG and cardiorespiratory monitoring, resulting in immediate seizure cessation and resolution of EEG abnormalities within hours, is diagnostic. As recent work has shown that some infants do not respond to the initial IV dose, a 3-day trial of oral pyridoxine (30 mg/kg/day) is recommended for nonresponders. If successful, supplementation is lifelong as seizures recur on withdrawal of the pyridoxine. The poorly understood disorder, **folinic acid-responsive seizures**, has recently been shown to be genetically and biochemically identical to pyri-doxine dependency. Previously, this disorder, initially identified by novel peaks in CSF chromatography, was treated by supplementation with folinic acid (3–5 mg/kg/day). This was effective in stopping seizures in some of these cases but did not prevent severe developmental sequelae. Similarly, many patients with pyridoxine dependency, although seizure free, had long-term develop-mental deficits. For this reason, and based on their allelic nature, it has been suggested that patients diagnosed with either of these disorders be treated with both supplements.

7. **Epilepsy syndromes.** These syndromes are rare, together accounting for about 1% of cases of seizures in the newborn period. **Benign familial neonatal convulsions** occur in otherwise well infants on day 2 or 3 of life. Seizures may be focal clonic or tonic (usually asymmetrical). Family history should be sought as it is often unreported. Seizures resolve after a variable period, usually within 6 months. This disorder is associated with abnormality of voltage-gated potassium channels, usually KCNQ2 and less frequently KCNQ3. Develop-mental outcome is normal, but 5% to 15% may have later nonfebrile convul-sions. **Benign infantile neonatal seizures** ("fifth day fits") present suddenly

on days 4 to 6 of life, often with frequent seizures leading to status epilepticus. Seizures are initially focal clonic often with apnea. Tonic seizures are not expected in this disorder. Seizures usually cease within 2 weeks. The etiology is unknown. More severe epilepsy syndromes are also seen, presenting in this period. These include the following:

a. Early myoclonic epilepsy (EME), often presenting in the first few days of life with focal motor seizures and myoclonus, which may be subtle and erratic and usually affects the face and limbs. Tonic seizure appear relatively late in this disorder. The seizures are very refractory to medications. The EEG is characterized by a burst-suppression pattern, which may only be seen in sleep, and, if present throughout the sleep–wake cycle, is exacerbated by sleep. This syndrome is often associated with underlying metabolic disorders, for instance, glycine encephalopathy (described above). Development is severely affected, and many infants die, often within their first year.

b. Early infantile epileptic encephalopathy (Ohtahara syndrome) is also associated with very refractory epilepsy. In contrast to EME, it is characterized by early onset of tonic spasms along with focal motor seizures. Myoclonus is rare in the early stages of this disorder. It is also associated with a burst-suppression pattern on EEG, which is relatively invariant. Whereas EME tends to be associated with underlying metabolic disorders, EIEE is more usually associated with structural lesions. Developmental prognosis is also poor in this syndrome with many evolving to a chaotic epileptiform pattern known as hypsarrhythmia on EEG, and accompanied by infantile spasms.

c. Malignant migrating partial seizures in infancy (Coppola syndrome) may present from the first to the tenth month of life. Focal motor seizures occur and escalate aggressively, shifting clinically and electrographically from side to side, and proving highly refractory to anticonvulsant medications. Developmental status is acutely affected and prognosis for normal outcome is poor, although cases with less than devastating outcome have now been described. The etiology is unknown.

IV. INVESTIGATIONS. The approach to investigations should be individualized with an emphasis on early identification of correctable disorders. It is directed by a detailed history of the pregnancy, labor and delivery, and subsequent course. It should proceed in parallel with stabilization of vital functions, including supported respiration if necessary, EEG confirmation of seizures if available, and with anticonvulsant treatment of ongoing seizures if present. General metabolic screening and assessment for evidence of sepsis (which may include lumbar puncture and/or screening for inborn errors of metabolism) should all be considered and the approach modified by the individual case history. Neuroimaging should be considered. Cranial ultrasound examination can be accomplished at the bedside and may identify intracranial hemorrhage, especially in the premature. However, its ability to identify convexity hemorrhages and cortical abnormalities is limited. Head CT, and especially brain MRI, are more helpful to confirm these disorders. However, they may not be available; and, if available, usually require transportation, with the risk of destabilization of ill infants and must often be deferred until after the infant is stabilized and treatment has been initiated.

V. TREATMENT. Seizures themselves and treatment with anticonvulsant medication may impair respiratory drive and the ability to maintain adequate circulation.

Therefore, supportive management to ensure maintenance of adequate ventilation and perfusion is imperative (see Table 56.2 for treatment of common acute metabolic derangements; see Chaps. 23 and 60).

The decision to treat neonatal seizures with anticonvulsant drugs depends on the risk of acute seizure-related respiratory or cardiac decompensation in a critically ill newborn, as well as the potential for long-term seizure-related neurologic injury balanced against the potential adverse effects of anticonvulsant medications. Some newborns may not need treatment with anticonvulsant medication, for instance, those with seizures due to reversible and appropriately treated metabolic derangements, or those with rare, short-lived events. However, in considering a decision not to treat, it is important to recognize that a significant proportion of newborns with electroclinical seizures have additional clinically silent ENS. In the setting of severe neonatal encephalopathy, these events may be prolonged and refractory to treatment, and efforts to eliminate them may be limited by systemic vulnerability to the circulatory effects of anticonvulsant medications.

Adverse effects of anticonvulsants, aside from respiratory and cardiovascular suppression, are also of concern in the developing brain. In studies of normal immature animals, many anticonvulsants, including phenobarbital, phenytoin, diazepam, clonazepam, valproic acid, and vigabatrin, increased the rate of apoptotic neuronal cell death, as do N-methyl-d-aspartate (NMDA) receptor antagonists. How this relates to the risk–benefit balance in human neonates with seizures is not known, and further study is required. The AMPA antagonist, topiramate, as well as the novel drug levetiracetam, do not appear to have this effect.

A number of factors alter the pharmacokinetics of the anticonvulsant drugs in neonates. Physiologic immaturity delays drug elimination, and asphyxial injury to the liver and kidney may further delay metabolism. Maturation of the various pathways involved in drug metabolism occurs at variable rates over the first weeks of life, and recovery from perinatal injury improves hepatic and renal function. Overall, there is a dramatic increase in the ability to eliminate the commonly used anticonvulsant drugs, so that changes in dosing are required to maintain therapeutic drug levels over the first weeks of life.

When anticonvulsant treatment is indicated, phenobarbital is the drug most commonly used as first-line therapy. Other first-line options include benzodiazepines (diazepam, lorazepam) and phenytoin or, if available, its prodrug fosphenytoin. There have been few studies comparing the efficacy of these drugs in the treatment of neonatal seizures. Painter et al. compared treatment with phenobarbital and phenytoin and found no difference in efficacy between the two drugs, with fewer than 50% of infants achieving control with either drug. Typical initial doses of the first-line drugs are provided in Table 56.3, and additional discussion of the individual drugs is given below.

A. **Phenobarbital** affects GABAA receptors to enhance GABA-related inhibition. It may also inhibit excitatory amino acid transmission and block voltage-activated calcium currents. It is a weak acid, with low lipid solubility. Phenobarbital is subject to protein binding, and it is the unbound (free), unionized fraction that is active. Alterations in acid–base balance in the newborn may affect efficacy of the drug for this reason. Phenobarbital is metabolized in the liver and excreted by the kidney. Its half-life is long, from 100 to 300 hours, or longer in premature infants, but declines to 100 hours or less over the first weeks of life. An initial intravenous (IV) loading dose of 20 mg/kg may be followed by increments of 5 to 10 mg/kg IV to a total of 40 mg/kg, with higher doses associated with improved efficacy. Careful monitoring of cardiac and respiratory function is required in vulnerable infants.

Table 56.3	Anticonvulsant Drug Doses for Initial Management of Neonatal Seizures	
Drug	**Initial Dose**	**Maintenance**
Phenobarbital	20 mg/kg IV Consider further 5–10 mg/kg increments to a total of 40 mg/kg	Check drug levels; may not need further doses for many days 3–4 mg/kg/day
Phenytoin	20 mg/kg IV Fosphenytoin: 20 mg PE/kg IV (see text)	3–4 mg/kg/day divided bid to qid
Benzodiazepines	Lorazepam: 0.05–0.1 mg/kg IV Diazepam: 0.3 mg/kg IV	

B. **Phenytoin/fosphenytoin.** Phenytoin acts by blockade of voltage-dependent sodium channels, probably by binding to inactivated channels and stabilizing the inactive state. This decreases the tendency of neurons to high frequency, repetitive firing, and therefore their excitability. Phenytoin is a weak acid and is poorly soluble in water. High lipid solubility results in rapid entry to the brain, but it is quickly redistributed and levels decline, requiring continued administration to restore brain levels. It is protein bound, although to a lesser degree in newborns than in older children and adults. Phenytoin is metabolized in the liver and eliminated in the kidney. Its half-life varies with concentration, increasing with higher concentrations due to decreased clearance as levels increase. An IV loading dose of 20 mg/kg of phenytoin administered at no greater than 1 mg/kg/minute (to avoid cardiac arrhythmia and hypotension) is followed by a maintenance dose of 2 to 3 mg/kg/day IV divided between 2 and 4 doses. Fosphenytoin is a prodrug of phenytoin. Its advantages are its higher water solubility and lower pH, which, in addition to the lack of toxic vehicles, required for its formulation, reduce local irritation of skin and blood vessels at the site of infusion. Fosphenytoin is converted to phenytoin by plasma phosphatase enzymes in neonates as in adults. Dosing is in "phenytoin equivalents" (PE), that is, a loading dose of fosphenytoin is 20 mg PE/kg IV.

C. **Benzodiazepines.** Diazepam, lorazepam, and midazolam, like other benzodiazepines, bind to the postsynaptic GABAA receptor to enhance GABA-activated inhibitory chloride currents. At high levels, benzodiazepines may also influence voltage-gated sodium channels and calcium channels. Benzodiazepines are lipid soluble. Differential lipid solubility confers some advantage on lorazepam, which is less lipid soluble and, therefore, is not redistributed away from the brain as rapidly as diazepam is. Benzodiazepines are metabolized in the liver, and the majority of the drug is excreted in the urine. The plasma half-life of both lorazepam and diazepam is approximately 30 hours and may be longer in premature and/or asphyxiated newborns. Onset of action is within minutes for both drugs; however, duration of action is longer for lorazepam (up to 24 hours). Diazepam may be more effective as a continuous infusion. Lorazepam is given IV at a dose of 0.05 to 0.1 mg/kg. Diazepam dose is 0.3 mg/kg IV. An infusion rate of 0.3 mg/kg/hour IV has been described. Midazolam is a short-acting benzo-diazepine that has been used as a continuous IV infusion (0.1–0.4 mg/kg/hour) after an initial loading dose (0.15 mg/kg). Benzodiazepines are typically used as second- or third-line agents in neonatal seizures, but may also be used as an initial treatment due to their earlier onset of action in anticipation of the effect of a con-current dose of phenobarbital.

Upward of 90% of neonatal seizures will ultimately be controlled by the combined use of the earlier mentioned anticonvulsant medications. The natural history and evolution/resolution of underlying brain injury in the first days of neonatal life may also contribute to a reduction in seizures.

Many other drugs have been used in an attempt to control refractory cases. Support for their use is based on reports of efficacy in small, uncontrolled series. Lidocaine has been used, mostly in Europe, as an IV infusion of 4 mg/kg/hour with decreasing doses over 4 to 5 days. This drug has a narrow therapeutic range and may induce seizures at higher levels.

Orally administered anticonvulsants that have been used adjunctively include carbamazepine (10 mg/kg initially, followed by 15–20 mg/kg/day), primidone (loading dose 15–25 mg/kg followed by 12–20 mg/kg/day), and valproic acid (three of 6 neonates developed hyperammonemia).

Of the new anticonvulsants, there is a case report of a single newborn with refractory seizures of unknown etiology that responded to the introduction of lamotrigine (4.4 mg/kg/day). There are a number of reports of the use of levetiracetam in single cases or small series. Surveys indicate that off-label use of levetiracetam and topiramate in this setting is not uncommon among child neurologists.

No guidelines exist as to appropriate duration of anticonvulsant treatment for newborns with seizures, and there is wide variation in practice. There is a trend toward shorter therapy, taking into account the short-lived nature of precipitating causes, the recovery from acute hypoxic-ischemic encephalopathy in many instances, and the possible detrimental effect of anticonvulsants on the immature brain. Newborns with persistent, difficult-to-control seizures, persistently abnormal EEG, and/or persistently abnormal neurologic examination should be considered for longer-term treatment following discharge from hospital.

VI. PROGNOSIS. Advances in obstetric management and in neonatal intensive care have yielded a reduction in mortality in infants with neonatal seizures from about 40% to <20%, with <10% mortality in term infants in one recent series. Morbidity rates have changed less, partly due to increased numbers of survivors among ill, premature newborns, who have a greater risk of neurologic sequelae. Long-term sequelae, including cerebral palsy and intellectual disabilities, still occur at a high rate of up to 30% to 35%, with postneonatal seizures occurring in up to 20%. The most important factor affecting outcome for infants with neonatal seizures is the **underlying etiology**. For instance, normal development can be expected in infants with benign idiopathic neonatal seizures and in 90% of those with primary subarachnoid hemorrhage, whereas only 50% of those with HIE, and even fewer with a developmental defect will have normal outcome. **Gestational age** is also an important factor with increasing mortality and morbidity with increasing immaturity.

Useful clinical indicators for a good outcome include a normal neonatal neurologic exam, normal or mildly abnormal neonatal EEG background activity, and normal neuroimaging or abnormalities limited to extraparenchymal injury.

Whether seizures themselves confer additional brain injury and adversely affect, the ultimate outcome in brain-injured neonates has been very controversial. Studies in immature animal models indicate that seizures in the developing brain are associated with age-specific alterations in hippocampal nerve cells and their synaptic connections. Other studies have shown that immature animals subjected to seizures have evidence of cognitive impairment (poorer performance in spatial learning tasks) when tested in adolescence or adulthood. These animals are more susceptible to epileptogenesis when encountering a brain injury in later life. There are as yet no studies in human survivors of neonatal seizures capable of addressing the questions raised by these findings.

Suggested Readings

Gallagher RC, Van Hove JLK, et al. Folinic acid-responsive seizures are identical to pyridoxine-dependent epilepsy. *Annals of Neurology* 2009;65:550–556.

Holmes GL. The long-term effects of neonatal seizures. *Clinics in Perinatology* 2009;36:901–914.

Mizrahi EM, Kellaway P. Characterization and classification of neonatal seizures. *Neurology* 1987;37:1837–1844.

Painter MJ, Scher MS, Stein AD, et al. Phenobarbital compared with phenytoin for the treatment of neonatal seizures. *NEJM* 1999;341:485–489.

Silverstein FS, Jensen FE. Neonatal seizures. *Annals of Neurology* 2007;62:112–120.

Tekgul H, Gauvreau K, Soul JS, et al. The current etiologic profile and neurodevelopmental outcome of seizures in term newborn infants. *Pediatrics* 2006;117:1270–1280.

Volpe JJ, ed. *Neonatal Seizures in Neurology of the Newborn.* 5th ed. Philadelphia: WB Saunders; 2008:203–244.

Neural Tube Defects

Joseph R. Madsen and Anne R. Hansen

I. DEFINITIONS AND PATHOLOGY. Since the central nervous system starts as a tube, which develops into the most complex structures in the body, it is no surprise that neural tube defects constitute one of the most serious congenital malformations in newborns. The term refers to a group of disorders that is heterogeneous with respect to embryologic timing, involvement of specific elements nervous system, clinical presentation, and prognosis.

A. Types of neural tube defects

1. **Primary neural tube defects** constitute the majority of neural tube defects and can be viewed as due to primary failure of closure of the neural tube or disruption of an already closed neural tube between 18 and 25 days' gestation. The resulting abnormality usually manifests in two anatomic lesions: (i) an exposed (open or *aperta*) neural placode along the midline of the back caudally and rostrally; and (ii) the Arnold-Chiari II (ACII) malformation (malformation of pons and medulla, with downward displacement of cerebellum, medulla, and fourth ventricle into the upper cervical region), with associated aqueductal stenosis and hydrocephalus.

   a. Myelomeningocele is the most common primary neural tube defect. It involves a saccular outpouching of neural elements (neural placode), typically through a defect in the bone and the soft tissues of the posterior thoracic, sacral, or lumbar regions, the latter comprising 80% of lesions. Dura and arachnoid are typically included in the sac (meningo-), which contains visible neural structures (myelo-), and the skin is usually discontinuous over the sac. Hydrocephalus occurs in 84% of these children; ACII malformation occurs in approximately 90%, although the link between hydrocephalus and the malformation has been significantly reevaluated in recent years, with therapeutic implications as will be discussed. Various associated anomalies of the central nervous system are noted, most importantly, cerebral cortical dysplasia in up to 92% of cases.

   b. Encephalocele. This defect of anterior neural tube closure is an outpouching of dura with or without brain, noted in the occipital region in 80% of cases, and less commonly in the frontal or temporal regions. It may vary in size from a few millimeters to many centimeters.

   c. Anencephaly. In the most severe form of this defect, the cranial vault and posterior occipital bone are defective, and derivatives of the neural tube are exposed, including both brain and bony tissue. The defect usually extends through the foramen magnum and involves the brain stem. It is not compatible with long-term survival.

2. **Secondary neural tube defects.** Five percent of all neural tube defects result from abnormal development of the lower sacral or coccygeal segments during secondary neurulation. This leads to defects primarily in the lumbosacral

spinal region. These heterogeneous lesions are rarely associated with hydrocephalus or the ACII malformation, and the skin is typically intact over the defect. Since the cerebellar abnormality of the ACII malformation is evident on prenatal scans, this radiographic finding is useful in distinguishing open from closed neural tube abnormalities.

a. Meningocele is an outpouching of skin and dura without involvement of the neural elements. Meningoceles may be associated with bone and contiguous soft tissue abnormalities.

b. Lipomeningocele is a lipomatous mass usually in the lumbar or sacral region, occasionally off the midline, typically covered with full-thickness skin. Adipose tissue frequently extends through the defect into the spine and dura and adheres extensively to a distorted spinal cord or nerve roots.

c. Sacral agenesis/dysgenesis, diastematomyelia, and myelocystocele, all may have varying degrees of bony involvement. Although rarely as extensive as with primary neural tube defects, neurologic manifestations may be present representing distortion or abnormal development of peripheral nerve structures. These lesions may be inapparent on physical examination of the child, resulting in the use of the term *occulta* to describe them.

B. Etiologies. The exact cause of failed neural tube closure remains unknown, and proposed etiologies for both primary and secondary neural tube defects are heterogeneous. Factors implicated include folic acid deficiency, maternal ingestion of the anticonvulsants carbamazepine and valproic acid and folic acid antagonists, such as aminopterin; maternal diabetes; and disruptive influences, such as prenatal irradiation and maternal hyperthermia. A genetic component is supported by the fact that there is concordance for neural tube defect in monozygotic twins and an increased incidence with consanguinity and with a positive family history. Neural tube defects can occur with trisomies 13 and 18, triploidy, and Meckel syndrome (autosomal recessive syndrome of encephalocele, polydactyly, polycystic kidneys, cleft lip and palate), as well as other chromosome disorders. Although specific genes (particularly those in the folate-homocysteine pathway) have been implicated as risk factors, the genetics are likely complex and multifactorial (see Chap. 10).

C. Epidemiology and recurrence risk. The incidence of neural tube defects varies significantly with geography and ethnicity. In the United States, the overall frequency of neural tube defects is approximately 1 in 2,000 live births. The literature may underestimate the true prevalence, because of the effects of prenatal diagnosis and termination of affected pregnancies. A well-established increased incidence is known among individuals living in parts of Ireland and Wales, and carries over to descendants of these individuals who live elsewhere in the world. This may be true also for other ethnic groups, including Sikh Indians and certain groups in Egypt. More than 95% of all neural tube defects occur to couples with no known family history. Primary neural tube defects carry an increased empiric recurrence risk of 2% to 3% for couples with one affected pregnancy, with the risk increasing further if more than one sibling is affected. Similarly, affected individuals have a 3% to 5% risk of having one offspring with a primary neural tube defect. Recurrence risk is strongly affected by the level of the lesion in the index case, with risks as high as 7.8% for lesions above T11. In 5% of cases, neural tube defects may be associated with uncommon disorders; some, such as Meckel syndrome, are inherited in an autosomal recessive manner, resulting in a 25% recurrence risk. Secondary neural tube defects are generally sporadic and carry no increased recurrence risk.

In counseling families for recurrence, however, it is critical to obtain a careful history of drug exposure and/or family history.

D. **Prevention.** Controlled, randomized clinical studies of prenatal multivitamin administration both for secondary prevention in mothers with prior affected offspring and for primary prevention in those without a prior history have shown a 50% to 70% reduced incidence of neural tube defects in women who take multivitamins for at least 3 months prior to conception and during the first month of pregnancy (1). The Centers for Disease Control and Prevention of the U.S. Public Health Service recommends that women of childbearing age who are capable of becoming pregnant should consume 0.4 mg of folic acid per day to reduce their risks of having a fetus affected with spina bifida or other neural tube defects. Higher doses are recommended for women with prior affected offspring. In addition, folate supplementation of enriched cereal-grain products has been mandated by the U.S. Food and Drug Administration (FDA); however, the level of folate intake from this source is not high enough to forgo additional supplementation in the large majority of women.

II. DIAGNOSIS

A. **Prenatal diagnosis.** The combination of maternal serum α-fetoprotein (AFP) determinations and prenatal ultrasonography and rapid-acquisition fetal MRI scans, along with AFP and acetylcholinesterase determinations on amniotic fluid where indicated, greatly improves the ability to make a prenatal diagnosis and to distinguish from abdominal wall defects. Maternal serum AFP measurements of 2.5 multiples of the median (MoM) in the second trimester (16–18 weeks) have a sensitivity of 80% to 90% for myelomeningocele. The exact timing of this measurement is critical as AFP levels change throughout pregnancy. Karyotype may also be performed at the time of amniocentesis to detect associated chromosomal abnormalities. Ultrasonographic diagnosis through direct visualization of the spinal defect or through indirect signs related to ACII malformation has a sensitivity of >90%. The Chiari malformation is seen as the "banana sign" or a flattened cerebellum and a transient frontal bone anomaly called a "lemon sign." Ultrasound can also demonstrate the level of termination of the normal cord and placode. Prenatal MRI may define the defect more accurately. Determining the prognosis based on prenatal ultrasonography remains difficult, except in obvious cases of encephalocele or anencephaly (see Chap. 1), but an appreciation of the level of disruption can be helpful in that higher spinal levels within the thoracolumbar range portend a correspondingly higher level of neurologic deficit. Some patients with higher thoracic or cervical lesions, however, have remarkable preservation of function; often, restitution of the spinal cord below the lesion is evident on the MRI in these cases.

B. **Postnatal diagnosis.** Except for some secondary neural tube defects, most neural tube defects, especially meningomyelocele, are immediately obvious at birth. Occasionally, some saccular masses, usually in the low sacrum, including sacrococcygeal teratomas, can be mistaken for a neural tube defect.

III. EVALUATION

A. **History.** Obtain a detailed family history. Ask about the occurrence of neural tube defects and other congenital anomalies or malformation syndromes. Note should be made of any of the risk factors described in the preceding text, including maternal medication use in the first trimester or maternal diabetes.

B. **Physical examination.** It is important to perform a thorough physical examination, including a neurologic examination. The following portions of the examination are likely to reveal abnormal conditions:

1. **Back.** Inspect the defect and note if it is leaking cerebrospinal fluid (CSF). Use a sterile nonlatex rubber glove when touching a leaking sac (in most circumstances, only the neurosurgeon needs to touch the back). Note the location, shape, and size of the defect and the thin "parchment-like" overlying skin, although it has little relation to the size of the sac. Often, the sac is deflated and has a wrinkled appearance. It is important to note the curvature of the spine and the presence of a bony gibbus underlying the defect. For suspected closed lesions, document hemangioma, hairy patch, deep dimple or sinus tract if present; ultrasonography of the lower spine can show the level of the conus and presence of normal root movement in cases where this is in question.

2. **Head.** Record the head circumference and plot daily until stable postoperatively. At birth, some infants will have macrocephaly because of hydrocephalus, and still, more will develop hydrocephalus after closure of the defect on the back. Ultrasonography is useful to assess ventricular size. Assess the intracranial pressure (ICP) with the baby sitting upright by palpating the anterior fontanel and tilting the head and torso forward until the midportion of the anterior fontanel is flat. The fontanels may be quite large and the calvarial bones widely separated (see Chap. 54).

3. **Eyes.** Abnormalities in conjugate movement of the eyes are common and include esotropias, esophorias, and abducens paresis.

4. **Neurologic examination.** Observe the child's spontaneous activity and response to sensory stimuli in all extremities. Predicting ambulation and muscle strength based on the "level" of the neurologic deficit can be misleading; and, very often, the anal reflex or "wink" will be present at birth and absent postoperatively, owing to spinal shock and edema.

5. **Lower extremities.** Look for deformities (e.g., club feet), as well as muscle weakness and limited range of motion. Look at thigh positions and skinfolds, and perform the Ortolani and Barlow maneuvers for evidence of congenital dysplasia of the hips. With open lesions, this exam should be deferred until after the repair of the meningomyelocele. Dislocation of the hips can also be diagnosed by ultrasonography (see Chap. 58).

   Repeated neurologic examinations at periodic intervals is more helpful in predicting functional outcome than a single newborn examination. Similarly, sensory examination of the newborn can be misleading because of the potential absence of a motor response to pinprick. Carefully examine deep tendon reflexes (see Table 57.1).

6. **Bladder and kidneys.** Palpate the abdomen for evidence of bladder distension or kidney enlargement. Observe the pattern of urination, and check the infant's response to the Credé maneuver by monitoring residual urine in the bladder.

C. **General newborn assessment.** Evaluate all newborns with neural tube defects for the presence of congenital heart disease (especially ventricular septal defect [VSD]), renal malformation, and structural defects of the airway, gastrointestinal tract, ribs, and hips. Although uncommon in primary neural tube defects, these

Table 57.1 Correlation between Segmental Innervation; Motor, Sensory, and Sphincter Function; Reflexes; and Ambulation Potential

Lesion	Segmental innervation	Cutaneous sensation	Motor function	Working muscles	Sphincter function	Reflex	Potential for ambulation
Cervical/ Thoracic	Variable	Variable	None	None	—	—	Poor, even in full braces
Thoracolumbar	T12	Lower abdomen	None	None	—	—	—
	L1	Groin	Weak hip flexion	Iliopsoas	—	—	Full braces, long-term ambulation unlikely
	L2	Anterior upper thigh	Strong hip flexion	Iliopsoas and sartorius	—	—	
Lumbar	L3	Anterior distal thigh and knee	Knee extension	Quadriceps	—	Knee jerk	
	L4	Medial leg	Knee flex- ion and hip abduction	Medial hamstrings	—	Knee jerk	May ambulate with braces and crutches

(continued)

Table 57.1 Correlation between Segmental Innervation; Motor, Sensory, and Sphincter Function; Reflexes; and Ambulation Potential *(Continued)*

Lesion	Segmental innervation	Cutaneous sensation	Motor function	Working muscles	Sphincter function	Reflex	Potential for ambulation
Lumbosacral	L5	Lateral leg and medial knee	Foot dorsiflexion and eversion	Anterior tibial and peroneals	—	Ankle jerk	—
	S1	Sole of foot flexion	Foot plantar	Gastrocnemius, soleus, and posterior tibial	—	Ankle jerk	Ambulate with or without short leg braces
Sacral	S2	Posterior leg and thigh	Toe flexion	Flexor hallucis	Bladder and rectum	Anal wink	—
	S3	Middle of buttock	—	—	Bladder and rectum	Anal wink	Ambulate without braces
	S4	Medial buttock	—	—	Bladder and rectum	Anal wink	—

Source: From Noetzel MJ. Myelomeningocele: current concepts of management. *Clin Perinatol* 1989;16(2):311–329.

can be encountered and should be considered before beginning surgical treatment or before discharge from the hospital. Other findings of associated chromosomal anomalies may be noted. In addition, plan an ophthalmologic examination and hearing evaluation during the hospitalization or following discharge.

IV. CARE TEAM. The care of an infant with a neural tube defect requires the coordinated efforts of a number of medical and surgical specialists, as well as specialists in nursing, physical therapy, and social service. Some centers have a myelodysplasia team to help coordinate the following specialists.

A. Specialty consultations

1. **Neurosurgery.** The initial care of the child with an open neural tube defect is predominantly neurosurgical. The neurosurgeon is responsible for assessment and surgical closure of the defect and for evaluation and treatment of elevated ICP.

2. **Neonatology/Pediatrics.** A thorough evaluation before surgical procedures is important, particularly to detect other abnormalities, such as congenital cardiac anomalies, that might influence surgical and anesthetic risk.

3. **Genetics.** A clinical geneticist should conduct a complete dysmorphology evaluation during the first hospitalization. Follow-up during outpatient visits should include genetic counseling.

4. **Urology.** Consult a urologist on the day of birth because of the risk of obstructive uropathy.

5. **Orthopedics.** The pediatric orthopedic surgeon is responsible for the initial assessment of musculoskeletal abnormalities and long-term management of ambulation, seating, and spine stability. Clubfeet, frequently encountered in these newborns, should be assessed and may be managed during this hospitalization.

6. **Physical therapy.** Involve physical therapists in planning for outpatient physical therapy programs.

7. **Social service.** Arrange for a social worker familiar with the special needs of children with neural tube defects to meet the parents as early as possible. Children with meningomyelocele may require a considerable amount of parents' time and resources, thereby placing considerable strain on both parents and siblings.

V. MANAGEMENT

A. Fetal surgery. *In utero* repair was first performed in 1994. Observational studies have found that *in utero* repair is associated with lower rates of ventriculoperitoneal (VP) shunting and consistent reversal of hindbrain herniation. Long-term effects remain uncertain. A multicenter, randomized controlled trial of *in utero* surgical correction with standard management was recently completed and found that performing prenatal surgery on fetuses with myelomeningocele may lead to better outcomes than if the surgery is performed postnatally. After 12 months, the 91 infants who had prenatal surgery were 30% less likely to die or need additional surgical procedures than the 92 infants who were treated postnatally. Follow up at 2 ½ years of age revealed that those treated prenatally demonstrated improved physical development and motor function, such as unassisted walking, compared with those treated after birth. However, prenatal surgery was associated with increased risk of complications during pregnancy, including premature delivery and tearing of the uterine wall from the surgical scar. When the diagnosis of myelomeningocele is made prenatally, *in utero* repair is an option that parents may consider.

B. Perinatal. Caesarean section prior to the onset of labor is the preferred mode of delivery because it decreases the likelihood of rupturing the meningeal sac and is associated with improved neurologic outcome (2).

C. Preoperative Management

1. **Neurology**

   a. Care of placode: At birth, the very thin sac is often leaking. Keep the newborn in the prone position with a sterile saline-moistened gauze sponge placed over the defect covered by plastic wrap. This reduces bacterial contamination and tissue damage related to dehydration.

   b. ACII malformation: A cranial ultrasound should generally be obtained soon after birth. ACII malformations result from premature fusion of the posterior fossa leaving insufficient space for the cerebrum, cerebellum, and brain stem. Brain stem and portions of the cerebellum may herniate through the foramen magnum into the upper cervical spinal canal. Obstructed flow of CSF results in hydrocephalus the majority of the time.

   c. Seizures: There is a 20% to 25% incidence of seizures in this population (3) due to brain anomalies in addition to Chiari malformations.

2. **Infectious disease.** Administer intravenous antibiotics (ampicillin and gentamicin) to diminish the risk of meningitis, particularly due to group B streptococci. Newborns with an open spinal defect can receive a massive inoculation of bacteria directly into the nervous system at the time of vaginal delivery or even *in utero* if the placental membranes rupture early. Meningitis is a particularly devastating complication.

3. **Fluids/nutrition.** Because insensible losses are minimized by covering the lesion with plastic wrap, standard maintenance fluids are generally appropriate.

4. **Urologic/renal**

   a. Clean intermittent catheterization is indicated to check postvoid residuals until urologic and renal function are assessed.

   b. If voiding pattern is abnormal, it is important to determine if the etiology is abnormal bladder emptying, renal function, or both. A serum creatinine level is useful in making this distinction.

5. **Latex allergy.** Because of the potential for development of a severe allergy to latex rubber, no latex equipment should be used.

6. **Surgical treatment.** Open defects must be urgently closed due to the risk of infection. Children whose defect is covered with skin and whose nervous system is therefore not at risk for bacterial contamination may undergo elective repair after 1 month of age.

   The initial neurosurgical treatment of an open meningomyelocele consists of (i) closing the defect to prevent infection and (ii) reducing the elevated ICP. The back should be closed on the first day of life or as soon thereafter as safely possible to minimize the risk of infection. Techniques are available to rapidly close even very large cutaneous defects without skin grafting. Intracranial hypertension can be initially controlled by continuous ventricular drainage, although this is rarely needed in actual practice. Because ICP often increases following closure of the back in unshunted patients, anterior fontanel tension and head circumference should be carefully monitored. A VP shunt catheter can be placed either at the time of back closure or as a second procedure after back closure. However, the experience with prenatal closure and an increasing desire to avoid permanent shunting in an infant who can be managed in another way has led many practitioners to delay placement of a shunt and consider such alternatives as endoscopic third ventriculocisternostomy with choroid plexus cauterization (ETV-CPC) (4). Regardless of planned strategy for dealing with hydrocephalus if it becomes symptomatic, close monitoring is important.

The surgical approach varies with the precise anatomy, but in brief, the thin, translucent tissue and skin too thin to use are trimmed away around the circumference of the defect, then the placode is rolled into a more normal shape and gently held in this configuration with fine sutures to the pial edge. The edges of what would have been dura mater are identified, isolated, and closed over the placode, then the skin is closed with the goal of attaining a well-vascularized, watertight closure.

7. **Management of hydrocephalus.** If the fluid pressure seems to put the integrity of the skin closure at risk, shunting of the ventricles (by a permanent VP shunt), or temporary external ventricular drainage, may be performed during the same operation. However, since the experience with prenatal closure has raised awareness that fewer patients need shunts than previously thought, watchful waiting in the hopes of avoiding a permanent shunt has become a more common approach. Indeed, Warf has shown that use of an internal rerouting of CSF flow (by endoscopic third ventriculostomy), sometimes accompanied by choroid plexus cauterization at the same endoscopic procedure, may diminish the need for shunts to about 25% of all infants with spina bifida (5).

D. Postoperative Management

1. **Neurology**
   a. The infant must remain prone or on the side until the wound heals. Head circumference needs to be measured daily, particularly in the infant who has not had shunt placement.
   b. **Magnetic resonance imaging (MRI) of the head** should generally be obtained post-op, even if there is no clinical evidence of hydrocephalus. It is particularly valuable in assessment of the posterior fossa and syringomyelia. **Computed tomography (CT) scans** should be avoided unless no other options are available because of the relatively high-radiation exposure.
   c. **Sensory impairment** can be associated with myelomeningocele. Strabismus is commonly associated with Chiari malformation. Hearing and vision screens should be performed prior to discharge.

2. **Nutrition.** Feeding difficulties are commonly associated with the ACII malformation. Growth and nutritional status must be watched closely as well as the infant's ability to suck and swallow. Acute deterioration in feeding skills may signal increased intracranial pressure, including a shunt malfunction in shunted patients.
   a. Monitor ICP, including daily weights, and input/output.
   b. Observe for spitting, gagging, choking, and hypoxia.

3. **Urologic/renal**

   a. Obtain urine culture, urinalysis, and serum creatinine as a baseline, if not already done preoperatively.

   b. Ultrasound of the urinary tract will detect associated renal anomalies, as well as possible hydronephrosis from vesicoureteral reflux.

   c. Postvoid residuals and urodynamic studies should be performed early in the hospitalization or shortly after discharge to document the status of the bladder, as well as urinary sphincter function and innervation. This study will serve as a basis for comparison later in life.

   d. Consider a voiding cystourethrogram to assess for vesicoureteral reflux if there is an abnormality seen on ultrasonographic or urodynamic study or in the setting of a rising serum creatinine level.

   e. Clean intermittent catheterization (CIC) is recommended for those infants who have large postvoid residuals, evidence of significant hydronephrosis and/or increased bladder pressure on urodynamics studies. CIC is started in the hospital and continued at discharge. Those infants who do not manifest these problems can safely be allowed to spontaneously void.

4. **Orthopedics**

   a. Obtain plain films of lower extremities if there is concern regarding club feet or other anomalies raised by physical exam.

   b. Obtain CXR. Rib deformities are common; cardiac malformations may also be identified.

   c. Obtain plain films of spine. Abnormalities in vertebral bodies, absent or defective posterior arches, and evidence of kyphosis are common.

   d. Evidence of dysplasia of hips is common, and some children with neural tube defects are born with dislocated hips. Ultrasonographic examination of the hips can be very helpful to the orthopedic surgeon (see Chap. 58).

5. **Family and social worker**

   a. Family care providers will need to play an active role in home management. It is critical for them to understand the child's condition and the implications for home care. The involvement of multiple specialists heightens the importance of the identification of a primary care provider (pediatrician or family practitioner) to coordinate the flow of information.

   b. The family stress of caring for a child with myelomeningocele cannot be underestimated. A social worker should be available for the family from the time of diagnosis. An excellent information and support resource is the Spina Bifida Association of America (phone number: [202] 944-3285; available at: www.sbaa.org).

VI. PROGNOSIS

A. **Survival.** Nearly all children with neural tube defects, even those severely affected, can survive for many years. In a recent large observational study, the 1-year survival rate for children with myelomeningocele was 91%, whereas for encephalocele it was 79%. Survival rates appear to have increased since folic acid fortification of the U.S. grain supply was started, possibly because of a general decrease in severity or location of lesions. Survival rates are significantly influenced by selection bias of prenatal diagnosis and termination of severely affected fetuses, and by decisions to intervene or to withhold aggressive medical and surgical care in the early neonatal period. Most deaths occur in the most severely affected children and are likely related to brain stem dysfunction.

B. Long-term outcome. There are a wide variety of medical and developmental issues associated with myelomeningocele. Children with myelomeningocele require a comprehensive multidisciplinary team of providers, including neurosurgery; orthopedic surgery; urology; physiatry; gastroenterology; endocrinology; pulmonary medicine; and physical, occupational, and speech language pathology.

   1. Neurosurgical issues. In one cohort study of myelomeningocele patients, 86% underwent VP shunt, the large majority of whom required additional shunt revision. Release of tethered cord was required in 32%, and scoliosis was diagnosed in 49%, of whom approximately half required a spinal fusion procedure (6). Approximately 5% of newborns with open neural tube defects develop symptoms related to the ACII malformation.

   a. Increased ICP can result from evolving hydrocephalus in the unshunted child or shunt malfunction or infection in the shunted child. Elevated ICP requires urgent assessment as symptoms may progress rapidly and can be fatal (7). It can present as pontomedullary symptoms from lower brain stem dysfunction:

   i. Headache, irritability, bulging fontanel, sixth nerve palsy, paralysis of upward gaze

   ii. New onset of respiratory complications, particularly stridor from vocal cord paralysis, central and/or obstructive apnea

   iii. Worsening oromotor function, vomiting, abnormal gag, and vomiting (often confused with gastroesophageal reflex)

   iv. Change in cognitive function

   These symptoms may indicate shunt malfunction but frequently disappear without treatment. In the shunted child, after ensuring that CSF drainage is adequate, surgical decompression of the Chiari malformation should be considered. If the symptoms persist, especially in association with cyanosis, the prognosis is poor, with the risk of respiratory failure and death. Tracheostomy is occasionally necessary. Posterior fossa decompression and cervical laminectomy are surgical options but are often not successful.

   b. Shunt infection should be suspected if symptoms of ICP are accompanied by fever and increased white blood cell count.

   i. A shunt tap is necessary to rule out a shunt infection.

   ii. A shunt series and CT scan may be necessary in conjunction with neurosurgical evaluation.

   c. Seizures remain a risk, and families should be familiar with signs and symptoms to monitor, as well as an initial treatment approach.

   2. Motor outcome. This depends more on the level of paralysis and surgical intervention than it does on congenital hydrocephalus. In a 12-year study of adult myelomeningocele patients, one-third experienced deterioration in their ambulatory capacity over the study period. All those with lesions at the L5 neurologic levels were community ambulators, except one who was a household walker. At the L4 level, there was a slight decrease in functional ambulators. For the L3 level patients, less than one-third were still community or household ambulators at the end of the 12 years of observations (8). Most children with neural tube defects will have a delay in motor progress, but appropriate bracing, physical therapy interventions, and monitoring and treatment of kyphosis and scoliosis can mitigate this. Factors, such as obesity, frequent hospitalizations, tethering of the spinal cord, and decubitus ulcers, may also contribute to motor delays.

3. **Intellectual outcome.** Approximately 75% of children with myelomeningocele have IQ scores >80. Many children with myelomeningocele require some sort of special education. Learning disabilities arise from challenges in language processing, visual/perceptual and fine motor deficits. A formal neurodevelopmental assessment should be obtained if any questions arise about a child's social and cognitive abilities.

An increased risk of cognitive delay is associated with high thoracic level lesions, severe hydrocephalus at birth, development of a CNS infection early in life, intracranial hypertension, and seizures. One study found that although 37% of individuals with myelomeningocele required additional assistance with school work or attended special education classes, 85% were attending or had graduated from secondary school or college (6).

4. **Hearing and vision** status must be formally reassessed to rule out any exacerbation of learning difficulties. Hearing loss has historically been a problem associated with antibiotic use in the setting of urinary tract infections, but has been dramatically reduced with the advent of clean intermittent catheterization.

5. **Urologic/renal issues**
   a. Approximately 85% of children require clean intermittent catheterization for bladder dysfunction; 80% achieve social bladder continence.
   b. **Urinary tract infections** are common. Prophylactic antibiotics may be indicated, especially if vesicoureteral reflux is present. Amoxicillin is commonly used in newborns and young infants. Other antibiotics, such as Bactrim and nitrofurantoin are used in older children (9).

6. **Growth and nutrition.** Failure to thrive is a common problem in infants and young children.
   a. Some children require gastrostomy tube placement secondary to aspiration risk or inability to take in adequate calories orally. A videofluoroscopic swallowing study can be helpful to assess risk of aspiration with oral feeds.
   b. Arm span may more accurately reflect growth, since growth below the waistline is usually disproportionately slow or distorted by lower extremity or spinal deformities.
   c. Skinfold thickness is a valuable measure of nutrition.
   d. Bowel incontinence and constipation are prominent problems. An aggressive, consistent bowel program is often required and may include laxatives, suppositories, enemas, or even antegrade colonic enemas (10).

7. **Orthopedic complications**
   a. Worsening scoliosis or kyphosis may cause restrictive lung disease.
   b. Osteopenia, particularly in the nonambulatory patient, increases the risk for pathologic fractures.
   c. Contractures of hips, knees, and ankles, and hip dislocation are common. Treatments include physical therapy, orthotics, neuromuscular blockades, and surgeries.
   d. Decubitus ulcers may develop, especially involving the feet, secondary to limited movement and diminished peripheral sensation. Secondary infection is an additional problem. Regular assessment of appropriate fit, padding, and positioning of wheelchairs and other seating systems minimizes ulcer risk.

8. **Endocrinopathies.** Children can develop precocious puberty and growth hormone deficiency, presenting as poor growth despite adequate nutrition.

9. **Rehabilitation** therapies, including physical, occupational, and speech/language services are critical to optimize the health and development of a child with myelomeningocele.

   a. Initially, services should be established through state Early Intervention (EI) programs, which are mandated under the Individuals with Disabilities Education Act (IDEA). EI referral should be made early during an infant's initial hospitalization as there can be a waiting list.

   b. After age 3, services are provided through the public school system.

10. **Latex allergy.** Despite trying to avoid latex exposure, latex hypersensitization is seen in approximately one-third of children with neural tube defects, and may be associated with life-threatening anaphylaxis. Risk is minimized by:

    a. Ongoing avoidance of latex-containing products

    b. Avoidance of foods that may cross-react with latex, such as avocado, banana, and water chestnuts

11. **The primary care physician** plays a critical role in coordinating the care of a child with myelodysplasia (11). The role includes general pediatric care, as well as surveillance for complications, communication with multiple subspecialists, and advocacy in school programs and the community.

REFERENCES

1. Padmanabhan R. Etiology, pathogenesis and prevention of neural tube defects. *Congenital Anomalies* 2006;46:55–67.
2. Luthy DA, Wardinsky T, Shurtleff DB, et al. Cesarean section before the onset of labor and subsequent motor function in infants with meningomyelocele diagnosed antenatally. *N Engl J Med* 1991;324:662–666.
3. Talwar D, Baldwin MA, Horbatt CI. Epilepsy in children with meningomyelocele. *Pediatr Neurol* 1995;13:29–32.
4. Warf BC, Campbell JW. Combined endoscopic third ventriculostomy and choroid plexus cauterization as primary treatment of hydrocephalus for infants with myelomeningocele: long-term results of a prospective intent-to-treat study in 115 East African infants. *J Neurosurg Pediatr* 2008;2:310–316.
5. Warf BC. Endoscopic third ventriculostomy and choroid plexus cauterization for pediatric hydrocephalus. *Clin Neurosurg* 2007;54:78–82.
6. Bowman RM, McLone DG, Grant JA, et al. Spina bifida outcome: a 25-year prospective. *Pediatr Neurosurg* 2001;34(3):114–120.
7. Madikians A, Conway EE Jr. Cerebrospinal fluid shunt problems in pediatric patients. *Pediatr Ann* 1997; 26:613–620.
8. Esterman N. Ambulation in patients with myelomeningocele: a 12-year follow-up. *Pediatr Phys Ther* 2001 Spring;13(1):50–51.
9. Bauer SB. The management of the myelodysplastic child: a paradigm shift. *BJU Int* 2003;92(suppl 1):23–28.
10. Leibold S, Ekmark E, Adams RC. Decision making for a successful bowel continence program. *Eur J Pediatr Surg* 2000;10(suppl 1):26–30.
11. Elias ER, Hobbs N. Spina bifida: sorting out the complexities of care. *Contemp Peds* 1998;25:156–171.

Suggested Readings

American Academy of Pediatrics, Committee on Genetics. Folic acid for the prevention of neural tube defects. *Pediatrics* 1999;104(2 pt 1):325–327.

Bol KA, Collins JS, Kirby RS. The National Birth Defects Prevention Network. Survival of infants with neural tube defects in the presence of folic acid fortification. *Pediatrics* 2006;117:803–813.

Czeizel AE, Dudás I. Prevention of the first occurrence of neural-tube defects by periconceptional vitamin supplementation. *N Engl J Med* 1992;327:1832–1835.

Elias ER, Sadeghi-Nejad A. Precocious puberty in girls with myelodysplasia. *Pediatrics* 1994;93:521–522.

Feuchtbaum LB, Currier RJ, Riggle S, et al. Neural tube defect prevalence in California (1990–1994): eliciting patterns by type of defect and maternal race/ethnicity. *Genet Test* 1999;3:265–272.

Fletcher JM, Barnes M, Dennis M. Language development in children with spina bifida. *Semin Pediatr Neurol* 2002;9(3):201–208.

Glader LJ, Elias ER, Madsen JR. Myelodysplasia. In: Hansen AR, Puder M, eds. *Manual of Neonatal Surgical Intensive Care*. 2nd ed. Philadelphia: BC Decker Inc.; 2009:459–472.

Goh YI, Bollano E, Einerson TR, et al. Prenatal multivitamin supplementation and rates of congenital anomalies: a meta-analysis. *J Obstet Gynaecol Can* 2006;28:680–689.

Jobe AH. Fetal surgery for myelomeningocele. *N Engl J Med* 2002;347:230–231.

Johnson MP, Gerdes M, Rintoul N, et al. Maternal-fetal surgery for myelomeningocele: neurodevelopmental outcomes at 2 years of age. *Am J Obstet Gynecol* 2006;194:1145–1150.

Kaufman BA. Neural tube defects. *Pediatr Clin North Am* 2004;51(2):389–419.

Mitchell LE, Adzick NS, Pasquariello PS, et al. Spina bifida. *Lancet* 2004;364(9448): 1885–1895.

Oakley GP Jr. The scientific basis for eliminating folic acid-preventable spina bifida: a modern miracle from epidemiology. *Ann Epidemiol* 2009;19(4):226–230.

Shaer CM, Chescheir N, Schulkin J. Myelomeningocele: a review of the epidemiology, genetics, risk factors for conception, prenatal diagnosis, and prognosis for affected individuals. *Obstet Gynecol Surv* 2007;62(7):471–479.

Thompson DN. Postnatal management and outcome for neural tube defects including spina bifida and encephalocoeles. *Prenat Diagn* 2009;29(4):412–419.

Walsh DS, Adzick NS. Foetal surgery for spina bifida. *Semin Neonatol* 2003;8(3):197–205.

58 Orthopaedic Problems
James R. Kasser

This chapter considers common musculoskeletal abnormalities that may be detected in the neonatal period. Consultation with an orthopaedic surgeon is often required to provide definitive treatment after the initial evaluation.

I. CONGENITAL MUSCULAR TORTICOLLIS

A. **Congenital muscular torticollis (CMT)** is a disorder characterized by limited motion of the neck, asymmetry of the face and skull, and a tilted position of the head. It is usually caused by shortening of the **sternocleidomastoid (SCM) muscle** but may be secondary to muscle adaptation from an abnormal *in utero* position of the head and neck.

   1. **The etiology** of the shortened SCM muscle is unclear; in many infants, it is due to an abnormal *in utero* position, and in some, it may be due to the stretching of the muscle at delivery. The result of the latter is a contracture of the muscle associated with fibrosis. One hypothesis is that the SCM abnormality is secondary to a compartment syndrome occurring at the time of delivery.

   2. **Clinical course.** The limitation of motion is generally minimal at birth, but increases over the first few weeks. At 10 to 20 days, a mass is frequently found in the SCM muscle. This mass gradually disappears, and the muscle fibers are partially replaced by fibrous tissue, which contracts and limits head motion. Because of the limited rotation of the head, the infant rests on the ipsilateral side of the face in the prone position and on the contralateral occiput when supine. The pressure from resting on one side of the face and the opposite occipital bone contributes to the facial and skull asymmetry. The ipsilateral zygoma is depressed and the contralateral occiput flattened.

   3. **Treatment.** Most infants will respond favorably to positioning the head in the direction opposite to that produced by the tight muscle. Padded bricks or sandbags can be used to help maintain the position of the head until the child is able to move actively to free the head. Passive stretching by rotating the head to the ipsilateral side and tilting it toward the contralateral side may also help. The torticollis in most infants resolves by the age of 1. Helmets are sometimes used to treat persistent head asymmetry after a few months of age. Patients who have asymmetry of the face and head and limited motion after 1 year should be considered for surgical release of the SCM muscle.

B. **Differential diagnosis.** Torticollis with limited motion of the neck may be due to a congenital abnormality of the cervical region of the spine. Some infants with this disorder also have a tight SCM muscle. These infants are likely to have significant limitation of motion at birth, which is not generally seen in CMT. Radiologic evaluation of the cervical region is necessary to make this diagnosis. Infection in the retropharyngeal area may present with torticollis. The neck mass seen in torticollis in the SCM muscle may be differentiated from other cervical lesions by ultrasound.

II. POLYDACTYLY

A. **Duplication of a digit** may range from a small cutaneous bulb to an almost perfectly formed digit. Treatment of this problem is variable. Syndromes associated with polydactyly include Laurence-Moon-Biedl syndrome, chondroectodermal dysplasia, Ellis-van Creveld syndrome, and trisomy 13. Polydactyly is generally inherited in an autosomal dominant manner with variable penetrance.

B. **Treatment**

1. The small functionless skin bulb without bone or cartilage at the ulnar border of the hand or lateral border of the foot can be ligated and allowed to develop necrosis for 24 hours. The part distal to the suture should be removed. The residual stump should have an antiseptic applied twice a day to prevent infection. Do not tie off digits on the radial side of the hand (thumb) or the medial border of the foot.

2. When duplicated digits contain bone or muscle attached by more than a small bridge of skin, treatment is delayed until the patient is evaluated by an orthopedist or hand surgeon. In general, polydactyly is managed surgically in the first year of life after 6 months of age. X-rays can be delayed until necessary for definitive management.

III. FRACTURED CLAVICLE (see Chap. 6)

A. **The clavicle** is the site of the most common fracture associated with delivery.

B. **Diagnosis** is usually made soon after birth, when the infant does not move the arm on the affected side or cries when that arm is moved. There may be tenderness, swelling, or crepitance at the site. Occasionally, the bone is angulated. Diagnosis can be confirmed by radiographic examination. A "painless" fracture discovered by radiography of the chest is more likely a congenital pseudarthrosis (nonunion). All pseudarthroses occur on the right side unless associated with dextrocardia.

C. **The clinical course** is such that clavicle fractures heal without difficulty. **Treatment** consists of providing comfort for the infant. If the arm and shoulder are left unprotected, motion occurs at the fracture site when the baby is handled. We usually pin the infant's sleeve to the shirt and put a sign on the baby to remind personnel to decrease motion of the clavicle. No reduction is necessary. If the fracture appears painful, a wrap to decrease motion of the arm is useful.

IV. CONGENITAL AND INFANTILE SCOLIOSIS

A. **Congenital scoliosis** is a lateral curvature of the spine secondary to a failure either of formation of a vertebra or of segmentation. Scoliosis in the newborn may be difficult to detect; by bending the trunk laterally in the prone position, however, a difference in motion can usually be observed. Congenital scoliosis is differentiated from **infantile scoliosis** in which no vertebral anomaly is present. Infantile scoliosis often improves spontaneously, although the condition may be progressive in infants who have a spinal curvature of >20 degrees. If the scoliosis is progressive, treatment is indicated and magnetic resonance imaging (MRI) of the spine looking for spinal cord pathology should be done. Rarely, severe congenital scoliosis may be termed *thoracic insufficiency syndrome* and be associated with pulmonary compromise.

B. **Clinical course.** Congenital scoliosis will increase in many patients. Bracing of congenital curves is usually not helpful. Surgical correction with chest expansion or limited fusion may be indicated before the curve becomes severe. Many patients with congenital curves have renal or other visceral abnormalities. Abdominal ultrasonography is used to screen all such patients.

V. DEVELOPMENTAL DISLOCATION OF THE HIP (DDH).

Most (but not all) hips that are dislocated at birth can be diagnosed by a careful physical examination (see Chap. 8). The U.S. Preventive Services Task Force has recommended against generalized ultrasound screening of infants for DDH. Such screening is common in Europe but not in the United States. Ultrasonographic examination of the hip is useful for diagnosis in high-risk cases. In general, ultrasonography is delayed as a screening technique until 1 month of age to avoid a high incidence of false-positive examinations. X-ray examination will not lead to a diagnosis in the newborn because the femoral head is not calcified but will reveal an abnormal acetabular fossa seen with hip dysplasia. There are three types of congenital dislocations.

A. The **classic DDH** is diagnosed by the presence of Ortolani sign. The hip is unstable and dislocates on adduction and also on extension of the femur but readily relocates when the femur is abducted in flexion. No asymmetry of the pelvis is seen. This type of dislocation is more common in females and is usually unilateral, but it may be bilateral. Hips that are unstable at birth often become stable after a few days. The infant with hips that are unstable after 5 days of life should be treated with a splint that keeps the hips flexed and abducted. The **Pavlik harness** has been used effectively to treat this group of patients, with approximately 80% success rate. Ultrasonography is used to monitor the hip during treatment as well as to confirm the initial diagnosis.

B. The **teratologic type of dislocation** occurs very early in pregnancy. The **femoral head does not relocate on flexion and abduction;** that is, Ortolani sign is not present. If the dislocation is unilateral, there may be asymmetry of the gluteal folds and asymmetric motion with limited abduction. In bilateral dislocation, the perineum is wide and the thighs give the appearance of being shorter than normal. This may be easily overlooked, however, and requires an extremely careful physical examination. Limited abduction at birth is a characteristic of this type of dislocation. Treatment of the teratologic hip dislocation is by open reduction. Exercise to decrease contracture is indicated, but the use of the Pavlik harness is not beneficial.

C. The **third type of dislocation** occurs late, is unilateral, and is associated with a **congenital abduction contracture** of the contralateral hip. The abduction contracture causes a pelvic obliquity. The pelvis is lower on the side of the contracture, which is unfavorable for the contralateral hip, and the acetabulum may not develop well. After the age of 6 weeks, infants with this type of dislocation develop an apparent short leg and have asymmetric gluteal folds. Some infants will develop a dysplastic acetabulum, which may eventually allow the hip to subluxate. Treatment of the dysplasia is with the Pavlik harness, but after the age of 8 months, other methods of treatment may be necessary.

VI. GENU RECURVATUM, or hyperextension of the knee, is not a serious abnormality and is easily recognized and treated. It must be differentiated, however, from subluxation or dislocation of the knee, which also may present with hyperextension of the knee. The latter two abnormalities are more serious and require more extensive treatment.

A. **Congenital genu recurvatum** is secondary to *in utero* position with hyperextension of the knee. This can be treated successfully by repeated cast changes, with progressive flexion of the knee until it reaches 90 degrees of flexion. Minor degrees of recurvatum can be treated with passive stretching exercises.

B. All infants with **hyperextension of the knee** should have a radiographic examination to differentiate genu recurvatum **from true dislocation of the knee**. In congenital genu recurvatum, the tibial and femoral epiphyses are in proper alignment except for the hyperextension. In the subluxated knee, the tibia is completely anterior or anterolateral to the femur. The tibia is shifted forward in relation to the femur and is frequently lateral as well.

Congenital fibrosis of the quadriceps is frequently associated with the fixed dislocated knee, and open reduction is essential, as attempted treatment of the dislocated knee by stretching or by repeated cast changes is hazardous and may result in epiphyseal plate damage.

C. **Treatment.** Hyperextended or subluxated knees are treated with manipulation and splinting after delivery with progressive knee flexion and reduction. Fixed dislocation of the knee will require open reduction but not in the neonatal period.

VII. DEFORMITIES OF THE FEET

A. **Metatarsus Adductus (MTA)** is a condition in which the metatarsals rest in an adducted position, but the appearance does not always reveal the severity of the condition. Whether treatment is necessary is determined by the difference in the degree of structural change in the metatarsals and tarsometatarsal joint.

1. Most infants with MTA have **positional deformities** that are probably caused by *in utero* position. The positional type of MTA is flexible, and the metatarsals can be passively corrected into abduction with little difficulty. **This condition does not need treatment.**

2. The **structural MTA** has a relatively fixed adduction deformity of the forefoot, and the metatarsals cannot be abducted passively. The etiology has not been definitely identified but is probably related to *in utero* position. This is seen more commonly in the firstborn infant and in pregnancies with oligohydramnios. Most infants with the structural types of MTA have a valgus deformity of the hindfoot. **The structural deformity needs to be treated with manipulation and immobilization in a shoe or cast** until correction occurs. Although there is no urgency to treat this condition, it is more easily corrected earlier than later and should be done before the child is of walking age.

B. **Calcaneovalgus deformities** result from an *in utero* position of the foot that holds the ankle dorsiflexed and abducted. At birth, the top of the foot lies up against the anterior surface of the leg. Structural changes in the bones do not seem to be present. The sequela to this deformity appears to be a valgus or pronated foot that is more severe than the typical pronated foot seen in toddlers. Whether this disorder is treated or not, it is variable, and no study supports either course. **Treatment consists of either exercise or application of a short leg cast** that will keep the foot plantar flexed and inverted. If the foot cannot be plantar flexed to a neutral position, casts are indicated. Casts are changed appropriately for growth and maintained until plantar flexion and inversion are equal to those of the opposite foot. Generally, the foot is held in plaster for approximately 6 to 8 weeks. Feet that remain in the calcaneovalgus position for several months may be more likely to have significant residual *pes valgus*; a fixed or rigid calcaneovalgus deformity probably represents a congenital vertical talus.

C. **Congenital clubfoot** is a deformity with a multifactorial etiology. A first-degree relative of a patient with this deformity has 20 times the risk of having a clubfoot than does the normal population. The risk in subsequent siblings is 3% to 5%. The more frequent occurrence in the firstborn and the association with oligohydramnios suggest an influence of *in utero* pressure as well. Sometimes, clubfoot is part of a syndrome. Infants with neurologic dysfunction of the feet (spina bifida) often have clubfoot.

1. **There are three and sometimes four components to the deformity.** The foot is in equinus, cavus, and varus position, with a forefoot adduction; therefore, the clubfoot is a talipes equinocavovarus with metatarsal adduction. Each of these deformities is sufficiently rigid to prevent passive correction to a neutral position by the examiner. The degree of rigidity is variable in each patient.

2. Treatment should be started early, within a few days of birth. An effective method of treatment consists of manipulation and application of either tapes or plaster or fiberglass casts that are changed weekly. The Ponseti method is the treatment of choice for idiopathic clubfoot in which the midfoot is sequentially corrected with casts, followed by a heel cord tenotomy to correct equinus after 6 to 8 weeks of cast correction. After tenotomy, the foot is immobilized in a corrected position for 3 weeks; braced full time for 3 months and a night bracing program is used until age 4 years. Physical therapy and splinting are used in a newborn with complex medical problems as initial management.

Suggested Readings

Cooperman DR, Thompson GH. Neonatal orthopaedics. In: Fanaroff AA, Martin RJ, eds. *Neonatal Perinatal Medicine.* 6th ed. St. Louis, MO: Mosby, 1997:1709.

Jones KL, Smith DW. *Smith's Recognizable Patterns of Human Malformation.* 5th ed. Philadelphia: WB Saunders, 1997.

Lovell WW, Winter RB. *Pediatric Orthopaedics.* 6th ed. Philadelphia: Lippincott Williams & Wilkins, 2006.

Osteopenia (Metabolic Bone Disease) of Prematurity

Steven A. Abrams

I. GENERAL PRINCIPLES

A. Definition

1. Osteopenia is defined as postnatal bone mineralization that is inadequate to fully mineralize bones. Osteopenia occurs commonly in very low birth weight (VLBW) infants. Prior to the use of high-mineral containing diets for premature infants, which is the current practice, significant radiographic changes were seen in about half of the infants with birth weight <1,000 g.

2. The current incidence is unknown and is likely closely associated with the severity of overall illness and the degree of prematurity. It may still be seen in as many as half of all infants with birth weight <600 g.

B. Etiology

1. **Deficiency of calcium and phosphorus are the principal causes.** Demands for rapid growth in the third trimester are met by intrauterine mineral accretion rates of approximately 120 mg of calcium and 60 mg of phosphorus/kg/day. Poor mineral intake and absorption after birth result in undermineralized new and remodeled bone.

   a. Diets low in mineral content. These diets predispose preterm newborns to metabolic bone disease.

   b. Unsupplemented human milk. In this circumstance, urinary calcium increases, suggesting a phosphorus deficiency that is greater than the calcium deficiency.

   c. Excessive fluid restriction. This may lead to low mineral intake.

   d. Long-term use of parenteral nutrition.

   e. Formulas that are not designed for use in preterm infants (e.g., full-term, elemental, soy-based, lactose-free). Soy-based formulas should be avoided after hospital discharge as well.

   f. Furosemide therapy. This causes renal calcium wasting, but is not likely the principal contributor to osteopenia for most preterm infants.

   g. Long-term steroid use.

2. **Vitamin D deficiency.** In mothers not supplemented with high amounts of vitamin D (e.g., >4,000 IU/day), human milk has a total vitamin D content of 25 to 50 IU/L, which is insufficient for maintaining 25-hydroxy-vitamin D (25[OH]D) levels in preterm infants at >20 ng/mL. However, when vitamin D intake is adequate, even VLBW newborns can synthesize

1,25-dihydroxyvitamin D (1,25[OH]$_2$D), although synthesis may be minimal in the first few weeks of life.

a. Maternal vitamin D deficiency can cause congenital rickets (uncommon) or hypocalcemia (more common).

b. Inadequate vitamin D intake or absorption produces nutritional rickets, but this is not the primary cause of osteopenia or rickets in preterm infants.

c. Vitamin D malabsorption and inadequate conversion of vitamin D to 25(OH)D can worsen osteopenia in infants with cholestatic liver disease.

d. Chronic renal failure (renal osteodystrophy).

e. Chronic use of phenytoin or phenobarbital increases 25(OH)D metabolism.

f. Hereditary pseudovitamin D deficiency: type I (abnormality or absence of 1-α-hydroxylase activity) or type II (tissue resistance to 1,25[OH]$_2$D). These are extremely rare.

II. DIAGNOSIS

A. Clinical presentation

1. Osteopenia (characterized by bones that are undermineralized or "washed out") develops during the first postnatal weeks. Signs of rickets (epiphyseal dysplasia and skeletal deformities) usually become evident after 6 weeks postnatal age or by term-corrected gestational age. The risk of bone disease is greatest for the sickest, most premature infants.

B. History

1. A history of VLBW, especially <26 weeks or 800 g birth weight, and use of fluid restriction, prolonged parenteral nutrition, or long-term steroid are very common.

2. Rapid increase in alkaline phosphatase value is common.

3. A history of a fracture noticed by caregivers or incidentally on x-rays taken for other purposes may be seen.

C. Physical examination

1. **Clinical signs** include respiratory insufficiency or failure to wean from a ventilator, hypotonia, pain on handling due to pathologic fractures, decreased linear growth with sustained head growth, frontal bossing, enlarged anterior fontanel and widened cranial sutures, craniotabes, posterior flattening of the skull, "rachitic rosary" (swelling of costochondral junctions), Harrison grooves (indentation of the ribs at the diaphragmatic insertions), and enlargement of wrists, knees, and ankles.

D. Laboratory studies

1. **Laboratory evaluation.** The earliest indications of osteopenia are often a decreased serum phosphorus concentration, typically <3.5 to 4 mg/dL (1.1–1.3 mmol/L), and an increased alkaline phosphatase activity. Alkaline phosphatase values >800 IU/L are worrisome, especially if combined with serum phosphorus values <4 mg/dL (1.3 mmol/L). However, it is often difficult to distinguish the normal rise in alkaline phosphatase activity associated with rapid bone mineralization from the pathologic increase related to early

osteopenia. In this circumstance, decreased bone mineralization observed on a radiograph confirms the diagnosis.

a. Serum calcium level (low, normal, or slightly elevated) is not a good indicator of the presence or severity of metabolic bone disease.

b. Serum alkaline phosphatase level (an indicator of osteoclast activity) is often but not invariantly correlated with disease severity (>1,000 IU/L in severe rickets).

c. Normal neonatal range of alkaline phosphatase is much higher than in adults. Values of 400 to 600 IU/L are common in VLBW infants with no evidence of osteopenia.

d. Hepatobiliary disease also elevates alkaline phosphatase level. Determining bone isoenzymes may be helpful but is not usually clinically necessary.

e. Solitary elevated alkaline phosphatase level rarely occurs in the absence of bone or liver disease (transient hyperphosphatasemia of infancy). This elevation can be >2,000 IU/L and persist for several months. It is not associated with any pathology, and the etiology is unknown.

f. Serum 25(OH)D levels do not need to be routinely assessed in preterm infants. Optimal levels in infants are unknown as are functional outcomes at any level. When assessed, targets of >20 ng/mL are reasonable based on very limited evidence. There is no evidence that levels of 12 to 20 ng/mL lead to worsened osteopenia in preterm infants.

E. Imaging

1. **Radiographic signs** include widening of epiphyseal growth plates; cupping, fraying, and rarefaction of the metaphyses; subperiosteal new-bone formation; osteopenia, particularly of the skull, spine, scapula, and ribs; and, occasionally, osteoporosis or pathologic fractures.

a. A loss of up to 40% of bone mineralization can occur without radiographic changes. Chest films may show osteopenia and sometimes rachitic changes.

b. Wrist or knee films can be useful. Generally, if marked abnormalities are present, films should be obtained again 4 to 6 weeks later after a clinical intervention.

c. Measurement of bone mineral content by densitometry or ultrasonography remains investigational in preterm infants.

III. TREATMENT

A. Management

1. In VLBW infants, early enteral feeding significantly enhances the establishment of full-volume enteral intake, leading to increased calcium accumulation and decreased osteopenia.

2. Mineral-fortified human milk or "premature" formulas are the appropriate diets for preterm infants weighing <1,800 to 2,000 g; their use at 120 kcal/kg/ day can prevent and treat metabolic bone disease of prematurity (see Chap. 21).

3. Bone formation is dependent on a combination of adequate calcium and phosphorus availability; supplementation of either calcium or phosphorus alone may not be enough to prevent rickets.

4. Infants small for gestation (weighing <1,800–2,000 g) will usually also benefit from human milk fortification or use of premature infant formula regardless of gestational age.

5. Elemental mineral supplementation of human milk is less desirable than the use of prepackaged fortifiers containing calcium and phosphorus because of concern over medication error and potential hyperosmolarity.

6. The long-term use of specialized formulas in VLBW infants, including soy and elemental formulas, should be discouraged as they may increase the risk of osteopenia.

7. In special circumstances, including babies with radiologic evidence of rickets not responding to fortified human milk or premature formula, smaller amounts of calcium (usually up to 40 mg of elemental calcium/kg/day) and/or sodium or potassium phosphate (usually up to 20 mg of elemental phosphorus) can be provided. This is usually needed in babies whose birth weights were <800 g or who had a prolonged hospital course, including long-term total parenteral nutrition (TPN), fluid restrictions, or bronchopulmonary dysplasia. Due to concerns about tolerance, it is usual to add the intravenous forms of phosphorus (sodium or potassium phosphate) orally to the diet. This may also be done when the serum phosphorus is persistently below 4.0 mg/dL, although evidence supporting this practice is lacking.

8. Ensure adequate vitamin D stores by an intake of 200 to 400 IU/day with at least 400 IU/day being provided by hospital discharge. This may require giving supplemental vitamin D to both breast milk and formula-fed infants at discharge.

9. High doses of vitamin D have not been shown to have short or long-term benefits. Some prefer to give 800 IU/day. This is unlikely to be harmful, but there is no evidence of benefit.

10. Rare defects in vitamin D metabolism may respond better to dihydrotachysterol (DHT) or calcitriol.

11. Furosemide-induced renal calcium wasting may be lessened by adding a thiazide diuretic or by alternate-day administration. Benefits of these approaches are not well established in neonates.

12. Avoid nonessential handling and vigorous chest physiotherapy in preterm infants with severely undermineralized bones. Recent data suggests that daily passive physical activity (range of motion, 5–10 minutes) may enhance both growth and bone mineralization.

13. Infants receiving human milk with added fortifier or premature formula should have serum calcium, phosphorus, and alkaline phosphate levels monitored periodically. Measurement of vitamin D metabolite levels and parathyroid hormone (PTH) levels are rarely useful in this setting. Once the alkaline phosphatase activity has peaked and is declining (usually to <500 IU/L), these no longer need to be measured in fully enterally fed infants if an appropriate feeding regimen is being provided.

14. Human milk fortification or the use of premature infant formula can usually be discontinued after the infant weighs approximately 2,000 to 2,200 g and is tolerating enteral feeds well. It may be continued longer for infants who are fluid restricted or have a markedly elevated alkaline phosphatase activity or radiologic evidence of osteopenia.

15. At hospital discharge, infants with birth weight <1,500 g who are formula-fed may benefit from the use of a transitional formula that has calcium and

phosphorus contents midrange between that of preterm formulas and formulas designed for full-term infants. Such infants may need additional vitamin D to achieve an intake of 400 IU/day.

16. Former VLBW infants discharged from hospital receiving unsupplemented mother's milk are at risk for persistent osteopenia. They, like all human milk-fed infants, should be provided with vitamin D supplementation based on American Academy of Pediatrics (AAP) guidelines for full-term infants (400 IU/day). Members of this patient population may be candidates for a follow-up measurement of serum phosphorus and alkaline phosphatase activity at 4 to 8 weeks postdischarge.

17. Consideration should be given to the use of 2 to 3 feedings per day of a transitional formula postdischarge for otherwise human milk-fed VLBW infants to provide adequate protein as well as minerals.

Suggested Readings

Atkinson SA, Tsang RC. Calcium, magnesium, phosphorus, and vitamin D. In: Tsang RC, Uauy R, Koletzko B, et al. eds. *Nutrition of the Preterm Infant: Scientific Basis and Practical Guidelines*. 2nd ed. Cincinnati, OH: Digital Educational Publishing; 2005:135.

Hawthorne KM, Abrams SA. Safety and efficacy of human milk fortification for very-low-birthweight infants. *Nutr Rev* 2004;62(12):482–485.

Hsu SC, Levine MA. Perinatal calcium metabolism: physiology and pathophysiology. *Semin Neonatol* 2004;9(1):23–36.

Mitchell SM, Rogers SP, Hicks PD, et al. High frequencies of elevated alkaline phosphatase activity and rickets exist in extremely low birth weight infants despite current nutritional support. *BMC Pediatr* 2009;9:47.

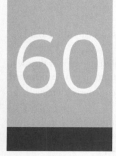

60 Inborn Errors of Metabolism

Ayman W. El-Hattab and V. Reid Sutton

I. INTRODUCTION. Infants with inborn errors of metabolism (IEM) are usually normal at birth with signs typically developing in hours to days after birth. The signs are usually nonspecific and may include respiratory distress, hypotonia, poor sucking, vomiting, lethargy, or seizures. These signs are common to several other neonatal conditions, such as sepsis and cardiopulmonary dysfunction; therefore, it is important to maintain a high index of suspicion of IEM in sick neonates, since most of these disorders can be lethal unless diagnosed and treated immediately.

Although IEM are individually rare, their overall incidence is as high as 1 in 2,000. About 100 different IEM may present clinically in the neonatal period. Most IEMs are transmitted as autosomal recessive genetic diseases. A history of parental consanguinity or previous sibling with unexplained neonatal death or severe illness should raise the suspicion for an IEM. Some IEM, such as the urea cycle disorder (UCD) or-nithine transcarbamylase (OTC) deficiency, are X-linked. As in any X-linked disorder, the severely affected family member could have been a maternal uncle, or a brother, or perhaps a mildly affected mother, sister, or maternal aunt.

II. CLINICAL PRESENTATION. Newborns with IEMs can present with one or more of the following clinical groups:

A. Neurologic deterioration (lethargy/coma). Poor sucking and decreased activity may progress to lethargy, coma, muscle tone changes, involuntary movements, apnea, bradycardia, and hypothermia. IEMs associated with neurologic deterioration may be subdivided as follows to narrow the differential diagnosis:

1. **IEMs with metabolic acidosis:** Maple syrup urine disease (MSUD), organic acidurias, fatty acid oxidation defects, and primary lactic acidemias (defects of gluconeogenesis, pyruvate metabolism, and mitochondrial respiratory chain function) (see IV.)

2. **IEMs with hypoglycemia:** Organic acidurias, defects of fatty acid oxidation, and defects of gluconeogenesis (see V.)

3. **IEMs with hyperammonemia:** UCD, propionic acidemia (PPA), and methyl-malonic acidemia (MMA) (see VI.)

B. Seizures may be the presenting symptom in pyridoxine-responsive seizures, pyridoxal phosphate-responsive seizures, nonketotic hyperglycinemia (NKH), sulfite oxidase/molybdenum cofactor deficiency, disorders of creatine biosynthesis and transport, and peroxisomal disorders (see VII.)

C. Hypotonia. Severe hypotonia is a common symptom in sick neonates. Few IEMs present as predominant hypotonia in the neonatal period. These disorders include mitochondrial respiratory chain defects, peroxisomal disorders, sulfite oxidase/molybdenum cofactor deficiency, and NKH (see VIII.).

D. **Liver dysfunction.** Galactosemia is the most common metabolic cause of liver disease in the neonate (see IX.). Three main clinical groups of hepatic symptoms can be identified.

1. **Hepatomegaly with hypoglycemia** suggest gluconeogenesis defects (e.g., glycogen storage diseases).

2. **Liver failure** (jaundice, coagulopathy, elevated transaminases, hypoglycemia, and ascites) occurs in hereditary fructose intolerance, galactosemia, tyrosinemia type I, fatty acid oxidation defects, and mitochondrial respiratory chain defects.

3. **Cholestatic jaundice with failure to thrive** is observed primarily in α1-antitrypsin deficiency, Byler disease, inborn errors of bile acid metabolism, peroxisomal disorders, citrin deficiency, and Niemann-Pick disease type C.

E. **Cardiac dysfunction.** Long-chain fatty acid oxidation defects and mitochondrial respiratory chain defects can present with cardiomyopathy, arrhythmias, and hypotonia in neonates. The neonatal form of Pompe disease, a lysosomal disorder with glycogen storage, presents with generalized hypotonia, failure to thrive, and cardiomyopathy (Table 60.1).

Table 60.1	Inborn Errors of Metabolism Associated with Neonatal Cardiomyopathy
Disorders of fatty acid oxidation	
Carnitine uptake deficiency	
Carnitine-acylcarnitine translocase (CAT) deficiency	
Carnitine palmitoyltransferase II (CPT II) deficiency	
Long-chain hydroxyacyl-CoA dehydrogenase (LCHAD) deficiency	
Trifunctional protein deficiency	
Very long chain acyl-CoA dehydrogenase (VLCAD) deficiency	
Mitochondrial respiratory chain disorders	
Tricarboxylic acid cycle defects	
α-Ketoglutarate dehydrogenase deficiency	
Glycogen storage diseases	
Pompe disease (glycogen storage disease type II)	
Phosphorylase b kinase deficiency	
Lysosomal storage disorders	
I-cell disease	

Table 60.2	Inborn Errors of Metabolism Associated with Abnormal Urine Odor in Newborns
Inborn error of metabolism	**Odor**
Glutaric acidemia type II	Sweaty feet
Isovaleric acidemia	Sweaty feet
Maple syrup urine disease	Maple syrup
Hypermethioninemia	Boiled cabbage
Multiple carboxylase deficiency	Tomcat urine

F. **Apnea** in the neonatal period can be the presenting sign in NKH and long-chain fatty oxidation defects.

G. **Abnormal urine odor.** An abnormal urine odor is present in some diseases in which volatile metabolites accumulate (Table 60.2).

H. **Dysmorphic features.** Several IEM can present with facial dysmorphism (Table 60.3).

I. **Hydrops fetalis.** Congenital disorders of glycosylation and most lysosomal storage diseases can present with hydrops fetalis (Table 60.4).

Table 60.3	Inborn Errors of Metabolism Associated with Dysmorphic Features
Disorder	**Dysmorphic features**
Peroxisomal disorders (Zellweger syndrome)	Large fontanelle, prominent forehead, flat nasal bridge, epicanthal folds, hypoplastic supraorbital ridges
Pyruvate dehydrogenase deficiency	Epicanthal folds, flat nasal bridge, small nose with anteverted flared alae nasi, long philtrum
Glutaric aciduria type II	Macrocephaly, high forehead, flat nasal bridge, short anteverted nose, ear anomalies, hypospadias, rocker-bottom feet
Cholesterol biosynthetic defects (Smith-Lemli-Opitz syndrome)	Epicanthal folds, flat nasal bridge, toe 2/3 syndactyly, genital abnormalities, cataracts
Congenital disorders of glycosylation	Inverted nipples, lipodystrophy
Lysosomal storage disorders (I-cell disease)	Hurler-like phenotype

Table 60.4	Inborn Errors of Metabolism Associated with Hydrops Fetalis
Lysosomal disorders	
Mucopolysaccharidosis types I, IVA, and VII	
GM1 gangliosidosis	
Gaucher disease	
Niemann-Pick disease type C	
Sialidosis	
Galactosialidosis	
Farber disease	
Hematologic disorders	
Glucose-6-phosphate dehydrogenase deficiency	
Pyruvate kinase deficiency	
Glucosephosphate isomerase deficiency	
Others	
Congenital disorders of glycosylation	
Neonatal hemochromatosis	
Mitochondrial respiratory chain defects	
Glycogen storage disease type IV	

III. EVALUATION OF A NEONATE WITH SUSPECTED IEM

The laboratory evaluation of a neonate with suspected IEM is summarized in Table 60.5. The initial laboratory studies should be obtained immediately once IEM is suspected. The results of these tests can help to narrow the differential diagnosis and determine which specialized tests are required. For neonatal seizures, additional tests are needed (Table 60.5).

A. **Complete blood cell count.** Neutropenia and thrombocytopenia may be associated with a number of organic acidemias. Neutropenia may also be found with glycogen storage disease type Ib and mitochondrial diseases such as Barth syndrome and Pearson syndrome.

B. **Electrolytes and blood gases** are required to determine whether an acidosis or alkalosis is present and, if so, whether it is respiratory or metabolic and if there is an increased anion gap. The organic acidemias and primary lactic acidosis cause

Table 60.5	Laboratory Studies for a Newborn Suspected of Having an Inborn Error of Metabolism
Initial laboratory studies	
Complete blood count with differential	
Serum glucose and electrolytes	
Blood gases	
Liver function tests and coagulation profile	
Plasma ammonia	
Plasma lactate and pyruvate	
Plasma amino acids, quantitative	
Plasma carnitine and acylcarnitine profile	
Urine reducing substances, pH, ketones	
Urine organic acids	
Additional laboratory studies considered in neonatal seizures	
Cerebrospinal fluid (CSF) amino acids	
Cerebrospinal fluid (CSF) neurotransmitters	
Sulfocysteine in urine	
Very long chain fatty acids	

metabolic acidosis with a raised anion gap in early stages. Most metabolic conditions result in acidosis in late stages as encephalopathy and circulatory disturbances progress. A persistent metabolic acidosis with normal tissue perfusion may suggest an organic acidemia or a primary lactic acidosis. A mild respiratory alkalosis in nonventilated babies suggests hyperammonemia. However, in late stages of hyperammonemia, vasomotor instability and collapse can cause metabolic acidosis. A flowchart for the investigation of metabolic acidosis in patients with suspected IEM is presented in Figure 60.1.

C. **Glucose.** Hypoglycemia is a critical finding in some IEMs. Ketones are useful in developing a differential diagnosis for newborns with hypoglycemia (Fig. 60.2). Nonketotic hypoglycemia is the hallmark of defects of fatty acid oxidation. Hypoglycemia associated with metabolic acidosis and ketones suggests an organic acidemia or defect of gluconeogenesis (glycogen storage disease type I or fructose-1,6-bisphosphatase deficiency).

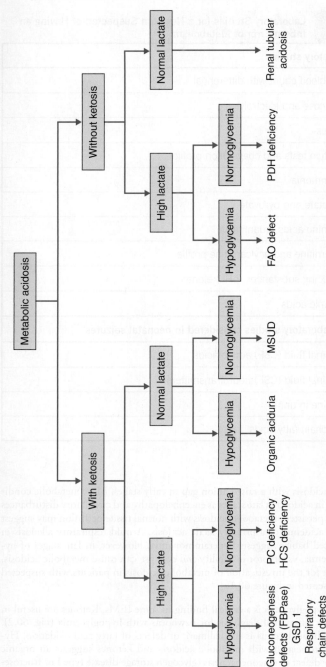

Figure 60.1. Approach to the investigation of neonatal metabolic acidosis. FBPase = fructose-1,6-bisphosphatase deficiency; GSD I = glycogen storage type I; PC = pyruvate carboxylase; HCS = holocarboxylase synthetase; MSUD = maple syrup urine disease; PDH = pyruvate dehydrogenase; FAO = fatty acid oxidation. Note that while a significant hyperlactatemia is more associated with mitochondrial respiratory chain defects and pyruvate metabolism disorders, milder lactate elevations can be seen in organic acidurias and MSUD.

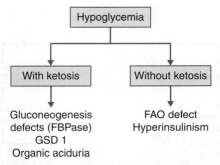

Figure 60.2. Approach to the investigation of persistent hypoglycemia in the newborn with suspected inborn errors of metabolism (IEM). FBPase = fructose-1,6-bisphosphatase deficiency; GSD I = glycogen storage disease type I; FAO = fatty acid oxidation.

D. Plasma ammonia level should be determined in all neonates suspected of having an IEM. Early recognition of severe neonatal hyperammonemia is crucial since irreversible damage can occur within hours. Hyperammonemia is the major indicator for urea cycle disorders. However, hyperammonemia with ketoacidosis suggests an underlying organic acidemia. Figure 60.3 summarizes the approach to neonatal hyperammonemia.

E. Plasma lactate level. A high plasma lactate can be secondary to hypoxia, cardiac disease, infection, or seizures, whereas primary lactic acidosis may be caused by disorders of gluconeogenesis, pyruvate metabolism, and respiratory chain defects. Some IEM (fatty acid oxidation disorders, organic acidemias, and urea cycle disorders) may also be associated with a secondary lactic acidosis. Persistent increase of plasma lactate above 3 mmol/L in a neonate who did not suffer from asphyxia and who has no evidence of other organ failure should lead to further investigation for an IEM. Specimens for lactate measurement should be obtained from a central line or through an arterial stick, since the use of tourniquet during venous sampling may result in a spurious increase in lactate.

F. Liver function tests (LFTs). Galactosemia is the most common metabolic cause of liver dysfunction in the newborn period. Other causes of abnormal LFTs in the newborn include tyrosinemia, α1-antitrypsin deficiency, neonatal hemochromatosis, mitochondrial respiratory chain disorders, and Niemann-Pick disease type C.

G. Urine for reducing substances, pH, and ketones. Reducing substances are tested by the Clinitest reaction that detects excess excretion of galactose and glucose but not fructose. A positive reaction with the Clinitest should be investigated further with the Clinistix reaction (glucose oxidase) that is specific for glucose. Reducing substances in urine can be used as screening for galactosemia; however, this test is not very reliable because of high false-positive and false-negative rates. Urine pH below 5 is expected in cases of metabolic acidosis associated with IEM; otherwise, renal tubular acidosis is a consideration. In neonates, the presence of ketonuria is always abnormal and an important sign of metabolic disease.

H. Plasma amino acid analysis is indicated for any infant suspected of having IEM. Recognition of patterns of abnormalities is important in the interpretation of the results.

I. Urine organic acid analysis is indicated for patients with unexplained metabolic acidosis, seizures, hyperammonemia, hypoglycemia, and/or ketonuria.

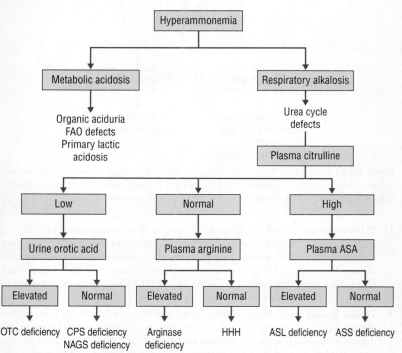

Figure 60.3. Approach to the investigation of neonatal hyperammonemia. UOA = urine organic acids; OTC = ornithine transcarbamylase; CPS = carbamyl phosphate synthetase; NAGS = N-acetyl glutamate synthase; HHH = hyperornithinemia, hyperammonemia, homocitrullinuria; ASA = argininosuccinic acid; ASL = argininosuccinic acid lyase; ASS = argininosuccinic acid synthetase.

J. Plasma carnitine and acylcarnitine profile. Carnitine transports long-chain fatty acids across the inner mitochondrial membrane. An elevation of carnitine esters may be seen in fatty acid oxidation defects, organic acidemias, and ketosis. In addition to patients with inherited disorders of carnitine uptake, low carnitine levels are common in preterm infants and neonates receiving total parenteral nutrition (TPN) without adequate carnitine supplementation. Several metabolic diseases may cause secondary carnitine deficiency.

IV. IEM WITH METABOLIC ACIDOSIS.
Metabolic acidosis with a high anion gap is an important laboratory feature of many IEM, including MSUD, organic aciduria, fatty acid oxidation defects, and primary lactic acidemias (defects of gluconeogenesis, pyruvate metabolism, and mitochondrial respiratory chain). The presence or absence of ketosis in metabolic acidosis can narrow the differential diagnosis (Fig. 60.1).

A. Maple syrup urine disease

1. An autosomal recessive disorder due to deficiency of branched-chain α-keto acid dehydrogenase (Fig. 60.4).

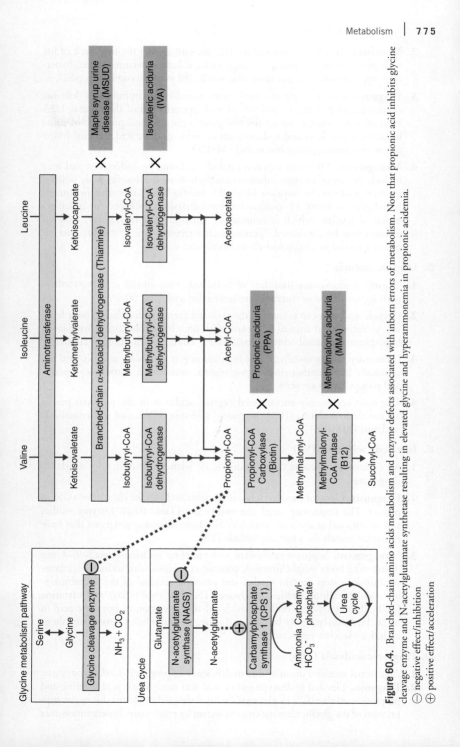

Figure 60.4. Branched-chain amino acids metabolism and enzyme defects associated with inborn errors of metabolism. Note that propionic acid inhibits glycine cleavage enzyme and N-acetylglutamate synthetase resulting in elevated glycine and hyperammonemia in propionic acidemia.
⊖ negative effect/inhibition
⊕ positive effect/acceleration

2. **Manifestations.** Severe form of MSUD presents during the first week of life with poor feeding, vomiting, lethargy, extreme ketosis, seizures, coma, hypertonicity, opisthotonus, and urine that smells like maple syrup (Table 60.2).

3. **Diagnosis.** Increased plasma levels of branched-chain amino acids (leucine, isoleucine, alloisoleucine, and valine) with perturbation of the normal 1:2:3 ratio of isoleucine:leucine:valine, low plasma alanine, and presence of urine branched-chain keto and hydroxyacids on urine organic acid analysis. Many newborn screening programs include MSUD.

4. **Management.** Efforts to suppress catabolism should be undertaken and may include the use of dextrose infusion (usually 6–8 mg dextrose/kg body weight/minute) and insulin infusion (0.05–0.1 unit/kg/hour) to maintain normal blood glucose levels. Hemofiltration/hemodialysis is indicated for quick removal of leucine, which is neurotoxic. Thiamine (10 mg/kg/day) trial for 3 weeks may be considered. Treatment after recovery from the acute state requires a special low branched-chain amino acid diet.

B. **Organic aciduria**

1. Organic acidurias are disorders of branched-chain amino acid metabolism with accumulation of intermediate carboxylic acids (Fig. 60.4).

2. Organic acidurias can present in the neonatal period with lethargy, poor feeding, vomiting, and truncal hypotonia with limb hypertonia, myoclonic jerks, hypothermia, unusual odor, cerebral edema, coma, and multiorgan failure.

3. Laboratory testing usually reveals high anion gap metabolic acidosis, and occasionally, hyperammonemia, hypoglycemia, neutropenia, thrombocytopenia, and pancytopenia are seen.

4. The most commonly encountered organic acidurias in the neonatal period are isovaleric acidemia (IVA), propionic acidemia (PPA), and methylmalonic acidemia (MMA).

C. **Isovaleric acidemia (IVA)**

1. An autosomal recessive disorder due to deficiency of isovaleryl-CoA dehydrogenase.

2. **Diagnosis.** Elevated isovalerylglycine in urine and isovalerylcarnitine (C5) in plasma. The urine may smell like sweaty feet (Table 60.2). Enzyme studies and mutational analysis are available. Newborn screening programs that have expanded metabolic screening include IVA.

3. **Management.** Suppress catabolism with dextrose infusion (usually 6–8 mg dextrose/kg body weight/minute), counteract acidosis with sodium bicarbonate infusion, stop protein intake, and promote removal of the excess isovaleric acid by administration of glycine (150–250 mg/kg/day) and carnitine (100–300 mg/kg/day), both of which enhance excretion of isovaleric acid in urine. Hemodialysis may be needed if above measures fail. Chronic treatment includes a leucine-restricted diet.

D. **Propionic acidemia (PPA)**

1. Autosomal recessive disorder due to deficiency of propionyl-CoA carboxylase.

2. **Diagnosis.** Elevated hydroxypropionic acid and methylcitric acid in urine and propionylcarnitine (C3) in plasma. Glycine is elevated in plasma due to the suppression of the glycine cleavage enzyme system by propionate; hyperammonemia

is due to propionate suppression of N-acetylglutamate synthetase (Fig. 60.4); and neutropenia may be seen and is caused by bone marrow suppression. Newborn screening programs that have expanded metabolic screening include PPA.

3. **Management.** Suppress catabolism with dextrose infusion (usually 6–8 mg dextrose/kg body weight/minute), counteract acidosis with sodium bicarbonate infusion, and stop protein intake. Supplementation with carnitine (100–300 mg/kg/day) to enhance excretion of propionic acid in urine. Biotin is a cofactor for propionyl-CoA carboxylase and may be beneficial in rare patients. Chronic treatment includes a diet low in amino acids that produce propionic acid (isoleucine, valine, methionine, and threonine).

E. **Methylmalonic acidemia (MMA)**

1. An autosomal recessive disorder due to deficiency of methylmalonyl-CoA mutase.

2. **Diagnosis.** Elevated methylmalonic and methylcitric acids in urine; and increased propionylcarnitine (C3) and glycine in plasma. Enzyme studies and mutational analysis are available. Newborn screening programs that have expanded metabolic screening include MMA.

3. **Management.** Suppress catabolism with dextrose infusion (usually 6–8 mg dextrose/kg body weight/minute), counteract acidosis with sodium bicarbonate infusion, stop protein intake, and supplement with carnitine (100–300 mg/kg/day) to enhance excretion of methylmalonic acid in urine. Vitamin B_{12} (adenosylcobalamin) is a cofactor for methylmalonyl-CoA mutase and hydroxycobalamin injection (1 mg daily) should be given as a trial or until a disorder of cobalamin transport or synthesis can be excluded (Note: a normal serum B_{12} level does **not** exclude these disorders). Chronic treatment includes a diet low in amino acids that produce propionic and methylmalonic acids (isoleucine, valine, methionine, and threonine).

F. **Defects of pyruvate metabolism** can present with severe neonatal metabolic acidosis with elevated lactate and pyruvate and include pyruvate dehydrogenase (PDH), pyruvate carboxylase (PC), and holocarboxylase synthetase (HCS) deficiencies.

1. **Pyruvate dehydrogenase deficiency**

a. The pyruvate dehydrogenase complex is encoded by genes on autosomes and on the X chromosome. A deficiency is usually X-linked with the most severe illness in male infants due to deficiency of PDH that catalyzes the conversion of pyruvate to acetyl-CoA.

b. **Manifestations.** Severe lactic acidosis, hypotonia, feeding and breathing abnormalities, seizures, encephalopathy, white matter abnormalities, brain malformation, and dysmorphic facial features (Table 60.3).

c. **Diagnosis.** Elevated lactate and pyruvate in various body fluids is suggestive. Enzyme studies and/or mutational analysis are necessary for a definitive diagnosis.

d. **Management.** Excess glucose may make the acidosis worse; therefore, a high fat diet (80%–85% of calories from fat) may be administered to reduce the lactic acidosis. The enzyme cofactor thiamine (500–2,000 mg/day) should be given. Treatment is usually not very effective, particularly when compared with urea cycle defects and organic acidurias.

2. **Pyruvate carboxylase deficiency**

a. An autosomal recessive disorder due to deficiency of PC that catalyzes the conversion of pyruvate to oxaloacetate.

   b. Manifestations. Severe neonatal lactic acidosis, encephalopathy, coma, seizures, and hypotonia.

   c. Diagnosis. Elevated lactate, pyruvate, ketones, and ammonia are suggestive. Enzyme studies and/or mutational analysis are necessary for a definitive diagnosis.

   d. Management. Usually not effective and include the enzyme cofactor biotin (10–40 mg/day) and carbohydrate-restricted diet.

3. **Holocarboxylase synthetase deficiency (multiple carboxylase deficiency)**

   a. An autosomal recessive disorder due to deficiency of HCS enzyme that catalyzes the binding of biotin with the inactive apocarboxylases; leading to carboxylase activation. Deficiency of this enzyme causes malfunction of all carboxylases, including propionyl-CoA, acetyl-CoA, 3-methylcrotonyl-CoA, and pyruvate carboxylases.

   b. Manifestations. Affected infants become symptomatic in the first few weeks of life with respiratory distress, hypotonia, seizures, vomiting, and failure to thrive. Skin manifestations include generalized erythematous rash with exfoliation and alopecia totalis. These infants may also have an immunodeficiency manifested by a decrease in the number of T cells.

   c. Diagnosis. Lactic acidosis, ketosis, organic acids (methylcrotonylglycine, 3-hydroxyisovaleric, 3-hydroxypropionic, and methylcitric acids), and hyperammonemia. Enzyme studies and mutational analysis are available.

   d. Management. Almost all patients respond to treatment with very large amounts of biotin (10–40 mg/day), although in some affected neonates, the response may be only partial.

V. IEM WITH HYPOGLYCEMIA. Hypoglycemia is a frequent finding in neonates.

The suspicion of an IEM should be raised if it is severe and persistent without any other etiology (see Chap. 24). Hypoglycemia associated with ketosis suggests an organic acidemia or a defect of gluconeogenesis such as glycogen storage disease type I or fructose-1,6-diphosphatase deficiency. Nonketotic or hypoketotic hypoglycemia is the hallmark of fatty acid oxidation defects (Fig. 60.2).

A. Defects of fatty acid oxidation

1. Fatty acid oxidation defects can present in neonatal period with hypoketotic hypoglycemia, lactic acidosis, cardiomyopathy, and hepatopathy. These include deficiencies of very long chain acyl-CoA dehydrogenase (VLCAD), long-chain hydroxyacyl-CoA dehydrogenase (LCHAD), medium chain acyl-CoA dehydrogenase (MCAD), carnitine palmitoyltransferases I and II (CPTI, CPTII), and systemic primary carnitine deficiency.

2. **Diagnosis.** Abnormal acylcarnitine profile (Table 60.6). Enzyme studies and mutational analysis are available.

3. **Management.** Glucose infusion, carnitine (50–100 mg/kg/day), and avoid fasting. For long-chain defects, such as VLCAD or LCHAD, a formula whose primary fat is medium chain triglycerides (MCT) is indicated.

B. Defect of gluconeogenesis

1. **Fructose-1,6-bisphosphatase deficiency** can present with neonatal lactic acidosis, ketosis, hypoglycemia, hepatomegaly, coma, and seizure. Treatment includes glucose and bicarbonate infusion.

2. **Glycogen storage disease type 1** may present as hypoglycemia in the newborn period, but more typically presents at 3 to 6 months of age with poor

Table 60.6	Acylcarnitine Profile in Fatty Acid Oxidation Defects
Fatty acid oxidation defect	**Acylcarnitine profile**
Very long chain acyl-CoA dehydrogenase (VLCAD) deficiency	Elevated C16 (hexadecanoylcarnitine), C14 (tertadecanoylcarnitine), C14:1 (tetradecenoylcarnitine), C12 (dodecanoylcarnitine), and ratio of C14:1/C12
Medium chain acyl-CoA dehydrogenase (MCAD) deficiency	Elevated C6 (hexanoylcarnitine), C8 (octanoylcarnitine), C10 (decanoylcarnitine), C10:1 (decenoylcarnitine), and ratio of C8/C10
Short-chain acyl-CoA dehydrogenase (SCAD) deficiency	C4 (butyrylcarnitine)
Long-chain hydroxyacyl-CoA dehydrogenase (LCHAD) deficiency	Elevated C14OH (hydroxytetradecenoylcarnitine), C16OH (hydroxyhexadecanoylcarnitine), C18OH (hydroxystearoylcarnitine), and C18:1OH (hydroxyoleylcarnitine)
Carnitine palmitoyltransferase I (CPTI) deficiency	Elevated total carnitine; and decreased C16 (hexadecanoylcarnitine), C18 (octadecanoylcarnitine), and C18:1 (octadecenoylcarnitine).
Carnitine palmitoyltransferase II (CPTII) deficiency	Decreased total carnitine; and elevated C16 (hexadecanoylcarnitine) and C18:1 (octadecenoylcarnitine).
Systemic primary carnitine deficiency	Decreased total carnitine

growth, hypoglycemia, and hepatomegaly. Laboratory findings include lactic acidosis, hypertriglyceridemia, and hyperurecemia. Treatment includes the avoidance of fasting through frequent and/or continuous feeding.

VI. IEM WITH HYPERAMMONEMIA.

It is essential to measure ammonia in every sick neonate whenever an IEM is considered. Hyperammonemia can be caused by urea cycle disorders (UCDs), organic acidurias (MMA and PPA), and liver failure. The presence of respiratory alkalosis or metabolic acidosis can help in guiding the evaluation (Fig. 60.3). Transient hyperammonemia can be seen in premature neonates with respiratory distress.

A. Urea cycle disorders

1. Urea cycle defects are among the most common IEMs. Most UCDs are inherited as autosomal recessive conditions, with the exception of the

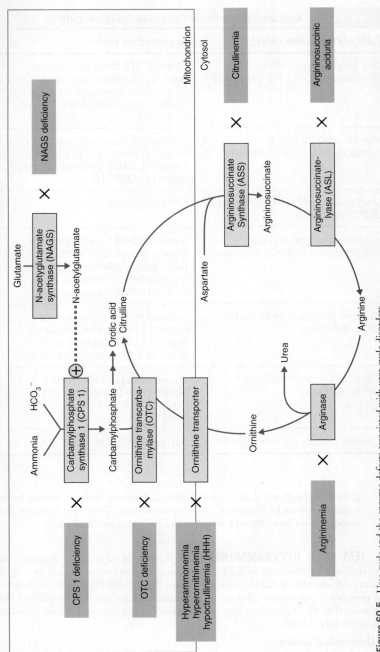

Figure 60.5. Urea cycle and the enzyme defects associated with urea cycle disorders.

X-linked disorder ornithine transcarbamylase (OTC) deficiency. Figure 60.5 represents the urea cycle and the specific enzyme deficiencies that lead to UCDs.

2. **Manifestations.** UCDs can present at any age. In neonates, rapidly progressive symptoms appear in the first few days of life after a short symptom-free interval. These include poor feeding, vomiting, lethargy, hypotonia, and hyperventilation. These patients may develop seizures, apnea, coma, coagulopathy, and increased intracranial pressure unless hyperammonemia is diagnosed and treated promptly.

3. **Diagnosis.** In neonatal-onset UCD, ammonia levels are usually higher than 300 μmol/L and are often in the range of 500 to 1,500 μmol/L. Respiratory alkalosis secondary to hyperventilation is an important initial clue for the diagnosis of a UCD. Other laboratory abnormalities may include mild serum liver enzyme elevations and coagulopathy. Plasma amino acid analysis and urinary orotic acid can pinpoint the metabolic defect and provide a diagnosis (Fig. 60.3). Newborn screening programs that have expanded metabolic screening include some, but not all, of the UCDs.

4. **Management**
   a. Suppression of catabolism. Efforts to suppress catabolism should be undertaken and may include the use of dextrose infusion (usually 6–8 mg dextrose/kg body weight/minute) and insulin infusion (0.05–0.1 unit/kg/hour) to maintain normal blood glucose levels.
   b. Decrease flux through the cycle. All feedings should be discontinued.
   c. Remove ammonia. Intravenous ammonia-scavenging drugs (Ammonul) should be started for ammonia levels above 300 μmol/L. Ammonul (sodium benzoate 100 mg/mL and sodium phenylacetate 100 mg/mL) is given as loading dose of 2.5 mL/kg in 25 mL/kg of 10% dextrose solution over a 60- to 120-minute period followed by the same dose over 24 hours as maintenance infusion. L-arginine hydrochloride is used with Ammonul in loading and maintenance. The L-arginine doses are 200 mg/kg from loading and similar dose for maintenance in carbamyl phosphate synthetase I (CPS) and OTC deficiency; and 600 mg/kg in argininosuccinate synthase (ASS) and argininosuccinate lyase (ASL) deficiencies. L-arginine hydrochloride is not used for arginase deficiency. A repeat loading dose of Ammonul can be given in neonates with severe illness not sooner than 24 hours of the first loading dose. Iatrogenic hypernatremia may be seen due to the high sodium load from Ammonul. Hemofiltration/hemodialysis is the only means for rapid removal of ammonia from blood in acute neonatal hyperammonemia. Hemodialysis is preferred over peritoneal dialysis because it is much more effective. Dialysis is considered in case of very high ammonia levels (>500). However, while preparing for dialysis, the dextrose, insulin, and ammonia scavenger therapy should be maintained.
   d. Enteral nutrition. After the patient is stabilized, oral feeding should be started in consultation with a nutritionist with expertise in managing UCDs. The diet prescription is a mix of formulas low in protein (typically around the RDA) and rich in essential amino acids.
   e. Long-term therapy. Oral medications that are used for long-term treatment includes arginine (up to 600 mg/kg/day for ASS and ASL deficiencies), citrulline (100–200 mg/kg/day for OTC and CPS deficiencies), and ammonia

scavengers sodium benzoate (250–400 mg/kg/day) and sodium phenylbutyrate (250–500 mg/kg/day).

VII. IEM WITH NEONATAL SEIZURES.
Seizures may be the presenting symptom in pyridoxine-responsive seizures, pyridoxal phosphate-responsive seizures, nonketotic hyperglycinemia, sulfite oxidase deficiency, and peroxisomal disorders.

A. Pyridoxine (B6)-responsive seizures

1. An autosomal recessive disorder of lysine metabolism pathway due to deficiency of α-aminoadipic semialdehyde (α-AASA) dehydrogenase, leading to accumulation of AASA and its metabolite piperidine carboxylic acid, which binds and inactivates pyridoxal phosphate.

2. **Manifestations.** Usually presents with encephalopathy and seizures started shortly after birth.

3. Diagnosis is established by demonstration of cessation of the seizure on pyridoxine supplementation (50–100 mg/day oral); this is typically documented with continuous electroencephalogram (EEG) monitoring. Abnormal laboratory results include increased pipecolic acid in CSF and plasma and increased AASA in CSF, plasma, and urine. Mutational analysis is available, as is plasma AASA and piperideine-6-carboxylate.

B. Pyridoxal phosphate-responsive seizures

1. An autosomal recessive disorder due to deficiency of pyridox(am)ine 5'-phosphate oxidase (PNPO).

2. **Manifestations.** Presents with refractory neonatal seizures not responsive to pyridoxine, microcephaly, and hypotonia.

3. Diagnosis is established by demonstration of cessation of the seizure on pyridoxal phosphate supplementation (30 mg/day oral in 3 doses); this is typically documented with continuous EEG monitoring. CSF amino acid analysis shows elevated glycine and threonine. CSF neurotransmitter analysis shows abnormalities in dopamine and seratonin metabolites. Mutational analysis is available, as is plasma AASA and piperideine-6-carboxylate.

C. Nonketotic hyperglycinemia (NKH)

1. An autosomal recessive disorder due to deficiency of the glycine cleavage complex characterized by defective glycine degradation and glycine accumulation in tissues.

2. **Manifestations.** Patients with neonatal form of NKH present with lethargy, hypotonia, and poor feeding within few days of birth. Seizures, hiccups, and apneic episodes are common. EEG shows a characteristic burst-suppression pattern. Many infants die within few weeks of life, typically from apnea; survivors develop profound psychomotor retardation. In transient NKH, which is secondary to the immaturity of glycine cleavage enzymes, laboratory and clinical abnormalities return to normal by 2 to 8 weeks of age.

3. **Diagnosis.** Elevated glycine levels on plasma amino acid analysis and CSF/plasma glycine ratio (samples of plasma and CSF should be obtained around the same time for accurate calculation of the ratio).

4. There is no known effective treatment for NKH. Sodium benzoate (250–750 mg/kg/day) to reduce glycine levels and dextromethorphan (5–20 mg/kg/day) or memantine can be used in an attempt to block the neuroexcitatory effects of glycine upon NMDA receptors, and possibly improve seizure control.

D. Sulfite oxidase deficiency

   1. An autosomal recessive disorder due to deficiency of sulfite oxidase enzyme.

   2. Manifestations. Can present with neonatal seizures, encephalopathy, microcephaly, and progressive psychomotor retardation.

   3. Diagnosis. Elevated sulfocysteine in urine and decreased uric acid, homocysteine, and cysteine in plasma. Enzyme studies and mutational analysis are available.

   4. There is no known effective treatment.

VIII.   IEM WITH HYPOTONIA. IEM that can present with predominant hypotonia include respiratory chain defects, peroxisomal disorders, sulfite oxidase deficiency, and NKH.

A. Respiratory chain defects

   1. The principal function of mitochondria is to produce adenosine triphosphate (ATP) from the oxidation of fatty acids and sugars through the electron transport chain. Therefore, tissues that are more dependent on aerobic metabolism, such as brain, muscle, and heart, are more likely to be affected in these disorders. The neonatal presentation of respiratory chain defects include the following:
   a. Hypotonia, lactic acidosis, hypoglycemia, and liver dysfunction as in mitochondrial DNA depletion syndromes.
   b. Anemia, neutropenia, and thrombocytopenia as in Pearson syndrome.
   c. Cardiomyopathy as in Barth syndrome.

B. Peroxisomal disorders

   1. Zellweger syndrome, neonatal adrenoleukodystrophy (ALD), and infantile Refsum disease represent a continuum, with the Zellweger syndrome being the most severe one. In all three disorders, the basic defect is the failure of peroxisomal biogenesis, that is, to assemble peroxisomes.

   2. Manifestations. Newborn infants with Zellweger syndrome have dysmorphic facial features (Table 60.3), severe weakness and hypotonia, neonatal seizures, eye abnormalities, hepatomegaly with hepatic dysfunction, short proximal limbs, and occasionally "stippled" epiphyses.

   3. Diagnosis. Elevated phytanic and very long chain fatty acids (VLCFAs). Enzyme studies and mutational analysis are available.

   4. There is no known effective treatment.

IX.   IEM WITH LIVER DYSFUNCTION

A. Hepatomegaly with hypoglycemia occurs in gluconeogenesis defects (fructose-1,6-bisphosphatase deficiency).

B. Liver failure occurs in galactosemia, hereditary fructose intolerance, tyrosinemia type I, fatty acid oxidation defects, and respiratory chain defects.

C. Cholestatic jaundice occurs in peroxisomal disorders, citrin deficiency, α1-antitrypsin deficiency, Byler disease, inborn errors of bile acid metabolism, and Niemann-Pick disease type C.

D. Galactosemia (see Chap. 26)

1. An autosomal recessive disease due to deficiency of galactose-1-phosphate uridyltransferase (GALT) that functions in the catabolic pathway of galactose.

2. Manifestations. Typical symptoms of galactosemia in the newborn develop after ingestion of lactose (glucose–galactose disaccharide) through a standard formula or breast milk. Clinical manifestations include vomiting, diarrhea, feeding difficulties, hypoglycemia, jaundice, hepatosplenomegaly, liver dysfunction, renal tubulopathy, lethargy, irritability, seizures, cataracts, and increased risk of *Escherichia coli* neonatal sepsis. Delayed diagnosis results in cirrhosis and mental retardation.

3. Diagnosis is established by enzyme or mutation analysis. Galactose is elevated in plasma, and galactose-1-phosphate is elevated in red blood cells. All newborn screening programs screen for galactosemia either by measuring GALT enzyme activity or galactose levels. Infants with galactosemia have galactose in their urine but not glucose. They have a positive clinitest test for reducing substance but a negative glucose oxidase test (see III.G.)

4. Management consists of substituting a soy-based formula for breastfeeding or for a standard formula, and later, a galactose-restricted diet.

E. Hereditary fructose intolerance

1. An autosomal recessive disorder due to deficiency of fructose-1,6-bisphosphate aldolase (aldolase B), which functions in the catabolic pathway of fructose.

2. Manifestations develop when the neonate is exposed to fructose from the sucrose (glucose–fructose disaccharide) in soy-based formulas or later from fruits. Early manifestations include vomiting, hypoglycemia, jaundice, lethargy, irritability, seizures, hepatosplenomegaly, liver dysfunction, renal tubulopathy, and coma.

3. Diagnosis. Enzyme assay in the liver and/or mutational analysis.

4. Management. Elimination of sucrose, fructose, and sorbitol from the diet.

F. Tyrosinemia type I

1. An autosomal recessive disorder due to deficiency of fumarylacetoacetate hydrolase, which functions in the catabolic pathway of tyrosine.

2. Manifestations. It can present in neonatal period with liver failure, vomiting, bleeding, septicemia, hypoglycemia, and renal tubulopathy.

3. Diagnosis. Elevated succinylacetone in urine and elevated tyrosine and methionine in plasma. Enzyme studies and mutational analysis are available. Newborn screening programs may screen for tyrosine and/or succinylacetone in the bloodspot to diagnose tyrosinemia; however, many cases may be missed when the screening uses tyrosine alone.

4. Management. Nitisinone (NTCB) (1–2 mg/kg/day in 2 doses), phenylalanine, and tyrosine-restricted diet.

G. Neonatal intrahepatic cholestasis caused by citrin deficiency (NICCD)

1. An autosomal recessive disorder due to deficiency of citrin, which is a mitochondrial aspartate–glutamate carrier.

2. **Manifestations.** It can present in the neonatal period with transient intrahepatic cholestasis, hepatomegaly, liver dysfunction, growth retardation, hemolytic anemia, and hypoglycemia. NICCD is generally not severe, and symptoms disappear by age 1 year with appropriate treatment. During adulthood, some individuals develop neuropsychiatric symptoms.

3. **Diagnosis.** Elevated plasma concentrations of citrulline, threonine, methionine, and tyrosine. Mutational analysis is available. Elevated citrulline on newborn screening may lead to the diagnosis.

4. **Management.** Supplementation with fat-soluble vitamins and use of lactose-free formula and high medium-chain triglycerides. Subsequently, a diet rich in lipids and protein and low in carbohydrates is recommended.

X. MANAGEMENT OF INFANT AT RISK FOR A METABOLIC DISORDER

A. Before or during pregnancy. When a sibling has a metabolic disorder or symptoms consistent with a metabolic disorder, the following steps should be taken:

1. Clinical reports and hospital charts should be reviewed.

2. Prenatal genetic counseling regarding possible diagnoses.

3. The parents and relatives should be screened for possible clues to diagnosis.

4. When a diagnosis is known, intrauterine diagnosis by measurement of abnormal metabolites in the amniotic fluid or by enzyme assay or DNA analysis of amniocytes or chorionic villus cells.

5. Planning to deliver the baby in a facility equipped to handle potential metabolic or other complications.

B. Initial evaluation

1. A careful physical examination seeking any of the signs of IEM.

2. Nonmetabolic causes of symptoms such as infection, asphyxia, or intracranial hemorrhage need to be evaluated.

3. The newborn screening program should be contacted for the results of the screening and for a list of the disorders screened.

4. Blood and urine tests should be obtained as summarized in Table 60.5. It is important to obtain these specimens at the time of presentation before starting treatment for metabolic disease. Enzyme assay and mutational analysis may be done for confirmation of diagnosis.

C. Management of acute metabolic decompensation

1. **Reversal of catabolism and promotion of anabolism.** The patient should be kept nothing by mouth (NPO) for 1 to 2 days, adequately hydrated, and provided with IV dextrose (6–8 mg dextrose/kg body weight/minute). Insulin is a potent anabolic hormone and it can be administered at dose of 0.05 to

0.1 unit/kg/hour if metabolic stability cannot be achieved. IV dextrose needs to be adjusted to maintain normal blood glucose levels. Ringer lactate should **not** be used for fluid or electrolyte therapy in a child with a known or suspected metabolic disorder as this can worsen lactic acidosis.

2. **Correction of metabolic acidosis.** If the infant is acidotic (pH <7.22) or the bicarbonate level is <14 mEq/L, sodium bicarbonate can be given at dose of 1 to 2 mEq/kg as a bolus followed by a continuous infusion. If hypernatremia is a problem, potassium acetate can be used in the maintenance fluid.

3. **Correction of hypoglycemia (see Chap. 24)**
   a. Calories. Caloric consumption during a period of decompensation, in order to support anabolism, should be at least 20% greater than that needed for ordinary maintenance. One must remember that withholding natural protein from the diet also eliminates this source of calories, which should be replaced using other dietary or nutritional (non-nitrogenous) sources.
   b. Lipids. To supply extra calories, the neonate can be supplied with lipids in the form of oral medium chain triglycerides (MCT) or parenteral intralipid. However, before feeding MCT, it is very important to be certain that the infant does not have a short chain or medium chain fatty acid oxidation disorder (SCADD or MCADD); otherwise, this could provoke a very severe metabolic reaction.
   c. Protein. All natural protein should be withheld for 48 to 72 hours while the patient is acutely ill. Afterward, amino acid supplementation may be very beneficial in facilitating clinical improvement by enhancing anabolism, but it should be implemented only under the supervision of a physician/nutritionist with expertise in IEMs. Special parenteral amino acid solutions and specialized formulas are available for many disorders.
   d. L-Carnitine. Free carnitine levels are low in the organic acidemias because of increased esterification with organic acid metabolites. Carnitine supplementation (100–300 mg/kg/day) may facilitate excretion of these metabolites. Diarrhea is the primary adverse effect of oral carnitine.
   e. Antibiotics. For certain organic acidemias (e.g., PPA, MMA), gut bacteria are a significant source of organic acid synthesis (e.g., propionic acid). Eradicating the gut flora with a short course of a broad-spectrum antibiotic (e.g., neomycin, metronidazole) orally or intravenously may speed the recovery of a patient in acute crisis.
   f. Elimination of toxic metabolites. Hydration promotes renal excretion of toxins. Hemofiltration/hemodialysis is indicated in cases of unresponsive hyperammonemia (>500 mg/dL) or hyperleucinemia (in MSUD).
   g. Cofactor supplementation. Pharmacologic doses of appropriate cofactors may be useful in cases of vitamin-responsive enzyme deficiencies (e.g., thiamine in MSUD).
   h. Treatment of precipitating factors. Infection should be treated as per usual protocols. Excess protein ingestion should be discontinued.

D. **Monitoring the patient.** The patient should be monitored closely for any mental status changes, overall fluid balance, evidence of bleeding (if thrombocytopenic), and symptoms of infection (if neutropenic). Biochemical parameters need to be followed, including electrolytes, glucose, ammonia, blood gases, complete blood cell count (CBC), and urine for ketones and specific gravity.

E. Recovery and initiation of feeding.

1. The patient should be kept NPO until his or her mental status is more stable. Anorexia, nausea, and vomiting during the acute crisis period make significant oral intake unlikely.

2. If the patient is not significantly neurologically compromised, consideration should be given to providing the patient (orally or by nasogastric tube) with a modified formula preparation containing all but the offending amino acids. When the infant is able to take oral feedings, a specific diet must be used. The diet will be individualized for each child and his or her metabolic defect; for example, in galactosemia, the infant should be fed a lactose-free formula.

XI. POSTMORTEM DIAGNOSIS.

If an infant is dying or has died of what may be a metabolic disease, it is important to make a specific diagnosis in order to help the parents with genetic counseling for future reproductive planning. Sometimes, families that will not permit a full autopsy will allow the collection of some premortem or immediately postmortem specimens that may help in diagnosis. Specimens that should be collected include the following:

A. Blood, both clotted and heparinized. The specimen should be centrifuged and the plasma frozen. Lymphocytes may be saved for culture.

B. Urine, frozen.

C. Spinal fluid, frozen.

D. Skin biopsy for fibroblast culture to be used for DNA analysis or enzyme assay. Two samples should be taken from a well-perfused area in the torso. The skin should be well cleaned, but any residual cleaning solution should be washed off with sterile water. The skin can be placed briefly in sterile saline until special media are available.

E. Liver and/or muscle biopsy samples. Both premortem samples and generous-size postmortem samples should be flash-frozen to preserve enzyme integrity as well as tissue histology.

F. Others. Depending on the nature of the disease, other tissues such as cardiac muscle, brain, and kidney should be preserved. Photographs can be taken as well as a full skeletal radiologic screening for infants with dysmorphic features. A full autopsy should be done if permitted.

XII. ROUTINE NEWBORN SCREENING.

Each state in the United States mandates the disorders evaluated in its own newborn screening program. Recent advances have enabled tandem mass spectrometry (MS/MS) to be applied to the newborn screening specimen. This technique is currently being used in all states to offer screening for many treatable IEMs. A list of what each state screens for may be found on the individual state governmental website or in aggregate on the national newborn screening and genetic resource center website (http://genes-r-us.uthscsa.edu/). Very useful information for follow-up of newborn screening ("ACT Sheets") and for confirmation of a disorder identified by newborn screening ("Algorithms") is available on the website of the American College of Medical Genetics: www.acmg.net/resources/policies/ACT/condition-analyte-links.htm. Table 60.7 includes the newborn screen analytes and the suspected diagnoses with each analyte.

Table 60.7	Newborn Screen Primary Analytes and the Suspected Diagnoses
Analyte	**Condition**
Biotinidase	Biotinidase deficiency
Elevated galactose and deficient GALT	Classical galactosemia
Elevated galactose and normal GALT	Galactokinase deficiency Galactose epimerase deficiency
C0	Systemic primary carnitine deficiency (carnitine uptake deficiency)
C0; C0/C16+C18	Carnitine palmitoyltransferase I (CPTI) deficiency
C3	Methylmalonic acidemias Propionic acidemia
C3DC	Malonic acidemia
C4	Short chain acyl-CoA dehydrogenase (SCAD) deficiency Ethylmalonic encephalopathy Isobutyryl-CoA dehydrogenase deficiency
C4OH	Medium/short chain hydroxyacyl-CoA dehydrogenase (M/SCHAD) deficiency
C4, C5	Glutaric acidemia 2 Ethylmalonic encephalopathy
C5	Isovaleric acidemia Short/branched chain acyl-CoA dehydrogenase deficiency
C5DC	Glutaric acidemia type I
C5OH	Beta-ketothiolase deficiency Biotinidase deficiency Holocarboxylase deficiency HMG-CoA lyase deficiency Methylcrotonyl-CoA carboxylase (MCC) deficiency
C8, C6, C10	Medium chain acyl-CoA dehydrogenase (MCAD) deficiency
C14:1	Very long chain acyl-CoA dehydrogenase (VLCAD) deficiency
C16, C18:1	Carnitine palmitoyltransferase II (CPTII) deficiency
	(continued)

Table 60.7	(Continued)
Analyte	**Condition**
C16OH, C18:1-OH	Long chain hydroxyacyl-CoA dehydrogenase (LCHAD) deficiency Trifunctional protein (TFP) deficiency
Arginine	Argininemia
Citrulline	Argininosuccinic aciduria Citrullinemia I Citrullinemia II Pyruvate carboxylase deficiency
Methionine	Homocystinuria Hypermethioninemia Glycine N-methyltransferase (GNMT) deficiency Adenosylhomocysteine hydrolase deficiency
Leucine	Maple syrup urine disease (MSUD) Hydroxyprolinuria
Phenylalanine	Phenylketonuria (PKU) Biopterin cofactor biosynthesis defect Biopterin cofactor regeneration defect
Elevated tyrosine and normal succinylacetone	Tyrosinemia II Tyrosinemia III
Tyrosine normal/elevated and succinylacetone elevated	Tyrosinemia I

GALT = galactose-1-phosphate uridyltransferase; DC = decraboxylic.

Suggested Readings

Behrman ER, Kliegman R, Jensen H, et al. eds. Metabolic diseases. In: *Nelson Textbook of Pediatrics*. 16th ed. Philadelphia: WB Saunders; 2000.

Browning MF, Levy HL, Wilkins-Haug LE, et al. Fetal fatty acid oxidation defects and maternal liver disease in pregnancy. *Obstet Gynecol* 2006;107(1):115–120.

Burton BK. Inborn errors of metabolism in infancy: a guide to diagnosis. *Pediatrics* 1998;102(6):e69.

Chakrapani A, Cleary MA, Wraith JE. Detection of inborn errors of metabolism in the newborn. *Arch Dis Child Neonatal Ed* 2001;84(3):205–210.

Enns GM, Packman S. Diagnosing inborn errors of metabolism in the newborn: clinical features. *NeoReviews* 2001;2:183–191.

Enns GM, Packman S. Diagnosing inborn errors of metabolism in the newborn: laboratory investigations. *NeoReviews* 2001;2:192–200.

Fernandes J, Saudubray JM, van de Berghe G, et al. eds. Inborn metabolic diseases. Germany: Springer; 2006.

James PM, Levy HL. The clinical aspects of newborn screening: importance of newborn screening follow-up. *Ment Retard Dev Disabil Res Rev* 2006;12(4):246–254.

Leonard JV, Morris AA. Inborn errors of metabolism around time of birth. *Lancet* 2000;356(9229):583–587.

Scaglia F, Longo N. Primary and secondary alterations of neonatal carnitine metabolism. *Semin Perinatol* 1999;23(2):152–161.

Scriver CR, Beaudet AL, Sly WS, et al. eds. *The metabolic and molecular bases of inherited disease.* 8th ed. Vols. I–IV. New York: McGraw-Hill; 2001.

Sue CM, Hirano M, DiMauro S, et al. Neonatal presentations of mitochondrial metabolic disorders. *Semin Perinatol* 1999;23(2):113–124.

Summar M, Tuchman M. Proceedings of a consensus conference for the management of patients with urea cycle disorders. *J Pediatr* 2001;138(suppl 1):S6–S10.

The Urea Cycle Disorders Conference Group. Consensus statement from a conference for the management of patients with urea cycle disorders. *J Pediatr* 2001;138(suppl 1):S1–S5.

Zinn AB. Inborn errors of metabolism. In: Fanaroff AA, Martin RJ, eds. *Neonatal-perinatal medicine.* 6th ed. St. Louis: Mosby; 1997.

61

Disorders of Sex Development

Ari J. Wassner and Norman P. Spack

I. DEFINITION AND NOMENCLATURE. The term *disorders of sex development* (DSD) is preferred over older terms such as *ambiguous genitalia, pseudohermaphroditism,* and *intersex* to denote atypical development of genetic, gonadal, and phenotypic sex (see Table 61.1). Examples of DSD presenting in the newborn period include infants with the following findings:

A. A penis and bilaterally nonpalpable testes.

B. Unilateral cryptorchidism with hypospadias.

C. Penoscrotal or perineoscrotal hypospadias, with or without microphallus, even if the testes are descended.

D. Apparently female appearance with enlarged clitoris or inguinal hernia.

E. Overtly abnormal genital development such as cloacal exstrophy.

F. Asymmetry of labioscrotal folds, with or without cryptorchidism.

G. Discordance of external genitalia with prenatal karyotype.
   Since internal genital anatomy, karyotype, and sex assignment cannot be determined from a baby's external appearance, a thorough evaluation is required. The evaluation must be expedited because of conditions such as salt-wasting congenital adrenal hyperplasia (CAH) that could be life threatening within the first weeks of life.

II. IMMEDIATE POSTNATAL CONSIDERATIONS PRIOR TO SEX ASSIGNMENT. While the rapid determination of sex assignment is essential for the parents' peace of mind, care must be taken to avoid drawing premature conclusions. Prompt consultation with a pediatric endocrinologist will facilitate the evaluation, and most causes of DSD can be clarified in 2 to 4 days, although some cases may take 1 to 2 weeks or longer. Sex assignment depends on anatomy, functional prenatal and postnatal endocrinology, and the potential for sexual functioning and fertility, which may be independent of genetic sex. Until a sex assignment is made, gender-specific names or references should be withheld. The physician should examine the infant's genitalia in the presence of the parents and then discuss with them the process of genital differentiation; that their child's genitalia are incompletely or variably formed; and that further tests will be required before a decision can be made regarding the infant's sex. Circumcision is contraindicated until a determination is made concerning the need for surgical reconstruction.

Table 61.1	Proposed Revised Nomenclature
Previous	**Proposed**
Intersex	DSD
Male pseudohermaphrodite	46,XY DSD
Undervirilization of an XY male	"
Undermasculinization of an XY male	"
Female pseudohermaphrodite	46,XX DSD
Overvirilization of an XX female	"
Masculinization of an XX female	"
True hermaphrodite	Ovotesticular DSD
XX male or XX sex reversal	46,XX testicular DSD
XY sex reversal	46,XY complete gonadal dysgenesis
DSD = disorder of sex development. From Hughes IA, Houk C, Ahmed SF, et al. Consensus statement on management of intersex disorders. *Arch Dis Child* 2006;91(7):554–563.	

III. NORMAL SEXUAL DEVELOPMENT.

The process of gonadal and genital differentiation is depicted in Figure 61.1. Sex determination progresses in stages. In general, early undifferentiated structures will develop down the normal female pathway by default, unless specific factors are present that direct differentiation down the male pathway.

A. **Genetic sex** is determined by the chromosomal complement of the zygote and the presence or absence of specific genes necessary for normal sexual development.

B. **Gonadal sex.** Undifferentiated gonads develop in the bilateral genital ridges around 6 weeks of gestation and begin to differentiate by 7 weeks. *SRY*, which encodes the primary testis-determining factor on the short arm of the Y chromosome, causes the undifferentiated gonads to develop into testes. Specific ovarian-determining genes have also been identified. Most 46,XX males and 46,XY females result from aberrant interchange between the X and Y chromosomes during paternal meiosis.

C. **Phenotypic sex** refers to the appearance of the genitalia. The fetal testis secretes two hormones critical for male genital formation: anti-müllerian hormone (AMH) is produced by Sertoli cells, and testosterone is produced by Leydig cells.

1. **Internal genitalia.** AMH causes regression of the müllerian ducts that would otherwise become the uterus, fallopian tubes, and upper vagina. Testosterone stabilizes the wolffian ducts and promotes their development into the vas deferens,

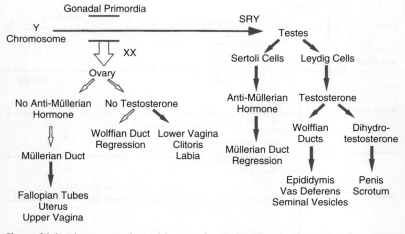

Figure 61.1. The process of gonadal, internal genital, and external genital differentiation. (From Holm IA. Ambiguous genitalia in the newborn. In: Emans SJ, Laufer M, Goldstein D, eds. *Pediatric and Adolescent Gynecology.* 4th ed. Philadelphia: Lippincott Williams & Wilkins; 1998:53.)

seminal vesicles, and epididymis. Müllerian duct regression and wolffian duct development require high *local* concentrations of AMH and testosterone, respectively. Failure of a testis to develop on one side may result in ipsilateral retention of müllerian structures and regression of wolffian structures.

2. **External genitalia.** The enzyme 5α-reductase, present in high concentration in genital skin, converts testosterone to dihydrotestosterone (DHT). DHT is the primary hormone responsible for masculinizing the external genitalia, including the genital tubercle and labioscrotal folds, which form the penis and scrotum, respectively. In the absence of DHT, these undifferentiated structures develop into the clitoris and labia. Testicular descent into the scrotum requires testosterone and generally occurs in the last 6 weeks of gestation.

Finally, formation of normal male internal and external genitalia under the influence of testosterone and DHT requires functional androgen receptors in the target tissues.

D. **Time Course.** The timeline of fetal sexual differentiation is depicted in Figure 61.2 and Table 61.2.

1. **First trimester.** Testicular synthesis of testosterone is stimulated by placental human chorionic gonadotropin (hCG) due to its activation of the luteinizing hormone (LH) receptor. The first trimester is the only period during which the labioscrotal folds are susceptible to fusion. If a female fetus is exposed to excess androgens during the first trimester, her clitoris and labioscrotal folds will virilize and may appear indistinguishable from a normal male penis and scrotum, although the latter will be empty.

2. **Second and third trimesters.** Testicular androgens are stimulated by gonadotropins (primarily LH) from the fetal pituitary and are responsible for increase in penile size, scrotal maturation, and testicular descent. In a female fetus,

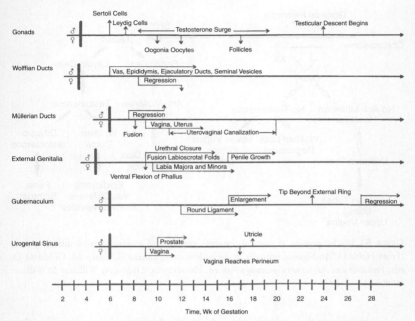

Figure 61.2. Timelines for six aspects of sexual differentiation. (From White PC, Speiser PW. Congenital adrenal hyperplasia due to 21-hydroxylase deficiency. *Endocr Rev* 2000;21(3):245–291. Adapted from Barthold JS, Gonzalez R. Intersex states. In: Gonzalez ET, Bauer SB, eds. *Pediatric Urology Practice.* Philadelphia: Lippincott Williams & Wilkins; 1999:547–578.)

Table 61.2	Timetable of Sexual Development
Days after conception	**Events of sexual development**
19	Primordial germ cells migrate to the genital ridge
40	Genital ridge forms an undifferentiated gonad
44	Müllerian ducts appear; testes develop
62	Anti-müllerian hormone (from testes) becomes active
71	Testosterone synthesis begins (induced by placental hCG)
72	Fusion of the labioscrotal swellings
73	Closure of the median raphe
74	Closure of the urethral groove
77	Müllerian regression is complete

exposure to excess androgens during the second or third trimester may lead to clitoral enlargement and darkening and rugation of the labioscrotal folds but not to labial fusion. Growth hormone also contributes to penile growth. High intrauterine concentrations of testosterone may influence brain development, possibly affecting later behavior and the formation of **gender identity**.

IV. NURSERY EVALUATION OF A NEWBORN WITH SUSPECTED DSD

A. History

1. **Family history** of CAH, hypospadias, cryptorchidism, infertility, pubertal delay, corrective genital surgery, genetic syndromes, or consanguinity.

2. **Neonatal death.** Death of a male sibling from vomiting or dehydration in early infancy may suggest undiagnosed CAH.

3. **Maternal drug exposure** during pregnancy, such as to androgens (e.g., testosterone, Danazol), antiandrogens (e.g., finasteride, spironolactone), estrogens, progestins, or antiseizure medications (e.g., phenytoin, trimethadione).

4. **Maternal virilization** during pregnancy due to maternal CAH, virilizing adrenal or ovarian tumor, or placental aromatase deficiency.

5. **Placental insufficiency.** First-trimester synthesis of testosterone in the fetal testis is dependent on placental hCG due to its activation of the LH receptor.

6. **Prenatal findings** suggesting associated conditions such as oligohydramnios or renal anomalies (genitourinary malformations) or skeletal abnormalities (campomelic dysplasia).

B. Physical examination

1. **External genitalia.** The examiner should note the stretched penile length, width of the corpora, engorgement, presence of chordee, position of the urethral orifice, presence of a vaginal opening, and pigmentation and symmetry of the scrotum or labioscrotal folds. The normal full-term male infant has a penile length of at least 2.5 cm, measured stretched from the pubic ramus to the tip of the glans (see Fig. 61.3). The normal full-term female infant has a clitoris <1 cm in length. Posterior fusion of the labioscrotal folds is defined as an increased **anogenital ratio**, which is the distance between the anus and the posterior fourchette divided by the distance between the anus and the base of the clitoris. An anogenital ratio >0.5 is indicative of first-trimester androgen exposure.

2. **Gonadal size, position, and descent** should be carefully noted. A gonad below the inguinal ligament is usually a testis, but an ovotestis or a uterus may present as an inguinal hernia. Abnormal genital development with clitoromegaly, or an apparently well-formed penis with an empty scrotum, should raise immediate concern that the infant is a female virilized by CAH.

3. **Bimanual rectal examination** may reveal müllerian structures (e.g., a cervix or uterus palpable in the midline).

4. **Associated anomalies** should be noted. Dysmorphic features suggest a more generalized disorder. Denys-Drash syndrome (Wilms tumor and nephropathy) or WAGR (**W**ilms tumor, **A**niridia, **G**enitourinary anomalies, and mental **R**etardation) syndrome, both due to the mutations of *WT1* (11p13), can cause DSD in both 46,XY and 46,XX infants. Other conditions associated

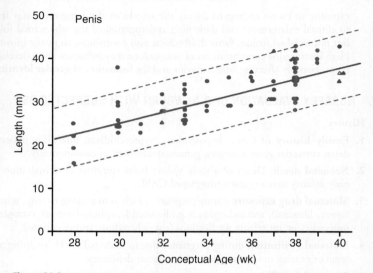

Figure 61.3. Stretched penile length of normal premature and full-term babies (closed circles), showing lines of mean ± 2 standard deviations. Correlation coefficient is .80. Superimposed are data for two small-for-gestational-age infants (open triangles), seven large-for-gestational-age infants (closed triangles), and four twins (closed boxes), all of whom are in the normal range. (From Feldman KW, Smith DW. Fetal phallic growth and penile standards for newborn male infants. *J Pediatr* 1975;86(3):395–398.)

with disorders of sex development include Smith-Lemli-Opitz, Robinow, and Goldenhar syndromes; campomelic dysplasia; and trisomy 13.

C. Diagnostic tests

  1. Laboratory tests are tailored to the differential diagnosis.

   a. First-line testing should generally include a karyotype, serum electrolytes, blood urea nitrogen (BUN), creatinine, 17-hydroxyprogesterone (17-OHP), and testosterone.

   b. Other tests such as plasma renin activity (PRA), LH, follicle-stimulating hormone (FSH), AMH, or levels of other adrenal hormones may be indicated in certain circumstances.

   c. Chromosome analysis on peripheral blood can be performed by karyotype within 48 hours and, more rapidly, by **fluorescent *in situ* hybridization (FISH)**. Although a standard karyotype may show 46,XX, FISH for *SRY* may reveal that it has been translocated to an X chromosome or an autosome. FISH for other genes involved in sex development may be indicated in specific circumstances. Any abnormal karyotype detected prenatally should be confirmed immediately after birth.

  2. Pelvic ultrasonography, especially when the bladder is full, can determine whether a uterus is present. However, this determination can be difficult and may require an experienced ultrasonographer. Testes can often be visualized by ultrasound, but ovaries are less likely to be identified. Given the association between urologic and genital malformations, ultrasonographic evaluation should include the kidneys, ureters, and bladder. Magnetic resonance imaging (MRI) may be needed to locate intra-abdominal testes or to confirm the presence of a uterus when ultrasonography is indeterminate.

3. **Voiding cystourethrogram (VCUG) or genitogram** may reveal a vagina with a cervix at its apex (indicating the presence of a uterus) or a utricle (a müllerian duct remnant). It may also reveal the presence of abnormal connections between the urinary and genital tracts (e.g., urethrovaginal fistula).

Table 61.3 summarizes causes and Figure 61.4 describes an approach to patients with disorders of sex development.

V. 46,XX DSD (VIRILIZED 46,XX FEMALES).
The infant has normally developed müllerian structures and no wolffian structures but has evidence of external genital virilization.

A. **Congenital adrenal hyperplasia.** The most common DSD presenting in the neonatal period is a female infant with CAH. The most common form of CAH (>90%) is due to deficiency of 21-hydroxylase (21-OH in Fig. 61.5) caused by mutations in *CYP21A2*. Virilization may occur in rarer forms of CAH due to deficiency of 11β-hydroxylase (11-OH or CYP11B1) or 3β-hydroxysteroid dehydrogenase (3β-HSD or HSD3B2).

1. **Epidemiology.** The incidence of 21-OH deficiency is 1:16,000 births based on data from worldwide newborn screening programs. Patients with salt wasting outnumber those without ("simple virilizing" CAH) by 3:1. The male:female sex ratio is 1:1. While females are easily detected at birth due to abnormal genital development, males have normal genitalia and may be missed on clinical exam (although hyperpigmentation of the scrotum can be a clue).

2. **Diagnosis.** In the United States, all state newborn screening programs include screening for 21-OH deficiency. Blood spots are obtained on filter paper, ideally between 48 and 72 hours of age, and 17-OHP is measured. Normal values must be determined for each individual screening program because they depend on the filter paper thickness and the immunoassay used. The 17-OHP is elevated on newborn screening in 99% of infants with 21-OH deficiency detected in the newborn period.

  a. False-positive results. Obtaining a blood sample before 48 hours of age can cause a false-positive result. Since normal values for 17-OHP are inversely related to gestational age and birth weight, false-positive results can occur in premature and low birth weight infants, as well as in infants who are acutely ill.

  b. False-negative results. Prenatal administration of steroids (e.g., betamethasone) may suppress 17-OHP levels and may cause false-negative results; newborns who received such medications should be rescreened after 3 to 5 days.

  c. Rapid evaluation of suspected 21-OH deficiency is critical to avert salt-wasting crises. Clinical suspicion or abnormal newborn screening results should be confirmed immediately by measurement of serum 17-OHP. An adrenocorticotropic hormone (ACTH) level may aid diagnosis, and measurement of plasma renin activity and aldosterone may help differentiate between salt wasting and simple virilizing forms. Serum electrolytes should be monitored at least every other day until salt wasting is confirmed or ruled out.

  d. Rare forms of CAH. In an infant with 11-OH deficiency, levels of 11-deoxycortisol and 11-deoxycorticosterone are elevated. An infant with 3β-HSD deficiency may have mildly elevated 17-OHP on newborn screen; 17-hydroxypregnenolone is markedly elevated in these infants.

Table 61.3	Causes of Disorders of Sex Development		

| Disorder | Phenotype | | Karyotype |
	External Genitalia	Gonads	
Disorders of gonadal differentiation			
Ovotesticular DSD	Ambiguous	Ovarian and testicular tissue	46,XX; 46,XY; 46,XX/46,XY
Mixed gonadal dysgenesis	Variable	Streak gonad and dysgenetic testis	45,X/46,XY; 46,XYp-
46,XY complete gonadal dysgenesis	Female or ambiguous	Dysgenetic testes or streak gonads	46,XY
46,XX testicular DSD	Male or ambiguous	Testes	46,XX
46,XX DSD (masculinization of the genetic female)			
Congenital adrenal hyperplasia			
21α-hydroxylase deficiency	Ambiguous	Ovaries	46,XX
11β-hydroxylase deficiency	Ambiguous	Ovaries	46,XX
3β-hydroxysteroid dehydrogenase deficiency	Ambiguous	Ovaries	46,XX
Placental aromatase deficiency	Ambiguous	Ovaries	46,XX
Maternal androgen excess	Ambiguous	Ovaries	46,XX
46,XY DSD (incomplete masculinization of the genetic male)			
Testicular unresponsiveness to hCG and LH (LH receptor mutation)	Ambiguous	Testes	46,XY

(continued)

Table 61.3	(Continued)		
	Phenotype		
Disorder	External Genitalia	Gonads	Karyotype
Disorders of testosterone synthesis			
Steroidogenic acute regulatory protein deficiency	Ambiguous	Testes	46,XY
Side-chain cleavage enzyme deficiency	Ambiguous	Testes	46,XY
3β-hydroxysteroid dehydrogenase deficiency	Ambiguous	Testes	46,XY
17α-hydroxylase deficiency	Ambiguous	Testes	46,XY
17,20-lyase deficiency	Ambiguous	Testes	46,XY
17β-hydroxysteroid dehydrogenase deficiency	Ambiguous	Testes	46,XY
Disorder of testosterone metabolism			
5α-reductase deficiency	Ambiguous	Testes	46,XY
End-organ resistance to testosterone			
Complete androgen insensitivity syndrome	Female	Testes	46,XY
Partial androgen insensitivity syndrome	Ambiguous	Testes	46,XY
Vanishing testes syndrome	Variable	Absent gonads	46,XY
Lack of anti-müllerian hormone or AMH receptor	Male	Testes, uterus, fallopian tubes	46,XY

Modified from Wolfsdorf JI, Muglia L. Endocrine disorders. In: Graef JW, ed. *Manual of Pediatric Therapeutics*. Philadelphia: Lippincott-Raven; 1997:381–413.
HCG = human chorionic gonadotropin; LH = luteinizing hormone.

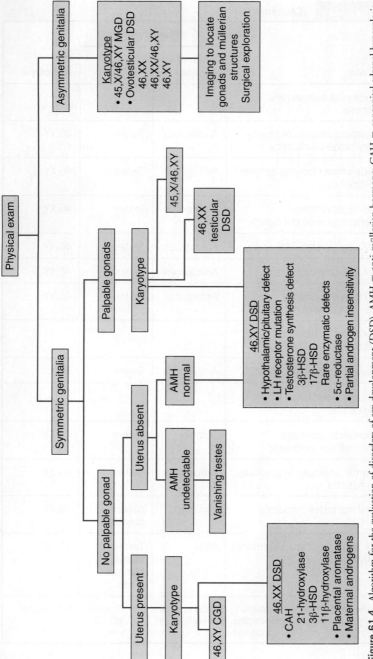

Figure 61.4. Algorithm for the evaluation of disorders of sex development (DSD). AMH = anti-müllerian hormone; CAH = congenital adrenal hyperplasia; CGD = complete gonadal dysgenesis; 3β-HSD = 3β-hydroxysteroid dehydrogenase; 17β-HSD = 17β-hydroxysteroid dehydrogenase; LH = luteinizing hormone; MGD = mixed gonadal dysgenesis.

e. Newborn screening may not detect infants with mild simple virilizing 21-OH deficiency. Therefore, in a virilized 46,XX female suspected of having a form of CAH, or who has equivocal 17-OHP levels, an **ACTH stimulation test** may be necessary to demonstrate the adrenal enzyme defect (Fig. 61.5).

3. Management. In an infant suspected of 21-OH deficiency, treatment should be started as soon as the laboratory tests above have been obtained.

a. Glucocorticoids. Hydrocortisone 20 mg/m²/day, divided into q8h dosing, should be given to all infants suspected of 21-OH deficiency.

$$\text{Body surface area (m}^2) = \sqrt{\frac{\text{Length (cm)} \times \text{weight (kg)}}{3600}}$$

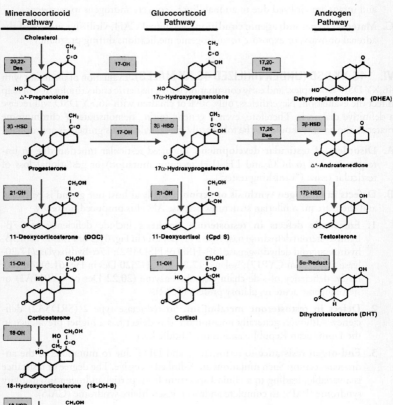

Figure 61.5. Pathways of steroid biosynthesis. (From Esoterix, 4301 Lost Hills Road, Calabasas Hills, CA 91301.)

b. Mineralocorticoids. In cases of salt-wasting CAH, fludrocortisone acetate (Florinef) 0.1 to 0.2 mg daily should be given. Salt-wasting crises usually develop between the 5th and 14th day of life but can occur as late as 1 month and may occur even in affected infants whose virilization is not severe. Weight, fluid balance, and electrolytes must be monitored closely, with blood samples at least every 2 days during the first few weeks of life to detect hyponatremia or hyperkalemia. If salt wasting occurs, salt loss should be replaced initially with intravenous normal saline with glucose added. Salt wasting due to aldosterone deficiency typically requires replacement of about 8 mEq/kg/day of sodium. Once the infant is stabilized, NaCl 1 to 2 grams daily, divided into q6h dosing, should be added to the formula (each gram of NaCl contains 17 mEq of sodium).

B. Placental aromatase deficiency. The hallmark of this disorder is that both mother and infant are virilized due to an inability to convert androgens to estrogens.

C. Maternal hyperandrogenic conditions. Maternal CAH, virilizing tumors of the adrenal or ovary, or exposure to androgenic medications during pregnancy.

VI. 46,XY DSD (UNDERVIRILIZED 46,XY MALES).

Evaluation of the infant with 46,XY DSD is complex, and early consultation with a pediatric endocrinologist will help direct the evaluation. Nevertheless, only 50% of children with 46,XY DSD will receive a definitive diagnosis. Therefore, even if genetic testing demonstrates Y chromosome material, the parents should not be told hastily that a male sex assignment is appropriate.

A. Disorders of testicular development. Impaired testicular function due to unresponsiveness to hCG and LH (LH receptor mutation) or gestational loss of testicular tissue ("vanishing testes").

B. Defects in androgen synthesis or action. Usually at least one gonad is palpable, and there are no müllerian structures because AMH is produced normally.

1. **Enzymatic defects in testosterone synthesis** include deficiency of 17β-hydroxysteroid dehydrogenase type 3 (17β-HSD in Fig. 61.5 or HSD17B3); 3β-hydroxysteroid dehydrogenase (3β-HSD or HSD3B2); 17α-hydroxylase/17,20-lyase (17-OH or CYP17); isolated 17,20-lyase (17,20 Des in Fig. 61.5); or, very rarely, deficiency of side-chain cleavage enzyme (20,22 Des or CYP11A1) or steroidogenic acute regulatory protein (StAR).

2. **Defect in testosterone metabolism.** 5α-reductase type 2 (SRD5A2) deficiency. Although generally uncommon, this defect has a higher prevalence in the Dominican Republic and in the Middle East.

3. **End-organ resistance** to testosterone and DHT due to mutations of the androgen receptor. Such mutations are X-linked recessive. The degree of resistance is a variable, leading to a clinical spectrum from partial androgen insensitivity syndrome (PAIS) to complete androgen insensitivity syndrome (CAIS).

C. Environmental disorders. Maternal drug ingestion (e.g., finasteride, spironolactone, phenytoin).

D. Evaluation focuses on establishing the presence or absence of testes and their ability to produce androgens.

1. **Presence of testes.** If testes are not palpable, their presence should be confirmed by imaging and/or AMH level (see VI.F. and VI.G.).

2. **Laboratory evaluation** is focused on determining whether the cause of undervirilization is due to a defect in testosterone synthesis, metabolism, or action. Blood samples should be obtained for measurement of electrolytes, FSH, LH, testosterone, DHT, androstenedione, dehydroepiandrosterone (DHEA), 17-OHP, 17-hydroxypregnenolone, and AMH. Serum electrolytes may reveal hyponatremia and hyperkalemia in 3β-HSD deficiency. Measurement of 11-deoxycorticosterone and plasma renin activity may help define the type of enzyme deficiency.

3. A **hCG stimulation test** may be necessary if the above results do not lead to a diagnosis.

   a. **Timing.** Testing should be performed within the first 2 to 3 months of life when the hypothalamic-pituitary-gonadal axis is active.

   b. **Technique.** HCG 500 IU is given intramuscularly every alternate day for a total of three doses. DHEA, androstenedione, testosterone, and DHT concentrations are measured 24 hours after the final dose of hCG.

   c. **Interpretation.** Inability to increase the testosterone level in response to hCG is a characteristic of LH receptor mutations, gestational loss of testicular tissue, or an enzymatic defect in testosterone synthesis. An elevated testosterone:DHT ratio (>20:1) after hCG stimulation suggests 5α-reductase deficiency, whereas a low testosterone:androstenedione ratio (<0.8:1) suggests 17β-HSD deficiency.

4. An **ACTH stimulation test** may be necessary to define defects in earlier enzymatic steps of testosterone synthesis such as deficiencies of 3β-HSD, side chain cleavage enzyme, StAR, or 17-OH, which also produce cortisol insufficiency and CAH (Fig. 61.5). The former three deficiencies are associated with salt wasting; 17-OH deficiency is associated with salt retention and hypertension, although these are often not present in the newborn period.

5. **Androgen insensitivity syndrome.** If the initial laboratory tests show high levels of testosterone that do not increase when hCG is given, and the ratios of testosterone:androstenedione and testosterone:DHT are normal, the infant probably has **PAIS**.

   a. **Further evaluation** may include monthly administration of 25 to 50 mg of intramuscular depo testosterone for 3 months. Failure of the stretched penile length to increase by 2.0 ± 0.6 cm supports the diagnosis of PAIS.

   b. **Genetic studies of the androgen receptor** will detect mutations in fewer than 25% of patients with PAIS.

   c. **Sex assignment** in cases of PAIS is particularly complex. In the past, infants with PAIS were routinely assigned female sex and underwent gonadectomy and feminizing genitoplasty, but this practice has become controversial. When a testis is retained, these patients will virilize to a variable degree during puberty, but will develop gynecomastia and will not achieve normal adult penile size on their own. It is not possible, however, to predict the extent to which an infant with PAIS will respond to endogenous or exogenous testosterone.

   d. Newborns with the **complete form of androgen resistance (CAIS)** have normal-appearing female external genitalia (including the lower third of the vagina) and absent müllerian and wolffian structures. They may be identified by an antepartum 46,XY karyotype or by the presence of an apparent inguinal hernia that proves to be a testis. More often, they present at puberty with primary amenorrhea. Infants with CAIS should be raised female, and their gender identities are invariably female.

E. Microphallus (<2.5 cm in a full-term infant) with or without cryptorchidism has many causes in addition to those above, including hypothalamic-pituitary disorders of gonadotropin production such as Kallmann syndrome, holoprosencephaly, septo-optic dysplasia, and other causes of multiple pituitary hormone deficiencies. Growth hormone deficiency is independently associated with microphallus. Infants with panhypopituitarism often have neonatal hypoglycemia and direct hyperbilirubinemia. Among the many other conditions associated with microphallus are CHARGE association; trisomy 21; and Prader-Willi, Robinow, Klinefelter, Carpenter, Meckel-Gruber, Noonan, de Lange, Fanconi, and fetal hydantoin syndromes. Treatment with testosterone enanthate 25 mg intramuscularly given monthly for 3 months may substantially increase penile length in these patients.

F. Bilateral cryptorchidism. Bilateral cryptorchidism at birth occurs in 3:1,000 infants, most of whom are premature. By 1 month of life, the testes are still undescended in 1:1,000 infants.

1. **Imaging.** Either ultrasonography or MRI may reveal inguinal or intra-abdominal testes, although MRI is more sensitive for locating the latter.

2. **Laboratory evaluation.** If testicular tissue cannot be found by exam or imaging, levels of serum FSH, LH, and testosterone should be measured. These hormones rise shortly after birth and are elevated until approximately 6 months of age in boys.
   a. If testosterone levels are low, the presence and responsiveness of testicular tissue can be assessed by **hCG stimulation test** (see VI.D.3.). Elevated serum gonadotropins with a low basal testosterone concentration that fails to rise in response to hCG suggest absent or nonfunctioning testes.
   b. Undetectable serum **AMH** is indicative of bilateral anorchia rather than undescended testes (see VI.G.).

3. **Management.** A urologist should be consulted and, if surgery is indicated, orchidopexy should be performed by 1 year of life. If intra-abdominal testes cannot be brought into the scrotum, they should be removed because of the 3- to 10-fold increased risk of germ cell cancer in cryptorchid testes.

4. **Persistent müllerian duct syndrome (PMDS)** in 46,XY infants is caused by defects in AMH or its receptor. Cryptorchidism is common in infants with PMDS, who, otherwise, have normal male genitalia but retain a uterus and fallopian tubes.

5. **Other conditions** associated with cryptorchidism include trisomy 21; congenital ichthyosis; neural tube defects; renal and urinary tract malformations; and numerous syndromes, including Prader-Willi, Bardet-Biedl, Aarskog, Cockayne, Fanconi, Noonan, Klinefelter, and fetal hydantoin syndromes.

6. **The presence of any of the following** physical findings also merits evaluation for a disorder of sex development:
   a. Unilateral cryptorchidism with hypospadias, especially proximal (e.g., perineoscrotal or penile) hypospadias.
   b. Unilateral cryptorchidism with microphallus.

G. Use of AMH. The hCG stimulation test is used to assess the presence and function of testicular tissue but it can be cumbersome and expensive and occasionally requires protracted dosing to stimulate a refractory testis. AMH is an alternative marker of the presence of testicular tissue. AMH is produced in a sexually dimorphic manner. Starting at birth, AMH from Sertoli cells rises to a peak of 115 ng/mL at 6 months of age, then declines during adolescence to an adult male level of 4 ng/mL. In contrast, granulosa cells of the ovary do not make significant amounts of AMH until puberty, when levels in girls also reach approximately 4 ng/mL. Thus, measuring AMH by enzyme-linked immunosorbent assay (ELISA) can distinguish whether testicular tissue is present or absent. AMH in the normal or detectable range has a 100% positive predictive value for the presence of testicular tissue; the predictive value for anorchia is 94% if AMH is undetectable.

VII. GONADAL DIFFERENTIATION DISORDERS

A. **Ovotesticular DSD (true hermaphroditism).** The chromosomal complement in this rare condition is variable: 70% of patients are 46,XX; less than 10% are 46,XY; and the remainder show mosaicism with a Y chromosome-containing cell line (most commonly 46,XX/46,XY).

1. **Physical findings.** The external genitalia may appear normal or may show incomplete labioscrotal fusion, asymmetric labioscrotal folds, or hypospadias. Whether the internal structures contain wolffian or müllerian elements depends on the local presence of testosterone and AMH on that side of the abdomen.

2. **Evaluation.** A hCG stimulation test that produces a rise in serum testosterone confirms the presence of Leydig cells, whereas a measurable AMH level indicates the presence of Sertoli cells.

3. **Diagnosis** is based on the histology of the gonads, which, by definition, contain both testicular and follicle-containing ovarian tissue. Laparotomy, gonadal biopsy, or both may be required for diagnosis.

4. **Management.** Dysgenetic Y chromosome-containing gonads should be removed. Sex assignment should be based on the external and internal genitalia and the degree of intrauterine androgen exposure. If male sex assignment is made, müllerian structures should be removed.

B. **Mixed gonadal dysgenesis (MGD).** The hallmark of MGD is the presence of a testis on one side of the body and either a streak gonad or dysgenetic testis on the other side. This disorder has a 45,X/46,XY chromosomal complement. Often, the Y chromosome is abnormal, or the Y chromosome material may be translocated to an autosome.

1. **Physical findings.** The combination of asymmetric external genitalia and one palpable testis in the labioscrotal fold is almost certainly MGD. However, the appearance of 45,X/46,XY mosaicism can range from normal male to normal female; in fact, 90% of 45,X/46,XY infants diagnosed prenatally are normal phenotypic males at birth. In patients with MGD, each gonad governs the differentiation of the ipsilateral internal genital structures. A fallopian tube and uterus are frequently present on one side, and these structures can herniate into the labioscrotal fold. Children with MGD may have features similar to Turner syndrome such as webbed neck, lymphedema, short stature, and, occasionally, cardiac defects (e.g., coarctation of the aorta).

2. **Management.** Sex assignment is discretionary because of the marked phenotypic and hormonal variability. Approximately two-thirds are raised as females. If AMH is measurable, or if a hCG stimulation test causes a significant rise in serum testosterone indicative of testicular tissue, the testis should be sought by

imaging and/or surgery. The testis should be removed if female sex assignment is made or brought into the scrotum for close observation if male sex assignment is made. Streak and dysgenetic gonads should be removed in infancy, since germ cell tumors may arise in up to 30% of these children, sometimes within the first few years of life. All children with MGD should be evaluated by a pediatric endocrinologist, as many will have poor linear growth and be candidates for growth hormone therapy.

C. **46,XY complete gonadal dysgenesis (CGD).** 46,XY CGD has also been referred to as *complete sex reversal*. Infants with 46,XY CGD fail to masculinize due to incomplete testicular differentiation, which is a result of abnormal functioning of SRY itself or of factors that regulate or are regulated by it. Bilateral streak gonads are present and internal genital structures are female due to inadequate production of AMH and testosterone. The external genitalia usually appear female, but clitoromegaly may occur if "gonadal" hilus cells secrete testosterone. These patients are usually raised female and may not be diagnosed until they fail to initiate puberty and exhibit high gonadotropins consistent with gonadal failure. Up to 30% of patients with 46,XY CGD may develop germ cell tumors, so their streak gonads should be removed in infancy.

D. **46,XX testicular DSD.** These individuals usually appear phenotypically male, but 20% have abnormal genital development. At puberty, they produce insufficient testosterone and resemble patients with Klinefelter syndrome (small testes, azoospermia, eunuchoid body habitus, gynecomastia). Cryptic mosaicism with a Y chromosome-bearing cell line or translocation of *SRY* to the X chromosome may be responsible. In *SRY*-negative individuals, duplication of *SOX9* (17q24) may be detected by FISH.

VIII. ISSUES OF SEX ASSIGNMENT. In the past, a primary criterion for male sex assignment was penile size adequate for sexual function. 46,XY infants born with little or no penile tissue have traditionally been given female sex assignment and surgically and hormonally feminized by means of genitoplasty early in life and estrogen treatment at the age of puberty. This practice remains under debate. Sex assignment is complicated by evidence that the prenatal hormonal environment may influence gender identity formation and gender role behavior. During the second trimester, the normal fetal testis produces levels of testosterone comparable to those of an adult male. A 46,XY neonate born with minimal penile tissue, who is not androgen resistant and who has been exposed to normal intrauterine testosterone concentrations, may retain a male-gender identity regardless of sex assignment. Fueling the debate are new techniques, such as intracytoplasmic sperm injection (ICSI), which make fertilization possible without penetration or ejaculation.

Likewise, under debate is the issue of sex assignment in the most severely virilized 46,XX newborns with CAH, who have completely fused with labioscrotal folds and a penile urethra. A minority opinion recommends male sex assignment and gonadectomy, thereby eliminating the need for feminizing genitoplasty. Nevertheless, many geneticists and endocrinologists continue to recommend female sex assignment to preserve fertility.

Whether and when to perform genital surgery, particularly clitoral reduction in virilized females, is also the subject of controversy. Whereas some adults with DSD view their genital surgery as mutilation, most parents prefer surgery so that their child's genitalia appear more consistent with the assigned sex. One-stage surgical procedures that preserve the neurovascular bundle can be done in infancy and are much improved compared with the clitorectomies routinely performed several decades ago.

Parents require a thorough explanation of their child's condition as the laboratory and imaging data become available. They should participate with the interdisciplinary team in decision making during assessment of the options for medical and surgical therapy and of the prospects for genital appearance, gender identity, sexual functioning, and fertility. The full medical team should include a pediatrician/neonatologist, pediatric endocrinologist, pediatric surgeon and/or pediatric urologist, geneticist, and a counselor experienced in dealing with DSD. Finally, long term, unbiased studies of gender identity and sexual functioning in individuals born with various forms of DSD are needed to provide insight into the difficult task of sex assignment for these infants.

Suggested Readings

Achermann JC, Hughes IA. Disorders of sex development. In: Kronenberg HM, Melmed M, Polonsky KS, et al., eds. *Williams Textbook of Endocrinology*. 11th ed. Philadelphia: Saunders; 2008.

American Academy of Pediatrics. Evaluation of the newborn with developmental anomalies of the external genitalia. *Pediatrics* 2000;106(1 pt 1):138–142.

Anhalt H, Neely EK, Hintz RL. Ambiguous genitalia. *Pediatr Rev* 1996;17(6):213–220.

Hughes IA, Houk C, Ahmed SF, et al. Consensus statement on management of intersex disorders. *Arch Dis Child* 2006; 91:554–563.

White PC, Speiser PW. Congenital adrenal hyperplasia due to 21-hydroxylase deficiency. *Endocr Rev*. 2000;21(3):245–291.

62 Surgical Emergencies in the Newborn

Steven A. Ringer and Anne R. Hansen

I. POTENTIAL SURGICAL CONDITIONS PRESENTING IN THE FETUS

A. **Polyhydramnios** (amniotic fluid volume >2L) occurs in 1 in 1,000 births.

1. Gastrointestinal (GI) obstruction (including esophageal atresia [EA]) is the most frequent surgical cause of polyhydramnios.

2. Other causes of polyhydramnios include abdominal wall defects (omphalocele and gastroschisis), anencephaly, diaphragmatic hernia (DH), maternal diabetes with consequent fetal hyperglycemia and glucosuria and other conditions impairing the fetus' ability to concentrate urine, tight nuchal cord and other causes of impaired fetal swallowing, and fetal death.

3. All women with suspected polyhydramnios should have an ultrasonographic examination. In experienced hands, this is the study of choice for the diagnosis of intestinal obstruction, abdominal wall defects, DH, as well as abnormalities leading to an inability of the fetus to swallow.

4. If intestinal obstruction is diagnosed antenatally and there is no concern for dystocia, vaginal delivery is acceptable. Pediatric surgical consultation should be obtained before delivery.

B. **Oligohydramnios** is associated with amniotic fluid leak, intrauterine growth restriction, postmaturity, fetal distress, renal dysgenesis or agenesis (Potter syndrome; see Chap. 28). If the duration of oligohydramnios is prolonged, it is important to anticipate respiratory compromise in these infants, as adequate amniotic fluid volume is generally necessary for normal pulmonary development, particularly during the second trimester of gestation. Severity of pulmonary hypoplasia correlates with degree and duration of oligohydramnios.

C. **Meconium peritonitis** can be diagnosed prenatally by ultrasonography, typically seen as areas of calcification scattered throughout the abdomen. Postnatally, calcifications are confirmed by plain film of the abdomen. It is usually due to antenatal perforation of the intestinal tract. Therefore, it is most commonly seen in association with a congenital lesion causing intestinal obstruction, either anatomic or functional (see IV.A.).

D. **Fetal ascites** is usually associated with urinary tract anomalies (e.g., lower urinary tract obstruction due to posterior urethral valves). Other causes include hemolytic disease of the newborn, any severe anemia (e.g., α-thalassemia), peritonitis, thoracic duct obstruction, cardiac disease, hepatic or portal vein obstruction, hepatitis, and congenital infection (e.g., TORCH infections; see Chaps. 48–53), as well as other causes of hydrops fetalis (see Chap. 26). After birth, ascites may be seen in congenital nephrotic syndrome. Accurate prenatal ultrasonography is important in light of the potential for fetal surgery to minimize renal parenchymal injury by decompressing either the bladder or a hydronephrotic kidney (see Chaps. 1 and 28).

E. Dystocia may result from fetal hydrocephalus, intestinal obstruction, abdominal wall defect, genitourinary anomalies, or fetal ascites (see I.D.).

F. Fetal surgery. The potential for surgical intervention during fetal life continues to develop. It depends heavily on the availability of precise prenatal diagnostic techniques and experience in accurately characterizing disorders, including the use of ultrasonography and fast magnetic resonance imaging (MRI).

Advances in obstetric and anesthesia management have also contributed to the feasibility of performing *in utero* procedures. The mother must be carefully managed through what is often a long and unpredictable anesthesia course. Medications that reduce uterine irritability have been developed that maximally ensure that the uterus can be maintained without contractions during and after the procedure. The criteria for consideration of a procedure include the following:

1. **Ethical considerations** are important, including balancing both the potential risk and benefit to the fetus with the potential pain or harm to the mother, as well as the impact on the family as a whole.

2. **Technical feasibility**

3. **Severity of fetal condition.** Initially, most cases dealt with conditions that were life threatening either because they caused death *in utero* or the inability to survive postnatal life if born unrepaired. Currently, cases are considered when a condition is not life threatening but is severe, and either the condition itself is progressive (such as the growth of a large tumor partially obstructing the fetal airway), or the consequences of the condition worsen progressively (such as worsening hydrops due to a large teratoma).

4. **Necessary resources.** The care of the mother, fetus, and potential baby during surgery in the immediate postoperative period, and after birth must all be available in seamless proximity to the institution where the surgery is performed.

   Fetal surgery has been successfully used for removal of an enlarging chest mass, such as an adenomatoid malformation of the lung or a bronchopulmonary sequestration. Other mass lesions, such as sacrococcygeal teratoma, when diagnosed *in utero*, have been treated with excision or by fetoscopically guided laser ablation of the feeder vessels, resulting in involution. Progressive fetal urethral obstruction has been ameliorated by the use of shunts or fulgaration of posterior urethral valves. Similar fetoscopic laser ablation of connecting vessels has been used successfully in the treatment of twin–twin transfusion syndrome or twin reversed arterial perfusion (TRAP). Fetal surgical correction of meningomyelocele is a rapidly evolving area of endeavor (see Chap. 57).

   Successful fetal procedures that we are currently performing include ***ex utero* intrapartum treatment** (EXIT) procedures for complex airway obstructions and complex congenital DH, aortic valve dilation for critical aortic stenosis, atrial septostomy, or stent placement for intact atrial septum with hypoplastic left heart syndrome, vascular photocoagulation for twin–twin transfusion syndrome or TRAP syndrome, and percutaneous bladder shunt for bladder outlet obstruction. Indications for fetal intervention continue to evolve and change.

II. POSTNATAL SURGICAL DISORDERS: DIAGNOSIS BY PRESENTING SYMPTOM

A. **Respiratory distress** (see III.B. and C.; Chaps. 29–39). Although most etiologies of respiratory distress are treated medically, some respiratory disorders do require surgical therapies.

  1. Choanal atresia (see III.C.1.).
  2. Laryngotracheal clefts (see III.C.3.).
  3. Tracheal agenesis
  4. EA with or without tracheoesophageal fistula (TEF) (see III.A.)
  5. Congenital lobar emphysema
  6. Cystic adenomatoid malformation of the lung, pulmonary sequestration
  7. DH (see III.B.)
  8. Biliary tracheobronchial communication (extremely rare)

B. **Scaphoid abdomen**

  1. DH (see III.B.)
  2. EA without TEF (see III.A.)

C. **Excessive mucus and salivation.** EA with or without TEF (see III.A.).

D. **Abdominal distention** can be due to pneumoperitoneum or intestinal obstruction (mechanical or functional).

  1. **Pneumoperitoneum.** Any perforation of the bowel may cause pneumoperitoneum (see Chap. 27).

     a. Any portion of the GI tract can potentially perforate for a variety of reasons, including poor bowel wall integrity (e.g., necrotizing enterocolitis or localized ischemia of the stomach or small bowel associated with some medications such as indomethacin) and excessive pressure (e.g., obstruction, TEF, or instrumentation [i.e., with a nasogastric tube]). Perforated stomach is associated with large amounts of free intra-abdominal air. Active GI air leak requires urgent surgical closure. It may be necessary to aspirate air from the abdominal cavity to relieve respiratory distress before definitive surgical repair.

     b. Air from a pulmonary air leak may dissect into the peritoneal cavity of infants receiving mechanical ventilation. Treatment of pneumoperitoneum transmitted from pulmonary air leak should focus on managing the pulmonary air leak.

  2. **Intestinal obstruction**

     a. EA with TEF (see III.A.) can present as abdominal distension. Obstruction of proximal bowel (e.g., complete duodenal atresia) causes rapid distension of the left upper quadrant. Obstruction of distal bowel causes more generalized distention, varying with location of obstruction.

     b. The normal progression of the air column seen on an x-ray film of the abdomen is as follows: 1 hour after birth, the air is past the stomach into the upper jejunum; 3 hours after birth, it is at the cecum; 8 to 12 hours after birth, it is at the rectosigmoid. This progression is slower in the premature infant.

E. **Vomiting.** The causes of vomiting can be differentiated by the presence or absence of bile.

1. **Bilious emesis.** The presence of bile-stained vomit in the newborn should be treated as a life-threatening emergency, with at least 20% of such infants requiring emergency surgical intervention after evaluation. Surgical consultation should be obtained immediately. Unless the infant is clinically unstable, a contrast study of the upper gastrointestinal tract should be obtained as quickly as possible.

   Intestinal obstruction may result from malrotation with or without midgut volvulus; duodenal, jejunal, ileal, or colonic atresias; annular pancreas; Hirschsprung disease; aberrant superior mesenteric artery; preduodenal portal vein; peritoneal bands; persistent omphalomesenteric duct; or duodenal duplication.

   Bile-stained emesis is occasionally seen in infants without intestinal obstruction who have decreased motility (see II.E.2.c.). In these cases, the bile-stained vomiting will only occur one or two times and will present without abdominal distention. However, a nonsurgical condition is a diagnosis of exclusion: bilious emesis is malrotation until proven otherwise.

2. **Nonbilious emesis**
   a. Feeding excessive volume
   b. Milk (human or formula) intolerance
   c. Decreased motility
      i. Prematurity
      ii. Antenatal exposure to $MgSO_4$ or antenatal, prenatal, or postnatal exposure to narcotics
      iii. Sepsis with ileus
      iv. Central nervous system (CNS) lesion
   d. Lesion above ampulla of Vater
      i. Pyloric stenosis
      ii. Upper duodenal stenosis
      iii. Annular pancreas (rare)

F. **Failure to pass meconium** can occur in sick and/or premature babies with decreased bowel motility. It also may be the result of the following disorders:

   1. Imperforate anus

   2. Microcolon

   3. Mucous plug

   4. Other causes of intestinal obstruction

G. **Failure to develop transitional stools** after the passage of meconium

   1. Volvulus, other intestinal destruction

   2. Malrotation

H. **Hematemesis and hematochezia**

   1. **Nonsurgical conditions.** Many patients with hematemesis and most patients with **hematochezia** (bloody stools) have a nonsurgical condition. Differential diagnosis includes the following:
      a. Milk intolerance/allergy (usually cow's milk protein allergy)
      b. Instrumentation (e.g., nasogastric tube, endotracheal tube)
      c. Swallowed maternal blood
         i. Maternal blood is sometimes swallowed by the newborn during labor and delivery. This can be diagnosed by an Apt test performed on blood aspirated from the infant's stomach (see XI.G. and Chap. 43).

    ii. In breastfed infants, either microscopic or macroscopic blood noted several days after birth in either emesis or stool may be due to swallowed blood during breastfeeding in setting of cracked maternal nipples. Inspecting the mother's breasts or expressed milk is usually diagnostic. If not, aspirate the contents of the baby's stomach after a feeding and send the recently swallowed milk for an Apt test.

    d. Coagulation disorders, including disseminated intravascular coagulation (DIC), lack of postnatal vitamin K injection (see Chap. 43).

2. Surgical conditions resulting in hematemesis and bloody stool.

    a. Necrotizing enterocolitis (most frequent cause of hematemesis and bloody stool in premature infants; see Chap. 27)

    b. Gastric or duodenal ulcers (due to stress, steroid therapy)

    c. GI obstruction: late sign, concerning for threatened or necrotic bowel

    d. Volvulus

    e. Intussusception

    f. Polyps, hemangiomas

    g. Meckel diverticulum

    h. Duplications of the small intestine

    i. Cirsoid aneurysm

I. Abdominal masses (see VIII.)

    1. Genitourinary anomalies, including distended bladder (see VII. and Chap. 28)

    2. Hepatosplenomegaly: may be confused with other masses; requires medical evaluation

    3. Tumors (see VII.)

J. Birth trauma (see Chap. 6)

    1. Fractured clavicle/humerus (see Chap. 58)

    2. Intracranial hemorrhage (see Chap. 54)

    3. Lacerated solid organs—liver, spleen

    4. Spinal cord transection with quadriplegia

III. LESIONS CAUSING RESPIRATORY DISTRESS

A. EA and TEF. At least 85% of infants with EA also have TEF. Pure EA and TEF with proximal TEF may be suspected on prenatal ultrasonography by the absence of a stomach bubble.

    1. Postnatal presentation depends on the presence or absence as well as on the location of a TEF.

    a. Infants often present with excessive salivation and vomiting soon after feedings. They may develop respiratory distress due to the following:

        i. Airway obstruction by excess secretions

        ii. Aspiration of saliva and milk

        iii. Compromised pulmonary capacity due to diaphragmatic elevation secondary to abdominal distension

        iv. Reflux of gastric contents up the distal esophagus into the lungs through the fistula

b. If there is no fistula, or if it connects the trachea to the esophagus proximal to the atresia, no GI gas will be seen on x-ray examination, and the abdomen will be scaphoid.

c. TEF without EA (H-type fistula) is extremely rare and usually presents after the neonatal period. The diagnosis is suggested by a history of frequent pneumonias or respiratory distress temporally related to meals.

2. **Diagnosis**

   a. **EA** itself is diagnosed by the inability to pass a catheter into the stomach. The catheter is inserted into the esophagus until resistance is met. Air is then injected into the catheter while listening (for lack of air) over the stomach. The diagnosis is confirmed by x-ray studies showing the catheter coiled in the upper esophageal pouch. Plain x-ray films may demonstrate a distended blind upper esophageal pouch filled with air that is unable to progress into the stomach. (The plain films may also show associated cardiac or vertebral anomalies of the cervical or upper thoracic region of the spine.) Pushing 50 mL of air into the catheter under fluoroscopic examination may show dilatation and relaxation of the upper pouch, thereby avoiding the need for contrast studies.

   b. **H-type fistula.** This disorder can often be demonstrated with administration of nonionic water-soluble contrast medium (Omnipaque) during cinefluoroscopy. The definitive examination is combined fiberoptic bronchoscopy and esophagoscopy with passage of a fine balloon catheter from the trachea into the esophagus. The H-type fistula is usually high in the trachea (cervical area).

3. **Associated issues and anomalies.** Babies with TEF and EA are often of low birth weight. Approximately 20% of these babies are premature (five times the normal incidence), and another 20% are small for gestational age (eight times the normal incidence). Other anomalies may be present, including chromosomal abnormalities and the VACTERL association (**V**ertebral defects, imperforate **A**nus, **C**ardiac defects, **T**EF with **E**A, **R**enal dysplasia or defects, and **L**imb anomalies).

4. **Management.** Preoperative management focuses on minimizing the risk of aspiration and avoiding gaseous distension of the GI tract with positive pressure crossing from the trachea into the esophagus.

   a. A multiple end-hole suction catheter (Replogle) should be placed in the proximal pouch and put to continuous suction immediately after the diagnosis is made.

   b. The head of the bed should be elevated 30 degrees to diminish reflux of gastric contents into the fistula and aspiration of oral secretions that may accumulate in the proximal esophageal pouch.

   c. If possible, mechanical ventilation of these babies should be avoided until the fistula is controlled because the positive pressure may cause severe abdominal distension compromising respiratory function. If intubation is required, the case should be considered an emergency. Guidelines for intubation are the same as for other types of respiratory distress (see Chap. 66). The endotracheal tube should be advanced to just above the carina in the hopes of obstructing airflow through the fistula. Most commonly, the fistula connects to the trachea near the carina. Care must be taken to avoid accidental intubation of the fistula. Optimally, if mechanical ventilation is required, it should be done using a relatively high rate and low pressure to minimize GI distension. Heavy sedation should be avoided because it compromises patient's spontaneous respiratory effort, which generates negative intrathoracic pressure, minimizing passage of air through the fistula into the esophagus.

d. Surgical therapy usually involves immediate placement of a gastrostomy tube. As soon as the infant can tolerate further surgery, the fistula is divided; and, if possible, the proximal and distal ends of the esophagus are anastamosed primarily.

e. Many infants with EA are premature or have other defects that make it advisable to delay primary repair. Mechanical ventilation and nutritional management may be difficult in these infants because of the TEF. These babies need careful nursing care to prevent aspiration and gastrostomy with G-tube feedings to allow growth until repair is possible. In some cases, the fistula can be divided, with deferral of definitive repair.

f. If the infant has cardiac disease that requires surgery, it is usually best to repair the fistula first. If not, the postoperative ventilatory management can be very difficult.

g. Patients with long-gap EA can be extremely challenging to manage. We have developed a referral center for such patients who are treated with innovative esophageal growth induction techniques that can allow for primary repairs, thereby avoiding the need for gastric, colonic, or jejunal interposition.

B. Diaphragmatic Hernia

1. **Anatomy.** The most common site is the left hemithorax, with the defect in the diaphragm being posterior (foramen of Bochdalek) in 70% of infants. It can also occur on the right, with either an anterior or a posterior defect. **Bilateral DH is extremely rare.**

2. **Incidence** occurs in approximately 1 in 4,000 live births. Fifty percent of these hernias are associated with other malformations, especially cardiac, neural tube, intestinal, skeletal, and renal defects. DH has been associated with trisomies 13 and 18, and 45,XO, and has been reported as part of Goldenhar, Beckwith-Wiedemann, Pierre Robin, Wolf-Hirschhorn (4 p deletion), Pallister-Killian (tetrasomy 12p), Fryns, Goltz-Gorlin, and congenital Rubella syndromes. In some cases, DH is familial.

3. **Symptoms.** Infants with large DHs usually present at birth with cyanosis, respiratory distress, a scaphoid abdomen, decreased or absent breath sounds on the side of the hernia, and heart sounds displaced to the side opposite the hernia. Small hernias, right-sided hernias, sac-type hernias, and substernal hernias of Morgagni may have a more subtle presentation, manifested as feeding problems and mild respiratory distress. Associated structural malformations include congenital heart disease (CHD), neural tube defects, skeletal anomalies, intestinal atresias, and renal anomalies.

4. **Diagnosis**

   a. Prenatal Diagnosis. DHs often occur after the routine 16-week prenatal ultrasonography; therefore, many of these cases are not diagnosed until postnatally. The development of polyhydramnios can prompt a later fetal ultrasonography that will detect DH. Diagnosis earlier in gestation may correlate with a poorer prognosis due to severity of condition. The prognostic advantage of prenatal diagnosis is that it generally leads to delivery in a center, equipped to optimize chances for survival. If delivery before term is likely, fetal lung maturity should be assessed to evaluate the need for maternal betamethasone therapy (see Chap. 33). Presence of liver in the thorax correlates with increased severity and poorer prognosis. Lung-to-head ratio (LHR) can be measured prenatally, and in skilled hands, can help predict severity of involvement and help guide initial therapy. In our institution, there are no reported survivors with an LHR <1. An LHR >1.4 has a 100% survival rate and a LHR between 1 and 1.4, has a 38% survival rate with a high need for extracorporeal membrane oxygenation (ECMO). Early work suggests that relative lung volumes, as measured by MRI, may have an important role in predicting the risk of morbidity and mortality. The lower the percent predicted lung volume (PPLV), the higher the risk.

b. Postnatal Diagnosis. The diagnosis is made or confirmed by radiograph. Because of the possibility of marked cardiothymic shift, a radiopaque marker should be placed on one side of the chest to aid interpretation of the x-ray film.

c. Differential diagnosis. Diaphragmatic eventration, congenital cystic adenomatoid malformation, pulmonary sequestration, and bronchogenic cyst.

5. Treatment

a. Severe cases that have been diagnosed before birth may be best managed with delivery by the EXIT procedure, with immediate institution of ECMO (see Chap. 39). This requires a multidisciplinary team consisting of obstetricians, specialized anesthesiologists, surgeons, neonatologists, nurses, respiratory therapists, and ECMO technicians to be assembled at a specialized center. Deep general anesthesia is established in the mother, ensuring fetal anesthesia. Maternal laparotomy is performed, with exposure of the uterus, which should be extremely hypotonic because of the anesthesia. Bleeding is minimized by using a special device to open the uterus that simultaneously cuts a full-thickness uterine incision and places hemostatic clips along the incision.

The fetus is then partially delivered through the uterine opening. A pulse oximeter probe is placed on the fetal hand to permit direct monitoring of heart rate and oxygen saturation, with the oxygen saturation maintained at fetal levels of approximately 60%. If the saturation gets too high, the umbilical vessels will constrict and the umbilical blood supply will diminish. Monitoring may be augmented by palpation of the umbilical pulse.

The fetus is then intubated and assessed. A decision is then made whether delivery should be completed at that point, and further care continued as detailed in (see III.B.5.b. and c.). If the fetal condition does not improve upon intubation or if the DH is known to be severe, the EXIT procedure may be used as a bridge to immediate initiation of ECMO. Once the fetus is partially delivered, the surgeons can expose the major vessels of the neck and insert the ECMO catheters. Portable ECMO equipment brought to the operating room is then used during transport to the intensive care unit or during subsequent surgery on the delivered newborn.

b. Intubation. All infants should be intubated immediately after delivery if the diagnosis has been made antenatally or at the time of postnatal diagnosis. Bag-and-mask ventilation is contraindicated. Immediately after intubation, a large sump nasogastric tube should be inserted and attached to **continuous** suction. Care must be taken with assisted ventilation to keep inspiratory pressures low to avoid damage or rupture of the contralateral lung. Peripheral venous and arterial lines are preferable, as umbilical lines may need to be removed during surgery However, if umbilical lines are the only practical access, these should be placed initially. Heavy sedation should be avoided as spontaneous respiratory effort enables the use of the pressure support mode of ventilation, which we have found to induce the least barotrauma.

c. Preoperative management is focused on avoiding barotrauma and minimizing pulmonary hypertension. That said, permissive hypercapnia is the preferred respiratory approach, although the mode of ventilation remains controversial, including the role for high-frequency ventilation. Avoidance of hypoxia and acidosis will aid in minimizing pulmonary hypertension. Inhaled nitric oxide has not been shown to reduce the need for ECMO, but its role in reducing right heart strain may be beneficial. The role of exogenous surfactant remains controversial.

6. **Surgical repair** is through either the abdomen or the chest, with reduction of intestine into the abdominal cavity.

7. **Mortality and prognosis**
   a. Mortality from DHs is largely related to associated defects, especially pulmonary hypoplasia and CHD. Our local survival is now >90% for infants without associated CHD. Repair of the defect itself is relatively straightforward; the underlying pulmonary hypoplasia and pulmonary hypertension are largely responsible for overall mortality (see Chap. 36).
   b. Prognosis. Factors associated with better prognosis are herniation of bowel into chest after 2nd trimester, absence of liver herniation, and absence of co-existing anomalies, especially cardiac. Early oxygen (PO_2) and carbon dioxide tension (PCO_2) are predictive of prognosis. In addition, the later the onset of postnatal symptoms, the higher the survival rate.

C. **Other mechanical causes for respiratory distress**

1. **Choanal atresia.** Bilateral atresia presents in the delivery room as respiratory distress that resolves with crying. Infants are obligate nasal breathers until approximately 4 months of age. An oral airway is effective initial treatment. Definitive therapy includes opening a hole through the bony plate, which can be accomplished with a laser in some settings.

2. **Robin anomaly** (Pierre Robin syndrome) consists of a hypoplastic mandible associated with a secondary, U-shaped midline cleft palate. Often, the tongue occludes the airway causing obstruction. Prone positioning or forcibly pulling the tongue forward will relieve the obstruction. These infants often improve after placement of a nasopharyngeal or endotracheal tube. If the infant can be supported for a few days, he or she will sometimes adapt, and aggressive procedures can be avoided. In some cases, a lip tongue adhesion or mandibular distraction can avoid the need for tracheostomy or enable earlier decannulation. A specialized feeder (Breck) facilitates PO feeding the infant, but sometimes, a gastrostomy is necessary. Severely affected babies will require tracheostomy and gastrostomy.

3. **Laryngotracheal clefts.** The length of the cleft determines the symptoms. The diagnosis is made by instillation of contrast material into the esophagus and is confirmed by bronchoscopy. Very ill newborns should undergo immediate bronchoscopy without contrast studies.

4. **Laryngeal web occluding the larynx.** Perforation of the web by a stiff endotracheal tube or bronchoscopy instrument may be lifesaving.

5. **Tracheal agenesis.** This rare lesion is suspected when a tube cannot be passed down the trachea. The infant ventilates by way of bronchi coming off the esophagus.

Diagnosis is by use of contrast material in the esophagus and by endoscopy. Prognosis is poor as tracheal reconstruction is difficult.

6. **Congenital lobar emphysema** may be due to a malformation, a cyst in the bronchus, or a mucous or meconium plug in the bronchus. These lesions cause air trapping, compression of surrounding structures, and respiratory distress. There may be a primary malformation of the lobe (polyalveolar lobe). Overdistension from mechanical ventilation may cause lobar emphysema. Extrinsic pressure on a bronchus can also cause obstruction. Lower lobes are generally relatively spared. Diagnosis is by chest x-ray.

   a. **High-frequency ventilation** may enable the lobar emphysema to recover (see Chap. 29).

   b. **Selective intubation.** After consultation with a surgeon, selective intubation of the opposite bronchus may be attempted in an effort to decompress the emphysematous lobe if overinflation is thought to be the cause. It should generally be viewed as a temporizing therapy and should not be employed for more than a few hours. Many infants will not tolerate this procedure due to both overdistension of the ventilated lung and profound V:Q mismatch; therefore, it must be carefully considered and monitored. Rarely, selective intubation is successful and the lobar emphysema does not recur. Much more commonly, even if the selective intubation is initially helpful, the baby goes on to develop recurrence and progression of the emphysema and further respiratory compromise. Occasionally, selective suctioning of the bronchus on the side of the emphysema may remove obstructing mucus or meconium.

   c. **Bronchoscopy, resection.** If the baby is symptomatic and conservative measures fail, bronchoscopy should be performed to remove any obstructing material or rupture a bronchogenic cyst. If this procedure fails, surgical resection of the involved lobe should be considered.

7. **Cystic adenomatoid malformation and pulmonary sequestration** may be confused with a DH. Respiratory distress is related to the effect of the mass on the uninvolved lung. This malformation can cause shifting of the mediastinal structures.

8. **Vascular rings.** The symptomatology of vascular rings is related to the anatomy of the ring. Both respiratory (stridor) and GI (vomiting, difficulty swallowing) symptoms may occur. Barium swallow radiography may be diagnostic. Computed tomography (CT) or MRI can be useful to more clearly delineate the anatomy, especially in the setting of double aortic arch. An echocardiogram may be necessary to rule out intracardiac anomalies. Bronchoscopy can be helpful if tracheal stenosis is suspected.

IV. LESIONS CAUSING INTESTINAL OBSTRUCTION.
The most critical lesion to rule out is malrotation with midgut volvulus. All patients with suspected intestinal obstruction should have a nasogastric sump catheter placed to continuous suction without delay. Any baby with a GI obstruction is at increased risk for exacerbated hyperbilirubinemia due to increased enterohepatic circulation.

A. **Congenital mechanical obstruction**

   1. Intrinsic types include atresia, stenosis, hypertrophic pyloric stenosis, cysts within the lumen of the bowel, and imperforate anus.

2. Extrinsic forms of congenital mechanical obstruction include congenital peritoneal bands with or without malrotation, annular pancreas, duplications of the intestine, aberrant vessels (usually the mesenteric artery or preduodenal portal vein), hydrometrocolpos, and obstructing bands (persistent omphalomesenteric duct).

B. Acquired mechanical obstruction

1. Malrotation with volvulus

2. Intussusception; unusual in neonatal period

3. Peritoneal adhesions
  a. After meconium peritonitis
  b. After abdominal surgery
  c. Idiopathic

4. Mesenteric thrombosis

5. Strictures secondary to necrotizing enterocolitis

6. Incarcerated inguinal hernia (relatively common in premature infants)

7. Formation of abnormal intestinal concretions not associated with CF

C. Functional intestinal obstruction constitutes the major cause of intestinal obstruction seen in the neonatal unit.

1. Immature bowel motility

2. Defective innervation (Hirschsprung disease) or other intrinsic defects in the bowel wall

3. Paralytic ileus
  a. Induced by medications
    i. Narcotics (prenatal or postnatal exposure)
    ii. Hypermagnesemia due to prenatal exposure to magnesium sulfate
  b. Septic ileus

4. Meconium ileus, meconium plug, and small left colon syndrome

5. Endocrine disorders (e.g., hypothyroidism)

D. The more **common etiologies** of GI obstruction warrant more detailed discussion.

1. Pyloric stenosis typically presents with nonbilious vomiting after the age of 2 to 3 weeks, but it has been reported in the first week of life. Radiographic examination will show a large stomach with little or no gas below the duodenum. Often, the pyloric mass, or "olive," cannot be felt in the newborn. The infant may have associated jaundice and hematemesis. Diagnosis can usually be confirmed by ultrasonography, which limits the need for an upper GI series and the consequent radiation exposure.

2. Duodenal atresia. 70% of cases have other associated malformations, including Down syndrome, cardiovascular (CVR) anomalies, and such GI anomalies as annular pancreas, EA, malrotation of the small intestine, small-bowel atresias, and imperforate anus.
  a. There may be a history of polyhydramnios.
  b. It is commonly diagnosed prenatally by ultrasonography.
  c. Vomiting of bile-stained material usually begins a few hours after birth.
  d. Abdominal distention is limited to the upper abdomen.

e. The infant may pass meconium in the first 24 hours of life; then bowel movements cease.

f. The diagnosis is suggested if aspiration of the stomach yields >30 mL of gastric contents before feeding.

g. A plain radiograph of the abdomen will show air in the stomach and upper part of the abdomen ("double bubble") with no air in the small or large bowel. Contrast radiographs of the upper intestine are not mandatory.

h. Preoperative management includes decompression with nasogastric suction.

3. Jejunal and ileal atresias. Most are the result of intrauterine vascular accidents, but as many as 15% to 30% are associated with CF; these patients should therefore be screened (see IV.D.4.c.).

4. Meconium ileus is a frequent cause of meconium peritonitis. Unlike most other etiologies of obstruction in which flat and upright x-ray films will demonstrate fluid levels, in cases of nonperforated meconium ileus, the distended bowel may be granular in appearance or may show tiny bubbles mixed with meconium.

a. No meconium will pass through the rectum, even after digital stimulation.

b. Ninety percent of babies with meconium ileus have CF. Blood sample or cheek brushing for DNA analysis can be used to screen for CF if newborn or antenatal screening has not been performed. If the results are negative or equivocal or if the baby weighs >2 kg and is older than 2 weeks ideally (but certainly older than 3 days), a sweat test should be performed. Sweat tests on babies who are younger or smaller risk both false-positive results due to the high NaCl content of the sweat of newborns and false-negative or uninterpretable results when an adequate volume of sweat cannot be obtained.

c. Rare cases (both familial and nonfamilial) of meconium ileus are not associated with CF.

d. Decompression with continuous nasogastric suction will minimize further distention. Contrast enemas can be both diagnostic and therapeutic. Meglumine diatrizoate (Gastrografin) or diatrizoate sodium (Hypaque) can be used in an adequately hydrated infant. Meglumine diatrizoate is often diluted 1:4 before use. Because these contrast agents are hypertonic, the baby should start the procedure well hydrated, and careful attention should be paid to fluid balance after the procedure. If the diagnosis is certain and the neonate is stable, repeat therapeutic enemas may be administered in an effort to relieve the impaction.

e. Surgical therapy is required if the contrast enema fails to relieve the obstruction.

f. Microcolon distal to the atresia will generally dilate spontaneously with use.

5. **Imperforate anus.** Fifty percent have anomalies, including those in the VACTERL association. Infants with imperforate anus may pass meconium if a rectovaginal or rectourinary fistula exists. A fistula is present in 80% to 90% of males and 95% of females. It may take 24 hours for the fistula to become evident. The presence or absence of a visible fistula at the perineum is the critical distinction in the diagnosis and management of imperforate anus.

a. Perineal fistula. Meconium may be visualized on the perineum. It may be found in the rugal folds or scrotum in boys and in the vagina in girls. This fistula may be dilated to allow passage of meconium to temporarily relieve intestinal obstruction. When the infant is beyond the newborn period, the imperforate anus can generally be primarily repaired.

b. No perineal fistula present. There may be a fistula that enters the urinary tract or, for girls, the vagina. The presence of meconium particles in the urine is diagnostic of a rectovesicular fistula. Vaginal examination with a nasal speculum or cystoscope may reveal a fistula. A cystogram may show a fistula and document the level of the distal rectum, which can also be defined by ultrasonography. A temporary colostomy may be necessary in neonates with an imperforate anus without a perineal fistula. Primary repair of these infants without a colostomy is now being performed at some institutions.

6. **Volvulus with or without malrotation of the bowel**

   a. Malrotation may be associated with other GI abnormalities such as DH, annular pancreas, and bowel atresias and is always seen with omphalocele.

   b. If this condition develops during fetal life, it may cause the appearance of a large midabdominal calcific shadow on x-ray examination; this results from calcification of meconium in the segment of necrotic bowel.

   c. After birth, there is a sudden onset of bilious vomiting in an infant who has passed some normal stools. Malrotation, as the cause of intestinal obstruction, is a surgical emergency because intestinal viability is at stake. **Bilious emesis equals malrotation until proved otherwise.**

   d. If the level of obstruction is high, there may not be much abdominal distension.

   e. Signs of shock and sepsis are often present.

   f. A radiograph of the abdomen will often show a dilated small bowel, although a normal radiograph does not rule out malrotation, which can be intermittent.

   g. If a malrotation is present, barium enema may show failure of barium to pass beyond the transverse colon or may show the cecum in an abnormal position.

   h. The test of choice is an upper GI series, specifically looking for an absent or abnormal position of the ligament of Treitz that confirms the diagnosis of malrotation.

7. **Annular pancreas** may be nonobstructing but associated with duodenal atresia or stenosis. It presents as a high intestinal obstruction.

8. **Hydrometrocolpos.** In this rare condition, a membrane across the vagina prevents fluid drainage and the consequent accumulation causes distension of the uterus and vagina.

   a. The hymen bulges.

   b. Accumulated secretions in the uterus may cause intestinal obstruction by bowel compression.

   c. This intestinal obstruction may, in turn, cause meconium peritonitis or hydronephrosis.

   d. Edema and cyanosis of the legs may be observed.

   e. If hydrometrocolpos is not diagnosed at birth, the secretions will decrease, the bulging will disappear, and the diagnosis will be delayed until puberty.

9. **Meconium and mucous plug syndrome** is seen in infants who are premature or sick (see II.F.), and those with functional immaturity of the bowel with a small left colon, as seen in infants of diabetic mothers or those with Hirschsprung disease (see IV.D.10.). CF should also be ruled out. Treatment may simply consist of a glycerin suppository, warm half-normal saline enemas (5 to 10 mL/kg), and rectal stimulation with a soft rubber catheter.

More typically, and if these maneuvers are unsuccessful, a contrast enema with a hyperosmolar contrast material may be both diagnostic and therapeutic. A normal stooling pattern should follow evacuation of a plug.

10. **Hirschsprung disease** should be suspected in any newborn who fails to pass meconium spontaneously by 24 to 48 hours after birth and who develops distension relieved by rectal stimulation. This is especially so if the infant is neither premature nor born to a diabetic mother. The diagnosis should be considered until future development shows sustained normal bowel function.

   a. When the diagnosis is suspected, every effort should be made to rule the condition in or out. If the diagnosis is considered but seems very unlikely, parents taking the newborn home must specifically understand the importance of immediately reporting any obstipation, diarrhea, poor feeding, distention, lethargy, or fever. Development of a toxic megacolon may be fatal.

   b. Contrast enema frequently does not show the characteristic transition zone in the newborn, but a follow-up radiograph 24 hours after the initial study may reveal retained contrast material.

   c. Rectal biopsy is obtained to confirm the diagnosis. If suspicion is relatively low, a suction biopsy is useful, as presence of ganglion cells in the submucosal zone rules out the diagnosis. If the index of suspicion is high or the suction biopsy is positive, formal full-thickness rectal biopsy is the definitive method for diagnosis. Absence of ganglion cells and hypertrophic nonmyelinated axons is diagnostic. Histochemical tests of biopsy specimens show an increase in acetylcholine.

   d. Obstipation can be relieved by gentle rectal irrigations with warm saline solution. If the patient has a barium enema, gentle rectal saline washes are helpful in removing trapped air and barium. Once the abdomen is decompressed, feedings may be offered.

   e. Babies require surgical intervention when the diagnosis is made. A primary pull-through procedure is usually possible for correction, avoiding the need for a colostomy. At many institutions, colostomy is the standard, and it is always indicated when there is enterocolitis or adequate decompression cannot be achieved. Definitive repair is postponed until the infant is of adequate size and stability.

   f. Even once the aganglionic segment is removed, the bowel that remains is not completely normal. These patients remain at risk for constipation, encopresis, and even life-threatening enterocolitis.

V. OTHER SURGICAL PROBLEMS

A. Appendicitis is extremely rare in newborns. Its presentation may be that of pneumoperitoneum. The appendix usually perforates before the diagnosis is made; therefore, the baby may present with intestinal obstruction, sepsis, or even DIC related to the intra-abdominal infection. Rule out Hirschsprung disease.

B. Omphalocele. The sac may be intact or ruptured. The diagnosis is often made by prenatal ultrasonography. Cesarean section may prevent rupture of the sac, but is not specifically indicated unless the defect is large (>5 cm) or contains liver.

1. **Intact sac.** Emergency treatment includes the following:

   a. Use latex-free products, including gloves.

   b. Provide continuous nasogastric sump suction

   c. It is preferable to encase intestinal contents in a bowel bag (e.g., Vi-Drape isolation bag) as it is the least abrasive. Otherwise, cover the sac with warm saline-soaked gauze, then wrap the sac on abdomen with Kling gauze and cover with plastic wrap to support the intestinal viscera on the abdominal wall, taking great caution to ensure no kinking of the mesenteric blood supply.

d. Do not attempt to reduce the sac because this can rupture it, interfere with venous return from the sac, or cause respiratory compromise.

e. Bowel viability may be compromised with a small abdominal wall defect and an obstructed segment of eviscerated intestine. In these circumstances, before transfer, the defect must be enlarged by incising the abdomen cephalad or caudad to relieve the strangulated viscera.

f. Keep the baby warm, including thoroughly wrapping in warm blankets to prevent heat loss.

g. Place a reliable intravenous line in an upper extremity.

h. Monitor temperature and pH.

i. Start broad-spectrum antibiotics (ampicillin and gentamicin).

j. Obtain a surgical consultation; definitive surgical therapy should be delayed until the baby is stabilized. In the presence of other more serious abnormalities (respiratory or cardiac), definitive care can be postponed as long as the sac remains intact.

2. **Ruptured sac.** As in the preceding text for intact sac except surgery is more emergent.

3. As up to 80% will have associated anomalies, physical examination should include a careful search for phenotypic features of chromosomal defects as well as CHD, genitourinary defects such as cloacal exstrophy, craniofacial, musculoskeletal, vertebral, or limb anomalies. The Beckwith-Wiedemann syndrome includes omphalocele, macroglossia, hemihypertrophy, and hypoglycemia.

C. Gastroschisis [15], by definition, contains no sac, and the intestine is eviscerated.

1. For uncomplicated gastroschisis, there is no advantage to a specific route of delivery, but a cesarean section is recommended for large lesions or those in which the liver is exposed. Preoperative management as per omphalocele with ruptured sac (see V.B.2.).

2. Obtain immediate surgical evaluation.

3. Eight percent to 16% of these infants will have other gastrointestinal anomalies, including volvulus, atresias, intestinal stenosis, or perforation.

4. Unlike omphalocele, gastroschisis is not commonly associated with anomalies unrelated to the GI tract.

VI. RENAL DISORDERS (see Chap. 28)

A. Genitourinary abnormalities. First void should be noted in all infants. Approximately 90% of babies void in the first 24 hours of life and 99% within the first 48 hours of life. Genitourinary abnormalities should be suspected in babies with abdominal distention, ascites, flank masses, persistently distended bladder, bacteriuria, pyuria, or poor growth. Male infants exhibiting these symptoms should be observed for the normal forceful voiding pattern.

1. Posterior urethral valves may cause obstruction.

2. Renal vein thrombosis should be considered in the setting of hematuria with a flank mass. It is more common among infants of diabetic mothers.

a. Renal ultrasonography will initially show a large kidney on the side of the thrombosis. Kidney will return to normal size over ensuing weeks to months.

b. Doppler ultrasonography will show diminished or absent blood flow to involved kidney.

c. Current treatment in most centers starts with medical support in the hope of avoiding surgery. Heparin is generally not indicated, but its use has been advocated by some (see Chaps. 28 and 44).

3. **Exstrophy of the bladder.** Ranges from an epispadias to complete extrusion of the bladder onto the abdominal wall. Most centers attempt bladder turn-in within the first 48 hours of life.

a. Preoperative management

    i. Use moist, fine-mesh gauze or petroleum jelly-impregnated gauze to cover the exposed bladder.

    ii. Transport the infant to a facility for definitive care as soon as possible.

    iii. Obtain renal ultrasonography.

b. Intraoperative management. Surgical management of an extrophied bladder includes turn-in of the bladder to preserve bladder function. The symphysis pubis is approximated. The penis is lengthened. Iliac osteotomies are not necessary if repair is accomplished within 48 hours. No attempt is made to make the bladder continent at this initial procedure.

4. **Cloacal exstrophy** is a complex GI and genitourinary anomaly that includes vesicointestinal fissure, omphalocele, extrophied bladder, hypoplastic colon, imperforate anus, absence of vagina in women, and microphallus in men.

a. Preoperative management

    i. Gender assignment. It is surgically easier to create a phenotypic female, regardless of genotype. Understanding of the long-term psychological effects of this practice has made this decision extremely controversial, and no one approach is correct for all patients. Endocrine consultation is critical when deciding phenotypic gender assignment (see Chap. 61), and decisions should be made only after a collaborative discussion, including the parents, urologist, surgeon, endocrinologist, neonatologist, and appropriate counselors.

    ii. Nasogastric suction relieves partial intestinal obstruction. The baby excretes stool through a vesicointestinal fissure that is often partially obstructed.

    iii. A series of complex operations is required in stages to achieve the most satisfactory results.

b. Surgical management

    i. The focus is first on separating the gastrointestinal from the genitourinary tract. The hemibladders are sewn together and closed. A colostomy is created and the omphalocele is closed.

    ii. Later stages focus on bladder reconstruction, often requiring augmentation using intestine or stomach.

    iii. Subsequent procedures are designed to reduce the number of stomas and create genitalia, although this remains controversial.

VII. TUMORS

A. Teratomas are the most common tumor in the neonatal period. Although they are most commonly found in the sacrococcygeal area, they can arise anywhere, including the retroperitoneal area or the ovaries. Approximately 10% contain malignant elements. Prenatal diagnosis is often made by ultrasonography. Dystocia and airway compromise should be considered prenatally. Masses compromising the airway have been successfully managed by the EXIT procedure (see III.B.5.a.), with establishment of an airway before complete delivery of the baby.

After delivery, evaluation may include rectal examination, ultrasonography, CT, MRI, as well as serum α-fetoprotein, and β-human chorionic gonadotropin measurements are used in evaluation. Calcifications are often seen on x-ray films. Excessive heat loss and platelet trapping are possible complications.

B. **Neuroblastoma** is the most common malignant neonatal tumor, accounting for approximately 50%. It is irregular, stony hard, and ranges in size from minute to massive. There are many sites of origin; the adrenal–retroperitoneal area is the most common. On rare occasions, this tumor can cause hypertension or diarrhea by the release of tumor by-products, especially catecholamines or vasointestinal peptides. Serum levels of catecholamines and their metabolites should be measured. Calcifications can often be seen on plain radiographs. Ultrasonography is the most useful diagnostic test. Prenatal diagnosis by ultrasonography is associated with improved prognosis. Of note, many neuroblastomas diagnosed prenatally resolve spontaneously before birth.

C. **Wilms tumor** is the second most common malignant tumor in the newborn. It presents as a smooth flat mass and may be bilateral. One should palpate gently to avoid rupture. Ultrasonography is the most useful diagnostic test.

D. **Sarcoma botryoides.** This grape-like tumor arises from the edge of the vulva or vagina. It may be small and therefore be confused with a normal posterior vaginal tag. Intravenous pyelogram (IVP) is an important test preoperatively, especially to avoid confusing the lesion with an obstructing ureterocele.

E. **Other** tumors include hemangiomas, lymphangiomas, hepatoblastomas, hepatomas, hamartomas, and nephromas.

VIII. ABDOMINAL MASSES

A. **Renal** masses (see VI. and Chap. 28) are the most common etiology: polycystic kidneys, multicystic dysplastic kidney, hydronephrosis, and renal vein thrombosis.

B. **Other** causes of abdominal masses include tumors (see VII.), adrenal hemorrhage, ovarian tumor or cysts, pancreatic cyst, choledochal cyst, hydrometrocolpos, mesenteric or omental cyst, and intestinal duplications, hepatosplenomegaly.

IX. INGUINAL HERNIA

is found in 5% of premature infants weighing <1,500 g, and as many as 30% of infants weighing <1,000 g at birth. It is more common in small-for-gestational-age infants and male infants. In females, the ovary is often in the sac.

A. **Surgical repair.** Inguinal hernia repair is the most common operation performed on premature infants. In general, hernias in this patient population can be repaired shortly before discharge home if they are easily reducible and cause no other problems.

1. **Repair before discharge.** In a term infant, repair should be scheduled when the diagnosis is made. For stable premature infants, repair is usually delayed until discharge is near, so that patients may leave the hospital without the risk of incarceration. An incarcerated hernia can usually be reduced with sedation,

steady firm pressure, and elevation of the feet. If a hernia has been incarcerated, it should be repaired as soon as the edema has resolved. The operation may be difficult and should be performed by an experienced pediatric surgeon. The use of spinal anesthesia has simplified the postoperative care of the infants with respiratory problems. As these infants often develop postoperative apnea, they should be monitored in hospital for at least 24 hours after surgery.

2. **Repair after discharge.** Infants with significant pulmonary disease, such as bronchopulmonary dysplasia, are often best repaired at a later time when their respiratory status has improved. We have occasionally had well-instructed parents bring their babies home, and then have them readmitted later for repair. The risks and benefits of this option must be weighed carefully as there is a real risk of the hernia incarcerating at home.

X. ACUTE SCROTAL SWELLING

A. Differential diagnosis includes the following:

1. **Testicular torsion.** Approximately 70% of the cases of testicular torsion that are diagnosed in the newborn period actually occur prenatally. In the newborn, testicular torsion is generally extravaginal (the twist occurs outside the tunica vaginalis) and is caused by an incomplete attachment of the gubernaculum to the testis, allowing torsion and infarction.

   a. Diagnosis is made by physical examination. The testicle is generally nontender, firm, indurated, and swollen with a slightly bluish or dusky cast of the affected side of the scrotum. If the torsion is acute, rather than longstanding, it will be extremely tender to palpation. The testicle can have a transverse lie or be high riding. The overlying skin, limited to the scrotum itself, may be erythematous or edematous. Transillumination is negative, and the cremasteric reflex is absent. Ultrasonography employing Doppler flow studies can be helpful if available, but testing should not delay referral for surgery if there is a possibility that the torsion is recent.

   b. Treatment. In the vast majority of cases, the torsed testicle is already necrotic at birth; therefore, surgical intervention will not salvage the testicle. However, if there is *any possibility* that the torsion occurred recently, and the infant is otherwise healthy, emergency surgical exploration and detorsion should be performed within 4 to 6 hours. This may result in salvage of the torsed testicle. Because there have been reports of bilateral testicular torsion, surgical exploration should include contralateral orchiopexy. Even if emergency exploration is not indicated because of definitive evidence of chronicity of torsion, exploration should be performed on a nonemergent basis to rule out a tumor with clinical and imaging findings identical to testicular torsion.

   c. Prognosis. Testicular protheses are available. Oligospermia has been reported after unilateral testicular torsion.

2. **Trauma/scrotal hematoma.** Most commonly secondary to breech delivery. This is generally bilateral, and may present with hematocele, scrotal swelling, and ecchymoses. Typically, transillumination is negative. Resolution is usually spontaneous but severe cases may require surgical exploration, evacuation of the hematocele, and repair of the testes.

3. **Torsion of the testicular appendage.** Swelling is usually less marked and may present on palpation or as a blue dot on the scrotum. The cremasteric reflexes

are preserved, and Doppler flow ultrasonography may be helpful in ruling out testicular torsion. No treatment is needed.

4. Incarcerated hernia

5. Spontaneous idiopathic scrotal hemorrhage. Most common in large-for-gestational-age (LGA) infants. Distinguishable from torsion by the appearance of a small but distinct ecchymosis over the superficial inguinal ring.

6. Tumor. These are usually nontender, solid, and firm. Transillumination is negative.

7. Meconium peritonitis

XI. COMMON TESTS used in the diagnosis of surgical conditions include the following:

A. **Abdominal x-ray examinations.** A flat plate radiograph of the abdomen kidney-ureter-bladder (KUB) is sufficient for assessing intraluminal gas patterns and mucosal thickness. A left lateral decubitus or cross table lateral radiograph is obtained to ascertain the presence of free air in the abdomen.

1. Contrast enema may be diagnostic in suspected cases of Hirschsprung disease. It may reveal microcolon in the infant with complete obstruction of the small intestine and may show a narrow segment in the sigmoid in the infant with meconium plug syndrome due to functional immaturity.

2. Upper GI series with meglumine diatrizoate may be used to demonstrate obstructions of the upper gastrointestinal tract.

3. In patients with suspected malrotation, a combination of contrast studies may be necessary, starting with a contrast swallow/upper GI. In combination with air or contrast media, an upper GI series will determine the presence or absence of the normally placed ligament of Treitz. A contrast enema may show malposition of the cecum but will not always rule out malrotation. Neonates with intestinal obstruction presumed secondary to malrotation require urgent surgery to relieve possible volvulus of the midgut.

B. Ultrasonography is the preferred method of evaluating abdominal masses in the newborn. It is useful for defining the presence of masses, together with their size, shape, and consistency.

C. CT is an excellent modality to evaluate abdominal masses as well as their relation to other organs, at the cost of a large radiation exposure. Contrast enhancement can outline the intestine, blood vessels, kidneys, ureter, and bladder.

D. MRI is useful to better define the anatomy and location of masses.

E. IVP should be restricted to evaluating genitourinary anatomy if other modalities (ultrasonography and contrast CT) are not available. The IVP dye is poorly concentrated in the newborn.

F. Radionuclide scan of the kidneys can aid in determining function. This is especially useful in assessing complex genitourinary anomalies and in evaluating the contribution of each kidney to renal function.

G. **The Apt test** differentiates maternal from fetal blood. A small amount of bloody material is mixed with 5 mL of water and centrifuged. One part 0.25N sodium hydroxide is added to five parts of the pink supernatant. The fluid remains pink in the presence of fetal blood but rapidly becomes brown if maternal blood is present. The test is useful only if the sample is not contaminated by pigmented material (e.g., meconium/stool) (see Chap. 43).

H. Screening for CF is usually done by measuring immunoreactive trypsin from Guthrie spots. More definitive genetic testing can be performed on DNA sampling obtained from **blood or cheek brush sampling**. When the test result is negative but clinical suspicion remains high, a sweat test should be done. Ideally, the baby should be older than 2 weeks (certainly older than 3 days) and weigh >2 kg to avoid both false-positive results due to the relatively high chloride content of newborns' sweat, as well as false negative or be uninterpretable results if <100 mg of sweat can be collected. It may be necessary to repeat the test when the infant is 3 to 4 weeks old if an adequate volume of sweat cannot be collected.

XII. PREOPERATIVE MANAGEMENT BY PRESENTING SYMPTOM

A. Vomiting without distention

1. The mechanics of feeding the baby should be observed. Rapid feeding, intake of excessive volume and lack of burping are all causes of nonbilious vomiting without distension.

2. Functional and mechanical causes must be ruled out. Often, a history, physical examination, and observation of feedings are sufficient. An abdominal x-ray may be useful.

3. If the baby's general condition is good, feedings of dextrose water should be attempted. If this is tolerated, milk should be tried again. If vomiting recurs and there is a family history of milk allergy, blood in the stool, or elevated percentage of eosinophils on the complete blood count (CBC), consider a trial of non–cow's milk-based formula (e.g., soy based or elemental).

B. Nonbilious vomiting with distention. An overall assessment of the well-versus-sick appearance of the baby, as well as the degree of the abdominal distension, is critical in determining the evaluation and management of nonbilious vomiting and distention. In general, there should be a low threshold to assess for mechanical and functional obstruction, starting with history, physical examination, abdominal radiographs, and $\pm$ contrast studies depending on the clinical presentation. If no source of obstruction is identified, many babies with nonbilious vomiting and mild distention respond to glycerin suppositories, half-strength saline enemas (5 mL/kg body weight), rectal stimulation with a soft rubber catheter, or a combination of these measures. Limited feedings, stimulation to the rectum, and care for the general condition of the baby will solve most of these problems.

C. Bilious vomiting and abdominal distention

1. Immediately arrange for appropriate diagnostic evaluation (generally upper gastrointestinal [UGI] series) to rule out malrotation with midgut volvulous.

2. **Enteral feedings should be discontinued.** Continuous gastric decompression with a sump catheter is mandatory if intestinal obstruction is suspected. All infants with presumed intestinal obstruction should be transported with a nasogastric suction catheter in place, attached to a catheter-tip syringe for continuous aspiration of gastric contents. Failure to decompress the stomach could lead to gastric rupture, aspiration, or respiratory compromise secondary

to excessive diaphragmatic convexity into the thorax. This is especially important in infants who are to be transported by air, because loss of cabin pressure would create a high-risk setting for the rupture of an inadequately drained viscous.

3. Shock, dehydration, and electrolyte imbalance should be prevented or treated if present (see Chaps. 23 and 40).

4. Broad-spectrum antibiotics (ampicillin and gentamicin) should be initiated if there is suspicion of volvulus or any question about bowel integrity. Clindamycin should be added or ampicillin and gentamicin should be substituted with piperacillin and tazobactam (Zosyn) if perforation is high risk or documented.

5. Studies that should be performed include the following:
   a. Monitoring of oxygen saturation, blood pressure, and urine output
   b. Blood tests as follows:
      i. CBC with differential and blood culture
      ii. Electrolytes
      iii. Blood gases and pH
      iv. Clotting studies (e.g., prothrombin time, partial thromboplastin time)
   c. Contrast study (start with upper GI) to rule out malrotation.

D. Masses. The following steps may be taken to determine the etiology of abdominal masses:

1. Complete blood cell count with differential

2. Determination of the level of catecholamines and their metabolites

3. Urinalysis

4. X-ray examination of the chest and abdomen with the infant supine and upright

5. Abdominal ultrasonography

6. Contrast-enhanced CT

7. MRI

8. Angiography; venous and arterial

9. Surgical consultation

XIII. GENERAL INTRAOPERATIVE MANAGEMENT

A. Monitoring devices

1. Temperature probe

2. Electrocardiogram (ECG) and/or CVR monitor

3. Pulse oximetry responds rapidly to changes in patient condition but is subject to artifacts.

4. Transcutaneous PO_2 (see Chap. 30) is helpful if pulse oximetry is unavailable but can be inaccurate in the setting of anesthetic agents that dilate skin vessels.

5. Arterial cannula to monitor blood gases and pressure

B. Well-functioning intravenous line. Babies with omphalocele or gastroschisis should have the intravenous line in the upper extremities, neck, or scalp.

C. Maintenance of body temperature

1. Warmed operating room
2. Humidified, warmed anesthetic agents
3. Warmed blood and other fluids used intraoperatively
4. Cover exposed parts of the baby, especially the head (with a hat).

D. Fluid replacement

1. Replace loss of >15% of total blood volume with warmed packed red blood cells.
2. Replace ascites loss with normal saline mL/mL to maintain normal blood pressure.
3. The neonate loses approximately 5 mL of fluid per kilogram for each hour that the intestine is exposed. This should generally be replaced by Ringer's lactate.

E. Anesthetic management of the neonate is reviewed in Chapter 67.

F. Postoperative pain management is discussed Chapter 67.

G. Postoperatively, the newborn fluid requirement must be monitored closely, including replacement of estimated losses due to bowel edema as well as losses through drains.

Suggested Readings

Achildi O, Grewal H. Congenital anomalies of the esophagus. *Otolaryngol Clin North Am* 2007;40(1):219–244.

Adzick NS, Nance ML. Pediatric surgery: Second of two parts. *N Engl J Med* 2000;342(23): 1726–1732.

American Academy of Pediatrics, Committee on Bioethics. Fetal therapy: ethical considerations. *Pediatrics* 1999;103(5 pt 1):1061–1063.

Chandler JC, Gauderer MW. The neonate with an abdominal mass. *Pediatr Clin North Am* 2004;51(4):979–997.

Glick RD, Hicks MJ, Nuchtern JG, et al. Renal tumors in infants less than 6 months of age. *J Pediatr Surg* 2004;39(4):522–525.

Hansen A, Puder M. *Manual of surgical neonatal intensive care.* 2nd ed. Hamilton: BC Decker; 2009.

Irish MS, Pearl RH, Caty MG, et al. The approach to common abdominal diagnosis in infants and children. *Pediatr Clin North Am* 1998;45(4):729–772.

Johnson MP, Burkowski TP, Reitleman C, et al. In utero surgical treatment of fetal obstructive uropathy: a new comprehensive approach to identify appropriate candidates for vesicoamniotic shunt therapy. *Am J Obstet Gynecol* 1994;170(6):1776–1779.

Jona JZ. Advances in neonatal surgery. *Pediatr Clin North Am* 1998;45(3):605–617.

Keckler SJ, St Peter SD, Valusek PA, et al. VACTERL anomalies in patients with esophageal atresia: an updated delineation of the spectrum and review of the literature. *Pediatr Surg Int* 2007;23(4):309–313.

Kunisaki SM, Barnewolt CE, Estroff JA, et al. Ex utero intrapartum treatment with extracorporeal membrane oxygenation for severe congenital diaphragmatic hernia. *J Pediatr Surg* 2007;42(1):98–104.

Liechty KW, Crombleholme TM, Flake AW, et al. Intrapartum airway management for giant fetal neck masses: the exit (ex utero intrapartum treatment) procedure. *Am J Obstet Gynecol* 1997;177(4):870–874.

Nakayama D, Bose C, Chescheir N, et al. *Critical care of the surgical newborn*. Armonk: Futura Publishing; 1997.

Nuchtern JG. Perinatal neuroblastoma. *Semin Pediatr Surg* 2006;15(1):10–16.

Parad RB. Buccal cell DNA mutation analysis for diagnosis of cystic fibrosis in newborns and infants inaccessible to sweat chloride measurement. *Pediatrics* 1998;101(5):851–855.

Reiner WG, Gearhart JP. Discordant sexual identity in some genetic males with cloacal exstrophy assigned to female sex at birth. *N Engl J Med* 2004;350(4):333–341.

Ringer SA, Stark AS. Management of neonatal emergencies in the delivery room. *Clin Perinatol* 1989;16(1):23–41.

Sheldon CA. The pediatric genitourinary examination: inguinal, urethral, and genital diseases. *Pediatr Clin North Am* 2001;48(6):1339–1380.

Stone KT, Kass EJ, Cacciarelli AA, et al. Management of suspected antenatal torsion: what is the best strategy? *J Urol* 1995;153(3 pt 1):782–784.

Skin Care
Caryn E. Douma

I. INTRODUCTION. The skin performs a vital role in the newborn period. It provides a protective barrier that assists in the prevention of infection, facilitates thermoregulation, and helps control insensible water loss and electrolyte balance. Other functions include tactile sensation and protection against toxins. The neonatal intensive care unit (NICU) environment presents numerous challenges to maintaining skin integrity. Routine care practices, including bathing, application of monitoring devices, intravenous (IV) catheter insertion and removal, tape application, and exposure to potentially toxic substances disrupt the normal barrier function and predispose both premature and term newborns to skin injury. This chapter will address basic physiologic differences that affect newborn skin integrity, describe skin care practices in the immediate newborn period and discuss common disorders.

II. ANATOMY. The three main layers of the skin are the epidermis, the dermis, and the subcutaneous layer. The epidermis is the outermost layer providing the first line of protection against injury. It performs a critical barrier function, retaining heat and fluid and providing protection from infection and environmental toxins. Its structural development has generally occurred by 24 weeks' gestation, but the epidermal barrier function is not complete until after birth. Maturation typically takes 2 to 4 weeks following exposure to the extrauterine environment. The epidermis is composed primarily of keratinocytes, which mature to form the stratum corneum. The dermis is composed of collagen and elastin fibers that provide elasticity and connect the dermis to the epidermis. Blood vessels, nerves, sweat glands, and hair follicles are another integral part of the dermis. The subcutaneous layer, composed of fatty connective tissue, provides insulation, protection, and calorie storage.

The premature infant has significantly fewer layers of stratum corneum than term infants and adults, which can be seen by the transparent, ruddy appearance of their skin. Infants born at <30 weeks may have <2 to 3 layers of stratum corneum compared with 10 to 20 layers in adults and term newborns. The maturation of the stratum corneum is accelerated following premature birth, and improved barrier function and skin integrity is generally present within 10 to 14 days. Other differences in the skin integrity of premature infants include decreased cohesion between the epidermis and the dermis, less collagen, and a marked increase in transepidermal water loss.

III. SKIN CARE PRACTICES. Routine assessment, identification, and avoidance of harmful practices combined with early treatment can eliminate or minimize neonatal skin injury. The identification of potential risk factors for injury and the development of skin care policies and guidelines are an essential part of providing care to both premature and term newborns.

An evidence-based neonatal skin care guideline was created through the collaboration of the National Association of Neonatal Nurses (NANN) and the Association of Women's Health, Obstetric and Neonatal Nurses (AWHONN) (2007) in an effort to provide clinical practice recommendations for practitioners caring for newborns from birth to 28 days of age. This guideline provides a comprehensive reference for developing unit-based skin care policies.

A. Assessment

   1. Daily inspection and assessment of all skin surfaces is an essential part of neonatal skin care. The utilization of a validated skin care assessment tool provides a standardized method to perform the assessment and develop the appropriate treatment plans. A widely used tool is the Neonatal Skin Condition Score (NSCS), developed and validated as part of the AWHONN/NANN skin care guideline (see Table 63.1).

   2. Identification of risk factors.
      a. Prematurity.
      b. Use of monitoring equipment.
      c. Adhesives used to secure central and peripheral access lines, endotracheal tubes.
      d. Edema.
      e. Immobility secondary to extracorporeal membrane oxygenation (ECMO), muscle relaxant, and high-frequency ventilation, which can cause pressure necrosis.

Table 63.1	AWHONN Neonatal Skin Condition Score (NSCS)
Dryness	
1 = Normal, no sign of dry skin	
2 = Dry skin, visible scaling	
3 = Very dry skin, cracking/fissures	
Erythema	
1 = No evidence of erythema	
2 = Visible erythema, <50% body surface	
3 = Visible erythema, ≥50% body suface	
Breakdown	
1 = None evident	
2 = Small, localized areas	
3 = Extensive	
Note: perfect score = 3, worst score = 9	

f. Use of high-risk medications, including vasopressors, calcium, and sodium bicarbonate.

g. Devices with potential for thermal injury such as radiant warmers. Temperature of any product in contact with the skin should not be higher than 41°C/105°F.

3. Avoidance of practices with potential to cause injury

B. Bathing

1. Initial bath should be performed 2 to 4 hours after admission, when temperature has been stabilized to prevent the risk of hypothermia. Provide a controlled environment utilizing warming lights and warm blankets. Bathing is often deferred for the first 24 hours in infants <36 weeks' gestation.

2. Use mild nonalkaline, preservative-free soap. Avoid the use of dyes or perfumes.

3. Daily bathing is not indicated. Warm sterile water is sufficient for premature infants during the first few weeks of life. No more than two or three times per week is preferred.

C. Adhesives

1. Minimize the use of adhesives and tape.

2. Use nonadhesive products in conjunction with transparent dressings and double-backed tape to secure IV catheters.

3. Avoid the use of adhesive bonding agents that can be absorbed easily through the skin.

4. Use warm sterile water to remove adhesives from the skin to prevent epidermal stripping. Adhesive removers contain hydrocarbon derivatives or petroleum distillates that can result in toxicity in the preterm population.

5. Pectin barriers should be applied to the skin before application of adhesives when securing umbilical lines, endotracheal tubes, feeding tubes, nasal cannulae, and urine bags. Remove carefully using soft gauze or cotton balls soaked in warm water.

D. Cord care

1. Clean the umbilical cord area with mild soap and water during the first bath. Keep it clean and dry. Wipe gently with water if the area becomes soiled with stool or urine.

2. Routine application of alcohol is not recommended and may delay cord separation.

3. The routine use of antibiotic ointments and creams are not recommended.

4. Assess for signs of swelling or redness at the base of cord.

E. Humidity

1. Consider the use of humidified incubator care in infants <32 weeks' gestation and/or <1,200 g to decrease transepidermal water loss, maintain skin integrity, decrease fluid requirements, and minimize electrolyte imbalance. Strict equipment cleaning protocols must be in place during humidification.

2. Recommended relative humidity (RH) is 75% to 80% for the first 7 days, decreasing to 50% to 60% RH during the second week until 30 to 32 weeks' postmenstrual age (PMA).

3. Most infants will require humidity only for the first 2 weeks of life.

F. Circumcision care

1. Maintain dressing with petroleum gauze for the first 24 hours.

2. Keep the site clean and dry using water for the first few days.

G. Disinfectants

1. Minimize the use of isopropyl alcohol and alcohol-based disinfectants in pre-term infants.

2. Use povidone-iodine or chlorhexidine, removing with sterile saline following a procedure to avoid the risk of chemical burns. Evidence is currently inconclusive for chlorhexidine use in low birth weight infants. Prolonged or frequent exposure to iodine-containing solutions in premature infants may affect thyroid function.

H. Emollients

1. Emollients are used to prevent and treat skin breakdown and dryness.

2. Emollients should not be used routinely in extremely premature infants because their use may increase the risk of systemic infection.

3. Single use or patient-specific containers should be used to minimize the risk of contamination.

4. Product should not contain perfumes, dyes, or preservatives.

IV. WOUND CARE. Wounds acquired in the immediate newborn period are most commonly related to surgical procedures, trauma, contact dermatitis, or excoriation. Skin care protocols and careful attention to positioning can prevent many of the common wounds requiring treatment. Epidermal stripping is common and can be avoided by minimizing adhesive use and utilizing protective barriers. Routine assessment and prompt treatment maximizes healing.

A. Common causes of neonatal wounds

1. Surgical procedures

2. Trauma

3. Pressure necrosis

4. IV extravasation

5. Prolonged contact with moisture or chemicals

6. Skin excoriation

B. Three phases of wound healing

1. **Inflammatory phase** occurs when the wound is created and is characterized by erythema, swelling, and warmth.

2. **Proliferative phase** is characterized by granulation and tissue regeneration.

3. **Maturation phase** includes contraction of the shape of the wound; scar tissue is visible.

C. Treatment. Accurate assessment followed by immediate, effective treatment promotes wound healing and prevents further damage. Individualized, multidisciplinary care plans should be developed and implemented, considering the etiology, the type of wound, and the gestational age of the infant. Most neonatal wounds are caused by trauma or surgical procedures. Optimal wound treatment is achieved through proper assessment, cleansing, and dressing choice. Multiple wound care products are currently available to optimize healing and prevent further injury.

1. **Wound assessment**

   a. Assess wound for color, thickness, and exudates using standardized tools to provide consistent and objective documentation.

2. **Wound cleansing**

   a. Avoid the use of antiseptics in open wounds. Sterile normal saline (NS) is the preferred cleanser to remove debris and necrosed tissue using gentle friction or irrigation. Moistening the wound every 4 to 6 hours until the wound surface is clear facilitates the healing process.

   b. Clinical signs of infection may require culture and treatment with local or systemic antibiotics.

3. **Common wound dressings and products**

   a. Occlusive, nonadherent dressings provide a moist environment to promote healing and protect the site from further injury.

   b. Gauze

   c. Hydrocolloids

   d. Hydrogels

   e. Barrier creams

V. INTRAVENOUS EXTRAVASATIONS AND INFILTRATION. IV extravasations and infiltration injuries can be prevented with frequent site assessment and prompt intervention.

A. **Prevention**

   1. Hourly site assessment and documentation of the integrity of the IV site.

   2. Peripheral IV infusions should not exceed 12.5% dextrose concentrations.

   3. Use central access whenever possible for vasopressors and other high-risk medications.

B. **Treatment**

   1. When an infiltration or extravasation occurs, stop the infusion immediately and elevate the extremity. Do not apply heat or cold as further tissue damage may occur. Pharmacologic intervention should be administered as soon as possible but no later than 12 to 24 hours from the time of injury.

   2. Hyaluronidase is used to treat infiltration or extravasation of hyperosmolar or extremely alkaline solutions. Administer as a solution diluted to 1 mL in NS. Refer to hospital formulary for concentration and dilution guidelines. Inject 0.2 mL subcutaneously in five separate sites around the leading edge of the infiltrate using a 25- or 27-gauge needle. Change the needle after each skin entry.

   3. Phentolamine is used to treat injury caused by extravasation of vasoconstrictive agents such as dopamine, epinephrine, or dobutamine. Use a 0.5 to 1 mg/mL solution of phentolamine diluted in NS. Consult hospital formulary for dosage. Inject 0.2 mL subcutaneously in five separate sites around the leading edge of the infiltrate using 25- or 27-gauge needle. Change the needle after each skin entry.

   4. Consider consultation with plastic surgery for severe injury.

VI. COMMON SKIN LESIONS. Transient cutaneous lesions are common in the neonatal period. Among the most common are the following:

A. **Erythema toxicum**

1. Scattering of macules, papules, and even some vesicles, or small white or yellow pustules that usually occur on the trunk and also frequently appear on the extremities and face. It occurs in up to 70% of term newborns; occurs rarely in premature infants.

2. Unknown etiology.

3. Vesicle contents when smeared and stained with Wright stain will show a predominance of eosinophils.

4. No treatment necessary.

B. **Diaper dermatitis**

1. Common skin disorder in infants and children most often affecting the groin, buttocks, perineum, and anal area. It is multifactorial, most often caused by sensitivity to the chemicals contained in detergent, clothing or diapers, and friction or exposure to urine and feces. The damp environment increases the skin pH, leading to impaired barrier function and skin breakdown.

2. Prevention is the best treatment, including maintaining normal (acidic) skin pH, frequent diaper changes, keeping diaper area clean with warm water, and applying barrier products if needed. There is no need to completely remove the barrier products with each diaper change. If condition worsens or persists beyond the first few days, antifungal treatment should be considered.

3. Use of powder is not recommended due to the risk of inhalation.

C. **Milia**

1. Multiple pearly white or pale yellow papules or cysts mainly found on the nose, chin, and forehead in term infants.

2. Consists of epidermal cysts up to 1 mm in diameter that develop in connection with the pilosebaceous follicle.
   a. Disappear within the first few weeks requiring no treatment.

D. **Sebaceous gland hyperplasia**

1. Similar to milia with smaller more numerous lesions primarily confined to the nose, upper lip, and chin.

2. Rarely occurs in preterm infants.

3. Related to maternal androgen stimulation.

4. Disappears within the first few weeks.

VII. VASCULAR ABNORMALITIES. Vascular abnormalities occur in up to 40% of newborns. Hemangiomas appear on 1% to 3% of newborns at birth and develop in another 10% within the first few weeks of life. Premature infants have a higher incidence of developing hemangiomas, especially those born at <1,000 g. Most completely resolve by age 12 and do not require intervention unless they interfere with vital functions.

A. **Cavernous hemangioma.** Deep strawberry hemangioma is often present at birth. The lesion grows during the first year, but regression is often not complete.

They can be associated with significant complications, including hemorrhage due to platelet trapping (Kasabach-Merritt syndrome), hypertrophy of involved structures (Klippel-Trenaunay syndrome), heart failure (due to arteriovenous anastomoses), and infection. Treatment may involve surgery, occlusion, laser therapy, steroids, propranolol, or α-interferon.

B. **Nevus simplex (salmon patch or macular hemangioma).** Flat, pink macular lesion found on the forehead, upper eyelid, nasolabial area, glabella, or nape of the neck. It is the most common vascular lesion found in the newborn, occurring in 30% to 40% of infants. Often referred to as a stork bite, it consists of distended dermal capillaries. Most resolve by 1 year of age, excluding those found on the neck.

C. **Nevus flammeus (port-wine stain).** Flat or mildly elevated, reddish-purple lesion; most commonly found on the face. The lesion is a vascular malformation of dilated capillary—like vessels that do not involute. They are often unilateral and may be associated with hemangiomas of the underlying structures. The association of nevus flammeus in the region of the first branch of the trigeminal nerve with cortical lesions of the brain is known as the Sturge-Weber syndrome.

D. **Strawberry hemangioma.** May be present at birth or present as a pale macule with irregular margins. More common in the head, neck, and trunk but they can occur anywhere. Most grow rapidly during the first 6 months and continue to grow for the first year. The majority involute completely by age 4 to 5.

E. **Disorders of lymphatic vessels**

   1. Lymphangiomas
   2. Cystic hygroma
   3. Lymphedema

VIII. PIGMENTATION ABNORMALITIES.

Pigmentary lesions may be present at birth and are most often benign. Some of the most common are briefly described in the subsequent text. A diffuse pattern of hyperpigmentation presenting in the newborn period is unusual and may indicate a variety of hereditary, nutritional, or metabolic disorders. Hypopigmentation presenting in a diffuse pattern may be linked to endocrine, metabolic, or genetic disease.

A. **Mongolian spots**

   1. Benign pigmented lesions found in 70% to 90% of Black, Hispanic, and Asian infants. The lesions may be small or large, grayish blue or bluish black in color.

   2. Caused by the increased presence of melanocytes, most commonly found in the lumbosacral region.

B. **Café au lait spots**

   1. Flat, brown, round, or oval lesions with smooth edges occurring in 10% of normal infants.

   2. Usually of little or no significance but may indicate neurofibromatosis if larger than 4 to 6 cm or >6 are present.

C. **Albinism.** Most commonly an autosomal recessive condition involving abnormal melanin synthesis leading to a deficiency in pigment production. The only effective treatment is protection from light.

D. Piebaldism (partial albinism). Autosomal dominant disorder present at birth characterized by off-white macules (depigmented lesions with hyperpigmented borders) on the scalp and forehead and on the trunk and extremities. The hair may be involved as well. A white "forelock," as in Waardenburg syndrome, is a feature of this disorder.

E. Junctional nevi. Brown or black, flat or slightly raised lesions present at birth occurring at the junction of the dermis and epidermis. They are benign lesions requiring no treatment.

F. Compound nevi. Larger than junctional nevi, involving the dermis and epidermis. Removal is recommended to decrease the possibility of later progression to malignant melanoma.

G. Giant hairy nevi. Present at birth, they may involve 20% to 30% of the body surface, with other pigmentary abnormalities frequently present. Brown to black and leathery in appearance, also known as bathing trunk nevi, they have a large amount of hair and may include central nervous system involvement. Surgical removal is indicated for cosmetic reasons and because they can progress to malignant melanoma.

IX. DEVELOPMENTAL ABNORMALITIES OF THE SKIN

A. Skin dimples and sinuses can occur on any part of the body, but they are most common over bony prominences such as the scapula, knee joint, and hip. They may be simple depressions on the skin of no pathologic significance or actual sinus tracts connecting to deeper structures.

1. A pilonidal dimple or sinus may occur in the sacral area. A sinus that is deep but does not communicate with the underlying structures is usually insignificant.

2. Some deep sinuses connect to the central nervous system. Occasionally, a dimple, sometimes accompanied by a nevus or hemangioma, may signify an underlying spinal disorder. These usually require neuroimaging scans for diagnosis.

3. Dermal sinuses or cysts along the cheek or jawline or extending into the neck, may represent remnants of the branchial cleft structures of the early embryo.

4. A preauricular sinus is the most common and may be unilateral or bilateral. It appears in the most anterior upper portion of the tragus of the external ear. They rarely cause problems in the newborn period, but may require later excision due to infection.

B. Small skin tags can occur on the chest wall near the breast and are of no significance.

C. Aplasia cutis (congenital absence of the skin) occurs most frequently in the midline of the posterior part of the scalp. Treatment involves protection from trauma and infection. Other malformations may be associated, including trisomy 13.

X. OTHER SKIN DISORDERS. Complete identification and description of all dermatologic disorders is beyond the scope of this chapter. Several of the more common developmental and hereditary disorders are mentioned below.

A. Scaling disorders

1. Most common causes of scaling in the neonatal period are related to desquamation found in postmature and dysmature infants. The condition is time limited and transient without long-term consequences.

2. Less common scaling disorders that occur within the first month of life include harlequin ichthyosis, collodion baby, X-linked ichthyosis, bullous ichthyosis, and others.

B. **Vesicobullous eruptions**

1. Epidermolysis bullosa is a group of genetic disorders characterized by lesions that appear at birth or within the first few weeks. Severity of symptoms ranges from simple, nonscarring bullae to more severe forms with large numerous lesions that result in scarring, contractions, and loss of large areas of the epidermis. Specific diagnosis requires skin biopsy. Prevention of infection and protection of the fragile skin surfaces is the goal of treatment.

C. **Infections** caused by bacterial (especially staphylococcal, pseudomonas, *Listeria*), viral (herpes simplex), or fungal (e.g., candidal) organisms may also cause vesicular, bullous, or other skin manifestations.

Suggested Readings

Association of Women's Health, Obstetric and Neonatal Nurses. *Neonatal skin care: evidence-based clinical practice guideline.* 2nd ed. Washington, DC: Association of Women's Health, Obstetric and Neonatal Nurses; 2007.

Eichenfield LF, Frieden IJ, Esterly NB. *Textbook of neonatal dermatology.* Philadelphia, PA: WB Saunders; 2001.

64 Retinopathy of Prematurity

Deborah K. VanderVeen and John A. F. Zupancic

GENERAL PRINCIPLES

I. DEFINITION. **Retinopathy of Prematurity (ROP)** is a multifactorial vasoproliferative retinal disorder that increases in incidence with decreasing gestational age. Approximately 65% of infants with a birth weight <1,250 g and 80% of those with a birth weight <1,000 g will develop some degree of ROP.

II. PATHOGENESIS

A. **Normal development.** After the sclera and choroid have developed, retinal elements, including nerve fibers, ganglion cells, and photoreceptors, migrate from the optic disc at the posterior pole of the eye and move toward the periphery. The photoreceptors have progressed 80% of the distance to their resting place at the ora serrata by 28 weeks of gestation. Before the retinal vessels develop, the avascular retina receives its oxygen supply by diffusion across the retina from the choroidal vessels. The retinal vessels, which arise from the spindle cells in the adventitia of the hyaloid vessels at the optic disc, begin to migrate outward at 16 weeks' gestation. Migration is complete by 36 weeks on the nasal side and by 40 weeks on the temporal side.

B. **Possible mechanisms of injury.** Clinical observations suggest that the onset of ROP consists of two stages.

1. The **first stage** involves an initial insult or insults, such as hyperoxia, hypoxia, or hypotension, at a critical point in retinal vascularization that results in vasoconstriction and decreased blood flow to the developing retina with a subsequent arrest in vascular development. The relative hyperoxia after birth is hypothesized to downregulate the production of growth factors such as vascular endothelial growth factor (VEGF) that are essential for the normal development of the retinal vessels.

2. During the **second stage**, neovascularization occurs. This aberrant retinal vessel growth is thought to be driven by excess angiogenic factors (such as VEGF) upregulated by the hypoxic avascular retina. New vessels grow through the retina into the vitreous. These vessels are permeable; thus, hemorrhage and edema can occur. Extensive and severe extraretinal fibrovascular proliferation can lead to retinal detachment and abnormal retinal function. In most affected infants, however, the disease process is mild and regresses spontaneously.

C. **Risk factors.** ROP has been consistently associated with low gestational age, low birth weight, and prolonged oxygen exposure. In addition, the potential or confirmed risk factors include lability in oxygen requirement as well as markers of neonatal illness severity, such as mechanical ventilation, systemic infection, blood transfusion, intraventricular hemorrhage, and poor postnatal weight gain.

III. DIAGNOSIS

A. **Screening.** Because no early clinical signs or symptoms indicate developing ROP, early and regular retinal examination is necessary. The timing of the occurrence of ROP is related to the maturity of retinal vessels and, therefore, postnatal age. In the cryotherapy for retinopathy of prematurity (CRYO-ROP) study, for infants <1,250 g, the median postnatal ages at the onset of stage 1 ROP, prethreshold disease, and threshold disease were 34, 36, and 37 weeks, respectively. At the time of the first examination, 17% of infants had ROP, and prethreshold ROP has been reported as early as 29 weeks of gestational age. Because ROP that meets treatment criteria may be reached at a later postnatal age, all preterm infants who meet screening criteria and are discharged before they show resolution of the ROP or have mature retinal vasculature must continue to have ophthalmologic examinations on an outpatient basis.

B. **Diagnosis.** ROP is diagnosed by retinal examination with indirect ophthalmoscopy; this should be performed by an ophthalmologist with expertise in ROP screening. The current recommendation is to screen all infants with a birth weight <1,500 g or with a gestational age <30 weeks. Infants who are born after 30 weeks of gestational age may be considered for screening if they have been ill (e.g., those who have had severe respiratory distress syndrome, hypotension requiring pressor support, or surgery in the first several weeks of life). Because the timing of ROP is related to postnatal age, infants who are born at <26 weeks of gestation are examined at the postnatal age of 6 weeks, those who are born at 27 to 28 weeks of gestation are examined at the postnatal age of 5 weeks, those born at 29 to 30 weeks of gestation are examined at the postnatal age of 4 weeks, and those >30 weeks of gestation are examined at the postnatal age of 3 weeks. Patients are examined every 2 weeks until their vessels have grown out to the ora serrata and the retina is considered mature. If ROP is diagnosed, the frequency of examination depends on the severity and rapidity of the progression of the disease.

IV. CLASSIFICATION AND DEFINITIONS

A. **Classification.** The International Classification of Retinopathy of Prematurity (ICROP) is used to classify ROP. This classification system consists of four components (see Fig. 64.1).

1. **Location** refers to how far the developing retinal blood vessels have progressed. The retina is divided into three concentric circles or zones.

   a. Zone 1 consists of an imaginary circle with the optic nerve at the center and a radius of twice the distance from the optic nerve to the macula.

   b. Zone 2 extends from the edge of zone 1 to the ora serrata on the nasal side of the eye and approximately half the distance to the ora serrata on the temporal side.

   c. Zone 3 consists of the outer crescent-shaped area extending from zone 2 out to the ora serrata temporally.

2. Severity refers to the **stage** of disease.

   a. Stage 1. A demarcation line appears as a thin white line that separates the normal retina from the undeveloped avascular retina.

   b. Stage 2. A ridge of fibrovascular tissue with height and width replaces the line of stage 1. It extends inward from the plane of the retina.

Children's Hospital Boston

**OPHTHALMOLOGIC CONSULTATION FOR
RETINOPATHY OF PREMATURITY (ROP)**

Gestational age (weeks) _____ Birth weight _____ gm

Date of exam _____ Adjusted age (weeks) _____

Ophthalmologist _____ MD
(PRINT NAME)

USE PLATE OR PRINT

NAME _____
LAST   FIRST

DATE _____ DIV _____

MED. REC. NO. _____

EXAMINATION:
☐ Pertinent record reviewed

Extended Ophthalmoscopy

Right Eye   **Left Eye**

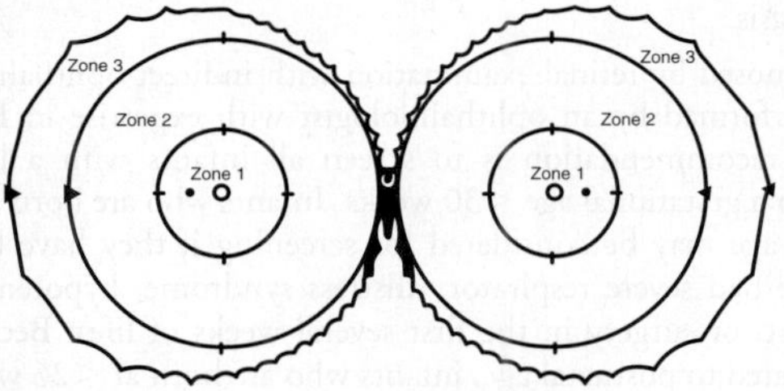

Penlight examination (both eyes)

☐ External   ☐ Anterior chamber
☐ Lids   ☐ Iris
☐ Conjunctiva   ☐ Lens
☐ Cornea   ☐ _____

COMMENTS: _____

_____

_____

Right eye	Other findings (mark with an "X")	Left eye
	Dilatation/Tortuosity	
☐	Mild	☐
☐	Moderate	☐
☐	Severe	☐
	Iris vessel dilatation	
	Pupil rigidity	
	Vitreous haze	
	Hemorrhages	
	Neovascular tufts posterior to ridge	
	Neovascular cylinders posterior to ridge	

Right eye	Summary diagnosis	Left eye
	Mature retina	
	Immature, no ROP	
Zone		Zone
	ROP	

Stage	Zone	Number of clock hours	Stage	Zone	Number of clock hours

Other: _____

_____

_____

Plan: Repeat exam in: _____

Examined by: _____ , M.D.
(Signature)

Physician I.D. #

03241 25/pkg 05/06

Figure 64.1. Sample of form for ophthalmologic consultation.

c. Stage 3. The ridge has extraretinal fibrovascular proliferation. Abnormal blood vessels and fibrous tissue develop on the edge of the ridge and extend into the vitreous.

d. Stage 4. Partial retinal detachment may result when scar tissue pulls on the retina. Stage 4A is partial detachment not involving the macula, so that there is still a chance for good vision. Stage 4B is partial detachment that involves the macula, thereby limiting the likelihood of good vision in that eye.

e. Stage 5. Complete retinal detachment occurs. The retina assumes a funnel-shaped appearance and is described as open or narrow in the anterior and posterior regions.

3. **Extent** refers to the circumferential location of the disease and is reported as clock hours in the appropriate zone.

4. **Plus disease** is an additional designation that refers to the presence of vascular dilatation and tortuosity of the posterior retinal vessels in at least two quadrants. This indicates a more severe degree of ROP and may also be associated with iris vascular engorgement, pupillary rigidity, and vitreous haze. **Preplus disease** describes vascular abnormalities of the posterior pole (mild venous dilatation or arterial tortuosity) that are present but are insufficient for the diagnosis of plus disease.

B. Definitions

1. **Aggressive posterior ROP** is an uncommon, rapidly progressing, severe form of ROP characterized by its posterior location (usually zone 1), and prominence of plus disease out of proportion to the peripheral retinopathy. Stage 3 ROP may appear as a flat, intraretinal network of neovascularization. When untreated, this type of ROP usually progresses to stage 5.

2. **Threshold ROP** is present if 5 or more contiguous or 8 cumulative clock hours (30-degree sectors) of stage 3 with plus disease in either zone 1 or 2 are present. This is the level of ROP at which the risk of blindness is predicted to be at least 50% and at which the CRYO-ROP study showed that the risk of blindness could be reduced to approximately 25% with treatment.

3. **Prethreshold ROP** is any ROP in zone 1 less than threshold ROP, and in zone 2, stage 2 ROP with plus disease, stage 3 without plus disease, or stage 3 with plus disease but fewer than the requisite clock hours that define threshold ROP.

   a. Type 1 prethreshold ROP includes:

   i. In zone 1, eyes with any ROP and plus disease or stage 3 with or without plus disease.

   ii. In zone 2, stage 2 or 3 ROP with plus disease.

   b. Type 2 prethreshold ROP includes:

   i. In zone 1, stage 1 or 2 without plus disease.

   ii. In zone 2, stage 3 without plus disease.

V. TIMING OF TREATMENT

A. Current recommendations are to consider treatment for eyes with **type 1 prethreshold ROP** based on the early treatment for ROP (ETROP) randomized trial that showed a significant benefit for treatment of eyes with type 1 ROP.

B. Close observation is currently recommended for **type 2 prethreshold ROP.** Treatment should be considered for an eye with type 2 ROP when progression to type 1 status or threshold ROP occurs. Approximately 15% of type 2 eyes progress to type 1 ROP.

VI. PROGNOSIS

A. **Short-term prognosis.** Risk factors for ROP requiring treatment include posterior location (zone 1 or posterior zone 2), presence of ROP on the first examination, increasing severity of stage, circumferential involvement, the presence of plus disease, and rapid progression of disease. Most infants with stage 1 or 2 ROP will experience spontaneous regression. If prethreshold ROP develops, about 77% of type 2 eyes regress without study treatment but only 31.5% of eyes with type 1 regress spontaneously. In ETROP study, treatment for type 1 ROP (compared to conventional timing at threshold) reduced unfavorable visual outcomes from 33% to 25%. Unfortunately, only 35% of patients maintained visual acuity at 6 years of age of 20/40 or better, suggesting more work to prevent development of ROP is important. Any zone 3 disease has an excellent prognosis for complete recovery.

B. **Long-term prognosis.** Infants with significant ROP have an increased risk of high myopia, anisometropia and other refractive errors, strabismus, amblyopia, astigmatism, late retinal detachment, and glaucoma. **Cicatricial disease** refers to residual scarring in the retina and may be associated with retinal detachment years later. The prognosis for stage 4 ROP depends on the involvement of the macula; the chance for good vision is greater when the macula is not involved. Once the retina has detached, the prognosis for good vision is poor even with surgical reattachment, although some useful vision may be preserved. All premature infants who meet screening criteria regardless of the diagnosis of ROP are at risk for long-term vision problems, from either ocular or neurologic abnormalities. We recommend a follow-up evaluation by an ophthalmologist with expertise in neonatal sequelae at approximately 1 year of age, or sooner if ocular or visual abnormalities have been noted.

VII. PREVENTION.

Currently, no proven methods are available to prevent ROP. Multiple large clinical trials to prevent ROP have been performed evaluating the use of prophylactic vitamin E therapy, reduction in exposure to bright light, and administration of penicillamine, but none of these have shown clear benefit. Nonrandomized studies have suggested that lower or more tightly regulated oxygen saturation limits early on in the neonatal course that may reduce the severity of ROP without adverse effects on mortality, bronchopulmonary dysplasia, or neurologic sequelae. In the recently reported SUPPORT study, preterm infants under 28 weeks of gestation who were randomized to lower oxygen ranges had lower rates of retinopathy but higher rates of mortality. Several other multicenter randomized trials to formally test this hypothesis are currently underway. Early nutritional support, normalization of IGF-1 levels, and adequate physiologic postnatal weight gain are associated with less severe ROP.

VIII. TREATMENT

A. **Laser therapy.** Laser photocoagulation therapy for ROP is the preferred initial treatment in most centers. Laser treatment is delivered through an indirect ophthalmoscope and is applied to the avascular retina anterior to the ridge of extraretinal fibrovascular proliferation for 360 degrees. An average of 1,000 spots are placed in each eye, but the number may range from a few hundred to approximately 2,000. Both argon and diode laser photocoagulation have been successfully used in infants with severe ROP. The procedure can be performed in the newborn intensive care unit and usually can be performed with local anesthesia and sedation, avoiding some of the adverse effects of general anesthesia. Clinical observations and comparative studies suggest that laser therapy is at least as effective as cryotherapy in achieving favorable visual outcomes. The development of cataracts, glaucoma, or anterior segment ischemia following laser surgery or cryotherapy have been reported.

B. **Cryotherapy.** A cryoprobe is applied to the external surface of the sclera and areas peripheral to the ridge of the ROP are frozen until the entire anterior avascular retina has been treated. Approximately, 35 to 75 applications are made in each eye. The procedure is usually done under general anesthesia. Cryotherapy causes more inflammation and requires more analgesia than laser therapy but may be necessary in special cases, such as when there is poor pupillary dilation or vitreous hemorrhage, both of which prevent adequate delivery of laser therapy.

C. **Anti-VEGF therapy.** Intravitreal injection of VEGF inhibitors is controversial for ROP treatment. Currently, two multicenter randomized trials are underway to establish safety and efficacy of intravitreal bevacizumab (off-label) for type 1 ROP compared to standard laser therapy. This treatment may be considered for selected cases, as salvage treatment, or in conjunction with vitrectomy surgery.

D. **Retinal reattachment.** Once the macula detaches in stage 4B or 5 ROP, retinal surgery is usually performed in an attempt to reattach the retina. This may include vitrectomy with or without lensectomy, and membrane peeling if necessary, to remove tractional forces causing the retinal detachment. A scleral buckling procedure may be useful for more peripheral detachments with drainage of subretinal fluid for effusional detachments. Reoperations for redetachment of the retina are common. Even if the retina can be successfully attached with rare exception, the visual outcome is in the range of legal blindness. Despite the low vision measure, however, children find any amount of vision useful, and untreated stage 5 ROP eventually leads to no light perception vision. The achievement of even minimal vision can result in a large difference in a child's overall quality of life.

Suggested Readings

Early Treatment for Retinopathy of Prematurity Cooperative Group, Good WV, Hardy RJ, et al. Final visual acuity results in the early treatment for retinopathy of prematurity study. *Arch Ophthalmol* 2010;128(6):663–671.

Early Treatment for Retinopathy of Prematurity Cooperative Group. Revised indications for the treatment of retinopathy of prematurity: results of the early treatment for retinopathy of prematurity randomized trial. *Arch Ophthalmol* 2003;121(12): 1684–1694.

International Committee for the Classification of Retinopathy of Prematurity. The International Classification of Retinopathy of Prematurity revisited. *Arch Ophthalmol* 2005;123(7): 991–999.

Section on Ophthalmology American Academy of Pediatrics, American Academy of Ophthalmology, American Association for Pediatric Ophthalmology and Strabismus. Screening examination of premature infants for retinopathy of prematurity. *Pediatrics.* 2006;117(2):572–576.

SUPPORT Study Group of the Eunice Kennedy Shriver NICHD Neonatal Research Network, Carlo WA, Finer NN, et al. Target ranges of oxygen saturation in extremely preterm infants. *N Engl J Med* 2010;362(21):1959–1969.

65

Hearing Loss in Neonatal Intensive Care Unit Graduates

Jane E. Stewart and Aimee Knorr

I. DEFINITION. Neonatal intensive care unit (NICU) graduates are at high risk for developing hearing loss. When undetected, hearing loss can result in delays in language, communication, and cognitive development. Hearing loss falls into four major categories:

A. Sensorineural loss is the result of abnormal development or damage to the cochlear hair cells (sensory end organ) or auditory nerve.

B. Conductive loss is the result of interference in the transmission of sound from the external auditory canal to the inner ear. The most common cause for the conductive hearing loss is accumulation of fluid in the middle ear or middle ear effusion. Less common are anatomic causes such as microtia, canal stenosis, or stapes fixation that often occur in infants with craniofacial malformations.

C. Auditory dyssynchrony or auditory neuropathy. In this less common type of hearing loss, the inner ear or cochlea appears to receive sounds normally; however, the transfer of the signal from the cochlea to the auditory nerve is abnormal. The etiology of this disorder is not well understood; however, babies who have a history of severe hyperbilirubinemia, prematurity, hypoxia, and immune disorders are at increased risk. There is also a reported genetic predisposition to auditory dyssynchrony.

D. Central hearing loss. In this type of hearing loss, despite an intact auditory canal and inner ear and normal neurosensory pathways, there is abnormal auditory processing at higher levels of the central nervous system.

II. INCIDENCE. The overall incidence of severe congenital hearing loss is 1 to 3 in 1,000 live births. However, 2 to 4 per 100 infants surviving neonatal intensive care have some degree of sensorineural hearing loss.

III. ETIOLOGY

A. Genetic. Approximately 50% of congenital hearing loss is thought to be of genetic origin (70% recessive, 15% autosomal dominant, and 15% with other types of genetic transmission). The most common genetic cause of hearing loss is a mutation in the **connexin 26 (Cx26) gene**, located on chromosome 13q11–12. The carrier rate for this mutation is 3% and it causes approximately 20% to 30% of congenital hearing loss. Deletion of the **mitochondrial gene** 12S rRNA, A1555G, is associated with a predisposition for hearing loss after exposure to aminoglycoside antibiotics.

Other mutations, such as those of the SLC26A4 gene and connexin 30 (Cx30) gene, are associated with newborn hearing loss. Approximately 30% of infants with hearing loss have other associated medical problems that are part of a **syndrome**. More than 400 syndromes are known to include hearing loss (e.g., Alport, Pierre Robin, Usher, Waardenburg syndromes, and trisomy 21).

B. **Nongenetic.** In approximately 25% of childhood hearing loss, a nongenetic cause is identified. Hearing loss is thought to be secondary to an injury to the developing auditory system in the intrapartum or perinatal period. This injury may result from infection, hypoxia, ischemia, metabolic disease, ototoxic medication, or hyperbilirubinemia. Preterm infants and infants who require newborn intensive care or a special care nursery are often exposed to these factors.

1. **Cytomegalovirus (CMV)** congenital infection is the most common cause of nonhereditary sensorineural hearing loss. Approximately 1% of all infants are born with CMV infection in this country. Of these (~40,000 infants/year), 10% have clinical signs of infection at birth (small for gestational age, hepatosplenomegaly, jaundice, thrombocytopenia, neutropenia, intracranial calcifications, and skin rash), and 50% to 60% of these infants develop hearing loss. Although most (90%) infants born with CMV infection have no clinical signs of infection, hearing loss still develops in 10% to 15% of these infants, and it is often progressive. Because there has not been an established treatment for CMV in the newborn, prevention of hearing loss is currently not possible. However, treatment with the antiviral agent ganciclovir (given intravenously) and valganciclovir (given orally) is being studied, and preliminary data indicate that these antiviral agents may prevent the development and/or progression of hearing loss.

C. **Risk factors.** The Joint Committee on Infant Hearing (JCIH) listed the following risk indicators associated with permanent congenital, progressive, or delayed-onset hearing loss in their 2007 position statement.

1. Caregiver concern[a] regarding hearing, speech, language, or developmental delay

2. Family history of permanent childhood hearing loss

3. Neonatal intensive care of more than 5 days or any of the following regardless of length of stay: ECMO[a], assisted ventilation, exposure to ototoxic medications (gentamicin and tobramycin) or loop diuretics (furosemide), and hyperbilirubinemia that requires exchange transfusion (some centers use a level of ≥20 mg/dL as a general guideline for risk)

4. *In utero* infections such as CMV[a], herpes, rubella, syphilis, and toxoplasmosis

5. Craniofacial anomalies, including those that involve the pinna, ear canal, ear tags, ear pits, and temporal bone anomalies

6. Physical findings, such as a white forelock, that are associated with a syndrome known to include a sensorineural or permanent conductive hearing loss

7. Syndromes associated with progressive or late-onset hearing loss such as neurofibromatosis, osteopetrosis, and Usher syndrome. Other frequently identified syndromes include Waardenburg, Alport, Pendred, and Jervell and Lange-Nielsen.

8. Neurodegenerative disorders[a] such as Hunter syndrome or sensory motor neuropathies such as Friedreich ataxia and Charcot-Marie-Tooth syndrome

---

[a]Risk indicators that are of greater concern for delayed hearing loss.

9. Culture-positive postnatal infections associated with sensorineural hearing loss[a] including bacterial and viral (especially herpes viruses and varicella) meningitis

10. Head trauma, especially basal skull/temporal bone fractures that require hospitalization

11. Chemotherapy[a]

12. Recurrent or persistent otitis media for at least 3 months

All infants with 1 or more risk factors should have ongoing, developmentally appropriate hearing screening, and at least 1 diagnostic audiology assessment by 24 to 30 months (the current recommendation of the JCIH). Risk factors that are highly associated with the late-onset hearing loss or progressive hearing loss such as congenital CMV or treatment with extracorporeal membrane oxygenation (ECMO) warrant earlier and more frequent follow-up.

D. **Detection.** Universal newborn hearing screening is recommended to detect hearing loss as early as possible. The JCIH and the American Academy of Pediatrics endorse a goal that 100% of infants be tested during their hospital birth admission. The percentage of infants screened in this country prior to 1 month of age has increased from 46.5% in 1999 to 97% in 2007.

IV. SCREENING TESTS.

The currently acceptable methods for physiologic hearing screening in newborns are auditory brainstem response (ABR) and evoked otoacoustic emissions (EOAE). A threshold of 35 dB has been established as a cutoff for an abnormal screen, which prompts further testing.

A. **Auditory brainstem responses (ABR)** measures the electroencephalographic waves generated by the auditory system in response to clicks through three electrodes placed on the infant's scalp. The characteristic waveform recorded from the electrodes becomes more well defined with increasing postnatal age. ABR is reliable after 34 weeks postnatal age. The automated version of ABR allows this test to be performed quickly and easily by trained hospital staff. Though the EOAE is acceptable for routine screening of low-risk infants, the AAP recommends the ABR over the EOAE in high-risk infants including NICU patients and graduates. This is because the ABR tests the auditory pathway beyond the cochlea and picks up neural hearing loss including auditory dyssynchrony. The automated version of ABR allows this test to be performed quickly and easily by trained hospital staff.

B. **EOAEs.** This records acoustic "feedback" from the cochlea through the ossicles to the tympanic membrane and ear canal following a click or tone burst stimulus. EOAE is even quicker to perform than ABR. However, EOAE is more likely to be affected by debris or fluid in the external and middle ear, resulting in higher referral rates. Furthermore, EOAE is unable to detect some forms of sensorineural hearing loss including auditory dyssynchrony. EOAE is often combined with automated ABR in a two-step screening system.

V. FOLLOW-UP TESTING.

Follow-up testing of infants who fail their newborn screen is critical. Despite the high success in screening (97%) of newborns, currently, 46% of infants who fail their initial screen are lost to follow-up. Infants who have failed the screen in both ears should have a diagnostic auditory brainstem

Table 65.1	Definitions of the Degree and Severity of Hearing Loss
Mild	15–40 dB
Moderate	40–60 dB
Severe	60–90 dB
Profound	90+ dB
Source: American Academy of Audiology	

response performed by a pediatric audiology specialist within 2 weeks of their initial test. Infants with unilateral abnormal results should have follow-up testing within 3 months. Testing should include a full diagnostic frequency-specific ABR to measure hearing threshold. Evaluation of middle ear function (tympanometry using a 1,000-hz probe tone), observation of the infant's behavioral response to sound, and parental report of emerging communication and auditory behaviors should also be included.

A. Definitions of the degree and severity of hearing loss are listed in Table 65.1

B. Infants who have risk factors for progressive or delayed-onset sensorineural and/or conductive hearing loss require continued surveillance even if the initial newborn screening results are normal.

C. Infants with **mild or unilateral hearing loss** should also be monitored closely with repeat audiology evaluations and provided with early intervention services as they are at increased risk for both progressive hearing loss and delayed and abnormal development of language and communication skills.

D. All infants should be monitored by their primary care providers for normal hearing and language development.

VI. MEDICAL EVALUATION. An infant diagnosed with true hearing loss should have the following additional evaluations:

A. Complete evaluation should be performed by an otolaryngologist or otologist who has experience with infants. Referral for radiologic imaging with computed tomography (CT) or magnetic resonance imaging (MRI) should occur when needed.

B. Genetic evaluation and counseling should be provided for all infants with true hearing loss.

C. Examination should be performed by a pediatric ophthalmologist to detect eye abnormalities that may be associated with hearing loss.

D. Developmental pediatrics, neurology, cardiology, and nephrology referral should be made as indicated.

VII. HABILITATION/TREATMENT. Infants with true hearing loss should be referred for early intervention services to enhance the child's acquisition of developmentally appropriate language skills. This should include therapy from speech and language pathologists, audiologists, and special educators. Infants who are appropriate

candidates and whose parents have chosen to utilize personal amplification systems should be fitted with hearing aids as soon as possible. Children with severe to profound bilateral hearing loss may be candidates for cochlear implants by the end of the first year of age. Early intervention resources and information for parents to make decisions regarding communication choices should also be provided as promptly as possible.

VIII. PROGNOSIS. The prognosis depends largely on the extent of hearing loss as well as the time of diagnosis and treatment. For optimal auditory brain development, normal maturation of the central auditory pathways depends on the early maximizing of auditory input. The earlier habilitation starts, the better the child's chance of achieving age-appropriate language and communication skills. Fitting of hearing aids by the age of 6 months has been associated with improved speech outcome. Initiation of early intervention services before 3 months of age has been associated with improved cognitive developmental outcome at 3 years. Language and communication outcomes for children receiving early cochlear implants and the accompanying intensive multidisciplinary team therapy are also extremely promising.

Suggested Readings

American Academy of Pediatrics, Joint Committee on Infant Hearing. Year 2007 position statement: principles and guidelines for early hearing detection and intervention programs. *Pediatrics* 2007;120(4):898–921.

Grosse SD, Ross DS, Dollard SC. Congenital cytomegalovirus (CMV) infection as a cause of permanent bilateral hearing loss: a quantitative assessment. *J Clin Virol* 2008;41(2):57–62.

Harlor AD Jr, Bower C, Committee on Practice and Ambulatory Medicine. Hearing assessment in infants and children: recommendations beyond neonatal screening. *Pediatrics* 2009;124(4):1252–1263.

Kaye CI, Committee on Genetics, Accurso F. Newborn screening fact sheets. *Pediatrics* 2006; 118(3):e934–e963.

Kral A, O'Donoghue GM. Profound deafness in childhood. *N Engl J Med* 2010;363(15): 1438–1450.

Morton CC, Nance WE. Newborn hearing screening—A silent revolution. *N Engl J Med* 2006;354(20):2151–2164.

Weichbold V, Nekahm-Heis D, Welzl-Mueller K. Universal newborn hearing screening and postnatal hearing loss. *Pediatrics* 2006;117(4):e631–e636.

Online Resources

American Academy of Audiology: http://www.audiology.org

American Speech-Language-Hearing Association: http://www.asha.org

Better Hearing Institute: http://www.betterhearing.org/

Boystown National Research Center: http://www.babyhearing.org/

Center for Disease Control and Prevention: http://www.cdc.gov/ncbddd/ehdi/default.htm

Hands & Voices: http://www.handsandvoices.org/

Harvard Medical School Center for Hereditary Deafness: http://hearing.harvard.edu/

Marion Downs National Center for Infant Hearing: http://www.colorado.edu/slhs/mdnc/

National Association of the Deaf: http://www.nad.org

National Center for Hearing Assessment and Management: http://www.infanthearing.org/

National Deaf Education Network/Clearinghouse: http://www.clerccenter.gallaudet.edu/ Clearinghouse/index.html

66

Common Neonatal Procedures

Steven A. Ringer and James E. Gray

Invasive procedures are a necessary but potentially risk-laden part of newborn intensive care. To provide maximum benefit, these techniques must be performed in a manner that both accomplishes the task at hand and maintains the patient's general well-being.

I. GENERAL PRINCIPLES

A. **Consideration of alternatives.** For each procedure, all alternatives should be considered, and risk–benefit ratios should be evaluated. Many procedures involve the placement of indwelling devices made of plastic. Polyvinylchloride-based devices leach a plasticizer, Di(2-ethylhexyl)-phthalate (DEHP), which may be toxic over a long-term exposure. Alternatives exist and devices that are DEHP-free should be used for procedures on neonates whenever possible.

B. **Monitoring and homeostasis.** Ideally, the operator should delegate another care provider to be responsible for the ongoing monitoring and management of the patient during a procedure. This person's primary focus should be on the patient rather than the procedure being performed. They must assess cardiorespiratory and thermoregulatory stability throughout the procedure and apply interventions when needed. For sterile procedures, a particularly important function is ensuring the integrity of the sterile field. Continuous monitoring can be accomplished through a combination of invasive (e.g., arterial blood pressure monitoring) or noninvasive (e.g., oximeter) techniques. This monitoring can most effectively be standardized through the use of a procedure checklist so that the monitoring caregiver can ensure that each step is appropriately completed and documented by sign-off on the part of all providers at the conclusion of the procedure.

C. **Pain control.** Treatment of procedure-associated discomfort can be accomplished with pharmacologic or nonpharmacologic approaches (see Chap. 67). The potential negative impact of any medication on the patient's cardiorespiratory status should be considered. Oral sucrose (e.g., 24% solution, 0.2–0.4 mL/kg) is very effective in reducing pain of minor procedures and blood drawing. It can also be used as an adjunctive therapy for more painful procedures when the patient can tolerate oral medication. Morphine or fentanyl is commonly administered before beginning potentially painful procedures. The use of neonatal pain scales to assess the need for medication is recommended.

D. **Informing the family.** Other than during true emergencies, we notify parents of the need for invasive procedures in their child's care before we perform them. We discuss the indications for and possible complications of each procedure. In addition, alternative procedures, where available, are also discussed. Informed consent should be obtained for procedures with a significant degree of invasiveness or risk.

E. **Precautions.** The operator should use universal precautions, including wearing gloves, impermeable gowns, barriers, and eye protection to prevent exposure to blood and bodily fluids that may be contaminated with infectious agents.

F. **The safety pause.** Before beginning any procedure, the entire team should take a "safety pause" or "time out" to ascertain that the correct procedure is to be performed on the correct patient and, if appropriate, on the correct side (e.g., thoracostomy tube, central venous catheter placement). This pause should be incorporated into the checklist for the procedure.

G. **Education and supervision.** Individuals should be trained in the conduct of procedures before performing the procedure on patients. This training should include a discussion of indications, possible complications and their treatment, alternatives, and the techniques to be used. For some procedures, there are mannequins or other options for simulation training, which also offer the opportunity to refine team skills. Experienced operators should be available at all times to provide further guidance and needed assistance.

H. **Documentation.** Careful documentation of procedures enhances patient care. For example, noting difficulties encountered at intubation or the size and positioning of an endotracheal tube used provides important information if the procedure must be repeated. We routinely write notes after all procedures, including unsuccessful attempts. We document the date and time, indications, performance of the safety pause, monitoring, premedication for pain control, the techniques used, difficulties encountered, complications (if any), and results of any laboratory tests performed.

II. BLOOD DRAWING. The preparations for withdrawing blood depend somewhat on the blood studies that are required.

A. **Capillary blood** is drawn when there is not a need for many serial studies in close succession.

1. **Applicable blood studies** include hematocrit, blood glucose (using glucometers or other point-of-care testing methods), bilirubin levels, electrolyte determinations, and, occasionally, blood gas studies.

2. **Techniques**
   a. The extremity to be used should be warmed to increase peripheral blood flow.
   b. **Spring-loaded lancets minimize pain** while ensuring a puncture adequate for obtaining blood. The blood should flow freely, with minimal or no squeezing. This will ensure the most accurate determination of laboratory values.
   c. **Capillary punctures of the foot should be performed on the lateral side of the sole of the heel,** avoiding previous sites if possible.
   d. **The skin should be cleaned carefully** with an antiseptic such as alcohol or povidone-iodine before puncture to avoid infection of soft tissue or underlying bone.

B. **Venous blood** for blood chemistry studies, blood cultures, and other laboratory studies can be obtained from a peripheral vein of adequate caliber to enable access and withdrawal of blood. The **antecubital and saphenous veins are often promising sites.** For blood cultures, the area should be cleaned with an alcohol or iodine-containing solution; if the position of the needle is directed by using a sterile-gloved finger, the finger should be cleaned in the same way. A new sterile needle should be used to insert the blood into the culture bottles.

C. **Arterial blood** may be needed for blood gases, some metabolic studies, and when the volume of blood needed would be difficult to obtain from a peripheral vein and no indwelling catheter is available. **Arterial punctures** are usually carried out by using the radial artery or posterior tibial artery. Rarely, the brachial artery is used when no other site is available. Radial artery punctures are most easily done using a 25- to 23-gauge butterfly needle and transillumination often aids in locating the vessel. After performing an Allen test to ensure collateral perfusion, the radial artery is visualized and entered with the bevel of the needle facing up and at a 15-degree angle against the direction of flow. (Recently, it has become controversial whether or not the Allen test should be considered the standard of care, especially regarding the interpretation of an abnormal test.) If blood is not obtained during the initial insertion of the needle, it can be advanced until the artery is transfixed, and then slowly withdrawn until blood flow occurs.

D. **Catheter blood samples**

1. **Umbilical artery or radial artery catheters** are often used for repetitive blood samples, especially for blood gas studies.

2. **Techniques**

   a. **A needleless system for blood sampling** from arterial catheters **should be used**. Specific techniques for use vary with the product and the manufacturer's guidelines should be followed.

   b. For **blood gas studies**, a 1-mL preheparinized syringe or a standard 1-mL syringe rinsed with 0.5 mL of heparin is used to withdraw the sample. The rate of sample withdrawal should be limited to 1.5 mL/minute to avoid altering downstream arterial perfusion.

   c. **The catheter must be adequately cleared of infusate** before withdrawing samples **to avoid false readings**. After the sample is drawn, blood should be cleared by infusing a small volume of heparinized saline-flushing solution.

III. INTRAVENOUS THERAPY. The insertion and management of intravenous catheters require great care. As in older infants, hand veins are used most often, but veins in the arms, foot, ankle, and scalp can be used. Transillumination of an extremity can help identify a vein, and newer devices that enhance the detection of veins may be even more useful.

IV. BLADDER TAP

A. Because bladder taps are most often used to obtain urine for culture, **a sterile technique is crucial**. Careful cleaning with an antiseptic such as alcohol or an iodine solution over the prepubic region is essential.

B. **Technique.** Bladder taps are done with a 5- to 10-mL syringe attached to a 22- or 23-gauge needle or to a 23-gauge butterfly needle. Before the tap, one should try to determine that the baby has not recently urinated. Ultrasonographic guidance is useful. One technique is as follows:

1. The pubic bone is located by touch.

2. The needle is placed in the midline, just superior to the pubic bone.

3. The needle is inserted and aimed at the infant's coccyx.

4. If the needle goes in >3 cm and no urine is obtained, one should assume that the bladder is empty and wait before attempting again.

V. LUMBAR PUNCTURE

A. Technique

1. The infant should be placed in the lateral decubitus position or in the sitting position with legs straightened. The assistant should hold the infant firmly at the shoulders and buttocks so that the lower part of the spine is curved. Neck flexion should be avoided so as not to compromise the airway.

2. A sterile field is prepared and draped with towels. Chlorhexidine should not be used to sterilize the skin prior to an LP as it is specifically not intended to be introduced into the central nervous system.

3. A 22- to 24-gauge spinal needle with a stylet should be used. Use of a nonstyleted needle, such as a 25-gauge butterfly needle, may introduce skin into the subarachnoid space and is to be avoided.

4. The needle is inserted in the midline into the space between the fourth and fifth lumbar spinous processes. The needle is advanced gradually in the direction of the umbilicus, and the stylet is withdrawn frequently to detect the presence of spinal fluid. Usually, a slight "pop" is felt as the needle enters the subarachnoid space.

5. The cerebrospinal fluid (CSF) is collected into three or four tubes, each with a volume of 0.5 to 1.0 mL.

B. Examination of the spinal fluid.
CSF should be inspected immediately for turbidity and color. In many newborns, normal CSF may be mildly xanthochromic, but it should always be clear.

1. **Tube 1.** Cell count and differential should be determined from the unspun fluid in a counting chamber. The unspun fluid should be stained with methylene blue; it should be treated with concentrated acetic acid if there are numerous red blood cells (RBCs). The centrifuged sediment should be stained with Gram and Wright stains.

2. **Tube 2.** Culture and sensitivity studies should be obtained.

3. **Tube 3.** Glucose and protein determinations should be obtained.

4. **Tube 4.** The cells in this tube should also be counted if the fluid is bloody. The fluid can be sent for other tests (such as polymerase chain reaction amplification for herpes simplex virus [HSV], etc.).

C. Information obtainable

1. When the CSF is collected in three or four separate containers, an **RBC count** can be measured on the first and last tubes to see if there is a decrease in the number of RBCs/mm^3 between the first and last specimens. In fluid obtained from a traumatic tap, the final tube will have fewer RBCs than the first; more equal numbers suggest the possibility of an intracranial hemorrhage. CSF in the newborn may normally contain up to 600 to 800 RBCs/mm^3.

2. **White blood cell (WBC) count.** The normal number of WBCs/mm^3 in newborns is a matter of controversy. We accept from 5 to 8 lymphocytes or monocytes as normal if there are no polymorphonuclear WBCs. Others accept up to 25 WBCs/mm^3 as normal, including several polymorphonuclear cells. Data obtained from high-risk newborns without meningitis (see Table 66.1) show 0 to 32 WBCs/mm^3 in term infants and 0 to 29 WBCs/mm^3 in preterm infants

Table 66.1	Cerebrospinal Fluid Examination in High-risk Neonates without Meningitis	
Determination	Term	Preterm
White blood cell count (cells/mL)		
No. of infants	87	30
Mean	8.2	9.0
Median	5	6
Standard deviation		
Range	0–32	0–29
± 2 Standard deviations	0–22.4	0–25.4
Percentage of polymorphonuclear cells	61.3%	57.2%
Protein (mg/dL)		
No. of infants	35	17
Mean	90	115
Range	20–170	65–150
Glucose (mg/dL)		
No. of infants	51	23
Mean	52	50
Range	34–119	24–63
Glucose in cerebrospinal fluid divided by blood glucose (%)		
No. of infants	51	23
Mean	81	74
Range	44–248	55–105

From Sarff LD, Platt LH, McCracken GH Jr. Cerebrospinal fluid evaluation in neonates: comparison of high-risk neonates with and without meningitis. *J Pediatr* 1976;88(3):473–477.

with approximately 60% polymorphonuclear cells to be within the normal range. Higher WBC counts are generally seen with gram-negative meningitis than with group B streptococcal disease; as high as 50% of the latter group will have 100 WBCs/mm^3 or less. Because of the overlap between normal infants and those with meningitis, the presence of polymorphonuclear leukocytes in CSF deserves careful attention. Ultimately, the diagnosis depends on culture results and clinical course.

3. Data on **glucose and protein levels** in CSF from high-risk newborns are shown in Table 66.1. Normally, the CSF glucose level is approximately 80% of the blood glucose level for term infants and 75% for preterm infants. If the blood glucose level is high or low, there is a 4- to 6-hour equilibration period with the CSF glucose.

   The normal level of CSF protein in newborns may vary over a wide range. In full-term infants, levels below 100 mg/dL are acceptable. In premature infants, the acceptable level can be as high as 180 mg/dL. Values for high-risk infants are shown in Table 66.1. The level of CSF protein in the premature infant appears to be related to the degree of prematurity.

   No single parameter can be used to rule out or rule in meningitis. Meningitis may occur in the absence of positive blood cultures (see Chap. 49).

VI. INTUBATION

A. **Endotracheal intubation.** In most cases, an infant can be adequately ventilated by bag and mask so that endotracheal intubation can be performed as a controlled procedure.

1. **Tube size and length.** The correct tube size (see Chap. 5) and depth of insertion (see Fig. 66.1) can be estimated from the infant's weight.

2. **Route.** Contradictory data exist over the preferred route for endotracheal intubation (i.e., oral vs. nasal). In most circumstances, local practice should guide this selection with two exceptions. First, oral intubation should be performed in all emergent situations, as it is generally easier and quicker than nasal intubation. In addition, oral intubation is preferable when significant coagulopathy (e.g., thrombocytopenia) exists. Second, a functioning endotracheal tube should never be electively changed simply to provide an alternate route.

3. **Technique**

   a. **The patient should be adequately ventilated using bag and mask** to ensure that the patient has normal oxygen saturations (appropriate for gestational age) before laryngoscopy. Laryngoscopy and intubation of an active, unmedicated patient is more uncomfortable for the patient and more difficult for the operator, and the risk of complications may be increased. Whenever possible, the patient should be premedicated with a narcotic or short-acting benzodiazepine, unless the patient's condition is a contraindication (see Chap. 67).

   b. Throughout the intubation procedure, **observation of the patient and monitoring of the heart rate are mandatory.** Pulse oximetry should also be used when available. Electronic monitoring with an audible pulse rate enables the team to be aware of the heart rate throughout the procedure. If bradycardia is observed, especially if accompanied by hypoxia, the procedure should be stopped, and the baby should be ventilated with bag and mask. An anesthesia bag attached to the tube adapter can deliver oxygen to the pharynx during the procedure. Alternatively, free-flow oxygen at 5 L/min can be given from a tube placed at one-half inch from the infant's mouth.

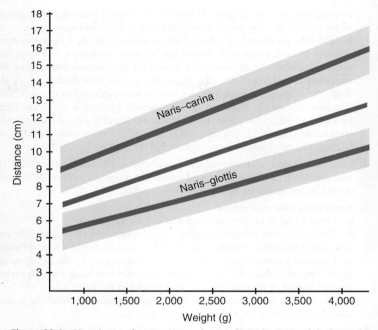

Figure 66.1. The relation of naris–carina and naris–glottis distance with body weight. The middle line represents the distance from naris to midtrachea. (Modified from Coldiron JS. Estimation of nasotracheal tube length in neonates. *Pediatrics* 1968;41[4]:823–828.)

c. The baby's neck should be slightly extended (the "sniffing" position) with the baby's body aligned straight. The operator should stand looking down the midline of the body.

d. The **laryngoscope** is held between the thumb and first finger of the left hand, with the second and third fingers holding the baby's chin and stabilizing the head.

e. The **laryngoscope blade** is passed into the right side of the mouth and then to the midline, sweeping the tongue up and out of the way. The blade tip should be advanced into the vallecula, and the handle of the laryngoscope raised to an angle of approximately 60 degrees, relative to the bed. The blade should then be lifted while maintaining the same angle, with care being taken not to rock or lever the laryngoscope blade. Visualization of the vocal cords may be improved by pushing down slightly on the larynx with the fourth or fifth finger of the left hand (or having an assistant do it) to displace the trachea posteriorly.

f. The **endotracheal tube** is held with the right hand and inserted between the vocal cords to approximately 2 cm below the glottis (less in extremely small infants). During nasotracheal intubation, the tube can be guided by moving the baby's head slightly or with small Magill-type forceps. If a finger is pressing on the trachea, the tube can be felt passing through.

g. The anatomic structures of the larynx and pharynx have different appearances. The esophagus is a horizontal posterior muscular slit. The glottis, in contrast, consists of an anterior triangular opening formed by the vocal cords meeting anteriorly at the apex. This orifice lies directly beneath the epiglottis, which is lifted away by gentle upward traction with the laryngoscope.

h. The **tube position** is checked by auscultation of the chest to ensure equal aeration of both lungs and observation of chest movement with positive-pressure inflation. An end-tidal CO_2 monitor is recommended to confirm the intratracheal position of the tube. If air entry is poor over the left side of the chest, the tube should be pulled back until it becomes equal to the right side. The insertion length of an oral tube is generally between 6 and 7 cm when measured at the lip for the smallest babies, and 8 and 9 cm for term or near-term babies (Fig. 66.1). The tube will "steam up" if it is correctly placed in the trachea. The baby should show improved oxygenation.

4. Once correct position is ascertained, the tube should be held against the palate with one finger until it can be taped securely in place; the position of the tube should be confirmed by radiograph when possible.

5. Commonly observed errors
  a. Focus is placed on the procedure and not on the patient.
  b. The baby's neck is hyperextended. This displaces the cords anteriorly and obscures visualization or makes the passing of the endotracheal tube difficult.
  c. Excessive pressure is placed on the infant's upper gum by the laryngoscope blade. This result from the tip of the laryngoscope blade being tilted or rocked upward instead of traction being exerted parallel to the baby.
  d. The tube is inserted too far and the position not assessed, resulting in continued intubation of the right main stem bronchus.

6. Laryngeal mask airway (LMA). Occasionally, it is not possible for a team to successfully insert an endotracheal tube despite multiple attempts. In these cases, the LMA can be a life-saving alternative to provide rescue ventilation until a more stable airway can be established. The size 1 LMA is appropriate and recommended for infants weighing 2.5 to 5 kg, although there are reports of its successful use in preterm babies as small as 0.8 kg.

  The LMA may be especially useful during the initial resuscitation after birth. It cannot, however, be used as a route for tracheal suctioning (e.g., for meconium-stained fluid).

B. Nasal continuous positive airway pressure (CPAP). Continuous distending pressure can be applied using nasal prongs as part of the ventilator circuit. These are simple to insert and are held on by a Velcro-fastened headset. In unusual circumstances, CPAP can be delivered through an appropriately sized endotracheal tube passed nasally and advanced to a pharyngeal position just inferior to the uvula. This tube is then connected to the ventilator circuit as in the preceding text.

VII. THORACENTESIS AND CHEST TUBE PLACEMENT (see Chap. 38)

VIII. VASCULAR CATHETERIZATION (see Figs. 66.2 and 66.3 for diagrams of the newborn venous and arterial systems).

A. Types of catheters
  1. Umbilical artery catheters (UACs) are used (i) for frequent monitoring of arterial blood gases, (ii) as a stable route for infusion of parenteral fluids, and (iii) for continuous monitoring of arterial blood pressure.

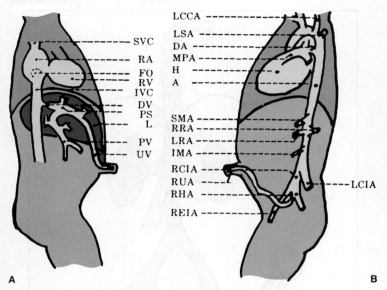

Figure 66.2. A: Diagram of the newborn umbilical venous system (SVC = superior vena cava; RA = right atrium; FO = foramen ovale; RV = right ventricle; IVC = inferior vena cava; DV = ductus venosus; PS = portal sinus; L = liver; PV = portal vein; UV = umbilical vein). **B:** Diagram of the newborn arterial system, including the umbilical artery (LCCA = left common carotid artery; LSA = left subclavian artery; DA = ductus arteriosus; MPA = main pulmonary artery; H = heart; A = aorta; SMA = superior mesenteric artery; RRA = right renal artery; LRA = left renal artery; IMA = inferior mesenteric artery; LCIA = left common iliac artery; RCIA = right common iliac artery; RUA = right umbilical artery; RHA = right hypogastric artery; REIA = right external iliac artery). (From Kitterman JA, Phibbs RH, Tooley WH. Catheterization of umbilical vessels in newborn infants. *Pediatr Clin North Am* 1970;17[4]:895–912.)

2. **Peripheral artery catheters** are used when frequent blood gas monitoring is still required and an umbilical artery catheter is contraindicated, cannot be placed, or is removed because of complications. Peripheral artery catheters must not be used to infuse alimentation solution or medications. They require that motion of the infant's extremity be kept restricted.

3. **Umbilical vein catheters (UVC)** are used for exchange transfusions, monitoring of central venous pressure, infusion of fluids (when passed through the ductus venous and near the right atrium), and emergency vascular access for infusion of fluid, blood, or medications.

4. **Central venous catheters** are used largely for prolonged parenteral nutrition and occasionally to monitor central venous pressure and can also be placed percutaneously. Preferred veins are the basilic or saphenous, the cephalic or lesser saphenous, or the median antecubital. Alternate veins are the brachial (with caution to avoid arterial cannulation), posterior auricular, superficial temporal, or external jugular.

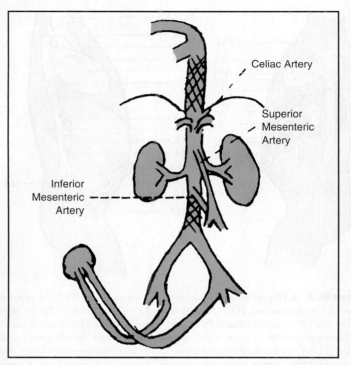

Figure 66.3. Localization of umbilical artery catheters. The cross-hatched areas represent sites in which complications are least likely. Either site may be used for placement of the catheter tip.

B. Umbilical artery catheterization

1. **Guidelines.** In general, only seriously ill infants should have an umbilical artery catheter placed. If only a few blood gas measurements are anticipated, peripheral arterial punctures should be performed together with noninvasive oxygen monitoring, and a peripheral intravenous route should be used for fluids and medications.

2. **Technique**

   a. Sterile technique is used. Before preparing cord and skin, make external measurements to determine how far the catheter will be inserted (see Figs. 66.3–66.5). For a high UAC, the distance is usually (umbilicus-to-shoulder) +2 cm plus the length of the stump. In a high setting, the catheter tip is placed between the sixth and tenth thoracic vertebrae; in a low setting, the tip is between the third and fourth lumbar vertebrae.

   b. The cord stump is suspended with forceps. It and the surrounding area are washed carefully with an antiseptic solution. In infants, the optimal agent is not clear. Chlorhexidine (for patients with mature skin) and alcohol are common choices. It is important to avoid chemical burns caused by iodine solution by carefully cleaning the skin (including the back and trunk) with sterile

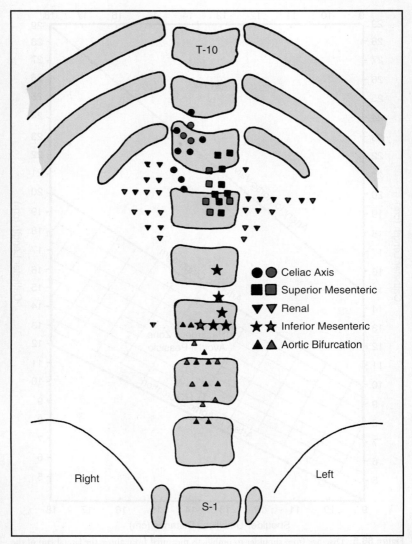

Figure 66.4. Distribution of the major aortic branches found in 15 infants by aortography as correlated with the vertebral bodies. Filled symbols represent infants with cardiac or renal anomalies (or both); open symbols represent those without either disorder. Major landmarks appear at the following vertebral levels: diaphragm, T12 interspace; celiac artery, T12; superior mesenteric artery, L1 interspace; renal artery, L1; inferior mesenteric artery, L3; aortic bifurcation, L4. (From Phelps DL, Lachman RS, Leake RD, et al. The radiologic localization of the major aortic tributaries in the newborn infant. *J Pediatr* 1972;81[2]:336–339.)

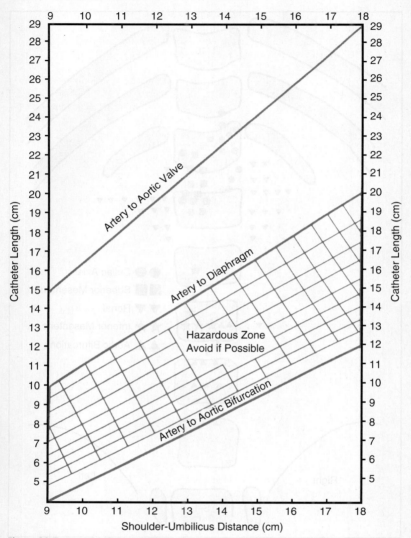

Figure 66.5. Distance from shoulder to umbilicus measured from above the lateral end of the clavicle to the umbilicus as compared with the length of umbilical artery catheter needed to reach the designated level. (From Dunn PM. Localization of the umbilical catheter by postmortem measurement. *Arch Dis Child* 1969;41:69.)

water after the solution has dried. For extremely preterm infants (<28 weeks), alcohol can also cause a chemical burn and should be washed off with sterile water as above. Following this, the abdomen is draped with sterile towels.

c. Umbilical (twill) tape should be placed as a simple tie around the base of the cord itself. In unusual circumstances, it is necessary to place the tape on the umbilical skin itself. If this is done, care must be taken to loosen the tie after the procedure. The tape is used to gently constrict the cord to prevent bleeding. The cord is then cut cleanly with a scalpel to a length of 1.0 to 1.5 cm.

d. **The cord is stabilized** with a forceps or hemostat, and the two arteries are identified.

e. The open tip of an iris forceps is inserted into the artery lumen and gently used to **dilate the vessel**; and then the closed tip is inserted into the lumen of an artery to a depth of 0.5 cm. Tension on the forceps tip is released, and the forceps is left in place to dilate the vessel for approximately 1 minute. This pause may be the most useful step in insertion of the catheter.

f. **The forceps is withdrawn**, and a sterile saline-filled 3.5F or 5F umbilical vessel catheter with an end hole is threaded into the artery. The smaller catheter is generally used for infants weighing <1,500 g. A slightly increased resistance will be felt as the catheter passes through the base of the cord and as it navigates the umbilical artery–femoral artery junction. The following problems with umbilical artery catheterization may occur.

  i. **The catheter will not pass into the abdominal aorta.** Sometimes, a double-catheter technique will allow successful cannulation in this situation, especially if the first catheter has made a false track and is no longer in the lumen of the umbilical artery. Leave the original catheter in place and gently pass a second catheter along side it.

  ii. **The catheter may pass into the aorta but then loop caudad back down the contralateral iliac artery** or out in one of the arteries to the buttocks. There may be difficulty in advancing the catheter and cyanosis or blanching of the leg or buttocks may occur. This happens more frequently when a small catheter (3.5 Fr) is placed in a large baby. Sometimes, using a larger, stiffer catheter (5 Fr) will allow the catheter to advance up the aorta. Alternatively, retracting the catheter into the umbilical artery, rotating it, and readvancing it into the aorta may result in aortic placement. If this fails, the catheter should be removed and placement attempted through the other umbilical artery. Sometimes, the catheter goes up the aorta and then loops back on itself. This also happens more frequently when a small catheter is used in a large baby. The catheter may also enter any of the vessels coming off the aorta. If the catheter cannot be advanced to the desired position, the tip should be pulled to a low position or the catheter should be removed.

  iii. **There is persistent cyanosis, blanching, or poor distal extremity perfusion.** This may be improved by warming the contralateral leg, but if there is no improvement, the catheter should be removed. **Hematuria** is also an indication for catheter removal.

g. When the catheter is advanced, the appropriate distance and placement should be confirmed by radiographic examination.

h. The catheter should be fixed in place with a purse-string suture using silk thread, and a tape bridge added for further stability (see Chap. 63).

3. Catheter removal

a. The umbilical artery catheter should be removed when either of the following criteria is met.

  i. The infant improves such that continuous monitoring and frequent blood drawings are no longer necessary.

   ii. A maximum dwell time of 7 days is recommended by the Centers for Disease Control and Prevention (CDC) to reduce infectious and thrombotic complications.

   iii. Complications are noted.

   b. Method of catheter removal. The catheter is removed slowly over a period of 30 to 60 seconds, allowing the umbilical artery to constrict at its proximal end while the catheter is still occluding the distal end. This usually prevents profuse bleeding. Old sutures should be removed. If bleeding should occur despite this method, pressure should be held at the stump of the umbilical artery until the bleeding ceases. This may take several minutes.

4. **Complications associated with umbilical artery catheterization.** Significant morbidity can be associated with complications of umbilical artery catheterization. These complications are mainly due to vascular accidents, including thromboembolic phenomena to the kidney, bowel, legs, or rarely the spinal cord. These may manifest as hematuria, hypertension, signs of necrotizing enterocolitis or bowel infarction, and cyanosis or blanching of the skin of the back, buttocks, or legs. Other complications seen are infection, disseminated intravascular coagulation, and vessel perforation. All these complications are indications for catheter removal. Close observation of the skin, monitoring of the urine for hematuria, measuring blood pressure, and following the platelet count may give clues to complications.

   a. We perform Doppler ultrasonographic examination of the aorta and renal vessels in infants in whom we are concerned about vascular complications. If thrombi are observed, the catheter is removed.

   b. If there are small thrombi without symptoms or with increased blood pressure alone, we usually remove the catheter, follow the resolution of the thrombi by ultrasonographic examination, and treat hypertension if necessary (see Chap. 28). If there are signs of emboli or loss of pulses, or coagulopathy, and no intracranial hemorrhage is present, we consider heparinization and maintaining the partial thromboplastin time (PTT) to double the control value. Published data to guide practice are limited. If there is a large clot with impairment of perfusion, we consider the use of fibrinolytic agents (see Chap. 44). Surgical treatment of thrombosis is not generally effective.

   c. Blanching of a leg following catheter placement is the most common complication noted clinically. Although this often occurs transiently, it deserves careful attention. One technique that may reverse this finding is to warm the opposite leg. If the vasospasm resolves, the catheter may be left in place. If there is no improvement, the catheter should be removed.

5. **Other considerations**

   a. Use of heparin for anticoagulation to prevent clotting. Whether the use of heparin in the infusate decreases the incidence of thrombotic complications is not known. We use diluted heparin 0.5 unit/mL of infusate.

   b. Positioning of the catheter tip. Little helpful information convincingly supports the choice between high and low placement of UACs. A higher complication rate has been reported in infants with the catheter tip at L3 to L4, compared with T6 to T10, owing to more episodes of blanching and cyanosis of one or both legs. No difference between the high- and low-position groups was seen in the rate of complications requiring catheter removal. Renal complications and emboli to the bowel may be more common with catheter tips placed at T6 to T10 while catheters placed low (L3–L4) are associated with complications such as cyanosis and blanching of the leg, which are easier to observe.

    c. Indwelling time. The incidence of complications associated with umbilical artery catheterization appears to be directly related to the length of time the catheter is left in place. The need for the catheter should be reassessed daily, and the catheter should be removed as soon as possible.

6. **Infection and use of antibiotics.** We do not use prophylactic antibiotics for placement of UACs. In infants with UACs, we use antibiotics whenever infection is suspected and after appropriate cultures have been obtained ensuring the coverage of coagulase-negative *Staphylococcus aureus*.

C. **Umbilical vein catheterization** (see Figs. 66.2 and 66.6).

1. **Indications.** We use umbilical vein catheterization for emergency vascular access and exchange transfusions; in these cases, the venous catheter is replaced by a peripheral intravenous catheter or other access as soon as possible. In critically ill and extremely premature infants, we also use an umbilical vein catheter to infuse vasopressors and as the primary route of venous access in the first several days after birth.

2. **Technique**

    a. The site is prepared as for umbilical artery catheterization after determining the appropriate length of catheter to be inserted (Fig. 66.6).

    b. Any clots seen are removed with forceps, and the umbilical vein is gently dilated as with the umbilical artery in VIII.C.

    c. The catheter (3.5 Fr or 5 Fr) is prepared by filling the lumen with heparinized saline solution and 1 unit/mL of saline solution through an attached syringe. The catheter should never be left open to the atmosphere because negative intrathoracic pressure could cause an air embolism.

    d. The catheter is inserted while gentle traction is exerted on the cord. Once the catheter is in the vein, one should try to slide the catheter cephalad just under the skin, where the vein runs very superficial. If the catheter is being placed for emergency (vascular access) or for an exchange transfusion, it should be advanced only as far as is necessary to establish good blood flow (usually 2–5 cm). If the catheter is being used for continuous infusion or to monitor central venous pressure, it should be advanced through the ductus venosus into the inferior vena cava and its position verified by x-ray.

    e. Only isotonic solutions should be infused until the position of the catheter is verified by x-ray studies. If the catheter tip is in the inferior vena cava, hypertonic solutions may be infused.

    f. If no other access is available, catheters may be left in place for up to 14 days; after which the increased risk of infectious or other complications is excessive. In very low birth weight infants, our practice is to change access to a peripherally placed central venous catheter by 10 days whenever possible.

D. **Multiple-lumen catheters for umbilical venous catheterization**

1. **Indications.** Placement of a double- or triple-lumen catheter into the umbilical vein provides additional venous access for administration of incompatible solutions (e.g., those containing vasopressor agents, sodium bicarbonate, or calcium). The use of a multiple-lumen catheter significantly reduces the need for multiple peripheral intravenous catheters and skin punctures and is preferred in very low birth weight infants.

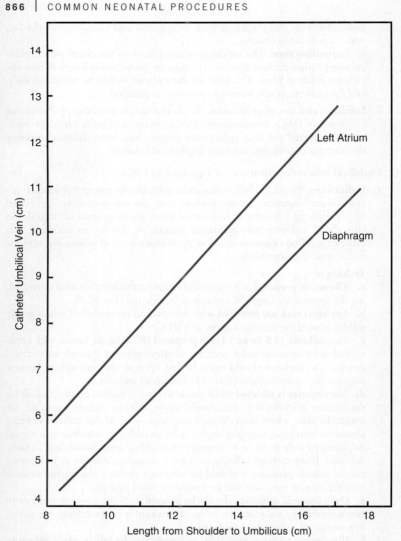

Figure 66.6. Catheter length for umbilical vein catheterization. The catheter tip should be placed between the diaphragm and the left atrium. (From Dunn PM. Localization of the umbilical catheter by postmortem measurements. *Arch Dis Child* 1966;41:69.)

2. Technique

a. Direct placement. Multiple-lumen catheters are inserted according to the same procedure as single-lumen catheters described above. The increased pliability of many of the multiple-lumen catheters makes inadvertent passage into the hepatic veins more likely.

b. Modified Seldinger technique. In patients with an indwelling single-lumen catheter, a wire exchange technique may be used to change to a multiple-lumen catheter. Although this method decreases the probability of catheter loss during exchange, it entails the risks of wire passage including cardiac dysrhythmias and perforation and should be attempted only by those familiar with the Seldinger technique.

3. Usage. All compatible continuous infusions should run through one port and a heparinized infusion of saline and/or dextrose as needed should run through the second port; it can be interrupted to give intermittent therapies such as antibiotics or blood products and can be accessed to draw blood for laboratory testing. The fewer times the line is entered, the lower the risk of introducing a catheter associated blood stream infection.

E. Percutaneous radial artery catheterization. Placement of an indwelling radial artery catheter is a useful alternative to umbilical artery catheterization for monitoring blood gas levels and blood pressure.

1. Advantages

a. Accessibility (when the umbilical artery is inaccessible or has been used for a long period).

b. Reflection of preductal flow (if the right radial artery is used).

c. Avoidance of thrombosis of major vessels, which is sometimes associated with umbilical vessel catheterization.

2. Risks are usually small if the procedure is performed carefully, but infection, air embolus, inadvertent injection of incorrect solution, and arterial occlusion may occur.

3. Equipment required includes a 22- or 24-gauge intravenous cannula with stylet, a T-connector, heparinized saline flushing solution (0.5–1.0 unit of heparin per milliliter of solution), and an infusion pump.

4. Method of catheterization

a. The adequacy of the ulnar collateral flow to the hand must be assessed. The radial and ulnar arteries should be simultaneously compressed, and the ulnar artery should then be released. The degree of flushing of the blanched hand should be noted. If the entire hand becomes flushed while the radial artery is occluded, the ulnar circulation is adequate.

b. The hand may be secured on an arm board with the wrist extended, leaving all fingertips exposed to observe color changes.

c. The wrist is prepared with an antiseptic such as alcohol or an iodine-containing solution, and the site of maximum arterial pulsation is palpated.

d. The intravenous cannula is inserted through the skin at an angle of <30 degrees to horizontal and is slowly advanced into the artery. Transillumination may help delineate the vessel and its course. If the artery is entered as the catheter is advanced, the stylet is removed and the catheter is advanced in the artery. If there is no blood return, the artery may be transfixed. The stylet is then removed, and the catheter is slowly withdrawn until blood flow occurs; then it is advanced into the vessel.

5. Caution. Only heparinized saline solution (0.45%–0.9%) is infused into the catheter. The minimum infusion rate is 0.8 mL/hour; the maximum is 2 mL/hour.

F. Percutaneous central venous catheterization is useful for long-term venous access for intravenous fluids, particularly parenteral nutrition.

1. **Peripheral vein catheterization** is useful in infants weighing <1,500 g. This is the primary method of central venous access.

   a. The equipment required includes sterile towels, a 1.1 Fr or 1.9 Fr silicone or double-lumen polyurethane catheter cut to the appropriate length, a splittable introducer needle, and iris forceps.

   b. Technique. Careful attention to sterile technique is required including the provision of adequate space for equipment. The operator should be assisted by another caregiver who can obtain additional equipment as needed, ensure integrity of the sterile field, and monitor the progress of the procedure using a specific checklist. The infant is sedated and placed supine. An appropriate vein of entry is selected. This may be a basilic, greater saphenous, or external jugular vein. The cephalic vein should be avoided, as central placement is more difficult. The site is prepared with an antiseptic solution such as chlorhexidine (for infants with mature skin) or alcohol, and the introducer needle is inserted into the vein until blood flows freely. The silicone catheter is inserted through the needle with forceps and is slowly advanced the predetermined distance for central venous positioning. The introducer needle is removed, the extra catheter length is coiled on the skin near the insertion site, and the site is covered with transparent surgical covering. The catheter tip is positioned at the junction of the vena cava and right atrium, as confirmed by radiography. Especially with the smaller gauge catheters, visualization is best accomplished by an oblique radiograph, so as to separate the catheter position from that of the cardiothymic silhouette. Some physicians inject a small amount of isotonic contrast material to make visualization easier.

   c. Complications include hemorrhage during insertion, infection, and thrombosis of the catheter, but these are unusual. Some babies will develop a thrombophlebitis, usually within 24 hours of catheter placement. Care must be taken when flushing or infusing to minimize the pressure on the catheter, which could cause catheter rupture. By using a larger syringe (10 mL), infusion pressure is reduced over that obtained with a smaller (3 mL) syringe.

2. **Subclavian vein catheterization** may occasionally be useful in infants weighing >1,200 g, although in general, a surgically placed central venous catheter is preferred when other access cannot be established. Operators should receive specific training in this procedure before performing it.

IX. ABDOMINAL PARACENTESIS FOR REMOVAL OF ASCITIC FLUID

A. Indications

1. Therapeutic indications include respiratory distress resulting from abdominal distension (e.g., hydropic infants, infants with urinary ascites) for which removal of ascitic fluid will ameliorate respiratory symptoms. In addition, interference with urine production or lower extremity perfusion resulting from increased intra-abdominal pressure may be improved by paracentesis.

2. Diagnostic indications include the evaluation of suspected peritonitis.

B. **Technique**

1. The equipment needed includes an 18- to 22-gauge intravenous catheter, three-way stopcock, and a 10- to 50-mL syringe.

2. The lower abdomen is prepared with antiseptic such as alcohol or povidone-iodine solution and the area is draped. If the bladder is distended, it is drained with manual pressure or a urinary catheter. A local anesthetic such as 1% lidocaine (Xylocaine) is infiltrated into the subcutaneous tissues when possible. The catheter should be inserted either in the midline or immediately lateral to the rectus sheath, at a level one-third of the distance between the umbilicus and the symphysis pubis. Once the tip is below the skin, the connected syringe should be aspirated as the catheter is advanced approximately 1 cm until the resistance of passing through the abdominal wall diminishes or fluid is obtained. Five to 10 mL of fluid is removed for diagnostic paracentesis while 10 to 20 mL/kg should be removed for therapeutic effects. The catheter is removed, and the site bandaged. Ultrasound guidance can be useful, especially in situations when the volume of intraperitoneal fluid is minimal enough that there is concern that the fluid may be difficult to locate or that an abdominal organ could accidentally be punctured during the procedure.

C. **Potential complications**

1. Cardiovascular effects, including tachycardia, hypotension, and decreased cardiac output may result from rapid redistribution of intravascular fluid to the peritoneal space following removal of large amounts of ascites.

2. Bladder or intestinal aspiration may occur more frequently in the presence of a dilated bladder or bowel. These puncture sites usually heal spontaneously and without significant clinical findings.

Suggested Readings

Barone JE, Madlinger RV. Should an Allen test be performed before radial artery cannulation? *J Trauma* 2006;61(2):468–470.

Fletcher MA, McDonald MG, Avery GB, eds. *Atlas of Procedures in Neonatology.* Philadelphia: JB Lippincott Co; 1994.

Garges HP, Moody MA, Cotten CM, et al. Neonatal meningitis: what is the correlation among cerebrospinal fluid cultures, blood cultures, and cerebrospinal fluid parameters? *Pediatrics* 2006;117(4):1094–1100.

Garland JS, Henrickson K, Maki DG. The 2002 Hospital Infection Control Practices Advisory Committee Centers for Disease Control and Prevention guideline for prevention of intravascular device-related infection. *Pediatrics* 2002;110(5):1009–1013.

Green R, Hauser R, Calafat AM, et al. Use of di(2-ethylhexyl) phthalate-containing medical products and urinary levels of mono(2-ethylhexyl) phthalate in neonatal intensive care unit infants. *Environ Health Perspect* 2005;113(9):1222–1225.

Latini G. Potential hazards of exposure to di-(2-ethylhexyl)-phthalate in babies. A review. *Biol Neonate* 2000;78(4):269–276.

Pronovost P, Needham D, Berenholtz S, et al. An intervention to decrease catheter-related bloodstream infections in the ICU. *N Engl J Med* 2006;355(26):2725–2732.

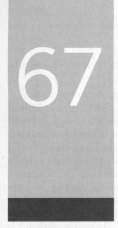

67 Preventing and Treating Pain and Stress among Infants in the Newborn Intensive Care Unit

Carol Spruill Turnage and Michelle A. LaBrecque

I. BACKGROUND. Recognition that both premature and full-term infants experience pain has led to increasing appreciation of the prevalent problem of undertreatment of stress and pain of infants who are hospitalized in the newborn intensive care unit (NICU). Both humanitarian considerations and scientific principles favor improved management strategies to prevent pain and stress whenever possible and, when discomfort is unavoidable, to provide prompt and appropriate treatment.

A. Fetal and neonatal physiologic responses to pain. Peripheral nerve receptors develop very early in gestation and are abundant by 22 weeks of gestation on most of the fetal body. Evidence of functional thalamocortical connections that are required for conscious perception of pain has been demonstrated as early as 29 weeks of gestation. Autonomic and endocrine responses to noxious stimuli are present even earlier in development. Although this stress response may not indicate fetal pain perception at a conscious level, it has harmful effects on the developing fetus, and the administration of analgesia has been shown to suppress these responses.

Early in development, overlapping nerve terminals create local hyperexcitable networks, enabling even low-threshold stimuli to produce an exaggerated pain response. Fetal wounds heal more quickly and with less scarring than those of infants, children, or adults. The process, in part, involves sprouting of sensory nerve endings in and near the site of tissue injury. Although it seems to enhance wound healing, hyperinnervation results in hypersensitivity to painful stimuli that persists after wound healing has occurred. Repeated noxious stimuli further alter sensitivity to painful stimuli and appear to lower the pain threshold, slow the recovery, and adversely affect long-term outcomes.

Physiologic responses to painful or stressful stimuli include increases in circulating catecholamines, increased heart rate and blood pressure, and elevated intracranial pressure. The fetus is capable of mounting a stress response at approximately 23 weeks of gestation. The autonomic and other markers of the stress response of the immature fetus or preterm infant, however, are less competent than that of the more mature infant or child. Therefore, among immature infants, neither the common vital sign changes associated with pain or stress (e.g., tachycardia, hypertension) nor behavioral cues (e.g., agitation) are reliable indicators of painful stimuli. Even when the infant's stress response is intact, persistence of painful stimuli for hours or days fatigues or deactivates the sympathetic nervous system response, obscuring the signs of pain or discomfort.

B. Medical and developmental outcomes

1. **Neonatal medical and surgical outcomes.** Neonatal responses to pain may worsen the compromised physiologic states such as hypoxia, hypercarbia, acidosis, hyperglycemia or respiratory distress. Early studies of surgical responses showed more stable intraoperative course and improved postoperative recovery among infants who received perioperative analgesia and anesthesia. Changes in intrathoracic pressure due to diaphragmatic splinting and vagal responses produced in response to pain following invasive procedures precipitate hypoxemic events and alterations in oxygen delivery and cerebral blood flow.

2. **Neurodevelopmental outcomes.** Behavioral and neurologic studies suggest that preterm infants who experience repeated painful procedures and noxious stimuli are less responsive to painful stimuli at 18 months corrected age. However, at 8 to 10 years of age, unlike their normal birth weight peers, infants who were born at or below 1,000 g birth weight rate medical pain intensity greater than measures of psychosocial pain. These data provide evidence that neonatal pain and stress influence neurodevelopment and affect later perceptions of painful stimuli and behavioral responses, and that prevention and control of pain are likely to benefit infants. There are few large randomized clinical trials of pain management. The Neurologic Outcomes and Preemptive Analgesia in Neonates (NEOPAIN) trial evaluated preemptive analgesia with morphine infusion up to 14 days among ventilated preterm infants and showed no overall difference in the primary composite outcome (neonatal death, severe intraventricular hemorrhage [IVH], or periventricular leukomalacia [PVL]) between placebo and preemptive morphine-treated groups. We use opioids to treat procedural or post operative pain but do not routinely use continuous opioid infusions for all ventilated preterm neonates. Morphine infusions should be used cautiously with extreme prematurity or preexisting hypotension. Analgesics or sedatives which have less cardiovascular effects, such as fentanyl or ketamine, may be better alternatives if required in these neonates.

II. PRINCIPLES OF PREVENTION AND MANAGEMENT OF NEONATAL PAIN AND STRESS

A. Principles of pain management in newborns include the following:

1. Neuroanatomic components and neuroendocrine systems of the neonate are sufficiently developed to allow transmission of painful stimuli.

2. Exposure to prolonged or severe pain may increase neonatal morbidity.

3. Infants who have experienced pain during the neonatal period respond differently to subsequent painful events.

4. Severity of pain and effects of analgesia can be assessed in the neonate using validated instruments.

5. Newborn infants usually are not easily comforted when analgesia is needed.

6. A lack of behavioral responses (including crying and movement) does not necessarily indicate the absence of pain.

   The pain intensity of the anticipated painful procedure from venipuncture to abdominal surgery differs dramatically. Careful thought and planning help the health care team to develop an appropriate pain management plan before a painful event.

B. **Current American Academy of Pediatrics (AAP) recommendations** for assessment and management of pain and stress in the newborn should be followed.

1. **Assessment of pain and stress in the newborn.** Newborns should be assessed for pain routinely, and before and after procedures, by caregivers who are trained to assess pain using multidimensional tools. The pain scales that were used should help guide caregivers to provide effective pain relief. Because small variations in scoring points can result in undertreatment or overtreatment, the proficiency of individual caregivers using the chosen pain scale should be reassessed periodically to maintain reliability in assessing pain. A video and case scenario is helpful.

2. **Reducing pain from bedside care procedures**

   a. Laboratory tests or procedures should be reviewed daily to reduce the number of unwarranted skin punctures and painful tests.

   b. The combination of either oral sucrose or glucose, breastfeeding, and other nonpharmacologic pain-reduction methods (nonnutritive sucking, kangaroo care, hand containment or facilitated tuck, and swaddling) are evidence-based interventions that reduce the pain response to heel stick or acutely painful events.

   c. Topical anesthetics can be used to reduce pain associated with venipuncture, lumbar puncture, and intravenous (IV) catheter insertion when time permits but are ineffective for heel-stick blood draws, and repeated use of topical anesthetics should be limited.

3. **Reducing pain from surgery.** Anticipation and planning for pain management is essential to the success of any pain management program. Information aids the planning process and includes postmenstrual age (PMA), acuity, comorbidities, type of procedure or surgery, and respiratory support along with standard hand-off communication to reduce variation in pain management.

   a. Health care facilities providing surgery for neonates should establish a protocol for pain management in collaboration with anesthesia, surgery, neonatology, nursing, and pharmacy. Such a protocol requires a coordinated, multidimensional strategy, and a priority in perioperative pain management.

   b. Sufficient anesthesia and analgesia is provided to prevent intraoperative pain and stress responses and decrease postoperative analgesic requirements.

   c. Surgical pain requires both preplanning and a well-defined "hand off" from physician to physician and recovery or operating room (OR) nurse to the NICU nurse. With specific attention to a review of medications received in the OR or recovery, a preemptive approach to pain management is more likely to succeed. Utilizing a written tool for the "hand off" report may decrease confusion from misinterpreted or lost information and delays in postoperative analgesia.

   d. Pain is routinely assessed using a valid, reliable scale designed for postoperative or prolonged pain in neonates.

   e. Opioids are the basis for postoperative analgesia after a major surgery in the absence of regional anesthesia. During the immediate postoperative period, opioids are most effective when scheduled at regular intervals. Although there is little evidence indicating a benefit of continuous opioid infusion over intermittent dosing, for safety and simplicity reasons, continuous infusions are recommended for major surgery in the neonate. Careful consideration to dosing and respiratory monitoring is essential. Dosing as needed (PRN) can lead to missed doses and fluctuating drug levels that do not provide adequate pain relief.

f. Postoperative analgesia is used for as long as pain assessment documentation indicates that it is required. Dosing intervals or dosages can be weaned if pain remains well controlled.

g. Elimination of opioids may be influenced by enterohepatic recirculation and elevated plasma concentrations, so monitoring for side effects should be maintained for several hours after opioids are discontinued.

h. Acetaminophen is sometimes used after surgery as an adjunct to regional anesthetics or opioids, but there are inadequate data on pharmacokinetics at gestational ages <28 weeks to permit calculation of appropriate dosages. Acetaminophen significantly reduces the pain response to tissue excision and pain scores during circumcision in some studies. Analgesic efficacy is disputed in other reports where acetaminophen did not relieve acute pain during heel stick or the postoperative pain from cardiac surgery.

4. Reducing pain from other major procedures

    a. Analgesia for chest drain insertion comprises all of the following:

        i. General nonpharmacologic measures

        ii. Systemic analgesia with a rapidly acting opiate such as fentanyl

        iii. Slow infiltration of the skin site with a local anesthetic before incision, unless there is life-threatening instability.

    b. Analgesia for chest drain removal comprises the following:

        i. General nonpharmacologic measures (especially positioning/swaddling)

        ii. Short-acting, rapid-onset systemic analgesia

    c. Data show anesthetic drops, oral sucrose administration, and containment reduce the pain response to eye exams for retinopathy of prematurity. There are no data on the effects of bright lighting following dilatation for eye exams. A thoughtful approach to minimize discomfort after an exam may be to decrease lighting or shield the infant's eyes from light for 4 to 6 hours.

    d. Retinal surgery should be considered as a major surgery, and effective opiate-based pain relief should be provided.

III. EVALUATING NEONATAL PAIN AND STRESS.

A number of validated and reliable scales of pain assessment are available. Behavioral indicators (e.g., facial expression, crying, body/extremity movement), as well as physiologic indicators (e.g., tachycardia or bradycardia, hypertension, tachypnea or apnea, oxygen desaturation, palmar sweating, vagal signs), are useful in assessing an infant's level of comfort or discomfort. Biochemical markers for pain and stress such as plasma cortisol or catecholamine levels are not typically used in the clinical setting but may be useful for research.

Physiologic responses to painful stimuli include release of circulating catecholamines, heart rate acceleration, blood pressure increase, and a rise in intracranial pressure. Because the stress response of the immature fetus or preterm infant is less robust than that of the more mature infant or child, gestational age at birth and PMA must be considered when evaluating the pain response. Among preterm infants who are experiencing pain, a change in vital signs associated with the stress response (e.g., tachycardia, hypertension) and agitation are not consistently evident. Even among infants with an intact response to pain, a painful stimulus that persists for hours or days exhausts the sympathetic nervous system output and obscures the clinician's ability to objectively assess the infant's level of discomfort.

Changes in vital signs are not specific to pain and may be unreliable when used alone to identify pain. Changes in facial activity and heart rate are the most sensitive measures of pain that were observed in term and preterm infants. By 25 to 26 weeks, the facial expression is the same as for children/adults. Before that, various facial components of a grimace may be observed separately such as eye squeeze. The premature infant pain profile (PIPP) scores the facial components separately to capture the lower birth weight infant who may be limited in the ability to produce and sustain a full grimace.

A. **Pain assessment.** Selecting the most appropriate tool for evaluating neonatal pain is essential to its management. Documentation of pain is just as crucial. In general, pain scores that are documented along with vital signs can be monitored more easily for trends and subtle patterns so pain, unrelieved pain, or opioid tolerance can be identified early. Physicians, nurses, and parents express different perceptions of pain cues when presented with the same infant pain responses. A caregiver's bias can influence both judgment and action when they are evaluating and treating pain. A pain-scoring tool with appropriate age range, acceptable psychometric properties, clinical utility, and feasibility may reduce bias even though none is perfect. Many tools exist and a few of the more common ones are shown in Table 67.1.

Table 67.1	Examples of Neonatal Pain Scoring Tools with Acceptable Psychometric Data		
Pain instrument	**Age range**	**Assessment items**	**Indications**
CRIES[1]	Neonates from 32–60 wk	**C**rying **R**equires increased oxygen **I**ncreased vital signs **E**xpression **S**leeplessness	Postoperative
Premature infant pain profile (PIPP)[2]	Tested in infants 27 wk to term	Gestational age Behavioral state Heart rate Oxygen saturation Brow bulge Eye squeeze Nasolabial furrow	Procedural postoperative up to 24 hours
Neonatal infant pain scale (NIPS)[3]	28–38 wk	Facial expression Crying Breathing pattern Arm movement Leg movement State of arousal	Procedural

[1]Krechel SW, Bildner J. CRIES: A new neonatal postoperative pain measurement score. Initial testing of validity and reliability. *Paediatric Anaesthesia* 1995;5:53–61.
[2]Stevens B, Johnston C, Petryshen P, Taddio A. Premature infant pain profile: Development and initial validation. *The Clinical Journal of Pain* 1996;12:13–22.
[3]Lawrence J, Alcock D, McGrath P, Kay J, MacMurray SB, Dulberg C. The development of a tool to assess neonatal pain. *Neonatal Network.* 1993;12:59–66.

1. **Critically ill infants.** Pain responses are influenced by the gestational age and behavioral state of an infant. Most pain scales that have been tested use acute pain for the stimulus (heel stick), and very few tools that measure acute-prolonged or chronic pain have been adequately tested. Critically ill infants may not be able to exhibit indicators of pain due to their illness acuity. Few scales include parameters of nonresponse that may be present when an infant is severely ill or extremely premature. A lack of response does not mean that an infant is not in pain. In that case, the caregiver will need to base treatment decisions on other data such as type of disease, health status, pain risk factors, maturity, invasive measures (i.e., chest tubes), medications that blunt response, and scheduled painful procedures. Existing pain instruments do not account for the extremely low birth weight infant whose immature physiologic and behavioral responses are challenging to interpret. Infants with neurologic impairment can mount a similar pain response as healthy term infants, although the intensity may be diminished. The pain response can be increased in individual infants based on prior pain history and handling before a painful event.

2. **Moderately ill or healthy infants.** Infants in intermediate or newborn nurseries experience painful procedures that require assessment and management. Pain scales that rely on many physiologic measures will not be appropriate for use in healthy newborns when cardiorespiratory monitoring is typically not used.

3. **Chronic or prolonged pain.** Physiologic and behavioral indicators can be markedly different when pain is prolonged. Infants may become passive with few or no body movements, little or no facial expression, less heart rate and respiratory variation, and, consequently, lower oxygen consumption. Caregivers may erroneously interpret these findings to indicate that these infants are not feeling pain due to their lack of physiologic or behavioral signs. Quality and duration of sleep, feeding, quality of interactions, and consolability combined with risk factors for pain may be more indicative of persistent pain. A promising tool for assessment of prolonged pain in preterm infants is the EDIN (*Échelle Douleur Inconfort Nouveau-Né*, neonatal pain and discomfort scale) (Debillon 2001), although psychometric evaluation is incomplete. There is evidence that repetitive and/or prolonged exposure to pain may increase the pain response (hyperalgesia) to future painful stimulation and may even result in pain sensation from nonpainful stimuli (allodynia).

Because no pain tool is completely accurate in identifying all types of pain in every infant, other patient data must be included in the assessment of pain. Pain that is persistent or prolonged, associated with end-of-life care, or influenced by medications cannot be reliably measured using current pain instruments.

IV. MANAGEMENT: PAIN PREVENTION AND TREATMENT.

Attention to the intensity of diagnostic, therapeutic, or surgical procedures that are commonly performed in the NICU is fundamental toward the development of strategies that are appropriate for mild, moderate, or severe pain levels. This should include consideration of the history, clinical status, and PMA of the patient. A decision matrix for pain management (Table 67.2) illustrates some options available based on anticipated pain level by procedure type. Diagnostic procedures such as heel lance, venipuncture,

Table 67.2 Pain Management Decision Matrix Based on Procedure Intensity

Procedure	Pacifier NNS*	Sucrose	Breast feed	Contain or Swaddle	Skin to Skin	Topical Anesthetic	Lidocaine Sub Q	Opioid	Other
Heel lance	+	+	+	+	+				Automated lance
IV insertion	+	+	+	+	+	+			
Eye exam	+	+		+		+ eye drops			
Lumbar puncture	+	+				+	+		Careful handling
Peripherally inserted central catheter (PICC) placement	+	+		+		+		+	Short-acting opioid (i.e., fentanyl) Guided ultrasound technique
Chest tube insertion/removal	+						+	+	Short-acting opioid
Endotracheal tube suctioning		+ / -		+				+	

Procedure							Treatment
Circumcision	+	+	+ (upper arms)	+/−	+		Mogen clamp preferred; dorsal penile nerve block, ring block, or caudal block; consider acetaminophen pre/post procedure
Ventriculoperitoneal shunt placement						+	General anesthesia + analgesia
Gastroschisis repair							Epidural anesthesia & analgesia
Ileostomy, colostomy closure							Epidural anesthesia & analgesia

*NNS = nonnutritive sucking

Procedure intensity legend: + = intervention appropriate; +/− = optional; Minimally invasive, acute, short duration = white; Invasive therapeutic procedures, acute-prolonged, moderate duration = light gray; Surgery, extended tissue injury; moderate to severe pain, prolonged duration = dark gray.

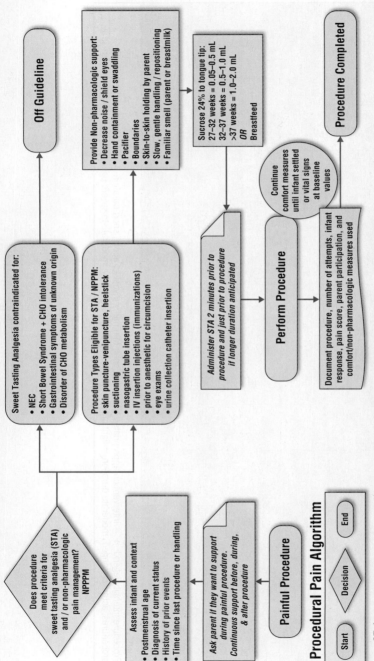

Figure 67.1. Procedural pain algorithm for sweet tasting analgesia or non-pharmacologic pain management.

or IV catheter insertion may depend on environmental, behavioral, and sweet tasting analgesia (sucrose, breastfeed) to decrease pain responses (Figure 67.1).

A. **Environmental and behavioral approaches.** Painful or stressful procedures should be reviewed daily and be limited to those based on medical necessity to decrease redundant or unwarranted blood sampling. Combining painful procedures with nonurgent routine care or prior handling may intensify the pain experience. The infant's eyes should be shielded when procedural lights are used or the infant is positioned where light is directed toward the face. Once the procedure is finished, a caregiver should stay to comfort and support the infant until physiologic and behavioral cues confirm recovery from the event.

B. **Physiologic interventions** consist of taste-mediated analgesia combined with nonpharmacologic strategies (e.g., environmental, hand containment or facilitated tucking, pacifier, skin-to-skin holding).

1. Sucrose analgesia 0.012 g to 0.12 g (0.05 mL to 0.5 mL of 24% solution) given orally 2 minutes before and just prior to the painful procedure is recommended for procedural pain and should be combined with other nonpharmacologic strategies such as nonnutritive sucking (e.g., pacifier), containment, eye protection from procedure lights, and decreased sound/activity around the bed. For procedures that last longer than 5 minutes, repeated dosing should be considered. Sweet-tasting solutions (sucrose and glucose) decrease the pain response in infants up to 12 months of age. Long-term outcomes from repeated dosing of sweet solutions in early infancy and in preterm infants are not known. Sucrose must be given on the tongue where taste buds for sweet taste are concentrated. Sucrose will not be effective if given by nasogastric tube.

2. Breast milk administered on the tongue before or during painful procedures is as effective as sucrose/glucose for single events. Repeated use of breastfeeding for pain has not been studied, so effects over time are unknown. Potential refusal of breast milk or breastfeeding, especially in preterm infants, should be considered until more is known about repeated use and whether the association with pain affects later feeding success.

C. **Pharmacologic management.** A number of considerations are relevant to the pharmacologic management of neonatal pain.

1. **Complementary therapies.** Environmental and behavioral interventions should be applied to all infants experiencing painful stimuli. These measures and sucrose analgesia are often useful in conjunction with pharmacologic treatments.

2. **Prophylaxis versus pain treatment.** Opioid analgesia given on a scheduled basis results in a lower total dose and improved pain control compared with "as needed" dosing.

3. **Gestational maturity.** Pain should be assumed and treatment should be initiated in the immature, acutely ill infant who may be incapable of mounting a stress response to signal his or her discomfort. The inability of the infant to mount an appropriate response is especially relevant when the infant is extremely immature or the painful stimulus is severe and/or prolonged.

4. The routine use of continuous infusions of morphine, fentanyl, or midazolam in chronically ventilated preterm neonates is not recommended by the AAP because of concern about short-term adverse effects and lack of long-term outcome data.

V. PHARMACOLOGIC TREATMENT OF PROCEDURE-RELATED PAIN

A. **Analgesia for minimally invasive procedures**

  1. **Sucrose.** Administration of 24% oral sucrose solution is an effective analgesic (see IV.B.1, in the preceding text).

  2. **Topical analgesia.** EMLA, a mixture of lidocaine and prilocaine, is safe and effective as a topical anesthetic and approved for use in neonates over 37 weeks of gestation. It is contraindicated in infants less than 1 year of age who concurrently take methemoglobin-inducing agents (i.e., sulfas, acetaminophen, phenobarbital).

B. **Analgesia for invasive procedures.** Opioids (e.g., morphine or fentanyl) and sedatives (e.g., midazolam or phenobarbital) are often used in treating critically ill newborns undergoing invasive or very painful diagnostic or therapeutic procedures (Table 67.2). Alleviating pain is the most important goal. Therefore, treatment with analgesics is recommended over sedation without analgesia.

  1. For the most invasive procedures, pharmacologic **premedication** is recommended. Except in instances of emergency intubation, newborns should be premedicated for invasive procedures. Examples of procedures for which premedication is indicated include elective intubation (Table 67.3), chest tube insertion or removal, peripheral arterial catheter placement, laser surgery, and circumcision.

  2. For **intubation**, the AAP recommends medication with fentanyl 1 to 3 mcg/kg. Fentanyl must be infused slowly (no faster than 1 mcg/kg/minute) to avoid complications of chest wall rigidity and impaired ventilation. Among infants at or near-term gestation undergoing an isolated procedure such as intubation, midazolam 0.1 mg/kg may be used in addition to opioid analgesia to lessen agitation, defensive movements, and potential trauma. For tracheal intubation, the addition of a short-acting muscle relaxant given after analgesia administration

Table 67.3	Premedication for Non-emergent Intubation: Preterm and Term Infant (see section V.B.2. and V.B.4.)
Medication Category	**Dose**
Opioid Analgesia	Fentanyl 0.5–4 mcg/kg IV infused over 2–5 minutes (preferred analgesia) Morphine 0.05–0.1 mg/mg IV
Sedative	Midazolam 0.05–0.1 mg/kg IV infused over 2–5 minutes (not recommended in preterm infants)
Anticholinergic agent	Atropine 0.02 mg/kg IV (for infants >2 kg) Acts by blocking vagal stimulation of heart
Neuromuscular Blocking agents (muscle relaxants)	Rocuronium 0.6–1.2 mg/kg IV Vecuronium 0.1 mg/kg IV

may decrease the procedure duration and number of attempts needed, thereby decreasing the potential for severe oxygen desaturation. Before adding a short-acting muscle relaxant (vecuronium, rocuronium) for intubation, airway control, and the ability to perform, effective bag-mask ventilation must be assured. **For the first few days of mechanical ventilation**, if analgesia is needed, medication with fentanyl 1 to 3 mcg/kg or morphine 0.05 to 0.15 mg/kg can be given every 4 hours. The AAP guideline on pain management does not recommend routine continuous opioid infusions in mechanically ventilated preterm neonates because of concern about short-term adverse effects and lack of data on long-term outcomes.

3. For **circumcision**, pretreatment includes both oral (24%) sucrose analgesia and acetaminophen 15 mg/kg preoperatively and, for the procedure, dorsal penile block or ring block with a maximum lidocaine dose of 0.5%, 0.5 mL/kg. Developmental positioning of the upper extremities using a blanket and restraining only the lower limbs may decrease the stress of a 4-point restraint. Following the procedure, an infant might benefit from acetaminophen.

4. Sedatives and opioids may cause respiratory depression and their use should be restricted to settings where respiratory depression can be promptly treated by medical staff experienced in airway management. Paradoxical reactions to benzodiazepines including seizure-like myoclonus have been reported, especially in preterm neonates. Limited data is available on the long term effects of benzodiazepines in preterm and term infants. Benzodiazepine exposure in rodent models extends cortical apoptosis, alters developing gamma-aminobutyric acid (GABA) receptors and results in long-term behavioral and cognitive impairment. Thus, cautious use of sedatives during early brain development is recommended.

C. **Postoperative analgesia.** Tissue injury, which occurs during all forms of surgery, elicits profound physiologic responses. The more marked these responses to surgery, the greater the morbidities. Thus, minimizing the endocrine and metabolic responses to surgery by decreasing pain has been shown to significantly improve the outcomes in neonatal surgery.

Improving pain management and improving outcomes in the neonate requires a team approach and coordinated strategy of multidimensional pain reduction. Factors considered in developing a postoperative pain management plan include:

1. Pain history and previous opioid/sedative use

2. Severity of procedure (invasiveness, anesthesia time, and amount of tissue manipulation)

3. Postoperative airway management (expected extended intubation, expected short-term intubation, and not intubated)

4. Postoperative desired level of sedation

The goal of postoperative pain management is preventive analgesia. Central sensitization is induced by noxious inputs, and the administration of postoperative analgesic drugs immediately (prior to "awakening" from general anesthesia) may prevent the spinal and supraspinal hyperexcitability caused by acute pain resulting in decreased analgesic use. Opioids are the basis for postoperative analgesia after moderate/major surgery in the absence of regional anesthesia. A postoperative pain algorithm clearly guides practice and provides a standard of care for most infants during the postoperative period (Figure 67.2).

Morphine and fentanyl provide a similar degree of analgesia. Morphine has greater sedative effects, less risk of chest wall rigidity, and produces less tolerance. Fentanyl has faster onset, shorter duration of action, fewer effects on GI motility, less hemodynamic instability, and less urinary retention.

Acetaminophen is routinely used as an adjunct to regional anesthetics or opioids in the immediate postoperative period. However, evidence is limited in newborns that acetaminophen given by enteral route is effective for analgesia or reduces total opioid administration following surgery. Reduced pain response 6 hours following circumcision has been reported. Use of IV acetaminophen may be effective, but it is not currently approved for use in term and preterm neonates in the United States.

Sedatives (i.e., benzodiazepines) do not provide analgesia but may be given to manage agitation related to other factors such as mechanical ventilation. Postoperative sedatives can be administered in combination with analgesia to reduce opioid requirements and associated adverse effects. Preservative free benzodiazepines should be used in neonates to prevent risk of benzyl alcohol toxicity. Caution should be used in administering benzodiazepines in patients less than 35 weeks PMA due to the potential for seizure-like myoclonus and limited evidence on the long term effects of these medications.

Postoperative analgesia is used as long as pain assessment scales and clinical judgment indicates that it is required. Nonpharmacologic methods of pain management should be optimized in addition to minimizing noxious stimuli. Using behavioral distraction techniques and comfort helps to decrease anxiety.

D. **Naloxone for reversal of opioid side effects.** Naloxone (Narcan) is used to treat the side effects of excessive opioid, most commonly respiratory depression, although pruritus and emesis may also occur in newborns. Pruritus may be exhibited by agitation and increased movement in an attempt to alleviate symptoms. In an infant receiving opioid analgesia, naloxone can be used in order to achieve the optimal goal of blocking the adverse effects without exacerbating pain. If the infant's clinical status permits, an approach is to titrate administration of naloxone, giving it in increments of 0.05 mg/kg until the side effects are reversed.

E. **Opioid tolerance.** Opioid administration that is prolonged may lead to tolerance and the need for a higher dose to relieve symptoms. Pain behaviors recur, sleep is disrupted, and an infant may exhibit a high-pitched cry or tremors during handling. Infants are not able to interact with their parent or caregiver as they did when pain was absent. Management is directed at increasing the dosage to an effective analgesic dose.

F. **Opioid and sedative weaning.** Prolonged use of opioids and sedatives can result in iatrogenic physical dependence. Long-term effects of exposure to these agents on neonatal neurodevelopment are not fully understood. Opioids and sedatives are weaned in a manner that shortens the length of exposure to these medications while easing the effects of withdrawal (see Chap. 12).

Neonates exposed to continuous or higher doses of opioids for >5 days are at increased risk for opioid withdrawal. Opioid withdrawal is more prevalent and may occur earlier in infants receiving fentanyl compared to morphine. Weaning rather than abrupt discontinuation is recommended. An overall opioid and sedative-weaning plan can be developed and individualized prior to

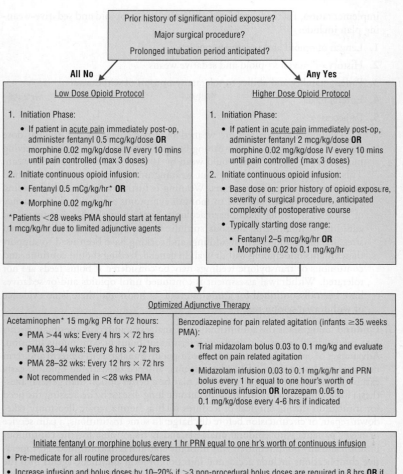

Figure 67.2. Postoperative pain management algorithm. Adapted from postopereative pain management protocol used at Children's Hospital Boston. (see section V.C.)

*Data are limited on post-operative use of high dose acetaminophen in newborns, including optimal dose and frequency. Institutions should develop protocols based on their populations and interpretation of the data.

implementation. Factors considered in developing an opioid and sedative-weaning plan include:

1. Length of opioid and sedative exposure
2. History of previous opioid and sedative weans
3. Patient stability and ability to tolerate symptoms of withdrawal
4. Enteral feeds
5. IV access

Opioids and sedatives are weaned by a percentage of the original dose that the patient is on when weaning begins. For example, a patient receiving morphine 0.2 mg/kg/hour would wean by 10% or 0.02 mg/kg at each wean. This strategy continues throughout weaning unless symptoms of withdrawal or a change in condition occurs. Weaning is further individualized by using a withdrawal assessment tool to monitor symptoms and guide the frequency of additional dosing. Nonpharmacologic comfort methods are essential in addition to minimizing noxious stimuli. Removing noxious environmental stressors, protecting sleep, swaddling, and rocking have been used to support these infants undergoing withdrawal. In general, feeding should continue, and continuous or transpyloric feedings may be considered if bolus feeds are not tolerated. Withdrawal assessment is continued until opioids and/or sedatives have been discontinued for a minimum of 72 hours and there is no evidence of withdrawal symptoms.

G. **Epidural analgesia** is the administration of analgesics and local anesthetic agents into the epidural space as a single or intermittent bolus or continuous infusion. Advantages of epidural anesthesia and postoperative analgesia in preterm and term neonates are lower doses of paralytic agents, absence of systemic opioids, early extubation, and effective analgesia. This may be a better option than general anesthesia for former preterm infants with chronic lung disease by decreasing the need for intubation during surgical procedures such as hernia repair, ileostomy take-down/repair, or circumcision before discharge. In some institutions, a pain service manages patients with epidural analgesia and is responsible for the continuous infusion and any bolus requirements until the epidural is discontinued. Postoperative complications include accidental injection of local anesthetic agents into the intravascular system, venous air embolism, local or systemic infection, meningitis, atelectasis, apnea, and hypoxemia. Cardiorespiratory monitoring and assessment of the infant's sensory responses, pain behaviors, respiratory status, integrity of the dressing, urine output, vital signs, and any changes in pump settings or additional bolus requirements are essential.

Suggested Readings

American Academy of Pediatrics Committee on Fetus and Newborn, American Academy of Pediatrics Section on Surgery, Canadian Paediatric Society Fetus and Newborn Committee. Prevention and management of pain in the neonate: an update. *Pediatrics* 2006;118(5):2231–2241.

Anand KJ, Aranda JV, Berde CB, et al. Summary proceedings from the neonatal pain-control group. *Pediatrics* 2006;117(3 pt 2):S9–S22.

Anand KJS, Stevens BJ, McGrath PJ, eds. *Pain in Neonates and Infants.* 3rd ed. Edinburgh: Elsevier; 2007:329.

Debillon T, et al. Development and initial Validation of the EDIN scale: a new tool for assessing prolonged pain in preterm infants. *Arch Dis Child Fetal Neonatal Ed.* 2001;85(1):F36–41.

Durrmeyer X, Vutskits L, Anand KJS, Rimensberger PC. Use of Analgesic and Sedative Drugs in the NICU: Integrating Clinical Trials and Laboratory Data. *Pediatr Res* 2010;67:117–127.

Kumar P, Denson SE, Mancuso TJ, et al. Premedication for nonemergency endotracheal intubation in the neonate. *Pediatrics* 2010;125(3):608–615.

Walden M, Gibbins S. *Pain Assessment and Management: Guideline for Practice.* 2nd ed. Glenview, IL: National Association of Neonatal Nurses (NANN); 2008:30.

Appendix A

Common Neonatal Intensive Care Unit (NICU) Medication Guidelines

Caryn E. Douma and Jennifer Schonen Gardner

ACETAMINOPHEN

Classification: Analgesic; antipyretic.

Indication: Analgesia.

Dosage/administration: <32 weeks postmenstrual age (PMA): 10 to 15 mg/kg/dose q12h orally (PO)/ rectally (PR) PRN; 32 through 36 weeks PMA: 10 to 15 mg/kg/dose q8h PO/PR PRN; ≥37 weeks: 10 to 15 mg/kg/dose q6h PO/PR PRN.

Precautions: Rectal suppositories associated with erratic release. G6PD deficiency. Elimination is prolonged in patients with liver dysfunction.

Monitoring: Complete blood count (CBC), liver function tests (LFTs).

Adverse reactions: Rash, Blood dyscrasias (thrombocytopenia, leukopenia, pancytopenia, and neutropenia). Adverse reactions are associated with excessive dosages.

Acute effects: Hepatic necrosis, transient azotemia, and renal tubular necrosis.

Chronic effects: Anemia, renal damage, and gastrointestinal (GI) disturbances.

Treatment of overdose/severe toxicity: N-Acetylcysteine (NAC).

ACYCLOVIR

Classification: Antiviral agent.

Indications: Treatment of herpes simplex infections, varicella zoster infections with central nervous system (CNS) and pulmonary involvement, and herpes simplex encephalitis.

Dosage/administration: (see Table A.1)

Table A.1	Acyclovir
Indication	**Dosage***
Localized HSV infection	20 mg/kg/dose IV q8h for 14 to 21 d Infusion concentration must be <7 mg/mL, usual concentration = 5 mg/mL
Disseminated or CNS infections	20 mg/kg/dose IV q8h for 21 d
HSV = herpes simplex virus; IV = intravenous; CNS = central nervous system; q8h = every 8 hours; q12h = every 12 hours. *use q12h interval for <30 wk PMA.	

Do not refrigerate due to precipitation of the drug. Infuse by syringe pump over ≥1 hour.

Precautions: Reduce dosage for impaired renal function.

Monitoring: Renal and hepatic function, CBC, intravenous (IV) site for phlebitis.

Adverse reactions: Nephrotoxicity, bone marrow suppression, fever, thrombocytosis, and transitory increase of serum creatinine and liver enzymes. Rare encephalopathy associated with rapid IV administration (lethargy, obtundation, agitation, tremor, seizure, and coma). Risk of crystalline nephropathy is minimized by slow infusion rates and adequate hydration.

ADENOSINE

Classification: Antiarrhythmic agent.
Indication: Acute treatment of paroxysmal supraventricular tachycardia (PSVT).
Dosage/administration:
Initial dose: 0.05 mg/kg/dose given rapid IV push. If not effective within 1 to 2 minutes, may increase dose by 0.05 mg/kg/dose increment every 1 to 2 minutes to a maximum single dose of 0.25 mg/kg or termination of PSVT. Administer over 1 to 2 seconds at peripheral IV (PIV) site closest to the patient's heart. Follow each dose with a normal saline (NS) flush.
Precautions: Transient arrhythmias may occur between supraventricular tachycardia (SVT) termination and onset of normal sinus rhythm. Recurrence of SVT occurs in approximately 30% of treated patients. Bronchoconstriction may occur in asthmatics.
Monitoring: Continuous electrocardiogram (EKG), heart rate, blood pressure, respirations.
Adverse reactions: Flushing, dyspnea, and irritability (usually resolves within 1 minute). Arrhythmias, bradycardia, heart block, and hyperventilation.

ALBUMIN

Classification: Plasma volume expander.
Indications: Hypovolemia, hypoproteinemia.
Dosage/administration: (see Table A.2)

Table A.2	Albumin	
Indication	**IV dosage**	**Administration**
Hypovolemia	0.5 g/kg/dose	Infuse **5% albumin** over >60 min, may be infused more rapidly (10–20 min) in hypovolemic shock, repeat PRN
Hypoproteinemia	0.5–1 g/kg/dose	Infuse **5% albumin** over >2 h, repeat q1–2d. Dilutions may be made with NS or D₅W in cases of sodium restriction
Maximum dose: 6 g/kg/day. If >6 g/kg/24 hour is required, consider blood products for treatment of hypovolemia.		
IV = intravenous; PRN = as needed; NS = normal saline.		

Precautions: *There is no clinical advantage to using albumin as a volume expander compared to using NS.* Infuse using a 5-micron filter or larger. Use within 4 hours after opening vial. Albumin is contraindicated in patients with severe anemia or congestive heart failure (CHF). **Albumin 25% is contraindicated in preterm neonates due to increased risk of intraventricular hemorrhage (IVH). Do not use sterile water to dilute albumin due to risk of hypotonic associated hemolysis. Use NS or D₅W. Sodium load: 130 mEq/L (5%), 160 mEq/L (25%).**
Monitoring: Observe for signs of hypervolemia, pulmonary edema, and cardiac failure.
Adverse reactions: Chills, fever, and urticaria. Rapid infusion (>1 g/minute) may precipitate CHF and pulmonary edema due to fluid overload.

ALPROSTADIL

Classification: Prostaglandin.

Indications: Temporary maintenance of patent ductus arteriosis (PDA), in neonates with ductal-dependent congenital heart disease.

Dosage/administration:

Initial: 0.05 mcg/kg/minute.

Maintenance: 0.01 to 0.4 mcg/kg/minute; titrate to effective dosage with therapeutic response. Maximal drug effect usually seen within 30 minutes in cyanotic lesions; may take several hours in acyanotic lesions. Administer as a continuous IV infusion on a syringe pump (central venous access preferred). Dilute with dextrose or NS. Recommended concentration is 10 mcg/mL. Doses above 0.4 mcg/kg/minute are not likely to produce additional benefits and have a higher incidence of side effects.

Precautions: Use cautiously in neonates with bleeding tendencies. If hypotension or pyrexia occurs, reduce infusion until symptoms subside. Severe hypotension or bradycardia requires drug discontinuation with cautious reinstitution at a lower dose. Apnea occurs in approximately 10% to 12% of neonates with congenital heart defects during alprostadil infusions (especially in those weighing <2 kg at birth) and usually appears during the first hour of drug infusion. **Be prepared to intubate and resuscitate.**

Adverse reactions: Apnea, respiratory depression, flushing, bradycardia, fever, seizure-like activity, systemic hypotension, hypocalcemia, hypokalemia, hypoglycemia, and cortical proliferation of long bones has been seen with long-term infusions; diarrhea, gastric-outlet obstruction secondary to antral hyperplasia (occurrence related to duration of therapy >120 hours and cumulative dose), inhibition of platelet aggregation.

AMPHOTERICIN-B (CONVENTIONAL)

Classification: Systemic antifungal agent.

Indication: Treatment of suspected or proven systemic fungal infections.

Dosage/administration: 1 to 1.5 mg/kg IV q24h infused over ≥2 hours. Average duration of therapy is 2 to 4 weeks. Maximum concentration for infusion is 0.1 mg/mL for peripheral line administration and 0.5 mg/mL for central line administration. Flush with dextrose.

Precautions: Concurrent use with other nephrotoxic medications may lead to additive nephrotoxicity. If renal dysfunction occurs as a result of amphotericin therapy, give dose every other day. Corticosteroids may increase the potassium depletion caused by amphotericin. May intensify toxicity to neuromuscular blocking agents (e.g., pancuronium) secondary to hypokalemia. Use with caution in patients with electrolyte instabilities. **Do not confuse with lipid-based forms of amphotericin.**

Contraindications: Incompatible with NS and TPN. Do not dilute/flush with NS or mix with any other medication that is diluted in NS. Do not mix with any other medication or electrolytes to avoid precipitation.

Adverse reactions: Hypokalemia, hypomagnesemia, nephrotoxicity, LFT abnormalities, thrombocytopenia, anemia, leukopenia, fever/chills, bronchospasm, and tachycardia.

Monitoring: Blood urea nitrogen (BUN), serum creatinine, LFTs, serum electrolytes, CBC, vitals, Hgb/Hct, inputs and outputs, monitor EKG changes for signs of hypokalemia, IV site for signs of phlebitis.

AMPHOTERICIN-B LIPID COMPLEX (ABLC)

Classification: Systemic antifungal agent.

Indication: Treatment of suspected or proven systemic fungal infections in patients resistant to conventional amphotericin B therapy or with renal/hepatic dysfunction.

Dosage/administration: 2.5 to 5 mg/kg IV q24h infused over ≥2 hours. Maximum concentration for infusion is 2 mg/mL. Average duration of therapy is 2 to 4 weeks. Flush with dextrose.

Precautions: Concurrent use with other nephrotoxic medications may lead to additive nephrotoxicity. Corticosteroids may increase the potassium depletion caused by amphotericin. May intensify toxicity to neuromuscular blocking agents (e.g., pancuronium) secondary to hypokalemia. Use with caution in patients with electrolyte instabilities. **Do not confuse with conventional amphotericin-B or other lipid-based forms of amphotericin.**

Contraindications: Incompatible with NS and TPN. Do not dilute/flush with NS or mix with any other medication that is diluted in NS. Do not mix with any other medication or electrolytes to avoid precipitation.

Adverse reactions: Hypokalemia, hypomagnesemia, nephrotoxicity, fever/chills, LFT abnormalities, renal dysfunction, thrombocytopenia, anemia, leukopenia, hypotension, arrhythmias, and tachycardia.

Monitoring: BUN, serum creatinine, LFTs, serum electrolytes, CBC, vitals, inputs and outputs, monitor EKG changes for signs of hypokalemia.

AMPHOTERICIN-B LIPOSOMAL (AMBISOME®)

Classification: Systemic antifungal agent.

Indication: Treatment of suspected or proven systemic fungal infections.

Dosage/administration: 5 to 7 mg/kg IV q24h infused over ≥2 hours. Maximum concentration for infusion is 2 mg/mL. Average duration of therapy is 2 to 4 weeks. Flush with dextrose.

Precautions: Concurrent use with other nephrotoxic medications may lead to additive nephrotoxicity. Corticosteroids may increase the potassium depletion caused by amphotericin. May intensify toxicity to neuromuscular blocking agents (e.g., pancuronium) secondary to hypokalemia. Use with caution in patients with electrolyte instabilities. **Do not confuse with conventional amphotericin-B or other lipid–based forms of amphotericin.**

Contraindications: Do not dilute with NS or mix with any other medication that is diluted in NS. Do not mix with any other medication or electrolytes to avoid precipitation. Not compatible with TPN.

Adverse reactions: Hypokalemia, nephrotoxicity, LFT abnormalities, thrombocytopenia, tachycardia, anemia, fever, and chills (acute infusion reactions).

Monitoring: BUN, serum creatinine, LFTs, serum electrolytes, CBC, vitals, inputs and outputs, monitor EKG changes for signs of hypokalemia.

AMPICILLIN

Classification: Semisynthetic penicillinase-sensitive penicillin with bactericidal activity.

Indications: Combined with either an aminoglycoside or cephalosporin for the prevention and treatment of infections with group B *streptococci*, *Listeria monocytogenes*, and susceptible *Escherichia coli* species.

Dosage/administration: (see Table A.3)

Table A.3	Ampicillin	
Postmenstrual age	Postnatal age	Dosing
<30 wk PMA	1–28 d of age	100 mg/kg/dose q12h
	>28 d of age	100 mg/kg/dose q8h
30–37 wk PMA	1–14 d of age	100 mg/kg/dose q12h
	>14 d of age	100 mg/kg/dose q8h
>37 wk PMA	1–7 d of age	100 mg/kg/dose q8h
	>7 d of age	75 mg/kg/dose q6h

q12h = every 12 hours; q8h = every 8 hours; q6h = every 6 hours.
Dose may be lowered to 50 mg/kg/dose if meningitis is ruled out.

Infused over ≥15 minutes on syringe pump. Maximum final concentration for administration is 100 mg/mL. IM administration associated with sterile abscess formation. Reconstituted solution must be used within 1 hour after mixing due to loss of potency.

Precautions: Dosage adjustment for renal impairment. **Not compatible with TPN.**

Drug interactions: Blunting of peak aminoglycoside concentration if administered simultaneously with ampicillin.

Adverse reactions: Diarrhea, hypersensitivity reaction (rubella-like rash and fever, although rare in neonatal population), nephritis (typically preceded by eosinophilia), elevated transaminases, penicillin encephalopathy (CNS excitation and seizure activity associated with large or rapidly administered doses), hemolytic anemia, and pseudomembranous colitis.

ATROPINE SULFATE

Classification: Anticholinergic agent.

Indication: Prolonged cardiopulmonary resuscitation unresponsive to epinephrine.

Dosage/administration: IV: 0.01 to 0.03 mg/kg/dose administered over 1 minute, every 5 to 15 minutes, for two to three doses with a maximum total dose of 0.04 mg/kg.

NOTE: Low doses (<0.1 mg) may cause paradoxical bradycardia secondary to central action.

Endotracheal tube (ETT) : 0.01 to 0.03 mg/kg/dose immediately followed by 1 mL NS. Administer undiluted form for IV and ETT administration.

Clinical considerations: Effective oxygenation and ventilation must precede atropine treatment of bradycardia. Monitor heart rate.

Contraindications: Tachycardia, narrow-angle glaucoma, thyrotoxicosis, GI or genitourinary obstruction.

Precautions: Spastic paralysis or CNS damage.

Adverse reactions: Tachycardia, mydriasis, cycloplegia, abdominal distention/ileus, urinary retention, arrhythmias, esophageal reflux, fever, hyperthermia, and elevated white blood cell (WBC) count.
Antidote: Physostigmine.

CAFFEINE CITRATE
Classification: Respiratory stimulant.
Indication: Apnea of prematurity.
Dosage/administration:
Loading dose: 20 mg/kg IV or orally. Infuse over ≥30 minutes on syringe pump.
Maintenance dose: 5 to 10 mg/kg IV or orally daily, starting 24 hours after loading dose. Minibolus: 5 to 10 mg/kg/dose. Infuse IV maintenance dose over ≥10 minutes on a syringe pump. Do not skip scheduled doses when administering a bolus. It takes approximately 1 week for caffeine citrate to reach steady-state levels due to its long half-life. **Do not push IV doses of caffeine citrate.**
Precautions: Do not use caffeine-based formulations because of different dosage requirements. Do not use caffeine preparations that contain sodium benzoate.
Adverse reactions: Cardiac arrhythmias, tachycardia (withhold dose for heart rate >180), insomnia, restlessness, irritability, nausea, vomiting, and diarrhea. Consider a decrease in dose to treat the CNS and/or GI side effects, diuresis, and increased urinary calcium excretion.
Monitoring parameters: Monitor heart rate, number and severity of apnea spells. Following serum levels is generally not indicated. Toxicity rarely occurs at levels <50 mcg/mL

CALCIUM
Classification: Electrolyte supplement; calcium salt.
Indication: Treatment and prevention of hypocalcemia.
Dosage/administration: Hypocalcemia (maintenance therapy): Calcium glubionate: 360 to 1,200 mg/kg/day, PO divided q4–6h. Maximum 9 g/day.
Symptomatic hypocalcemia (acute treatment): Calcium gluconate: 100 mg/kg/dose (equal to approximately 10 mg/kg/dose elemental calcium). Infuse over 10 to 30 minutes on a syringe pump. May need to slow down or stop infusion for persistent bradycardia. Not for intramuscular (IM) or subcutaneous (SC) administration, for IV administration only.
Precautions: IV: Rapid administration is associated with bradycardia. Extravasation may cause tissue necrosis. Use hyaluronidase to treat extravasation. Bolus infusion by umbilical arterial catheter (UAC) has been associated with intestinal bleeding and lower extremity tissue necrosis.
PO: solution is hypertonic; use with caution in infants at high risk for NEC.
Contraindications: Hypercalcemia, renal calculi, and ventricular fibrillation.
Adverse reactions: IV: Arrhythmias and deterioration of cardiovascular function/bradycardia. Extravasation may cause skin sloughing.
PO: gastric irritation/diarrhea.
Monitoring parameters: Monitor serum calcium and phosphorus levels. Monitor vitamin D levels when indicated. Avoid hypercalcemia during treatment and correct hypomagnesemia if present. Observe IV infusion site closely for extravasation.

CAPTOPRIL

Classification: Angiotensin-converting enzyme inhibitor.
Indication: Moderate to severe hypertension, afterload reductions in CHF.
Dosage/administration:
Initial dose:
Premature newborns: 0.01 to 0.05 mg/kg/dose PO q8–12h.
Term newborns: 0.05 to 0.1 mg/kg/dose PO q8–24h.
Maximum recommended dose: 0.5 mg/kg/dose PO q6–24h. Titrate dose and frequency to effect. Administer on an empty stomach 1 hour before or 2 hours after feedings, if possible. Food decreases absorption by approximately 50%. Administration times need to be consistent.
Precautions: Use with caution and modify dosage in patients with renal impairment.
Contraindications: Angioedema, bilateral renal artery stenosis, hyperkalemia, renal failure.
Adverse reactions: Hypotension, rash, fever, eosinophilia, neutropenia, GI disturbances, cough, dyspnea, acute renal failure, hyperkalemia, and proteinuria. Development of jaundice or elevated hepatic enzymes is a reason for immediate drug withdrawal. Severe hypotension may occur in patients who are sodium or volume depleted. Lower or half doses may be used.
Monitoring parameters: Monitor blood pressure (BP) for hypotension within 1 hour after first dose or after a new higher dose, BUN, serum creatinine, renal function, urine dipstick for protein, CBC with differential, serum potassium.

CEFOTAXIME SODIUM

Classification: Third-generation cephalosporin.
Indications: Reserved for suspected or documented gram-negative meningitis or sepsis. Combine with ampicillin or vancomycin for empiric therapy.
Dosage/administration: (see Table A.4)

Table A.4	Cefotaxime Sodium	
Age	**Weight**	**Dosage (IV/IM)**
All neonates (0–4 wk)	<1,200 g	50 mg/kg/dose IV/IM q12h
Postnatal age ≤7 d	1,200–2,000 g	50 mg/kg/dose IV/IM q12h
Postnatal age ≤7 d	>2,000 g	50 mg/kg/dose IV/IM q8h
Postnatal age >7 d	1,200–2,000 g	50 mg/kg/dose IV/IM q8h
Postnatal age >7 d	>2,000 g	50 mg/kg/dose IV/IM q6h
IM = intramuscularly; IV = intravenously; q6h = every 6 hours; q8h = every 8 hours; q12h = every 12 hours.		

Maximum concentration for infusion is 100 mg/mL in dextrose 5% water (D_5W), dextrose 10% water (D10W), or NS. Infuse over >30 minutes on syringe pump. Maximum concentration for IM dose is 300 mg/mL.

Precautions: Dosage modification for impaired renal function.
Monitoring: CBC, BUN, creatinine, LFTs.
Drug interactions: Blunting of peak aminoglycoside concentration if administered over <2 hours before/after cefotaxime.
Adverse reactions: Leukopenia, granulocytopenia, pseudomembranous colitis, serum–sickness-like reaction, and transient elevation of BUN, creatinine, eosinophils, liver enzymes, and rash.
Clinical considerations: Routine or frequent use of cephalosporins in the neonatal intensive care unit may quickly result in the emergence of resistant enteric organisms.

CEFTAZIDIME

Classification: Third-generation cephalosporin.
Indications: Broad-spectrum cephalosporin with antipseudomonal activity. Treatment of gram-negative meningitis.
Dosage/administration: (see Table A.5)

Table A.5	Ceftazidime	
Age	**Weight**	**Dosage (IV/IM)**
All neonates	<1,200 g	50 mg/kg/dose IV/IM q12h
Postnatal age ≤7 d	1,200–2,000 g	50 mg/kg/dose IV/IM q12h
Postnatal age ≤7 d	>2,000 g	50 mg/kg/dose IV/IM q8h
Postnatal age >7 d	>1,200 g	50 mg/kg/dose IV/IM q8h

IM = intramuscularly; IV = intravenously; q8h = every 8 hours; q12h = every 12 hours.

Final concentration for infusion is 100 mg/mL in dextrose 5% water (D_5W) or NS. Infuse over >30 minutes on syringe pump.
Clinical considerations: Treat serious pseudomonal infections with ceftazidime in combination with an aminoglycoside. **Routine or frequent use of cephalosporins in the neonatal intensive care unit will quickly result in the emergence of resistant enteric organisms.**
Precautions: Modify dosage for renal impairment.
Drug interaction: Blunting of peak aminoglycoside concentration if administered simultaneously with ceftazidime.
Monitoring: CBC, renal, and LFTs.
Adverse reactions: Transient leukopenia and bone marrow suppression, rash, false-positive direct Coombs test, candidiasis, hemolytic anemia, pseudomembranous colitis, and transient elevation of eosinophils, platelets, renal, and LFTs.

CEFTRIAXONE SODIUM

Classification: Third-generation cephalosporin.
Indications: Good activity against both gram-negative and gram-positive organisms except for *Pseudomonas* spp., *enterococci*, methicillin-resistant *Staphylococci*, and *L. monocytogenes*. Indicated for treatment of gonococcal meningitis and conjunctivitis. Not recommended for use in neonates with hyperbilirubinemia. Use cefotaxime instead.

Dosage/administration: (see Table A.6)

Table A.6	Ceftriaxone Sodium	
Age	Weight	Dosage (IV/IM)
Postnatal age ≤7 d	All weights	50 mg/kg/dose IV/IM q24h
Postnatal age >7 d	≤2,000 g	50 mg/kg/dose IV/IM q24h
Postnatal age >7 d	>2,000 g	75 mg/kg/day IV/IM q24h
IM = intramuscularly; IV = intravenously; q24h = every 24 hours.		

Gonococcal prophylaxis: 25 to 50 mg/kg IV/IM as a single dose (dose not to exceed 125 mg).

Disseminated gonococcal infection: 25 to 50 mg/kg/day (maximum dose: 125 mg) IV/IM q24h for 7 days, up to 10 to 14 days if meningitis is documented.

Nondisseminated infections including ophthalmia neonatorum: 25 to 50 mg/kg IV/IM (maximum dose: 125 mg) single dose.

Maximum concentration for IV administration is 100 mg/mL in dextrose or saline. Infused over >30 minutes on syringe pump. IM doses can be reconstituted with 1% lidocaine without epinephrine to reduce pain at injection site but is not recommended in small infants due to possible lidocaine-related cardiac adverse effects. Maximum concentration for IM administration is 350 mg/mL. Avoid administration of calcium-containing solutions or products within 48 hours of the last administration of ceftriaxone (IV).

Precautions: Do not use in gallbladder, biliary tract, liver, or pancreatic disease. Consider cefotaxime or ceftazidime instead.

Clinical considerations: Do not use as sole therapy for staphylococcal or pseudomonal infections. Combine with ampicillin for initial empirical therapy of meningitis. Ceftriaxone displaces bilirubin from albumin-binding sites, leading to increased free-serum bilirubin levels. In newborns with hyperbilirubinemia, use cefotaxime instead of ceftriaxone.

Monitoring: CBC, electrolytes, BUN, creatinine, AST, ALT, and bilirubin.

Adverse reactions: Leukopenia, anemia, GI intolerance, and rash. Transient increase in eosinophils, platelets, bleeding time, free serum bilirubin concentration, and renal/LFTs. Transient formation of gallbladder precipitates characterized by vomiting and cholelithiasis. GI tract bacterial or fungal overgrowth.

CHLORAL HYDRATE

Classification: Sedative, hypnotic.

Indications: Sedative/hypnotic.

Dosage/administration: 25 to 50 mg/kg/dose PO or PR, q6–8h as needed.

Maximum dose: 50 mg/kg/dose. To reduce gastric irritation, dilute in feedings or administer after feedings.

Precautions: Rectal suppositories are not recommended because of unreliable release characteristics. Use caution with concurrent administration of furosemide and anticoagulants.

Clinical considerations: No analgesic properties. Excitation may occur instead of sedation in infants with pain. Assess level of sedation. Toxic metabolites (trichloroethanol) have long half-lives in neonates and accumulate with repeated doses. Oral onset of action: 10 to 15 minutes.

Contraindications: Significant hepatic or renal impairment.

Adverse reactions: Paradoxical excitation, GI intolerance, allergic manifestations, leukopenia, eosinophilia, vasodilation, cardiopulmonary depression (especially when coadministered with barbiturates and opiates), cardiac arrhythmias, CNS depression, ileus and bladder atony, and indirect bilirubin.

CHLOROTHIAZIDE

Classification: Thiazide diuretic.

Indications: Fluid overload, pulmonary edema, BPD, CHF, and hypertension.

Dosage/administration: 20 to 40 mg/kg/day PO, divided q12h. IV: 2 to 8 mg/kg/day, divided q12h. Variable absorption from GI tract. IM and SC administration not recommended because of local pain and irritation.

Contraindications: Anuria or significant hepatic dysfunction.

Drug interactions: Reduced antihypertensive effect with concurrent nonsteroidal anti-inflammatory drug use.

Monitoring: Serum electrolytes, calcium, phosphorus, blood glucose, urine output, BP, and daily weight.

Adverse reactions: Hypochloremic alkalosis, prerenal azotemia, volume depletion, blood dyscrasias, decreased serum potassium and magnesium levels, and increased levels of glucose, uric acid, lipids, bilirubin, and calcium.

CITRATE MIXTURES, ORAL

Classification: Electrolyte supplement.

Indication: Metabolic acidosis.

Dosage/administration: 0.5 to 1 mEq/kg/dose, PO 3 or 4 times/day. Give with feedings. Adjust dose to maintain desired bicarbonate or urine pH. One mEq citrate equivalent to 1 mEq bicarbonate (see Table A.7).

Table A.7	Content (mEq) in Each mL of Citrate Mixture		
Citrate mixtures	**Na$^+$**	**K$^+$**	**Bicarbonate**
Polycitra®	1	1	2
Polycitra®-K	0	2	2
Bicitra®	1	0	1
Oracit®	1	0	1

Precautions: Use with caution in infants receiving potassium supplements.

Adverse reaction: Laxative effect.

CLINDAMYCIN

Classification: Anaerobic antibiotic.

Indications: Treatment of *Bacteroides fragilis* septicemia, peritonitis, necrotizing enterocolitis (NEC). Not indicated for meningitis.

Dosage/administration: (see Table A.8)

Table A.8	Clindamycin	
Postnatal age	Weight	Dosage
Postnatal age ≤7 d	≤2,000 g	10 mg/kg/day divided q12h
	>2,000 g	15 mg/kg/day divided q8h
Postnatal age >7 d	<1,200 g	10 mg/kg/day divided q12h
	1,200–2,000 g	15 mg/kg/day divided q8h
	>2,000 g	20–30 mg/kg/day divided q6–8h
IV = intravenously; q6–8h = every 6 to 8 hours; q8h = every 8 hours; q12h = every 12 hours.		

Infuse over >30 minutes on syringe pump. Maximum concentration for infusion is 18 mg/mL in dextrose 5% water or NS. IM administration is associated with sterile abscess formation.

Contraindication: Hepatic impairment.

Warnings: Can cause severe and possibly fatal pseudomembranous colitis characterized by severe persistent diarrhea and possibly the passage of blood and mucus.

Drug interactions: May potentiate the level and effects of neuromuscular-blocking agents.

Adverse reactions: *Pseudomembranous colitis*, Stevens-Johnson syndrome, glossitis, pruritus, granulocytopenia, thrombocytopenia, hypotension, and increased LFTs.

DEXAMETHASONE SODIUM PHOSPHATE

Classification: Glucocorticoid.

Indications: Anti-inflammatory glucocorticoid used to facilitate extubation and improve lung mechanics. The American Academy of Pediatrics strongly discourages the use of dexamethasone for treatment or prevention of bronchopulmonary dysplasia.

Dosage/administration: Acetate injection is not for IV use. Administer IV on syringe pump over >5 minutes. Maximum concentration 1 mg/mL. Maximum dose: 1 mg/kg/day IV/PO.

Extubation/airway edema dosing: 0.25 to 0.5 mg/kg × 1. May repeat q8h for a total of four doses.

Begin dosing 4 hours before extubation.

Precautions: Hyperglycemia and glycosuria occur frequently after the first few doses. Increase in BP is common. Edema, hypertension, pituitary–adrenal axis suppression, growth suppression, glucose intolerance, hypokalemia, alkalosis, Cushing syndrome, peptic ulcer, immunosuppression.

Monitoring: Hemoglobin, occult blood loss, BP, serum potassium and glucose; IOP with systemic use >6 weeks; weight and height. Echocardiogram if receiving longer than 7 days.

Adverse reactions: Facial flushing, ↑ BP, tachycardia, agitation, hyponatremia, hyperglycemia, poor growth, bone demineralization, protein catabolism, secondary adrenal suppression, nausea, dyspepsia, vomiting, pain at injection site, itchy or light-sensitive eyes, rhinitis, upper respiratory infections, leukocytosis, nose bleed, nasal congestion.

Dexamethasone given for treatment or prevention of BPD has been associated with a higher risk of cerebral palsy and neurodevelopmental abnormalities. Its use should be avoided except under exceptional clinical circumstances (maximal ventilatory support or high risk of mortality).

DIAZOXIDE

Classification: Antihypoglycemic agent.
Indication: Hyperinsulinemic hypoglycemia.
Dosage/administration: 8 to 15 mg/kg/day, PO, divided q8–12h.
Clinical considerations: Used only for glucose-refractory hypoglycemia. Positive responses are usually seen within 48 to 72 hours and occur in less than 50% of neonates.
Contraindications: Compensatory hypertension associated with aortic coarctation or arteriovenous (AV) shunts.
Precautions: Diabetes mellitus, renal, or liver disease. May displace bilirubin from albumin.
Monitoring: BP, CBC, serum uric acid levels.
Drug interactions: Phenytoin.
Adverse reactions: Hyperglycemia (insulin reverses diazoxide-induced hyperglycemia), ketoacidosis, sodium and water retention, hypotension, thrombocytopenia, hyperosmolar coma, and GI irritation.

DIGOXIN

Classification: Antiarrhythmic agent, inotrope.
Indications: Heart failure, paroxysmal atrioventricular nodal tachycardia, atrial fibrillation/flutter, SVT.
Dosage/administration: (see Table A.9)

Table A.9	Digoxin			
	Total digitalizing (total loading) dose		**Maintenance dose**	
Age	**PO**	**IV**	**PO**	**IV**
≤29 wk	20 mcg/kg	15 mcg/kg	5 mcg/kg q24h	4 mcg/kg q24h
30–36 wk	25 mcg/kg	20 mcg/kg	6 mcg/kg q24h	5 mcg/kg q24h
≥37 wk	40 mcg/kg	30 mcg/kg	5 mcg/kg q12h	4 mcg/kg q12h
IV = intravenously; PO = orally; q12h = every 12 hours; q24h = every 24 hours.				

Reserve total digitalizing dose (TDD) for treatment of life-threatening arrhythmias and acute CHF. Administer over 24 hours in three divided doses: first dose is one-half TDD, second dose is one-fourth TDD administered 8 hours after first dose, and third dose is one-fourth TDD administered 8 hours after second dose. Administer IV doses over >10 minutes on syringe pump. Utilize maintenance dose schedule for nonacute arrhythmia and CHF conditions. Do not administer IM. Oral doses should be 25% greater than IV doses. The pediatric IV formulation (100 mcg/mL) may be given undiluted. The pediatric oral elixir is 50 mcg/mL.

Precautions: Reduce dose for renal and hepatic impairment. Cardioversion or calcium infusion may precipitate ventricular fibrillation in the digoxin-treated neonate (may be prevented by lidocaine pretreatment).

Monitoring: Heart rate/rhythm for desired effects and signs of toxicity, serum calcium, magnesium, potassium (especially in neonates receiving diuretics and amphotericin-B, both of which predispose to digoxin toxicity), and renal function.

Therapeutic levels: 0.8 to 2 ng/mL. Neonates may have falsely elevated digoxin levels as a result of maternal digoxin-like substances.

Contraindications: Atrioventricular block, idiopathic hypertrophic subaortic stenosis, ventricular dysrhythmias, atrial fibrillation/flutter with slow ventricular rates, or constrictive pericarditis.

Drug interactions: Amiodarone, erythromycin, cholestyramine, indomethacin, spironolactone, quinidine, verapamil, and metoclopramide.

Adverse reactions: Persistent vomiting, feeding intolerance, diarrhea, and lethargy, shortening of QT_c interval, sagging ST segment, diminished T-wave amplitude, bradycardia, prolongation of PR interval, sinus bradycardia or S-A block, atrial or nodal ectopic beats, ventricular arrhythmias. Toxicity enhanced by hypokalemia, hyper- and hypomagnesemia, hypercalcemia. Treat life-threatening digoxin toxicity with digoxin immune fab.

DOBUTAMINE

Classification: Sympathomimetic, adrenergic agonist agent.

Indications: Treatment of hypoperfusion, hypotension, short-term management of cardiac decompensation. Has more effect on cardiac output than dopamine but less effect on blood pressure.

Dosage/administration: 2 to 25 mcg/kg/minute continuous IV infusion on syringe pump. Begin at a low dose and titrate to obtain desired mean arterial pressure. Central *venous* access is preferred. **Do not administer through UAC.**

Precautions: Hypovolemia should be corrected before use. Infiltration causes local inflammatory changes. Extravasation may cause dermal necrosis. Use phentolamine to treat extravasation.

Contraindications: Idiopathic hypertrophic subaortic stenosis.

Adverse reactions: Hypotension if hypovolemic, arrhythmias, tachycardia (with high doses), cutaneous vasodilation, increased BP, and dyspnea.

Monitoring: Continuous heart rate, arterial BP, and IV site.

DOPAMINE

Classification: Sympathomimetic, adrenergic agonist agent.

Indications: Treatment of hypotension.

Dosage/administration: 2 to 25 mcg/kg/minute through continuous IV infusion on syringe pump. Once 20 to 25 mcg/kg/minute is reached, consideration should be given to adding a second pressor. Clinical benefits have been noted at doses of up to 40 mcg/kg/minute. Begin at a low dose and titrate to obtain desired mean arterial pressure. Central *venous* access preferred. **Do not administer through UAC.**

Precautions: Hypovolemia should be corrected before use. Extravasation may cause tissue necrosis. Treat dopamine extravasation with phentolamine.

Contraindications: Pheochromocytoma, tachyarrhythmias, or hypovolemia may increase pulmonary artery pressure. Use with caution in neonates with pulmonary hypertension.

Adverse reactions: Arrhythmias, tachycardia, vasoconstriction, hypotension, widened QRS complex, bradycardia, hypertension, excessive diuresis and azotemia, reversible suppression of prolactin and thyrotropin secretion, increased pulmonary artery pressure.
Monitoring parameters: Continuous heart rate and arterial BP, urine output, peripheral perfusion, and IV site.

ENALAPRILAT/ENALAPRIL

Classification: Angiotensin-converting enzyme inhibitor, antihypertensive.
Indications: Hypertension, CHF.
Dosage/administration:
Enalaprilat: 5 to 10 mcg/kg/dose (0.005–0.01 mg/kg/dose), IV q8–24h.
Enalapril maleate: Initial dose: 0.1 mg/kg/day PO q24h; may be given without regard to feeding times; increase dose and/or interval according to response, every few days. Oral suspension prepared by dissolving a crushed 2.5-mg tablet in 25 mL of isotonic citrate buffer yielding a final concentration of 100 mcg/mL. Suspension is stable for 30 days refrigerated.
Precaution: Impaired renal function.
Monitoring: BP, renal function, serum electrolytes, especially potassium. Hold for mean arterial pressure <30 and heart rate <100.
Adverse reactions: Transient or prolonged episodes of hypotension, oliguria, mild nonoliguric renal failure, hypotension in volume-depleted neonates, and hyperkalemia in neonates receiving potassium supplements and/or potassium-sparing diuretics.

ENOXAPARIN

Classification: Low-molecular-weight heparin, anticoagulant.
Indication: Prophylaxis and treatment of thromboembolic disorders.
Dosage/administration: Prophylaxis: 0.75 mg/kg/dose SC q12h. Treatment:
Premature neonates: 2 mg/kg/dose SC q12h
Full-term neonates: 1.7 mg/kg/dose SC q12h.
Clinical considerations: Adjust dose to maintain antifactor Xa level between 0.5 and 1 unit/mL for treatment and 0.2 to 0.4 unit/mL for prophylaxis. Peak antifactor Xa activity is obtained 4 hours after dose (see Table A.10).

Table A.10	Enoxaparin		
Antifactor Xa treatment	**Antifactor Xa prophylaxis**	**Dose titration**	**Time to repeat antifactor Xa level**
<0.35 unit/mL	<0.15 unit/mL	↑ dose by 25%	4 h after next dose
0.35–0.49 unit/mL	0.15–0.19 unit/mL	↑ dose by 10%	4 h after next dose
0.5–1 unit/mL	0.2–0.4 unit/mL	Keep same dose	Next day, then 1 week later (4 h after dose) Adjust dose for weight gain

(continued)

Table A.10	Enoxaparin *(Continued)*		
Antifactor Xa treatment	Antifactor Xa prophylaxis	Dose titration	Time to repeat antifactor Xa level
1.1–1.5 units/mL	0.41–1 unit/mL	↓ dose by 20%	4 h after next dose
1.6–2 units/mL	1.1–2 units/mL	Hold dose for 3 h then ↓ dose by 30%	4 h after next dose
>2 units/mL	>2 units/mL	Repeat level: Hold all doses until antifactor Xa is 0.5 unit/mL; then ↓ dose by 40%	Before next dose and q12h until antifactor Xa is <0.5 unit/mL
↑ = increase; ↓ = decrease; q12h = every 12 hours.			

For SC administration only. To minimize bruising, do not administer IM or IV; do not rub injection site.

Precaution: Reduce dose by 30% in severe renal impairment.

Contraindications: Avoid or hold in infants who require lumbar puncture to minimize risk of epidural/spinal hematoma.

Adverse effects: Fever, edema, hemorrhage, thrombocytopenia, pain/erythema at injection site.

EPINEPHRINE

Classification: Adrenergic agent.

Indications: Cardiac arrest, refractory hypotension, bronchospasm.

Dosage/administration: (see Table A.11)

Table A.11	Epinephrine	
Indication	Dose	Comments
Severe bradycardia and hypotension	**IV push:** 0.1–0.3 mL/kg of **1:10,000** concentration (equal to 0.01–0.03 mg/kg or 10–30 mcg/kg)	May repeat q 3–5 min as needed
	Endotracheal tube: 0.3–1 mL/kg of **1:10,000** concentration (equal to 0.03–0.1 mg/kg or 30–100 mcg/kg)	
Continuous IV	Start at 0.05–0.1 mcg/kg/min. Adjust dose to desired response to a maximum of 1 mcg/kg/min.	Use the **1:1,000** formulation for mixing continuous IV preparations.
IV = intravenous; q = every.		

Monitoring: Continuous heart rate and BP monitoring.
Drug interactions: Incompatible with alkaline solutions (sodium bicarbonate).
Precautions: Note the differences in concentration for emergency administration and continuous IV epinephrine doses. High doses of preservative-containing epinephrine will necessitate caution in selection of epinephrine preparations. Always use a 1:10,000 concentration (0.1 mg/mL) for individual doses, ETT doses, and for emergency administration (IV and endotracheal). Use the 1:1,000 concentration for preparation of continuous infusions. Correction of acidosis before administration of catecholamines enhances their effectiveness.
Contraindications: Hyperthyroidism, hypertension, and diabetes.
Adverse reactions: Ventricular arrhythmias, tachycardia, pallor and tremor, severe hypertension with possible IVH, myocardial ischemia, hypokalemia, and decreased renal and splanchnic blood flow. IV infiltration may cause tissue ischemia and necrosis (consider treatment with phentolamine).

EPINEPHRINE RACEMIC
Classification: Adrenergic agonist.
Indication: Treatment of postextubation stridor.
Dosage/administration: 0.25 to 0.5 mL of 2.25% **racemic epinephrine** solution diluted with NS to total volume of 3 mL given by nebulizer q2–4h PRN over 15 minutes.
Clinical considerations: Observe closely for rebound airway edema. Closely monitor heart rate (hold for heart rate >180 beats/minute) and BP during administration.
Adverse reactions: Tachyarrhythmias, hypokalemia, arrhythmias.

ERYTHROMYCIN
Classification: Macrolide antibiotic.
Indications: Treatment of infections caused by *Chlamydia*, *Mycoplasma*, and *Ureaplasma*; treatment and prophylaxis of *Bordetella pertussis* and ophthalmia neonatorum; also used as a prokinetic agent.
Dosage/administration: (see Table A.12)

Table A.12	Erythromycin	
Indication	**Dosage**	**Comment**
Systemic infections	Erythromycin ethylsuccinate (E.E.S., EryPed): 10 mg/kg/dose PO ≤7d: q12h >7d, >2 kg: q6–8h >7d, ≥1.2 kg: q8h >7d, <1.2 kg: q12h	Administer with feeding to enhance absorption and to reduce possible GI upset
Severe systemic infections or PO route unavailable (erythromycin lactobionate)	5–10 mg/kg/dose, IV q6h (Dilute to 1–5 mg/mL and infuse >1 h)	Use only preservative free IV erythromycin formulations

(continued)

Table A.12	Erythromycin *(Continued)*	
Indication	**Dosage**	**Comment**
Opthalmia neonatorum	Prophylaxis: 0.5–1 cm ribbon of 0.5% ointment into each conjunctival sac × 1	Administered at birth
Prokinetic agent	**Initial:** 3 mg/kg IV over 60 minutes, followed by 20 mg/kg/day PO in 3–4 divided doses 30 min before meals	
Ureaplasma urealyticum (erythromycin lactobionate)	5–10 mg/kg/dose IV q6h; treat for 10–14 d	
Chlamydia conjunctivitis and pneumonia (erythromycin ethylsuccinate)	12.5 mg/kg/dose PO q6h × 14 d	

GI = gastrointestinal; IV = intravenously; PO = orally; q6h = every 6 hours; q8h = every 8 hours; q12h = every 12 hours.

Precautions: Do not administer IM (causes pain and necrosis). A 10-fold increased risk of hypertrophic pyloric stenosis is seen in neonates under 2 weeks who receive oral erythromycin for pertussis prophylaxis. In infants <1 month, use azithromycin. Hepatotoxicity can occur with preexisting liver impairment.
Contraindication: Pre-existing hepatic dysfunction.
Drug interactions: Increased blood levels of carbamazepine, digoxin, cyclosporine, warfarin, methylprednisolone, and theophylline.
Test interactions: False-positive urine catecholamines.
Monitoring: LFTs, CBC (eosinophilia), HR, and BP (during IV administration), IV site.
Adverse reactions: Anaphylaxis, rash, stomatitis, candidiasis, hepatotoxicity, reversible ototoxicity (high-dose erythromycin), intrahepatic cholestasis, vomiting, diarrhea, bradycardia, and hypotension (during IV administration).

FAMOTIDINE
Classification: H_2 blocker.
Indications: Short-term therapy and treatment of duodenal ulcer, gastric ulcer, gastroesophageal reflux disease (GERD), control of gastric pH in critically ill patients (similar to ranitidine, famotidine does not significantly interfere with cytochrome P450, thereby reducing its potential for drug interactions). Famotidine has little antiandrogenic effect.
Dosage/administration:
IV: 0.25 to 0.5 mg/kg/dose, q24h. Administer IV dose over >10 minutes on syringe pump.
PO: 0.5 to 1 mg/kg/dose, q24h.
Precautions: Use with caution and modify dose in patients with renal impairment. Avoid injection formulations that contain benzyl alcohol.
Monitoring: Gastric pH, BUN, creatinine, urine output, bilirubin, LFTs, and CBC.

Adverse reactions: Dry mouth, constipation, thrombocytopenia, agranulocytosis, neutropenia, and elevated liver enzymes. Use of H_2 blockade in very low birth weight (VLBW) infants has been associated with a higher risk of nectrotizing enterocolitis. Use of H_2 blockers in preterm neonates has been associated with an increased risk of fungal and late-onset bacterial sepsis.

FENTANYL CITRATE

Classification: Narcotic analgesic.
Indication: Analgesia, sedation, anesthesia.
Dosage/administration:
Sedation/analgesia: 1to 2 mcg/kg/dose q2–4h. Administer slow IV push over 3 to 5 minutes. Larger IV bolus doses (>5 mcg/kg) should be administered over 5 to 10 minutes. Consider using syringe pump for administration. If used for rapid sequence intubation in combination with paralytic agent, it may be given as IV bolus. Continuous infusion: 1 to 2 mcg/kg; then 1 to 2 mcg/kg/hour. Titrate as needed. Tolerance may develop quickly.
Anesthesia: 5 to 50 mcg/kg/dose.
Dilution instructions: Mix 1 mL of 100 mcg/2 mL fentanyl in 9 mL NS. Mixture: 5 mcg/mL.
Precautions: Rapid IV infusion may result in apnea and chest wall rigidity. May require nondepolarizing skeletal muscle relaxant to reverse effect.
Contraindications: Increased intracranial pressure, severe respiratory depression, and severe liver or renal insufficiency.
Adverse reactions: CNS and respiratory depression, skeletal/thoracic muscle rigidity, vomiting, constipation, peripheral vasodilation, miosis, biliary or urinary tract spasms, and antidiuretic hormone release; tolerance develops in association with continuous IV infusions for >5 days.
Monitoring: Respiration rate (RR), heart rate, BP, abdominal status, and muscle rigidity. Adherence to extracorporeal membrane oxygenation (ECMO) membranes and tubing may necessitate increased dose. Fewer cardiovascular effects than morphine.

FERROUS SULFATE

Classification: Oral mineral supplement.
Indication: Prophylaxis for prevention of iron-deficiency anemia in preterm newborns.
Dosage/administration: 2 to 4 mg of elemental iron/kg/day PO. Administer in 1 or 2 divided doses per day. Patients receiving erythropoietin require 6 mg/kg/day of elemental iron. Concentration of elemental iron/mL may vary based on manufacturer. When ordering, specify the exact amount in mg and clarify whether it is mg of elemental or salt form to avoid over- or under dosing. 1 mg elemental iron = 5 mg ferrous sulfate. Iron supplementation may increase hemolysis if adequate vitamin E therapy is not supplied. Start iron therapy not later than 2 months of age.
Clinical considerations: Absorption is variable.
Contraindications: Peptic ulcer disease, ulcerative colitis, enteritis, hemochromatosis, and hemolytic anemia.
Drug interactions: Decreased absorption of both iron and tetracycline when given together. Antacids and chloramphenicol decrease iron absorption.
Monitoring: Hemoglobin and reticulocyte counts during therapy. Observe stools (may color the stool black and may cause false-positive guaiac test for blood), and monitor for constipation.

Adverse reactions: Constipation, diarrhea, and GI irritation.

Overdose: Serum iron level >300 mcg/dL usually requires treatment because of severe toxicity; acute GI irritation, erosion of GI mucosa, hematemesis, lethargy, acidosis, hepatic and renal dysfunction, circulatory collapse, coma, and death. Antidote is deferoxamine chelation therapy. Gastric lavage with 1% to 5% sodium bicarbonate or sodium phosphate solution prevents additional absorption of iron.

FLUCONAZOLE

Classification: Systemic antifungal agent.

Indications: Treatment of systemic fungal infections, meningitis, and severe superficial mycoses. Alternative to amphotericin-B in patients with preexisting renal impairment or when concomitant therapy with other potentially nephrotoxic drugs is required. Recently used as prophylaxis against invasive fungal infections in VLBW infants in NICU with high fungal infection rates.

Dosage/administration: Daily dose of fluconazole is the same for oral and IV administration. See Table A.13 for interval.

Table A.13	Flucanozole Dosing Interval for Invasive Candidiasis	
Gestational Age (Weeks)	**Postnatal Age (Days)**	**Interval (Hours)**
≤29	0 to 14 >14	48 24
30 and Older	0 to 7 >7	48 24

Systemic infections, including meningitis: 12 mg/kg loading dose, then 6 to 12 mg/kg/dose q24h. Administer IV dose on syringe pump over >60 minutes or PO.

Thrush: 6 mg/kg on day 1, then 3 mg/kg/dose q24h PO.

Prophylaxis: 3 mg/kg/dose once daily, 2 times/week for the first 2 weeks, then every other day for a total of 4 to 6 weeks (longer duration for infants with birth weight <1,000 g). Consider 6 mg/kg/dose twice weekly if targeting *Candida* strains with higher MIC. Administer IV dose on syringe pump for 60 minutes.

Clinical considerations: Well-absorbed orally. Good cerebrospinal fluid penetration by both IV and oral routes.

Precaution: Adjust dosage for impaired renal function.

Drug interactions: Warfarin, phenytoin, rifampin. Possible interference with metabolism of caffeine, midazolam, barbiturates, and phenytoin.

Food interaction: Food decreases the rate but not its extent of absorption.

Monitoring: Renal, LFTs (AST, ALT, direct bilirubin), and CBC for eosinophilia.

Adverse reactions: Vomiting, diarrhea, exfoliative skin disorders, and reversible increased AST, ALT, alkaline phosphatase.

FOLIC ACID

Classification: Vitamin, mineral, nutritional supplement.

Indication: Treatment of megaloblastic and macrocytic anemias as a result of folate deficiency.

Dosage/administration: 0.1 mg/day. May be given PO/IM/IV/SC. Administer deeply if an IM route is used. The oral form may be given without regard to feeds.

Clinical considerations: May mask hematologic defects of vitamin B_{12} deficiency but will not prevent progression of irreversible neurologic abnormalities, despite the absence of anemia.

Precautions: The injection contains benzyl alcohol (1.5%) as a preservative; avoid using in preterm infants.

Contraindications: Pernicious, aplastic, and normocytic anemias.

Drug interactions: May decrease phenytoin serum concentrations.

Monitoring parameters: Hematocrit, hemoglobin, and reticulocyte.

Adverse effects: GI upset, pruritus, rash, slight flushing but generally well tolerated.

FOSPHENYTOIN

Classification: Anticonvulsant.

Indications: Management of generalized convulsive status epilepticus refractory to phenobarbital. For short term ($<$5 days) parenteral (IV or IM) administration when other means of phenytoin administration are unavailable, inappropriate, or less advantageous.

Dosage/administration: Should always be dosed in PE: phenytoin equivalent. Fosphenytoin 1 mg PE = phenytoin 1 mg = fosphenytoin 1.5 mg.

Loading dose: 15 to 20 mg PE/kg IM or IV. Infuse loading dose over $>$10 minutes on syringe pump. Initial loading dose up to 30 mg/kg has been reported for status epilepticus.

Maintenance dose: Initial: 5 mg/kg/day in two divided doses. Usual: 5 to 8 mg/kg/day in two divided doses. Some infants $>$7 days of age may require up to 8 mg/kg/dose q8h. Begin maintenance dose 12 to 24 hours after the loading dose. Modify dose in infants with hepatic or renal impairment. Maximum concentration for IV or IM administration is 25 mg PE/mL. Flush IV line with NS before/after administration.

Precautions: To avoid medication errors, always prescribe and dispense fosphenytoin in milligram of PE. Consider the amount of phosphate delivered by fosphenytoin in infants who require phosphate restriction. Each 1 mg PE fosphenytoin delivers 0.0037 mmol of phosphate. Use with caution in infants with hyperbilirubinemia. Fosphenytoin and bilirubin compete with phenytoin and displace phenytoin from plasma protein-binding sites. This results in an increased serum concentration of free phenytoin. Use with caution in hypotension and myocardial insufficiency.

Contraindications: Heart block, sinus bradycardia.

Adverse reactions: Hypotension, vasodilation, tachycardia, bradycardia, fever, hyperglycemia, neutropenia, thrombocytopenia, megaloblastic anemia, osteomalacia, and serious skin reactions.

Monitoring considerations: Monitor BP, EKG during IV loading doses.

Monitoring parameters: Therapeutic levels: 10 to 20 mg/L total phenytoin **or** 1 to 2 mg/L unbound (free) phenytoin only. Toxic levels at 30 to 50 mg/L total phenytoin.

Guidelines for obtaining levels: Obtain phenytoin levels 2 hours after the end of IV infusion or 4 hours after IM dose for status epilepticus. Obtain the first level 48 hours after the loading dose. For maintenance dosing, check through just before dose.

FUROSEMIDE

Classification: Loop diuretic.

Indications: Management of pulmonary edema. To provide diuresis and improve lung function when a greater diuretic effect than produced by chlorothiazide (Diuril®) is needed.

Dosage/administration:

IV: 1 to 2 mg/kg/dose q12–24h.

PO: 2 to 4 mg/kg/dose q12–24h. For long-term use, consider alternate day therapy or longer (dosing interval q48 to 72 h) in order to prevent toxicities. Give with feeds to reduce GI irritation. Give the alcohol and sugar-free product to neonates. IV form may be used orally.

Monitoring: Follow daily weight changes, urine output, serum phosphate, and serum electrolytes. Closely monitor potassium levels in neonates receiving digoxin.

Precautions: Use with caution in hepatic and renal disease.

Adverse reactions: Fluid and electrolyte imbalance, hyponatremia, hypokalemia, hypocalcemia/ hypercalciuria, hypochloremic alkalosis, nephrocalcinosis (associated with long-term therapy), potential ototoxicity (especially if receiving aminoglycosides), prerenal azotemia, hyperuricemia, agranulocytosis, anemia, thrombocytopenia, interstitial nephritis, pancreatitis, and cholelithiasis (in BPD or CHF and long-term total parenteral nutrition and furosemide therapy).

GANCICLOVIR

Classification: Antiviral agent.

Indication: Treatment or prophylaxis of cytomegalovirus (CMV) infections.

Dosages/administration: For congenital CMV infection, 6 mg/kg/dose q12h for 6 weeks; infuse over >1 hour on syringe pump. Maximum concentration for infusion must not exceed 10 mg/mL in dextrose or NS. **Administer through central line to minimize the risk of phlebitis if available.** May be administered through peripheral line if central line is not available. Do not administer IM or SC to avoid severe tissue irritation that is due to its high pH.

Precautions: Treat ganciclovir as a **cytotoxic** drug. **Avoid all contact** with skin and mucous membranes. Wear impervious protective gown, nonlatex procedure gloves, and mask. Priming of IV set should not allow any drug to be released into the environment. For infants with neutropenia, an absolute neutrophil count <500 or thrombocytopenia with a platelet count <25,000, use a decreased dose. Consider treatment with granulocyte colony-stimulating factor (G-CSF) (Neupogen®) in patients with neutropenia. Adjust dose in renal impairment. Avoid dehydration during therapy.

Adverse reactions: Neutropenia, leukopenia, granulocytopenia, thrombocytopenia, and anemia. Thrombocytopenia is usually reversible and responds to a decreased dose, inflammation at IV site, increased LFTs, increased BUN/serum creatinine, fever, and diarrhea. Decrease dosage if renal function worsens.

Monitoring considerations: Obtain daily CBC with differential and platelet count. Obtain weekly BUN and serum creatinine. At the first sign of significant renal dysfunction, the dose of ganciclovir should be adjusted by either reducing the number of mg/dose or by prolonging the dosing interval.

GENTAMICIN SULFATE

Classification: Aminoglycoside, antibiotic.

Indications: Active against gram-negative aerobic bacteria, some activity against coagulase-positive staphylococci, ineffective against anaerobes, streptococci.

Dosage/administration: (see Table A.14)

Table A.14	Gentamicin Sulfate		
PMA	**Postnatal**	**Dose**	**Interval**
≤29 wk*	0–7 d	5 mg/kg	48 h
	8–28 d	4 mg/kg	36 h
	≥29 d	4 mg/kg	24 h
30–34 wk	0–7 d	4.5 mg/kg	36 h
	≥8 d	4 mg/kg	24 h
≥35 wk	ALL	4 mg/kg	24 h
*Or significant asphyxia, PDA, or treatment with indomethacin.			

Administer IV infusion on a syringe pump over >30 minutes. IV route preferred because IM absorption is variable.

Precaution: Modify dosage interval in patients with renal impairment.

Drug interactions: Indomethacin decreases gentamicin clearance and prolongs its half-life. Increased neuromuscular blockade is observed when aminoglycosides are used with neuromuscular blocking agents (e.g., pancuronium). The risk of aminoglycoside-induced ototoxicity and/or nephrotoxicity is increased when used concurrently with loop diuretics (e.g., furosemide, bumetanide) or vancomycin. Neuromuscular weakness or respiratory failure may occur in infants with hypermagnesemia.

Adverse reactions: Vestibular and irreversible auditory ototoxicity (associated with high trough levels) and renal toxicity (occurs in the proximal tubule, associated with high trough levels, usually reversible). Treat extravasation with hyaluronidase around periphery of an affected area.

Monitoring: Renal function (creatinine, urine output), drug peak, and trough levels.

Guidelines for obtaining levels: Draw trough levels within 30 minutes before the next dose. Draw peak levels at 30 minutes after the end of a 30-minute infusion or 1 hour after an IM injection. For all infants, **obtain blood levels pre- and post-third dose.**

Trough: Less than 1.5 mcg/mL.

Peak: 6 to 12 mcg/mL (dependent upon indication).

Dose adjustment: For trough levels between 1.5 and 2 mcg/mL, obtain another trough with next dose. Aminoglycosides exhibit linear kinetics. Decreasing the dose by a specified percentage will result in an equal decrease in percentage of peak level.

GLUCAGON

Classification: Antihypoglycemic agent.

Indication: Treatment of hypoglycemia in cases of documented glucagon deficiency or refractory to IV dextrose infusions.

Dosage/administration: 25 to 200 mcg/kg/dose (0.025–0.2 mg/kg/dose) IV push/IM/SC every 20 minutes as needed.

Maximum dose: 1 mg.

Continuous IV: Administer in dextrose 10% water solution, 0.5 to 1 mg infused over 24 hours. (Doses >0.02 mg/kg/hour did not produce additional benefit.) Add hydrocortisone if no response occurs within 4 hours. Slowly taper over at least 24 hours after desired effect has been reached.

Dosing Considerations: Wide variation in recommended dosage exists between manufacturer's labeling and published case reports.

Contraindications: Should not be used in small-for-gestational-age infants.

Precautions: Do not delay starting glucose infusion while awaiting effect of glucagon. Use caution in infants with history of insulinoma or pheochromocytoma.

Monitoring: Serum glucose, sodium. Rise in serum glucose will last approximately 2 hours after bolus.

Adverse reactions: Vomiting, tachycardia, hypertension, hyponatremia, thrombocytopenia, ileus, and GI upset. May result in rebound hypoglycemia.

HEPARIN SODIUM

Classification: Anticoagulant.

Indications: To maintain patency of single- and double-lumen central catheters, thrombosis treatment.

Clinical considerations: Neonates have low-antithrombin plasma concentrations and may require boluses of antithrombin III for heparin to be effective.

Dosage/administration: (see Table A.15)

Table A.15	Heparin Sodium	
Indication	Dosage	Comment
Heparin lock for central lines	1–2 mL of 10 unit/mL solution q4–6h and PRN	To maintain patency
Continuous infusion for the maintenance of central venous and/or arterial line	Add heparin to make a final concentration of 0.5–1 unit/mL	To maintain patency
Continuous heparin drip	75 unit/kg bolus over 10 minutes, then 28 units/kg/hour. Titrate to maintain desired PTT and heparin level	Do not bolus in critically ill neonates
IV = intravenous; PRN = as needed; q4–6h = every 4 to 6 hours.		

Contraindications: Platelet count <50,000/mm^3, suspected intracranial hemorrhage, GI bleeding, shock, severe hypotension, and uncontrolled bleeding.

Precautions: Risk factors for hemorrhage include IM injections, venous and arterial blood sampling, and peptic ulcer disease. Use preservative-free heparin in neonates. To avoid systemic heparinization in small neonates, use more dilute (0.5 unit/mL) heparin flush concentrations.

Monitoring for therapeutic heparin: Follow platelet counts every 2 to 3 days. Assess for signs of bleeding and thrombosis. Heparin level (0.3–0.7 unit/mL), PTT (70–100 seconds).

Drug interactions: Thrombolytic agents and IV nitroglycerin.

Adverse reactions: Heparin-induced thrombocytopenia reported in some heparin-exposed newborns. Other adverse reactions include hemorrhage, fever, urticaria, vomiting, increased LFTs, osteoporosis, and alopecia.

Antidote: Protamine sulfate (1 mg/100 units of heparin given in the previous 4 hours).

HYALURONIDASE

Classification: Antidote, extravasation.

Indications: Prevention of tissue injury caused by IV extravasation of hyperosmolar or extremely alkaline solutions.

Dosage/administration: SC or intradermal: May use concentrations from 15 to 150 units/mL. Inject five separate 0.2-mL injections into the leading edge of the infiltrate. Use a 25 or 27 gauge needle, and change after each injection. Elevate the extremity. Do not apply heat and do not administer IV. Best results are obtained when used within 1 hour of extravasation. May repeat if necessary. Add overfill in syringe upon dispensing for drug remaining in needle during frequent changes.

Clinical considerations: Some agents for which hyaluronidase is effective include aminophylline, amphotericin, calcium, diazepam, erythromycin, gentamicin, methicillin, nafcillin, oxacillin, phenytoin, potassium chloride, sodium bicarbonate, tromethamine, vancomycin, total parenteral nutrition, and concentrated IV solutions.

Warnings: Hyaluronidase is neither effective nor indicated for treatment of extravasations of vasoconstrictive agents (phentolamine is the preferred agent for the treatment of extravasation with vasoconstrictive agents).

HYDRALAZINE

Classification: Antihypertensive, vasodilator.

Indication: BP reduction in neonatal hypertension. After load reduction in CHF.

Dosage/administration:

Initial dose: 0.1 to 0.5 mg/kg/dose IV q6–8h. Increase gradually to a maximum of 2 mg/kg/dose IV q6h as required for BP control. Usual concentration for IV administration is 1 mg/mL. Maximum concentration for IV administration is 20 mg/mL.

Oral dose: 0.25 to 1 mg/kg/dose PO q6–8h. Administer with food to enhance absorption. Double the dose when changing from IV to oral solution because hydralazine is only, approximately, 50% absorbed.

Precautions: Use with caution in severe renal and cardiac disease. Adjust dosing interval in renal impairment.

Clinical considerations: May cause reflex tachycardia. Concurrent β-blocker therapy recommended to reduce the magnitude of reflex tachycardia and to enhance antihypertensive effect. Maximum effect occurs in 3 to 4 days. Tachyphylaxis reported with chronic therapy.

Drug interactions: Concurrent use with other antihypertensives allows reduced dosage requirements of hydralazine to <0.15 mg/kg/dose.

Monitoring: Daily monitoring of heart rate, BP, urine output, and weight. Perform guaiac test on all stools and obtain CBC at least twice weekly.

Adverse reactions: Tachycardia, vomiting, diarrhea, orthostatic hypotension, salt retention, edema, GI irritation and bleeding, anemia, and temporary agranulocytosis.

HYDROCHLOROTHIAZIDE

Classification: Thiazide diuretic.

Indications: Fluid overload, pulmonary edema, BPD, CHF, and hypertension.

Dosage/administration: 1 to 2 mg/kg/dose PO q12h.
Contraindications: Anuria or renal failure.
Monitoring: Serum electrolytes, calcium, phosphorus, blood glucose, bilirubin, urine output, BP, and daily weight.
Adverse reactions: Hypochloremic alkalosis, volume depletion, displacement of bilirubin, blood dyscrasias, decreased serum potassium, sodium and magnesium levels, and increased levels of glucose, uric acid, and calcium.

HYDROCORTISONE

Classification: Adrenal corticosteroid with mostly glucocorticoid effects.
Indication: Vasopressor-resistant hypotension; treatment of cortisol insufficiency; based on two retrospectively matched cohort studies of the cognitive and motor neurodevelopmental outcomes at school age, hydrocortisone maybe a "safer" alternative to dexamethasone for treatment of CLD in "exceptional clinical circumstances."
Dosage/administration: Initial dose may be given as a slow IV push in over >3 to 5 minutes. Administer subsequent doses in over >30 minutes on syringe pump.
Vasopressor-resistant hypotension: (see Table A.16)

Table A.16	Hydrocortisone for Vasopressor-resistant Hypotension
Day	**Dose/frequency**
Day 1 initial dose	1 mg/kg/dose IV q8h × 3 doses
Day 2 follow in 12 h with	0.5 mg/kg/dose IV q12h × 2 doses
Day 3 follow in 12 h with	0.25 mg/kg/dose IV q12h × 2 doses
Day 4 follow in 24 h with	0.125 mg/kg/dose IV × 1 dose
IV = intravenous; q8h = every 8 hours; q12h = every 12 hours.	

If BP improves and other vasopressors have been weaned off, treatment may stop after 24 hours. Final concentration for infusion is 1 mg/mL in dextrose or saline. Use preservative-free hydrocortisone sodium succinate formulation for IV dosing.
CAH: Oral 10 to 20 mg/m^2/day in 3 divided doses. Stress dose 30 to 50 mg/m^2/dose.
BPD: A suggested regimen for BPD is a starting dose of 5 mg/kg/day of hydrocortisone tapered over 7 to 10 days.
Precautions: Acute adrenal insufficiency may occur with abrupt withdrawal following long-term therapy or during periods of stress.
Adverse reactions: Hypertension, salt retention, edema, cataracts, peptic ulcer, immunosuppression, hypokalemia, hyperglycemia, dermatitis, Cushing syndrome, and skin atrophy. Risk of GI perforation when given concurrently with indomethacin.

IBUPROFEN

Classification: Nonselective cyclooxygenase enzyme inhibitor. Inhibitor of prostaglandin synthesis. Nonsteroidal anti-inflammatory agent.
Indications: Pharmacologic closure of clinically significant ductus arteriosus.
Dosage/administration: (Calculate all doses based on birth weight)

Initial dose: 10 mg/kg IV × 1, then 5 mg/kg IV at 24 and 48 hours after initial dose. Infuse over 15 minutes at a port closest to insertion site (do not infuse in the same line with TPN).

Precautions: Avoid using together with steroids to decrease incidence of GI bleeding. Use with caution in patients with decreased renal or hepatic function, dehydration, CHF, hypertension, history of GI bleeding, or those receiving anticoagulants.

Monitoring: BUN and serum creatinine, CBC, occult blood loss, liver enzymes; echocardiogram, heart murmur, urine output (hold doses if output <0.6 mL/kg/hour).

Adverse reactions: Edema, peptic ulcer, GI bleed, GI perforation, neutropenia, anemia, agranulocytosis, inhibition of platelet aggregation, and acute renal failure.

IMMUNE GLOBULIN

Classification: Immune globulin.

Indications: Alloimmune thrombocytopenia and isoimmune hemolytic disease of the newborn causing hyperbilirubinemia.

Dosage/administration: 0.5 to 1 g/kg IV over >2 to 3 hours. May repeat in 12 hours if necessary. Usual concentration for IV administration is 5% to 10% (50–100 mg/mL).

Precautions: Response to live vaccines may be reduced following the treatment.

Monitoring: Continuous heart rate and BP monitoring during administration. Decreasing rate or stopping infusion may help relieve some adverse effects (flushing, changes in pulse rate, and blood pressure fluctuation).

Adverse reactions: Transient hypoglycemia, tachycardia, and hypotension (resolved with cessation of infusion). Tenderness, erythema, and induration at injection site and allergic manifestations. Rare hypersensitivity reactions reported with rapid IV administration.

INDOMETHACIN

Classification: Cardiovascular agent.

Indication: Pharmacologic alternative to surgical closure of PDA.

Dosage/administration: (see Table A.17)

Table A.17	Indomethacin		
Age at first dose	First dose (mg/kg/dose IV)	Second dose (mg/kg/dose IV)	Third dose (mg/kg/dose IV)
<48 h	0.2	0.1	0.1
2–7 d	0.2	0.2	0.2
>7 d	0.2	0.25	0.25
IV = intravenous.			

IV dosing only—oral dosing is not recommended. Give by IV syringe pump over >30 minutes, three doses/course with a usual maximum of two courses, given at 12- to 24-hour intervals. Some infants require a longer treatment course.

Clinical considerations: Hold enteral feeds until 12 hours after last indomethacin dose.

Contraindications: Impaired renal function (urine output <0.6 mL/kg/hour for the preceding 8 hours, or significant renal dysfunction), active bleeding, ulcer disease, NEC or stool heme test >3+, platelet count <60,000/mm^3, and coagulation defects.

Precautions: Use with caution in neonates with cardiac dysfunction and hypertension. Because indomethacin causes a decrease in renal and GI blood flow, withhold enteral feedings during therapy. Reduction in cerebral flow reported with IV infusions of <5 minutes in duration. Should not use in combination with glucocorticoids if possible, given an increased risk of spontaneous intestinal perforation.

Monitoring: Urine output (keep >0.6 mL/kg/hour), serum electrolytes, serum BUN and creatinine, and platelet count. Closely assess pulse pressure, cardiopulmonary status, and PDA murmur for evidence of success/failure of therapy. Guaiac test all stools and test gastric aspirates to detect GI bleeding. Observe for prolonged bleeding from puncture sites.

Drug interactions: Concurrent administration with digoxin and/or with aminoglycosides results in increased plasma concentrations of these respective agents. Spontaneous intestinal perforation is increased when used in combination with glucocorticoids.

Adverse reactions: Decreased platelet aggregation, ulcer, GI intolerance, hemolytic anemia, bone marrow suppression, agranulocytosis, thrombocytopenia, ileal perforation, transient oliguria, electrolyte imbalance, hypertension, hypoglycemia, indirect hyperbilirubinemia, and hepatitis.

INSULIN, REGULAR

Classification: Pancreatic hormone, hypoglycemic agent.
Indication: Hyperglycemia, hyperkalemia.
Dosage/administration: (see Table A.18)

Table A.18	Insulin		
Indication	Dosage	Administration	Comment
Bolus	0.05–0.2 unit/kg q6h PRN	Give as IV bolus	Monitor glucose every 15–30 min
Continuous IV infusion	0.01–0.1 unit/ kg/hour	If BG remains >180 mg/dL, titrate in increments of 0.01 unit/kg/hour	Before start of infusion, purge IV tubing with minimum of 25 mL of the infusion solution to saturate plastic binding sites. Titrate to maintain euglycemia
		If hypoglycemia occurs, D/C insulin infusion and give D$_{10}$W at 2 mL/kg (0.2 g/kg)	
Hyperkalemia	First administer calcium gluconate 50 mg/kg/dose IV then sodium bicarbonate 1–2 mEq/kg/dose IV	Follow with dextrose 500 mg/kg/dose + regular insulin 0.1 unit/kg/dose IV	

(continued)

Table A.18	Insulin *(Continued)*		
Indication	Dosage	Administration	Comment
	Calcium gluconate *is not compatible* with NaHCO$_3$ Flush IV lines between infusions		

IV = intravenously; PRN = as needed; BG = blood glucose; D/C = discontinue; q6h = every 6 hours.

For IV bolus and IV infusion, use regular human insulin. Mix 15 units of regular insulin in 150 mL IV bag NS or dextrose 5% water (D$_5$W) = 10 units/100 mL or 0.1 unit/mL. Maximum recommended concentration is 1 unit/mL.

Monitoring: Follow blood glucose concentration every 30 minutes to 1 hour after starting infusion and after changes in infusion rate. Follow these parameters q2–4h after achieving a stable euglycemic state.

Clinical considerations: Reduce loss of insulin that is due to adsorption to the plastic tubing by flushing tubing with a minimum of 25 mL of insulin solution before beginning the infusion.

Precaution: Only regular insulin may be administered IV.

Adverse reactions: Hyperglycemic rebound, urticaria, anaphylaxis; may rapidly induce hypoglycemia, hypokalemia. Insulin resistance may develop with prolonged use and necessitate an increased dose.

LEVOTHYROXINE SODIUM

Classification: Thyroid hormone.

Indications: Replacement or supplementary therapy for hypothyroidism.

Dosage/administration: To avoid differences in bioavailability, use the same brand of thyroid hormone (100 mg levothyroxine = 65 mg thyroid USP).

Initial oral dose: 10 to 15 mcg/kg/day q24h; adjust in 12.5 mcg increments every 2 weeks until T$_4$ is 10 to 15 mcg/dL and thyroid-stimulating hormone (TSH) is <15 mU/L.

Term infant average oral dose: 37.5 to 50 mcg/day. Administer oral dose on an empty stomach. When starting IV or switching from PO to IV route, IV dose should be 50% to 75% of the oral dose/day. Use only NS to reconstitute IV preparations. Use immediately after mixing. Do not add to any other solution. Usual concentration for infusion is 20 to 40 mcg/mL. Maximum concentration for infusion is 100 mcg/mL. Administer as a slow IV push. May also be given IM.

Clinical considerations: Oral route preferred: use IV when oral route is unavailable or with myxedema stupor/coma.

Contraindications: Thyrotoxicosis and uncorrected adrenal insufficiency.

Precautions: Use with caution in infants receiving anticoagulants. In infants with cardiac disease, begin with one-fourth of usual maintenance dose and increase weekly. Do not use the IV form orally because it crystallizes when exposed to acid. **Do not administer iron or zinc within 4 hours of levothyroxine dose.**

Monitoring: Adjust dosage based on clinical status and serum T$_4$ and TSH. Serum T$_4$ and TSH levels should be measured every 1 to 2 months or 2 to 3 weeks after any change in dose. Obtain serum T_4, free T_4 index, and TSH levels. Adequate therapy should suppress TSH values to 15 mU/L within 3 to 4 months of starting therapy. Assess for signs of hypothyroidism: lethargy, poor feeding, constipation, intermittent cyanosis, and prolonged neonatal jaundice. In addition, closely assess for signs of thyrotoxicosis: hyperreactivity, tachycardia, tachypnea, fever, exophthalmos, and goiter. Periodically assess growth and bone-age development.

Adverse reactions: Hyperthyroidism, rash, weight loss, diarrhea, tachycardia, cardiac arrhythmias, tremors, fever, and hair loss. Prolonged over treatment can produce premature craniosynostosis and acceleration of bone age.

LINEZOLID

Classification: Antibiotic, oxazolidinone.

Indications: Treatment of bacteremia caused by susceptible vancomycin-resistant *Enterococcus faecium* (VREF).

Dosage/administration: 10 mg/kg/dose IV/PO q8h. Preterm newborns <7 days old: 10 mg/kg/dose IV/PO q12h. Infuse IV dose over >60 minutes.

Precautions: There have been reports of VREF and *Staphylococcus aureus* (methicillin-resistant) developing resistance to linezolid during its clinical use.

Monitoring: CBC; platelet counts and hemoglobin, particularly in patients at increased risk for bleeding, patients with preexisting thrombocytopenia or myelosuppression, or concomitant medications that decrease platelet count or function or produce bone marrow suppression, and in patients requiring >2 weeks of therapy; number and type of stools/day for diarrhea, AST, ALT.

Adverse reactions: Elevated ALT; diarrhea; thrombocytopenia, anemia.

LORAZEPAM

Classification: Benzodiazepine, anticonvulsant, sedative hypnotic.

Indication: Status epilepticus refractory to conventional therapy; sedation.

Dosage/administration:

Initial dose: 0.05 to 0.1 mg/kg/dose IV over >5 minutes; (repeat in 10–15 minutes if necessary for status epilepticus).

Maximum dose: 4 mg/dose.

Maintenance dose: 0.05 mg/kg/dose IV/IM/PO/PR, q6–8h, depending on response. Reduce dosage in hepatic or renal impairment. The IV formulation may be given orally. May administer with feeds to decrease GI distress.

Contraindication: Preexisting CNS depression or severe hypotension.

Warning: Rhythmic myoclonic jerking movements have been observed in preterm infants.

Precautions: Some preparations contain 2% benzyl alcohol and may be hazardous to neonates in high doses. Dilute before IV use with equal volume of NS or sterile water. Use with caution in infants with renal or hepatic impairment or myasthenia gravis.

Monitoring: Respiratory status during and after administration.

Adverse reactions: CNS depression, bradycardia, circulatory collapse, respiratory depression, BP instability, and GI symptoms. Discontinue therapy if syncope and paradoxic CNS stimulation occurs.

METHADONE

Classification: Narcotic, analgesic.

Indication: Treatment of neonatal opiate withdrawal.

Dosage/administration:
Initial dose: 0.05 to 0.2 mg/kg/dose PO or slow IV push. Give q8h for 2 to 3 doses, then q12–24h. Titrate dose based on neonatal abstinence score (NAS). Wean dose by 10% to 20% per week over 4- to 6-week period.
Clinical considerations: Tapering is difficult because of its long elimination half-life (16–25 hours). Consider alternative agents.
Monitoring: Respiratory and cardiac status.
Drug interactions: Methadone metabolism accelerated by rifampin and phenytoin; this may precipitate withdrawal symptoms.
Adverse reactions: Respiratory depression, ileus, delayed gastric emptying, QTc prolongation.

METOCLOPRAMIDE
Classification: Antiemetic, prokinetic agent.
Indications: Improve gastric emptying and GI motility.
Dosage/administration: GI dysmotility: 0.4 to 0.8 mg/kg/day divided q6h IV/PO; orally administer 30 minutes before feeds. Oral solution available as 0.1 mg/mL and 1 mg/mL. Administer IV over ≥30 minutes on syringe pump. Maximum concentration for IV infusion is 5 mg/mL (usual concentration: 1 mg/mL) in NS or dextrose. IV form may be given orally.
Contraindications: GI obstruction, pheochromocytoma, history of seizure disorder.
Monitoring: Measure gastric residuals, monitor complete blood count weekly.
Adverse reactions: Warnings: May cause tardive dyskinesia (often irreversible). Treatment duration and total dose are associated with an increased risk. Drowsiness, restlessness, agitation, diarrhea, methemoglobinemia, agranulocytosis, leukopenia, neutropenia, and extrapyramidal symptoms (may occur following IV administration of large doses and within 24–48 hours of starting therapy; responds rapidly to Benadryl® and subsides within 24 hours after stopping metoclopramide).
Overdose: Associated with doses greater than 1 mg/kg/day, characterized by drowsiness, ataxia, extrapyramidal reactions, seizures, and methemoglobinemia (treat with methylene blue).

MIDAZOLAM
Classification: Benzodiazepine, sedative hypnotic, anticonvulsant.
Indication: Sedation.
Dosage/administration: IV dose: 0.05 to 0.15 mg/kg/dose q2–4h as needed. Administer over ≥15 minutes on syringe pump. Severe hypotension and seizures have been reported with rapid infusion in neonates. Final infusion concentration is 0.5 mg/mL in NS or dextrose. Intranasal: 0.2 mg/kg/dose (using injectable formulation).
Contraindications: Preexisting CNS depression or shock.
Precautions: CHF and renal impairment. Some formulations may contain 1% benzyl alcohol.
Monitoring: RR, heart rate, BP.
Drug interactions: CNS depressants, anesthetic agents, cimetidine, and theophylline. Decrease midazolam dose by 25% during prolonged concurrent narcotic administration.
Adverse reactions: Sedation, respiratory arrest, apnea, cardiac arrest, hypotension, bradycardia, and seizures (following rapid bolus administration and in neonates with underlying CNS disorders). Encephalopathy reported in several infants sedated for 4 to 11 days with midazolam and fentanyl.

MILRINONE

Classification: Phosphodiesterase inhibitor.

Indications: Effective inotropic agent indicated for the short-term IV treatment of CHF. In infants with decreased myocardial function, milrinone increases cardiac output, decreases pulmonary capillary wedge pressure, and decreases vascular resistance. It increases myocardial contractility and improves diastolic function by improving left ventricular diastolic relaxation without increasing myocardial oxygen consumption.

Dosage/administration: Administer with a loading dose followed by a continuous infusion. A pilot study recommends different dosing in premature infants <30 weeks GA due to longer half-life.

Loading dose >30 wks GA: 50 to 75 mcg/kg administered through syringe pump over >15 minutes (**Loading doses are generally not given to newborn infants**).

Loading dose <30 wks GA 0.75 mcg/kg/minute for 3 hours, then 0.2 mcg/kg/minute.

Maintenance dose: 0.25 to 0.75 mcg/kg/minute. Titrate dose to effect.

Maximum infusion rate: 1 mcg/kg/minute. Usual concentration for infusion is 100 mcg/mL. Maximum is 250 mcg/mL in NS or dextrose. Central line preferred. **Do not administer through UAC.**

Monitoring parameters: EKG, BP, CBC, electrolytes. Volume expanders may be needed to counteract the vasodilatory effect and potential decrease in filling pressures.

Adverse effects: Thrombocytopenia, arrhythmias, hypotension.

MORPHINE SULFATE

Classification: Opiate, narcotic analgesic.

Indication: Analgesia, sedation, treatment of opiate withdrawal.

Dosage/administration:

Analgesia/sedation: 0.05 to 0.1 mg/kg/dose IV/IM/SC q4–8h as needed for pain. Administer bolus over >5 minutes on syringe pump.

Continuous IV infusion: Following administration of loading dose, start continuous infusion: 0.01 to 0.02 mg/kg/hour. Titrate for clinical indications. Use only preservative-free formulation.

Concentration for administration: 0.1 to 1 mg/mL in NS or dextrose.

Treatment of opiate withdrawal: (see Tables A.19 and A.20)

For treatment of opiate withdrawal, monitor NAS scores closely to avoid infant becoming obtunded due to overdosage. Discontinue when dose is <25% of maximum dose. Administration of oral morphine solution with food may increase bioavailability.

Table A.19	Morphine Sulfate
For NAS score	**Initial oral dose**
8–10	0.32 mg/kg/day divided q4h
11–13	0.48 mg/kg/day divided q4h
14–16	0.64 mg/kg/day divided q4h
>17	0.8 mg/kg/day divided q4h
NAS = neonatal abstinence score; q4h = every 4 hours.	

Table A.20	Morphine Sulfate
For NAS score	**Maintenance oral dose**
>8 × 3 successive scores	↑ dose by 0.16 mg (0.4 mL/kg/day) divided q4h to max dose
<8 × 3 successive scores	Wean by 10% of the max daily dose. If infant has been weaned too quickly, go back to last effective dose.
NAS = neonatal abstinence score; q4h = every 4 hours; ↑ = increasing.	

Precautions: Fentanyl is preferred over morphine in neonates with cardiovascular and hemodynamic instability. Morphine causes histamine release leading to increased venous capacitance and suppression of adrenergic tone. Hypotension and chest wall rigidity may occur with rapid IV administration. Tolerance may develop following prolonged use (>96 hours).

Contraindications: Increased intracranial pressure. Use with caution in severe hepatic, renal impairment.

Adverse reactions: Hypotension, CNS depression, respiratory depression, bradycardia, transient hypertonia, ileus, delayed gastric emptying, constipation, and urinary retention. Naloxone should be available to reverse adverse effects.

Monitoring: Monitor RR, heart rate, and BP closely; observe for abdominal distention and loss of bowel sounds; monitor input and output to evaluate urinary retention.

NAFCILLIN

Classification: Semisynthetic penicillinase-resistant antistaphylococcal penicillin.

Indications: Primarily active against *staphylococci*. Reserve for penicillin-resistant *S. aureus* infections.

Dosage/administration: (see Table A.21)

Table A.21	Nafcillin	
Age	**Birth weight**	**IV dosage and interval**
0–4 wk	<1,200 g	25 mg/kg/dose q12h
≤7 d	1,200–2,000 g	25 mg/kg/dose q12h
>7 d	1,200–2,000 g	25 mg/kg/dose q8h
≤7 d	>2,000 g	25 mg/kg/dose q8h
>7 d	>2,000 g	25–35 mg/kg/dose q6h
IV = intravenous; q6h = every 6 hours; q8h = every 8 hours; q12h = every 12 hours.		

IV: Final concentration of 100 mg/mL infused over >30 minutes on syringe pump.

Precautions: Dosing interval increased with hepatic dysfunction. Oral route not recommended because of poor absorption. Avoid IM administration if possible.

Monitoring: CBC, BUN, creatinine, and LFTs. Observe for hematuria and proteinuria.
Clinical considerations: Better cerebrospinal fluid penetration than methicillin. Decrease dose by 33% to 50% in infants with combined renal/hepatic impairment.
Drug interactions: Blunting of peak aminoglycoside concentration when administered simultaneously with nafcillin.
Adverse reactions: Agranulocytosis hypersensitivity, granulocytopenia, vein irritation, and nephrotoxicity (eosinophilia may precede renal damage). Treat extravasation with hyaluronidase.

NALOXONE

Classification: Narcotic antagonist.
Indications: Used concurrently during neonatal resuscitation for narcotic-induced CNS depression. Not recommended as part of initial resuscitation of newborn with respiratory depression in the delivery room.
Dosage/administration:
0.1 mg/kg bolus IV/IM/SC; endotracheally at higher dose (see below). **Doses as low as 0.01 to 0.03 mg/kg may be effective for reversing narcotic-induced depression.** May repeat every 2 to 3 minutes if needed. Multiple doses may be necessary because of its short duration of action (every 20–60 minutes). IV or ETT route preferred, IM or SC route may lead to delayed onset of action. Recommended ETT dose is 2 to 10 times the IV dose.
Contraindications: Use with caution in infants with chronic cardiac disease, pulmonary disease, or coronary disease. Do not administer to newborns of narcotic dependent mothers, as it may precipitate seizures.
Adverse reactions: Use caution in infants receiving medication for pain control.
Will produce narcotic withdrawal syndrome in newborns with chronic dependence. Abrupt reversal may result in vomiting, diaphoresis, tachycardia, hypertension, and tremors.
Monitoring: Heart rate, respiratory rate, BP, neurologic status.

NOREPINEPHRINE

Classification: Adrenergic agonist agent, α-adrenergic agonist, sympathomimetic.
Indications: Treatment of shock that persists after adequate fluid volume replacement; severe hypotension; cardiogenic shock.
Dosage/administration:
Initial: 0.05 to 0.1 mcg/kg/minute, titrate to desired effect; maximum dose: 1 to 2 mcg/kg/minute. Usual concentration 0.1 mg/mL. Dilute with D_5W; dilution in NS is not recommended. **Central venous access is preferred. Do not administer through UAC.**
Precautions: Blood/volume depletion should be corrected, if possible, before norepinephrine therapy; extravasation may cause severe tissue necrosis; do not give to patients with peripheral or mesenteric vascular thrombosis because ischemia may be increased and the area of infarct extended; use with caution in patients with occlusive vascular disease.
Monitoring: BP, heart rate, urine output, peripheral perfusion.
Adverse reactions: Cardiac arrhythmias, bradycardia, tachycardia, dyspnea, hypertension, pallor; organ ischemia (due to vasoconstriction of renal and mesenteric arteries), ischemic necrosis, and sloughing of superficial tissue after extravasation. If extravasation occurs, administer phentolamine as soon as possible.

NYSTATIN

Classification: Nonabsorbed antifungal agent.

Indications: Treatment of susceptible cutaneous, mucocutaneous, and oropharyngeal fungal infections caused by *Candida* species.

Dosage/administration:

Oral: Preterm infant: 1 mL (100,000 units) q6h. Term infant: 2 mL (200,000 units) q6h. Apply half of dose with swab to each side of mouth q6h after feedings.

Topical therapy: Apply powder, ointment, or cream to the affected area q6h. Powder should be used for moist lesions.

Continue oral therapy and topical application for 2 to 3 days beyond resolution of fungal infection.

Clinical considerations: Combination therapy for candidal perineal infections with oral and topical nystatin is possible because of nystatin's poor absorption in the GI tract and because the GI tract serves as the reservoir for fungi causing perineal infection. Eliminate factors contributing to fungal growth (wet, occlusive diapers, and the use of contaminated nipples). Breastfeeding mothers should be concurrently treated topically.

Adverse reactions: Irritation, contact dermatitis, diarrhea, and vomiting.

OCTREOTIDE

Classification: Antisecretory agent, somatostatin analog.

Indications: Pharmacologic management of persistent hyperinsulinemic hypoglycemia of infancy (nesidioblastosis), adjunct treatment of congenital and postoperative chylothorax.

Dosage/administration: Hyperinsulinemic hypoglycemia: 2 to 10 mcg/kg/day IV or SC, initially divided q12h; increase dosage depending upon patient response by either using a more frequent interval (q6–8h) or larger dose.

Maximum dose: 10 mcg/kg/dose q6h.

Chylothorax: 1 to 7 mcg/kg/hour continuous infusion; start low and titrate dose to effect (decreased chyle production).

Clinical considerations: Glucose response should occur within 8 hours. Chyle production should decrease within 24 hours.

Precautions: Glucose tolerance; use with caution in patients with renal impairment. Suppression of growth hormone with long-term therapy.

Monitoring: Cholelithiasis, blood sugar, thyroid function tests, fluid and electrolyte balance, and fecal fat.

Adverse reactions: hyperglycemia, galactorrhea, hypothyroidism, flushing, edema, hypertension, palpitations, CHF, bradycardia, arrhythmias, conduction abnormalities, diarrhea, constipation, fat malabsorption, growth hormone suppression, vomiting, abdominal distension, biliary sludge.

OMEPRAZOLE

Classification: Proton-pump inhibitor; gastric acid secretion inhibitor, GI agent, gastric or duodenal ulcer treatment.

Indications: Short-term (<8 weeks) treatment of documented reflux esophagitis or duodenal ulcer refractory to conventional therapy.

Dosage/administration: 0.5 to 1.5 mg/kg/dose PO daily through nasogastric tube, or jejunostomy tube daily for 4 to 8 weeks. Maximum effective dose: 3.5 mg/kg/day divided BID.

Precautions: Mild transaminase elevations have been reported in children who received omeprazole for extended periods. Use with caution in infants with respiratory alkalosis due to high content of sodium bicarbonate in the oral suspension; avoid use in infants on sodium restriction.

Contraindications: Hypersensitivity to omeprazole or any component.

Adverse reactions: Tachycardia, bradycardia, palpitations, altered sleeping patterns, hemifacial dysesthesia, fever, irritability, dry skin, rash, hypoglycemia, diarrhea, vomiting, constipation, discoloration of tongue and feces, feeding intolerance because of anorexia, irritable colon, urinary frequency, agranulocytosis, pancytopenia, thrombocytopenia, anorexia, leukocytosis, hepatitis, increased LFTs, jaundice, hematuria, pyuria, proteinuria, glycosuria, cough, and epistaxis. Use of H_2 blockade in VLBW infants has been associated with a higher risk of bacterial/fungal sepsis and NEC; omeprazole has not been studied in neonatal population.

Monitoring: Observe for symptomatic improvement within 3 days. Edema, hypertension, weight gain, and metabolic alkalosis. Consider esophageal pH monitoring to assess for efficacy (pH >4). Aspartate aminotransferase/ALT if duration of therapy is >8 weeks.

PALIVIZUMAB

Classification: A humanized monoclonal antibody to respiratory syncytial virus (RSV).

Indications: Prophylaxis for the prevention of RSV in high-risk infants
  * Infants <24 months with chronic lung disease (CLD) receiving medical therapy for CLD within 6 months before start of RSV season. Severe CLD patients may benefit from prophylaxis during a second RSV season. (5 doses)
  * Infants <24 months of age with congenital heart disease (CHD) based on the degree of physiologic cardiovascular compromise (5 doses)
  * <12 months of age with history of prematurity (≤28 weeks) (5 doses)
  * <35 weeks gestation, <12 months of age with history of congenital abnormalities of the airway or neuromuscular condition that compromises the ability to manage secretions (5 doses)
  * Neonates <6 months of age, born between 29 and 31 weeks and 6 days gestation (5 doses)
  * Neonates <3 months of age, born between 32 to 35 weeks without CLD who attend childcare or live with a sibling <5 years of age (3 doses)

Refer to AAP policy statement for the full guideline

Dosage/administration: 15 mg/kg/dose IM, given every 30 days for up to 5 doses (depending on indication) during the RSV season (i.e., October/November through March/April).

Precautions: History of hypersensitivity related to the use of other immunoglobulin preparations, blood products, or other medications. Efficacy has not been demonstrated in the treatment of established RSV infection. Give with caution to patients with thrombocytopenia or any coagulation disorder. Not recommended for children with cyanotic congenital heart disease.

Adverse effects: Vomiting, diarrhea, rash, rhinitis, arrhythmia, fever, otitis media, upper respiratory infection and erythema, and moderate induration at the injection site.

PANCURONIUM BROMIDE

Classification: Nondepolarizing neuromuscular blocking agent.

Indications: Skeletal muscle relaxation, increased pulmonary compliance during mechanical ventilation, facilitates endotracheal intubation.

Dosage/administration: 0.05 to 0.15 mg/kg/dose IV (may be administered undiluted by slow IV push) q1–2h as needed. Usual dose: 0.1 mg/kg/dose.

Clinical considerations: Should not be used in tachycardic infants or some cardiac conditions due to tachycardia side effect. Because sensation remains intact, administer concurrent sedation and analgesia as needed. Apply ophthalmic lubricant.

Precautions: Preexisting pulmonary, hepatic, or renal impairment. In neonates with myasthenia gravis, small doses of pancuronium may have profound effects (may need to decrease dosage).

Monitoring: Continuous cardiac, BP monitoring, assisted ventilation status.

Table A.22	Factors Influencing the Duration of Neuromuscular Blockade
Potentiation	Antagonism
Acidosis, hypothermia, neuromuscular disease, hepatic disease, renal failure, cardiovascular disease, aminoglycosides, succinylcholine, hypermagnesemia, and hypokalemia- or potassium-depleting drugs (e.g., amphotericin-B, corticosteroids), furosemide, hyponatremia, hypocalcemia	Pyridostigmine, neostigmine, or edrophonium in conjunction with atropine, alkalosis, epinephrine, theophylline, hyperkalemia, hypercalcemia

Adverse reactions: Tachycardia, hypertension, hypotension, excessive salivation, rashes, bronchospasm.

Antidote: Neostigmine 0.04 mg/kg IV (with atropine 0.02 mg/kg given 30–60 seconds before neostigmine administration).

PENICILLIN G PREPARATIONS

Classification: Antibiotic. Penicillin G potassium, or Penicillin G sodium.

Caution: Do not confuse with benzathine penicillin; used for IM injections only.

Indications: Treatment of neonatal meningitis and bacteremia, group B streptococcal infections, and congenital syphilis.

Dosage/administration: IM, IV (IV route is preferred to avoid muscle fibrosis and atrophy). Only aqueous Penicillin G should be used IV. Final concentration for IV infusion is 50,000 units/mL infused >30 minutes on syringe pump. When treating bacteremia, use the meningitis dose until meningitis is ruled out.

Group B streptococcal meningitis in neonates:
≤7 days postnatal age: 250,000 to 450,000 units/kg/day divided q8h.
>7 days postnatal age: 450,000 to 500,000 units/kg/day divided q4–6h.

Other Group B streptococcal infections in neonates:
200,000 units/kg/day divided q6h.

Meningitis and serious infections in infants and children:
300,000 to 500,000 units/kg/day divided q4–6h. Maximum dose: 24 million units/day.

Mild to moderate infections in neonates:
Postnatal age 0 to 7 days, <2,000 g: 25,000 to 50,000 units/kg/dose q12h
Postnatal age 8 to 30 days, <2,000 g: 25,000 to 50,000 units/kg/dose q8h
Postnatal age 0 to 7 days, >2,000 g: 25,000 to 50,000 units/kg/dose q8h
Postnatal age 8 to 30 days, >2,000 g: 25,000 to 50,000 units/kg/dose q6h

Monitoring: Serum potassium and sodium for renal failure and high-dose therapy. Weekly CBC, BUN, creatinine.

Precautions: Dosage adjustment for renal failure. Use only aqueous penicillin G for IV administration.
Drug interactions: Blunting of peak aminoglycoside serum concentration if administered simultaneously with Penicillin G preparations.
Test interactions: Positive direct Coombs test.
Adverse reactions: Bone marrow suppression, neutropenia, granulocytopenia, anaphylaxis, hemolytic anemia, interstitial nephritis, Jarisch–Herxheimer reaction, change in bowel flora (candida superinfection, diarrhea), CNS toxicity, pseudomembranous colitis, renal tubular damage.

PHENOBARBITAL

Classification: Anticonvulsant, sedative, hypnotic.
Indications: Management of neonatal seizures, neonatal withdrawal.
Dosage/administration:
Seizures: Loading dose: 20 mg/kg/dose, administer IV loading dose over >15 minutes (<1 mg/kg/minute) on syringe pump. Administer additional doses of 5 to 10 mg/kg every 5 minutes until cessation of seizures or a total dose of 40 mg/kg is administered. Use the IV route if possible because of unreliable IM absorption.
Maintenance therapy: 3 to 5 mg/kg/day IV/IM/PO daily. Begin maintenance therapy 12 to 24 hours after loading dose. Parenteral dose preferred for seriously ill neonate.
Neonatal withdrawal syndrome: Administer loading dose, then titrate based on NAS. Loading dose: 15 to 20 mg/kg/dose. Maintenance dose: 1 to 4 mg/kg/dose PO q12h. Closely follow blood levels after stabilization of abstinence symptoms for 24 to 48 hours, decrease the daily dose by 10% to 20% per day.
Clinical considerations: Long half-life (40–200 hours).
Warnings: Abrupt discontinuation in infants with seizures may precipitate status seizures.
Precaution: Hepatic or renal impairment.
Monitoring: Therapeutic serum concentration 20 to 40 mcg/mL (20–30 mcg/mL for NAS). Obtain trough levels just before the next dose. Monitor respiratory status.
Drug interactions: Benzodiazepines, primidone, warfarin, corticosteroids, and doxycycline. Increased serum concentrations with concurrent phenytoin or valproate.
Adverse reactions: Respiratory depression (with serum concentrations >60 mcg/mL), hypotension, circulatory collapse, paradoxical excitement, megaloblastic anemia, hepatitis, and exfoliative dermatitis. Sedation reported at serum concentrations >40 mcg/mL.

PHENTOLAMINE MESYLATE

Classification: Extravasation antidote, vasodilator, α-adrenergic blocking agent.
Indication: Local treatment of dermal necrosis caused by extravasation of vasoconstrictive agents (e.g., dopamine, dobutamine, epinephrine, norepinephrine, and phenylephrine).
Dosage/administration: Do not exceed 0.1 mg/kg or 2.5 mg total. Using a 27- to 30-gauge needle, inject 0.2 mL of solution (prepared by diluting 2.5–5 mg in 10 mL of preservative-free NS) subcutaneously at five separate sites around edge of infiltration (1 mL total volume); change needle between each skin entry. Repeat if necessary. Best results if used within 12 hours after extravasation occurrence.
Clinical considerations: Topical 2% nitroglycerin ointment may be used for significantly swollen extremity.
Contraindication: Renal impairment.
Precaution: Gastritis or peptic ulcer.
Monitoring: Assess affected area for reversal of ischemia. Closely monitor BP, heart rate/rhythm. Normal skin color should return to blanched area within 1 hour.

Adverse reactions: Hypotension, tachycardia, arrhythmias, nasal congestion, vomiting, diarrhea, and exacerbation of peptic ulcer.

PHENYTOIN

Classification: Anticonvulsant.

Indication: Treatment of seizures refractory to phenobarbital.

Dosage/administration:

Loading dose: 15 to 20 mg/kg/IV infusion on syringe pump over 30 to 40 minutes. Dilute to 5 mg/mL with NS. Use a 0.22 micron in-line filter. Start infusion immediately after preparation. Observe for precipitates. **Avoid using in central lines because of the risk of precipitation. If must use a central line, then flush catheter with 1 to 3 mL NS before and after administration because of heparin incompatibility.**

Maintenance dose: 4 to 8 mg/kg q24h IV infusion on syringe pump over >30 minutes. May increase to 8 mg/kg/dose q8–12h after 1 week of age. Maintenance doses usually start 12 hours after loading dose. Avoid IM route because of erratic absorption, pain on injection, and precipitation of drug at injection site. Oral absorption is erratic.

Precautions: Rapid IV administration has resulted in hypotension, cardiovascular collapse, and CNS depression. May cause local irritation, inflammation, necrosis, and sloughing with or without signs of infiltration.

Contraindications: Heart block, sinus bradycardia.

Adverse reactions: Hypersensitivity reaction, arrhythmias, hypotension, hyperglycemia, cardiovascular collapse, liver damage, blood dyscrasias, hypoinsulinemia, SJS/TEN; extravasation may cause tissue necrosis and may be treated with hyaluronidase around the periphery of affected site.

Monitoring: Heart rate, rhythm, hypotension during infusion, and IV site for extravasation.

Monitoring parameters: Obtain trough level 48 hours after IV loading dose. Therapeutic serum concentration: 8 to 15 mcg/mL for first 3 weeks of life, then 10 to 20 mcg/mL secondary to changes in protein binding. Tube feedings decrease oral phenytoin bioavailability. Check for drug interactions.

PIPERACILLIN AND TAZOBACTAM

Classification: Antibiotic, β-lactam and β-lactamase inhibitor combination.

Indications: Treatment of non-CNS infections caused by susceptible β-lactamase producing bacteria, NEC.

Dosage/administration: 50 to 100 mg/kg/dose piperacillin component IV over 30 minutes. (see Table A.23 for interval). Note: Each 3.375 g vial contains 3 g piperacillin sodium and 0.375 g tazobactam sodium.

Table A.23	Piperacillin and Tazobactam	
PMA (weeks)	**Postnatal (days)**	**Interval (hours)**
≤29	0–28	12
	>28	8
		(continued)

Table A.23	Piperacillin and Tazobactam *(Continued)*	
PMA (weeks)	**Postnatal (days)**	**Interval (hours)**
30–36	0–14	12
	>14	8
37–44	0–7	12
	>7	8
≥45	ALL	8

Precautions: Caution in patients with hypernatremia (sodium content is 2.79 mEq/g of piperacillin) and preexisting seizure disorders. Decrease dose in renal dysfunction.
Monitoring: CBC, electrolytes, bleeding time, serum creatinine, LFTs, IV site.
Adverse reactions: Blood dyscrasias, hyperbilirubinemia, hypokalemia, arrhythmias, tachycardia, elevations in LFTs, BUN, and serum creatinine.

RANITIDINE
Classification: Histamine-2 receptor antagonist.
Indications: Duodenal and gastric ulcers, gastroesophageal reflux disease, and hypersecretory conditions.
Dosage/administration:
Oral dose: 2 to 4 mg/kg/day PO divided q8–12h to maximum 6 mg/kg/day.
IV dose: 1 mg/kg/dose IV q12h infused over 30 minutes on syringe pump. Usual concentration for infusion is 1 mg/mL mixed with dextrose or NS. Maximum concentration for IV infusion is 2.5 mg/mL.
Continuous IV dose: 1.5 to 2.5 mg/kg/day. Titrate dose to maintain a gastric pH >4.
Clinical considerations: Because of the absence of possible endocrine toxicity and drug interactions, ranitidine is preferred over cimetidine. Ranitidine effectively increases gastric pH. Increased gastric pH may promote the development of gastric colonization with pathogenic bacteria or yeast.
Precautions: Use with caution in infants with liver and renal impairment. IV formulation contains 0.5% phenol; no short-term toxicity has been reported. Manufacturer's oral solution contains 7.5% alcohol.
Drug interactions: May increase serum levels of theophylline, warfarin, and procainamide.
Monitoring: Monitor gastric pH to assess ranitidine efficacy.
Adverse reactions: GI disturbance, sedation, thrombocytopenia, hepatotoxicity, vomiting, bradycardia, or tachycardia. Use of H_2 blockade in VLBW infants has been associated with a higher risk of NEC, bacterial, and fungal sepsis.

SODIUM BICARBONATE
Classification: Alkalinizing agent.
Indications: Treatment of documented or assumed metabolic acidosis during prolonged resuscitation after establishment of effective ventilation. Treatment of bicarbonate deficit caused by renal or GI losses. Adjunctive treatment of hyperkalemia.

Dose/administration:
Replacement: Infuse over >20 to 30 minutes on syringe pump.
Resuscitation: 1 to 2 mEq/kg slow IV push over at least 2 minutes. **Administer more slowly in premature infants to decrease risk of IVH.**
Correction of metabolic acidosis: HCO_3 needed (mEq) = HCO_3 deficit (mEq/L) × (0.3 × body weight [kg]). Administer half of calculated dose, and then assess the need for remainder.
Maximum concentration for infusion is 0.5 mEq/mL (4.2%—osmolarity is 1,000 mOsm/L).
For continuous IV infusion: Use 50 mEq sodium bicarbonate (8.4% concentration) and add to 50 mL of appropriate diluent (e.g., dextrose, maximum 10%; NS; or sterile water). Concentration is 0.5 mEq/mL. Maximum infusion rate for continuous IV administration is 1 mEq/kg/hour.
Precautions: Rapid injection of hypertonic sodium bicarbonate (1 mEq/mL) solution has been linked to IVH.
Adverse effects: Pulmonary edema, respiratory acidosis, local tissue necrosis, hypocalcemia, hypernatremia, metabolic alkalosis, hypokalemia.
Monitoring: Follow acid–base status; arterial blood gases; serum electrolytes, including calcium; and urinary pH. Use hyaluronidase to treat IV extravasation.

SPIRONOLACTONE
Classification: Potassium-sparing diuretic.
Indications: Mild diuretic with potassium-sparing effects. Used in conjunction with thiazide diuretics in the treatment of CHF, hypertension, edema, and BPD when prolonged diuresis is desirable.
Dosage/administration: 1 to 3 mg/kg/day PO divided q12–24h.
Clinical considerations: Offers little to no additional benefit when included as part of the regimen to treat BPD. Only commercially available in tablet form. Solution may be made by crushing eight 25 mg tablets and suspending powder in 50 mL of simple syrup (stable for 28 days, refrigerated).
Contraindications: Renal failure, anuria, hyperkalemia.
Monitoring: Serum sodium and urine potassium and renal function.
Drug interactions: May potentiate ganglionic blocking agents and other antihypertensive agents.
Adverse reactions: Hyperkalemia, vomiting, diarrhea, hyperchloremic metabolic acidosis, dehydration, hyponatremia, decrease in renal function.

SURFACTANTS
Classification: Natural, animal-derived exogenous surfactant agent.
Indications:
Prophylaxis: Infants with high risk for respiratory distress syndrome (RDS), defined in clinical trials as a birth weight <1,250 g, and larger infants with evidence of pulmonary immaturity.
Rescue therapy: Infants with moderate to severe RDS, defined in clinical trials as requirement for mechanical ventilation and fractional concentration of inspired oxygen (FiO_2) higher than 40%.
Treatment: Full-term infants with respiratory failure that is due to meconium aspiration, pneumonia, or persistent pulmonary hypertension.

Dosage/administration: (see Table A.24)

Table A.24	Surfactant	
Surfactant	**Doses**	**Comments**
Beractant (Survanta®)	4 mL/kg/dose	Bovine lung surfactant Divided into four aliquots, with up to three additional doses (four total), administered q6h if needed
Calfactant (Infasurf®)	3 mL/kg/dose	Bovine lung surfactant Divided into two aliquots, with up to two additional doses, administered q12h if needed
Poractant alfa (Curosurf®)	Initial dose = 2.5 mL/kg/dose Subsequent doses = 1.25 mL/kg/dose	Porcine lung surfactant Divided into two aliquots, followed by up to two additional doses of 1.25 mL/kg/dose, administered q12h if needed.

q6h = every 6 hours; q12h = every 12 hours.
Aliquots should be administered with infant in different positions to facilitate spreading of surfactant.

Administered intratracheally by instillation using a 5-French end-hole catheter or similar device inserted into the infant's ETT with the tip of the catheter protruding just beyond the end of the ETT and above the infant's carina.

Prophylactic therapy: Intratracheally as soon as possible after birth.

Rescue therapy: Intratracheally immediately following the diagnosis of RDS.

Clinical considerations: Suction ETT before administration. Delay suctioning post-administration as long as possible (minimum of 1 hour). Repeat doses are usually determined by evidence of continuing respiratory distress or if patient requires >30% inspired oxygen.

Monitoring: Assess ETT patency and correct anatomic location before administration of surfactant. Monitor oxygen saturation and heart rate continuously during administration of doses. Rapid improvement in lung oxygenation and compliance may occur and require a decrease in support. After administration of each dose, monitor arterial blood gases frequently to detect and correct postdose abnormalities of ventilation and oxygenation.

Precautions: A videotape demonstrating surfactant administration procedure is available from Ross Laboratories and Forest Laboratories and should be viewed before use of their products.

Adverse reactions: Transient bradycardia, hypoxemia, pallor, vasoconstriction, hypotension, ETT blockage, hypercapnia, apnea, pulmonary hemorrhage, and hypertension may occur during the administration process.

URSODIOL

Classification: Gallstone dissolution agent.

Indications: Facilitates bile excretion in infants with biliary atresia, and TPN cholestasis. Improves hepatic metabolism of essential fatty acids in infants with cystic fibrosis.

Dosages/administration:

Biliary atresia: 10 mg/kg/dose PO q12h.

Cholestasis: 10 mg/kg/dose q8h.

Cystic fibrosis: 15 mg/kg/dose orally q12h.

Administration: Administer with food. Must be refrigerated.

Precautions: Obtain baseline ALT, aspartate aminotransferase, alkaline phosphate, direct bilirubin. Use with caution in infants with chronic liver disease.

Adverse reactions: Hepatotoxicity, nausea, vomiting, abdominal pain, and constipation.

Monitoring: Hepatic transaminases, direct bilirubin.

VANCOMYCIN HYDROCHLORIDE

Classification: Antibiotic.

Indications: Drug of choice for serious infections caused by methicillin-resistant staphylococci, penicillin-resistant pneumococci, and coagulase-negative *staphylococcus.* The oral route is used for the treatment of *Clostridium difficile,* if metronidazole has failed.

Dosage/administration: (see Table A.25)

Table A.25	Vancomycin	
Postnatal age	Weight (kg)	Dose
≤7 d	<1.2 kg	15 mg/kg/dose IV q24h
≤7 d	1.2–2 kg	10–15 mg/kg/dose IV q12–18h
≤7 d	>2kg	10–15 mg/kg/dose IV q8–12h
>7 d	<1.2 kg	15 mg/kg/dose IV q24h
>7 d	1.2–2kg	10–15 mg/kg/dose IV q8–12h
>7 d	>2kg	15 mg/kg/dose IV q8h
IV = intravenous; q8h = every 8 hours; q8–12h = every 8 to 12 h; q12–18h = every 12 to 18 hours; q24h = every 24 hours.		

IV infusion over >60 minutes on syringe pump. Final concentration for infusion is 5 mg/mL. Mix in NS or dextrose.

Precautions: Use with caution in patients with renal impairment or those receiving other nephrotoxic or ototoxic drugs; dosage modification required in patients with impaired renal function.

Adverse reactions: Red man syndrome (erythema multiform-like reaction with intense pruritus; tachycardia; hypotension; rash involving face, neck, upper trunk, back, and upper arms) usually develops during a rapid infusion of vancomycin or with doses >15 to 20 mg/kg/hour and usually dissipates in 30 to 60 minutes. Lengthening infusion time usually eliminates the risk of subsequent doses. Cardiac arrest, fever, chills, eosinophilia, and neutropenia reported after prolonged administration (>3 weeks); phlebitis may be minimized by slow infusion and more dilution of the drug. If extravasation occurs, consider using hyaluronidase around periphery of an affected area. Also reported are ototoxicity and nephrotoxicity, especially if administered concurrently with other nephrotoxic or ototoxic medications. Associated with elevated serum concentrations.

Monitoring: Assess renal function. Therapeutic serum concentrations: Trough 10 to 15 mcg/mL (15–20 mcg/mL when treating pneumonia, meningitis, endocarditis, or bone infections. Sample should be drawn 30 minutes to just before next dose. Peak levels should be monitored when treating meningitis, 30 minutes after end of infusion (30–40 mcg/mL).

VECURONIUM

Classification: Nondepolarizing neuromuscular blocking agent.

Indications: Skeletal muscle relaxation, increased pulmonary compliance during mechanical ventilation, and facilitates endotracheal intubation.

Dosage/administration: 0.1 mg/kg (range: 0.03 to 0.15 mg/kg/dose) IV push q1–2h as needed.

Precautions: Preexisting pulmonary, hepatic impairment. Premature neonates may be more sensitive to vecuronium effects. Commercially available diluent contains benzyl alcohol; use sterile water for reconstitution in neonates.

Monitoring: Continuous cardiac, BP monitoring, assisted ventilation status.

Clinical considerations: Because sensation remains intact, administer concurrent sedation and analgesia as needed. Apply ophthalmic lubricant.

Factors influencing duration of neuromuscular blockade: (see Table A.22)

Adverse reactions: Arrhythmias, tachycardia (to a lesser degree than pancuronium), hypotension, hypertension, rash, and bronchospasm.

Antidote: Neostigmine 0.025 mg/kg IV (with atropine 0.02 mg/kg).

VITAMIN A INJECTION

Classification: Nutritional supplement, fat-soluble vitamin.

Indication: To minimize incidence of CLD in high risk, preterm newborns.

Dosage/administration: 5,000 IU, IM 3 times/week for 12 doses total. Start within 72 hours of birth in infants with birth weights <1,000 g. Administer with a 25- to 29-gauge needle.

Caution: Do not use concurrently with glucocorticoids.

Contraindications: Do not administer IV.

Adverse effects: Full fontanel, hepatomegaly, edema, mucocutaneous lesions, bony tenderness.

VITAMIN B₁

Classification: Water-soluble vitamin supplement.

Indications: Treatment of thiamine deficiency

Table A.26	Vitamin B$_1$
Indications	**Dosage/administration (for preterm and term infants)**
Thiamine AI	200 mcg/day
Thiamine deficiency	Preventive dose 0.5–1 mg/day PO
Thiamine deficiency	Therapeutic dose 5–10 mg/day, PO daily or divided q8h
PO = orally; q8h = every 8 hours; AI = Adequate Intake.	

Thiamine sources: 1 mL of PolyviSol® or Vi-Daylin® supplies 400 mcg and 500 mcg respectively. Human milk supplies 56 mcg/day.

Dosage/administration: (see Table A.26)

Drug interactions: Thiamine requirements increased with high-carbohydrate diets or high-concentration IV dextrose solutions.

Test interactions: Large doses may interfere with spectrophotometric determination of serum theophylline.

Adverse reactions: Allergic reaction, angioedema, and cardiovascular collapse. Severity and frequency of adverse reactions increases with parenteral route of administration.

VITAMIN B$_6$

Classification: Water-soluble vitamin supplement.

Indications: Prevention and treatment of pyridoxine-dependent seizures.

Dosage/administration: 50 to 100 mg IV over >1 minute, or IM as a single test dose; followed by 30-minute observation period. IV route is preferred. If response seen, begin maintenance dose of 50 to 100 mg PO every day (range: 10–200 mg). The injectable form may be given PO. Mix with feedings if desired.

Monitoring: Electroencephalogram monitoring recommended during initial therapy for pyridoxine-dependent seizures, RR, heart rate, BP.

Precautions: Risk of profound sedation and respiratory depression; ventilatory support may be required.

Adverse reactions: Sedation, increased aspartate aminotransferase, decreased serum folic acid level, allergic reaction, respiratory distress, and burning/stinging sensation at the injection site. Seizures reported following IV administration of very large doses.

VITAMIN D

Classification: Fat-soluble vitamin.

Indications: Vitamin D supplementation/deficiency, refractory rickets

Dosage/administration:
Supplementation in breastfed babies: 400 IU PO daily
Treatment of vitamin D deficiency: 1,000 IU PO daily

Clinical considerations: Vitamin D supplements available in two forms: vitamin D$_2$ (ergocalciferol) and vitamin D$_3$ (cholecalciferol). Ergocalciferol formulations are very concentrated and have high potential for dosing error. Cholecalciferol is available as individual supplements and also in many multivitamin formulations.

Contraindications: Hypercalcemia, evidence of vitamin D toxicity.

Monitoring: Serum calcium, phosphorus, alkaline phosphatase levels. Excessive doses may lead to hypervitaminosis D manifested by hypercalcemia, azotemia, increased serum creatinine, mild hypokalemia, diarrhea, polyuria, metastatic calcification, and nephrocalcinosis.

Adverse reactions: Polyuria, nephrocalcinosis, hypertension, and arrhythmias.

VITAMIN E

Classification: Fat-soluble vitamin.

Indications: Prevention and treatment of vitamin E deficiency.

Dosage/administration:

Prevention: Usual dose: 5 IU PO every day. **Range:** 5 to 25 IU PO every day.

Treatment of Vitamin E deficiency: 25 to 50 IU/day (normal levels should occur within 1 week)

Clinical considerations: Requirements for vitamin E increase as the intake of poly-unsaturated fatty acids increases.

Precautions: Aquasol E is very hyperosmolar (3,000 mOsm); a 1:4 dilution with sterile water or feedings is required. Poorly absorbed in malabsorption disorders; use water-soluble forms.

Monitoring: Physiologic serum levels for preterm infants are 0.8 to 3.5 mg/dL and should be monitored during administration of pharmacologic doses of vitamin E.

Adverse reactions: Feeding intolerance, NEC, increased incidence of sepsis.

VITAMIN K$_1$

Classification: Fat-soluble vitamin.

Indications: Prevention and treatment of hemorrhagic disease of the newborn, hypoprothrombinemia caused by drug-induced or anticoagulant-induced vitamin K deficiency.

Dosage/administration:

Hemorrhagic disease of the newborn:

- Prophylaxis: (administered at birth).
  - **Less than 1.5 kg:** 0.5 mg IM **1.5 kg or more:** 1 mg IM.
- Treatment: 1 to 2 mg/day IM

Vitamin K deficiency: PO: 2.5 to 5 mg/day; SC, IV, IM: 1 to 2 mg/day administered as a single dose.

Warnings: Ineffective in hereditary hypoprothrombinemia or hypoprothrombinemia caused by severe liver disease. Severe hemolytic anemia or hyperbilirubinemia reported in neonates following administration of doses >20 mg. IM administration is not associated with an increased risk of childhood cancer.

Precautions: Despite proper dilution and rate of administration, severe anaphylactoid or hypersensitivity-like reactions (including shock and cardiac/respiratory arrest) have been reported to occur during or immediately after IV administration. IV administration is restricted to emergency use, should not exceed 1 mg/minute, and should occur with a physician in attendance. Use with caution in neonates with severe hepatic disease.

Drug interactions: Antagonizes action of warfarin.

Monitoring: Prothrombin time/partial thromboplastin time (PT/PTT) if giving a maintenance therapy. Allow a minimum of 2 to 4 hours to detect measurable improvement in these parameters.

ZIDOVUDINE

Classification: Antiretroviral agent, nucleoside analog reverse transcriptase inhibitor.

Indications: Treatment of neonates born to human immunodeficiency virus (HIV)-infected women.

Administration: May be administered with feedings but the manufacturer recommends administration within 30 minutes before or 1 hour after feedings. Initiate therapy within 12 hours after birth and continue for 6 weeks, with subsequent therapy that should be dependent on clinical status and results of HIV studies.

Final concentration for IV administration: 4 mg/mL.

Dosage/administration: (see Table A.27)

Table A.27	Zidovudine	
Age	Dose/Route	Comments
GA at birth: <30 wk	▪ Oral: 2 mg/kg/dose q12h ▪ IV: 1.5 mg/kg/dose q12h	Change interval to q8h at 4 wk of age
GA at birth: ≥30 and <35 wk	▪ Oral: 2 mg/kg/dose q12h ▪ IV: 1.5 mg/kg/dose q12h	Change interval to q8h at 2 wk of age
GA at birth: ≥35 wk	▪ Oral: 2 mg/kg/dose q6h ▪ IV: 1.5 mg/kg/dose q6h	

GA = gestational age; IV = intravenously; q6h = every 6 hours; q8h = every 8 hours; q12h = every 12 hours.

IV dose is administered over >1 hour on syringe pump. Conversion from oral to IV dose: IV dose = 3/4 of oral dose. Do not administer IM.

Clinical considerations: Use IV route only until oral therapy can be given.

Precautions: Use with caution in patients with bone marrow compromise or renal or hepatic impairment.

Adverse reactions: Anemia, leukopenia, granulocytopenia, thrombocytopenia, lactic acidosis, hepatomegaly, and neutropenia.

Drug interactions: Acetaminophen, acyclovir (increased toxicity), ganciclovir (increased hematological toxicity), cimetidine, indomethacin, and lorazepam. Coadministration with other drugs metabolized by glucuronidation increases toxicity of either drug and increases granulocytopenia. Fluconazole and methadone reduces metabolism—dosing interval should be lengthened.

Monitoring considerations: Weekly CBC, renal, LFTs, CD4 cell count, HIV, and RNA plasma levels.

ZINC ACETATE ORAL SOLUTION

Classification: Mineral supplement.

Indication: Prevention and treatment of zinc deficiency states.

Dosage/administration: Treatment of zinc deficiency: 0.5 to 1 mg of elemental Zn/kg/day PO in divided doses administered 1 to 3 times/day.

Clinical consideration: May administer with food if GI upset occurs.

Drug interactions: Iron and agents that increase gastric pH (e.g., H_2 blockers, proton pump inhibitors) may decrease zinc absorption.

Monitoring: Periodic serum copper, zinc levels.

Adverse effects: Nausea, vomiting, leukopenia, diaphoresis, and GI disturbances. At excessive doses: hypotension, tachycardia, neutropenia, and gastric ulcers.

Appendix B

Effects of Maternal Drugs on the Fetus

Stephanie Dukhovny

I. INTRODUCTION

A. In most instances, the **risk** of adverse fetal effects from drugs taken by the mother is not known. Properly designed scientific studies cannot be performed ethically; since they would require that women must take drugs even when they did not need them in order to eliminate the confounding effect of maternal disease or disorder. The current investigational methods (retrospective analysis, cohort studies, and case reports) often cannot differentiate the cause of the malformation or other adverse outcomes. When a problem occurs in association with a history of maternal drug ingestion, any of the following can be the cause:

1. The drug itself

2. The maternal disease state (e.g., diabetes, maternal infection, or environmental toxicity)

3. Preexistent physical disorders (e.g., amniotic bands) producing deformation and disruption

4. Unrecognized illness (e.g., unrecognized viral illness)

5. An already anomalous pregnancy may have produced symptoms that led to drug ingestion.

6. Genetic aberration

7. A spontaneous malformation rate of 2% to 3%, a stillbirth risk of 1%, and a spontaneous abortion rate of 25%

8. Other or unknown cause. In addition, maternal drug histories are extremely unreliable, and findings often depend on how the interview was conducted.

B. **Teratogenic effects.** Because of tremendous variability in maternal elimination and drug disposition characteristics, very little predictability comes from knowing the maternal dose. Timing of drug exposure is important. Drugs that are taken when the embryo is extremely undifferentiated are unlikely to produce physical malformation unless the drug persists in the body or alters the gamete. The most critical period for the induction of physical defects is believed to be 15 to 60 days after conception. Because the timing of this event is rarely known with certainty, however, one cannot exclude the possibility of malformation in any clinical situation. Drugs that are taken after organogenesis can affect the growth and development of the fetus. The brain, in particular, continues to grow and develop in the latter trimesters and beyond. A drug that is taken during gestation also can act as a transplacental carcinogen. In short, there is no "guaranteed safe" time for a pregnant woman to take a drug.

C. Even when a drug is associated with a statistically significant increase in the risk of a birth defect, the actual risk may remain low. For example, a birth defect that naturally occurs in 1 in every 1,000,000 births may be made 1,000 times more likely to occur by drug exposure, and still would be seen in only 0.1% of the drug exposures. A real example of this is with phenytoin exposure. This drug produces a 200% to 400% increase in the risk of common birth defects (cleft lip, heart defects); however,

85% of children born to women who take phenytoin are normal or have minor effects of exposure. Numerical risks cannot be stated with certainty for most drugs because the data have been collected retrospectively. Where a risk is stated, the value should be interpreted with caution. For a given pregnancy, a studied risk may not accurately reflect the risk to the fetus; genetic factors may have a strong influence on susceptibility to certain teratogens.

D. Manufacturer's recommendations and package inserts should be checked before the fetus is exposed to any drug or chemical agent.

II. EFFECTS OF COMMON MATERNAL DRUGS ON THE FETUS (SEE TABLE B.1)

A. References that are used to create the summary table are stated at the end of this appendix.

B. Pregnancy risk category

1. The **Food and Drug Administration** has offered a classification system to assign the risk of a particular drug to the fetus during pregnancy. The classification system is as follows:

a. Category A. Controlled studies show no risk. Adequate, well-controlled studies in pregnant women have not demonstrated a risk to the fetus in the first trimester of pregnancy, and there is no evidence of risk in later trimesters.

b. Category B. No evidence of risk in humans. Animal studies have not demonstrated a risk to the fetus, but there are no adequate studies in pregnant women; or animal studies have shown an adverse effect, but adequate studies in pregnant women have not demonstrated a risk to the fetus during the first trimester of pregnancy, and there is no evidence of risk in later trimesters.

c. Category C. Risk cannot be ruled out. Animal studies have shown an adverse effect on the fetus, but there are no adequate studies in humans; or there are no animal reproduction studies and no adequate studies in humans.

d. Category D. There is evidence of human fetal risk, but the potential benefits from the use of the drug in pregnant women may be acceptable despite its potential risks.

e. Category X. Contraindicated in pregnancy. Studies in animals or humans demonstrate fetal abnormalities or adverse reaction; reports indicate evidence of fetal risk. The risk of use in pregnant women clearly outweighs any possible benefit to the patient.

2. The risk category was assigned by referencing the textbook by Briggs et al. or by using the manufacturer's ratings. If Briggs et al. and the manufacturer's ratings differed from one another, both categories were listed (Briggs = subscript B; Manufacturer = subscript M).

3. Briggs et al. provided additional information beyond what was provided by the manufacturer that is helpful to the reader.

4. Manufacturer's recommendations and package inserts should be checked, before the fetus is exposed to these agents, for the most current information.

5. Additional information can be found at the Pregnancy Environmental Hotline (800-322-5014 or 617-466-8471, fax 617-487-2361) sponsored by the National Birth Defects Center and the Genesis Fund.

Table B.1 Effects of Common Maternal Drugs on the Fetus

Class	Drug	Risk category (see Sec. II)	Pharmacokinetics/reported effects on fetus
Analgesics/ antipyretics and NSAIDs	**Acetaminophen**	B	Crosses placenta
			Not implicated as a teratogen
			When used within dosing recommendations and for short-term use, acetaminophen is considered safe.
			Continuous use or high-toxic dosages have been associated with maternal anemia, maternal hepatorenal failure, maternal death, fetal hepatorenal failure, fetal death.
	Acetylsalicylic acid (aspirin)	C	Crosses placenta
		D—full-dose aspirin in third trimester	Not implicated as a teratogen
			No fetal or newborn effects have been shown with *low-dose* aspirin therapy.
			Full-dose aspirin associated with delayed onset and prolonged duration of labor (inhibition of prostaglandin synthesis)

		Full-dose ingestion within 5 d of delivery is associated with an increased risk of bleeding in both mother and baby.
		Platelet dysfunction has been described (see Chaps. 43 and 47).
		Association between **full-dose** maternal aspirin, near-term, and premature closure of the ductus arteriosus (inhibition of prostaglandin synthesis) and the syndrome of pulmonary hypertension in the newborn (see Chap. 36)
Ibuprofen	C	Increased risk of miscarriage in first trimester
	D—full-dose ibuprofen in third trimester	Not implicated as a teratogen. When used as a tocolytic agent, use is associated with reduced amniotic fluid volume.
		Like aspirin, another prostaglandin synthesis inhibitor, use is associated with delayed onset and prolonged duration of labor, premature closure of the ductus arteriosus, and pulmonary hypertension in the newborn.
Anesthetic agents used during labor and delivery		(See Chap. 12)
Atropine (anesthetic premedication)	C	Parasympatholytic/anticholinergic
		Rapidly crosses the placenta with fetal uptake

(continued)

Table B.1	Effects of Common Maternal Drugs on the Fetus *(Continued)*		
Class	Drug	Risk category (see Sec. II)	Pharmacokinetics/reported effects on fetus
			May directly effect fetal heart rate
			When used for premedication at 0.01 mg/kg, no fetal effects on heart rate or variability, and no effects on uterine activity were reported.
	Benzodiazepines		See psychotherapeutic agents, antipsychotics in the subsequent text
	Induction agents		
	Ketamine	B	Rapidly crosses the placenta
			Not implicated as a teratogen
			Rapid-acting IV general anesthetic agent
			When used in high doses (1.5–2.2 mg/kg), ketamine is associated with an increase in maternal blood pressure, increased uterine tone and contractions, newborn depression, and increased muscle tone in the infant.
			Can decrease beat-to-beat variability without changing fetal acid/base status
			These maternal/newborn effects were rarely observed with lower doses (0.2–0.5 mg/kg), which are commonly used today.

Propofol	B	Rapidly crosses the placenta
		Hypnotic agent
		Not implicated as a teratogen
		Associated with decreased APGAR scores and decreased neurobehavioral scores compared to infants born by spontaneous vaginal delivery Changes noted at 1 hour, resolved within 4 hours.
Thiopental	C	Rapidly crosses the placenta
		Rapid and ultrashort-acting IV general anesthetic agent
		Not implicated as a teratogen
		Decreased fetal heart rate variability has been observed.
Inhalation agents		
Enflurane	B	Rapid fetal uptake
		No adverse effects on APGAR scores or neurobehavioral status in the newborn
Halothane	C	Associated with uterine muscle relaxation and increased blood loss; however, low-dose halothane (0.5%) was not shown to have adverse maternal or newborn effects.
Isoflurane	C	Preferred agent in patients receiving beta-adrenergic therapy because of a reduced incidence of arrhythmias

(continued)

Table B.1	Effects of Common Maternal Drugs on the Fetus *(Continued)*		
Class	**Drug**	**Risk category (see Sec. II)**	**Pharmacokinetics/reported effects on fetus**
	Nitrous oxide	?	Short-term use as an obstetric anesthetic is considered safe
	Local anesthetics		
	Bupivacaine	C	Long-acting local anesthetic
			Reports of associated neonatal depression, hypoxia, fetal acidosis, and bradycardia
	Chloroprocaine	C	
	Lidocaine	C_B, B_M	Not implicated as a teratogen
			Injection into paracervical tissues or uterine cavity results in fetal heart rate decelerations.
			Epidural use is associated with maternal hypotension
	Ropivacaine	B	Rapidly crosses the placenta
			Use as an obstetric anesthetic is considered safe
	Scopolamine	C	Crosses the placenta
			Used to prevent nausea and vomiting associated with anesthesia and surgery

				Parasympatholytic/anticholinergic
				Fetal effects may include tachycardia and decreased heart rate variability.
				Report of newborn toxicity with fever, tachycardia, and lethargy; symptoms reversed with physostigmine.
	Skeletal muscle relaxants		C	Cross the placenta in small amounts near term, placenta transfer early in pregnancy has not been reported.
	Pancuronium		C	Short-term use has shown no demonstrable adverse effects on the fetus.
	Vecuronium		C	Repetitive or large doses have been associated with neonatal depression and transient fetal heart rate changes, which do not seem to correlate or indicate fetal compromise.
Anticoagulants	Heparin		C	Does not cross the placenta
				Not implicated as a teratogen
				Maternal complications include bleeding
	Warfarin and other coumarin derivatives		D_B, X_M	Oral anticoagulant
				Crosses the placenta
				Considered a teratogen

(continued)

Table B.1	Effects of Common Maternal Drugs on the Fetus *(Continued)*		
Class	Drug	Risk category (see Sec. II)	Pharmacokinetics/reported effects on fetus
			Fetal effects include:
			Embryopathy (fetal warfarin syndrome)—growth restriction, blindness, optic atrophy, microphthalmia, nasal hypoplasia, hypoplasia of the extremities, stippled epiphyses, mental deficiency, seizures, hearing loss, congenital heart disease, scoliosis, and death.
			Central nervous system defects
			Spontaneous abortion
			Stillbirth
			Prematurity
			Hemorrhage
	Enoxaparin (Lovenox)	B	Does not cross the placenta
			Not implicated as a teratogen
Anticonvulsants	**Carbamazepine**	D	Crosses the placenta
			Considered a teratogen

		Associated with spina bifida, craniofacial defects, fingernail hypoplasia, and developmental delay
Ethosuximide (Zarontin)	C	Used for the treatment of petit mal epilepsy
		Not well studied, making the conclusions regarding teratogenicity difficult
		Some reported newborn associations in a limited number of exposures include: patent ductus arteriosus, cleft lip/palate, mongoloid facies, altered palmar crease, accessory nipple, and hydrocephalus.
		Spontaneous hemorrhage in the newborn has been reported.
Lamotrigine (Lamictal)	C	Not implicated as a teratogen
		Suspicion of increased risk of oral cleft in one pregnancy registry, but not confirmed in other registries
Levetiracetam (Keppra)	C	Crosses the placenta
		Associated with low birth weight
Phenobarbital	D	Crosses the placenta
		Considered a teratogen

(continued)

Table B.1 Effects of Common Maternal Drugs on the Fetus *(Continued)*

Class	Drug	Risk category (see Sec. II)	Pharmacokinetics/reported effects on fetus
			No specific phenotype (in contrast to phenytoin)
			Studies confounded by combination use with phenytoin
			Associated findings: cardiovascular defects, cleft lip/palate, early hemorrhagic disease of the newborn (induction of fetal liver microsomal enzymes, depleting vitamin K and suppressing vitamin K-dependent coagulation factors), barbiturate withdrawal, impaired cognitive development
	Phenytoin (Dilantin)	D	Crosses the placenta
			Considered a teratogen, some suggest that this is dose-related
			Recognizable pattern of malformations known as *fetal hydantoin syndrome,* features include:
			Craniofacial anomalies: broad nasal bridge, wide fontanel, low-set hairline, broad alveolar ridge, metopic ridging, short neck, ocular hypertelorism, microcephaly, cleft lip/palate, abnormal or low-set ears, epicanthal folds, ptosis of eyelids, coloboma, and coarse scalp hair;
			Limb defects: small or absent nails, hypoplasia of distal phalanges, altered palmar crease, digital thumb, dislocated hip, and impaired growth;
			Other: congenital heart defects, CNS malformations, mental deficiency, and reported association with neuroectodermal tumors in newborn.

		May cause early hemorrhagic disease of the newborn (induction of fetal liver microsomal enzymes depleting vitamin K and suppressing vitamin K-dependent coagulation factors)
Primidone (Mysoline)	D	Structural analog of phenobarbital
		Considered a teratogen
		May see hemorrhagic disease of the newborn (vitamin K depletion)
Valproic acid (Depakene)	D	Readily crosses the placenta
		Considered a teratogen
		Associated fetal/newborn complications include: congenital abnormalities—valproic acid syndrome: neural tube defects (lumbar meningomyelocele), craniofacial, microcephaly, abnormal digits, hypospadias, congenital heart disease (atrial septal defects), delayed psychomotor development, and growth restriction.
		Other: hyperbilirubinemia, hepatotoxicity, transient hyperglycinemia, and withdrawal
Antihistamines		
First-generation		Not implicated as a teratogen
Diphenhydramine	B_M	
Chlorpheniramine	C	

(continued)

Table B.1	Effects of Common Maternal Drugs on the Fetus *(Continued)*		
Class	Drug	Risk category (see Sec. II)	Pharmacokinetics/reported effects on fetus
	Tripelennamine	B	
	Second-generation		Not implicated as a teratogen
	Loratadine	B_M	Unknown if it crosses the placenta; however, with a low molecular weight, some passage is expected.
Anti-infectives	**Amebicides**		
	Metronidazole	B	Crosses the placenta
			Contraindicated in the 1st trimester unless alternative treatment is inadequate
			Although mutagenic and carcinogenic in bacteria and rats, no clear association of these properties in humans.
			Most evidence suggests that there is no significant risk to the fetus.
	Aminoglycosides		
	Amikacin	C_B, D_M	Rapidly crosses the placenta
			Not implicated as a teratogen
			Theoretical risk of ototoxicity

Gentamicin	C (opthomological and topical preparations)	Rapidly crosses the placenta
	D (systemic preparations)	Used intrapartum for maternal infection: 2–3 doses
		Theoretical risk of ototoxicity, nephrotoxicity
Neomycin	C (opthomological and topical preparations)	Not implicated as a teratogen
	D (systemic preparations)	
		Theoretical risk of ototoxicity
Tobramycin	C (opthomological and topical preparations)	Theoretical risk of ototoxicity
	D (systemic preparations)	Neonatal potentiation of MgSO$_4$-induced neuromuscular weakness has been reported.
Streptomycin	D	Ototoxicity has been reported.

(continued)

Table B.1 Effects of Common Maternal Drugs on the Fetus *(Continued)*

Class	Drug	Risk category (see Sec. II)	Pharmacokinetics/reported effects on fetus
	Antibiotics: general		
	Chloramphenicol	C	Crosses the placenta at term
			Not implicated as a teratogen
			Cardiovascular collapse (gray baby syndrome) reported in one infant born to a mother who received a dose of chloramphenicol during labor.
	Clindamycin	B	Crosses the placenta
			Not implicated as a teratogen
	Erythromycin	B	Crosses the placenta, but in very low concentrations
			Not implicated as a teratogen
	Pentamidine	C	Crosses the placenta
			Embryocidal when given early in pregnancy, but not teratogenic
	Trimethoprim	C	Crosses the placenta
			Folate antagonist, suggestive association with neural tube, cardiovascular defects, also facial clefts
			May be used alone or in combination with sulfonamides

Antifungals		
Amphotericin B	B	Crosses the placenta
		Not implicated as a teratogen
		Drug of choice for the treatment of systemic fungal infections in pregnancy
Griseofulvin	C	Crosses the placenta
		Associated with an increased risk of fetal malformations
Ketoconazole	C_M	Not recommended for use during pregnancy due to congenital anomalies noted in animal studies
Flucytosine	C_M	Teratogenic in animal studies
Miconazole	C	Topical antifungal agent
		No reports documenting associated congenital malformations. Theoretical effects on fetal androgen synthesis
Antiviral—		
Acyclovir	B	Crosses the placenta
		No documented reports of adverse effects to the fetus or newborn

(continued)

Table B.1 Effects of Common Maternal Drugs on the Fetus *(Continued)*

Class	Drug	Risk category (see Sec. II)	Pharmacokinetics/reported effects on fetus
	Cephalosporins	B	Cephalosporins, as a class of drug, are generally considered safe to use during pregnancy. Many have been shown to cross the placenta
	Moxalactam	C	Some reports of possible cardiovascular malformations and oral cleft defects with cefaclor, ceftriaxone, cephalexin, and cephadrine
	Povidone–iodine (Betadine)	C	Readily cross the placenta
			May cause transient hypothyroidism in the newborn (topical and vaginal use)
	Penicillins	B	Many penicillin derivatives have been shown to readily cross the placenta
			As a class of drug, penicillins are not considered teratogenic
	Quinolones	C	Unknown in many quinolone derivatives whether transplacental passage occurs; although, the molecule is small enough for this to theoretically be possible.
			Norfloxacin and ciprofloxacin have been documented to cross the placenta.
			Animal evidence suggests association with cartilage damage and arthropathy; although, this has never been shown in human studies.
			No strong or convincing evidence that quinolone use is associated with congenital abnormalities.

		However, some small reports of possibly associated birth defects; although, a consistent pattern has not been identified.
		Most recommend not to use quinolones during pregnancy as safer alternatives exist.
Sulfonamides	C	Readily crosses the placenta
	D—if administered near term	When close to term, documented associated toxicities include increased bilirubin toxicity (competes with bilirubin for albumin binding sites) and hemolytic anemia.
		No strong evidence to suggest an association with congenital abnormalities
Tetracyclines (Doxycycline, Tetracycline)	D	Cross the placenta
		Associated with maternal hepatotoxicity in setting of azotemia or pyelonephritis
		Associated with disruption of fetal mineralized structures such as teeth (intense yellow-staining) and bones
		Possible risk for minor fetal anomalies
Urinary germicides Nitrofurantoin	B	Not considered a teratogen
		Caution with use in women who are close to term secondary to reports of newborn hemolytic anemia in women with glucose-6-phosphate dehydrogenase deficiency.

(continued)

Table B.1 Effects of Common Maternal Drugs on the Fetus *(Continued)*

Class	Drug	Risk category (see Sec. II)	Pharmacokinetics/reported effects on fetus
Antimalarials	**Chloroquine**	C	Crosses the placenta
			Drug of choice for prophylaxis and treatment of sensitive malaria during pregnancy
	Hydroxychloroquine (Plaquenil)	C	Crosses the placenta
			It is generally considered safe to use during pregnancy; however, studies and the number of exposures are limited.
	Quinine	D_B, X_M	Considered a teratogen
			Reported associated congenital anomalies including: CNS anomalies, limb defects, facial defects, heart defects, digestive organ anomalies, urogenital anomalies, hernias, and vertebral anomalies
			Reports of maternal and neonatal thrombocytopenia purpura
			Reports of neonatal hemolysis in G-6-PD deficient newborns
Antiparasitics	**Crotamiton 10%** (Eurax)	C	No toxicity reported in pregnancy and infants
	Lindane (gamma benzene hydrochloride, Kwell)	B	Possible association with hypospadias

			Theoretical concern for neurotoxicity, convulsions, and aplastic anemia
	Mebendazole (Vermox)	C	No strong evidence to suggest association with congenital malformations
	Paromomycin	C	Limited data, no linkage to congenital malformations
	Pyrethins piperonyl butoxide (A-200, RID, RTC)	C	Little data to assess safety
			Poorly absorbed; should have minimal potential toxicity
	Thiabendazole	C	No reports of human teratogenicity, reports of limb defects in animal studies
Antituberculars (see Chap. 52)	**Ethambutol**	B	Crosses the placenta
			No reports of associated congenital defects
			Recommended by the CDC along with isoniazid and rifampin as initial treatment regimen for pregnant women with tuberculosis
	Ethionamide	C	One case report of increased congenital anomalies
	Isoniazid	C	Crosses the placenta
			No strong association with congenital anomalies

(continued)

Table B.1	Effects of Common Maternal Drugs on the Fetus *(Continued)*		
Class	Drug	Risk category (see Sec. II)	Pharmacokinetics/reported effects on fetus
	Rifampin	C	Recommended by the CDC along with rifampin and ethambutol as initial treatment regimen for pregnant women with tuberculosis
			Crosses the placenta
			No strong association with congenital anomalies
			Association with hemorrhagic disease of the newborn
			Recommended by the CDC along with isoniazid and ethambutol as initial treatment regimen for pregnant women with tuberculosis
Cardiovascular	**ACE inhibitors** (Captopril, Enalapril)	C	No apparent increased human fetal risk when used in first trimester
		D—if used in second or third trimester	Second and third trimester use associated with fetal teratogenicity secondary to fetal hypotension and reduced renal blood flow resulting in anuria, renal dysgenesis, and renal failure. Anuria-associated oligohydramnios may result in fetal growth restriction, pulmonary hypoplasia, limb contractures, craniofacial deformation, and neonatal death.
	Antiarrhythmic agents		
	Lidocaine	B	Rapidly crosses the placenta

		Limited data with use as an antiarrhythmic during pregnancy; the few reports available do not suggest a significant risk to the fetus
Procainamide	C	Has not been linked to congenital anomalies or adverse fetal or newborn effects
Quinidine	C_B, B_M	Crosses the placenta
		Has not been linked to congenital anomalies
		Report of neonatal thrombocytopenia after maternal use
β-blockers Propranolol, Labetolol	C (first trimester)	Cross the placenta
	D (second or third trimester)	
		In late pregnancy, reports of fetal and neonatal effects including hypoglycemia, bradycardia, neonatal apnea, and respiratory distress
		Reports of intrauterine growth restriction (IUGR)
Calcium channel blockers	C	Cross the placenta
		Theoretical risk on calcium dependent processes of embryogenesis
Diltiazem	C	Linked to limb, tail malformation in mice, no definitive reports in humans

(continued)

Table B.1 Effects of Common Maternal Drugs on the Fetus *(Continued)*

Class	Drug	Risk category (see Sec. II)	Pharmacokinetics/reported effects on fetus
	Nifedipine	C	Commonly used for tocolysis in preterm labor and as an antihypertensive agent in pregnancy
			No definitive data of increased risk of congenital anomalies in humans
	Verapamil	C	Has not been linked to congenital anomalies
	Digoxin	C	Used for treatment of maternal or fetal arrhythmias
			Transplacental passage and uptake by the fetus increased with advancing gestational age
			No linkage to congenital anomalies
			Neonatal death has been reported after maternal overdose
Diuretics			
	Acetazolamide	C	No linkage to congenital anomalies in humans
	Thiazide diuretics		Cross the placenta
	Chlorothiazide, chlorthalidone, hydrochlorothiazide	C/D if used in pregnancy-induced hypertension (PIH)	Cross the placenta

			Can induce maternal hyperglycemia Recommendation that infant be observed for hypoglycemia
			Conflicting reports exist regarding association with congenital abnormalities; possible linkage to congenital heart defects with chlorthalidone with first trimester use.
			Neonatal thrombocytopenia, hemolytic anemia, and electrolyte imbalances have been reported
Furosemide		C	Crosses the placenta
			May decrease placental perfusion; use is only indicated in pregnancy if there is adequate support of intravascular volume in cases of congestive heart failure or chronic renal disease.
			Associated with increased fetal urine production
			No strong association with major congenital anomalies
Spironolactone		C/D if used in PIH	May decrease placental perfusion
			No strong association with major congenital anomalies; however, concern that the anti-androgenic effect caused feminization in male rat fetuses.

(continued)

Table B.1	Effects of Common Maternal Drugs on the Fetus *(Continued)*		
Class	Drug	Risk category (see Sec. II)	Pharmacokinetics/reported effects on fetus
	Other Antihypertensives		
	Diazoxide	C	Crosses the placenta
			May cause a rapid decrease in maternal blood pressure, decreased placental perfusion, and fetal bradycardia; less effects were seen with small doses at frequent intervals
			Uterine relaxant and therefore, may inhibit uterine contractions
			Use associated with neonatal hyperglycemia
	Methyldopa	B	Crosses the placenta
			Antihypertensive agent that does not alter blood flow to the uterus
			Not implicated as a teratogen
			Reports of neonatal decreased intracranial volume and reduced systolic blood pressure; neither considered clinically significant
	Nitroprusside	C	Crosses the placenta
			Not implicated as a teratogen

Drug	Category	Notes
		May see transient fetal bradycardia
		Standard maternal dosing does not appear to increase the risk for excessive cyanide accumulation in the fetus.
Prazosin	C	Crosses the placenta
		α1-adrenergic blocking agent
		Not implicated as a teratogen
Vasodilators		
Dipyridamole	B	Case series and case reports show no association with congenital abnormalities.
Disopyramide	C	Crosses the placenta
		No association to congenital abnormalities
		Reports of induction of uterine contractions near term leading to theoretical concern for preterm delivery
Hydralazine	C	Crosses the placenta
		Animal studies demonstrated skeletal anomalies when administered in the 1st trimester. Use in the third trimester is common and safe if maternal hypotension is avoided.

(continued)

Table B.1	Effects of Common Maternal Drugs on the Fetus *(Continued)*		
Class	Drug	Risk category (see Sec. II)	Pharmacokinetics/reported effects on fetus
			Neonatal reports of thrombocytopenia and bleeding; however, this may be related to severe maternal hypertension rather than the drug exposure, also case reports of fetal arrhythmia.
	Nitroglycerin	B_B, C_M	Rapid-onset, short-acting
			Reports, although limited in number, suggest no significant harm to the fetus.
			Some reports of fetal bradycardia and loss of beat-to-beat variability in response to a reduction in maternal blood pressure; these fetal cardiac effects are apparently of no lasting clinical significance.
Chemotherapy agents			Use of most antineoplastic agents are associated with low birth weight
			Limited exposures with often multiple agents used at once makes final interpretation of observations difficult.
			Congenital anomalies of virtually all organ systems have been described, but the risks of not treating the mother with cancer must be weighted against the risks of treatment.
Chemotherapy agents	Cytarabine	D	Early use in the first and second trimester is associated with a variety of chromosomal and congenital abnormalities. Risk of malformation is approximately 1 in 8.

Cyclophosphamide	D	Case reports of first trimester miscarriage and malformation of limbs and eyes. Considered to not increase the risk of congenital malformation if used in the 2nd and 3rd trimesters. Impaired fetal growth seen.
Dactinomycin	D/C	Limited reports of use during pregnancy; congenital anomalies of virtually all organ systems have been described.
		One report of six exposed pregnancies did not reveal an association with congenital anomalies.
Doxorubicin	D	Safe use in pregnancy is not established—embryotoxic and teratogenic in rats—embryotoxic and teratogenic in rabbits. Use should be limited to the 2nd and 3rd trimesters. Pancytopenia in the newborn has been reported with use during the third trimester.
5-Fluorouracil	D_B, X_M	Teratogenic effects in all animal species were studied. Reported associations with spontaneous abortions, cleft lip/palate, and VSD; report of 40 exposed pregnancies in the 2nd and 3rd trimesters as a combination regimen reported no stillbirths and 2 congenital anomalies (club foot, urethral reflux).
Daunorubicin	D	*1st trimester:* reports of spontaneous abortion, also of normal pregnancies; two case reports of fetuses with multiple anomalies
		2nd–3rd trimester: One report of 40 infants exposed demonstrated no adverse effects; a second report of 40 infants demonstrated 2 with congenital anomalies. In one series of 29 exposed pregnancies, newborn complications included anemia, hypoglycemia, electrolyte disturbances, and transient neutropenia. Risk of malformation is approximately 1 in 8.

(continued)

Table B.1		Effects of Common Maternal Drugs on the Fetus *(Continued)*	
Class	Drug	Risk category (see Sec. II)	Pharmacokinetics/reported effects on fetus
	6-Mercaptopurine	D	Congenital anomalies were seen in exposed mice, rats, hamsters, and rabbits; embryotoxic and teratogenic in rats—embryotoxic in rabbits. No malformation syndrome has been identified in humans. Neonatal pancytopenia and hemolytic anemia have been reported. Safe use in pregnancy is not established; however, several normal outcomes in human pregnancies have been reported.
	Mechlorethamine	D	Case reports of both normal and abnormal outcomes after chemotherapy regimens, including mechlorethamine, were used.
	Methotrexate	XD_B, X_M	Folic acid antagonist. Teratogenic effects in all animal species studied. Reported association with spontaneous abortions, cleft lip/palate, and VSD.
	Procarbazine	D	Congenital anomalies that were seen in exposed rats may be avoided with folic acid treatment. Case series of 22 exposed human infants demonstrated no anomalies. There are case reports of exposed infants with congenital defects. Associated with congenital abnormalities. Folic acid antagonist
			May produce gonadal dysfunction. Crosses the placenta
	Thioguanine	D	Purine analog interrupting nucleic acid biosynthesis. Crosses the placenta. Considered a teratogen
			Congenital anomalies were seen in exposed rats. Case reports of distal limb defects in exposed human infants. Associated with severe newborn myelosuppression

Other Chemo-therapeutic Agents	Vinca alkaloids Vincristine, vinde-sine, vinblastine, vinorelbine	D	Antimitotic. Congenital abnormalities were observed in animal studies; however, there are several reports of normal human pregnancy outcome. May produce gonadal dysfunction
	Bleomycin	D	Case reports exist of both normal children and children with congenital anoma-lies who were exposed in utero.
	Dacarbazine	C	Case reports of normal outcomes in children exposed in utero
Drugs of habit or abuse	**Caffeine**	B	Moderate to heavy consumption may be associated with the increased risk of late first and second trimester spontaneous abortion; although, no risk of mis-carriage with intake less than 200 mg/day. May produce gonadal dysfunction
			In mothers who have experienced a prior loss, even light use has been shown to increase the risk of fetal loss.
			Demonstration of increased fetal breathing and decreased heart rate after caffeine consumption. Crosses the placenta

(continued)

Table B.1 Effects of Common Maternal Drugs on the Fetus *(Continued)*

Class	Drug	Risk category (see Sec. II)	Pharmacokinetics/reported effects on fetus
			Fetuses of mothers with high caffeine consumption have been shown to have less time in active sleep and a greater time in arousal. No association with congenital anomalies
			High caffeine consumption with cigarette smoking increases the risk for low birth weight more than with cigarette smoking alone. Moderate to heavy consumption may be associated with the increased risk of late first and second trimester spontaneous abortion; although, no risk of miscarriage with intake less than 200 mg per day.
			Newborn cardiac arrhythmias have been described to be possibly related to caffeine withdrawal.
	Cocaine	C	See Chap. 12
		X if non-medicinal	
	Ethanol	D	See Chap. 12
		X if excessive or prolonged use	
	Marijuana	C	See Chap. 12
	Tobacco	C	See Chap. 12

Gastrointestinal	Anti-inflammatory		
	Sulfasalazine	B	No strong linkage to congenital abnormalities; however, there are reports of potential associations including cleft lip/palate, hydrocephalus, VSD, coarctation of the aorta, and genitourinary abnormalities. Caution near term due to the association between sulfonamides and newborn bilirubin toxicity. (See Chap. 26)
		D if used near term	
Antilipemic	Cholestyramine	B	Resin that binds bile acids
			One report of fetal subdural hematomas thought to be secondary to vitamin K deficiency caused by the drug or mother's underlying cholestasis. No strong linkage to congenital abnormalities; however, there are reports of potential associations including cleft lip/palate, hydrocephalus, VSD, coarctation of the aorta, and genitourinary abnormalities.
Antisecretory	Cimetidine	B	H_2-receptor antagonist inhibiting gastric acid secretion
			Crosses the placenta. Resin that binds bile acids
			Not implicated as a teratogen. No linkage to congenital malformations
			Antiadrenergic activity in animals; although, not shown in humans.
			No increased risk of congenital malformations

(continued)

Table B.1	Effects of Common Maternal Drugs on the Fetus *(Continued)*		
Class	Drug	Risk category (see Sec. II)	Pharmacokinetics/reported effects on fetus
	Ranitidine	B	Like cimetidine, however, ranitidine does not show antiadrenergic activity in animal or human studies with H_2-receptor antagonist inhibiting the gastric acid secretion.
Laxative			
	Docusate	C	Crosses the placenta
			One report of maternal and neonatal hypomagnesemia thought to be secondary to docusate sodium. No increased risk of congenital malformations
	Metoclopramide	B	Used in pregnancy for antiemetic effect and to increase gastric emptying time. No linkage to fetal toxicity or malformations
	Zofran (Ondansetron)	B	Crosses the placenta. Not implicated as a teratogen
Narcotics (see Chap. 12)	**Butorphanol**	C	
	Meperidine	B	
	Pentazocine	C	
	Propoxyphene	C for all, D if excessive or prolonged use at term	

Psychothera-peutic agents	Antipsychotics/tranquilizers		General comments:
	For schizophrenia:		For drugs in this class that are used for schizophrenia, there are reports of newborn toxicity when used close to term. Two clinical syndromes described:
			1. Syndrome more commonly seen with low-potency agents (e.g., chlorpromazine, prochlorperazine, thioridazine)—neonatal depression, lethargy, gastrointestinal dysfunction, and hypotension. These symptoms may last a few days.
			2. Syndrome more commonly seen with high-potency agents (e.g., haloperidol)—extrapyramidal signs including tremors, increased tone, spasticity, posturing, arching of the back, hyperactive deep tendon reflexes, and shrill crying. These symptoms may last for several months.
	Chlorpromazine	C	Crosses the placenta
			Considered safe when used in smaller antiemetic dosages
			When used for analgesia during labor, marked drop in maternal blood pressures have been noted.
			Most studies report no linkage to congenital anomalies.
	Haloperidol	C	Conflicting reports regarding an association with limb reduction defects

(continued)

Table B.1 Effects of Common Maternal Drugs on the Fetus *(Continued)*

Class	Drug	Risk category (see Sec. II)	Pharmacokinetics/reported effects on fetus
			Possible association with cardiovascular defects
			Use during labor at suggested dosages has not been linked with neonatal effects.
	Prochlorperazine, Thioridazine	C	Cross the placenta
			Use for nausea and vomiting is considered safe
			Although there are conflicting results, most studies suggest that phenothiazines are safe when used in low doses.
	For bipolar disease:		
	Lithium	D	Crosses the placenta
			Serum half-life in newborns are longer compared to the adult values.
			Strong association with congenital anomalies, especially cardiovascular defects (Ebstein anomaly)
			Reported fetal and newborn toxicities including: cyanosis, hypotonia, bradycardia, thyroid depression and goiter, cardiomegaly, and diabetes insipidus
			Most neonatal toxic effects are self-limited.

	Benzodiazepines		Most documented to readily cross the placenta with fetal accumulation of levels.
	Alprazolam	D	No linkage to congenital anomalies with alprazolam; however, reported associations with other drugs in this class:
	Clonazepam	D	Clonazepam—congenital heart defects
	Diazepam	D	Diazepam—cleft lip/palate (controversial, no linkage with more recent large cohort and case-control studies), inguinal hernia, dysmorphic features, fetal growth restriction, CNS defects
	Lorazepam	D	Lorazepam has been associated with anal atresia
			Risk of newborn toxicity and withdrawal especially with increased dosages or prolonged use; described clinical presentation of toxicity and withdrawal include:
			1. "Floppy infant syndrome"—hypothermia, hypotonia, lethargy, sucking difficulties, apnea, and cyanosis
			2. "Withdrawal syndrome"—tremors, irritability, inconsolable crying, restlessness, abnormal sleep pattern, hypertonicity, hyperreflexia, seizures, diarrhea, vomiting, and vigorous sucking. These symptoms may present up to 3 weeks after delivery and last for several months.
			Long-term neurobehavioral consequences controversial and inadequately studied.
	Tricyclic antidepressants		Cross the placenta

(continued)

Table B.1 Effects of Common Maternal Drugs on the Fetus *(Continued)*

Class	Drug	Risk category (see Sec. II)	Pharmacokinetics/reported effects on fetus
	Amitriptyline	C	Conflicting reports regarding association with limb reduction defects
	Imipramine	D	Although there are small number of exposures, possible association with cardiovascular defects with imipramine and nortriptyline
	Nortriptyline	D	The following newborn effects have been described with imipramine and nortriptyline use: periodic apnea, cyanosis, tachypnea, respiratory distress, irritability, seizures, feeding difficulties, heart failure, tachycardia, myoclonus, and urinary retention.
			Long-term neurodevelopmental studies lacking, one report of no lasting neurodevelopmental effect (see Nulman et al., 1997)
Selective serotonin reuptake inhibitors (SSRI)			Recent studies suggest a possible increase in congenital malformations, especially with early first trimester use (see Thormahlen, 2006 and Wogelius et al., 2006). Use of SSRI's late in pregnancy has been associated with a mild transient neonatal syndrome involving the central nervous, respiratory, and gastrointestinal systems.
	Fluoxetine (Prozac)	C	A neonatal withdrawal syndrome has been described. Onset may occur up to few days after delivery and last for several months. Symptoms similar to those described for benzodiazepines. Not associated with any major congenital anomalies. Use of fluoxetine after 20 weeks gestation has been associated with neonatal pulmonary hypertension. Long term neurodevelopmental studies demonstrated no differences in developmental outcomes.

Fluvoxamine (Luvox)	C	SSRI-exposed infants are also more likely to be low birth weight and experience respiratory distress including persistent pulmonary hypertension. Not associated with any major congenital anomalies.
Paroxetine (Paxil)	C	Paroxetine has been associated with cardiovascular anomalies but studies are not consistent. Use of paroxetine after 20 weeks gestation has been associated with risk of neonatal pulmonary hypertension. Long term neurodevelopmental studies demonstrated no differences in developmental outcomes. American College of Obstetrics and Gyncology currently recommends paroxetine use be avoided in pregnant women and women planning pregnancy (see Suggested Readings, Nulman et al., 1997)
Sertraline (Zoloft)	B	Animal studies do not demonstrate an association with any major congenital anomalies, although there are reports of various malformations associated with sertraline. Use of setraline after 20 weeks gestation has been associated with risk of neonatal pulmonary hypertension. Long term neurodevelopmental studies demonstrated no differences in developmental outcomes.
Venlafaxine (Effexor)	C	Animal studies have not demonstrated an increased risk of congenital anomalies. A published abstract suggested an increased risk in some malformations.
Thyroid medications (see Chap. 3)		
Thyroid supplementation		
Levothyroxine	A	Not associated with congenital anomalies.

(continued)

Table B.1	Effects of Common Maternal Drugs on the Fetus *(Continued)*		
Class	Drug	Risk category (see Sec. II)	Pharmacokinetics/reported effects on fetus
Antithyroid			
	Methimazole	D	Has been associated with aplasia cutis and choanal atresia, but recent studies have refuted this. Both methimazole and propylthiouracil can be used to treat pregnant women with hyperthyroidism.
	Propylthiouracil	D	Not associated with congenital anomalies. Both methimazole and propylthiouracil can be used to treat pregnant women with hyperthyroidism.

*Risk Categories are defined in II.
B = Briggs (see II.B.2); M = (see II.B.2);
M = Manufacturer (see II.B.4).

ACE = angiotensin-converting enzyme; CNS = central nervous system; IV = intravenous; NSAIDs = nonsteroidal anti-inflammatory drugs; PD = phosphate dehydrogenase; PIH = pregnancy-induced hypertension; SSRI = selective serotonin reuptake inhibitors; VSD = ventricular septal defect.

Suggested Readings

Berkovitch M, Elbirt D, Addis A, et al. Fetal effects of metoclopramide therapy for nausea and vomiting of pregnancy. *N Engl J Med* 2000;343(6):445–446.

Berlin CM Jr. Effects of drugs on the fetus. *Pediatr Rev* 1991;12(9):282–287.

Bodendorfer TW, Briggs GG, Gunning JE. Obtaining drug exposure histories during pregnancy. *Am J Obstet Gynecol* 1979;135(4):490–494.

Boyle RJ. Effects of certain prenatal drugs on the fetus and newborn. *Pediatr Rev* 2002;23(1):17–24.

Briggs GG, Freeman RK, Yaffe SJ. *Drugs in pregnancy and lactation: a reference guide to fetal and neonatal risk*, 6th ed. Philadelphia: Lippincott Williams & Wilkins, 2002.

Chambers CD, Hernandez-Diaz S, Van Marter LJ, et al. Selective serotonin-reuptake inhibitors and risk of persistent pulmonary hypertension of the newborn. *N Engl J Med* 2006;354(6):579–587.

Dean JC, Hailey H, Moore SJ, et al. Long term health and neurodevelopment in children exposed to antiepileptic drugs before birth. *J Med Genet* 2002;39(4):251–259.

Food and Drug Administration. Labeling and prescription drug advertising: content and format for labeling for human prescription drugs. *Fed Regist* 1980;44:37434–37467.

Holmes LB, Harvey EA, Coull BA, et al. The teratogenicity of anticonvulsant drugs. *N Engl J Med* 2001;344(15):1132–1138.

Kalter H, Warkany J. Congenital malformations (second of two parts). *N Engl J Med* 1983;308(9):491–497.

Kalter H, Warkany J. Medical progress. Congenital malformations: etiologic factors and their role in prevention (first of two parts). *N Engl J Med* 1983;308(8):424–431.

Koren G, Florescu A, Costei AM, et al. Nonsteroidal antiinflammatory drugs during third trimester and the risk of premature closure of the ductus arteriosus: A meta-analysis. *Ann Pharmacother* 2006;40(5):824–829.

Koren G, Pastuszak A, Ito S. Drugs in pregnancy. *N Engl J Med* 1998;338(16):1128–1137.

Levy G. Pharmacokinetics of fetal and neonatal exposure to drugs. *Obstet Gynecol* 1981;58(suppl 5):9S–16S.

Lusskin SI, Misri S. Infants with antenatal exposure to serotonin reuptake inhibitors (SSRI). In: Feigin RD, ed. UpToDate. Waltham, MA: UpToDate, 2007.

Moretti ME, Caprara D, Coutinho CJ, et al. Fetal safety of loratadine use in the first trimester of pregnancy: a multicenter study. *J Allergy Clin Immunol* 2003;111(3):479–483.

Moudgal VV, Sobel JD. Antifungal drugs in pregnancy: a review. *Expert Opin Drug Saf* 2003;2(5):475–483.

Murray L, Seger D. Drug therapy during pregnancy and lactation. *Emerg Med Clin North Am* 1994;12(1):129–149.

Neubert D, Chahoud I, Platzek T, et al. Principles and problems in assessing prenatal toxicity. *Arch Toxicol* 1987;60(1–3):238–245.

Nordeng H, Lindemann R, Perminov KV, et al. Neonatal withdrawal syndrome after in utero exposure to selective serotonin reuptake inhibitors. *Acta Paediatr* 2001;90(3):288–291.

Nulman I, Rovet J, Stewart DE, et al. Neurodevelopment of children exposed in utero to antidepressant drugs. *N Engl J Med* 1997;336(4):258–262.

Oberlander TF, Warburton W, Misri S, et al. Neonatal outcomes after prenatal exposure to selective serotonin reuptake inhibitor antidepressants and maternal depression using population-based linked health data. *Arch Gen Psychiatry* 2006;63(8):898–906.

Szeto HH. Kinetics of drug transfer to the fetus. *Clin Obstet Gynecol* 1993;36(2):246–254.

Szeto HH. Maternal-fetal pharmacokinetics and fetal dose-response relationships. *Ann N Y Acad Sci* 1989;562:42–55.

Szeto HH. Maternal-fetal pharmacokinetics: summary and future directions. *NIDA Res Monogr* 1995;154:203–217.

Thormahlen GM. Paroxetine use during pregnancy: is it safe? *Ann Pharmacother* 2006;40(10):1834–1837.

Use of psychoactive medication during pregnancy and possible effects on the fetus and newborn. Committee on drugs. American Academy of Pediatrics. *Pediatrics* 2000;105(4 pt 1):880–887.

Ward RM. Drug therapy of the fetus. *J Clin Pharmacol* 1993;33(9):780–789.

Ward RM. Maternal-placental-fetal unit: unique problems of pharmacologic study. *Pediatr Clin North Am* 1989;36(5):1075–1088.

Wogelius P, Nørgaard M, Gislum M, et al. Maternal use of selective serotonin reuptake inhibitors and risk of congenital malformations. *Epidemiology* 2006;17(6):701–704.

Appendix C

Maternal Medications and Breastfeeding

Karen M. Puopolo

I. **BACKGROUND.** Questions commonly arise regarding the safety of maternal medication use during breastfeeding. A combination of the biologic and chemical properties of the drug and the physiology of the mother and infant determines the safety of any individual medication. Consideration is given to the amount of drug that is found in breast milk, the half-life of the drug in the infant, and the biologic effect of the drug on the infant.

A. **Drug properties that affect entry into breast milk.** Molecular size, pH, acid-base dissociation constant (pKa), lipid solubility, and protein-binding properties of the drug all affect the **milk-to-plasma (M/P) concentration ratio,** which is defined as the relative concentration of the protein-free fraction of the drug in milk and maternal plasma. Small molecular size, slightly alkaline pH, non-ionization, high lipid solubility, and lack of binding to serum proteins all favor entry of a drug into breast milk. The half-life of the medication and frequency of drug administration are also important; the longer the cumulative time that the drug is present in the maternal circulation, the greater the opportunity for it to appear in breast milk.

B. **Maternal factors.** The total maternal dose and mode of administration (intravenous vs. oral), as well as maternal illness (particularly renal or liver impairment), can affect the persistence of the drug in the maternal circulation. Medications taken in the first few days postpartum are more likely to enter breast milk as the mammary alveolar epithelium does not fully mature until the end of the first postpartum week.

C. **Infant factors.** The maturity of the infant is the primary factor in determining the persistence of a drug in the infant's system. Preterm infants and term infants in the first month after birth metabolize drugs more slowly because of renal and hepatic immaturity. The total dose of a drug that the infant is exposed to is determined by the volume of milk ingested (per kg of body weight), as well as the frequency of feeding (or frequency of milk expression in the case of preterm infants).

II. **DETERMINATION OF DRUG SAFETY DURING BREASTFEEDING.** A number of available resources evaluate the risk of individual medications to the breastfed infant. Ideally, direct measurements of the entry of a drug into breast milk and the level and persistence of the drug in the breastfed infant, as well as experience with exposure of infants to the drug, are all used to make a judgment regarding drug safety. Unfortunately, this type of information is available for relatively few medications. In the absence of specific data, a judgment is made on the basis of both the known pharmacologic properties of the drug and the known or predicted effects of the drug on the developing infant. Clinicians providing advice to the nursing mother about the safety of a particular medication should be aware of the following points:

A. **Resources may differ in their judgment of a particular drug.** Information about some medications (especially newer ones) is in flux, and safety judgments may change over a relatively short period. Different resources approach the question of medication use in breastfeeding with different perspectives. For example, The *Physicians' Desk Reference* is a compendium of commercially supplied drug information. In the absence of specific data regarding the entry of a drug into the breast milk, drug manufacturers, generally, do not make a definitive statement about the safety of drugs in breastfeeding. Other resources, such as *Medications in Mother's Milk* (MMM) and the National Library of Medicine's toxicology data network (TOXNET) program, take the available data and make a judgment about relative safety of the drug.

B. **The safety of a drug in pregnancy may not be the same as the safety of the drug during breastfeeding.** Occasionally, a medication that is contraindicated in pregnancy (e.g., warfarin or ibuprofen) is safe to use while breastfeeding.

C. **Definitive data are not available for most medications or for specific clinical situations.** There is a need for individualized clinical judgment in many cases, taking into account the available information, the need of the mother for the medication, and the risk to the infant of both exposure to the drug and of exposure to breast milk substitutes. Consultation with the **Breastfeeding and Human Lactation Study Center** at the University of Rochester can aid the clinician in making specific clinical judgments.

III. RESOURCES. Resources listed as items III.A–D served as resource material for this appendix.

A. **LactMed is the Drugs and Lactation Database, part of the National Library of Medicine's TOXNET.** It is found at http://toxnet.nlm.nih.gov/cgi-bin/sis/htmlgen?LACT. This database includes information on the expected transfer of substances in breast milk, anticipated absorption of substances by the infant, data on maternal and infant blood levels, and possible adverse effects in the nursing infant. Suggested therapeutic alternatives are listed where appropriate. This resource does not offer a specific rating system but provides summary guidance based on available data (or lack of data). All data are derived from the scientific literature and fully referenced; links to PubMed are provided for cited literature.

B. **Hale T. *Medications and Mother's Milk*, 14th ed.** Amarillo, TX: Hale Publishing, 2010. This book is a comprehensive listing of hundreds of prescription and over-the-counter medications, radiopharmaceuticals, contrast agents, contraceptives, vitamins, herbal remedies, and vaccines, with primary references cited for most. The Food and Drug Administration's (FDA) Pregnancy Risk Category and AAP rating are provided for each drug (see text below about these sources). The author's own lactation risk category is as follows:

1. **L1:** safest
2. **L2:** safer
3. **L3:** moderately safe. Many drugs fall into this category, which are defined as follows: "There are no controlled studies in breastfeeding women; however, the risk of untoward effects to a breastfed infant is possible or controlled studies show only minimal and nonthreatening adverse effects. Drugs should be given only if the potential benefit justifies the potential risk to the infant."
4. **L4:** possibly hazardous
5. **L5:** contraindicated

C. **Briggs GG, Freeman RK, Yaffe SJ, eds. *Drugs in Pregnancy and Lactation*, 8th ed.** Philadelphia: Lippincott Williams & Wilkins, 2008. This book lists primary references and reviews data on more than 1,000 medications with respect to the risk to the developing fetus and the risk in breastfeeding. For drug use in pregnancy, the book provides a recommendation from 16 potential categories based on available human and animal reproduction data. For drug use in lactation, the book provides a recommendation from six potential categories based on available human and pharmacologic data.

D. Lawrence RA, Lawrence RM. *Breastfeeding: A Guide for the Medical Profession,* **7th ed.** Philadelphia: Elsevier, 2010. This book includes an extended discussion of the pharmacology of drug entry into breast milk. An appendix contains a listing of more than 600 drugs that are listed by drug category (analgesics, antibiotics, etc.) with the AAP safety rating, the Hale Lactation Risk Category, and the Weiner Code of Breastfeeding Safety listing, given when available. The appendix also contains extensive pharmacokinetic data for each drug including values for the M/P ratio and maximum amount (mg/mL) of drug found in breast milk.

E. **The Breastfeeding and Human Lactation Study Center.** The study center maintains a drug data bank that is regularly updated. Health professionals may call (585) 275–0088 to talk to staff members regarding the safety of a particular drug in breastfeeding. The study center will only take calls from health care professionals (not parents). The center is part of the Division of Neonatology, Golisano Children's Hospital at the University of Rochester Medical Center.

F. **The FDA's Pregnancy Risk Categories.** The FDA currently categorizes drugs using the following system:

1. **Category A.** Controlled studies in women fail to demonstrate a risk to the fetus.

2. **Category B.** Either animal-reproduction studies have not demonstrated a fetal risk or, if such a risk was found, it was not confirmed in later controlled studies in women.

3. **Category C.** Either studies in animals have revealed adverse effects on the fetus and there are no controlled studies in women, or studies in women and animals are not available. Drugs should be given only if the potential benefit justifies the potential risk to the fetus.

4. **Category D.** There is positive evidence of human fetal risk, but the benefits from use in pregnant women may be acceptable despite the risk (e.g., in a life-threatening situation or for a serious disease).

5. **Category X.** Studies in animals or human beings have demonstrated fetal abnormalities, and the risk of the use of the drug in pregnant women clearly outweighs any possible benefit.

   In 2008, the FDA proposed **eliminating** these categories. The agency is proposing to require that labeling should include a summary of the risks of using a drug during pregnancy and lactation, and a discussion of the data supporting that summary. The proposed labeling would also include relevant clinical information to help health care providers make prescribing decisions and counsel women about the use of drugs during pregnancy and/or lactation.

G. **American Academy of Pediatrics (AAP), Committee on Drugs. The transfer of drugs and other chemicals into human milk.** This AAP Pediatrics Policy Statement on medication use and breastfeeding (Pediatrics 2001;108(3):776–789) was retired in May 2010. Although still widely cited, this information is now outdated.

IV. INFORMATION ON COMMON MEDICATIONS.

Following are tables of medications commonly prescribed to breastfeeding women (Tables C.1–C.7). They are organized by category and are listed alphabetically within each category. Provided for each is the LactMed assessment and the Hale's MMM rating (L1–L5).

Table C.1	Antibiotics	
Medication	**LactMed**	**MMM**
Acyclovir	Acceptable	L2
Amikacin	Acceptable	L2
Amoxicillin	Acceptable	L1
Amphotericin B	Acceptable	L3
Ampicillin/Unasyn	Acceptable	L1
Augmentin	Acceptable	L1
Azithromycin	Acceptable	L2
Aztreonam	Acceptable	L2
Carbenicillin	Acceptable	L1
Cephalosporins:		
*List 1:	Acceptable	L1
†List 2:	Acceptable	L2
Chloramphenicol	Not advised	L4
Ciprofloxacin	Of concern; alternates are preferred	L3
Clarithromycin	Acceptable	L1
Clindamycin	May be of concern	L2
Doxycycline	Short-term use is acceptable	L3 (acute), L4 (chronic)
Erythromycin	Acceptable	L3 (<3 months), L2
Famciclovir	No data; alternates are preferred	L2
Fluconazole	Acceptable	L2
Gentamicin	Acceptable	L2
Griseofulvin	No data	L2
Imipenem-cilastatin	Acceptable	L2
		(continued)

Table C.1	*(Continued)*	
Medication	**LactMed**	**MMM**
Isoniazid	Should be discouraged	L3
Itraconazole	No data	L2
Kanamycin	Acceptable	L2
Ketoconazole	Limited data; alternates are preferred	L2
Loracarbef	No data; likely acceptable	L2
Meropenem	No data; likely acceptable	L3
Methicillin	Acceptable	L3
Metronidazole	Long-term use may be of concern	L2
Minocycline	Short-term use is acceptable	L2 (acute), L4 (chronic)
Mupirocin	Acceptable	L1
Nafcillin	No data; likely acceptable	L1
Nitrofurantoin	Not advised	L2
Norfloxacin	Short-term use is acceptable	L3
Ofloxacin	Short-term use is acceptable	L2
Penicillin G	Acceptable	L1
Piperacillin/Zosyn	Acceptable	L2
Sulfamethoxazole	Acceptable for healthy term infants; contraindicated for sick and premature infants	L3
Tetracycline	Short-term use is acceptable	L2
Trimethoprim	Acceptable	L2
Valacyclovir	Acceptable	L1

LactMed = National Library of Medicine Drugs and Lactation Database;
MMM = Medications in Mother's Milk.
*List 1: cefaclor, cefadroxil, cefazolin, cefdinir, cefoxitin, cefprozil, ceftazidime, ceftriaxone, cephalexin, cephalothin, cephapirin, cephradine.
†List 2: ceftibuten, cefepime, cefixime, cefoperazone, cefotaxime, cefotetan, cefpodoxime, cefuroxime.

Table C.2	Analgesics	
Medication	**LactMed**	**MMM**
Acetaminophen	Acceptable	L1
Aspirin	Unacceptable	L3
Butorphanol	Limited data; alternates are preferred	L2
Codeine	Of concern; alternates are preferred	L3
Fentanyl	Short-term intravenous or epidural use is acceptable. Long-term use is of concern; alternates are preferred	L2
Hydrocodone	Of concern; alternates are preferred	L3
Hydromorphone	Of concern; alternates are preferred	L3
Ibuprofen	Acceptable	L1
Indomethacin	Acceptable	L3
Ketorolac	Unacceptable due to FDA black box warning against use in lactation	L2
Meperidine	Unacceptable	L2/L3 (early postpartum)
Methadone	Acceptable if mother is on maintenance during pregnancy. Of concern if initiated after delivery	L3
Morphine	Short-term intravenous or epidural use is acceptable. Long-term use is of concern; alternates are preferred	L3
Nubain	Acceptable	L2
Naproxen	Limited data; alternates are preferred	L3/L4 (chronic use)
Oxycodone	Of concern; alternates are preferred	L3
LactMed = National Library of Medicine Drugs and Lactation Database; MMM = Medications in Mother's Milk.		

Table C.3	Antihypertensive and Cardiac Medications	
Medication	LactMed	MMM
Amiodarone	Of significant concern; cardiac and thyroid effects are likely	L5
Atenolol	Of concern to newborn and preterm infants; acceptable in infants >3 months of age	L3
Captopril	Acceptable	L2
Clonidine	Of concern; alternates are preferred	L3
Digoxin	Acceptable	L2
Diltiazem	Acceptable	L3
Dopamine/ dobutamine	No data; unlikely to be of concern. Likely to decrease milk production	L2
Enalapril	Acceptable	L2
Ephedrine	No data	L4
Epinephrine	Acceptable	L1
Flecainide	Limited data; likely acceptable	L3
Hydralazine	Acceptable	L2
Labetalol	Acceptable; alternates may be preferred for preterm infants	L2
Magnesium sulfate	Acceptable	L1
Methyldopa	Acceptable	L2
Nifedipine	Acceptable	L2
Nimodipine	Limited data; likely acceptable	L2
Procainamide	Limited data; likely acceptable	L3
Propranolol	Acceptable	L2
LactMed = National Library of Medicine Drugs and Lactation Database; MMM = Medications in Mother's Milk.		

Table C.4	Allergy and Respiratory Medications	
Medication	**LactMed**	**MMM**
Albuterol	Acceptable	L1
Beclomethasone	Acceptable	L2
Betamethasone	Limited data; likely not acceptable	L3
Budesonide	Acceptable	L1 (inhaled) L3 (oral)
Cetirizine (Zyrtec)	Acceptable at lower doses	L2
Clemastine (Tavist)	Of concern; alternates preferred	L4
Cromolyn sodium	Acceptable	L1
Dexamethasone	No data; alternates preferred	L3
Dextromethorphan	No data; likely acceptable	L1
Diphenhydramine	Acceptable at lower doses; alternates are preferred	L2
Fexofenadine (Allegra)	Acceptable at lower doses; could decrease milk production; alternates are preferred	L2
Flunisolide	No data but likely acceptable	L3
Hydrocortisone (topical)	Acceptable; do not use on nipples or other skin with direct infant contact	L2
Loratadine (Claritin)	Acceptable; could decrease milk production; use lower doses	L1
Methylprednisolone	Acceptable; of some concern at high intravenous doses	L2
Montelukast (Singulair)	No data; likely acceptable but alternates preferred	L3
Phenylephrine	Limited data; alternates are preferred. Could decrease milk production	L3
Prednisone	Acceptable at all but highest doses	L2
Pseudoephedrine	Unacceptable; acutely impairs milk production	L3/L4
Theophylline	Acceptable; use lower doses and serum levels	L3
LactMed = National Library of Medicine Drugs and Lactation Database; MMM = Medications in Mother's Milk.		

Table C.5	Psychoactive Medications	
Medication	LactMed	MMM
Alprazolam	Of concern; alternates preferred	L3
Amitryptyline	Acceptable	L2
Bupropion	Acceptable; alternates may be preferred	L3
Caffeine	Acceptable; intake should be minimized	L2
Carbamazepine	Of concern; alternates preferred	L2
Chloral hydrate	Of concern; alternates preferred for chronic use	L3
Chlordiazepoxide	No data	L3
Chlorpromazine	Acceptable; of concern when used in combination with other antipsychotic medication	L3
Citalopram (Celexa)	Acceptable but alternates may be preferred	L2
Clomipramine	Acceptable	L2
Clonazepam	Acceptable; of concern when used in combination with other antipsychotic medication	L3
Clozapine	Of concern; alternates preferred	L3
Desipramine	Acceptable	L2
Diazepam	Unacceptable	L3/L4 (chronic use)
Duloxetine (Cymbalta)	Acceptable; alternates may be preferred	L3
Escitalopram (Lexapro)	Acceptable	L2
Fluoxetine (Prozac)	Acceptable but alternates may be preferred	L2
Gabapentin	Acceptable; of concern when used in combination with other antipsychotic medication	L2
Haloperidol	Acceptable; of concern when used in combination with other antipsychotic medication	L2
		(continued)

Table C.5	Psychoactive Medications *(Continued)*	
Medication	**LactMed**	**MMM**
Lithium*	Of significant concern; likely unacceptable in preterm, newborn or dehydrated infants	L3*
Lorazepam (Ativan)	Acceptable	L3
Methylphenidate (Ritalin)	Limited data; likely acceptable; may decrease milk production	L3
Midazolam	Acceptable; chronic use may be of concern	L2
Oxazepam (Serax)	Acceptable	L3
Paroxetine (Paxil)	Acceptable; a preferred antidepressant for lactation	L2
Pentobarbital	Limited data; alternates are preferred	L3
Phenobarbital	Of concern; sedation can occur and monitoring infant serum levels may be required	L3
Phenytoin	Acceptable; of concern when used in combination with other anticonvulsant medication	L2
Prochlorperazine	No data; short-term use likely acceptable	L3
Sertraline (Zoloft)	Acceptable	L2
Valproic acid	Acceptable; monitor infant for hepatotoxicity	L2

LactMed = National Library of Medicine Drugs and Lactation Database;
MMM = Medications in Mother's Milk.
* Infant's serum lithium levels are 30% to 40% of the mother's level. Infant must be closely monitored by a pediatrician if used during breastfeeding, as drug has potential effects on infant neurodevelopment, cardiac rhythm, and thyroid function. It is recommended that the pediatrician periodically monitor the infant's BUN, creatinine, lithium level, and thyroid function; hydration status should also be closely monitored.

Table C.6	Gastrointestinal Medications	
Medication	**AAP**	**MMM**
Bismuth subsalicylate	Of concern; alternates preferred	L3
Cimetidine	Acceptable	L1
Docusate	Acceptable	L2
Domperidone	Little transfer into milk but not FDA approved for any use in the United States	L1
Famotidine	Acceptable	L1
Kaolin-pectin	No data	L1
Loperamide	Acceptable	L2
Metoclopramide	Likely acceptable; of some concern when used as galactagogue	L2
Nizatidine	Acceptable	L2
Omeprazole	Acceptable	L2
Ondansetron	No data	L2
Ranitidine	Acceptable	L2

LactMed = National Library of Medicine Drugs and Lactation Database; MMM = Medications in Mother's Milk.

Table C.7	Medications Contraindicated in Breastfeeding
Amiodarone	
Antineoplastic agents	
Bromocriptine	
Drugs of abuse	
Diethylstilbestrol	
Disulfiram	
Radioisotopes—usually require only temporary cessation of breastfeeding†	
Tamoxifen	

Note on oral contraceptives: Estrogen-containing preparations can reduce milk supply. Progestin-only oral contraceptives are safer with respect to milk production; depot injections of medroxyprogesterone (Depo-Provera) are also acceptable.

†*Note:* ^{131}Na-I treatment requires complete cessation of breastfeeding due to the concentration of this agent in the breast and in breast milk for weeks following completion of treatment.

Suggested Readings

Briggs GG, Freeman RK, Yaffe SJ, eds. *Drugs in Pregnancy and Lactation*. 8th ed. Baltimore: Lippincott Williams & Wilkins; 2008.

The CDC Guide to Breastfeeding Interventions. Available at: http://www.cdc.gov/breastfeeding.

Hale T. *Medications and Mother's Milk*. 14th ed. Amarillo, Tx: Hale Publishing; 2010.

Lawrence RA, Lawrence RM. *Breastfeeding: A Guide for the Medical Profession*, 7th ed. Philadelphia: Elsevier; 2010.

The United States Breastfeeding Committee (USBC). Available at: http://www.usbreastfeeding.org.

The United States National Library of Medicine Drugs and Lactation Database. Available at: http://toxnet.nlm.nih.gov/cgi-bin/sis/htmlgen?LACT.

Index

Note: Page numbers followed by an "*f*" denote figures; those followed by a "*t*" denote tables.

A

abdomen
  distention, 810, 827
  intra-abdominal injuries, 71–72
  masses, 353, 354*t*, 824
  masses, surgery, 812, 828
  newborn examination, 96
  paracentesis procedure, 868-869
ABO hemolytic disease, 338–339
abortion, spontaneous, 126
abrasions, 63, 72
acardia, multiple gestations, 128
acetazolamide, MH/IVH treatment, 700–701
acid handling, 352
acid-base physiology, 277, 331
acidosis, metabolic
  fluid, electrolyte management,
    277–278, 278*t*
  IEM, 770–771, 772*f,* 774–778, 775*f,* 786
acquired heart disease, 513–517.
  See also cardiac disorders
acquired syphilis, 664. *See also* syphilis
acquired thrombophilias, 548
ACTH stimulation test, 801, 803
activated protein C (APC), 628
acute lung injury. *See* pulmonary disorders
adenosine, tachycardias, 527
adrenal hemorrhage, 72
aEEG. *See* amplitude-integrated EEG
afterload reducing agents, 519–520
air embolism, systemic, 453
air leak
  mechanical ventilation, 390, 392
  meconium aspiration syndrome, 433
  neonatal resuscitation, 60–61
  PIE, 450–451
  pneumomediastinum, 451
  pneumopericardium, 451–452
  pneumothorax, 447–450
  RDS, 415
  risk factors, pathogenesis, 446
  types of, 447–453
air transport/travel, 186, 201, 202*t*
AKI. *See* acute kidney injury
albinism, 837
alkalosis, metabolic
  CLD, 283
  fluid, electrolyte management, 278–279,
    279*t*
  PPHN, 440–441

allergic colitis, 344
allergic transfusion reactions, 532
alpha-fetoprotein, maternal serum, 1–2
alternatives, considering, 851
ambiguous genitalia. *See* disorders of sex
    development
amblyopia, 187
AMH. *See* anti-müllerian hormone
Amicar®, EMCO, 459
amniocentesis, 3–4
amnioinfusion, MAS, 431
amniotic fluid analysis, 4
amphotericin B, 649, 650
amplitude-integrated EEG (aEEG),
    732, 733*f*
anaerobic bacterial infections, 645
analgesia, 880-884
androgen synthesis, 802
anemia 563
  blood loss, 565–566
  diagnosis, 566–568, 567*t*
  etiology, 565–566
  hemolysis, 566
  of infancy, 563
  of prematurity, 563–564, 564*t*
  prophylaxis, 570
  RBC production, 566
  therapy, 568–570
  transfusion, 568–570, 569*t*
  VLBW infants, 186
anencephaly, 743. *See also* neural tube defects
aneuploidy
  chromosome microdeletion, 118–119*t*
  common anomalies, 117*t,* 120–121*t*
  multiple gestations, 129
  prenatal screening, 2–3
anisometropia, 187
antepartum tests, 6–8
antibiotics
  LOS prevention, 644
  MAS, 433
  sepsis, meningitis, 625, 626*t*
anticoagulation, EMCO, 458–459
antihypertensive medications, preeclampsia,
    43, 45
anti-müllerian hormone (AMH), 792, 793*f,*
    794*t,* 804–805 803–804
antithyroid drugs, 25, 31
aorta
  arch, interrupted, 494–495, 495*f*

aorta *(Continued)*
coarctation of, 493–494, 493*f*
thrombosis, 550–552
aortic stenosis, 491–493, 492*f*
APC. *See* activated protein C
apgar scores, 52*t*, 61
apnea
definition, classification, incidence, 397
mechanical ventilation, 391
monitoring, evaluation, 399–400, 399*t*
neonatal resuscitation, 47, 53–55
pathogenesis, 398
persistent, 401
preventing SIDS, 401–402
primary, 47, 53
secondary, 47, 53
treatment, 400–401
apoptosis, asphyxia, 714
appendicitis, 821
Apt test, surgical emergencies, 826
arrhythmias
differential diagnosis, management,
521–526
emergency treatment, 526–528
evaluation, 521
ART. *See* assisted reproductive technology
arteries. *See also* blood
blood drawing, 852
catheterization, 860–865, 860*f*, 862*f*, 867
great, parallel circulation/transposition,
504–506, 505*f*
major arterial thrombosis, 550–552
measurements, 393
middle cerebral, assessment, 8
ascites, fetal, 808–809
ascitic fluid, abdominal paracentesis
procedure, 868–869
asphyxia, perinatal. *See* perinatal asphyxia
brief, 713
neuronal death, 714
aspirin, preeclampsia treatment, 45
assisted reproductive technology (ART), 132
associations, defined, 111
ativan. *See* lorazepam
atresia
biliary, 333
choanal, 816
esophageal, 813–814
pulmonary, 499–500, 500*f*
tricuspid, 501–502, 501*f*
atrioventricular block. *See* cardiac disorders
atrioventricular canal, 510–512, 510*f*, 511*t*
auditory dyssynchrony, 846. *See also* hearing,
hearing loss
auditory neuropathy, 846. *See also* hearing,
hearing loss

autoimmune thrombocytopenia, 583–584
autonomic seizures, 730. *See also* seizures
autonomic system, examination, 100
azithromycin, 422

B

babesiosis, blood transfusions, 529
Bacillus Calmette-Guérin (BCG)
vaccination, 682
bacterial infections, 624
anaerobic, 645–646
EOS, 624–625, 627–630, 632–637
focal, 651, 653–655
LOS, 637–345
sepsis, meningitis, 624–633, 635–639,
641–642, 646
bacterial sepsis. *See* early-onset sepsis; late-
onset sepsis
β-adrenergic blocking agents, 25
Ballard examination, 76, 77*f*
barometric pressure, 201, 202*t*
bathing newborns, 104, 833
β-blockers, cardiac disorders, 520
beat-to-beat variability, 9
behavioral health, 189, 425
Bell staging, NEC, 343
benzodiazepines, seizures, 739–741
bereavement follow-up. *See* end-of-life care
betamethasone, 42
bicarbonate handling, 352
bile ducts, 332–333
biliary atresia, 333
bilious emesis, 811, 820
bilirubin, 304–339. *See also*
hyperbilirubinemia
drugs that cause displacement of, 305*t*
encephalopathy, acute/chronic, 317
metabolism, 304–306
nomogram, 313*f*
source of, 304
toxicity, 317–318
biophysical profile, 8
bipyridine, cardiac disorders, 519
birth defects
anatomic pathology, 123
aneuploidies, 117*t*, 120–121*t*
chromosome microdeletion, 118–119*t*
etiology, 112
follow-up, 123
incidence of, 111–112
laboratory studies, 116–122
physical evaluation, 115–116
teratogens, 113–114*t*
birth weight
classification, 76
mortality, 81*f*

bladder tap procedure, 853
bleeding, 538
  anemia, 565–566
  autosomal dominant, 539
  diagnosis, 540–543, 541t, 542t
  etiology, 538–540
  transitory deficiencies, 538
  treatment, 543–545
blood
  banking, 89, 105
  drawing procedures, 852-853
  extravascular, hyperbilirubinemia, 315
  granulocytes, 534–535
  IVIG, newborn use, 535–536
  packed RBC, 530–533
  plasma product use, 533–534
  platelets use, 534
  priming, EMCO, 457–458
  whole, component transfusions,
    529–530
blood donor, designated, 530
blood gas
  arterial measurements, 393
  capillary determination, 393–394
  continuous analysis, 394
  mechanical ventilation effects, 382–385
blood gas monitoring
  EMCO, 458
  introduction to, 393
  mechanical ventilation, 391
  oxygen, noninvasive, 394–395
  pulmonary ventilation, 395–396
  RDS, 408
blood pressure
  ELBW infants, 163
  newborn examination, 94
  renal conditions, 366–368, 367t, 368t,
    369–370t, 371t
blood products, 529
blood transfusions
  anemia, 568–570, 569t
  BPD, 425
  component, 529–530
  ELBW infants, 163
  infections, 529, 530f
  reactions, 532–533
blood urea nitrogen (BUN), 360
bone injuries, 70–71
Borrelia burgdorferi, 683. *See also* Lyme
    disease
BPD. *See* bronchopulmonary dysplasia
brachial plexus injury, 69–70
bradycardias
  defined, 524–525
  emergency treatment, 527–528
  transient fetal, 44

breastfeeding, 266. *See also* feeding; milk;
    nutrition
  contraindications, 267–268
  hyperbilirubinemia, 313–314
  hypoglycemia, 293
  infant conditions, 265–266
  jaundice, 313
  LOS prevention, 644
  management, support, 263–264
  maternal conditions, 266
  maternal drug use, 140
  maternal thyroid medications, 38
  milk care, handling, 267
  newborn care, 107
  problem management, 264–265
  rationale for, 263
  SIDS, 402
  term infant recommendations, 263
bronchopulmonary dysplasia (BPD)
  associated complications, 425–426
  bronchodilators, 423
  clinical presentation, 419
  definition, epidemiology, 417
  discharge planning, 426–427
  fluid, electrolyte management, 283
  inpatient treatment, 419–425
  mechanical ventilation, 389–391
  medications, 422–424
  nutrition, 260–261
  outcome, 427–428
  outpatient therapy, 427
  pathogenesis, 417–418
"bronze baby" syndrome, 326
BUN. *See* blood urea nitrogen

C

café au lait spots, 837
caffeine
  BPD, 422
  ELBW infants, 161
  persistent apnea, 401
calcium, 297
  channel blockers, cardiac disorders, 520
  deficiency, osteopenia, 782
  IDMs, 17
  serum, 397–303
Candida, 647–650
candidal diaper dermatitis, 648
candidiasis
  late-onset invasive, 649
  oral, 647–648
  systemic, 648–650
capillary blood drawing, 852
capnography, 395–396
caput succedaneum, 64, 72, 99
carbapenemase-producing organisms, 643

carbohydrates, infant nutrition, 241, 242*f*
cardiac disorders, 469–528
  acquired heart disease, 513–517
  arrhythmias, 521–528
  bradycardia, 524–525
  cardiac massage, neonatal resuscitation, 56
  cardiac surgery, lesions, 513, 514–516*t*
  cardiomyopathies, 517
  cardiovascular support, ELBW infants, 163
  catheterization, 489–491, 489*t*, 490*f*
  congenital, clinical presentations, 471–476
  congenital, evaluation, 476–491
  congestive heart failure, 472, 475–476*t*
  dysfunction, IEM, 768, 768*t*
  ECG examination, 479, 483–484*t*, 485, 485*t*
  failure, EMCO, 454
  fetal monitoring, 8–10
  heart block, 524–525
  heart murmur, 472–474
  hyperoxia test, 485–486
  incidence, survival, 469–471
  introduction to, 469
  irregular rhythms, 525–526
  lesion-specific care, 491–513
  neonatal transport, 201
  newborn examination, 91–95
  perinatal asphyxia, 718
  pharmacology, 517–521
  stabilization, transport, 486–488
  top diagnoses, age, 470*f*
cardiac, great arteries, parallel circulation/
    transposition, 504–506, 505*f*
cardiogenic shock, 464. *See also* shock
carnitine, PN, 247
catheterization
  cardiac, 489–491, 489*t*, 490*f*
  catheter blood samples, 852
  catheter types, 858-859
  multiple-lumen catheters, 865–867
  percutaneous central venous, 868
  percutaneous radial artery, 867
  umbilical artery procedure, 860-865,
    860*f*, 862*f*
  umbilical vein, 865, 866*f*
  vascular, procedure, 858–868
catheters, multiple-lumen, 865–867
cavernous hemangioma, 836-837
cellulitis, 651
central hearing loss, 846. *See also* hearing,
    hearing loss
central nervous system (CNS) dysfunction,
    426
central-line associated bloodstream
    infections, 643, 645, 646*t*

cephalohematoma, 64, 99
cerebral dysgenesis, 736
cerebral hemorrhage. *See* intracranial
    hemorrhage; intraparenchymal
    hemorrhage
cerebral palsy (CP), 132, 725–726
cerebral perfusion, EMCO, 457
cerebral sinovenous thrombosis,
    552–553
cerebrospinal fluid (CSF) examination,
    854-856, 854*t*
cervical nerve root injury, 69
cesarean delivery, multiple births, 127
Chagas disease, 529
chemoreceptor response, apnea, 398
chest tube drainage, pneumothorax air leak,
    448–450
chickenpox. *See* varicella-zoster virus
Chlamydia trachomatis, 652–653
chlorpromazine, 148
choanal atresia, 816
cholestasis, 332
cholestasis neonate, intrahepatic, 785
chorionic villus sampling (CVS), 3
chorioretinitis, 315
chromosome anomalies. *See* aneuploidy
chromosome microdeletion, 118–119*t*
chronic lung disease (CLD). *See*
    bronchopulmonary dysplasia (BPD)
circumcision, 107–108
  medication, 881
  skin care, 834
clavicular fracture, 70–71, 758
clitoris, examination, 97. *See also* disorders of
    sex development (DSD)
clotting, 538–539, 544
clubfoot, 761
coagulase-negative *staphylococcus* (CONS),
    638–640
cocaine, maternal use, 149
cognitive delay, follow-up care, 188–189
cold injury, stress, 178–179
congenital adrenal hyperplasia (CAH), 797,
    798*t*, 800*f*, 801–802
congenital anomalies
  breastfeeding, 265–266
  clubfoot, 761
  IDMs, 20
  major, minor, 111
  multiple pregnancy, 128–129
  scoliosis, 758–759
congestive heart failure, 472, 475–476*t*.
    See also cardiac disorders
conjoined twins, 125, 129
conjunctivitis, 652–653
convulsions, benign neonatal, 737

continuous positive airway pressure (CPAP), 377–378. *See also* intubation
MAS, 433
procedure, 858
RDS, 408–409
contraction stress test (CST), 7–8
Coppola syndrome, 738
corticosteroids, 423–424, 433
CP. *See* cerebral palsy
cranial nerve injury, 67
creatinine, serum, normal values, 360*f*
Creutzfeldt-Jakob disease (vCJD), 529
cromolyn, BPD, 424
cryoprecipitate (CRYO), 529
cryptorchidism, 804
bilateral, 804
CSF. *See* cerebrospinal fluid
CST. *See* contraction stress test
CVS. *See* chorionic villus sampling
cyanosis, 51, 53–54
differential diagnosis, 473–474*t*
heart disease, 471–472
cysteine, PN, 247
cystic adenomatoid malformation, 817
cytokines, EOS, 627–628
cytomegalovirus (CMV)
blood transfusion, 529
clinical disease, 590–591
diagnosis, 591–592
epidemiology, 588–590
hearing loss, 847–848
prevention, 593–594
treatment, 592–593

D

DDH. *See* developmental dislocation of the hip
Death
neonatal bereavement, 225
decision making. *See* ethical decision making
deformations, 112, 128. *See also* birth defects
dehydration management, 273
delivery, labor conditions, 75–76
dental problems, VLBW infants, 188
deoxyribonucleic acid. *See* DNA analysis, sequencing; DNA typing, zygosity
dermatology, 832
transient pustular melanosis neonatorum, 97–98
developmental dislocation of the hip (DDH), 759
developmental follow-up programs, 189–190
developmentally supportive care, 173–174
goals of, 172

IDMs, 17
introduction, 166
neurobehavioral organization, facilitation, 167–171*t*
pain, stress, 175–176
parent support, education, 176
practices, 174–175
self-regulating behavior, 172
stress responses, 166
supportive environment, 173–174
diabetes, pregnancy, 11. *See also* infants of diabetic mothers
classifications, 12*t*
complications, 13
definition, epidemiology, 11
diabetic control, 14
genetics, 22
gestational, management, 13–14
hyperglycemia, 294
hypertrophic cardiomyopathy, 517
labor, delivery, 14–16
outcome, 11
pathophysiology, 11–12
perinatal survival, 22
types 1, 2 management, 13
dialysis, AKI management, 365
diaper dermatitis, 836
diaphragmatic hernia, 814
diastematomyelia, 744. *See also* neural tube defects
diazepam, 148
diazoxide, hypoglycemia, 292
DIC. *See* disseminated intravascular coagulation
dietary supplements, oral, 257*t*
digoxin, tachycardias, 520, 522–523
direct hyperbilirubinemia. *See* hyperbilirubinemia
discharge, discharge planning
bereavement follow-up, 229
community provider communication, 215, 216–217*t*
comprehensive plan goals, 203
developmentally supportive care, 176
discharge readiness, 205–206
discharge screening, 206, 207–211*t*
family assessment, 203–204
family instruction sheets, 206, 212*f*, 213*f*
follow-up care, 215
home discharge alternatives, 215–218
newborns, 108–110
nutrition, 261–262
preparing home services, 214
preparing the family, 206–214
system assessment, 204–205
disinfectants, skin care, 834

disorders of sex development (DSD)
46,XX, 797, 798t, 800f, 801
46,XY, 802–805
causes of, 798t–799t
defined, nomenclature, 791, 792t
gonadal differentiation disorders, 805–806
males, undervirilized 46,XY, 802–805
newborn evaluation, 795–797, 796f, 800f
normal sexual development, 792–795,
793, 794, 794t
sex assignment, 791, 806–807
disruptions, defined, 111–112
disseminated intravascular coagulation
(DIC), 544
diuretics, 422–423, 521
dizygotic (DZ) twins, 124–125.
See also multiple births
DNA analysis, sequencing, 4–5
DNA, free fetal, 5
DNA typing, zygosity, 125–126
documentation of procedures, 851
drug use/abuse, maternal, 134
addicted infant management, 142–143f
diagnostic tests, 135–139
history diagnosis, 134–135
infant care, treatment, 139–140
infant disposition, 152–153
infant withdrawal, 136–138t, 141–149
introduction to, 134
narcotics, pregnancy exposure, 140–141
neonatal abstinence syndrome, 145–145f
non-narcotics, 149–151
psychotropic medications, 151–152
referral, 139
DTO. *See* neonatal opium solution
Duchenne-Erb palsy, 69–70
ductus arteriosus, 471
dystocia, fetal surgery, 809

E

early-onset sepsis (EOS)
antibiotics, 625, 626t
asymptomatic infant evaluation, 628–630
clinical presentation, 624–625
epidemiology, risk factors, 624, 633t
evaluation, 625
evaluation algorithm, 630–632, 631f
organisms causing, 632–637
treatment, 625–628, 626t
ears, 66, 100
Ebstein anomaly, 503–504, 503f
ecchymoses, 72
echocardiography, 474–476, 477–478t,
488–489. *See also* cardiac disorders
eclampsia, 39, 44
eclamptic seizures, 44. *See also* seizures

ECMO, 460. *See* extracorporeal membrane
oxygenation
cannulation, 458
edema
hydrops, 334–337
management, 273
nondependent, 40
pulmonary, 41
ELBW infants. *See* extremely low birth
weight (ELBW) infants
electrocardiogram (ECG), 479, 483–484t,
485t
electroencephalogram (EEG)
perinatal asphyxia, 719–720
seizures, 730–732, 731f
EMCO, saline priming, 457
emesis, 810, 819
nonbilious, 811
emollients, skin care, 834
emotional health, follow-up care, 189
emphysema, subcutaneous, 453
enalapril, cardiac disorders, 520
encephalocele, 743. *See also* neural tube
defects
encephalopathy. *See also* hypoxic-ischemic
encephalopathy; perinatal asphyxia
acute/chronic, bilirubin, 317
neonatal, 711, 714
endocrine diseases, breastfeeding, 266
end-of-life care
bereavement follow-up, 228–229
care coordination, 226–228
family-centered principles, 225–226
introduction to, 225
end-tidal carbon monoxide (ETCOc), 316
energy, nutrient recommendations, 240,
240t
enteral feeding, 248
minimal, 248
enteral nutrition
caloric-enhance feedings, 255
early feeding, 248
feeding methods, 257–258
indications for formula use, 256–257t
iron, 258
milk, formula compositions, 251–254t
nutrients, 258–259
oral dietary supplements, 257t
preterm infants, 248–250
specialized formulas, 255
term infants, 250
tube feeding, 250, 250t
Enterobacter, 642
Enterococci, 641
enterocolitis, infectious, 344

enteroviruses, 618–619
epidural hemorrhage (EH), 689
epilepsy, 737–738
epinephrine, neonatal resuscitation, 56
Epstein pearls, 100
erythema toxicum, 97, 836
Escherichia coli, 635–636
esophageal atresia (EA), 812–814
ETCOc. *See* end-tidal carbon monoxide
ethanol, maternal use, 149–150
ethical decision making
  background, 219–220
  developing a process for, 220–221
  premature infants, 222
  principles, 219
  withdrawing life-sustaining treatment,
    222–224, 226–228
ethics, committee, 224
ex utero intrapartum treatment (EXIT),
  455–456, 809. *See also* surgical
  emergencies
examination of newborn. *See* newborn
  examination
exchange transfusion, hyperbilirubinemia,
  322*f,* 329–332
EXIT. *See ex utero* intrapartum treatment
exstrophy, 823
extracellular fluid (ECF), 269, 270*f*
extracorporeal membrane oxygenation
  (ECMO)
  background, 454
  complications, 461
  indications, contraindications, 454–455
  management, 457–460
  MAS, 433
  membranes, 124–126
  neurodevelopment, 462
  outcomes, 455*t,* 461–462, 462*t*
  physiology, 456–457
  PPHN, 440
  support, special situations, 460–461
  survival, 461
extracranial hemorrhage, 64
extremely low birth weight (ELBW) infants,
  160–165. *See also* prematurity, follow-up
  care; prematurity, premature infants
  cardiovascular support, 163
  delivery room care, 158–160
  fluid, electrolyte management, 161–162,
    162*t,* 281–283
  hearing loss, 187
  hyperglycemia, 294
  infection, 163–164
  intensive care, 160–165
  introduction to, 154
  nutritional support, 164–165

parents' desires, 158
post-resuscitation care, 160
prenatal considerations, 154–158
respiratory support, 159–161
shock, 467
standardized care protocols, 154–156*t*
survival, 154–157, 160
extremities, newborn examination, 98
eyes, 66, 100

F

facial fracture, 65
facial nerve injury, 67–68
family
  decision making, 223, 226–228
  developmentally supportive care, 176
  end-of-life care, bereavement follow-up,
    225–226
  genetic disease history, 3–5
  keeping informed, 851
  prematurity, follow-up care, 190
  preparing for discharge, 206–214
Fanconi syndrome, 374
fat necrosis, subcutaneous, 73
fatty acid oxidation, 778–779, 779*t*
feeding. *See also* breastfeeding; nutrition
  developmentally supportive care, 174–175
  early enteral, 248
  gastronomy, 258
  hypoglycemia, 293
  newborn care, 107
  orogastric, 257–258
  tubal, 250, 250*t*
feet deformities, 760–761
females. *See also* disorders of sex development
  (DSD)
  newborn examination, 97
  virilized 46,XX, 797, 798*t,* 800*f,* 801–802
femoral fractures, 71
FENa. *See* fractional excretion of Na
fetal alcohol syndrome (FAS), 150
fetal assessment, 1. *See* prenatal diagnosis
fetal lung maturity (FLM), 406–407
fetal monitoring, intrapartum, 63
fetal surgery, 809. *See also* surgical emergencies
fetus
  cell analysis, 4
  characteristics, associated risks, 75
  disease diagnosis, 1–5
  electronic monitoring, 8–10
  goiter, 27
  growth discordance, 127
  hypothyroidism, hyperthyroidism, 26
FFP. *See* fresh frozen plasma
fiberoptic blankets, 327
FLM. *See* fetal lung maturity

Florinef, 802
fluconazole, 647–650
fluids, electrolytes 269–283
    AKI management, 365
    body water distribution, 269–270
    BPD, 421–422, 424
    CLD, 283
    ECF, 269, 270*f*
    ELBW infants, 161–162, 162*t*, 281–283
    hypernatremic disorders, 275
    hyponatremic disorders, 273–275, 274*t*
    isonatremic disorders, 273
    IWL, 269–270, 270*f*
    K balance disorders, 279–281
    management, 272, 272*t*
    metabolic acid-base disorders, 277–279,
        278*t*, 279*t*
    nutrition, 231–240, 243
    oliguria, 275–277, 276*t*
    RDS, 414–415
    status assessment, 271–272
folinic acid, 659, 737
follow-up care. *See* discharge, discharge
    planning; prematurity, follow-up care
formulas
    discharge planning, 261
    indications for use, 256–257*t*
    nutrition compositions, 251–254*t*
    preterm, 249
    specialized, 255
    term infants, 250
46,XX, 797, 798*t*, 800*f*, 801
46,XX testicular DSD, 806
46,XY, 802–805
46,XY complete gonadal dysgenesis
    (CGD), 806
    fosphenytoin, 722, 739–740, 740*t*
fractional excretion of Na (FENa), 271
fractures
    clavicular, 70–71, 758
    humeral, 71
    long bone, 71
    skull, facial, mandibular, 65
frozen plasma, 533–534
fructose intolerance, IEM, 784
fungal infections, 646
    Malassezia furfur, 650
    Mucocutaneous candidiasis, 647–648
    systemic candidiasis, 648–650
furosemide
    AKI management, 365
    cardiac disorders, 521

G

galactosemia, 267, 784
gastroesophageal reflux (GER), 259, 426

gastrointestinal effects, perinatal asphyxia,
    718, 723
gastronomy feedings, 258
gastroschisis, surgery, 822
GBS. *See* group B *Streptococcus*
G-CSD. *See* granulocyte-colony stimulating
    factor
genetic disease, family history, 3–5, 22
genetic problems, 111. *See* birth defects
genetic sex, 792
genitalia, 96–97, 793, 793*f*, 795. *See also*
    disorders of sex development (DSD)
genitourinary abnormalities, 822–823
gentian violet, 647
genu recurvatum, 760
GER. *See* gastroesophageal reflux
germinal matrix hemorrhage/intraventricular
    hemorrhage (GMH/IVH)
    clinical presentation, 695
    complications, pathogenesis, 694–695
    diagnosis, 695–697, 696*t*
    etiology, pathogenesis, 692–694, 693*t*
    management, prognosis, 697–698, 699*f*,
        700–702
gestational age (GA)
    assessment, 1
    Ballard examination, 76, 77*f*
    large for, 88–89
    mortality, 82*f*
    seizures, 741
    small for, 86–88
giant hairy nevi, 838
Gilbert syndrome, 306
glomerular filtration, 351, 351*t*
glucagon, hypoglycemia, 292–293
glucocorticoids, GMH/IVH prevention, 697
glucose
    blood, 15, 17–18
    hyperglycemia, 295
    infant nutrition, 241, 242*f*
    intolerance, 14
    rate calculator, hypoglycemia, 289*f*
    tolerance, VLBW infants, 282
glutamine, 247, 258
glycine encephalopathy, 737
glycosuria, renal conditions, 358
glycosylated hemoglobin, diabetes, 13
goiter, fetal/neonatal, 27
gonadal differentiation disorders,
    805–806
gonadal dysgenesis, mixed, 805–806
gonadal sex, 792, 793*f*
graft-*versus*-host disease, 331
    transfusion-associated, 533
gram-negative organisms, 634–635, 638,
    641–642

granulocyte-colony stimulating factor
(G-CSF), 644
granulocytes, 534–535
Graves' disease
fetal/neonatal goiter, 27
hyperthyroidism, 25–26
group B *Streptococcus* (GBS). *See also* early-
onset sepsis (EOS)
current status of, 634
epidemiology, risk factors, 624, 633, 633*t*
evaluation, treatment, 634–635
microbiology, pathogenesis, 632
prevention, 633–634
growth, intrauterine curves, 232–235*f*
growth failure, BPD, 426
growth restriction, multiple births, 131–132

H

H2 blockers, 342
hCG. *See* human chorionic gonadotropin
hearing, hearing loss, 846
BPD, 426
conductive, 846
defined, incidence, 846
ELBW infants, 187
etiology, 846–848
follow-up testing, 848–849, 849*t*
habilitation/treatment, 849–850
medical evaluation, 849
NICU graduates, 846–850, 849*t*
prognosis, 850
screening tests, 848
heart. *See* cardiac disorders
heart block, 525
HELLP syndrome, 41
hemangiomas, 31
strawberry, 837
hematemesis, 811–812
hematochezia, 811–812
hematuria, 358, 372-373, 373*t*
hemolysis, exchange transfusion, 331
hemolysis, microangiopathic, 41
hemolytic disease. *See also*
hyperbilirubinemia
ABO, 338–339
antigens involved in, 323*t*, 324–325*t*
bilirubin toxicity, 317–318
infants with, 319
isoimmune, 337–338
hemolytic transfusion reaction, 532
hemophilia, 539
hemorrhage. *See also* intracranial
hemorrhage; pulmonary hemorrhage
adrenal, 72
extracranial, 64
subgaleal, 99

hemorrhagic disease of the newborn (HDN),
544–545
heparin, 45, 555–557, 556*t*, 557*t*, 558*t*
low-molecular-weight (LMW), 556–557,
557*t*, 558*t*
hepatic injury, 71–72
hepatitis
B virus, 610–613
blood transfusions, 529, 530*t*
C virus, 613–614
E virus, 614–615
G virus, 615
introduction to, 610
vaccine doses, 612*t*
hepatocellular dysfunction, 41
hepatosplenomegaly, 315
hernia
BPD, 426
diaphragmatic, 814–816
inguinal, 824–825
herpes simplex virus (HSV)
clinical manifestations, 595–596
diagnosis, 596–597
epidemiology, 594–595
prevention, management, 597–599, 598*t*
transmission, 595
treatment, 597
herpes zoster virus. *See* varicella-zoster virus
heterotaxy syndrome, 507
high-frequency oscillatory ventilation
(HFOV), 161
high-frequency ventilation (HFV), 380–381
high-risk newborns, 63
Ballard examination, 76, 77*f*
cord blood banking, 89
defined, 74–76
GA, birth weight classification, 76, 77*f*
LGA, 88–89
postterm infants, 82–86
preterm birth, 78–82
SGA, IUGR infants, 86–88
Hirschsprung disease, 821
HLA. *See* human leukocyte antigen
home care, 214. *See also* discharge, discharge
planning
hospice care, 218
HPT axis. *See* hypothalamic-pituitary-
thyroid axis
HSV. *See* herpes simplex virus
HTLV I/II. *See* human T-lymphotropic
virus I/II
human chorionic gonadotropin (hCG),
24, 803–805
human immunodeficiency virus (HIV)
blood transfusions, 529, 530*t*
breastfeeding contraindications, 268

human immunodeficiency virus *(Continued)*
  clinical disease, 605–607
  defined, 603
  diagnosis, 607–608
  epidemiology, 603–604
  prevention, 609–610
  transmission, 604–605
  treatment, 608–609
human leukocyte antigen (HLA), 530, 532
human T-lymphotropic virus I/II
    (HTLV I/II), 529, 530*t*
humeral fractures, 71
humidity, skin care, 833
hydralazine, 520
hydrocele, 96
hydrocortisone
  CAH, 801
  hypoglycemia, 292
  replacement, shock, 467
hydrometrocolpos, 820
hydronephrosis, 361–362
hydrops, 334–337
hydrops fetalis, 769, 770*t*
hyperammonemia, 773, 774*f,* 779–782,
    780*f*
hyperbilirubinemia. *See also* bilirubin
  ABO hemolytic disease, 338–339
  background, 304–306
  bilirubin nomogram, 313*f*
  bilirubin toxicity, 317–318
  breastfeeding, 313–314
  causes of, 309–310*t*
  conjugated, direct, 332–334
  etiology diagnosis, 308*f*
  exchange transfusion, 322*f,* 329–332
  family history, 307–314
  follow-up, 311*t,* 312*f*
  hemolytic disease, antigens involved in,
    323*t,* 324–325*t*
  hydrops, 334–337
  isoimmune hemolytic disease, 337–338
  neurotoxicity, risk factors, 322*t*
  nonphysiologic, 307–317
  phototherapy, 314*f,* 325–329
  physiologic, 306–307
  serum bilirubin levels, 320–321*f*
  severe, risk factors, 311*t*
hypercalcemia
  definition, etiology, 300–301
  diagnosis, 301–302
  treatment, 302–303
hyperglycemia
  defined, 293
  diabetes, pregnancy, 11
  etiology, 293–295
  treatment, 295–296

hyperkalemia
  exchange transfusion, 331
  fluid, electrolyte management, 279–281,
    282*f*
  packed RBC, 533
  VLBW infants, 283
hyperlipidemia, 246
hypermagnesemia, 45, 303
hypernatremic disorders, 275, 281–282
hyperosmolar formula, 295
hyperoxia testing, 485–486
hypertension, hypertensive disorders
  BPD, 425
  categories, 39
  preeclampsia, 40, 44
  renal conditions, 366–367, 369–370*t,*
    371*t*
  risk factors, 40*t,* 44
hyperthermia, 62, 179, 184
hyperthyroidism
  hypercalcemia, 301
  maternal, 25–26
  neonatal, 26, 37–38
hypertriglyceridemia, 246
hyperviscosity, 572. *See also* polycythemia
hypocalcemia
  definition, pathophysiology, etiology,
    297–298
  diagnosis, 298–299
  exchange transfusion, 331
  IDMs, 20
  packed RBC, 532
  seizures, 736
  treatment, 299–300
hypoglycemia
  defined, 284–285
  diabetes, pregnancy, 11
  diagnosis, 288–290
  etiology, 286–288
  exchange transfusion, 331
  follow-up, evaluation, 293
  glucose rates, 289*f*
  hyperinsulinemic, 286–287
  IDMs, 17–19
  IEM, 771, 773*f,* 778-779, 779*t,* 786
  incidence, 284
  knowledge gaps, 286
  management, 290–293
  neonatal, 17
  operational threshold, 285
hypokalemia, 279
hypomagnesemia
  defined, treatment, 303
  exchange transfusion, 331
  IDMs, 21
  seizures, 736

hyponatremic disorders, 273–275, 274t, 283
hypoosmolar hyponatremia. *See*
    hyponatremic disorders
hypoplastic left heart syndrome, 495–498,
    496f
hypoplastic right heart syndrome,
    499–500, 500f
hypotension, 468, 488
hypothalamic-pituitary hypothyroidism, 30
hypothalamic-pituitary-thyroid (HPT) axis,
    24
hypothermia, therapeutic, 724–725
hypothyroidism
    central, 30
    hyperbilirubinemia, 315
    maternal, 26–27
    neonatal, 26
hypotonia, 767-768, 783
hypovolemic shock, 463–464. *See also* shock
hypoxia
    hypoxic insult, NEC, 341
    respiratory failure, 201
hypoxic-ischemic encephalopathy (HIE).
    See also perinatal asphyxia
    defined, 711–712
    PVL, 704
    Sarnat stages, 716t–717t
    seizures, 732–734, 734t

I

ICH. *See* intracranial hemorrhage
ICROP. *See* International Classification of
    Retinopathy of Prematurity
IDMs. *See* infants of diabetic mothers
immunizations, prematurity, 186
immunoglobulin, hyperimmune, 536
immunoglobulin, intravenous (IVIG)
    EOS, 627
    LOS prevention, 643–645
    newborn use, 535–536
    parvovirus treatment, 601–602
inborn errors of metabolism (IEM), 767
    clinical presentation, 767-769
    hyperammonemia, 779–782, 780f
    hypoglycemia, 778-779, 779t
    hypotonia, 783
    infant management, 785–786
    introduction to, 767
    liver dysfunction, 783-785
    metabolic acidosis, 770–771, 772f,
        774-778, 775f
    neonate evaluation, 770–774, 771t
    postmortem diagnosis, 787
    routine newborn screening, 787,
        788–789t
    seizures, 736–737, 767, 782-783

infantile epileptic encephalopathy, 737
infants of diabetic mothers (IDMs).
    See also diabetes, pregnancy
    evaluation of, 16–17
    frequent problems, 20–22
    hypoglycemia, 17–19
    malformations, 20
    respiratory distress, 19–20
infections. *See also* perinatal infections
    blood transfusion, 529, 530f
    BPD, 418, 425–426
    ELBW infants, 163–164
    exchange transfusion, 331
    skin, 651–652, 839
infections, bacterial. *See* bacterial infections
infections, congenital
    CMV, 588–594
    CNS, 735
    defined, 588
    enteroviruses, 618–619
    hepatitis, 610–615
    HIV, 603–610
    parvovirus, 599–603
    rubella, 619–622
    V-ZV, 615–618
infections, fungal. *See* fungal infections
infections, viral. *See* viral infections
infectious enterocolitis, 344
injuries, soft tissue, 72–73
inotropes, 466, 487
insensible water loss (IWL), 269–270, 270f
inspissated bile syndrome, 333
insulin
    AKI management, 365
    hyperkalemia, 280–281
    infusions, hyperglycemia, 295–296
    lispro, hyperglycemia, 296
    PN, 247
    requirements, pregnancy, 13
intersex. *See* disorders of sex development
intestinal obstructions, surgery, 810,
    817–821
intestinal perforation (IP), 344
intra-abdominal injuries, 71–72
intracranial hemorrhage (ICH), 686
    EH, 689
    GMH/IVH, 692–702, 693, 696, 699
    intraparenchymal hemorrhage, 690–692
    introduction to, 686–687, 687
    IPH, 690–692
    PVL, 703–706
    SAH, 689–690
    SDH, 686–689
    seizure, 734–735, 734t
intrauterine fetal demise (IUFD),
    127–128

intrauterine growth curves, 232–235f
intrauterine growth restriction (IUGR)
  causes, diagnosis, 5–6
  multiple pregnancy, 127
  preeclampsia, 41, 45
  risks, management, 86–88
intravenous extravasations, 835
intravenous therapy, 853
intubation
  medication, 880, 880–881
  neonatal resuscitation, 55
  PPHN, 439
  procedure, 856–858, 857
inulin clearance GFR, 360t
iodine
  clearance increase, 24
  excess, 31
  hyperthyroidism treatment, 25–26
  maternal medication, breastfeeding, 38
  preparation, 37
  radioactive, 25–26
  worldwide deficiency, 31
iron, nutrition, 258
irradiation, blood transfusions, 529–530
isoimmune hemolysis, 4
isoimmune hemolytic disease, 337–338
isonatremic disorders, 273
isovaleric acidemia, 776

J

jaundice, 21, 98, 313–314.
    See also hyperbilirubinemia
joints, examination, 98

K

kangaroo care, 175
Kayexalate, 281, 365
kernicterus, 317
ketoacidosis, 13
kidneys. See also renal conditions
  acute kidney injury (AKI), 362–366,
      363–364t
  congenital anomalies, 366
  cystic disease, 376
  perinatal asphyxia, 718
Klumpke palsy, 70

L

labor, delivery conditions, 75–76
lacerations, 63, 72
lactoferrin, 644
lamellar bodies, 407
large for gestational age (LGA), 88–89
laryngeal web, 816
laryngotracheal clefts, 816

latent syphilis, 664. See also syphilis
late-preterm infants. See prematurity,
    premature infants
LCPUFAs. See long-chain polyunsaturated
    fatty acids
lecithin-sphingomyelin (L/S) ratio, 15t,
    406–407
left-to-right shunt lesions, 509–513
leukoreduction, blood transfusions,
    529–530
Lewis antigen, 338
LFTs. See liver function tests
LGA. See large for gestational age
life-sustaining treatment, withdrawing/
    withholding, 222–224, 226–228
lipids, nutrition, 243
lipomeningocele, 744. See also neural tube
    defects
Listeria monocytogenes, 636–637
liver
  dysfunction, IEM, 768, 783–785
  dysfunction, newborn bleeding, 539
  perinatal asphyxia, 718
liver function tests (LFTs), 773
lobar emphysema, 817
long-chain polyunsaturated fatty acids
    (LCPUFAs), 258–259
lorazepam, 148–149
LOS. See late-onset sepsis
L/S ratio. See lecithin-sphingomyelin ratio
lumbar puncture, 853
lung maturity, 6
lungs. See pulmonary disorders
Lyme disease, 683
lymph nodes, examination, 98
lymphatic vessels disorders, 837

M

macrosomia
  in high-risk newborns, 75
  IDMs, 21
  prenatal diagnosis, 6
macular hemangioma, 837
magnesium disorders, 303
magnesium sulfate, 43
magnetic resonance angiography (MRA),
    122
magnetic resonance spectroscopy (MRS),
    122
malaria, blood transfusions, 529
Malassezia furfur, 650
malformations, 111–112. See also birth
    defects
  major, 111
  minor, 111
malpractice insurance coverage, 194

mandibular fractures, 65
MAP. *See* mean airway pressure
maple syrup urine disease, 774, 775
marijuana, maternal use, 150
MAS. *See* meconium aspiration syndrome
maturation phase, 834
MDROs. *See* multiply drug-resistant organisms
mean airway pressure (MAP), 383–384
mechanical ventilation
  adjuncts to, 391
  air leak, 390, 392
  apnea, 391
  blood gas effects, 382–385
  BPD, 389–391, 419–420
  complications, sequelae, 391–392
  CPAP, 377–378
  disease states, 385–391, 386*t*
  HFV, 380–381
  introduction to, 377
  MAP, 383–384
  MAS, 389, 433
  medication, 881
  negative pressure, 381
  oxygenation, 382, 382*t*, 383*f*
  PPHN, 439
  pressure-limited, time-cycled, continuous flow, 378
  pulmonary mechanics, 385, 385*t*
  RDS, 385–389, 412–414
  respiration support indications, 381
  synchronized, patient triggered, 378–379
  volume-cycled ventilators, 379–380
meconium aspiration syndrome (MAS), 433
  cause, incidence, 429
  management, 431–434
  mechanical ventilation, 389
  medications, 433
  neonatal resuscitation, 60
  pathophysiology, 429–430, 430*f*
  prevention, 430–431
meconium passing, 811, 819–821
meconium peritonitis, 808
meconium-stained amniotic fluid (MSAF). *See* meconium aspiration syndrome
medications, 104–105, 887
meningitis, 624, 626*t*. *See also* early-onset sepsis; late-onset sepsis
meningocele, 744. *See also* neural tube defects
metabolic bone disease. *See* osteopenia
metabolism. *See also* inborn errors of metabolism
  acute disorders, seizure management, 735–736, 735*t*
  testing, birth defects, 122
  testing, PN, 246, 246*t*

metatarsus adductus (MTA), 760
methadone, 140–141, 148
methamphetamine, maternal use, 150
Methicillin-resistant *Staphylococcus aureus* (MRSA), 640
methylmalonic acidemia, 777
miconazole, 647
microcephaly, 315
microphallus, 804
microvascular disease, 15
middle cerebral artery, assessment, 8
milia, 97, 836
milk. *See also* breastfeeding
  care, handling of, 267
  discharge planning, 261
  fortified, 248–249
  jaundice, 314
  nutrition compositions, 251–254*t*
  term infants, 250
milrinone, cardiac disorders, 519
minerals, nutrition, 243–245
Mongolian spots. *See* dermal melanosis
monochorionic diamniotic, 124–125
monochorionic monoamniotic, 124–125
monozygotic (MZ) twins, 124–125.
  See also multiple births
morbidity, multiple births, 131–132
morphine, 147–148
motor system, examination, 101
mouth, examination, 100
MRA. *See* magnetic resonance angiography
MRI
  brain, 122
MRS. *See* magnetic resonance spectroscopy
MRSA. *See* Methicillin-resistant *Staphylococcus aureus*
MSAF (meconium-stained amniotic fluid). *See* meconium aspiration syndrome
MSAFP. *See* maternal serum alpha-fetoprotein
MTA. *See* metatarsus adductus
Mucocutaneous candidiasis, 647–648
mucous plug syndrome, 820–821
mucus/salivation, postnatal surgical disorders, 810
multiple births, 125, 129
  classification, 124
  diagnosis, 125–126
  epidemiology, 124–125
  etiology, 125
  fetal, neonatal complications, 127–131
  long-term morbidity, 131–132
  maternal complications, 126–127
  outcomes, 131–133
multiply drug-resistant organisms (MDROs), 643

multizygous pregnancy. *See* dizygotic (DZ) twins
muscle relaxation, mechanical ventilation, 391
Mycobacterium tuberculosis. See tuberculosis
myelocystocele, 744. *See also* neural tube defects
myelomeningocele, 743. *See also* neural tube defects
myocardial dysfunction
   IDMs, 21–22
   PPHN, 437
   transient, 517
myocarditis, 513
myoclonic epilepsy, 737
myoclonic seizures, 730. *See also* seizures
MZ. *See* monozygotic twins

N

NAIT. *See* neonatal alloimmune thrombocytopenia
narcotics
   addicted infant management, 142–143f
   infant withdrawal, 141–149
   neonatal abstinence syndrome, 145–145f
   pregnancy exposure, 140–141
nasogastric feedings, 257–258
neck, 63–67, 100
necrotizing enterocolitis (NEC)
   diagnosis, 342–344
   epidemiology, 340–341
   management, 345–348, 345t
   nutrition, 260
   pathogenesis, 341–342
   prevention, 349
   prognosis, 348–349
negative pressure, 381
Neisseria gonorrhoeae, 652–653
neonatal abstinence syndrome, 145–145f
neonatal alloimmune thrombocytopenia (NAIT), 581–583
neonatal morphine solution (NMS), 146
neonatal opium solution (NOS), 146–147
neonatal resuscitation. *See* resuscitation, neonatal
Neonatal Skin Condition Score (NSCS), 832, 832t
nephrocalcinosis, 375, 426
neural tube defects
   definition, pathology, 743–745
   diagnosis, 745
   evaluation, 745–749, 747–748t
   management, 749–752
   prevention, 745
   prognosis, 752–755
   types of, 743–744
   in utero repair, 749–750

neuroblastoma, 824
neurodevelopmental outcomes
   developmentally supportive care, 167–171t
   pain, stress management, 871
   prematurity, follow-up care, 188–189
neurologic deterioration, IEM, 767
neurologic examination, 100–101
neuromotor problems, 188
neurosyphilis, 664. *See also* syphilis
neutral thermal environment, 179, 180–182t
nevi, junctional, 838
nevus
   flammeus, 837
   simplex, 97, 837
newborn care
   assessments, 106–107
   circumcision, 107–108
   discharge, 108–110
   family, social issues, 107
   feedings, 107
   follow-up, 110
   nursery admission, 103
   routine care, 104
   routine medications, 104–105
   screening, 105–106
   skin care, 831–839
   transitional care, 103–104
newborn examination
   abdomen, 96
   birth defects, 115–116
   cardiorespiratory system, 94–95
   extremities, joints, spine, 98–99
   family history, 91, 92–93t
   general examination, 91
   genitalia, rectum, 96–97
   head, 99–100
   neurologic, 100–101
   screening, IEM, 787, 788–789t
   skin, 97–98
   thorax, 95–96
   vital signs, measurements, 91–94
NICU. *See* neonatal intensive care unit
nitric oxide, 161
   inhaled, 422–423, 439–440
nitroglycerine, 519–520
NMS. *See* neonatal morphine solution
nonstress test (NST), 6–7
NOS. *See* neonatal opium solution
nose, 65–66, 100
NSCS. *See* Neonatal Skin Condition Score
NST. *See* nonstress test
nuchal lucency, 2, 126
nursery admission, 103
nutrition, 230–262
   BPD, 260–261, 424

discharge planning, 261–262
ELBW infants, 164–165
enteral, 248–259
GER, 259
growth, 230–231, 232–235f
NEC, 260
oral dietary supplements, 257t
parenteral, 240–247
RDS, 414–415
recommendations, 231–240, 236–239t
nystatin, 647

O

octreotide, hypoglycemia, 292
ocular. *See* eyes
Ohtahara syndrome, 738
OI. *See* oxygenation index
oligohydramnios, 41, 808
oliguria, 41, 275–277, 276t
omphalitis, 652
omphalocele, 821–822
operational threshold, hypoglycemia, 285
ophthalmia neonatorum. *See* conjunctivitis
ophthalmologic care, ELBW infants, 187
opioids, 881–884
organic aciduria, 776
orogastric feedings, 257–258
orthopaedic problems, 757
    congenital, infantile scoliosis, 758–759
    DDH, 759–760
    feet deformities, 760–761
    fractured clavicle, 758
    genu recurvatum, 760
    polydactyly, 758
    torticollis, 757–758
osteomyelitis, 655
osteopenia
    defined, etiology, 762–763
    diagnosis, 763–764
    PN, 246
    treatment, 764–766
ovotesticular DSD, 805
oxygen
    BPD, 420, 421f
    noninvasive monitoring, 394–395
    oxygenation, 382, 382t, 383f
    PPHN, 439
    RDS, 408
    therapy, MAS, 432
    use, monitoring, 393–395
oxygenation index (OI), 454

P

PACs. *See* premature atrial contractions
pain, stress, 871
    assessment, 874–875, 874t
    background, 870–869
    control, 851
    decision matrix, procedure intensity, 875, 876–877t
    developmentally supportive care, 175–176
    evaluation, 873–875
    management, 875–879
    medical, developmental outcomes, 871
    pharmacologic management, 879–884
    physiologic responses to, 870
    postoperative, 881–882, 883f
    principles of, 871–873
    procedural pain algorithm, 875, 878f
pancreas, annular, 820
pancreatic lesions, 294
paregoric, 147
parenteral nutrition (PN), 240–247
parents. *See* family
parvovirus
    clinical manifestations, 600–601
    defined, 599
    diagnosis, 601
    epidemiology, 600
    prevention, 602–603
    transmission, 600
    treatment, 601–602
patent ductus arteriosus (PDA)
    BPD, 418
    ELBW infants, 163
    left-to-right shunt lesions, 509–510
    pulmonary hemorrhage, 444
    RDS, 415–416, 420
    shock, 468
Pavlik harness, 759–760
PCP. *See* phencyclidine
PDA. *See* patent ductus arteriosus
pediatric nursing homes, rehabilitation hospitals, 215
PEEP. *See* positive end-expiratory pressure
Pendred syndrome, 30
penis, 96. *See also* disorders of sex development (DSD)
percutaneous umbilical blood sampling (PUBS), 4–5
perinatal asphyxia
    brain imaging, 719
    defined, 711–712
    diagnosis, 714–715
    EEG, 719–720
    etiology, 712–713
    incidence, 712
    laboratory evaluation, 718–719
    multiorgan dysfunction, 717–718
    neurologic signs, 715–717
    neuroprotective strategies, 723–725
    outcome, 725–726

perinatal asphyxia *(Continued)*
  pathologic findings, 720
  pathophysiology, 713–714
  Sarnat stages, 716–717t
  seizures, 715–717, 722, 726, 732–734
  treatment, 720–723
perinatal depression, 467, 711
perinatal infections. *See also* infections
  CMV, 588–594
  defined, 588
  hepatitis, 610–615
  HIV, 603–610
  HSV, 594–599
  V-ZV, 615–618
periventricular hemorrhagic infarction
    (PVHI), 694. *See also* germinal matrix
    hemorrhage/intraventricular hemorrhage
periventricular leukomalacia (PVL)
  clinical presentation, diagnosis, 704–705
  etiology, pathogenesis, 703–704
  management, 705–706
  prognosis, 706
peroxisomal disorders, IEM, 783
persistent pulmonary hypertension of the
    newborn (PPHN)
  defined, 435
  diagnosis, 437–438
  epidemiologic associations, 435–436
  management, 438–442
  MAS, 434
  multiple births, 131
  pathology, pathophysiology, 436–437
  postneonatal outcomes, 442
petechiae, 72, 315
PG. *See* phosphatidylglycerol
PGE₁, cardiac disorders, 517, 518t
pharyngeal injury, 67
phencyclidine (PCP), 150–151
phenobarbital
  hyperbilirubinemia, 332
  infant narcotic withdrawal, 147–148
  perinatal asphyxia, 722
  seizure treatment, 739
phenytoin, 722, 739
PHH (posthemorrhagic hydrocephalus).
    See posthemorrhagic ventricular dilation
phosphatidylglycerol (PG), 407
phosphodiesterase inhibitors, 519
phosphorus, 352–353, 782
photoisomerization, 326
photo-oxidation, 326
phototherapy
  guidelines, hyperbilirubinemia, 314f
  hyperbilirubinemia, 325–326
  indications for, 326
  photochemical reactions, 326

side effects of, 328–329
  technique of, 326–328
phrenic nerve injury, 69
physical examination of newborn, 91
PIE. *See* pulmonary interstitial edema
piebaldism, 838
PIH. *See* pregnancy-induced hypertension
placenta
  abruption, 126
  aromatase deficiency, 802
  multiple births, 124–125
  pathological examination, 126
  polycythemia, 572–574
  thyroid disorders, 24–25
plasma
  fresh frozen, 533–534, 543
  frozen, 533–534
  levels, IEM, 773–774
  thawed, 533–534
plastic leaching, 851
platelet activating factor (PAF), 342
platelets, 534, 539, 584–585, 585t
PN. *See* parenteral nutrition
pneumomediastinum, 451
pneumonia
  diagnosis, 653–654
  EOS, 625
  nosocomial, 654
  ventilator-associated, 654
pneumopericardium, 451–452
pneumoperitoneum, 452, 810
pneumothorax air leak, 447–450
  needle aspiration, 447–448
polycystic kidney
  autosomal recessive polycystic kidney
    disease (ARPKD), 376
polycythemia, 572
  causes, 572–574
  clinical findings, 574
  defined, 572
  diagnosis, 575
  hypoglycemia, 287
  IDMs, 21
  incidence, 572
  management, 575–576
  outcome, 576
  PPHN, 442
  screening, 574–575
polydactyly, 758
polyhydramnios, 13, 808
portal vein thrombosis (PVT), 552
port-wine stain. *See* nevus
positive end-expiratory pressure (PEEP),
    445
posthemorrhagic hydrocephalus (PHH).
    See posthemorrhagic ventricular dilation

posthemorrhagic ventricular dilation
(PVD), 694–695, 699f. *See also*
germinal matrix hemorrhage/
intraventricular hemorrhage
postmaturity syndrome, 85
postterm infants, 82–86
potassium, 279–281, 352
PPHN. *See* persistent pulmonary
hypertension of the newborn
precautions, procedures, 851
prednisone, 37, 659
preeclampsia, 41–46
chronic hypertension risk, 44
delivery, 41
diagnosis, 40–41
etiologies, 39–40
hypertensive disorder categories, 39
incidence, epidemiology, 39
innovations, treatments, 45
management, 41–44
multiple gestations, 127
newborn implications, 45
recurrence risk, 44
pregnancy-induced hypertension (PIH), 127
preimplantation genetic diagnosis (PGD), 5
premature atrial contractions (PACs), 525,
526f
premature ventricular contractions (PVCs),
525–526, 527f
prematurity, follow-up care
cognitive delay, 188–189
dental problems, 188
emotional, behavioral health, 189
growth, 186–187
immunizations, 186
introduction to, 185
neuromotor problems, 188
parent function, support, 190
programs, 189–190
respiratory issues, 185–186
sensory issues, 187
prematurity, premature infants.
See also extremely low birth weight
(ELBW) infants
anemia, 563–564, 564t, 570
bilirubin, 318, 321f
BPD, 426
breastfeeding, 266
discharge, late-preterm infants, 109–110
discharge readiness, 205–206
enteral nutrition, 248–250
ethical decision making, 222
etiology, 78
fluid, electrolyte management, 272, 272f
hyperbilirubinemia, 315, 325
hypocalcemia, 297

incidence of, 78
management of, 79–80
multiple births, 126–127, 131–132
NEC, 340
neonatal resuscitation, 61
problems, 78–79
problems, long-term, 81–82, 83f, 84f
serum creatinine values, 360f
shock, 467–468
survival of, 80, 81f, 82f
temperature maintenance, 178, 183
urine/renal values, 359t
prenatal diagnosis
antepartum tests, 6–8
fetal disease, 1–5
fetal size, growth-rate, 5–6
fetal well-being, 6–10
GA assessment, 1
genetic disease, 3–5
intrapartum assessment, 8–10
IUGR, 5–6
lung maturity, 6
macrosomia, 6
maternal serum analysis screening, 1–3
prerenal azotemia, 362
pressure-limited, time-cycled, continuous
flow, 378
preterm labor, spontaneous, 14
prethreshold ROP, 843. *See also* retinopathy
of prematurity
primary syphilis, 664. *See also* syphilis
probiotics, 349, 644
procedures, 851–869
propionic acidemia, 776–777
propranolol, 37, 523
proteinuria, 40–41, 372
pseudohermaphroditism. *See* disorders of sex
development
pseudohypoparathyroidism, 298
Pseudomonas aeruginosa, 641–642
psychotropic medications, maternal use,
151–152
PUBS. *See* percutaneous umbilical blood
sampling
pulmonary air leak. *See* air leak
pulmonary atresia, 499–500, 500f
pulmonary disorders
lung biopsy, ECMO, 460
lung injury, BPD, 417–418
perinatal asphyxia, 718
prenatal diagnosis, 6
pulmonary hemorrhage, 443–445
pulmonary hypertension, 201, 425
pulmonary hypoplasia, 437
pulmonary interstitial edema (PIE),
450–451

pulmonary stenosis, 498–499, 499*f*
pulmonary vascular resistance, 471
pulmonary vasospasm, 437
pulmonary veins, 507, 508*f*
pulse oximetry, 94, 394
purpura fulminans, 548
pustulosis, 651–652
PVCs. *See* premature ventricular contractions
PVD. *See* posthemorrhagic ventricular
 dilation
PVHI. *See* periventricular hemorrhagic
 infarction
PVL. *See* periventricular leukomalacia
pyridoxine dependency, 737
pyrimethamine, 659
pyruvate metabolism defects, 777–778

R

radioactive iodine, 25–26
radionuclide scintigraphy, 361
RDS. *See* respiratory distress syndrome
rectum examination, 96–97
recurrent laryngeal nerve injury, 68
red blood cells (RBCs)
 diminished production, anemia, 566
 hemoglobin, bilirubin, 304
 packed, 530–533
refractive errors, ELBW infants, 187
renal blood flow (RBF), 350–351
renal conditions, 350–376
 abdominal masses, 354*t*
 AKI, 362–366, 363–364*t*
 ARPKD, 376
 assessment, 353–361
 blood pressure, 367–368, 367*t*, 368*t*,
  369–370*t*, 371*t*
 common problems, 361–376
 congenital syndromes, 355–358*t*
 embryogenesis, functional development,
  350–353
 hematuria, 372–373, 373*t*
 inulin clearance GFR, 361*t*
 normal serum creatinine values, 360*f*
 normal values, 359*t*
 perfusion, EMCO, 457
 proteinuria, 372
 surgical emergencies, 822–823
 tubular disorders, 374–375
 ultrasonography, 361–362
 UTI, 374
 vascular thrombosis, 368–372
renal tubular acidosis (RTA), 374–375
renal vein thrombosis (RVT), 22, 547, 552
reperfusion, asphyxia, 714
respiration
 apnea pathogenesis, 398

failure, EMCO, 454
newborn examination, 94
prematurity, follow-up care, 185–186
support, ELBW infants, 159–161
support, indications, 381
system distress, IDMs, 19–20
respiratory chain defects, 783
respiratory distress syndrome (RDS)
 acute complications, 415–416
 CPAP, 408–409
 diabetes, pregnancy, 15*t*, 16*t*
 identification, 406–407
 introduction to, 406
 lesions, surgical emergencies, 812–817
 long-term complications, 416
 mechanical ventilation, 385–389,
  412–414
 oxygen, 408
 postnatal surgical disorders, 810
 supportive therapy, 414–415
 surfactant replacement, 409–412, 411*t*
 transport, 201
respiratory syncytial virus (RSV), 185–186,
 622–623
resuscitation, neonatal, 47
 air leak, 60–61
 apgar scores, 52*t*, 61
 delivery, 50–59
 ELBW infants, 157–160
 evolving practices, 62
 general principles, 47–48
 meconium aspiration, 60
 medication, 55–59, 57–58*t*
 prematurity, 61
 preparation, 48–50
 shock, 60
 TTTS, 131
 withdrawing/withholding, 62
retinopathy of prematurity (ROP), 840
 aggressive posterior, 843
 BPD, 426
 classification, definitions, 840–843
 diagnosis, 840
 ICROP, 841, 842*f*
 pathogenesis, 840
 prevention, 844
 prognosis, 844
 treatment, 843–845
Rhesus D hemolytic disease, 337–338
rickets, VLBW infants, 186–187
Robin anomaly, 816
ROP. *See* retinopathy of prematurity
RSV. *See* respiratory syncytial virus
RTA. *See* renal tubular acidosis
rubella, 619–622
RVT. *See* renal vein thrombosis

S

sacral agenesis/dysgenesis, 744.
  See also neural tube defects
"safety pause," 851
SAH. *See* subarachnoid hemorrhage
sarcoma botryoides, 824
Sarnat stages of HIE, 716–717*t*
saturated phosphatidylcholine level, 15*t*
scaphoid abdomen, 810
SCM injury. *See* sternocleidomastoid injury
scoliosis, 758–759
  infantile, 758–759
screening, newborn care, 105–106
scrotal swelling, 825–826
scrotum examination, 96
SDH. *See* subdural hemorrhage
sebaceous hyperplasia, 97, 836
security of newborns, 103
seizures
  asphyxia, 715–717, 722, 726, 732–734
  diagnosis, 729–732, 731*f*
  drug doses, 740*t*
  eclamptic, 44
  etiology, 732–738, 734*t*
  IEM, 767, 782–783
  investigations, 738
  prognosis, 741–742
  treatment, 738–740
seizures clonic, focal, 729
seizures tonic, focal, 730
selective serotonin reuptake inhibitors
  (SSRIs), 151–152
sensorineural loss, 846. *See also* hearing,
  hearing loss
sepsis
  hyperglycemia, 294
  NEC, 343
  PN, 247
  skin infection, 651
sepsis, late-onset
  defined, 637–638
  epidemiology, risk factors, 638, 639*t*
  microbiology, 638–642
  prevention, 643–645
  symptoms, evaluation, 642
  treatment, 643
septic arthritis, 655
septic shock, 468. *See also* shock
sex assignment, 791, 806–807.
    See also disorders of sex development
sexual development, 792–795, 793*f*,
    794*f*, 794*t*. *See also* disorders of sex
    development
SGA. *See* small for gestational age
shingles. *See* varicella-zoster virus

shock
  clinical scenarios, management, 467–468
  defined, 463
  diagnosis, 464–465
  distributive, 463
  etiology, 463–464
  investigations, 465
  neonatal resuscitation, 60
  obstructive, 464
  treatment, 465–467
SIDS. *See* sudden infant death syndrome
single ventricles, complex, 507–508
sinus bradycardia, tachycardia, 524
skin care
  anatomy, 831
  common lesions, 836
  developmental abnormalities, 838
  dryness, newborn examination, 97
  infections, 651–652, 839
  intravenous extravasations, infiltration, 835
  introduction to, 831
  newborn examination, 97–98
  pigmentation abnormalities, 837–838
  practices, 831–834
  scaling disorders, 838–839
  vascular abnormalities, 836–837
  vesicobullous eruptions, 839
  wounds, 834–835
skull fracture, 65
sleep problems, follow-up care, 189
small for gestational age (SGA), 86–88, 315
small left colon syndrome, 22
smoking, SIDS, 402
social development, follow-up care, 189
sodium
  bicarbonate, AKI management, 365
  FENa, 271
  handling, 351–352
spine, 68–69, 98–99
spiramycin, 658
splenic injury, 72
SSRIs. *See* selective serotonin reuptake
    inhibitors
Staphylococcus aureus, 640
state system examination, 101
sternocleidomastoid injury, 66–67
steroids, CAH, 801, 801*f*
strabismus, ELBW infants, 187
subarachnoid hemorrhage (SAH), 689–690
subdural hemorrhage (SDH), 685–689
subgaleal hematoma, 64–65
subgaleal hemorrhage, 99
sucking blisters, 98
sudden infant death syndrome (SIDS),
    401–402
sulfadiazine, 659

sulfonylureas, hyperglycemia, 296
supraventricular tachycardia (SVT), 521–524
surface area formula, 801
surfactant(s)
  MAS, 433
  replacement, BPD, 420
  replacement, RDS, 409–412, 411*t*
  therapy, ELBW infants, 161
  therapy, pulmonary hemorrhage, 444–445
surgical emergencies, 809
  abdominal masses, 824
  appendicitis, 821
  fetus, surgical conditions, 808–809
  gastroschisis, 822
  inguinal hernia, 824–825
  intraoperative management, 828–829
  lesions, intestinal obstruction, 817–821
  lesions, respiratory distress, 812–817
  omphalocele, 821–822
  postnatal disorders, 810–812
  preoperative management, 827–828
  renal disorders, 822–823
  scrotal swelling, 825–826
  tests, 826–827
  tumors, 823–824
SVT. *See* supraventricular tachycardia
sympathomimetic amine infusions,
    517–518, 518*t*
syphilis, 664
  blood transfusions, 529, 530*t*
  congenital, 664–665
  diagnosis, 665–667
  epidemiology, 665
  evaluation, treatment, 668–670
  follow-up, 670
  infection control, 671
  maternal screening, treatment, 667–668
  pathophysiology, 664–665
  tertiary, 664
systemic hypertension, 425

T

tachycardia
  emergency treatment, 527
  narrow QRS complex, 521–524, 522*f*
  sinus, 524
  transient fetal, 44
  ventricular, 524
  wide-complex, 524
TB. *See* tuberculosis
TBG. *See* thyroxine-binding globulin
TcB. *See* transcutaneous bilirubin
TDD. *See* total digitalizing dose
TEF. *See* tracheoesophageal fistula
temperature
  conduction, temperature control, 179

control method hazards, 184
  heat loss, 179
  heat production, 178
  maintenance, 178–179
  neutral thermal environments, 179,
    180–182*t*
  newborn examination, 91
  preventing heat loss, 179–183
teratogens, 113–114*t*
teratomas, 823–824
term infants
  apnea, 397
  bilirubin, 318, 320*f*
  breastfeeding, 263
  enteral nutrition, 250
  fluid, electrolyte management, 272
  hyperbilirubinemia, 319–325
  serum creatinine values, 360*f*, 360*t*
  urine/renal values, 359*t*
testes, 96, 802. *See also* disorders of sex
    development
tetanus, neonatal, 647
tetralogy of Fallot, 502–503, 502*f*
threshold ROP, 843. *See also* retinopathy of
    prematurity
thrombin, 546
thrombocytopenia, 578
  early onset, 578–580, 579*f*
  immune, 581–584
  introduction to, 578
  late onset, 580–581, 581*f*
  platelet transfusions, 584–585, 585*t*
thromboembolic disorders, venous, 548–550
thrombolysis, 557–560, 560*t*
thrombophilias, acquired. *See* acquired
    thrombophilias
thrombophilias, inherited, 547–548
thromboses, 546
  aortic, major arterial, 550–552
  central catheter, 560–561, 561*t*
  cerebral sinovenous, 552–553
  IDMs, 22
  PVT, 552
  venous thromboembolic disorders,
    548–550
thrombosis, neonatal, 546
  arterial, 550–552
  catheter, 560–561, 561*t*
  diagnosis, 553
  epidemiology, risk factors, 547–548
  management, 553–561
  physiology, 546
  specific clinical conditions, 548–553
thyroid, thyroid disorders, 24
  antithyroid drugs, 25, 31
  congenital hypothyroidism, 28–37

diagnosis, 34–36
dysgenesis, 28
embryogenesis, 27–28
fetal/neonatal goiter, 27
hormone reference ranges, 29–30*t*
hypothyroxinemia, 31–34
maternal hyperthyroidism, 25–26
maternal hypothyroidism, 26–27
maternal medications, breastfeeding, 38
neonatal hyperthyroidism, 37–38
newborn screening follow-up, 35*f*
permanent, causes of, 28–30
physiology, fetus/newborn, 27–28
physiology, pregnancy, 24–25
prognosis, 36–37
test, imaging interpretation, 32–33*t*
thyroidectomy, 25
transient, causes of, 31
treatment, monitoring, 36
thyroiditis
autoimmune, 26
thyroid-stimulating hormone (TSH), 24–38
thyroxine, 36, 38
thyroxine-binding globulin (TBG), 24
tidal volume, measuring, 396
"time out," 851
tobacco, maternal use, 150
torticollis, 757
total digitalizing dose (TDD), 520
toxoplasmosis, 655
epidemiology, 656
maternal/fetal infection, 657–659
neonatal infection, 659
outcomes, 663
pathophysiology, 656
trace elements, nutrition, 245
tracheal agenesis, 816–817
tracheoesophageal compression, 27
tracheoesophageal fistula (TEF), 812–814
transcutaneous bilirubin (TcB), 315
transcutaneous oxygen, 395
transesophageal pacing, 527
transfusion reactions, 532–533
febrile, 533
transfusion-associated acute lung injury
(TRALI), 532
transfusion-associated graft-*versus*-host
disease (TA-GVHD), 533
transfusions, blood. *See* blood transfusions
transient tachypnea of the newborn (TTN),
403–407
transillumination, 447
transitional care, 103–104
transport, neonatal
air transport, 186, 201, 202*t*
cardiac disorders, 488

fixed-wing, 193
ground, 193
indications for, 192–193
introduction to, 192
legality, 193
medications used, 198–199*t*
NICU arrival, 200–201
organization of services, 193–195
prior management, 200
referring hospital responsibilities,
195–197
simulation, 202
specific conditions, 201
supplies for, 196–197*t*
transport teams, 193
equipment, 195*t*
responsibilities, 197–199
supplies, 196–197*t*
transpyloric feedings, 258
trauma, birth
bone injuries, 70–71
head, neck injuries, 63–67
intra-abdominal injuries, 71–72
introduction to, 63
nerve, spinal cord injuries, 67–70
newborn bleeding, 539
soft tissue injuries, 72–73
Treponema pallidum, 664. *See also* syphilis
tricuspid atresia, 501–502, 501*f*
trisomy 21 screening, 2–3
trophic feedings. *See* minimal enteral feeding
true hermaphroditism. *See* ovotesticular
DSD
truncus arteriosus, 506–507, 506*f*
TTTS. *See* twin-to-twin transfusion
syndrome
tube feeding, 250, 250*t*
tuberculosis (TB), 672
BCG vaccination, 680–681
congenital, 677–678
breastfeeding contraindications,
267–268
common medications, 679*t*
of fetus, newborn, 677–680, 679*t*
incidence, 672
maternal, 673–677, 676*f*
transmission, pathogenesis, 672–673
tubular disorders, 374–375
tubular function, 351–353
tumors, surgery, 823–824
twins. *See* multiple births
recipient, 129
twin-to-twin transfusion syndrome (TTTS),
129–131
type 1, 2 diabetes. *See* diabetes, pregnancy
tyrosinemia, 784

U

UCB. *See* umbilical cord blood
UCDs. *See* urea cycle disorders
ultrasonographic examinations
  birth defects, 122
  multiple births, 126
  renal conditions, 361–362
umbilical cord
  artery blood flow, 8
  artery catheterization procedure, 860–865,
    860*f*, 862*f*
  care, 104
  delayed clamping, polycythemia, 572–573
  multiple-lumen catheters, 865–867
  PUBS, 4–5
  vascular catheterization procedure,
    858–868
  vein catheterization, 865, 866*f*
  venous system, 859*f*
umbilical cord blood (UCB), 536
undervirilized 46,XY males, 802–805
urea cycle disorders (UCDs), 779–782, 780*f*
Ureaplasma urealyticum, 654
urinary tract infection (UTI), 374, 654–655
urine
  abnormal odor, IEM, 769, 769*t*
  analysis, IEM, 773
  electrolytes, 271
  normal values, 359*t*
uterine activity assessment, 8–9

V

VA EMCO. *See* venoarterial ECMO
vacuum caput, 64
valium. *See* diazepam
vancomycin, 640–641, 644
vanishing twin, 126
varicella-zoster virus (V-ZV)
  diagnosis, 616
  epidemiology, 615–616
  introduction to, 615
  prevention, 617–618
  treatment, 616–617
vasa previa, 131
vascular abnormalities, 836–837
vascular catheterization, 858–868.
    See also catheterization
vascular disruption syndromes, 128
vascular rings, 817
vasodilators, 519–520
vasopressor therapy, 466–467
vCJD. *See* Creutzfeldt-Jakob disease
VCUG. *See* voiding cystourethrography
velamentous cord insertion, 131
venoarterial (VA) ECMO, 456

venous blood drawing, 852
venous thromboembolic disorders, 548–550
venovenous (VV) ECMO, 456
ventilation. *See also* mechanical ventilation
  blood gas effects, 384–385, 384*t*
  ELBW infants, 160–161
  MAS, 433
  pulmonary, 395–396
ventilator-associated pneumonia, 654
ventilators, volume-cycled, 379–380
ventricular fibrillation, 524
ventricular septal defect, 512–513, 512*f*
ventricular tachycardia, 524
verapamil, SVT, 523
very low birth weight (VLBW) infants. *See*
  extremely low birth weight (ELBW)
  infants; prematurity, follow-up care;
  prematurity, premature infants
vesicobullous eruptions, 839
viral infections, 588
  CMV, 588–594
  enteroviruses, 618–619
  hepatitis, 610–615
  HIV, 603–610
  HSV, 594–599
  introduction to, 588, 589*t*
  parvovirus, 599–603
  RSV, 622–623
  rubella, 619–622
  V-ZV, 615–618
virilized 46,XX females, 797–802
vitamin(s)
  A, 161, 247, 422
  D, 45, 300, 782–783
  E, 258
  infant nutrition, 243, 244*t*
  K, 538, 543
  supplementation, discharge planning,
    261–262
VLBW (very low birth weight) infants. *See*
  extremely low birth weight (ELBW)
  infants; prematurity, follow-up care;
  prematurity, premature infants
voiding cystourethrography (VCUG), 361
volume-cycled ventilators, 379–380
vomiting, 810–811, 827–828
VV EMCO. *See* venovenous ECMO
V-ZV. *See* varicella-zoster virus

W

warfarin, newborn bleeding, 538
warmer, radiant, 49
well newborn care. *See* newborn care;
  term infants
West Nile virus (WNV), 529, 530*t*

whole blood. *See also* blood
  bleeding treatment, 543
  component transfusions, 529–530
  newborn use, 535
Wilms tumor, 824
WNV. *See* West Nile virus

Wolff-Parkinson-White (WPW) syndrome,
  522–524, 523*f*
wound care, 834–835

Z

zygosity, 124. *See also* multiple births